CLINICAL TEXTBOOK OF ADDICTIVE DISORDERS

Also Available

Women and Addiction: A Comprehensive Handbook
Edited by Kathleen T. Brady, Sudie E. Back,
and Shelly F. Greenfield

Clinical Textbook of Addictive Disorders

FOURTH EDITION

edited by
Avram H. Mack
Kathleen T. Brady
Sheldon I. Miller
Richard J. Frances

THE GUILFORD PRESS
New York   London

Copyright © 2016 The Guilford Press
A Division of Guilford Publications, Inc.
370 Seventh Avenue, Suite 1200, New York, NY 10001
www.guilford.com

Printed in the United States of America

This book is printed on acid-free paper.

Last digit is print number: 9   8   7   6   5   4

The authors have checked with sources believed to be reliable in their efforts to
provide information that is complete and generally in accord with the standards
of practice that are accepted at the time of publication. However, in view of the
possibility of human error or changes in behavioral, mental health, or medical
sciences, neither the authors, nor the editors and publisher, nor any other party
who has been involved in the preparation or publication of this work warrants
that the information contained herein is in every respect accurate or complete,
and they are not responsible for any errors or omissions or the results obtained
from the use of such information. Readers are encouraged to confirm the
information contained in this book with other sources.

Library of Congress Cataloging-in-Publication Data

Names: Mack, Avram H., editor.
Title: Clinical textbook of addictive disorders / edited by Avram H. Mack
   [and three others].
Description: Fourth edition. | New York : The Guilford Press, [2016] |
   Includes bibliographical references and index.
Identifiers: LCCN 2015037303| ISBN 9781462521685 (paperback) | ISBN
   9781462521692 (hardcover)
Subjects: LCSH: Substance abuse. | Alcoholism. | BISAC: PSYCHOLOGY /
   Psychopathology / Addiction. | MEDICAL / Psychiatry / General. | SOCIAL
   SCIENCE / Social Work. | PSYCHOLOGY / Psychotherapy / Counseling. |
   MEDICAL / Nursing / Psychiatric.
Classification: LCC RC564 .C55 2016 | DDC 362.29—dc23
LC record available at *http://lccn.loc.gov/2015037303*

IN MEMORIAM
Sheldon I. Miller

During the writing of this textbook, the field mourned the loss of Sheldon I. Miller, MD, who was involved with the conception of each edition of the *Clinical Textbook of Addictive Disorders*, including this one. In his last conversation with Richard J. Frances, he said he was hoping to read and edit chapters as they came in. This and earlier editions of this volume are among his great contributions to our field. Dr. Miller worked long and hard to improve the lives of patients suffering from addictions and was among the greatest leaders in the addictions field in the last half century. He was past president and cofounder of the American Academy of Addiction Psychiatry, the founder and editor of *The American Journal on Addictions*, the leader in developing added qualifications in addiction psychiatry for the American Board of Psychiatry and Neurology, and Emeritus Professor and Chairman of Psychiatry at Northwestern University Feinberg School of Medicine. Dr. Miller's wife, Sarah Miller, has generously directed The Guilford Press to donate his share of royalties from this book to an educational fund for the American Academy of Addiction Psychiatry.

About the Editors

Avram H. Mack, MD, is Associate Chair for Quality and Safety at the Children's Hospital of Philadelphia, where he is a practicing psychiatrist with a focus on substance use disorders and forensic, child, adult, and consultation–liaison psychiatry. Dr. Mack leads efforts on quality and patient safety and has had extensive experience as a teacher and administrator in undergraduate and graduate medical education for trainees and staff at the University of Pennsylvania, The Children's Hospital of Philadelphia, and previously at Georgetown University. He is board certified in general psychiatry, child and adolescent psychiatry, forensic psychiatry, and addiction medicine and presents, publishes, and testifies extensively regarding substance abuse. A past president of the Washington Psychiatric Society, he served on the board of directors of the American Psychiatric Association and on the Impaired Physicians Committee of the Medical Society of the District of Columbia. A distinguished Fellow of the American Psychiatric Association and a Fellow of the American College of Psychiatrists, Dr. Mack is a recipient of the Education Award presented by the Association for Academic Psychiatry in recognition of his efforts in advancing the patient safety movement within psychiatry.

Kathleen T. Brady, MD, PhD, is Distinguished University Professor and Associate Provost for Clinical and Translational Science at the Medical University of South Carolina. Her interests include drug and alcohol abuse/addiction and comorbid conditions. A board-certified psychiatrist, Dr. Brady leads numerous research projects and served as president of the American Academy of Addiction Psychiatry, a member of the Scientific Advisory Council of the National Institute on Drug Abuse, and a board member of the College on Problems of Drug Dependence. She has authored over 300 publications; presented at conferences, grand rounds, and symposia; and received numerous awards.

Sheldon I. Miller, MD, until his death in 2011, was Emeritus Professor of Psychiatry and former Chairman of the Department of Psychiatry and Behavioral Sciences at Northwestern University Feinberg School of Medicine. Recognized as a national leader in addiction psychiatry, he was a cofounder of the American Academy of Addiction Psychiatry. Dr. Miller was the author of more than 100 publications and Editor-in-Chief of the *American Journal on Addictions*. He served on the board of directors of the Accreditation Council for Graduate Medical Education and of the American Board of Emergency Medicine and was a Distinguished Fellow of the American Psychiatric Association and a member of the Group for the Advancement of Psychiatry.

Richard J. Frances, MD, is Clinical Professor of Psychiatry at New York University School of Medicine and Adjunct Professor at Rutgers New Jersey Medical School. He maintains a private practice in New York and was instrumental in the recognition of addiction psychiatry as a medical subspecialty. Board certified in psychiatry and addiction psychiatry, Dr. Frances was a cofounder and first president of the American Academy of Addiction Psychiatry, Director of Education at the University of Medicine and Dentistry of New Jersey (now part of Rutgers Biomedical and Health Sciences), Chair of the Department of Psychiatry at Hackensack University Medical Center, and President and Medical Director of Silver Hill Hospital. He has also held leadership positions at New York Hospital–Cornell Medical Center and has a special interest in addiction, with a focus on impaired professionals.

Contributors

Evaristo Akerele, MD, MPH, DFAPA, Department of Psychiatry, Columbia University Medical Center, New York, New York; Interfaith Medical Center, Brooklyn, New York

Sudie E. Back, PhD, Department of Psychiatry and Behavioral Sciences, Medical University of South Carolina, and Ralph H. Johnson Veterans Affairs Medical Center, Charleston, South Carolina

Nicolas Badre, MD, San Diego Central Jail, San Diego, California

D. Andrew Baron, MS, Pasadena, California

David A. Baron, DO, Department of Psychiatry, University of Southern California, Los Angeles, California

Kelly S. Barth, DO, Department of Psychiatry and Behavioral Sciences, Medical University of South Carolina, Charleston, South Carolina

Judith S. Beck, PhD, Beck Institute for Cognitive Behavior Therapy, and Department of Psychiatry, University of Pennsylvania School of Medicine, Philadelphia, Pennsylvania

Kathleen T. Brady, MD, PhD, Department of Psychiatry and Behavioral Sciences, Medical University of South Carolina, and Ralph H. Johnson Veterans Affairs Medical Center, Charleston, South Carolina

Christina Brezing, MD, Department of Psychiatry, Columbia University Medical Center, and Division on Substance Abuse, New York State Psychiatric Institute, New York, New York

Oscar G. Bukstein, MD, Department of Psychiatry, Boston Children's Hospital, Boston, Massachusetts

Kenneth M. Carpenter, PhD, Department of Psychiatry, Columbia University Medical Center, and Division on Substance Abuse, New York State Psychiatric Institute, New York, New York

Kathleen M. Carroll, PhD, Department of Psychiatry, Yale School of Medicine, New Haven, Connecticut

Joseph DiFranza, MD, Department of Community Medicine and Family Health, University of Massachusetts Medical School, Worcester, Massachusetts

Lance M. Dodes, MD (retired), Department of Psychiatry, Harvard Medical School, Boston, Massachusetts

Caroline M. DuPont, MD, The Institute for Behavior and Health, Inc., Rockville, Maryland

Robert L. DuPont, MD, The Institute for Behavior and Health, Inc., Rockville, Maryland

John Franklin, MD, MSc, Department of Psychiatry and Behavioral Sciences, Northwestern University, Chicago, Illinois

Marc Galanter, MD, Division of Alcoholism and Drug Abuse, Department of Psychiatry, NYU School of Medicine, NYU Langone Medical Center, New York, New York

Robert Gorney, MD, Richard J. Donovan Correctional Facility, California Department of Corrections and Rehabilitation, San Diego, California

Jon E. Grant, MD, Department of Psychiatry and Behavioral Neurosciences, University of Chicago, Chicago, Illinois

William M. Greene, MD, Division of Addiction Medicine, Department of Psychiatry, University of Florida College of Medicine, Gainesville, Florida

Shelly F. Greenfield, MD, MPH, Department of Psychiatry, Harvard Medical School, Boston, Massachusetts; Division of Alcohol and Drug Abuse and Division of Women's Mental Health, McLean Hospital, Belmont, Massachusetts

Colin N. Haile, MD, PhD, Department of Psychiatry and Behavioral Sciences, Baylor College of Medicine, and Michael E. DeBakey VA Medical Center, Houston, Texas

Deborah L. Haller, PhD, ABPP, Department of Public Health Sciences, University of Miami Miller Medical School, Miami, Florida

Amy Harrington, MD, Department of Psychiatry, University of Massachusetts Medical School, Worcester, Massachusetts

Deborah Hasin, PhD, Department of Psychiatry, Columbia University Medical Center, New York, New York

Abigail J. Herron, DO, The Institute for Family Health and Department of Psychiatry, Icahn School of Medicine at Mount Sinai, New York, New York

Dorian Hunter, PhD, private practice, Seattle, Washington

Dilip V. Jeste, MD, Department of Psychiatry and the Stein Institute for Research on Aging, UC San Diego Health Sciences, San Diego, California

Laura M. Juliano, PhD, Department of Psychology, American University, Washington DC

David Kalman, PhD, Department of Psychiatry, University of Massachusetts Medical School, Worcester, Massachusetts

Yifrah Kaminer, MD, Department of Psychiatry, University of Connecticut School of Medicine, Farmington, Connecticut

Edward Kaufman, MD, Northbound Treatment Services, Newport Beach, California

Cheryl Ann Kennedy MD, DFAPA, Department of Psychiatry and Department of Preventive Medicine and Community Health, Rutgers New Jersey Medical School, Newark, New Jersey

Edward J. Khantzian, MD, Department of Psychiatry, Harvard Medical School, Boston, Massachusetts

Bari Kilcoyne, MPH, New York Institute of Technology College of Osteopathic Medicine, Old Westbury, New York

Brian D. Kiluk, PhD, Department of Psychiatry, Yale School of Medicine, New Haven, Connecticut

Steve Koh, MD, MPH, MBA, Department of Psychiatry, UC San Diego Health Sciences, San Diego, California

Thomas R. Kosten, MD, Department of Psychiatry and Behavioral Sciences, Baylor College of Medicine, Houston, Texas

Frances R. Levin, PhD, Division on Substance Abuse, New York State Psychiatric Institute, New York, New York

Petros Levounis, MD, Department of Psychiatry, Rutgers New Jersey Medical School, Newark, New Jersey

Bruce S. Liese, PhD, Department of Psychology, University of Kansas, Lawrence, Kansas

Marsha M. Linehan, PhD, Behavioral Research and Therapy Clinics, University of Washington, Seattle, Washington

Walter Ling, MD, UCLA Integrated Substance Abuse Programs, Los Angeles, California

Thomas R. Lynch, PhD FBPsS, School of Psychology, University of Southampton, Southampton, United Kingdom

Avram H. Mack, MD, Department of Child and Adolescent Psychiatry and Behavioral Sciences, Children's Hospital of Philadelphia, Philadelphia, Pennsylvania

Elinore F. McCance-Katz, MD, State of Rhode Island Department of Behavioral Healthcare, Developmental Disabilities and Hospitals, Providence, Rhode Island

Jenna L. McCauley, PhD, Department of Psychiatry and Behavioral Sciences, Medical University of South Carolina, Charleston, South Carolina

Larissa J. Mooney, MD, Department of Psychiatry and Biobehavioral Sciences, University of California, Los Angeles, and UCLA Integrated Substance Abuse Programs, Los Angeles, California

Alicia R. Murray, DO, private practice, White Plains, New York

Ed Nace, MD, Department of Psychiatry, University of Texas Southwestern Medical Center at Dallas, Dallas, Texas

Niru Nahar, MD, Department of Psychiatry, Harlem Hospital, Columbia University Medical Center, New York, New York

Lisa M. Najavits, PhD, Department of Psychiatry, Boston University School of Medicine, and Veterans Affairs Healthcare System, Boston, Massachusetts

Edward V. Nunes, MD, Department of Psychiatry, Columbia University Medical Center, and Division on Substance Abuse, New York State Psychiatric Institute, New York, New York

Lori Pbert, PhD, Department of Medicine, University of Massachusetts Medical School, Worcester, Massachusetts

Marc N. Potenza, MD, PhD, Departments of Psychiatry and Neuroscience and Child Study Center, Yale School of Medicine, New Haven, Connecticut

Greta Bielaczyc Raglan, MA, Department of Psychology, American University, Washington DC

Richard Rawson, PhD, UCLA Integrated Substance Abuse Programs, Los Angeles, California

M. Zachary Rosenthal, PhD, Department of Psychiatry and Behavioral Sciences and Department of Psychology and Neuroscience, Duke University, Durham, North Carolina

Richard N. Rosenthal, MD, Center for Addictive Disorders, Department of Psychiatry, Icahn School of Medicine at Mount Sinai, New York, New York

Stephen Ross, MD, Department of Psychiatry, NYU School of Medicine, NYU Langone Medical Center, New York, New York

Steven J. Schleifer, MD, Department of Psychiatry, Rutgers New Jersey Medical School, Newark, New Jersey

Sidney H. Schnoll, MD, PhD, Pinney Associates, Inc., Bethesda, Maryland

Liana R. N. Schreiber, MPH, Department of Psychiatry, University of Minnesota, Minneapolis, Minnesota

Benjamin C. Silverman, MD, Department of Psychiatry, Harvard Medical School, and Partners Human Research Committee, Partners HealthCare, Boston, Massachusetts

Jennifer L. Smith, PhD, Department of Psychiatry, Columbia University Medical Center, and Division on Substance Abuse, New York State Psychiatric Institute, New York, New York

Dawn E. Sugarman, PhD, Department of Psychiatry, Harvard Medical School, Boston, Massachusetts; Division of Alcohol and Drug Abuse and Division of Women's Mental Health, McLean Hospital, Belmont, Massachusetts

R. Morgan Wain, PhD, Division on Substance Abuse, New York State Psychiatric Institute, New York, New York

Roger D. Weiss, MD, Department of Psychiatry, Harvard Medical School, Boston, Massachusetts; Division of Alcohol and Drug Abuse, McLean Hospital, Belmont, Massachusetts

Joseph Westermeyer, MD, PhD, Department of Psychiatry, University of Minnesota, and Minneapolis VA Medical Center, Minneapolis, Minnesota

Laurence Westreich, MD, Department of Psychiatry, NYU School of Medicine, NYU Langone Medical Center, New York, New York

Douglas Ziedonis, MD, Department of Psychiatry, University of Massachusetts Medical School, Worcester, Massachusetts

Preface

The *Clinical Textbook of Addictive Disorders, Fourth Edition*, is designed to inform the clinical practice of addiction psychiatry with developing scientific advances in order to broaden evidence-based treatment approaches. Our goal is to enhance our readers' skills, attitudes, and knowledge so they can provide the best in patient care. We have expanded the original contents and author base of this edition to include the latest research. As such, it is our hope that this volume can serve as a primary textbook in undergraduate programs, as well as a guide for graduate and lifelong learning programs that train clinicians in the treatment of addictive disorders. The target audience is broad: medical students, psychiatry residents, and general psychiatrists; addiction psychiatry fellows, addiction psychiatrists, and other primary care physicians; and those who practice addiction medicine, including nurses, social workers, psychologists, addiction counselors, and rehabilitation therapists. It may also be useful to individuals from a wide variety of other disciplines, including teachers, the criminal justice system workforce (e.g., lawyers, judges, police officers, and correctional officers), family members, and anyone interested in learning more about addictions and addiction-related disorders.

When we began work on the previous edition over a decade ago, vaccine therapy for addiction had not been explored, few drugs were in development, and little knowledge had been published about gender differences in addictive disorders. There had been little study of the effectiveness of 12-step facilitation, family, and network treatments. Prescription of buprenorphine and naltrexone was just beginning to be disseminated. Since then, remarkable progress has been made in basic biological understanding of addictions, matched by attempts to broaden treatment efforts with earlier identification of substance-related problems, greater involvement of primary care practitioners, efforts at harm reduction, broadening of culturally sensitive and gender-based approaches, the development of drug courts, increased access of care to the previously uninsured, and many areas of refinement of treatment techniques.

One of the great frontiers of neuroscience and psychiatry is understanding the biological, psychological, and social bases of addictive disorders and developing better ways to prevent, diagnose, and treat these disorders. Are the roots of addictions localized in various brain regions, specific nerve cells, neurotransmitters, and neural networks, and governed by genetics, or are they the result of infinitely more complex behavioral and social conditioning effects on the brain? What are the most important psychological, social, and cultural factors that contribute to substance-related disorders and their treatment, and how do these factors affect various brain functions? It is critical to understand addiction at multiple levels and develop a variety of strategies to help patients recover and to manage addiction-related problems.

While progress in understanding the genetics and neurobiology of addictions and related comorbidities has been great, translation of new findings to the development of more effective prevention and treatments strategies has been slow. All drugs of abuse and addictive behaviors increase dopamine levels and have effects on reducing D_2 receptor reward sensitivity in the limbic system, central tegmentum, and prefrontal cortex, leading to decreased inhibitory control. This helps explain the power of craving in driving addiction-related behaviors. Promising imaging studies of heavy cocaine users have found a correlation between low levels of central D_2 receptors and poor treatment response. This may help in the search for new and better ways to treat substance-related disorders.

The problems that patients with addictive disorders present to clinicians are usually complicated. Disentangling diagnostic issues related to intoxication, withdrawal, the chronic effects of use, and multiple substance use interacting with comorbid medical and psychiatric problems is indeed a challenge. Our authors review research that has helped us better approach and understand addiction at many systems levels: molecular, cellular, synaptic, genetic, pharmacological, behavioral, psychological, group, family, network, anthropological, social, political, and spiritual.

The introduction of DSM-5 is the culmination of 7 years of effort in incorporating new scientific findings and analysis of large pools of data. This work has led to major changes in the way substance use disorders (SUDs) are diagnosed. In DSM-5, the diagnostic term "substance-related and addictive disorders" is introduced and for the first time includes a non-substance-related disorder, gambling. Including the words "substance-related and addictive disorders" in the DSM-5 chapter heading leaves open the future addition of other, non-substance-related addictive disorders, such as Internet gaming, sex and food addictions, and shopping addictions, if evidence supporting their inclusion continues to grow. Internet gaming disorder, a global problem that is recognized as a disease in China, has been added to "Conditions for Further Study" in the Appendices of DSM-5, indicating that there is not sufficient evidence to include this as an addictive disorder at present, but it is under consideration for inclusion in future editions. Caffeine use disorder and caffeine withdrawal have also been added to the DSM-5 Appendices.

The major changes in DSM-5 diagnostic criteria for substance-related disorders are that legal problems were dropped and craving was added as a new criterion. Legal problems were not found to contribute substantially to diagnosis and variations in laws related to substance use further complicate validity. Craving was found to be diagnostically relevant in clinical practice and research, and may be particularly valuable in diagnosing tobacco use disorders. The terms "abuse" and "dependence" have been eliminated in DSM-5, because data indicate a continuum from abuse to dependence that is subsumed under the term "substance use disorder" containing 11 criteria, with demarcation of symptoms as mild (2–3), moderate (4–6), and severe (7–11). Recommended uses of severity criteria include placing a patient on methadone or buprenorphine only if his or her level of addiction is moderate to severe. Field studies exploring equivalence to the DSM-IV term "alcohol dependence" (often equated with the commonly used lay term "alcoholism"), or common use of the term "addiction," have not been conducted. However, epidemiological studies suggest that the equivalent to the commonly used term "alcoholism" or "drug addiction" will, in the long term, probably be seen as "severe" in DSM-5, requiring seven to 11 positive criteria. The text also makes it clear that tolerance is a normal physiological response in those requiring analgesic or antianxiety medications. Many patients require controlled substances to manage pain, and they develop tolerance and potential withdrawal but do not have other manifestations of addiction, such as escalation of dosing. These patients are not "addicted," although they have sometimes been labeled as "pseudodependent."

The term "addictive diorders" in the title of this book has been widely used by scientists and the lay public. However, this term has not been used in the DSM-5 nomenclature for fear of stigmatizing a population and given a lack of operational criteria. There was controversy about whether or not to use the term "addiction" in DSM-5. The term "dependence," as used in the DSM system, has caused confusion, because individuals can have physical dependence on drugs and not have the full spectrum of DSM dependence criteria. It was decided to use the term "substance-related disorders" in DSM-5, with the term "addictive" limited to nonsubstance reward system disorders such as gambling. The use of the term "addiction" in scientific circles has increased in journal titles (*American Journal of Addictions*) and organizational names (American Academy of Addiction Psychiatry; American Society of Addiction Medicine).

As always in science and life, we advise readers to evaluate everything, including the information in this textbook, with a healthy skepticism. Advances in neuroscience are increasingly impacting many aspects of treatment. However, even with a decade of progress in understanding genetics, the mechanisms of addictions, brain imaging, and brain neurochemistry, we are in the infancy of truly understanding how substances affect the vast complexity of brain functioning. Though the speed of sophisticated research is increasing, translating these advances in a way that impacts clinical practice is slow. Even bench-to-patient advances, such as the use of naltrexone to reduce craving, have variable and modest effectiveness. We hope that we will soon see the fruits of advances in translating genetic understanding into new and more personalized treatments. This book covers refinements and advances in psychotherapeutic approaches to substance-related and comorbid disorders, including motivational interviewing, cognitive-behavioral therapy, dialectical behavior therapy, 12-step facilitation approaches, relapse prevention, family therapy, psychodynamic-informed treatments, and psychopharmacology. Integrating self-help facilitation, cognitive-behavioral, motivational, psychodynamic, network, family, and group treatments, and understanding which treatment is best for which patients at what point in recovery, are issues that require further investigation. The role of nonspecific elements of treatment, faith, and support systems in enhancing effectiveness is also underexplored.

Crafting an effective treatment approach tailored to the specific needs of the individual patient requires great skill, knowledge, and wisdom. Although there are many theoretically based and researched manualized treatment approaches to addictions and comorbid conditions, the science of differential therapeutics in treating addicted patients is still early in its development. Studies have found a variety of approaches helpful, without clearly differentiating treatment results based on differential treatment approaches, or defining the best approach for each patient. Experienced clinicians will often blend the techniques described in this book and tailor them to patients' needs. Patient preferences and characteristics play a role in timing and treatment choices. Key issues in all treatments for addictions include forming a therapeutic alliance, improving motivation for change, increasing self-efficacy and self-care, use of collateral data and supports, medication use where indicated, and facilitation of group, family, network, and mutual-help programs when possible. Additionally, synchronous evaluation and treatment of comorbid psychiatric and medical problems, evaluation of level and staging of care, and attention to prevention and cost-effectiveness are important. While we emphasize the use of evidence-based approaches, how best to combine and use the treatments described in this book is still a combination of art and science. It may take a village of effective teamwork among patients, families, clinicians, police, courts, teachers, public policymakers, and other community supports to help prevent and treat addictions. The biopsychosocial challenges that SUDs and other addictive behaviors present—with new legal, illegal, designer, and performance-enhancing drugs being developed—as well as challenges related to new technologies, are likely to be with us well into the future. The need to educate primary care doctors, psychiatrists, and addiction psychiatrists to prepare them to deal effectively with addictions in the future should be a major national priority.

The proper diagnosis and tailored treatment planning for patients with substance-related disorders requires a firm knowledge and skills base that is acquired by reading, supervised clinical experience, sharing with colleagues, and attending educational meetings. In addition to acquiring knowledge and skills, approaching treatment of those with addictions with respect, empathy, compassion, and a sense of humor can help. The critical reader will glean the nuggets from all of our authors and integrate approaches with their own personalities and approaches for maximum effectiveness.

We are grateful to our diligent contributors for their hard work on these chapters, and we thank our spouses and the staff at The Guilford Press for all their support throughout the process. We hope this edition of our textbook will provide an update that will improve our readers' ability to provide high-quality care to individuals suffering with addictions and their loved ones.

Contents

PART IV. SPECIAL POPULATIONS

Contents   xix

CLINICAL TEXTBOOK OF ADDICTIVE DISORDERS

PART I

Foundations of Addiction

CHAPTER 1

Neurobiology of Substance Use Disorders

Implications for Treatment

THOMAS R. KOSTEN
COLIN N. HAILE

Advances in neuroscience, neuroimaging, pharmacology, and genetics have provided the tools needed to understand neurobiological aspects of the substance-related disorders. While the individual patient, rather than his or her disease, is the appropriate focus of treatment, an understanding of the neurobiology helps clarify the rationale for treatment methods and goals. More importantly, knowledge of brain effects or abnormalities allows for the use of medications that specifically target and reverse known neurochemical problems (Haile & Kosten, 2013). That a substance use disorder (SUD) is indeed a brain disease with neurochemical effects should be conveyed to the patient, in addition to the possibility that certain medications may be helpful.

Chronic substance use eventually results in structural and functional brain abnormalities that, for some, lead to the need to keep taking drugs to avoid a withdrawal syndrome (substance-induced disorder). Another component of SUDs is characterized by intense drug craving and compulsive use that is unique to a particular drug class. As we describe later in this chapter, elements of drug withdrawal and drug craving are mediated by different, yet overlapping, brain circuits. Many abnormalities associated with drug withdrawal resolve within days or weeks after the substance use stops. The abnormalities that mediate craving and compulsion, however, are structural changes that are more wide-ranging, complex, and long-lasting. Structural changes lead to abnormal brain function that may be amplified by environmental effects—for example, stress, social context of initial drug use, and psychological conditioning. Genetics also plays a significant role due to aberrant brain pathways that were abnormal even before the first dose of a particular drug was taken. These pathways predispose an individual to develop an SUD (Russo et al., 2010). Such abnormalities can produce craving that leads to relapse months or years after the individual has stopped using.

In this chapter we describe, in a simplified way, how drugs affect brain processes that underlie the motivational drive associated with drug use. Basic concepts such as drug tolerance and specific neurobiological processes and mechanisms that relate to withdrawal and intoxication are also addressed. Whereas these processes are highly complex, we try to explain them in terms that can be presented to patients. We also discuss the treatment implications of these concepts. Current models that help describe the development of an SUD are also noted. In the final section we review pharmacological therapy along with mechanism(s) of action in the brain. These actions attempt to offset directly or reverse some of the brain changes associated with a particular disorder. Studies have shown that pharmacotherapy greatly enhances the effectiveness of behavioral therapies. Although researchers do not yet have a comprehensive understanding about how these medications work, it is clear that they often renormalize brain abnormalities that have been induced by either genetic predisposition or chronic administration of high doses of a given substance.

NEUROBIOLOGICAL SUBSTRATES OF DRUG REINFORCEMENT

Many factors, both individual and environmental, influence whether a certain individual who experiments with a drug will continue taking it long enough to develop an SUD. For individuals who do continue, the drug's ability to provide intense feelings of pleasure is a critical reason.

Substances are consumed through many different routes (e.g., snorting, smoking, intravenous injection), and those that penetrate the brain more quickly are more often associated with compulsive use than those that enter the brain slowly (Fowler et al., 2008). In addition to the rapidity with which a drug enters the brain, all drugs associated with SUDs increase the neurotransmitter dopamine (DA) to supraphysiological levels within specific brain reward circuitry (Figure 1.1). The subsequent rise in synaptic DA then binds to unique DA-ergic receptor proteins on the surface of pre- and postsynaptic neurons (Figure 1.2). Another example is the opiate heroin that binds to mu opioid receptors, which are on the surfaces of opiate-sensitive neurons and induce their effects by inhibiting the cyclic adenosine monophosphate (AMP) second messenger system. Inhibition occurs through a G-protein mediated coupling leading to a series of changes in phosphorylation for a wide range of intraneuronal proteins (Nestler, 2012). The ability of heroin to bind to mu opioid receptors imitates the action of endogenous opioids such as beta-endorphin, initiating the same biochemical brain processes that are associated with positive subjective feelings from activities that are normally pleasurable (e.g., eating and sexual activity). Opioids such as oxycodone or methadone are prescribed therapeutically to relieve pain, but when these exogenous opioids activate the reward processes in the absence of significant pain, they can usurp normal brain reward circuitry and motivate repeated use of the drug simply for pleasure.

The mesocorticolimbic (midbrain and cortex) reward system consists of brain circuits activated to a degree by all drugs associated with compulsive use (Figure 1.2).

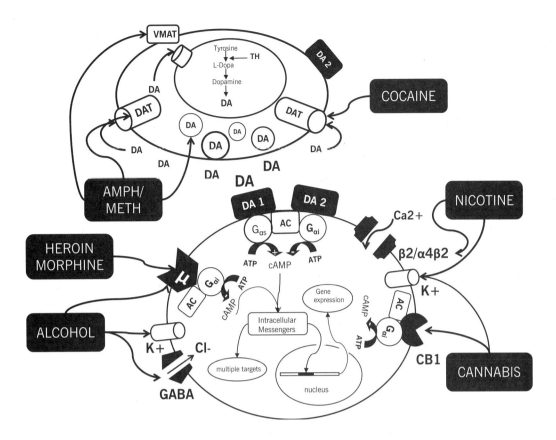

FIGURE 1.1. Hypothetical representation of a dopamine (DA) neuron, its target neuron, receptors, and transduction mechanisms implicated in the actions of various SUDs. Cocaine increases DA levels by blocking reuptake of the neurotransmitter through the dopamine transporter (DAT) back into the presynaptic cell for recycling. Supraphysiological levels of DA then activate their respective DA receptors (DA_1, DA_2). Cocaine-induced enhancement of dopamine activates D_1 receptors. Cyclic AMP levels are then increased via adenylate cyclase (AC) through $G_{\alpha s}$, whereas AC activity is decreased through $G_{\alpha i}$ G proteins. Cyclic AMP can enhance or decrease the action of intracellular messengers that have numerous targets including acting on DNA to initiate or suppress gene expression that alters cell activity. Amphetamine and methamphetamine (AMPH/METH) potently induces mobilization and release of vesicular DA increasing neurotransmitter levels in the synapse. AMPH/METH also prevents the inactivation of DA by altering the DAT and blocking reuptake. These drugs also alter the VMAT preventing normal repackaging of DA into vesicles. Opioids such as morphine and heroin bind to mu receptors on inhibitory GABA neurons in the VTA linked to inhibitory $G_{\alpha i}$ G proteins, subsequently decreasing intracellular cyclic AMP formation. Disinhibition of VTA DA neurons results in increased DA release in the NAc. The exact mechanisms responsible for alcohol's ability to increase DA are unknown; however, evidence suggests GABA, mu receptors, and potassium channels play a role. Nicotine can affect DA levels by at least two mechanisms: (1) increase VTA DA firing by direct activation of $beta_2$ receptors or through (2) receptors on GABA-ergic neurons that lead to disinhibition and increased DA release. Cannabinoids such as THC activate CB_1 receptors on GABA neurons linked to inhibitory $G_{\alpha i}$ G proteins that inhibit AC and cyclic AMP production. The G protein directly couples the CB_1 receptor to presynaptic voltage-dependent Ca^{2+} channels, which are inhibited, whereas inward rectifying K^+ channels are activated. It is hypothesized that inhibition of presynaptic release of GABA in the VTA disinhibits DA neurons, facilitating its release. Evidence also implicates opioid receptors in the ability of cannabinoids to facilitate DA release. TH, tyrosine hydroxylase; DBH, dopamine beta-hydroxylase; DAT, dopamine transporter; DA, dopamine; DA1, dopamine D_1 receptor; DA2, dopamine D_2 receptor; cAMP, cyclic adenosine 3′,5′-monophosphate; $G_{\alpha s}$, stimulatory G protein; $G_{\alpha i}$, inhibitory G protein; VMAT, vesicular monoamine transporter; Ca^{2+}, calcium; K^+, potassium; GABA, gamma-aminobutyric acid; THC, delta-9-tetrahydrocannabinol.

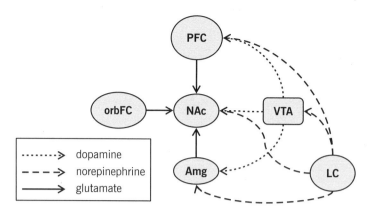

FIGURE 1.2. Representation of neurobiological circuitry that contributes to the reinforcing effects of different substances. Focus is given to neural connections and neurotransmitters DA, NE, and glutamate within mesocorticolimbic circuitry and other important brain structures involved in motor learning and conditioned behavior. Drugs of abuse activate the VTA–NAc pathway, then engage structures involved in learned stimulus–response behavior associated with drug taking. Conditioned reinforcement also involves the Amg, hippocampus (not shown), and NAc. Goal-directed behaviors, self-control, emotional regulation, and working memory involve the PFC and orbFC that send glutamatergic inputs into the NAc. The orbFC has also been linked to drug- and cue-induced "craving" states, along with the Amg and anterior cingulate cortex (not shown). The LC is the primary cell body region that gives rise to NE projections that affect either directly or indirectly most circuits that mediate the various aspects of drug reinforcement and withdrawal. LC NE inputs into the NAc and PFC play an especially important role in stimulant reinforcement, whereas the LC and associated circuits are responsible for withdrawal symptoms from opiates. Conceptually derived from Goldstein and Volkow (2011), Everitt and Robbins (2005), and Koob and Volkow (2010). Amg, amygdala; VTA, ventral tegmental area; NAc, nucleus accumbens; PFC, prefrontal cortex; orbFC, orbitofrontal cortex; LC, locus coeruleus.

This system generates signals in a part of the brain called the ventral tegmental area (VTA) that result in DA release in another brain structure into which VTA neurons project, the nucleus accumbens (NAc). This release of DA into the NAc is associated with positive subjective drug effects (Volkow et al., 2010). Other areas of the brain create a lasting record or memory that associates these good feelings with the circumstances and environment in which they occur (hippocampus). These memories, called "conditioned associations," have a neurocircuitry that often leads to the craving for drugs (amygdala, Amg). For example, when an individual with a SUD reencounters persons, places, or things (orbitofrontal cortex, orbFC) associated with drug use they may trigger the individual to make poor decisions and seek out more drugs in spite of many obstacles and detriment to themselves (prefrontal cortex, PFC) (Goldstein & Volkow, 2011).

Other substances activate this same brain circuitry but via different mechanisms and by stimulating or inhibiting different neurons within these circuits (Figure 1.1, Table 1.1). For example, opioids and cannabinoids can directly inhibit NAc activity, while stimulants such as cocaine and amphetamine (AMPH)-type substances such

TABLE 1.1. Drug Targets and Mechanism of Action

Drug	Target	Primary mechanism of action
Cocaine	DAT/NET/SERT	Binds to presynaptic monoamine transporters and blocks their reuptake, thereby increasing synaptic levels.
Amphetamine/ methamphetamine	NET/DAT, VMAT2, MAO	Induces NE and DA presynaptic release, reverses transporters.
Nicotine	nAChR agonist	Increases firing of VTA DA neurons through nicotinic beta$_2$ receptors; disinhibits DA neurons via alpha$_4$ beta$_2$ receptors on VTA GABA-ergic neurons.
Opioids (morphine, heroin)	Mu receptor agonist	Increases DA release by disinhibition of inhibitory GABA-ergic neurons through mu receptors.
Cannabis	CB$_1$ receptors	Increases DA by disinhibition of VTA DA neurons through CB$_1$ receptors on GABA-ergic neurons.
Alcohol	Undefined	Increases DA either by direct action or possibly by disinhibition via GABA-ergic receptors.

Note. VTA, ventral tegmental area; DAT, dopamine transporter; NET, norepinephrine transporter; SERT, serotonin transporter; VMAT2, vesicular monoamine transporter; MAO, monamine oxidase; nAChR, nicotinic acetylcholine receptor.

as methamphetamine (METH) act indirectly by binding to various DA transporters and either inhibiting the reuptake of DA back into the VTA neurons for recycling (cocaine) or actively pumping DA out of the VTA neuron (AMPH, METH; Figure 1.2). Although cocaine, AMPH, and METH bind DA transporter (DAT) sites all over the brain, the DAT sites in the VTA terminals that synapse with neurons in the NAc play a significant role in the positive subjective effects of these drugs. Since stimulation of the DA D$_2$ receptors inhibits the cyclic AMP cascade, this increase in DA in the synapse leads to relative inhibition of NAc neurons. The mechanism is more complex than this, however, since stimulation of D$_1$ receptors has the opposite effect on cyclic AMP (e.g., increases), and both D$_1$ and D$_2$ receptors are present on NAc neurons. D$_2$ receptors are also located on presynaptic neurons, where they serve as autoreceptors that, when stimulated, decrease release of presynaptic DA. The presumption is that D$_2$ receptor effects predominate perhaps simply due to more D$_2$ receptors or to a higher affinity of the D$_2$ than the D$_1$ receptors for DA. Activation of the cyclic AMP system results in myriad effects, including phosphorylation of intracellular proteins, receptors, receptor channels, sites on DNA that induce the expression of multiple genes, some related to synaptic plasticity that is long-lasting (Paulzen, Veselinovic, & Gründer, 2014). Other substances may be even more indirect in their stimulation of DA. For example, nicotine and benzodiazepines stimulate ion channels for calcium/sodium and chloride, respectively (Sulzer, 2011). The Ca^{2+}/sodium channel is a nicotinic receptor that normally binds acetylcholine, while the chloride channel is associated with gamma-aminobutyric acid (GABA) receptors. Activation of these ion channels can lead to depolarization of VTA neurons and release of DA from NAc neuron terminals either directly (nicotine) or indirectly (GABA). Entry of Ca^{2+} into the VTA neuron is required to facilitate the fusion of synaptic vesicles—that contain packaged neurotransmitter—in the VTA with the cell membrane that leads to release of DA from these vesicles. Similarly, the primary active constituent in cannabis, delta-9-tetrahydrocannabinol (THC), inhibits the inhibitory action of GABA on VTA neurons (through CB_1 receptors), thereby increasing synaptic DA levels at terminal sites within the NAc. For some substances, however, such as alcohol, we do not yet have a clear idea of the biochemical mechanisms that mediate reinforcement. Evidence does suggest that alcohol acts, in part, through mu opioid receptors such as heroin, or GABA receptors such as the sedative/hypnotic drugs (benzodiazepines). The active ingredient in the inhalant toluene increases neurotransmission directly by stimulating VTA neurons leading to DA release in NAc terminals. Inhalant use disorders are associated with profound neurotoxicity (Sulzer, 2011).

The ability of a substance to activate brain reward circuitry potently and produce positive subjective effects is one reason that individuals continue to use a given substance, particularly in the early stages. However, the continued desire and compulsion to use drugs builds over time and extends beyond simple pleasure seeking. This increased compulsion is related to enhanced incentive to procure and take drugs despite recurrent interpersonal problems or having to give up important social or occupational roles. Drug use in situations that may be physically harmful or continued use knowing a physical or psychological problem is directly related to the particular drug consumed are also criteria related to SUDs. Chronic drug consumption eventually leads to synaptic plasticity, which is responsible for tolerance and withdrawal upon cessation of drug use. The intensity of tolerance and withdrawal varies greatly across different drug classes but undoubtedly contributes to continued use. Although it may seem an almost insurmountable objective, reversal or normalization of altered neurotransmission, usually with behavioral treatments and/or pharmacotherapies, is essential to produce a positive clinical outcome.

DRUG TOLERANCE AND WITHDRAWAL

From a clinical standpoint, withdrawal can be one of the most powerful factors driving dependence or addictive behaviors. This seems particularly true for opioids, alcohol, benzodiazepines, nicotine, and, to a lesser extent, stimulants such as cocaine and METH. For hallucinogens or inhalants, however, withdrawal symptoms seem to have more limited importance. Treatment of the patient's withdrawal symptoms is based on understanding how withdrawal is related to aberrant brain chemistry and neuroadaptations in response to chronic repeated high doses of these drugs (Everitt & Robbins, 2005; Goldstein & Volkow, 2011; Kalivas & O'Brien, 2008; Koob & Volkow, 2010; Robison & Nestler, 2011).

Consistent with the concept of drug-induced neuroadaptations, repeated exposure to escalating dosages of most drugs alters brain physiology. Two clinically important consequences of these neuroadaptive effects include drug tolerance (the need to take higher and higher dosages of drugs to achieve the same effect) and withdrawal (a syndrome that occurs once drug use is decreased or discontinued). The neurobiological substrates responsible for tolerance and withdrawal symptoms overlap, since withdrawal symptoms occur only in patients who have developed tolerance.

Tolerance occurs because the brain cells that have receptors or transporters on them gradually become less responsive to the stimulation by the exogenous substances. For example, more heroin or morphine is needed to inhibit cyclic AMP and downstream second messenger systems within the VTA–NAc circuit, as well as to stimulate VTA neurons to release the same amount of DA in NAc terminals. Therefore, more opioid is needed to produce pleasurable subjective effects compared to that produced in previous drug-taking episodes. The mechanisms responsible for this reduced response are related to altered intracellular cyclic AMP–protein kinase A and cyclic AMP response element-binding protein (CREB) that lead to subsequent changes in gene expression of various proteins (Figure 1.2). Altered gene expression results in long-term structural changes not only in genes responsible for neuron integrity (brain-derived neurotrophic factor [BDNF], glia-derived neurotrophic factor [GDNF]) and sensitivity but also changes in amount of receptors and transporters. Indeed, chronic cocaine-induced inhibition of the DAT is associated with decreased DA D_2/D_3 receptors, whereas the DAT, norepinephrine transporter (NET), and serotonin transporter (SERT) are increased presumably to compensate for cocaine's effects (Table 1.2). These alterations, along with changes in other proteins and neurotransmitters associated with tolerance, may be considered an attempt by the brain to attain relative homeostasis in response to drug-induced disruption of normal neurotransmission. Tolerance to alcohol may be due to a more complex series of yet to be determined

TABLE 1.2. Neuroimaging Studies That Reveal Neurobiological Abnormalities Associated with Chronic Substance Use

	Cocaine	AMPH/ METH	Nicotine	Opioids	Cannabis	Alcohol
Baseline DA	↓	↓	—	—	—	↓
DA release	↓	↓	—	↓	↓	↓
D_2/D_3	↓	↓	↓	↓	NC	↓
DAT	↑	↓	↓	↓	↓	↓
NET	↑	—	—	—	—	—
SERT	↑	↓	—	NC	—	NC
VMAT2	↓	↓	—	—	—	—
Glutamate	↑	↓	NC	↓	↓	↑
GABA	↓	—	↓	—	—	NC↓
GABA-alpha$_5$R	—	—	—	—	—	↓
Mu receptor	↑	—	—	NC	—	↑

Note. Data from Albrecht et al. (2013); Buchert et al. (2004); Chang and Haning (2006); Cosgrove et al. 2009, 2010); Ding et al. (2010); Ernst and Chang (2008); Fehr et al. (2008); Gorelick et al. (2005); Heinz et al. (1998, 2005); Hietala et al. (1994); Hou et al. (2011); Jacobsen et al. (2000); Leroy et al. (2012); Licata and Renshaw (2010); Lingford-Hughes et al. (2012); Malison et al. (1998); Martinez et al. (2005, 2007, 2009, 2012); Moszczynska et al. (2004); Narendran et al. (2012); Reneman et al. (2002); Rominger et al. (2012); Sevy et al. (2008); Shi et al. (2008); Urban et al. (2012); Volkow et al. (1990, 1993, 1997, 2001, 2002); Wang et al. (1997, 2012); Yang et al. (2009). DA, dopamine; DAT, dopamine transporter; NET, norepinephrine transporter; SERT, serotonin transporter; VMAT2, vascular monoamine transporter; ↑, increase; ↓, decrease; NC, no change.

neurobiological changes at neuronal and molecular levels. Evidence suggests tolerance to alcohol involves GABA, opioid, DA and other neurochemical systems, including excitatory amino acid neurotransmitters such as glutamate and its multiplicity of receptor subtypes (Sulzer, 2011). Tolerance to cannabinoids/THC probably has a similar mechanism to that of opioids, since the cannabinoid CB1 receptor is also coupled to inhibitory G-proteins that decrease cyclic AMP levels and is associated with low D_2/D_3 receptor numbers. In contrast to cocaine, however, yet common to most other substances, chronic cannabinoid use is associated with decreased DAT levels (Table 1.2). Neurobiological mechanisms that relate tolerance following chronic hallucinogen administration such as lysergic acid diethylamide (LSD) are complex and presently unknown but probably involve changes in serotonergic 5-HT$_2$ receptors linked to the phosphoinositol phosphate (PIP) second messenger system.

TABLE 1.3. Medications Assessed and Indicated for SUDs

Addiction	Medication	Mechanism	Action
Cocaine	Disulfiram	Dopamine beta-hydroxylase	↓NE
	Doxazosin	Alpha$_1$ receptors	↓NE
	Lofexidine	Alpha$_2$ receptors	↓NE
	Modafinil	DAT, alpha receptors	↑DA, glutamate, orexin, ↓ GABA
	Topiramate	Na$^+$,Ca^{2+}, GABA	↓ glutamate
	Gabapentin	Na$^+$,Ca^{2+}, GABA	↓ glutamate
	N-Acetylcysteine	Cystine–glutamate exchanger	↑ glutamate
	Methylphenidate	DAT	↑ DA
Amphetamine/ methamphetamine/ MDMA	Bupropion	DAT, NET	↑DA, NE
	Naltrexone	Mu opioid receptors	↓ mu receptor activation
	Rivastigmine	Acetylcholinesterase	↑ acetylcholine
	Perindopril	ACE	↑ DA
	Modafinil	DAT, alpha receptors	↑ DA, glutamate, orexin, ↓ GABA
	Varenicline	Alpha$_4$ beta$_2$ receptors	↑ cholinergic effects
Nicotine	Nicotine[a]	Nicotinic cholinergic receptor	↑ DA
	Varenicline[a]	Alpha$_4$ beta$_2$ receptors	↑ cholinergic effects
	Bupropion[a]	DAT, NET	↑ DA, NE
	N-Acetylcysteine	Cystine–glutamate exchanger	↑ glutamate
	D-Cycloserine	NMDA	↑ glutamate function
Opioids (morphine, heroin)	Methadone[a]	Mu opioid receptors	↑ mu receptor activation
	Buprenorphine[a]	Mu, delta, kappa opioid receptors	↑↓ opioid receptor activation
	Naltrexone[a]	Mu opioid receptors	↓ mu receptor activation
Cannabis	Dronabinol	CB receptors	↑ CB receptor stimulation
Alcohol	Disulfiram[a]	Aldehyde dehydrogenase	↑ acetaldehyde
	Naltrexone[a]	Mu opioid receptors	↓ mu receptor activation
	Acamprosate[a]	NMDA receptors	glutamate/GABA modulation
	Topiramate	Na$^+$,Ca^{2+}, GABA	↓ glutamate

[a]FDA indication for SUD.

Opioids provide an outstanding example to illustrate how neuroadaptations associated with tolerance relate to withdrawal symptoms. Opioid withdrawal symptoms stem from changes in another important brain system, involving NE-ergic cell bodies located at the base of the brain—the locus coeruleus (LC; Figure 1.1). Neurons in the LC produce NE and widely distribute it to other parts of the brain, including the PFC, NAc, VTA, brainstem, and various subcortical regions, where it stimulates wakefulness, breathing, blood pressure, and general alertness, among other functions. When opioid molecules bind to mu receptors on neurons in the LC, they suppress NE release, resulting in drowsiness, slowed respiration, and low blood pressure—familiar depressant effects associated with opioid intoxication. Upon repeated exposure to opioids, however, LC neurons adapt to counter these depressant effects by increasing NE neurotransmission. Logically, when opioids are present, their suppressive impact is offset by increased NE, and the patient feels more or less normal, aside from the euphoric effects of the drug. When opioids are not present to suppress increased NE neurotransmission, withdrawal symptoms such as tremors, anxiety, muscle cramps, and diarrhea are triggered. Other brain areas within meso-limbocortical circuitry, in addition to the LC, also contribute to the production of opiate withdrawal symptoms. For example, patients may not be inclined to eat, since opioid-induced tolerance results in reduced VTA–NAc DA neurotransmission that is essential to the motivational and pleasurable characteristics associated with natural rewards such as food. At least in the case of opioids, and possibly other substances, neuroadaptive changes due to chronic drug consumption results in compensatory changes that in the absence of the drug also produce psychological (craving) withdrawal symptoms that contribute to continued drug use. Indeed, decreased baseline DA levels, compromised DA neurotransmission, and altered D_2/D_3 numbers within the NAc are associated with chronic substance use across many drug classes. As Table 1.3 illustrates, numerous medications have been tested as possible treatments for various SUDs. Many of the medications increase DA neurotransmission aimed at reversing abnormally low neurotransmitter levels.

PROGRESSION TO SUBSTANCE USE DISORDER

As we have seen, the initial pleasure from drugs is derived through the brain's natural reward system and promotes continued use. This may be viewed as the beginning stage in the development of an SUD. Limited or occasional use may then transition to active daily, even compulsive drug administration. Subsequently, repeated exposure to these drugs may result in a transition to compulsive and unremitting chronic drug taking characterized by intense craving, tolerance, and a withdrawal syndrome upon cessation of drug use. Often physical and/or psychological withdrawal occurs upon stopping drug intake and further contributes to relapse risk. In the case of opiates, use is essential to avert the unpleasant symptoms associated with withdrawal syndrome, whereas withdrawal symptoms from other drugs may be minimal and contribute little to relapse after discontinuation. Emerging evidence indicates that neuroplastic changes occur at each stage in the development of SUDs. These changes recruit and strengthen connections between specific brain areas, while reducing the influence of other areas. As noted earlier, long-lasting neuroadaptive brain changes may underlie compulsive drug-seeking behavior and are related to adverse consequences (societal, occupational, and physical) that are the hallmarks of SUDs (Everitt, 2014). Importantly, research indicates that the development of an SUD is also greatly influenced by an interaction between an individual's genetic makeup and environmental factors (stress in particular). Several models have been generated to help explain how occasional drug use produces changes in the brain that may lead to compulsive use. In reality, this process probably involves many different factors that have yet to be recognized or explained.

THE "CHANGED SET POINT" MODEL

The "changed set point" model of substance use has several variants based on altered neurobiology of DA neurons in the VTA and NA neurons in the LC during early phases of withdrawal and abstinence. The basic premise is that drug use alters a biological or physiological setting or baseline. One variant, by Koob and LeMoal (2001), is based on the idea that neurons of the mesolimbic reward pathways are naturally "set" to release enough DA in the NAc to produce a normal level of pleasure. Koob and LeMoal suggest that drug consumption leads to a vicious cycle that involves changing this set point to the degree that the release of DA is reduced when normally pleasurable activities occur and drugs are not present. Similarly, a change in set point occurs in the LC, but in the opposite direction, such that NE release is increased during withdrawal in particular, as described earlier. This model accounts for both the positive (drug-liking) and negative aspects (drug withdrawal syndrome) associated with SUDs.

A specific way that the DA neurons can become dysfunctional relates to an alteration in their baseline ("resting") levels of electrical activity and DA release (Grace, 2000). In this second variant of the changed set point model, baseline DA levels are regulated by two factors that influence the amount of basal DA release in the NAc: cortical excitatory (glutamate) neurons that drive the VTA DA neurons to release DA, and autoreceptors ("brakes") that shut down further release when DA concentrations become excessive. Activation of different receptor subtypes by various substances, such as mu opiate receptors by heroin, initially bypasses these brakes, and this leads to the release of high levels of DA in the NAc. However, with repeated chronic drug use, the brain responds to augmented DA by increasing the number and strength of the brakes on DA-ergic VTA neurons. Eventually, inhibitory autoreceptor control leads to decreased basal DA that is insufficient for normal neurotransmission. When this occurs, the individual will increase the total amount of drug consumed, such as heroin, in order to counteract reduced resting DA levels. When the individual stops taking a sufficient amount of drug to maintain a certain level of DA, deficient DA neurotransmission may result. This DA deficiency produces dysphoria (pain, agitation, malaise) coupled with other withdrawal symptoms that can lead to a cycle of chronic relapse to drug use.

A third variation of the set point change theory emphasizes drug-induced sensitization. "Sensitization" in this context relates to altered sensitivity to drug-associated environmental cues (incentive salience) that leads to drug "wanting" (pathological incentive motivation). This theory also states that craving for drugs may have greater influence in perpetuating use than reinforcement (drug "liking") or withdrawal (Berridge, Robinson, & Aldridge, 2009). In fact, incentive sensitization theory posits that the pleasurable aspects of drugs decrease as a full-blown SUD is established and drugs are "liked" less. The way the theory explains this is that only brain circuits that mediate the motivational aspect of incentive salience (drug "wanting") are sensitized, not circuits that mediate "liking" (drug-associated euphoria). The interactions between the mechanisms that mediate incentive salience and those responsible for learning or conditioning are essential to this theory. During periods of abstinence, when the drug is not available, memory of drug use and desire (wanting) or craving for the drug can be a major factor leading to drug-seeking behavior and subsequent relapse. Craving may represent increased activity of cortical (orbFC/PFC) excitatory (glutamate) projections, which can regulate DA in the NAc. NE-ergic neurons from the LC that project to and influence neurons in the VTA, NAc, and PFC may also play a role. Glutamate activity may increase, thereby increasing DA neurotransmission in the NAc and generating drug wanting or craving. In addition to glutamatergic input from the PFC (Figure 1.1), NE regulates VTA and NAc DA neurotransmission. Although drug withdrawal is not emphasized by this theory, NE projections from the LC also play an important role in withdrawal symptoms, particularly with opiates such as heroin. Consistent with the proposed circuitry, medications that show promise as pharmacotherapy for SUDs block or normalize glutamate and attenuate NE neurotransmission. Furthermore, as we discuss in the next section, studies also consistently show that individuals with SUDs have compromised PFC/orbFC activity responsible for normal impulse control, executive functioning, and memory processes. Accordingly, medications that increase PFC/orbFC function and memory also show promise as treatments.

The Cognitive Deficits Model

The cognitive deficits model proposes that individuals who develop SUDs have abnormalities within the PFC. The PFC is important for regulation of judgment, planning, impulse control, and other executive functions. To help us overcome some of our impulses for immediate gratification in favor of more important or ultimately more rewarding long-term goals, the PFC sends inhibitory signals to the mesolimbic reward system.

The cognitive deficits model proposes that PFC signaling to the mesolimbic reward system is compromised in individuals with substance use disorders, as a result, they have reduced ability to use judgment to restrain their impulses and are predisposed to compulsive drug-taking behaviors (Goldstein & Volkow, 2011). Consistent with this model, PFC deficits are common among individuals with a history of chronic drug use. Indeed, the longer individuals have been using, the greater the amount of damage and the worse their executive functioning. Furthermore, drug-associated deficits do not fully reverse upon stopping drug use. More specifically, chronic alcohol abusers have abnormally low levels of the inhibitory neurotransmitter GABA, the neurochemical in which glutamatergic neurons from the PFC regulate DA release within the VTA and NAc (Table 1.2). Interestingly, individuals with heroin use disorder may have PFC damage that is independent of their opioid use, which they may have inherited genetically or that is caused by some other factor or event in their lives. Pre-existing PFC damage may predispose individuals because they lack impulse control; this, coupled with further drug-induced PFC damage from chronic repeated drug use, increases the severity of these problems (Goldstein & Volkow, 2011).

THE IMPORTANT ROLE OF STRESS

The notion that patients with SUDs are more vulnerable to stress than the general population is a clinical truism. Numerous preclinical studies have documented that physical stressors (e.g., foot-shock or restraint stress) and psychological stressors can cause animals to reinstate drug seeking and self-administration (Epstein, Preston, Stewart, & Shaham, 2006). Furthermore, stressors can trigger drug craving in humans with SUDs (Sinha, 2013). One potential explanation for these observations is that drugs including opiates and stimulants increase levels of cortisol, a hormone that plays a primary role in responses to stress. Cortisol in turn increases the sensitivity of the mesolimbic reward system (Koob & Zorrilla, 2010). By these mechanisms, in certain individuals stress may contribute both to drug craving and the compulsion for continued drug use.

PHARMACOLOGICAL INTERVENTIONS AND TREATMENT IMPLICATIONS

Opioid Use Disorder

We next illustrate how long-term pharmacotherapies for opioid use disorder such as methadone, naltrexone, and buprenorphine can counteract or reverse the abnormalities underlying this disease (Table 1.3). These agents are particularly informative because they have agonist, antagonist, and partial agonist activity respectively. We do not review short-term treatments for relieving the withdrawal syndrome associated with abruptly stopping drug use, but we do refer readers elsewhere for detailed neurobiological explanations for various abstinence initiation approaches (Kosten & Haile, 2015; Kosten & O'Connor, 2003).

Methadone is a long-acting opioid medication with effects that last for days. Methadone can be associated with a use disorder, but because of its sustained stimulation of the mu receptors, it alleviates craving and compulsive drug seeking and use. In addition, methadone therapy tends to normalize many aspects of the hormonal disruptions linked to chronic opioid consumption (Kling et al., 2000; Schluger, Borg, Ho, & Kreek, 2001). For example, it moderates the exaggerated cortisol stress response (discussed earlier) that increases the danger of relapse in stressful situations.

Naltrexone is used to help patients avoid relapse after they have been detoxified from opioids. Its main therapeutic action is to occupy mu opioid receptors in the brain with a 100-fold higher affinity than agonists such as methadone or heroin, so that opioids taken exogenously cannot activate the receptor and in turn stimulate the brain's reward system. An individual who is adequately dosed with naltrexone does not experience the euphoric effects of opioids and is therefore less motivated to use them. An interesting neurobiological effect is that naltrexone appears to increase the number of available mu opiate receptors, which may help to renormalize the imbalance between the receptors and G (guanine nucleotide-binding) protein coupling to cyclic AMP (Kosten, 1990). Naltrexone is also sometimes used to detoxify patients rapidly from opioids. In this situation, while naltrexone blocks mu receptor activation, another drug, clonidine, suppresses opioid-induced excessive NE output that contributes to withdrawal symptoms (Kosten, 1990). Clonidine prevents withdrawal symptoms by activating alpha$_2$-adrenergic autoreceptors responsible for preventing release of NE. These receptors are co-localized with mu opiate receptors on LC neurons, and both receptor types inhibit cyclic AMP synthesis through similar inhibitory G proteins (Mazei-Robison & Nestler, 2012). Interestingly, unique to naltrexone's pharmacology, very low doses have been shown to produce agonist-like effects such as analgesia (Younger & Mackey, 2009). Preclinical studies also show that low-dose naltrexone blocks opioid-induced NE overproduction during withdrawal (Van Bockstaele, Qian, Sterling, & Page, 2008). Consistent with this, low-dose naltrexone in combination with an opioid medication during detoxification reduces withdrawal symptoms and craving (Mannelli et al., 2009).

Buprenorphine's action on the mu opioid receptors elicits two different therapeutic responses within neural circuits affected by chronic opioid consumption that are dose-dependent like naltrexone. At low doses, buprenorphine has agonist effects, but at high doses, it behaves like naltrexone, blocking the receptors so strongly that it can precipitate withdrawal in individuals who take high doses of opiates (e.g., those maintained on more than 40 mg of methadone daily). Because of its unique mechanism of action, chronic treatment with buprenorphine also prevents changes in the sensitivity of the mu receptor that likely play a role in relapse (Virk, Arttamangkul, Birdsong, & Williams, 2009). Several clinical trials have shown that buprenorphine is as effective as methadone when used at sufficient doses (Stotts, Dodrill, & Kosten, 2009). Buprenorphine has a safety advantage over methadone, since high doses precipitate withdrawal rather than the suppression of consciousness and respiration seen in overdoses of methadone and heroin. Thus, buprenorphine has less overdose potential than methadone, since it blocks other opioids and even itself as the dosage increases. Finally, buprenorphine can be given three times per week, simplifying observed ingestion during the early weeks of treatment (Kosten & Fiellin, 2004).

Stimulant Use Disorder

Next we review potential medications for stimulant use disorders and how they may exert therapeutic actions on neural circuitry adversely affected by chronic drug use. Because there are presently no U.S. Food and Drug Administration (FDA)-approved medications for stimulant use disorder, development is of the utmost importance. Fortunately, recent studies assessing medications specifically targeting NE show promise. For example, prazosin and doxazosin are alpha$_1$-adrenergic receptor antagonists, and currently both medications are indicated for the treatment of hypertension. Prazosin also has shown some benefit in treating symptoms associated with posttraumatic stress disorder (PTSD; Cukor, Spitalnick, Difede, Rizzo, & Rothbaum, 2009) likely because these individuals display increased NE release and receptor sensitivity linked to disruption in sleep and vivid nightmares. Several clinical trials have shown that prazosin significantly improves these symptoms (Raskind et al., 2007; Taylor, Freeman, & Cates, 2008). By extension, prazosin's ability to improve PTSD symptoms suggests that it may attenuate stress associated with relapse to drug use (Kosten, Rounsaville, & Kleber, 1988).

Evidence continues to indicate that alpha$_1$-adrenergic receptors are particularly crucial in mediating the behavioral effects produced by stimulants. NE in the PFC can activate alpha$_1$-adrenergic receptors that then enhance DA effects of stimulants in the NAc. This NE enhancement is blocked by prazosin directly infused into the PFC or administered peripherally (Blanc et al., 1994; Darracq, Blanc, Glowinski, & Tassin, 1998; Drouin et al., 2002). Prazosin also blocks drug-induced reinstatement of cocaine-seeking behavior in an animal model of relapse (Zhang & Kosten, 2005).

Prazosin's short half-life of 2–3 hours in humans may limit its use as a treatment for cocaine use disorder. In contrast, doxazosin has a much longer half-life (22 hours). Similar to the effects seen in animal studies with prazosin, doxazosin blocks the behavioral effects of cocaine in rodents (Haile, Hao, O'Malley, Newton, & Kosten, 2012). Moreover, Newton and colleagues (2012) showed that doxazosin (4 mg/day for 9 days) decreased cocaine's (20 and 40 mg) positive subjective effects, including "desire" for cocaine in non-treatment-seeking individuals with cocaine use disorder. Consistent with these results, a pilot outpatient clinical trial indicated that doxazosin (8 mg daily) significantly reduced cocaine use compared to placebo (Shorter, Lindsay, & Kosten, 2013). Prazosin and doxazosin have also shown potential in treating alcohol use disorder (Verplaetse, Rasmussen, Froehlich, & Czachowski, 2012). Although preliminary, these studies suggest that the alpha$_1$ receptor may be a viable therapeutic target for various SUDs. Large outpatient clinical trials are needed to extend and confirm these promising preliminary findings.

SUMMARY

SUDs are most appropriately understood as chronic, relapsing medical conditions. The neurobiology of these disorders is becoming well understood, but much remains unknown about the genomic mechanisms that predispose individuals to developing long-term drug use. The mesolimbic reward system involving many different interrelating neurotransmitter systems is central to clinical consequences of chronic drug use, including tolerance and withdrawal. Other brain areas, neurochemicals, and peripheral hormones such as cortisol also are relevant to continued drug use. Pharmacological interventions are highly effective for opiates, and we have illustrated three different approaches using an agonist, an antagonist, or a partial agonist. We also discussed promising medications for AMPH-like and cocaine use disorders for which we have no pharmacotherapies. Given the complex biological, psychological, and social aspects of these diseases, they must be accompanied by appropriate psychosocial treatments. Clinician awareness of the neurobiological basis that underlies the action of these drugs, and information sharing with patients can provide insight into patient behaviors and problems, and clarify the rationale for treatment methods and goals.

ACKNOWLEDGMENT

This work was supported by National Institute on Drug Abuse Grant Nos. P50-DA18827, R01-DA25223, and DP1DA33502.

REFERENCES

Albrecht, D. S., Skosnik, P. D., Vollmer, J. M., Brumbaugh, M. S., Perry, K. M., Mock, B. H., et al. (2013). Striatal D(2)/D(3) receptor availability is inversely correlated with cannabis consumption in chronic marijuana users. *Drug Alcohol Depend, 128*, 52–57.

Berridge, K. C., Robinson, T. E., & Aldridge, J. W. (2009). Dissecting components of reward: "Liking," "wanting," and learning. *Curr Opin Pharmacol, 9*, 65–73.

Blanc, G., Trovero, F., Vezina, P., Hervé, D., Godeheu, A. M., Glowinski, J., et al. (1994). Blockade of prefronto-cortical alpha$_1$-adrenergic receptors prevents locomotor hyperactivity induced by subcortical D-amphetamine injection. *Eur J Neurosci, 6*, 293–298.

Buchert, R., Thomasius, R., Wilke, F., Petersen, K., Nebeling, B., Obrocki, J., et al. (2004). A voxel-based PET investigation of the long-term effects of "Ecstasy" consumption on brain serotonin transporters. *Am J Psychiatry, 161*, 1181–1189.

Cao, J. L., Vialou, V. F., Lobo, M. K., Robison, A. J., Neve, R. L., Cooper, D. C., et al. (2010). Essential role of the cAMP–cAMP response-element binding protein pathway in opiate-induced homeostatic adaptations of locus coeruleus neurons. *Proc Natl Acad Sci USA, 107*, 17011–17016.

Chang, L., & Haning, W. (2006). Insights from recent positron emission tomographic studies of drug abuse and dependence. *Curr Opin Psychiatry, 19*, 246–252.

Cosgrove, K. P., Krantzler, E., Frohlich, E. B., Stiklus, S., Pittman, B., Tamagnan, G. D., et al. (2009). Dopamine and serotonin transporter availability during acute alcohol withdrawal: Effects of comorbid tobacco smoking. *Neuropsychopharmacol, 34*, 2218–2226.

Cosgrove, K. P., Tellez-Jacques, K., Pittman, B., Petrakis, I., Baldwin, R. M., Tamagnan, G., et al. (2010). Dopamine and serotonin transporter availability in chronic heroin users: A I-125 beta-CIT SPECT imaging study. *Psychiatry Res, 184*, 192–195.

Cukor, J., Spitalnick, J., Difede, J., Rizzo, A., & Rothbaum, B. O. (2009). Emerging treatments for PTSD. *Clin Psychol Rev, 29*, 715–726.

Darracq, L., Blanc, G., Glowinski, J., & Tassin, J. P. (1998). Importance of the noradrenaline-dopamine coupling in the locomotor activating effects of D-amphetamine. *J Neurosci, 18*, 2729–2739.

Ding, Y. S., Singhal, T., Planeta-Wilson, B., Gallezot, J. D., Nabulsi, N., Labaree, D., et al. (2010). PET imaging of the effects of age and cocaine on the norepinephrine transporter in the human brain using (S,S)-[(11)C]O-methylreboxetine and HRRT. *Synapse (New York, NY), 64*, 30–38.

Drouin, C., Darracq, L., Trovero, F., Blanc, G., Glowinski, J., Cotecchia, S., et al. (2002). Alpha$_{1b}$-adrenergic receptors control locomotor and rewarding effects of psychostimulants and opiates. *J Neurosci, 22*, 2873–2884.

Epstein, D. H., Preston, K. L., Stewart, J., Shaham, Y. (2006). Toward a model of drug relapse: An assessment of the validity of the reinstatement procedure. *Psychopharmacol, 189*, 1–16.

Ernst, T., & Chang, L. (2008). Adaptation of brain glutamate plus glutamine during abstinence from chronic methamphetamine use. *J Neuroimmun Pharmacol, 3*, 165–172.

Everitt, B. J. (2014). Neural and psychological mechanisms underlying compulsive drug seeking habits and drug memories—indications for novel treatments of addiction. *Eur J Neurosci, 40,* 2163–2182.

Everitt, B. J., & Robbins, T. W. (2005). Neural systems of reinforcement for drug addiction: From actions to habits to compulsion. *Nat Neurosci, 8,* 1481–1489.

Fehr, C., Yakushev, I., Hohmann, N., Buchholz, H. G., Landvogt, C., Deckers, H., et al. (2008). Association of low striatal dopamine d2 receptor availability with nicotine dependence similar to that seen with other drugs of abuse. *Am J Psychiatry, 165,* 507–514.

Fowler, J. S., Volkow, N. D., Logan, J., Alexoff, D., Telang, F., Wang, G. J., et al. (2008). Fast uptake and long-lasting binding of methamphetamine in the human brain: Comparison with cocaine. *NeuroImage, 43,* 756–763.

Goldstein, R. Z., & Volkow, N. D. (2011). Dysfunction of the prefrontal cortex in addiction: Neuroimaging findings and clinical implications. *Nat Rev Neurosci, 12,* 652–669.

Gorelick, D. A., Kim, Y. K., Bencherif, B., Boyd, S. J., Nelson, R., Copersino, M., et al. (2005). Imaging brain mu-opioid receptors in abstinent cocaine users: Time course and relation to cocaine craving. *Biol Psychiatry, 57,* 1573–1582.

Grace, A. A. (2000). The tonic/phasic model of dopamine system regulation and its implications for understanding alcohol and psychostimulant craving. *Addiction, 95*(Suppl. 2), S119–S128.

Haile, C. N., Hao, Y., O'Malley, P., Newton, T. F., & Kosten, T. A. (2012). The α1 antagonist doxazosin alters the behavioral effects of cocaine in rats. *Brain Sci, 2,* 619–633.

Haile, C. N., & Kosten, T. R. (2013). Pharmacotherapy for stimulant-related disorders. *Curr Psychiatry Rep, 15,* 415.

Heinz, A., Ragan, P., Jones, D. W., Hommer, D., Williams, W., Knable, M. B., et al. (1998). Reduced central serotonin transporters in alcoholism. *Am J Psychiatry, 155,* 1544–1549.

Heinz, A., Siessmeier, T., Wrase, J., Buchholz, H. G., Grunder, G., Kumakura, Y., et al. (2005). Correlation of alcohol craving with striatal dopamine synthesis capacity and D2/3 receptor availability: A combined [^{18}F]DOPA and [^{18}F]DMFP PET study in detoxified alcoholic patients. *Am J Psychiatry, 162,* 1515–1520.

Hietala, J., West, C., Syvalahti, E., Nagren, K., Lehikoinen, P., Sonninen, P., et al. (1994). Striatal D2 dopamine receptor binding characteristics *in vivo* in patients with alcohol dependence. *Psychopharmacol, 116,* 285–290.

Hou, H., Yin, S., Jia, S., Hu, S., Sun, T., Chen, Q., et al. (2011). Decreased striatal dopamine transporters in codeine-containing cough syrup abusers. *Drug Alcohol Depen, 118,* 148–151.

Jacobsen, L. K., Staley, J. K., Malison, R. T., Zoghbi, S. S., Seibyl, J. P., Kosten, T. R., et al. (2000). Elevated central serotonin transporter binding availability in acutely abstinent cocaine-dependent patients. *Am J Psychiatry, 157,* 1134–1140.

Kalivas, P. W., & O'Brien, C. (2008). Drug addiction as a pathology of staged neuroplasticity. *Neuropsychopharmacol, 33,* 166–180.

Kling, M. A., Carson, R. E., Borg, L., Zametkin, A., Matochik, J. A., Schluger, J., et al. (2000). Opioid receptor imaging with positron emission tomography and [^{18}F]cyclofoxy in long-term, methadone-treated former heroin addicts. *J Pharmacol Exp Ther, 295,* 1070–1076.

Koob, G. F., & Le Moal, M. (2001). Drug addiction, dysregulation of reward, and allostasis. *Neuropsychopharmacol, 24,* 97–129.

Koob, G. F., & Volkow, N. D. (2010). Neurocircuitry of addiction. *Neuropsychopharmacol, 35,* 217–238.

Koob, G. F., & Zorrilla, E. P. (2010). Neurobiological mechanisms of addiction: Focus on corticotropin-releasing factor. *Curr Opin Investig Drugs, 11,* 63–71.

Kosten, T. R. (1990). Neurobiology of abused drugs. Opioids and stimulants. *J Nerv Ment Dis, 178,* 217–227.

Kosten, T. R., & Fiellin, D. A. (2004). Buprenorphine for office-based practice: Consensus conference overview. *Am J Addict, 13*(Suppl. 1), S1–S7.

Kosten, T. A., & Haile, C. N. (2015). Opioid-related disorders. In D. Kasper et al. (Eds.), *Harrison's principles of internal medicine* (19th ed., pp. 468–472). New York: McGraw-Hill Professional.

Kosten, T. R., & O'Connor, P. G. (2003). Management of drug and alcohol withdrawal. *New Eng J Med, 348*, 1786–1795.

Kosten, T., Rounsaville, B., & Kleber, H. (1988). A 2.5 year follow-up of abstinence and relapse to cocaine abuse in opioid addicts. *NIDA Res Monogr, 81*, 231–236.

Leroy, C., Karila, L., Martinot, J. L., Lukasiewicz, M., Duchesnay, E., Comtat, C., et al. (2012). Striatal and extrastriatal dopamine transporter in cannabis and tobacco addiction: A high-resolution PET study. *Addict Biol, 17*, 981–990.

Licata, S. C., & Renshaw, P. F. (2010). Neurochemistry of drug action: Insights from proton magnetic resonance spectroscopic imaging and their relevance to addiction. *Ann NY Acad Sci, 1187*, 148–171.

Lingford-Hughes, A., Reid, A. G., Myers, J., Feeney, A., Hammers, A., Taylor, L. G., et al. (2012). A [^{11}C]Ro15 4513 PET study suggests that alcohol dependence in man is associated with reduced alpha$_5$ benzodiazepine receptors in limbic regions. *J Psychopharmacol, 26*, 273–281.

Malison, R. T., Best, S. E., van Dyck, C. H., McCance, E. F., Wallace, E. A., Laruelle, M., et al. (1998). Elevated striatal dopamine transporters during acute cocaine abstinence as measured by [^{123}I] beta-CIT SPECT. *Am J Psychiatry, 155*, 832–834.

Mannelli, P., Patkar, A. A., Peindl, K., Gorelick, D. A., Wu, L. T., & Gottheil, E. (2009). Very low dose naltrexone addition in opioid detoxification: A randomized, controlled trial. *Addict Biol, 14*, 204–213.

Martinez, D., Gil, R., Slifstein, M., Hwang, D. R., Huang, Y., Perez, A., et al. (2005). Alcohol dependence is associated with blunted dopamine transmission in the ventral striatum. *Biol Psychiatry, 58*, 779–786.

Martinez, D., Greene, K., Broft, A., Kumar, D., Liu, F., Narendran, R., et al. (2009). Lower level of endogenous dopamine in patients with cocaine dependence: Findings from PET imaging of D(2)/D(3) receptors following acute dopamine depletion. *Am J Psychiatry, 166*, 1170–1177.

Martinez, D., Narendran, R., Foltin, R. W., Slifstein, M., Hwang, D. R., Broft, A., et al. (2007). Amphetamine-induced dopamine release: Markedly blunted in cocaine dependence and predictive of the choice to self-administer cocaine. *Am J Psychiatry, 164*, 622–629.

Martinez, D., Saccone, P. A., Liu, F., Slifstein, M., Orlowska, D., Grassetti, A., et al. (2012). Deficits in dopamine D(2) receptors and presynaptic dopamine in heroin dependence: Commonalities and differences with other types of addiction. *Biol Psychiatry, 71*, 192–198.

Mazei-Robison, M. S., & Nestler, E. J. (2012). Opiate-induced molecular and cellular plasticity of ventral tegmental area and locus coeruleus catecholamine neurons. *Cold Spring Harb Perspect Med, 2*, a012070.

Moszczynska, A., Fitzmaurice, P., Ang, L., Kalasinsky, K. S., Schmunk, G. A., Peretti, F. J., et al. (2004). Why is parkinsonism not a feature of human methamphetamine users? *Brain, 127*, 363–370.

Narendran, R., Lopresti, B. J., Martinez, D., Mason, N. S., Himes, M., May, M. A., et al. (2012). In vivo evidence for low striatal vesicular monoamine transporter 2 (VMAT2) availability in cocaine abusers. *Am J Psychiatry, 169*, 55–63.

Nestler, E. J. (2012). Transcriptional mechanisms of drug addiction. *Clin Psychopharmacol Neurosci, 10*, 136–143.

Newton, T. F., De La Garza, R., II, Brown, G., Kosten, T. R., Mahoney, J. J., III, & Haile, C. N. (2012). Noradrenergic alpha(1) receptor antagonist treatment attenuates positive subjective effects of cocaine in humans: A randomized trial. *PLoS ONE, 7*, e30854.

Paulzen, M., Veselinovic, T., & Gründer, G. (2014). Effects of psychotropic drugs on brain plasticity in humans. *Restor Neurol Neurosci, 32*, 163–181.

Raskind, M. A., Peskind, E. R., Hoff, D. J., Hart, K. L., Holmes, H. A., Warren, D., et al. (2007). A parallel group placebo controlled study of prazosin for trauma nightmares and sleep disturbance in combat veterans with post-traumatic stress disorder. *Biol Psychiatry, 61*, 928–934.

Reneman, L., Booij, J., Lavalaye, J., de Bruin, K., Reitsma, J. B., Gunning, B., et al. (2002). Use of amphetamine by recreational users of ecstasy (MDMA) is associated with reduced striatal dopamine transporter densities: A [123I]beta-CIT SPECT study—preliminary report. *Psychopharmacol, 159*, 335–340.

Robison, A. J., & Nestler, E. J. (2011). Transcriptional and epigenetic mechanisms of addiction. *Nat Rev Neurosci, 12*, 623–637.

Rominger, A., Cumming, P., Xiong, G., Koller, G., Boning, G., Wulff, M., et al. (2012). [18F]Fallypride PET measurement of striatal and extrastriatal dopamine D 2/3 receptor availability in recently abstinent alcoholics. *Addict Biol, 17*, 490–503.

Russo, S. J., Dietz, D. M., Dumitriu, D., Morrison, J. H., Malenka, R. C., & Nestler, E. J. (2010). The addicted synapse: Mechanisms of synaptic and structural plasticity in nucleus accumbens. *Trends Neurosci, 33*, 267–276.

Schluger, J. H., Borg, L., Ho, A., & Kreek, M. J. (2001). Altered HPA axis responsivity to metyrapone testing in methadone maintained former heroin addicts with ongoing cocaine addiction. *Neuropsychopharmacol, 24*, 568–575.

Sevy, S., Smith, G. S., Ma, Y., Dhawan, V., Chaly, T., Kingsley, P. B., et al. (2008). Cerebral glucose metabolism and D2/D3 receptor availability in young adults with cannabis dependence measured with positron emission tomography. *Psychopharmacol, 197*, 549–556.

Shi, J., Zhao, L. Y., Copersino, M. L., Fang, Y. X., Chen, Y., Tian, J., et al. (2008). PET imaging of dopamine transporter and drug craving during methadone maintenance treatment and after prolonged abstinence in heroin users. *Eur J Pharmacol, 579*, 160–166.

Shorter, D., Lindsay, J. A., & Kosten, T. R. (2013). The alpha-1 adrenergic antagonist doxazosin for treatment of cocaine dependence: A pilot study. *Drug Alcohol Depend, 131*, 66–70.

Sinha, R. (2013). The clinical neurobiology of drug craving. *Curr Opin Neurobiol, 23*, 649–654.

Stotts, A. L., Dodrill, C. L., & Kosten, T. R. (2009). Opioid dependence treatment: Options in pharmacotherapy. *Exp Opin Pharmacother, 10*, 1727–1740.

Sulzer, D. (2011). How addictive drugs disrupt presynaptic dopamine neurotransmission. *Neuron, 69*, 628–649.

Taylor, H. R., Freeman, M. K., & Cates, M. E. (2008). Prazosin for treatment of nightmares related to posttraumatic stress disorder. *Am J Health Syst Pharm, 65*, 716–722.

Urban, N. B., Slifstein, M., Thompson, J. L., Xu, X., Girgis, R. R., Raheja, S., et al. (2012). Dopamine release in chronic cannabis users: A [11C]raclopride positron emission tomography study. *Biol Psychiatry, 71*, 677–683.

Van Bockstaele, E. J., Qian, Y., Sterling, R. C., & Page, M. E. (2008). Low dose naltrexone administration in morphine dependent rats attenuates withdrawal-induced norepinephrine efflux in forebrain. *Prog Neuro-Psychopharmacol Biol Psychiatry, 32*, 1048–1056.

Verplaetse, T. L., Rasmussen, D. D., Froehlich, J. C., & Czachowski, C. L. (2012). Effects of prazosin, an alpha1-adrenergic receptor antagonist, on the seeking and intake of alcohol and sucrose in alcohol-preferring (P) rats. *Alcohol Clin Exp Res, 36*, 881–886.

Virk, M. S., Arttamangkul, S., Birdsong, W. T., & Williams, J. T. (2009). Buprenorphine is a weak partial agonist that inhibits opioid receptor desensitization. *J Neurosci, 29*, 7341–7348.

Volkow, N. D., Chang, L., Wang, G. J., Fowler, J. S., Leonido-Yee, M., Franceschi, D., et al. (2001). Association of dopamine transporter reduction with psychomotor impairment in methamphetamine abusers. *Am J Psychiatry, 158*, 377–382.

Volkow, N. D., Fowler, J. S., Wang, G. J., Hitzemann, R., Logan, J., Schlyer, D. J., et al. (1993). Decreased dopamine D2 receptor availability is associated with reduced frontal metabolism in cocaine abusers. *Synapse (New York, NY), 14*, 169–177.

Volkow, N. D., Fowler, J. S., Wolf, A. P., Schlyer, D., Shiue, C. Y., Alpert, R., et al. (1990). Effects of chronic cocaine abuse on postsynaptic dopamine receptors. *Am J Psychiatry, 147*, 719–724.

Volkow, N. D., Wang, G. J., Fischman, M. W., Foltin, R. W., Fowler, J. S., Abumrad, N. N., et al. (1997). Relationship between subjective effects of cocaine and dopamine transporter occupancy. *Nature, 386*, 827–830.

Volkow, N. D., Wang, G. J., Fowler, J. S., Thanos, P. P., Logan, J., Gatley, S. J., et al. (2002). Brain DA D2 receptors predict reinforcing effects of stimulants in humans: Replication study. *Synapse (New York, NY), 46*, 79–82.

Volkow, N. D., Wang, G. J., Fowler, J. S., Tomasi, D., Telang, F., & Baler, R. (2010). Addiction: Decreased reward sensitivity and increased expectation sensitivity conspire to overwhelm the brain's control circuit. *Bioessays, 32*, 748–755.

Wang, G. J., Smith, L., Volkow, N. D., Telang, F., Logan, J., Tomasi, D., et al. (2012). Decreased dopamine activity predicts relapse in methamphetamine abusers. *Mol Psychiatry, 17*, 918–925.

Wang, G. J., Volkow, N. D., Fowler, J. S., Logan, J., Abumrad, N. N., Hitzemann, R. J., et al. (1997). Dopamine D2 receptor availability in opiate-dependent subjects before and after naloxone-precipitated withdrawal. *Neuropsychopharmacol, 16*, 174–182.

Yang, S., Salmeron, B. J., Ross, T. J., Xi, Z. X., Stein, E. A., & Yang, Y. (2009). Lower glutamate levels in rostral anterior cingulate of chronic cocaine users—A (1)H-MRS study using TE-averaged PRESS at 3 T with an optimized quantification strategy. *Psychiatry Res, 174*, 171–176.

Younger, J., & Mackey, S. (2009). Fibromyalgia symptoms are reduced by low-dose naltrexone: A pilot study. *Pain Med, 10*, 663–672.

Zhang, X. Y., & Kosten, T. A. (2005). Prazosin, an alpha-1 adrenergic antagonist, reduces cocaine-induced reinstatement of drug-seeking. *Biol Psychiatry, 57*, 1202–1204.

CHAPTER 2

Historical and Social Context of Psychoactive Substance Use Disorders

JOSEPH WESTERMEYER

Historical and social factors are key to understanding the epidemiology of addictive disorders. These factors affect the rates of addictive disorders in the community, the types of substances abused, the characteristics of abusive users, the course of these disorders, and the efficacy of treatment. These background features can also help in comprehending the genesis of these disorders, their treatment outcome, and preventive approaches.

Psychoactive substances have long helped people cope with difficulties in their lives. On the individual level, these substances can relieve adverse mental and emotional states (from social fears at a party to terror before battle), physical symptoms (e.g., pain and diarrhea), and burdensome social roles ("time out" from day-to-day existence through altered states of consciousness). Rituals and ceremonies can even require substance use, from alcohol in Jewish Passover rites and the Roman Catholic Mass, to peyote in the Native American Church (Albaugh & Anderson, 1974), to serving opium at certain Hindu marriages. Consumption of psychoactive substances parallels the evolution of human civilization.

Paradoxically, these substances that bless and benefit our existence can torment and decivilize us. Individuals and societies began learning this disturbing truth millennia ago. We continue to rediscover this harsh reality today and tomorrow, as though each new generation must learn afresh for itself. As our societies become more complex, so too do our psychoactive substances, our means of consuming them, and the problems associated with them.

ORIGINS OF PSYCHOACTIVE SUBSTANCE USE

Prehistory

Archaeological data document the importance of alcohol commerce in prehistorical times, both in the Mediterranean (where wine vessels have been discovered in numerous shipwrecks) and in China (where wine vessels have been found in burial sites). Neolithic farming technology not only developed the specialization needed for complex society but also provided excess carbohydrates for alcohol fermentation. In addition, incised poppy capsules in the prehistoric headdresses of Cretan priestesses indicate awareness of opium harvest methods (Westermeyer, 1999).

Anthropological studies of preliterate societies have shown the almost universal use of psychoactive substances. Prior to Columbus's travel to the New World, North and South American societies focused on the development of stimulant drugs (e.g., coca leaf, tobacco leaf, coffee bean) and hallucinogenic drugs (e.g., peyote, mushrooms). They used hallucinogens for ritual purposes and stimulant drugs for secular purposes, such as hard labor or long hunts. New World peoples discovered diverse modes of administration, such as chewing, nasal insufflation or "snuffing," pulmonary inhalation or "smoking," and rectal clysis (DuToit, 1977). African and Middle Eastern ethnic groups produced a smaller number of stimulants, such as qat and cannabis (Kennedy, Teague, et al., 1980). Groups across Africa and the Eurasian land mass obtained alcohol from numerous sources, such as honey, grains, tubers, fruits, and mammalian milk. A few specific drugs were also used across vast distances, such as opium across Asia and the stimulant betel from South Asia to Oceania. Old World peoples primarily consumed drugs by ingestion prior to 1500 C.E.

Early History

Written records of alcohol, opium, and other psychoactive substances appear with the earliest Egyptian and Chinese ideographic writings. Opium was described as an ingested medication in these first documents. Mayan, Aztec, and Incan statues and glyphs described ritual drug use (Furst, 1972). Medieval accounts across the Eurasian land mass recorded alcohol and drug use. Travelers of that era often viewed psychoactive substance use patterns in other areas as unusual, aberrant, or problematic. Examples include reports of Scandinavian "beserker" drinkers by the English and reports by Crusaders of Islamic military units or "assassins" intoxicated on cannabis. Along with animal sacrifice and the serving of meat, the provision of alcohol, betel, opium, tobacco, or other psychoactive substances came to have cultural, ritual, or religious symbolic meaning, including hospitality toward guests (Smith, 1965).

Substance use and social affiliation have long been associated with specific ethnic groups, social classes, sects, and castes. For example, one group in India consumed alcohol but not cannabis, whereas an adjacent group consumed cannabis but not alcohol (Carstairs, 1954). Religious identities can be tied to alcohol or drug consumption, or to abstinence from alcohol or drugs. As the problems from or associated with alcohol excess became known, ancient Hindu and Buddhist sects, as well as latter-day Islamic and fundamentalist Christian sects, prohibited alcohol drinking (Hippler, 1973). In addition to distinguishing people from one another, transcultural drinking has promoted cooperation and communication across ethnic groups and social classes, from Africa (Wolcott, 1974) to the Americas (Heath, 1971).

Culture and Social Change

Political, commercial, and technical advances have influenced the types of substances consumed, along with their supply, cost, availability, and modes of administration (Westermeyer, 1987). Cottage industry production of alcohol, tobacco, and other substances morphed into the purchase of mass-produced beverage alcohol and tobacco-based products, reflecting comparable economic changes (Caetano, 1987). International commerce, built on cheaper and more efficient transportation, facilitated drug production and distribution. Greater disposable income favored recreational intoxication (Caetano, Suzman, et al., 1983). Development of parenteral injection for medical purposes spread to recreational drug self-administration in the mid-1800s, within several years of its invention. Purification and modification of plant compounds (e.g., cocaine from the coca leaf, morphine and heroin from opium, and hashish oil from the cannabis plant) produced substances that were more potent and more easily transported, smuggled, or sold illicitly. Laboratory synthesis over the last century has produced addictive drugs that closely mimic naturally occurring substances (e.g., amphetamines, sedatives, opioids, and hallucinogens) but are more potent and sometimes cheaper than purified plant compounds.

Pharmacokinetics and pharmacodynamics of psychoactive substances may affect their social use. A case in point is the flushing reaction from alcohol consumption observed among a greater-than-expected number of Asians and Native Americans (but it is neither universal in these peoples nor limited to them). Absence of alcohol use among the northern Asian peoples who subsequently peopled much of East Asia and the Americas is a likely explanation, but the exact reason is unknown. The flushing reaction associated with alcohol (Johnson & Nagoshi, 1990) has been offered as a reason for two opposite phenomena:

1. The low rates of alcoholism among Asian peoples, who presumably find the reaction aversive and hence drink little—although rates are increasing across much of Asia (Ohmori, Koyama, et al., 1986).
2. The high rates of alcoholism among certain Native American groups, who presumably must "drink through" their flushing reaction to experience other alcohol effects.

Flushing may be more or less desirable, depending on how the culture values this biological effect. Among many East and Southeast Asian peoples influenced by Buddhist precepts, flushing is viewed as the emergence of cupidity or rage, with implied loss of emotional control. Modal differences in alcohol metabolism have also been observed among ethnic groups, and these differences support arguments in favor of biological causation. However, the intraethnic differences in alcohol metabolism greatly exceed the interethnic differences (Fenna, Mix, et al., 1971). Despite some minimal pharmacokinetic differences among people of different races, the observed differences appear to be due more to pharmacodynamics. That is, the influence of people vis-à-vis the drug (i.e., their traditions, taboos, expectations, and patterns of use) appears to exert greater influence than the drug vis-à-vis the people (e.g., rates of absorption and catabolism, and flushing reactions). Both pharmacodynamic factors related to culture and pharmacokinetic factors related to biological inheritance probably play roles in the individual's experience with psychoactive substances.

Social control measures arose as psychoactive substance abuse surfaced in advanced civilizations. One consistent approach was to enact and enforce laws. For example, pre-Columbian Aztecs limited the frequency and amount of drinking (Anawalt & Berdan, 1992). Later, in the post-Columbian period, England countered its "gin plague" with a tax on imported alcohol-containing beverages (Thurn, 1978) and its later "opium epidemic" with medical–pharmaceutical prescribing laws (Kramer, 1979). Another method to limit alcohol consumption was religious stricture (Hippler, 1973). Perhaps the first organized religion to prescribe abstinence from alcohol was Hinduism. Early Buddhist leaders counseled abstinence from alcohol as a means of quitting earthly bondage, achieving contentment in this life, and earning Nirvana after death. Islam became the third great religion to adopt abstinence from alcohol, reportedly when a town was sacked because of a drunken nighttime guard. The "gin plague" in England spawned several abstinence-oriented Christian sects, despite the earlier status of wine as a Christian sacramental substance (Johnson & Westermeyer, 2000).

Patterns of Psychoactive Substance Use

Episodic patterns of psychoactive substance use have been traditional in most societies at times of personal celebrations (e.g., birth and marriage), rituals (e.g., arrivals, departures, and changes in social status), and seasonal celebrations (e.g., harvest and New Year). Socially sanctioned, episodic psychoactive substance consumption may involve heavy use, with marked intoxication or drunkenness (Bunzel, 1940). Even in a low-technology environment, this pattern may cause problems. For example, psychotomimetic drugs such as cannabis can cause toxic psychosis (Chopra & Smith, 1974). Binge-type alcohol problems include fights, sexually transmitted disease, and falls. In a high-technology environment, with modern methods of transportation and industrial machinery, even occasional binges may pose threats to life and limb (Stull, 1972).

Daily or frequent use of alcohol may involve its use as a foodstuff (e.g., wine in Mediterranean regions). Daily stimulant use may accompany long, hard labor (e.g., paddy rice or taro farming, mining). Daily beer or wine drinking is not without its problems, even when socially sanctioned. Hepatic cirrhosis and other organ damage (e.g., to brain, bone marrow, neuromuscular system, and pancreas) may result from long-term, daily use of more than 2–4 ounces of alcohol, depending on body weight (Baldwin, 1977). Daily use of stimulants can lead to biomedical or psychosocial problems, such as oral cancers and other pathologies in the case of betel–areca chewing (Ahluwalia & Ponnampalam, 1968) or psychobehavioral changes in the case of coca-leaf chewing (Negrete, 1978).

Substance abuse epidemics began around five centuries ago, with some persisting over centuries as endemics. In the pre-Columbian era, sporadic cases of acute and chronic substance abuse problems were well known. However, relatively sudden, massive substance abuse problems appeared in the post-Columbian era. One of these was the English *gin epidemic* or "gin plague" (Thurn, 1978), which began in the late 1600s, spread to other areas of Europe, and continued for several decades. Transatlantic, intercontinental trade and the beginnings of the Industrial Revolution were its immediate precipitants. Around the same time, *opium epidemics* broke out in several Asian countries. The origins of these two continentwide epidemics were different, although they occurred around the same time, flamed by both internal forces and external influences. The post-Columbian spread of tobacco smoking to Asia introduced the inhabitants to inhalation as a new mode of drug administration. This new route of administration applied to an old drug, opium, produced a combination more addictive than the old opium-eating tradition. Imperial pressures against tobacco smoking (which was viewed as wasteful and associated with seditious elements) probably accelerated the popularity of opium smoking. Subsequently, European colonialism and international trade contributed to the import of Indian opium to several East Asian countries. Opium epidemics also occurred somewhat later in Europe and North America (Kramer, 1979). Although East Asian countries have largely controlled their opium problems, opiate endemics continue in Southeast and South Asia, the Middle East, parts of Europe, and North America. Numerous other drug epidemics have occurred in the last century: the tobacco pandemic related to cigarette smoking, amphetamine epidemics on most continents since the 1940s, and cocaine epidemics in Europe and North America.

SOCIAL FUNCTIONS OF SUBSTANCES OVER TIME

Social and socially approved purposes for which people use substances can differ across time and space. However, the list of functions associated with alcohol and drug use has remained small and fairly consistent through the centuries. Awareness of these functions can be important for clinicians, public health interveners, and patients themselves to appreciate. In many instances, non-drug interventions may substitute for drug use; examples include meditation, self-relaxation, exercise, song or dance in social gatherings, and mandatory limitations on daily hours of work.

Ceremonial use is widely known for alcohol, but ceremonial use of drugs is not so well-known. Peyote buttons are a sacramental substance in the Native American Church (Bergman, 1971). Hallucinogen use for religious purposes still occurs in many South American ethnic groups (DuToit, 1977). Supernatural sanctions, both prescribing use within certain bounds and prohibiting use outside these bounds, inveigh against abuse of these substances by devotees. Thus, ceremonial or religious use tends to be relatively safe. Examples of abuse do occur, however, such as the occasional Catholic priest whose alcoholism begins with abuse of sacramental wine.

Secular social use of alcohol and drugs occurs in numerous quasi-ritual contexts. Drinking may occur at annual events, such as New Year or harvest ceremonies (e.g., Thanksgiving in the United States). Weddings, births, funerals, and other family rituals are occasions for alcohol or drug use in many cultures. Marking of friendships, business arrangements, or intergroup competitions can virtually require substance use in some groups. For example, the *dutsen* in German-speaking Central Europe is a brief ritual in which friends or associates agree to address each other by the informal *du* ("thou") rather than by the formal *sie* ("you"). Participants, holding an alcoholic beverage in their right hands, link their right arms, toast each other, and drink with arms linked. The use of betel or areca, pulque or cactus beer, coca leaf, and other intoxicants has accompanied group work tasks, such as harvests or community *corvée* obligations (e.g., maintaining roads, bridges, and irrigation ditches). Although substance use may be heavy at ceremonial events, even involving intoxication, the social control of the group over dosage and the brief duration of use augurs against chronic abuse (although problems related to acute abuse may occur). Problems accrue if the group's central rationale for existence rests heavily on substance use (e.g., habitués of opium dens, taverns and cocktail lounges, crack houses, college party houses). In these latter instances, group norms for heavy alcohol or drug use may foster rather than prevent substance abuse (Dumont, 1967).

Medicinal use has prevailed in one place or another with virtually all psychoactive substances, including alcohol, opium, cannabis, tobacco, stimulants, and hallucinogens (Hill, 1990). Insofar as substances are prescribed or administered solely by licensed physicians, abuse had been rare or absent. For example, the prescribing of oral opium by Chinese physicians over many centuries prior to the opium epidemic had few or no adverse social consequences. On the other hand, self-prescribing of habit-forming or addictive drugs for medicinal purposes carries risks. Self-prescribing of opium by poppy farmers likewise antedates opium addiction in a majority of cases (Westermeyer, 1982). Thus, professional control over medicinal use had been relatively benign (prior to the recent U.S. iatrogenic opioid epidemic), whereas individual control over medicinal use of psychoactive compounds has often been problematic.

Dietary use of substances falls into two general categories: (1) the use of alcohol as a source of calories and (2) the use of herbal intoxicants to enhance taste. Fermentation of carbohydrates into alcohol has been a convenient way of storing calories that would otherwise deteriorate. Unique tastes and eating experiences associated with beverage alcohol (e.g., various wines) have further fostered their use, especially at ritual, ceremonial, or social meals. Cannabis and other intoxicating herbs have also been used from the Middle East to the Malay Archipelago as a means of enhancing soups, teas, pastries, and sweets.

Recreational use can presumably occur in either social or individual settings. Much substance use today occurs in recreational or "party" settings that have some psychosocial rationales (e.g., social "time out" and meeting friends) but minimal or no ritual or ceremonial aspects. So-called "recreational" substance use in these social contexts may in fact be quasi-medicinal (i.e., to reduce symptoms associated with social phobia, low self-esteem, boredom, or chronic dysphoria). Even solitary psychoactive substance use can be recreational (i.e., to enhance an enjoyable event) or medicinal (i.e., to relieve loneliness, insomnia, or pain).

Other purposes exist but are not as widespread as those described previously. In the 19th century, young European women took belladonna before social events in order to give themselves a ruddy, blushing complexion. Children may inhale household or industrial solvents as a means of mimicking adult intoxication (Kaufman, 1973). Intoxication may simply serve as a means for continuing social behaviors that existed previously without intoxication, for example, fights among men in some groups (Levy & Kunitz, 1969). Group patterns of alcohol/drug production or use may represent rebellion against prevailing norms by disenfranchised groups (Connell, 1961; Lurie, 1970).

HISTORY OF SUBSTANCE ABUSE TREATMENT AND PREVENTION

Ceasing substance use and finding satisfaction in a substance-free lifestyle has been an age-old strategy to treat and prevent substance abuse. Substance-focused strategies have included gradual decrease in dosage, isolation from the substance (in a monastary or a remote asylum), or relocation away from fellow users (in a halfway house or recovery farm). Other modalities have focused on the miseries associated with attempting abstinence, such as symptomatic use of nonaddicting medications, religious conversion (replacing narcotomania with religiomania), group support, residence in a substance-free environment, and expectant treatment with a variety of shamanistic, spiritual, dietary, herbal, and medicinal methods (Westermeyer, 1991).

Galenic medicine, with roots going back beyond two millennia, used a syndromal or symptom-focused approach. In the case of substance abuse, the strategy consisted of early identification of symptions associated with alcohol and drug abuse (e.g., craving, withdrawal, secondary problems). Another purpose of this model was to identify disorders not obviously associated with substance abuse, such as delirium tremens (i.e., alcohol and sedative withdrawal), withdrawal seizures, morphinism (i.e., opioid withdrawal), cannabis-induced acute psychosis, stimulant psychosis, and fetal alcohol syndrome. Once the etiology was determined, the specific treatment (i.e., cessation of substance abuse) could be prescribed. Description of pathophysiological and psychopathological processes has been a logical historical step in developing early recognition and intervention for substance use disorders (SUDs; Rodin 1981).

Progressive symptoms of addiction comprise a means of observing the early-to-late symptoms and signs of addiction, so that clinicians might classify the severity of the disorder and recommend interventions linked to that severity. Benjamin Rush, a physician from the Revolutionary War era, developed such a progressive classification for alcoholism. Parenthetically, Rush also promoted "asylum," away from access to alcohol, to take place in a family-like rural setting in a milieu of respect, consideration, and social support (Johnson & Westermeyer, 2000).

Pharmacological treatments can interact constructively with social factors to facilitate recovery. For example, disulfiram can act as an acceptable excuse for Native American alcoholics (and others) to resist peer pressures to drink (Savard, 1968). Recovering opioid addicts can take maintenance naltrexone as a mean of avoiding a relapse if social pressures might lead to an epsiode of unplanned use. Naltrexone, disulfiram, and other agents might be appended to contingency contracting, which is a social intervention.

Ethnic identity of the patient vis-à-vis the clinical setting can affect outcomes—an important issue in multiethnic socities such as the United States. Ethnic similarity between patients and staff may be more critical to the treatment process of substance disorders than in other medical or psychiatric conditions (Shore & Von Fumetti, 1972). Strong ethnic affiliation supports optimal treatment outcomes. Occasionally, ethnic or religious affiliation may change during the recovery process (Westermeyer & Lang, 1975).

National governmental involvement in addiction began with the appointment of an anti-opium ministry in China in the 1800s. Similar federal-level initiatives spread to the United States, where treatment for drug abuse (largely opiate dependence) began with the Harrison Act of 1914, outlawing nonmedical use of opiate drugs. For a time throughout the 1920s, heroin maintenance was dispensed in several clinics around the country. Despite case reports indicating beneficial outcomes from maintenance doses of heroin, these clinics lost funding due to political opposition. Two long-term prison-like hospitals for opiate addicts were established in Kentucky and Texas. Research in these institutions contributed greatly to understanding addiction, including the inefficacy of prison treatment for most cases of addiction. These legal sanctions beginning in 1914 did effectively reduce opiate dependence in the societal mainstream. However, certain groups continued to use drugs made illicit by the Harrison Act (i.e., seamen, musicians, certain minority groups, and inhabitants of coastal–border areas involved in smuggling).

Federal initiatives also led to prohibition of the production and commerce in alcohol beverages beginning in 1920. Prohibition failed in its goals, however, leading to its repeal in 1933. By 1950, the early antinarcotic successes of the Harrison Act were also starting to wane. Thus, following World War II, medical and social leaders were more aware of widespread addiction-related disabilities in the country. This led to the establishment of the National Institute of Mental Health (NIMH), which had divisions of alcoholism and drug abuse. By the 1970s, it became apparent that SUDs were widely prevalent. Numerous indices of alcohol abuse and alcoholism had been increasing since World War II, including hepatic cirrhosis and violence-related mortality. Endemic abuse of cocaine and opiates exploded into an epidemic in the late 1960s, followed by the appearance of stimulant and hallucinogen abuse. It was evident that NIMH was not adequately addressing either the alcohol or the drug epidemic. This led to the formation of the National Institute on Alcohol Abuse and Alcoholism (NIAAA) and the National Institute on Drug Abuse (NIDA), both of which have equal status with the NIMH under the Alcohol, Drug Abuse, and Mental Health Administration (ADAMHA). Located within the Department of Health and Human Services, ADAMHA funded the development of substance abuse research, training, clinical services, and prevention. Recent forces have favored the reintegration of drug and alcohol treatment.

SOCIAL AND SELF-HELP MOVEMENTS

Abstinence-oriented social movements first appeared among organized religions, as described earlier. South Asian sects arising from early Persian religions abstained from alcohol over 2 millennia ago. These movements continue today in some schools, Indian reservations, and health clubs (Jilek-Aall, 1978).

Religiomania has long served as a cure for dipsomania and narcotomania, as described previously. Children raised in these sects are taught the importance of life-long abstinence from alcohol and other drugs of abuse. Despite this childhood social-ization, those leaving these sects as adults can develop SUDs. Thus, the anti-SUD effects of various religions appear to persist only as long as one is actively affiliated with the group (Mariz, 1991).

Abstinent societies not tied to specific religions began to appear in the 18th and 19th centuries. Examples include the Anti-Opium Society in China and the Women's Christian Temperance Union in the United States. These groups engaged in political action, public education, social pressure against addiction or alcoholism, and support for abstinence. These societies led eventually to prohibition movements that sought legal strictures against the production, sale, and/or consumption of psychoactive sub-stances.

Self-help groups consisted of individuals who banded together to meet their com-mon financial, social, or personal needs (Lieberman & Borman, 1976). Movements have differed in several important aspects from earlier abstinence-oriented groups as follows:

- Individuals could remain in their homes, families, and jobs rather than joining a separate sect or relocating to an asylum or special group.
- Structure consisted of sponsorship, readings, meetings, and phased "step" recovery activities.
- The concept of a recovery process over time was introduced, as distinct from a sudden cure or conversion; this had biological, psychological, social, and spiritual dimensions.
- Organization was kept predominantly atomistic (i.e., autonomous, small groups) rather than hierarchical.
- Membership required self-identity as an alcoholic or addict, so that supportive or concerned persons were excluded from membership.

Like earlier movements, these self-help groups emphasized the importance of abstinence from psychoactive substance abuse, reliance on spiritual forces, and social affiliation or "fellowship." Alcoholics Anonymous served as a model for similar groups (i.e., Narcotics Anonymous, Cocaine Anonymous, Overeaters Anonymous, Gamblers Anonymous, and Emotions Anonymous). Groups for those personally affected by alcoholism have also appeared, such as Alateen for the teenage offspring of parents with alcoholism and Al-Anon for the spouses, parents, and other con-cerned associates of persons with alcoholism. The Adult Children of Alcoholics and Addicts (ACOAA) movement has also evolved to meet the needs of those distressed or maladaptive adults raised by alcoholic parents. Mothers Against Drunk Drivers (MADD) was originally formed to meet the support needs of parents whose children were killed by drunken auto drivers. MADD has since expanded its activities as a "watchdog" group that follows the records of legislators and judges in regard to alcohol-related legal offenses.

FACTORS ABETTING ALCOHOL–DRUG EPIDEMICS

Novel substances, new forms, or new routes of administration have presaged epidemics. Consequently, traditional sanctions against the substance were missing. For example, at the time of their gin epidemic, the English had sanctions regarding drinking mead and ale but not gin or rum. Likewise, Asian societies had traditions governing prescription of oral opium pills for medical purposes but not for opium smoking in recreational settings. Recently, in the United States, there was no social opposition to iatrogenic opioid addiction or "medical marijuana" when these venues for addiction appeared. In summary, social "immunity" against the neoaddictive force was lacking. In addition, as noted below, the substance must lend itself to profiteering.

Social upheaval has sometimes provided a favorable environment for substance use epidemics. Around the time of the gin epidemic, the Industrial Revolution in England, and later across Europe, forever altered the playing field between individuals and their social institutions. During the opium epidemics, imperial regimes in Asia and later in Europe were failing in their responsibilities to the governed and becoming outdated. Recently, in the United States, financial and organizational changes in the health care system have undermined the physician–patient relationship, as well as people's trust in health care generally.

Profiteering contributes a *sine qua non* for meeting the tremendous demand for substance imposed by the epidemic. In the gin epidemic, English merchant ships returning from trips to its colonies loaded gin, rum, and other alcohol-containing beverages as ballast before returning to England. Rum was derived from sugar cane grown with slave labor, and gin, from grains grown with indentured labor. With no import tax, calories of these alcohol-containing beverages were literally cheaper than calories of bread in London. In the opium epidemic, economic imperialism of Western powers provided a means of producing opium in one country (India) and selling it to others (especially China), and buying, transporting, and selling millions of pounds of opium annually. Likewise, today in the United States, an extensive and expanding capacity exists to produce, market, and distribute billions of opioid doses per year to addicted patients. In those states with laws supporting "medical marijuana," the expansion of productivity has been phenomenal (building on decades of experience from illicit production). Retail outlets have exploded over a short period, with several hundred retail outlets in Los Angeles alone. All of these epidemics have depended on venture capital, banks, corporate-level organizers, marketing opportunists, elected officials, and security rendered by the police and courts. Without profiteering, epidemics would fizzle.

Political and industrial corruption inevitably accompany substance abuse epidemics, as vested interests strategize to maintain their economic advantages. In the English gin epidemic, politicians allowed extended hours of business for pubs near factories. Factory owners paid workers in gin and rum. In the Asian opium epidemics, local petty chiefs (later termed "war lords") became involved in the trade as a means to obtain wealth and power. In the United States today, pharmaceutical companies, lobbies, "chronic pain" programs, and clinician–profiteers have delayed governmental and professional efforts to address the epidemic. In states with "medical marijuana," chronic users, formerly illicit cannabis farmers and marketing opportunists, have ramped up production and distribution to meet the large and growing demand.

HISTORICAL TRENDS IN OUR TIME

Anti-authority symbolism of certain drugs or modes of drug administration may displace the issue from psychoactive substance use per se to associated issues of ethnic identity, cultural change, political upheaval, class struggle, or intergenerational conflict (Robbins, 1973). For example, alcohol abuse among indigenous peoples has acted as an ongoing "protest" among conquered peoples, including the Irish in English-dominated Ireland and Native Americans in the United States (Thompson, 1992). Illicit raising of poppy as a cash crop and opium smuggling by ethnic minorities in Asia have provided a means of accessing wealth and funding political opposition (Westermeyer, 1982). Cannabis and hallucinogen use served as anti-authority symbols in the United States during the 1960s and 1970s.

Third-world economic profiteering yielded by drug and alcohol commerce has led to entrenched economic interests of producers, financiers, transport companies, security workers, community leaders, and elected or appointed officials, who then profit from people's misery. Numerous backward areas in the world today maintain their participation in world markets through illicit drug production and commerce (e.g., opium and heroin: Afghanistan, Burma, Laos, Mexico, Pakistan, and Thailand; cannabis and cocaine: the Caribbean nations and Mexico; cocaine: several South and Central American countries). Since the 1980s, financially challenged states in the United States have counted cannabis as a major cash crop, including North Carolina, Tennessee, Kentucky, Kansas, Nebraska, New Mexico, California, and Hawaii (Culhane, 1989). Large-scale substance abuse epidemics cannot exist with a political-economic-security system that permits, protects, and propagates alcohol/drug commerce and alcohol/drug use. To continue these rich profit sources, leaders are drawn into blocking development and progress of these drug-producing areas.

Government instability ensues gradually from drug-related corruption. The resulting inefficiency causes unstable countries and inchoate state governments to become hostage to epidemic economic forces. Societal breakdown results, contributing to a backlash of unsavory political movements aimed at opposing corrupt regimes (e.g., religious fundamentalism, rebellion, armed extragovernmental "war lords").

Industrialization and technological advances have fostered a redefinition of substance abuse (Stull, 1972). An intoxicated or "hungover" ox-cart driver can create limited damage, other than to cart, ox, and self. The alcohol- or drug-affected driver of a modern high-speed bus, captain of a ferry boat, or pilot of a jet transport can kill scores of people and destroy equipment and material worth millions of dollars. Handicraft artisans under the influence of drugs or alcohol can do little damage, whereas workers in a factory can harm many others, as well as destroy expensive machinery and bring production to a halt. Likewise, these advances have produced psychoactive compounds at lower cost; developed new compounds (e.g., the amphetamine and benzodiazepine epidemics); and enhanced the rapid, low-cost transport and sale of addictive substances.

Adolescent-onset substance abuse has escalated from rare sporadic cases to high prevalence in many communities over the last several decades (Cameron, 1968). Elements cited as reasons for this early onset have included widespread parental substance abuse, societal neglect of adolescents, poverty, rapid social changes, family breakdown, and political upheaval. Whatever the cause, the consequences are remarkably similar around the world: undermining of normal adolescent psychosocial development; poor socialization of children to assume adult roles; lack of job skills; emotional immaturity; and increased rates of adolescent psychiatric morbidity and adolescent mortality from suicide, accidents, and homicide.

MODERN TRENDS IN TREATMENT AND PREVENTION

Two central themes in the treatment of behavioral and mental disorders emerged during the late 1700s. One was the concept of *moral treatment*, consisting of a civil, respectful consideration for the recovering person. The other concept was *asylum*, a supportive environment away from drinking and drug access. Both methods persist today and remain basic cornerstones for treatment (Johnson & Westermeyer, 2000).

Detoxification became prevalent in the mid-1900s. Public detoxification facilities, established first in Eastern Europe, spread throughout the world. For many patients, this resource has offered an entree into recovery. For others, "revolving door" detoxification may actually produce lifelong institutionalization on the installment plan (Gallant, Bishop, et al., 1973). The conundrum of the treatment-resistant public inebriates exists today in all parts of the United States.

Drug substitution—replacing one drug for another—has been a recurrent approach in treatment. For example, laudanum (combined alcohol and opiates) was once prescribed for alcoholism. Morphine, and later heroin, was recommended for opium addiction during the mid-1800s. This approach is not extinct, as exemplified by the the 1970s shibboleth that alcoholics can safely substitute cannabis smoking for alcohol. Currently, methadone and buprenorphine are used for chronic opiate addicts who have failed attempts at drug-free treatment. Nicotine products have reduced the withdrawal effects experienced by tobacco-dependent people.

More sophisticated pharmacotherapy methods have evolved slowly over the decades, although these remain few in comparison with other areas of medicine. Disulfiram and metronidazole produce a noxious, toxic reaction from acetaldehyde accumulation if alcohol is consumed. Naltrexone, an opioid antagonist, prevents opiate agonist effects if an opioid is consumed. Moreover, it can reduce craving for alcohol. Acamprosate may accomplish the same end. Methadone reduces opioid craving in opioid-dependent patients, and its long half-life minimizes its agonist effects. Buprenorphine, with both agonist and antagonist actions, replicates actions of both naltrexone and methadone. Other medications are currently being investigated for use with other drugs or for special purposes.

The so-called *Minnesota model* of treatment developed from several sources: a state hospital program (at Wilmar, Minnesota) and a later private program (at Hazelden in Center City, Minnesota), supplemented by the first Veterans Administration program for alcoholism (at the Minneapolis Veterans Administration Hospital). The characteristics of this model varied over time as treatment evolved and changed. Definitions for this model still differ from one person to the next. Still, several core characteristics can be generally ascribed to the model. It begins with a periof of intensive, often residential care, ranging from weeks to months. The focus is on abstinence from alcohol and drugs; comorbid psychiatric disorder and healthful living receive minimal or no attention. Group sessions emphasize self-help, especially the Twelve Steps of Alcoholics Anonymous. Individualization is nil. Once this phase (often called "primary treatment") is completed, the next step is referral to a a self-help group. Pharmacotherapy or psychotherapy has almost no place in this model. Readmission is anathema; people are expected to recover from the initial exposure. At the time of its evolution in the 1950s and 1960s, this model served to bridge the formerly separate hospital programs and self-help groups—a laudable achievement. By the 1970s, it was becoming obsolete. Nowadays, many treatment programs employ selected aspects of the old "Minnesota model," integrating them flexibly with newer methods, in a more individualized and patient-centered manner.

Workplace programs have become a locus of prevention, early recognition, referral for treatment, and ongoing monitoring and rehabilitation. Following World War II, Hudolin and coworkers in Yugoslavia established factory- and commune-based recovery groups, with ties to treatment facilities (Hudolin, 1982). In the 1970s, similar "employee assistance programs" (EAPs) emerged in the United States.

Concurrent treatment for SUDs and other behavioral, emotional, and mental disorders evolved as the high prevalence of comorbid conditions was recognized. For certain chronic conditions—such as mild mental retardation, borderline intelligence, organic brain syndrome, or chronic schizophrenia—substance abuse treatment, rehabilitation, and self-help procedures need to be modified. Intensive outpatient programs, conducted during the day, evening, or weekend, help certain patients to recover when other measures fail. These intensive outpatient programs are modeled after similar psychiatric programs. Much of the treatment time is spent in groups of various sizes, although individual and family sessions may occur as well. Staff members are typically multidisciplinary and include counselors, nurses, occupational and recreational therapists, psychologists, psychiatrists, and social workers.

Monitoring of recovery in several contexts and by several sources (e.g., employers, licensing agencies, unions, treatment programs) enhances outcome (Westermeyer, 1989). This strategy supports the efforts of recovering people themselves. It can also aid in early recognition of relapse. Since this strategy assumes that some people relapse, this strategy provides ready access to crisis intervention and timely return to recovery.

Preventive techniques, first applied to the gin epidemic in Europe, the opium epidemic in Asia, and the Aztecs' abuse of alcohol, remain useful today. Control over hours and location of sales, taxes or duties to increase cost, changing of public attitudes via the mass media, education, and abstinence-oriented religion have all reduced prevalence rates of SUDs in modern times (Smart, 1982). The prolonged Asian opium epidemic demonstrated that laws alone are ineffective unless accompanied by socially integrated treatment and recovery programs, and compulsory abstinence in identified cases; law enforcement pressure against drug production, commerce, and consumption; and follow-up monitoring. Experience with anti-alcohol prohibition laws in Europe and North America demonstrated the futility of outlawing substance use that is supported by the citizenry at large. Adverse results from the Prohibition era in the United States included increased criminality associated with bootlegging alcohol, lack of quality control (e.g., methanol and lead contaminants), and development of unhealthy drinking patterns (e.g., surreptitious, rapid, without food, and in an unfavorable setting). Public interest groups (e.g., MADD) have reduced alcohol- and drug-related problems in high-use areas such as Indian reservations and college–university campuses. The United States has expended several 10s of billions of dollars since 1970 to reduce the supply of and demand for drugs. But mortality from hepatic cirrhosis, alcohol-related accidents, and suicide continue at an unprecedented level, especially among young American males. Our remaining work includes learning from history (our own, as well as that of others) and honing statecraft aimed at eliminating our endemic substance abuse.

Recent social experiments are apt to affect substance use prevalence and treatment in the coming decade or two. *Increased opioid prescribing* for chronic subjective complaints over the last two decades has produced the largest opioid epidemic yet observed in the United States. Iatrogenc opioid addiction has changed the demography, clinician–patient relationships, and access of youth and other family members to opioids. *Legalized "medical marijuana"* reduced the legal impasse in more than a dozen states in which local production, commerce, and/or sales in cannabis have produced a massive norm conflict regarding what the law states and what people do vis-à-vis cannabis. Although the norm conflict has been reduced, the prevalence of cannabis dependence, early exposure among youth, and cannabis-related traffic accidents has increased in early reports following legal production and use. *"Housing first,"* the strategy of housing substance abusers who are homeless before treating them, was aimed at reducing the huge number of homeless people in the United States. Early evaluations indicated that the experiment increased mortality and medical costs in substance abusers, produced an even higher rate of people without shelter, and undermined subsequent interventions tied to abstinence (Westermeyer & Lee, 2013).

COMMENT

Preventive and treatment efforts, age-old and wrought at great cost, are our forebearers' gift to us for dealing with psychoactive substance use gone astray. We ignore their costly bequests at our peril. To our credit, we continue to add to this compendium, from deeper understanding of psychoactive substance use to new social experiments in governing their use.

Historical and literary accounts have long documented individual attempts to draw back from the abyss of alcohol and drug disasters. At various times autobiographical, biographical, journalistic, and anecdotal, these descriptions list centuries-old recovery methods. Most of them are still employed today in lay and professional settings.

Three current social experiments in the United States (i.e., iatrogenic opioid addiction, "medical marijuana," and "housing first") were undertaken without adequate long-term research. Early indications are that they will be hugely destructive and costly to society but not be easily abated due to massive profiteering and political appropriation. At worst, they raise specters of *Soylent Green*, the cinematic society in which deluded people received brief benefits before being sacrificed to manufacture Soylent Green, the dietary stable. At best, like other social–substance use experiments before them, these movements will ultimately enlighten and guide us.

Despite missteps of empires and democracies along the way, the historical inclination has been gradual but salutary. Progress has been slow, built on mountains of misery, but ultimately beneficial. Much is known today, and more will be understood in the future.

REFERENCES

Ahluwalia, H. S., & Ponnampalam, J. T. (1968). The socioeconomic aspects of betel-nut chewing. *J Trop Med Hyg, 71,* 48–50.

Albaugh, B., & Anderson, P. (1974). Peyote in the treatment of alcoholism among American Indians. *Am J Psychiatry, 131,* 1247–1256.

Anawalt, P. R., & Berdan, F. F. (1992). The Codex Mendoza. *Sci Am, 266*(6), 70–79.

Baldwin, A. D. (1977). Anstie's alcohol limit: Francis Edmund Anstie 1833–1874. *Am J Public Health, 67*(7), 679–681.

Bergman, R. L. (1971). Navaho peyote use: Its apparent safety. *Am J Psychiatry, 128,* 695–699.

Bunzel, R. (1940). The role of alcoholism in two Central American cultures. *Psychiatry, 3,* 361–387.

Caetano, R. (1987). Acculturation and drinking patterns among U.S. Hispanics. *Brit J Addict, 82,* 789–799.

Caetano, R., & Suzman, R. M., et al. (1983). The Shetland Islands: Longitudinal changes in alcohol consumption in a changing environment. *Brit J Addict, 78,* 21–36.

Cameron, D. C. (1968). Youth and drugs: A world view. *JAMA, 206,* 1267–1271.

Carstairs, G. M. (1954). Daru and bhang: Cultural factors in the choice of intoxicant. *Q J Stud Alcohol, 15,* 220–237.

Chopra, G. S., & Smith, J. W. (1974). Psychotic reactions following cannabis use in East Indians. *Arch Gen Psychiatry, 30,* 24–27.

Connell, K. H. (1961). Illicit distillation: An Irish peasant industry. *Hist Stud Ireland, 3,* 58–91.

Culhane, C. (1989). Pot harvest gains across country. *USJ, 13*(8), 14.

Dumont, M. (1967). Tavern culture: The sustenance of homeless men. *Am J Orthopsychiatry, 37,* 938–945.

DuToit, B. M. (1977). *Drugs, rituals and altered states of consciousness.* Rotterdam: Balkema Press.

Fenna, D. L., Mix, O., et al. (1971). Ethanol metabolism in various racial groups. *CMAJ, 105,* 472–475.

Furst, P. T. (1972). *Flesh of the gods: The ritual use of hallucinogens.* New York: Praeger.

Gallant, D. M., Bishop, M. P., et al. (1973). The revolving door alcoholic. *Arch Gen Psychiatry, 28,* 633–635.

Heath, D. (1971). Peasants, revolution, and drinking: Interethnic drinking patterns in two Bolivian communities. *Hum Organ, 30,* 179–186.

Hill, T. W. (1990). Peyotism and the control of heavy drinking: The Nebraska Winnebago in the early 1900s. *Hum Organ, 49*(3), 255–265.

Hippler, A. E. (1973). Fundamentalist Christianity: An Alaskan Athabascan technique for overcoming alcohol abuse. *Transcult Psychiatry Res Rev, 10,* 173–179.

Hudolin, V. (1982). *Klubovi lijec alkoholicura (Clubs of treated alcoholics).* Zagreb, Croatia: Jumena.

Jilek-Aall, L. (1978). Alcohol and the Indian–White relationship: A study of the function of Alcoholics Anonymous among coast Salish Indians. *Confin Psychiatry, 21,* 195–233.

Johnson, D. R., & Westermeyer, J. (2000). Psychiatric therapies influenced by religious movements. In J. Boehnlein (Ed.), *Psychiatry and religion: The convergence of mind and spirit* (pp. 87–108). Washington, DC: American Psychiatric Press.

Johnson, R., & Nagoshi, C. (1990). Asians, Asian-Americans and alcohol. *J Psychoactive Drugs, 22*(1), 45–52.

Kaufman, A. (1973). Gasoline sniffing among children in a Pueblo Indian village. *Pediatrics, 51,* 1060–1065.

Kennedy, J. G., Teague, J., et al. (1980). Quat use in North Yemen and the problem of addiction: A study in medical anthropology. *Cult Med Psychiatry, 4,* 311–344.

Kramer, J. C. (1979). Opium rampant: Medical use, misuse and abuse in Britain and the west in the 17th and 18th centuries. *Brit J Addict, 74,* 377–389.

Levy, J. E., & Kunitz, S. J. (1969). Notes on some White Mountain Apache social pathologies. *Plateau, 42,* 11–19.

Lieberman, M. A., & Borman, L. D. (1976). Self-help groups. *J Appl Behav Sci, 12,* 261–303.

Lurie, N. O. (1970). The world's oldest on-going protest demonstration: North American Indian drinking patterns. *Pac Hist Rev, 40,* 311–332.

Mariz, C. L. (1991). Pentecostalism and alcoholism among the Brazilian poor. *Alcohol Treat Q, 8*(2), 75–82.

Negrete, J. C. (1978). Coca leaf chewing: A public health assessment. *Brit J Addict, 73,* 283–290.

Ohmori, T., & Koyama, T., et al. (1986). The role of aldehyde dehydrogenase isozyme variance in alcohol sensitivity, drinking habits formation and the development of alcoholism in Japan, Taiwan and the Philippines. *Prog Neuro-Psychopharmacol Biol Psychiatry, 10,* 229–235.

Robbins, R. H. (1973). Alcohol and the identity struggle: Some effects of economic change on interpersonal relations. *Am Anthropol, 75,* 99–122.

Rodin, A. E. (1981). Infants and gin mania in 18th century London. *JAMA, 245,* 1237–1239.

Savard, R. J. (1968). Effects of disulfiram therapy in relationships within the Navaho drinking group. *Q J Stud Alcohol, 29,* 909–916.

Shore, J. H., & Von Fumetti, B. (1972). Three alcohol programs for American Indians. *Am J Psychiatry, 128,* 1450–1454.

Smart, R. G. (1982). The impact of prevention legislation: An examination of research findings. In A. K. Kaplan (Ed.), *Legislative approaches to prevention of alcohol-related problems* (pp. 224–246). Washington, DC: Institute of Medicine.

Smith, W. R. (1965). Sacrifice among the Semites. In W. A. Lessa & E. Z. Vogt (Eds.), *Reader in comparative religion* (pp. 39–48). New York: Harper & Row.

Stull, D. D. (1972). Victims of modernization: Accident rates and Papago Indian adjustment. *Hum Organ, 31,* 227–240.

Thompson, J. W. (1992). Alcohol policy considerations for Indian people. *Am Indian Alsk Native Ment Health Res, 4*(3), 112–119.

Thurn, R. J. (1978). The gin plague. *Minn Med, 61,* 241–243.

Westermeyer, J. (1982). *Poppies, pipes and people: Opium and its use in Laos.* Berkeley: University of California Press.

Westermeyer, J. (1987). Cultural patterns of drug and alcohol use: An analysis of host and agent in the cultural environment. *UN Bull Narcotics, 39*(2), 11–27.

Westermeyer, J. (1989). Monitoring recovery from substance abuse: Rationales, methods and challenges. *Adv Alcohol Subst Abuse, 8*(1), 93–106.

Westermeyer, J. (1991). Historical–social context of psychoactive substance disorders. In R. Francis & S. Miller (Eds.), *Clinical textbook of addiction disorders* (pp. 23–40). New York: Guilford Press.

Westermeyer, J. (1999). The role of cultural and social factors in the cause of addictive disorders. *Psychiatr Clin N Am, 22*(2), 253–273.

Westermeyer, J., & Lang, G. (1975). Ethnic differences in use of alcoholism facilities. *Int J Addict, 10,* 513–520.

Westermeyer, J., & Lee, K. (2013). Residential placement for addicted veterans: ASAM criteria versus a veterans homeless program. *J Nerv Ment Dis, 201,* 567–571.

Wolcott, H. F. (1974). *African Beer Garden of Bulawayo: Integrated drinking in a segregated society.* New Brunswick, NJ: Rutgers Center of Alcoholism Studies.

PART II

Assessment of Addiction

CHAPTER 3

Diagnostic Assessment of Substance Abusers

DEBORAH HASIN
BARI KILCOYNE

Since the publication of DSM-III (American Psychiatric Association, 1980), standardized assessment procedures using specific diagnostic criteria have been available for diagnosing psychiatric disorders. The criteria for substance use disorders (SUDs) and comorbid psychiatric disorders have been operationalized through multiple diagnostic instruments (Samet, Waxman, Hatzenbuehler, & Hasin, 2007). These instruments provide several benefits over unstructured clinical interviews. While unstructured clinical interviews allow clinicians to obtain the most detailed information about individual symptoms, diagnoses using this method are often unreliable, since they are highly subjective and depend in large part on the clinician's expertise (Regier et al., 2013). In addition, clinicians do not typically ask about all disorders in a systematic order, which leaves the possibility that certain diagnoses will be missed (Regier et al., 2013; Hasin et al., 2013). Because of this, there is often a lack of agreement in diagnostic assessment (Andrews & Peters, 1998). The goal for diagnostic interviews in research is to obtain the highest reliability and validity of diagnoses while maintaining simplicity and ease of use. Semistructured and fully structured interviews increase the reliability and validity of diagnoses and can be used for clinical assessment and treatment decisions, as well as research purposes.

While reliability and validity are both important factors for a diagnostic instrument, reliability is a necessary condition for validity and is therefore often established before validity is investigated. "Reliability" refers to the replicability of a diagnostic assessment and is typically measured as joint or test–retest reliability. A diagnostic instrument is considered reliable if there is diagnostic concordance between two different raters of the same interview (joint reliability) or between interviews of the same participant interviewed independently at two different time points (test–retest reliability). Agreement of binary diagnoses can be measured using the kappa coefficient, whose values range from –1 to 1 and represents the degree of agreement, corrected for chance. A kappa of 1 represents perfect agreement; a kappa of 0 indicates agreement only at a chance level; and a kappa of –1 represents perfect disagreement (Cohen, 1960). While guidelines for kappa values vary (Spitzer, Williams, & Endicott, 2012), a kappa of .75+ is generally accepted as excellent agreement; .60–.74 indicates good agreement; .4–.59 indicates fair agreement; and a kappa of .39 or less indicates poor agreement (Landis & Koch, 1977; Fleiss, 1981).

If a diagnostic assessment is not reliable, it is more difficult to establish accurate and replicable diagnoses. This is important, because it may affect whether individuals qualify for inclusion in a study or are identified as eligible for a treatment procedure.

There are many factors that influence the result of a reliability study. These factors include study design (joint vs. test–retest reliability), subject population, interviewer training, and disorder base rates. Better reliability is often found among those with more severe psychopathology (i.e., clinical populations), although among substance abusers, comorbidity may also work against finding reliability (Bryant, Rounsaville, Spitzer, & Williams, 1992; Kranzler et al., 1995). Rare disorders are often found to have lower reliability than more common disorders. Reliability is particularly important in research on substance abusers because of the high degree of co-occurrence of SUDs and other psychiatric disorders (Hasin et al., 1996) and the necessity for studies to distinguish between them. For example, researchers often want to differentiate between symptoms related to substance intoxication or withdrawal and symptoms that present in similar ways (e.g., insomnia) but are associated with other psychiatric disorders (e.g., depression).

"Validity" refers to the significance of a diagnostic assessment and is a more complex phenomenon to measure than reliability. Validity studies usually involve comparing diagnoses from the assessment procedure in question with a "gold standard" and evaluating whether these agree in theoretically predicted ways. While a "gold standard" remains somewhat elusive for psychiatric diagnoses, diagnostic instruments are often compared with diagnoses made through clinical assessment, using strategies such as the LEAD (longitudinal, expert, all data) procedure. However, they can also be compared with other assessment procedures in widespread use, or other variables or measures such as clinical correlates or longitudinal course (Korsmeyer & Kranzler, 2009).

There are many ways to define validity, with the adjectives "face," "content," "concurrent," "convergent," and "predictive" representing some of the many terms used. *Face validity* refers to the common-sense meaning of a diagnosis or criterion and is based on whether the instrument appears to assess the construction in question. *Content validity* refers to whether the items included in the questionnaire provide coverage of all relevant domains. *Concurrent validity* refers to the ability of a criterion or diagnosis to predict other current clinical characteristics or whether the diagnoses obtained agree with some "gold standard." *Convergent validity* refers to whether measures correlate as expected with external validators. *Predictive validity* refers to the ability of a criterion or diagnosis to predict the natural course of an illness or its response to treatment (Rush, First, & Blacker, 2008; Korsmeyer & Kranzler, 2009). It is difficult to establish an interview with the highest reliability and validity across all disorders, since there is no "gold standard" to use as a basis of comparison.

Two types of research diagnostic interviews are available: semistructured and fully structured. Semistructured interviews give the interviewer some flexibility and allow more detailed responses to be recorded. Fully structured interviews, on the other hand, limit flexibility but may be administered by lay (nonclinician) interviewers. The following sections detail several of the diagnostic interviews available. Each was created to address issues or gaps in clinical psychiatric research and to establish more uniform diagnostic procedures. These interviews differ in types of psychiatric conditions assessed, as well as the level of training required for administration. Semistructured questionnaires such as the Psychiatric Research Interview for Substance and Mental Disorders (PRISM) and the Structured Clinical Interview for DSM (SCID) can be administered by clinicians or by lay interviewers with sufficient training and supervision. Fully structured questionnaires such as the Alcohol Use Disorders and Associated Disabilities Interview Schedule (AUDADIS) require less training and supervision and have been shown to have good test–retest reliability for alcohol and drug use disorders.

Current interviews are available in computer-assisted format offering the opportunity to download interviews directly to a central database. This not only makes the process of interviewing easier and shorter, but it eliminates rater errors previously seen with paper interviews. In addition, checks can be programmed directly into interview questionnaires to ensure that answers from later sections match up with answers obtained earlier in the interview or to automatically skip or adjust wording for subsequent questions based on patients' previous responses (Pierucci-Lagha et al., 2005; Samet et al., 2007).

DISTINGUISHING BETWEEN PRIMARY AND SUBSTANCE-INDUCED DISORDERS

Current diagnoses often distinguish between primary and substance-induced psychiatric disorders. These terms were introduced by DSM-IV and help to guide treatment options. "Primary disorders" arve those that are fully established prior to the onset of substance abuse or that occur during extended periods of abstinence. "Substance-induced disorders," on the other hand, are defined as those that occur during periods of substance use but exceed the expected effects of intoxication or withdrawal and/or those that remit within 1 month after substance use ends (Hasin & Kilcoyne, 2013). Different strategies are used by many of these diagnostic interviews to differentiate between the two disorder types (Samet et al., 2007) with each producing similar results.

ASSESSMENT MEASURES

Alcohol Use Disorders and Associated Disabilities Interview Schedule

The Alcohol Use Disorders and Associated Disabilities Interview Schedule (AUDADIS) is a fully structured questionnaire that can be administered by lay interviewers. It was developed by the National Institute on Alcohol Abuse and Alcoholism (NIAAA). It has been used in major national surveys of alcohol, drug, and psychiatric conditions in the United States (National Longitudinal Alcohol Epidemiologic Survey [NLAES]; National Endangered Species Act Reform Coalition [NESARC]), in community longitudinal surveys (Hasin, Van Rossem, McCloud, & Endicott, 1997d; Hasin & Paykin, 1998; Hasin, Keyes, Hatzenbuehler, Aharonovich, & Alderson, 2007) and in an Israeli household survey (Shmulewitz et al., 2010, 2011). The version of the AUDADIS used in studies published to date includes diagnoses of abuse and dependence on 10 classes of psychoactive substances according to DSM-III-R (American Psychiatric Association, 1987) and DSM-IV (American Psychiatric Association, 1994), as well as diagnoses of affective, anxiety, and personality disorders. The AUDADIS has been translated into multiple languages, including Spanish (Canino et al., 1999), Hebrew, Russian (Shmulewitz et al., 2010), Romanian (Vrasti et al., 1998) and others (Chatterji et al., 1997; Cottler et al., 1997; Hasin et al., 1997b; Pull et al., 1997; Ustun et al., 1997).

Diagnoses are assessed at two main time points: current (past 12 months) and past (prior to the last 12 months). These time points cover the lifetime history of the participant. Personality disorders are the only disorders assessed solely on a lifetime basis, since they are considered to be lifelong, stable patterns of thoughts and behaviors. In order to distinguish between substance-induced and primary disorders, questions include age at onset, as well as other clinically relevant features such as number of episodes and duration of the longest episode.

The AUDADIS is a highly reliable diagnostic instrument for a wide range of psychiatric diagnoses. Test–retest reliability for substance use and dependence diagnoses is good to excellent in clinical (Hasin et al., 1997b) and general population samples (Grant, Hartford, Dawson, Chou, & Pickering, 1995; Chatterji et al., 1997; Hasin, Van Rossem, McCloud, & Endicott, 1997c; Ustun et al., 1997; Canino et al., 1999; Grant et al., 2003; Ruan et al., 2008). There is also a range of fair to excellent reliability for other psychiatric sections (Canino et al., 1999; Grant et al., 2003; Ruan et al., 2008). Good concordance was found between the AUDADIS and the Composite International Diagnostic Interview (CIDI) for most diagnoses of substance dependence, with the exception of amphetamines. Agreement was poor for categories of substance abuse, though this is a common finding across a number of other assessments as well (Cottler et al., 1997). Convergent, discriminative, and construct validities of criteria and diagnoses of alcohol use disorders are good to excellent (Hasin, Grant, & Endicott, 1990; Hasin et al., 1994, 1997c; Canino et al., 1999; Hasin & Paykin, 1999; Hasin et al., 2003) and have been found to be valid relative to clinical diagnoses (Canino et al., 1999). The considerable agreement between the AUDADIS and clinical diagnoses generally suggests that the diagnoses produced by AUDADIS are valid (Canino et al., 1999).

Composite International Diagnostic Interview

The Composite International Diagnostic Interview (CIDI), based on the Diagnostic Interview Schedule (Robins et al., 1988; Cottler, Robins, & Helzer, 1989), was developed by investigators at Washington University in St. Louis. A CIDI modification was carried out by the World Health Organization for cross-cultural assessment of mental disorders following definitions and criteria from the *International Classification of Diseases* (ICD) and DSM (Ustun et al., 1997). As such, the CIDI is available in many languages and multiple versions (Wittchen et al., 1991). Although it was developed primarily for surveys in the general population (Robins et al., 1988), researchers have also used this instrument in clinical samples (e.g., Langenbucher, Morgenstern, Labouvie, & Nathan, 1994). It is fully structured for usc by trained nonclinician interviewers and allows investigators the option of establishing either ICD or DSM computer-generated diagnoses (Andrews & Peters, 1998).

The CIDI diagnoses both substance and psychiatric disorders. A specially created substance abuse module can be used alone or substituted for the less detailed coverage of drugs of abuse in the CIDI proper (Cottler et al., 1989; Cottler & Keating, 1990). Similar to other instruments, this section provides the opportunity to assess not only the presence or absence of dependence or abuse, but also the quality, severity, and predicted course. An early version of the CIDI, which was used in multiple studies, skipped questions about past dependence symptoms if the participant did not endorse any abuse symptoms (Hasin & Grant, 2004; Hasin, Hatzenbueler, Smith, & Grant, 2005), potentially leading to artificially low and biased estimates of dependence (Cottler, 2007; Grant et al., 2007); this problem has since been corrected to increase diagnostic accuracy.

The highly structured nature of the CIDI makes the collection of data easier when diagnosing a large number of subjects. Selection of 40 DSM-III diagnoses for inclusion in the original version was based on the availability of sufficient detail to produce appropriate questions for each criterion (Robins et al., 1988). In addition, the CIDI is modular, allowing use in both broad epidemiological surveys and narrower studies assessing only one or two diagnoses or a singular diagnostic category (anxiety, mood, etc.; Robins et al., 1988).

Researchers found good to excellent reliability for DSM-IV diagnoses of any substance use disorder (SUD) or substance dependence, with fair to good reliability for the abuse category (Langenbucher et al., 1994; Horton, Compton, & Cottler, 2000). Cross-instrument concordance comparing CIDI to the AUDADIS-ADR (Alcohol/ Drug Revised edition) found good concordance for most diagnoses of dependence, but lower concordance for abuse or harmful use categories (Chatterji et al., 1997; Cottler et al., 1997; Hasin et al., 1997b; Pull et al., 1997; Ustun et al., 1997). Additionally, a large, international field trial found excellent reliability for substance use questions and high cross-cultural acceptability (Cottler et al., 1991).

Psychiatric Research Interview for Substance and Mental Disorders

The Psychiatric Research Interview for Substance and Mental Disorders (PRISM) is a semistructured diagnostic interview developed by Columbia University investigators to address the lack of empirical evidence on the reliability or validity of psychiatric diagnoses among heavy drinkers or drug users (Hasin et al., 1996). Many features of the PRISM were designed to overcome problems related to making psychiatric diagnoses when individuals also drink alcohol or use drugs heavily (Hasin et al., 1996, 2006b). The current version assesses DSM-IV alcohol, drug, and psychiatric disorders and is most useful for research purposes, intake assessment, or treatment planning. Alcohol and seven other drug categories, including cocaine, heroin, cannabis, hallucinogens, sedatives, stimulants, and opiates, are assessed (Hasin et al., 2006b).

The PRISM has been used in cross-sectional and longitudinal studies in different populations (Hasin et al., 2002, 2006b; Aharonovich et al., 2005; Caton et al., 2005, 2007; Nunes, Liu, Samet, Matseoane, & Hasin, 2006; Drake et al., 2011; Samet et al., 2013). As with many semistructured questionnaires, the PRISM is modular, which allows interviewers to choose between modules depending on diagnostic aims, assessment needs, or research questions. What differentiates it from other diagnostic interviews is the placement of substance screening questions at the beginning of the assessment rather than in the middle of the interview. Thus, subsequent sections can refer to the substance screening questions to differentiate between substance-induced disorders and primary disorders, as well as expected effects of intoxication and withdrawal. In addition, this placement allows interviewers to obtain a thorough knowledge of the subject's drinking and drug use patterns and history of alcohol or drug use disorders before diving into other psychiatric sections (Hasin et al., 1996). The PRISM also provides current and lifetime diagnoses that commonly occur with heavy substance use.

The PRISM was found to have good to excellent reliability for DSM-III-R diagnoses, including affective disorders, SUDs, eating disorders, some anxiety disorders, and psychotic symptoms (Hasin et al., 1996). Since criterion variance is often found to be one of the principal contributors to unreliable diagnoses, significant efforts were made to reduce criterion variance and better anchor the criteria to improve reliability in the transition from DSM-III to DSM-IV. A 2006 reliability study of DSM-IV diagnoses of anxiety, affective disorders, and SUDs, in which heavy substance users were interviewed in multiple clinical settings, revealed good to excellent test–retest reliability for most substance dependence diagnoses, as well as current and lifetime major depression diagnoses. Also, fair to good reliability was found for anxiety disorders (Hasin et al., 2006b). Higher reliability was found in substance abusers using the PRISM than in other semistructured or fully structured interviews (Hasin et al., 1996, 2006b; Torrens, Serrano, Astals, Perez-Dominguez, & Martin-Santos, 2004; Morgello et al., 2006; Ramos-Quiroga et al., 2012). An independent validity study compared diagnoses using the Spanish version of the PRISM, the SCID-IV, and expert diagnosis made by an experienced clinician using all available data (LEAD). Higher concordance occurred between PRISM and LEAD for diagnoses of current depression, past substance-induced major depression, and borderline personality disorder than between SCID and LEAD (Torrens et al., 2004).

The PRISM assessment is now available in computerized form, with built-in logic checks designed to guide the interviewer through the assessment with reduced error. Translations of the complete assessment are also available in Spanish (Spain) and Norwegian.

Structured Clinical Interview for DSM

The Structured Clinical Interview for DSM (SCID), a semistructured diagnostic instrument, was originally based on DSM-III (Spitzer, Williams, Gibbon, & First, 1992), and has been updated to reflect DSM-IV criteria (First, Spitzer, Gibbon, &

Williams, 1996, 2002; First, Gibbon, Spitzer, & Williams, 1997). There are two main interviews, SCID-I and SCID-II. SCID-I was used to diagnose the major DSM-IV Axis I diagnoses, whereas SCID-II covered the assessment of personality disorders. The SCID uses a different approach from that of many other diagnostic instruments (Spitzer et al., 1992). Rather than inquire about all symptoms of diagnostic relevance, the SCID omits questions about the associated features of a disorder if the essential criteria are not met (Kranzler & Rounsaville, 1998). This allows interviewers to make diagnoses as the interview progresses rather than summarize symptom data into individual diagnoses at the end of the interview (Spitzer et al., 1992). The advantage of this approach is a briefer interview that more closely approximates clinical practice. The disadvantage is that complete symptom information is not produced, which is a limitation for studies that require such variables.

The eight classes of substances assessed during the interview include alcohol, sedatives–hypnotics–anxiolytics, cannabis, stimulants, opioids, cocaine, hallucinogens, and amphetamines. Drugs that do not fall into any of these categories are assessed as a separate category (e.g., inhalants, atropine). Diagnoses of alcohol dependence and abuse are conducted, followed by an assessment for the remaining categories, since alcohol use is found to be much more prevalent than use of other substances. For all remaining drug categories, assessment of an overall diagnosis of substance dependence or abuse occurs before diagnosing individual drug use disorders. SUDs are assessed in a single section, whereas the substance-induced and primary disorders are covered in their respective psychiatric sections.

Multiple studies assessing the interrater reliability of SCID using DSM-III-R diagnoses have found good reliability for a majority of categories in patient samples. Higher kappa coefficients were found for individual drug use disorders when enrollment was based on a likelihood of substance dependence. Lower kappa coefficients, ranging from fair to good, were found in nonpatient and substance-abusing patient samples (Williams et al., 1992). More recent studies assessing interrater or joint reliability using DSM-IV criteria found moderate to excellent agreement for Axis I disorders, with SCID-II personality disorders also showing excellent interrater agreement (Zanarini et al., 2000; Zanarini & Frankenburg, 2001; Lobbestael, Leurgans, & Arntz, 2011). Interrater reliability of substance dependence diagnoses and combined diagnoses of dependence/abuse was good to excellent, whereas reliability for abuse diagnoses was inconsistent.

The SCID (2013) has a variety of applications, including diagnostic evaluation, research, and training of mental-health professionals. The SCID-I has a modular structure that allows it to be adapted to the needs of particular studies. Sections can be removed for diagnoses that are irrelevant or not of interest to the study (Spitzer et al., 1992). There are three basic versions of the SCID-I: the research version (SCID-I-RV), the clinician version (SCID-CV) and a clinical trials version (SCID-CT). The research version covers the full complement of disorders, subtypes, and specifiers of interest to researchers. The research and clinical trial versions can be obtained through the Biometrics Research Department at Columbia University. The research version is provided as an unbound packet of pages, so that the investigator has the ability to leave out pages covering disorders or subtypes not relevant to a particular study. A computer-assisted version of the SCID-CV and SCID-II is available.

Semi-Structured Assessment for the Genetics of Alcoholism

The Semi-Structured Assessment for the Genetics of Alcoholism (SSAGA) was developed specifically for studies involving the genetics of substance use and psychiatric disorders.

The SSAGA was developed for the Collaborative Study on the Genetics of Alcoholism and borrows several features from the Schedule for Affective Disorders and Schizophrenia (SADS), Diagnostic Interview Schedule (DIS), SCID, and others (Bucholz et al., 1994). It is designed for use by lay interviewers and allows investigators to obtain a detailed psychiatric history of current and past health problems in adults, ages 18 and older (Bucholz et al., 1994). Major Axis I psychiatric disorders, as well as Antisocial Personality Disorder (ASPD), are covered during the interview. There is also a section that assesses demographics, medical history, suicidality, and home environment—factors that may be associated with an individual's psychiatric issues. One distinguishing feature is the inclusion of assessments for the alcohol dependence syndrome, the alcohol withdrawal syndrome, and the flushing response, in addition to assessments of alcohol abuse and dependence, and treatment history.

Similar to many other diagnostic interviews, the SSAGA allows investigators to establish temporality of diagnoses for those with multiple psychiatric disorders and SUDs by focusing on time periods of onset–offset. This distinction is necessary when determining primary and substance-induced diagnoses and directions for treatment, but is particularly useful in genetic studies in which the aim of part of the study is to distinguish between genes that contribute to multiple disorders and those that are unique to specific disorders (Bucholz et al., 1994). SSAGA also provides phenotyping (age of onset, drinking patterns, severity, etc.) of disorders, which allows investigators to analyze specific populations, since some genetic effects may be relevant only within particular subgroups (Bucholz et al., 1994).

The SSAGA was found to have good intra- and interrater reliability for a large number of diagnoses using DSM-III criteria (Bucholz et al., 1994). Good to excellent reliability was found for most substance dependence diagnoses with kappa values ranging from .70 to .90. SSAGA also showed good reliability for lifetime depression (kappa = .65) and ASPD (kappa = .70). Reliability for diagnoses of substance abuse ranged from poor to fair (Bucholz et al., 1994). An additional study that documented the reliability of individual criterion items for psychoactive substance dependence found good to excellent reliability for cocaine and alcohol. and lower reliability for the criteria of stimulant and sedative dependence (Bucholz et al., 1995). Validity of SSAGA was also confirmed in a study that compared SSAGA to another diagnostic instrument, SCAN, producing similar diagnoses (Hesselbrock, Easton, Bucholz, Schuckit, & Hesselbrock, 1999).

Semi-Structured Assessment for Drug Dependence and Alcoholism

The Semi-Structured Assessment for Drug Dependence and Alcoholism (SSADDA), a diagnostic instrument based on the SSAGA, was developed to acquire detailed information on drug dependence and commonly co-occurring DSM-IV disorders. While it was created specifically for use in genetic studies, its computer-assisted format and detailed coverage of a wide range of disorders make it suitable for a variety of applications that require careful diagnostic assessment (Pierucci-Lagha et al., 2005, 2007). It can be used by a trained (nonclinician) interviewer, and its computer-assisted format allows interviewers to enter subjects' responses directly. The data from these responses are directly uploaded to a database, eliminating time-consuming data entry and verification. In addition, the program includes cross-checking to identify inconsistent responses.

SSADDA includes diagnostic assessment for major drugs of abuse, as well as attention-deficit/hyperactivity disorder (ADHD) and gambling, which theoretically and clinically are relevant to drug dependence (Pierucci-Lagha et al., 2005). Environmental factors and adverse childhood experiences are also covered due to their likely impact on the risk of drug and alcohol dependence. One feature retained from SSAGA is the temporal assessment of disorders to distinguish those that are primary from those that are substance-induced (Bucholz et al., 1994).

SSADDA produces reliable diagnoses for alcohol and drug dependence disorders, as well as a variety of other psychiatric disorders in multiple population subtypes. Particularly high reliability was found for cocaine and opioid dependence (Pierucci-Lagha et al., 2005) similar to that which has been found for AUDADIS, CIDI, and PRISM (Hasin et al., 1997a, 2006b; Pull et al., 1997; Ustun et al., 1997). Individual diagnostic criteria for substance dependence have also been found to demonstrate fair to excellent reliability, with the most unreliable criteria associated with stimulants and sedative dependence (Pierucci-Lagha et al., 2007).

DISCUSSION

Many available diagnostic interviews have been found to be reliable and valid in different populations. We stress the importance of this because societies often differ in how they view substance consumption, thereby affecting the prevalence of diagnoses and manifestation of symptoms (Canino et al., 1999). In addition, each of the diagnostic instruments reviewed here incorporate questions that allow diagnosticians and interviewers to distinguish between comorbid diagnoses and establish whether psychiatric symptoms are related to substance use or independent of use. Semistructured interviews, while more expensive to administer in research studies, may be preferred over fully structured interviews, because they allow interviewers to phrase questions to fit the subject's understanding and to ask additional questions (probes) to clarify differential diagnoses (Spitzer et al., 1992). The diagnostic assessment selected for research depends primarily on the research question given that some diagnostics delve into certain topic areas more than others.

The use of semi- or fully structured diagnostic interviews standardizes the content of the diagnostic assessment, reducing criterion variance as a source of measurement error. However, the use of any semi- or fully structured diagnostic interview also requires adequate training of interviewers, since the lack of such standardization of interview practices has been established as a large source of information variance leading to diagnostic disagreement. The use of well-known methodology helps to minimize these two types of error variance (Spitzer & Fleiss, 1974; Spitzer, Endicott, & Robins, 1975; Endicott & Spitzer, 1978).

FUTURE DIRECTIONS

DSM-5 was published in May 2013. While a major paradigm shift did not occur in psychiatric diagnoses in DSM-5 (Frances, 2009, 2010; Kupfer & Regier, 2011), many changes were made in the criteria of many disorders. For SUDs, the DSM-IV distinction between two disorders, dependence and abuse, has been removed, with criteria collapsed into a single SUD category, which includes the seven dependence criteria, three of the four former abuse criteria (all but legal problems), and one new criterion (craving) (Hasin & Kilcoyne, 2013). DSM-5 requires that two or more criteria of the new combined total of eleven criteria be endorsed for a diagnosis of SUD. In addition, a scale of severity has been added. Endorsement of two to three criteria is categorized as mild, four to five criteria as moderate, and of six or more criteria as severe. The consolidation of abuse and dependence into a single disorder was based on indications from a large body of research (Hasin et al., 2013). The reliability and validity of the new combined disorder, relative to DSM-IV dependence, which was highly reliable and valid (Hasin, Muthuen, Wisnicki, & Grant, 1994; Hasin et al., 2006a; Hasin et al., 2013), has yet to be determined.

The PRISM and the AUDADIS have been updated to provide alcohol, drug, and psychiatric diagnoses based on DSM-5 (American Psychiatric Association, 2013), and the SCID is currently undergoing such a revision. The new DSM-5 version of the AUDADIS was used in a large, NIH-sponsored U.S. national survey of alcohol, drug, and psychiatric conditionsand was recently validated using the DSM-5 version of the PRISM. Results from this study provide support for the dimensional measure of SUD in DSM-5, with the AUDADIS and PRISM showing excellent concordance on dimensional scales of the majority of SUDs (Hasin et al., 2015). Researchers will be aided in the continuing evaluation of new DSM-5 criteria by reliable and valid diagnostic measures as the mental health and substance abuse fields await a better understanding of how the implementation of DSM-5 will impact both research and clinical work.

REFERENCES

Aharonovich, E., Liu, X., Samet, S., Nunes, E., Waxman, R., & Hasin, D. (2005). Postdischarge cannabis use and its relationship to cocaine, alcohol, and heroin use: A prospective study. *Am J Psychiatry, 162*(8), 1507–1514.

American Psychiatric Association. (1980). *Diagnostic and statistical manual of mental disorders* (3rd ed.). Washington, DC: Author.

American Psychiatric Association. (1987). *Diagnostic and statistical manual of mental disorders* (3rd ed., rev.). Washington, DC: Author.

American Psychiatric Association. (1994). *Diagnostic and statistical manual of mental disorders* (4th ed.). Washington, DC: Author.

American Psychiatric Association. (2013). *Diagnostic and statistical manual of mental disorders* (5th ed.). Arlington, VA: Author.

Andrews, G., & Peters, L. (1998) The psychometric properties of the Composite International Diagnostic Interview. *Soc Psychiatry Psychiatr Epidemiol, 33*(2), 80–88.

Bryant, K. J., Rounsaville, B., Spitzer, R. L., & Williams, J. B. (1992). Reliability of dual diagnosis: Substance dependence and psychiatric disorders. *J Nerv Ment Dis, 180*(4), 251–257.

Bucholz, K. K., Cadoret, R., Cloninger, C. R., Dinwiddie, S. H., Hesselbrock, V. M., Nurnberger, J. I., Jr., et al. (1994). A new, semi-structured psychiatric interview for use in genetic linkage studies: A report on the reliability of the SSAGA. *J Stud Alcohol, 55*(2), 149–158.

Bucholz, K. K., Hesselbrock, V. M., Shayka, J. J., Nurnberger, J. I., Jr., Schuckit, M. A., Schmidt, I., et al. (1995). Reliability of individual diagnostic criterion items for psychoactive substance dependence and the impact on diagnosis. *J Stud Alcohol, 56*(5), 500–505.

Canino, G., Bravo, M., Ramirez, R., Febo, V. E., Rubio-Stipec, M., Fernandez, R. L., et al. (1999). The Spanish Alcohol Use Disorder and Associated Disabilities Interview Schedule (AUDA-DIS): Reliability and concordance with clinical diagnoses in a Hispanic population. *J Stud Alcohol, 60*(6), 790–799.

Caton, C. L., Drake, R. E., Hasin, D. S., Dominguez, B., Shrout, P. E., Samet, S., et al. (2005). Differences between early-phase primary psychotic disorders with concurrent substance use and substance-induced psychoses. *Arch Gen Psychiatry, 62*(2), 137–145.

Caton, C. L., Hasin, D. S., Shrout, P. E., Drake, R. E., Dominguez, B., First, M. B., et al. (2007). Stability of early-phase primary psychotic disorders with concurrent substance use and substance-induced psychosis. *Br J Psychiatry, 190,* 105–111.

Chatterji, S., Saunders, J. B., Vrasti, R., Grant, B. F., Hasin, D., & Mager, D. (1997). Reliability of the alcohol and drug modules of the Alcohol Use Disorder and Associated Disabilities Interview Schedule—Alcohol/Drug-Revised (AUDADIS-ADR): An international comparison. *Drug Alcohol Depend, 47*(3), 171–185.

Cohen, J. (1960). A coefficient of agreement for nominal scales. *Educ Psychol Meas, 20,* 37–46.

Cottler, L. B. (2007). Drug use disorders in the National Comorbidity Survey: Have we come a long way? *Arch Gen Psychiatry, 64*(3), 380–381; author reply 381–382.

Cottler, L. B., Grant, B. F., Blaine, J., Mavreas, V., Pull, C., Hasin, D., et al. (1997). Concordance of DSM-IV alcohol and drug use disorder criteria and diagnoses as measured by AUDADIS-ADR, CIDI and SCAN. *Drug Alcohol Depend, 47*(3), 195–205.

Cottler, L. B., & Keating, S. K. (1990). Operationalization of alcohol and drug dependence criteria by means of a structured interview. *Recent Dev Alcohol, 8,* 69–83.

Cottler, L. B., Robins, L. N., Grant, B. F., Blaine, J., Towle, L. H., Wittchen, H. U., et al. (1991). The CIDI-core substance abuse and dependence questions: Cross-cultural and nosological issues: The WHO/ADAMHA Field Trial. *Br J Psychiatry, 159,* 653–658.

Cottler, L. B., Robins, L. N., & Helzer, J. E. (1989). The reliability of the CIDI-SAM: A comprehensive substance abuse interview. *Br J Addict, 84*(7), 801–814.

Drake, R. E., Caton, C. L., Xie, H., Hsu, E., Gorroochurn, P., Samet, S., et al. (2011). A prospective 2-year study of emergency department patients with early-phase primary psychosis or substance-induced psychosis. *Am J Psychiatry, 168*(7), 742–748.

Endicott, J., & Spitzer, R. L. (1978). A diagnostic interview: The Schedule for Affective Disorders and Schizophrenia. *Arch Gen Psychiatry, 35*(7), 837–844.

First, M. B., Gibbon, M., Spitzer, R. L., & Williams, J. B. W. (1997). *Structured Clinical Interview for DSM-IV Axis II Personality Disorders (SCID-II).* Washington, DC: American Psychiatric Press.

First, M. B., Spitzer, R. L., Gibbon, M., & Williams, J. B. W. (1996). *Structured Clinical Interview for DSM-IV Axis I Disorders, Clinician Version (SCID-CV).* Washington, DC: American Psychiatric Press.

First, M. B., Spitzer, R. L., Gibbon, M., & Williams, J. B. W. (2002). *Structured Clinical Interview for DSM-IV-TR Axis I Disorders, Research Version, Patient Edition (SCID-I/P).* New York: Biometrics Research, New York State Psychiatric Institute.

Fleiss, J. L. (1981). *Statistical methods for rates and proportions.* New York: Wiley.

Frances, A. (2009). Whither DSM-V? *Br J Psychiatry, 195*(5), 391–392.

Frances, A. (2010). The first draft of DSM-V. *BMJ, 340,* c1168.

Grant, B. F., Compton, W. M., Crowley, T. J., Hasin, D. S., Helzer, J. E., Li, T. K., et al. (2007). Errors in assessing DSM-IV substance use disorders. *Arch Gen Psychiatry, 64*(3), 379–380; author reply 381–372.

Grant, B. F., Dawson, D. A., Stinson, F. S., Chou, P. S., Kay, W., & Pickering, R. (2003). The Alcohol Use Disorder and Associated Disabilities Interview Schedule-IV (AUDADIS-IV): Reliability of alcohol consumption, tobacco use, family history of depression and psychiatric diagnostic modules in a general population sample. *Drug Alcohol Depend, 71*(1), 7–16.

Grant, B. F., Harford, T. C., Dawson, D. A., Chou, P. S., & Pickering, R. P. (1995). The Alcohol Use Disorder and Associated Disabilities Interview schedule (AUDADIS): Reliability of alcohol and drug modules in a general population sample. *Drug Alcohol Depend, 39*(1), 37–44.

Hasin, D., Carpenter, K. M., McCloud, S., Smith M., & Grant, B. F. (1997a). The Alcohol Use Disorder and Associated Disabilities Interview Schedule (AUDADIS): Reliability of alcohol and drug modules in a clinical sample. *Drug Alcohol Depend, 44*(2–3), 133–141.

Hasin, D. S., & Grant, B. F. (2004). The co-occurrence of DSM-IV alcohol abuse in DSM-IV alcohol dependence: Results of the National Epidemiologic Survey on Alcohol and Related Conditions on heterogeneity that differ by population subgroup. *Arch Gen Psychiatry, 61*(9), 891–896.

Hasin, D., Grant, B. F., Cottler, L., Blaine, J., Towle, L., Ustun, B., & Sartorius, N. (1997b). Nosological comparisons of alcohol and drug diagnoses: A multisite, multi-instrument international study. *Drug Alcohol Depend, 47*(3), 217–226.

Hasin, D. S., Grant, B., & Endicott, J. (1990). The natural history of alcohol abuse: Implications for definitions of alcohol use disorders. *Am J Psychiatry, 147*(11), 1537–1541.

Hasin, D. S., Greenstein, E., Aivadyan, C., Stohl, M., Aharonovich, E., Saha, T., et al. (2015). The Alcohol Use Disorder and Associated Disabilities Interview Schedule-5 (AUDADIS-5): Procedural validity of substance use disorders modules through clinical re-appraisal in a general population sample. *Drug Alcohol Depend, 148,* 40–46.

Hasin, D., Hatzenbuehler, M. L., Keyes, K., & Ogburn, E. (2006a). Substance use disorders: *Diagnostic and Statistical Manual of Mental Disorders,* fourth edition (DSM-IV) and *International Classification of Diseases,* tenth edition (ICD-10). *Addiction, 101*(Suppl. 1), 59–75.

Hasin, D. S., Hatzenbuehler, M., Smith, S., & Grant, B. F. (2005). Co-occurring DSM-IV drug abuse in DSM-IV drug dependence: Results from the National Epidemiologic Survey on Alcohol and Related Conditions. *Drug Alcohol Depend, 80*(1), 117–123.

Hasin, D. S., Keyes, K. M., Hatzenbuehler, M. L., Aharonovich, E. A., & Alderson, D. (2007). Alcohol consumption and posttraumatic stress after exposure to terrorism: Effects of proximity, loss, and psychiatric history. *Am J Public Health, 97*(12), 2268–2275.

Hasin, D. S., & Kilcoyne, B. (2013). Comorbidity of affective and substance use disorders. In M. B. Keller, W. H. Coryell, J. Endicott, & A. C. Leon (Eds.), *Clinical guide to depression: Findings from the Collaborative Depression Study.* Washington, DC: American Psychiatric Press.

Hasin, D., Liu, X., Nunes, E., McCloud, S., Samet, S., & Endicott, J. (2002). Effects of major depression on remission and relapse of substance dependence. *Arch Gen Psychiatry, 59*(4), 375–380.

Hasin, D. S., Muthuen, B., Wisnicki, K. S., & Grant, B. (1994). Validity of the bi-axial dependence concept: A test in the US general population. *Addiction, 89*(5), 573–579.

Hasin, D. S., O'Brien, C. P., Auriacombe, M., Borges, G., Bucholz, K., Budney, A., et al. (2013). DSM-5 criteria for substance use disorders: Recommendations and rationale. *American Journal of Psychiatry, 170*(8), 834–851.

Hasin, D., & Paykin, A. (1998). Dependence symptoms but no diagnosis: Diagnostic "orphans" in a community sample. *Drug Alcohol Depend, 50*(1), 19–26.

Hasin, D., & Paykin, A. (1999). Alcohol dependence and abuse diagnoses: Concurrent validity in a nationally representative sample. *Alcohol Clin Exp Res, 23*(1), 144–150.

Hasin, D., Samet, S., Nunes, E., Meydan, J., Matseoane, K., & Waxman, R. (2006b). Diagnosis of comorbid psychiatric disorders in substance users assessed with the Psychiatric Research Interview for Substance and Mental Disorders for DSM-IV. *Am J Psychiatry, 163*(4), 689–696.

Hasin, D. S., Schuckit, M. A., Martin, C. S., Grant, B. F., Bucholz, K. K., & Helzer, J. E. (2003). The validity of DSM-IV alcohol dependence: What do we know and what do we need to know? *Alcohol Clin Exp Res, 27*(2), 244–252.

Hasin, D. S., Trautman, K. D., Miele, G. M., Samet, S., Smith, M., & Endicott J. (1996). Psychiatric Research Interview for Substance and Mental Disorders (PRISM): Reliability for substance abusers. *Am J Psychiatry, 153*(9), 1195–1201.

Hasin, D. S., Van Rossem, R., McCloud, S., & Endicott, J. (1997c). Alcohol dependence and abuse diagnoses: Validity in community sample heavy drinkers. *Alcohol Clin Exp Res, 21*(2), 213–219.

Hasin, D. S., Van Rossem, R., McCloud, S., & Endicott, J. (1997d). Differentiating DSM-IV alcohol dependence and abuse by course: Community heavy drinkers. *J Subst Abuse, 9*, 127–135.

Hesselbrock, M., Easton, C., Bucholz, K. K., Schuckit, M., & Hesselbrock, V. (1999). A validity study of the SSAGA—a comparison with the SCAN. *Addiction, 94*(9), 1361–1370.

Horton, J., Compton, W., & Cottler, L. B. (2000). Reliability of substance use disorder diagnoses among African-Americans and Caucasians. *Drug Alcohol Depend, 57*(3), 203–209.

Korsmeyer, P., & Kranzler, H. R. (2009). *Encyclopedia of drugs, alcohol and addictive behavior.* Detroit, MI: Macmillan.

Kranzler, H. R., Kadden, R. M., Burleson, J. A., Babor, T. F., Apter, A., & Rounsaville B. J. (1995). Validity of psychiatric diagnoses in patients with substance use disorders: Is the interview more important than the interviewer? *Compr Psychiatry, 36*(4), 278–288.

Kranzler, H. R., & Rounsaville, B. J. (1998). *Dual diagnosis and treatment: Substance abuse and comorbid medical and psychiatric disorders.* New York: Marcel Dekker.

Kupfer, D. J., & Regier, D. A. (2011). Neuroscience, clinical evidence, and the future of psychiatric classification in DSM-5. *Am J Psychiatry, 168*(7), 672–674.

Landis, J. R., & Koch, G. G. (1977). The measurement of observer agreement for categorical data. *Biometrics, 33*(1), 159–174.

Langenbucher, J., Morgenstern, J., Labouvie, E., & Nathan, P. E. (1994). Lifetime DSM-IV diagnosis of alcohol, cannabis, cocaine and opiate dependence: Six-month reliability in a multisite clinical sample. *Addiction, 89*(9), 1115–1127.

Lobbestael, J., Leurgans, M., & Arntz, A. (2011). Inter-rater reliability of the Structured Clinical Interview for DSM-IV Axis I Disorders (SCID I) and Axis II Disorders (SCID II). *Clin Psychol Psychother, 18*(1), 75–79.

Morgello, S., Holzer, C. E., III, Ryan, E., Young, C., Naseer, M., Castellon, S. A., et al. (2006). Interrater reliability of the Psychiatric Research Interview for Substance and Mental Disorders in an HIV-infected cohort: Experience of the National NeuroAIDS Tissue Consortium. *Int J Methods Psychiatr Res, 15*(3), 131–138.

Nunes, E. V., Liu, X., Samet, S., Matseoane, K., & Hasin, D. (2006). Independent versus substance-induced major depressive disorder in substance-dependent patients: Observational study of course during follow-up. *J Clin Psychiatry, 67*(10), 1561–1567.

Pierucci-Lagha, A., Gelernter, J., Chan, G., Arias, A., Cubells, J. F., Farrer, L., et al. (2007). Reliability of DSM-IV diagnostic criteria using the Semi-Structured Assessment for Drug Dependence and Alcoholism (SSADDA). *Drug Alcohol Depend, 91*(1), 85–90.

Pierucci-Lagha, A., Gelernter, J., Feinn, R., Cubells, J. F., Pearson, D., Pollastri, A., et al. (2005).

Diagnostic reliability of the Semi-Structured Assessment for Drug Dependence and Alcohol-ism (SSADDA). *Drug Alcohol Depend, 80*(3), 303–312.

Pull, C. B., Saunders, J. B., Mavreas, V., Cottler, L. B., Grant, B. F., Hasin, D. S., et al. (1997). Concordance between ICD-10 alcohol and drug use disorder criteria and diagnoses as mea-sured by the AUDADIS-ADR, CIDI and SCAN: Results of a cross-national study. *Drug Alcohol Depend, 47*(3), 207–216.

Ramos-Quiroga, J. A., Diaz-Digon, L., Comin, M., Bosch, R., Palomar, G., Chalita, J. P., et al. (2012). Criteria and concurrent validity of Adult ADHD Section of the Psychiatry Research Interview for Substance and Mental Disorders. *J Atten Disord.* [Epub ahead of print]

Regier, D. A., Narrow, W. E., Clarke, D. E., Kraemer, H. C., Kuramoto, S. J., Kuhl, E. A., et al. (2013). DSM-5 field trials in the United States and Canada: Part II. Test–retest reliability of selected categorical diagnoses. *Am J Psychiatry, 170*(1), 59–70.

Robins, L. N., Wing, J., Wittchen, H. U., Helzer, J. E., Babor, T. F., Burke, J., et al. (1988). The Composite International Diagnostic Interview: An epidemiologic instrument suitable for use in conjunction with different diagnostic systems and in different cultures. *Arch Gen Psychia-try, 45*(12), 1069 –1077.

Ruan, W. J., Goldstein, R. B., Chou, S. P., Smith, S. M., Saha, T. D., Pickering, R. P., et al. (2008). The Alcohol Use Disorder and Associated Disabilities Interview Schedule–IV (AUDADIS-IV): Reliability of new psychiatric diagnostic modules and risk factors in a general population sample. *Drug Alcohol Depend, 92*(1–3), 27–36.

Rush, A. J., First, M. B., & Blacker, D. (Eds.). (2008). *Handbook of psychiatric measures* (2nd ed.). Washington, DC: American Psychiatric Press.

Samet, S., Fenton, M. C., Nunes, E., Greenstein, E., Aharonovich, E., & Hasin, D. (2013). Effects of independent and substance-induced major depressive disorder on remission and relapse of alcohol, cocaine and heroin dependence. *Addiction, 108*(1), 115–123.

Samet, S., Waxman, R., Hatzenbuehler, M., & Hasin, D. S. (2007). Assessing addiction: Concepts and instruments. *Addict Sci Clin Pract, 4*(1), 19–31.

Shmulewitz, D., Keyes, K., Beseler, C., Aharonovich, E., Aivadyan, C., Spivak, B., et al. (2010). The dimensionality of alcohol use disorders: Results from Israel. *Drug Alcohol Depend, 111*(1–2), 146–154.

Shmulewitz, D., Keyes, K. M., Wall, M. M., Aharonovich, E., Aivadyan, C., Greenstein E., et al. (2011). Nicotine dependence, abuse and craving: Dimensionality in an Israeli sample. *Addic-tion, 106*(9), 1675–1686.

Spitzer, R. L., Endicott, J., & Robins, E. (1975). Clinical criteria for psychiatric diagnosis and DSM-III. *Am J Psychiatry, 132*(11), 1187–1192.

Spitzer, R. L., & Fleiss, J. L. (1974). A re-analysis of the reliability of psychiatric diagnosis. *Br J Psychiatry, 125*, 341–347.

Spitzer, R. L., Williams, J. B., & Endicott, J. (2012). Standards for DSM-5 reliability. *Am J Psy-chiatry, 169*(5), 537; author reply 537–538.

Spitzer, R. L., Williams, J. B., Gibbon, M., & First, M. B. (1992). The Structured Clinical Inter-view for DSM-III-R (SCID): I. History, rationale, and description. *Arch Gen Psychiatry, 49*(8), 624–629.

Structured Clinical Interview for DSM Disorders (SCID). Retrieved February 25, 2013, from *www.scid4.org/index.html.*

Torrens, M., Serrano, D., Astals, M., Perez-Dominguez, G., & Martin-Santos, R. (2004). Diag-nosing comorbid psychiatric disorders in substance abusers: Validity of the Spanish versions of the Psychiatric Research Interview for Substance and Mental Disorders and the Structured Clinical Interview for DSM-IV. *Am J Psychiatry, 161*(7), 1231–1237.

Ustun, B., Compton, W., Mager, D., Babor, T., Baiyewu, O., Chatterji, S., et al. (1997). WHO study on the reliability and validity of the alcohol and drug use disorder instruments: Over-view of methods and results. *Drug Alcohol Depend, 47*(3), 161–169.

Vrasti, R., Grant, B. F., Chatterji, S., Ustun, B. T., Mager, D., Olteanu, I., et al. (1998). Reliability of the Romanian version of the alcohol module of the WHO Alcohol Use Disorder and Associated Disabilities: Interview Schedule–Alcohol/Drug—Revised. *Eur Addict Res, 4*(4), 144–149.

Williams, J. B., Gibbon, M., First, M. B., Spitzer, R. L., Davies, M., Borus, J., et al. (1992). The Structured Clinical Interview for DSM-III-R (SCID): II. Multisite test–retest reliability. *Arch Gen Psychiatry, 49*(8), 630–636.

Wittchen, H. U., Robins, L. N., Cottler, L. B., Sartorius, N., Burke, J. D., & Regier, D. (1991). Cross-cultural feasibility, reliability and sources of variance of the Composite International Diagnostic Interview (CIDI): The multicentre WHO/ADAMHA field trials. *Br J Psychiatry, 159*, 645–653, 658.

Zanarini, M. C., & Frankenburg, F. R. (2001). Attainment and maintenance of reliability of Axis I and II disorders over the course of a longitudinal study. *Compr Psychiatry, 42*(5), 369–374.

Zanarini, M. C., Skodol, A. E., Bender, D., Dolan, R., Sanislow, C., Schaefer, E., et al. (2000). The Collaborative Longitudinal Personality Disorders Study: Reliability of Axis I and II diagnoses. *J Pers Disord, 14*(4), 291–299.

CHAPTER 4

Laboratory Testing for Substances of Abuse

D. ANDREW BARON
DAVID A. BARON

In November 1988, President Ronald Reagan enacted a law, the Drug-Free Workplace (DFW) Act, that forever changed the landscape and mindset of drug testers. It brought drug testing to the general public, which began to develop awareness of an increasing problem in the workplace: drug abuse. Over time, substance abuse has evolved from ethanol to steroids, to cannabinoids, and now to opiates and synthetics, and with each evolution, more of the general population becomes involved. The costs for substance abuse and its treatment are at all time highs. Substance abuse is no longer the doping athlete or the common addict; it now includes all ages. Gil Kerlikowske, Director of the White House Office of National Drug Control Policy (ONDCP), agrees: "Prescription drug abuse is a silent epidemic that is stealing thousands of lives and tearing apart communities and families across America."

For the professionals working in clinical settings and in consultative roles (including sports, criminal/forensic and occupational settings), there will always be a need for corroborative sources of information. Testing of human tissues usually provides invaluable, albeit not definitive, diagnostic and therapeutic information in working with substance-using individuals. Testing plays an important role, because most drugs of abuse are illegal, and drug-abusing individuals who present often are in denial about their problem and have comorbid psychiatric symptoms. Drug testing aids in determining whether presenting symptoms are primarily psychiatric or substance-induced. Drug testing may be utilized as part of an initial treatment contract between the patient and treating clinician. Coercion often helps improve treatment outcomes. In methadone maintenance programs, testing is typically mandatory. Evidence to suggest that testing deters use can be seen in this example. Prior to testing in 1981, 48% of military personnel used drugs, but that rate declined to 5% after 3 years of implemented testing (Willette, 1986).

Mentioning drug abuse in athletes tends to yield a common denominator: performance enhancers/steroids. Many people will be familiar with the issues in Major League Baseball and some of its past and current prominent athletes surrounding the use of designer steroids or human growth hormone (HGH). Blood doping (erythropoietin [EPO]) has also become increasingly popular among athletes, shedding light on what was once thought to be undetectable by current testing methods. As the list of controlled substances increases, so does our ability to detect even the smallest evidence of substance use in an individual (an athlete recently was given a lengthy suspension by his league for testing positive for a steroid metabolite detected in his urine at 7 ppt [parts per trillion]). In an attempt to reclaim control over their particular sport, commissioners are cracking down increasingly hard on athletes caught doping and are now beginning to target "wellness centers," where purported performance enhancers may have been doled out.

WHAT ARE THE BENEFITS OF DRUG TESTING?

While substance abuse via high-profile situations (e.g., celebrities, athletes, and incidents recorded on news outlets) is quite commonplace, what is less commonly discussed is the general cost of substance abuse. According to the national Center on Addiction and Substance Abuse (CASA), during a 2009 study, the total cost of substance abuse was $374 billion, of which 98% was spent on consequences, with the remaining 2% spent on prevention and treatment, whereas drug overdose deaths (methadone accounted for nearly one-third of opiate-related deaths) in the United States eclipsed highway crash fatalities (37,485 vs. 33,808). The founder of CASA and former Secretary of Health Education and Welfare, Joseph Califano, now estimates the total cost of all consequences of drug abuse totals more than $1 trillion/year. These costs include, but are not limited to, lower productivity, absenteeism, low morale, accidents, health care costs, theft, on-the-job trafficking, and higher rates of turnover. In addition, according to the Center for Substance Abuse Research (CESAR), 9% of high school students have reported using marijuana 20 times or more in a given month (Center for Substance Abuse Research, 2012b). CESAR describes the shifting trend in opioid abuse, where buprenorphine has supplanted methadone as the number-one drug seized by law enforcement (Center for Substance Abuse Research, 2012a). The United States (currently 4.5% of the world population) uses an astounding 90% of hydrocodone (Vicodin) and 80% of oxycodone (OxyContin) manufactured. Understanding regional and/or national trends in drug abuse may aid in administering lower-cost testing that is both focused and effective.

TESTING METHODOLOGIES

There are a multitude of methods available to aid in the detection of drug use in humans. Given all the available tests, how does an individual or an agency decide on which test to administer? A number of questions may be posed before settling on a final decision:

1. For what drugs should one test?
2. How much time and money should be spent on testing?
3. How fast are the results needed?
4. What biological sample should be tested (urine, blood, sweat, saliva, hair, etc.)?

If there is no clinical indication to test for a specific compound, a "comprehensive drug screen" may be performed. The most commonly used analytic technique for a "comprehensive drug screen" is thin-layer chromatography (TLC), which is also the least expensive test available. TLC utilizes the differences in polarity and chemical interaction with developing solvents to produce different visualizations on a thin-layer coating. The visualizations are highlighted using ultraviolet (UV) or fluorescent lighting, or by color reactions created after being sprayed with chemical dyes. Identical molecules cluster in the same area, yielding specific color reactions. Unfortunately, while TLC is the least expensive test, it is somewhat insensitive to detection of controlled substances. A drug screen using TLC will only detect high levels of the following compounds: amphetamine, barbiturates, cocaine, codeine, dextromethorphan, diphenylhydantoin, morphine, diphenylpropanolamine, methadone, propoxyphene, or quinine (a heroin diluent). TLC does not detect the following compounds: 3,4-methlyenedioxyamphetamine (MDA), 3,4-methylenedioxymethamphetamine (MDMA), fentanyl, lysergic acid diethylamide (LSD), marijuana, mescaline, and PCP.

A preferred type of testing in recent years has been the implementation of on-site screening immunoassays. On-site testing has a variety of features that make it better suited for companies than its counterpart TLC. For example, most agencies prefer that testing be conducted quickly and with as little error as possible, obtaining desired results as expediently as humanly possible. Unlike TLC, in which samples are submitted to laboratories to determine results, on-site testing can produce significantly accurate results in as little as 10 minutes, making it the preferred method in hospitals, employment agencies, and clinics.

Of the more than half-dozen on-site testing kits available, two kits offer interesting approaches. The first, the Triage Panel for Drugs of Abuse plus Tricyclic Antidepressants (Biosite Diagnostics, Inc., San Diego, California) is based on the usage of Ascend MultImmunoassay (AMIA) technology for the simultaneous detection of multiple analytes in a sample. In the triage kit, the urine sample is placed in a reaction cup, which contains lyophilized reagents, and equilibrates for 10 minutes. The chemically labeled drugs compete with drugs that may be present in the urine for antibody binding sites. The mixture is then transferred to a solid phase membrane in the detection area containing various immobilized antibodies in discrete drug-class-specific zones. After a washing step, the operator visually examines each zone for the presence of a red bar. The method incorporates preset threshold concentrations that are independent for each drug. The assay response is proportional to the concentration of the unbound drug conjugate, so that no signal is observed at drug concentrations less than the threshold concentrations (Buechler et al., 1992). A positive sample can be identified by the formation of a distinct red-colored bar in the drug detection zone adjacent to the drug's abbreviated name, whereas a negative sample does not produce a colored bar. This process to determine the outcome of the sample usually takes between 10 and 12 minutes. The triage kit is available for the following drugs: amphetamines/methamphetamines, barbiturates, benzodiazepines, cocaine, PCP, THC, and tricyclic antidepressants.

Another testing device is the OnTrak TesTcup Collection/Urinalysis Panel (Roche Diagnostic Systems, Inc., Somerville, New Jersey). Unlike the triage kit, OnTrak screens for the following compounds *simultaneously*: amphetamine, cocaine, morphine, and THC. It will soon have the capability for the screening five different drugs. The OnTrak TesTcup is based on the principle of microparticle capture inhibition, relying on the competition between drug and drug conjugate immobilized on a membrane in the test chamber. The urine sample is collected directly in the TesTcup, which eliminates the need for collection site handling of the sample (a common source of error in previous testing methods). After closing the TesTcup and moving it to the test position, the sample reservoir is filled by tilting the cup for 5 seconds. The urine proceeds down immunochromatographic strips by capillary action and reacts with antibody-coated microparticles and drug conjugate present on the membrane. In approximately 3 to 5 minutes, the test-valid bars appear, a decal is removed from the detection window, and the results are interpreted as positive or negative. In the absence of drug, the antibody is free to interact with the drug conjugate, causing the formation of a blue band. When a drug is present in the specimen, it binds to the antibody-coated microparticles and no blue band is formed, causing the membrane to remain white, indicating a positive test (OnTrak TesTcup, 1998).

To keep pace with the increasing and expanding use of illicit drugs, testing beyond the "NIDA-5," the National Institute on Drug Abuse's five drugs of abuse, to include synthetics and synthetic opiates (buprenorphine) has become increasingly important. One such company, Express Diagnostics, offers comprehensive urine testing that includes a kit that tests for 17 controlled substances, as well as other kits to test for synthetic marijuana (K2, Spice) and alcohol.

Becoming increasingly popular are "at-home" kits that can be administered in the privacy of one's residence. One particular website offers a kit for $8.95 that covers 10 controlled substances (THC, cocaine, methamphetamine, antidepressants, opiates, barbiturates, methadone, amphetamines, benzodiazepines, and PCP). Another site offers a five-panel kit for as little as $1.99. Performing a generic Internet search for "Urine Drug Test Kit" yields a multitude of results with various prices. One can also enter the local dollar store and purchase a marijuana detection kit, if one is so willing.

Alcohol testing, which is done routinely by law enforcement officers during traffic stops, has now evolved into the home and workplace. While breath-testing devices are readily available for purchase on the Internet, a growing trend in laboratory testing of alcohol is testing for metabolites, particularly ethyl glucuronide (EtG) and ethyl sulfate (EtS). EtG can be detected in hair and nails. According to Dahl, Carlsson, Hillgren, and Helander (2011), "although EtG and EtS account for only < 0.1% of the ingested ethanol dose, they remain detectable in urine for several hours up to some days longer than ethanol, the time-lag largely depending on the amount consumed. . . . A positive finding of EtG and/or EtS is thus indicative of recent drinking, also when this is denied and the ethanol itself cannot be detected" (p. 1). While EtG and EtS are biomarkers for ethanol use (Center for Substance Abuse

Research, 2012c), the U.S. Substance Abuse and Mental Health Services Administration (SAMHSA) advises caution, as "Biomarkers, however, should not be used as the sole screening tool in light of their low-to-moderate sensitivity and specificity, and in the case of EtG, because of exposure to alcohol from sources other than drinking." (p. 4). Phosphatidyl ethanol (PEth), a direct serum-based biomarker, may prove more promising as PEth can remain in the blood for as long as 3 weeks after only about four drinks per day. EtG, EtS, and PEth demonstrate that new technology may be the link to better and accurate detection.

Despite the popularity of on-site kits and the fact that these kits have demonstrated greater than 97% agreement with gas chromatography/mass spectroscopy GC/MS) tests, these kits provide only *preliminary* results. For optimal results, it is recommended that a complete, thorough analysis of the sample be performed in a controlled, accredited laboratory setting.

The most common drug-testing locations are listed in Table 4.1.

LABORATORY ISSUES

The initiation of drug testing has created three rapidly growing cottage industries: (1) drug-testing laboratories, (2) private drug-testing companies, and (3) creation of products to beat drug tests.

The number of private laboratories conducting drug tests has grown dramatically since 1990. The industry even has its own trade organization, the Drug and Alcohol Testing Industry Association (DATIA). The major concern in drug testing occurs with the reporting of laboratory results. Unlike NIDA-certified testing of the Standard Drug Panel (see Table 4.2), clinical drug testing for drugs of abuse currently has no standard technical criteria, no standard screening cutoffs for positive tests, no confirmation cutoffs, no chain-of-custody requirements, no blind proficiency

TABLE 4.1. Summary of Test Locations

Place	Tested population	Tester	Pros	Cons
Home	Individuals (most commonly children or people entering workforce)	Individual (little experience)	Convenient; quick results; inexpensive	Variable results; lower sensitivity
Laboratory	Anyone who submits a sample	Lab tech (experienced)	Controlled environment; low error rate	Expensive; time consuming
Workplace	Generally new employees (pre-screening measure)	Lab tech (experienced, can be done in-house or sent to lab)	Same as lab; government regulated, decreases workplace incidents	Limited tested substance; does not ensure productivity
Athletics	Athletes (can be before, during, or after events)	Authorized laboratory	Ensures level playing field	Problems with COC; testing lags behind doping

TABLE 4.2. "NIDA 5" Standard Drug Panel	
Drug	Cutoffs (ng/ml)
Cocaine	300/150
Cannabinoids	50/15
PCP	25/25
Opiates	2,000/2,000
Amphetamines	1,000/500

TABLE 4.3. The Most Common Drug-Testing Technologies

- Thin-layer chromatography
- Radio immunoassay, enzyme immunoassay, fluorescent polarization immunoassay, enzyme-linked immunosorbent assay
- Gas chromatograpy
- Gas chromatography/mass spectroscopy
- Liquid chromatography

submission requirements, and no certification programs. As a result, a sample testing positive in laboratory A may be reported as negative by laboratory B based on different cutoff levels. Hansen, Caudill, and Boone's article, "Crisis in Drug Testing," published in the *Journal of the American Medical Association* in 1985, highlighted this problem. Unfortunately, little progress has been made in correcting it over the past 17 years. The issue is not the type of test administered or poor-quality laboratories, but the nonstandardized threshold for reporting a test as positive.

The most common drug-testing technologies are listed in Table 4.3. The most popular initial test screen is an enzyme immunoassay (EIA) analysis of a urine sample. If this is positive, a confirmatory GC/MS test is performed on the split sample. Given the greater sensitivity of GC/MS over EIA, the cutoff levels are reduced. There are settings and instances when it is important to contact the laboratory to ensure that there is a means to test for the substance, or to prompt the laboratory to test for the substance. It is common for general hospital laboratories to screen for only a limited number of substances. Many do not screen, for example, for gamma-hydroxybutryic acid (GHB). Although methods for testing for GHB continue to undergo refinement, reliable methods do exist (Chappell, Meyn, & Ngim, 2004).

FALSE-POSITIVE AND FALSE-NEGATIVE TESTS

The primary purpose of drug testing is to identify individuals using illegal or illicit drugs. Falsely accusing someone of using illegal substances is highly problematic, and it undermines the entire Drug-Free Program. Similarly, not being able to identify active drug users because of false-negative results renders a program of limited value. It does not deter use or identify users. For nonusers who are subject to drug testing, issues related to false-positive results are of great concern. Questions addressing which foods, prescribed medications, dietary supplements, or the potential for secondhand marijuana smoke that could result in a positive test are common.

An example of this issue is the concern that eating poppy seed bagels will result in a positive opiate test. Of particular interest is the cutoff level for opiates at 2,000 ng/ml for both EIA and GC/MS. Originally (1990), the cutoff level for opiates was only 300 ng/ml. The infamous poppy seed bagel saga, which resulted in the level being raised by over 300% in the NIDA-5 profile, is as follows: A number of New

York police officers tested positive for opiates. All denied ever using drugs and all had excellent job records inconsistent with drug use. An investigation revealed all had eaten bagels from the same deli. Analysis of the poppy seeds demonstrated an usually high level of opiates. The poppy seeds in question were discovered to be an unwashed, Iranian variety. To avoid future false-positive results, the Department of Transportation (DOT) raised the level for a positive test to 2,000 ng/ml, a level that cannot be reached by eating a few bagels.

Although urinalysis is the most widely used and best overall body fluid to screen for drug use, other body fluids can be measured as well. Hair testing (see Table 4.4) is growing in popularity but is not as sensitive to marijuana use as urinalysis. Despite commercial success, the scientific foundation for using hair analysis is limited. Its primary utility might be as a tool in the diagnosis and treatment of drug abuse disorders, particularly cocaine dependence. Salivary measurements offer the advantage of ease of collection but only detect recent drug use, which limits their utility. A number of drugs, including cocaine, morphine, amphetamine, and ethanol, have been detected in sweat. Unfortunately, there is a wide intersubject variability of drug concentration in sweat, resulting in a significant disadvantage when sweat is compared with other body fluids. Adding to the problem, sweat collection takes several days to several weeks and requires the use of a sweat patch (Cone, 2001). In deciding a testing methodology, the cost of each test and the cost–benefit ratio should also be considered (see

TABLE 4.4. Hair Testing

Detection range:	90 days
Sample size:	20+ mg (~50–70 strands) up to 3.9 cm (most recent 3.9 cm tested)
Where to cut:	As close to body as possible
Hair type:	Scalp most common, but any body hair can be used
Do hair products alter use?	No
First drug detection in hair:	5–10 days after first use

TABLE 4.5. Common Testing Modalities

Modality	Cost	Notes
Urine	~$4–50	Most common and inexpensive modality; commonly used in workplace, athletic, and medical settings
Blood	Variable	Most expensive testing modality, cost varies by drugs being detected; frequently used in athletes and medical settings
Sweat	~$35–350	Wide intersubject variability of drug concentration, takes several days–weeks and requires wearing patch
Saliva	~$15–75	Ease of collection; can only detect recent drug use
Hair	~$100–150	Growing in popularity; not as sensitive to THC as urine

(see Table 4.5). Urine tests are the most common and most inexpensive (~$4–50), followed by saliva (~$15–75), sweat (~$35–350), and hair (~$100–150), with blood tests (Table 4.6) being the most expensive and variable in cost depending on tests ordered. (See Tables 4.7–4.10 for drug test cutting levels for urine, hair, and saliva.)

CHAIN OF CUSTODY AND THE MEDICAL REVIEW OFFICER

A critical component of all drug-testing protocols (sports and workplace) is "chain of custody," which refers to the policy in which the collected sample (usually urine) never leaves the direct observation of a member of the drug-testing team until it arrives at the laboratory. Once collected, the processed sample remains under the direct observation of the testing team until it is hand-delivered to the shipping company, which also maintains direct observation until the sample is hand-delivered to the certified laboratory. The goal is to eliminate any potential tampering with the specimen. The MRO (medical review officer) is a licensed physician who interprets laboratory results and is responsible for reviewing the chain-of-custody form to ensure no potential tampering (Sgan & Hanzlick, 2003; Smith et al., 2003). If chain-of-custody cannot be verified, the test result is considered invalid. The overarching goal and philosophy of the Drug-Free Program is to *deter* drug use in the workplace, not merely detect it. The role of the MRO is to advocate for the employee/athlete donor and ensure the ongoing integrity of the testing program. One recent example of MRO and chain-of-custody significance can be found in the case of a prominent athlete who purportedly tested failed a drug test, which would have resulted in a suspension; the result was later overturned due to mishandling by the MRO and supposed contamination of said urine sample.

EVASION OF TRUE POSITIVE RESULTS

Drug users are highly motivated to "produce" a clean sample, whether it be to avoid job termination, litigation, or simple detection. In response to this need, an industry has emerged to provide products whose sole purpose is to create a false-negative test result. These products include pretested and certified drug-free urine substitution kits, a variety of adulterants, and—my personal favorite for originality—the Whizzinator (an artificial penis used to deliver a known drug-free urine sample under direct observation conditions). All of these products are readily available over the Internet and include disclaimers stating they should only be used in accordance with all federal, state, and local laws, and that the seller assumes no responsibility or liability associated with the use of their products. In addition to advertising their products, many of these Internet sites provide information for their customer. For example, one online vendor provides a nontechnical description of: how blood and urine drug tests work, information on how long-banned drugs are detectable in blood and urine after initial ingestion, and an accurate description of hair drug testing. It correctly points out that hair follicle drug testing is growing rapidly, but it does not report hair testing as being a poor method for marijuana detection compared to urine testing.

TABLE 4.6. Blood Drug Screen

Drug	Detection period
Amphetamines	12 hours
Methamphetamine	24 hours
Phenobarbital	4–7 days
Benzodiazepines	6–48 hours
Cannabis	2 days
Cocaine	24 hours
Codeine	12 hours
Cotinine	2–4 days
Morphine	6 hours
Heroin	6 hours
LSD	0–3 hours
Methadone	15–55 hours
PCP	24 hours

TABLE 4.7. Drug Test Workplace Cutoff Levels for Initial Urine (EMIT) Screen

Drug	Cutoffs (ng/ml)
Marijuana metabolite	50
Cocaine metabolite	150
Opiate metabolites[a]	2,000
Phencyclidine (PCP)	25
Amphetamines[b]	500

[a]Labs are permitted to initially test all specimens for 6-acetylmorphine at a 10 ng/ml cutoff.
[b]Target analyte must be d-methamphetamine and the test must significantly cross-react with MDMA, MDA, and MDEA.

TABLE 4.8. Drug Test Workplace Cutoff Levels for the Urine Confirmatory (GC/MS) Test

Drug	Cutoffs (ng/ml)
Marijuana metabolite[a]	15
Cocaine metabolite[b]	100
Morphine	2,000
Codeine	2,000
6-Acetylmorphine[c]	10
Phencyclidine (PCP)	25
Amphetamine	250
Methamphetamine[d]	250
MDMA	250
MDA	250
MDEA	250

[a]Delta-9-tetrahydrocannabinol-9-carboxylic acid.
[b]Benzoylecgonine.
[c]Labs test for 6-acetylmorphine when the morphine concentration exceeds 2,000 ng/ml.
[d]Specimen must also contain d-amphetamine at a concentration > 100 ng/ml.

TABLE 4.9. Drug Test Workplace Cutoff Levels for the (GC/MS) Hair Follicle Test

Drug	Cutoffs (pg/ml)
Marijuana metabolite[a]	1
Cocaine metabolite[b]	300
Opiates	500
Phencyclidine (PCP)	300
Amphetamines/methamphetamine[c]	300
MDMA (Ecstasy)	300

[a]Delta-9-tetrahydrocannabinol-9-carboxylic acid.
[b]Benzoylecgonine.
[c]Specimen must also contain d-amphetamine at a concentration ≥ 100 ng/ml.

TABLE 4.10. Drug Test Workplace Cutoff Levels for Saliva Swab Testing

Drug	Cutoffs (ng/ml)
Marijuana (THC)[a]	2
Cocaine metabolite[b]	30
Opiates/morphine	30
Phencyclidine (PCP)	50
Amphetamines/methamphetamine[c]	50
MDMA (Ecstasy)	50

[a]Delta-9-tetrahydrocannabinol-9-carboxylic acid.
[b]Benzoylecgonine.
[c]Specimen must also contain *d*-amphetamine at a concentration ≥ 100 ng/ml.

Those who interpret test results should be aware that addicts can be highly creative in their efforts to thwart detection and monitoring, usually by using a type of adulterant. "Adulterants" are substances placed in a sample to alter the results of a drug test. They accomplish this by physically altering the characteristics of the sample, such as temperature, pH, and specific gravity, which disrupts the mechanisms of the assay. Adulterants range from inexpensive household products such as soap, salt, bleach, lemon juice, or vinegar to expensive additives specifically marketed to produce a negative test. One Internet product selling for over $100 comes with a 300% money-back guarantee. As a result of adulterant use, drug testers must now employ techniques to screen for these additives. If the sample does not fall within established physiological parameters at the time of collection, it is voided on the spot and another sample must be produced and sent to the laboratory for analysis. One "do-it-yourself" kit, available on the Internet, includes a concealed intravenous (IV) bag with tubing (to be strapped to the lower abdomen or upper thigh) and two heating elements with temperature strips—all in an attempt to mask the use of adulterants. Do commercial adulterants really work? A study by Cody and Valtier (2001) tested the effectiveness of Stealth (an Internet-marketed adulterant) in masking a known positive urine sample spiked with THC. Stealth is provided in two vials: peroxidase and peroxide. These are combined in a urine sample to provide a robust oxidation potential. Although the peroxidase activity can be detected in urine samples, it is rarely tested for. The results of the controlled experiment revealed that adulterating an authentic, positive sample for marijuana with Stealth caused the sample to screen negative (false-negative result) using standard immunoassay techniques used by many drug-testing laboratories.

TESTING PROGRAMS FOR ATHLETES

Drugs have been used for thousands of years for enhancement of athletic performance, increasing work endurance, recreation, and as self-medication for pain and psychopathology. "Doping," the term used to describe the use of drugs to increase athletic performance, has been documented back to the ancient Greeks. Throughout history, the use of drugs to gain an advantage over one's competitors has been considered morally wrong and worthy of severe sanctions. Fair competition was the keystone of competitive sports. The Creed of the Olympics states that the most important factors are taking part and giving one's best effort, not winning. Fighting well and honorably took precedent over conquering the opponent, thus separating sport from war (in which all is fair). Cheaters disgraced not only themselves and their families but also the sport itself. Dopers in ancient times were stripped of their winnings and often ended up as slaves, attempting to pay back their debt to the sporting world. These drastic measures, including use of victory awards from cheaters to build statues to honor the Gods ringing the Olympic Stadium, were intended to deter drug use and other forms of cheating (casting spells on competitors) by producing a constant reminder to every athlete who entered the arena of the potential perils of attempting to gain an unfair advantage. Unfortunately, the spoils of victory and the cost of defeat, combined with an overwhelming drive to win at any cost, have kept doping a major issue in sports at every age and at every level of competition.

The ongoing "cat and mouse" game between cheaters and drug-testing agencies has become more sophisticated over the years. Despite an enormous investment of time and money in attempts to make competitive sports drug-free, the pressure to win keeps doping an integral (albeit negative) component of sports. Although not as well documented, the role of drug use and abuse in the workplace has had a greater negative impact on society in terms of personal and societal costs.

Despite the long history of drug abuse in sports and in the workplace, laboratory testing to detect drug use is a modern phenomenon. In 1967 the International Olympic Committee Medical Commission began banning certain drugs and testing for their use. Full scale drug testing for doping by athletes began in the 1972 Munich Games. Since 1967, the number of banned substances has grown every year, and the sophistication of laboratory analysis and testing protocols has advanced.

Sports doping control is not federally regulated in the United States, as it is in Australia, but typically it is closely monitored by the specific sports' governing bodies. The National Collegiate Athletic Association (NCAA) closely monitors the testing of collegiate athletes, while the U.S. Anti-Doping Agency (USADA) monitors and conducts all Olympics-related events in the United States. In sports testing, as in workplace programs, there are two types of testing programs: in-competition and out-of-competition programs. No advance notice (NAN) out-of-competition testing is the preferred method of the USADA, and it is reported by athletes themselves to be the best deterrent to drug use. As its name implies, this form of testing involves approaching an athlete at any time, without prior notice, and obtaining a urine sample. Olympic-caliber athletes must consent to participate in the program, which includes providing a personal log of their whereabouts at all times. Failure to comply leads to sanctions by the individual sport's (e.g., track and field, swimming, boxing) governing body. Major advances in doping control have also taken place recently in most professional sporting leagues (Major League Baseball [MLB], Fédération Internationale de Football Association [FIFA], National Football League [NFL]) to crack down on athletes trying to gain an unfair advantage by using designer drugs to increase performance. While the athletes still hold a slight advantage over their governing bodies, increased fines and penalties for positive testing and newer, specific tests are closing the gap toward fair play.

To help illuminate the problem drug testers face, see Table 4.11 for a small portion of what certain governing bodies test for and a list of substances that fall under the categories "steroids" and "stimulants," respectively. It is important to note that while this list may seem extensive, it is by no means complete. And with new synthetic agents being created regularly to help avoid detection and stay ahead of the drug testing curve, one can see which testing agencies have their hands full trying to keep a level playing field.

TABLE 4.11. List of Tested Substances

Grouping	Drugs tested
NIDA-5	THC, cocaine, amphetamines, opiates, PCP
NCAA (National Collegiate Athletics Association)	Anabolic agents, stimulants, alcohol, beta blockers (for rifle only), diuretics, street drugs, peptide hormones and analogues, anti-estrogens, beta$_2$ agonists
FDA (Food and Drug Administration)	Amphetamines, barbiturates, benzodiazepines, cannabinoids, cocaine and metabolites, methadone, methamphetamine, opiates, phencyclidine, phenobarbital, propoxyphene, TCA
MLB (Major League Baseball)	Cannabinoids, synthetic THC and cannabimimetics (K2, Soice, etc.), cocaine, LSD, opiates, MDMA, GHB, PCP, steroids, stimulants
Steroids	Androstadienedione, androstanediol, androstatrienedione (ATD), androstenediol, androstenedione, androstenetrione (6-OXO), bolandiol, bolasterone, boldenone, boldione, calusterone, clenbuterol, clostebol, danazol, dehydrochloromethyl testosterone, desoxy-methyl-testosterone, 1-testosterone, 4-dihydrotestosterone, drostanolone, epi-dihydrotestosterone, epitestosterone, ethylestrenol, fluoxymesterone, formebolone, furazol, 13a-ethyl-17a-hydroxygon-4-en-3-one, gestrinone, 4-hydroxy testosterone, 4-hydroxy-19-nortestosterone, mestanolone, mesterolone, methandieone, methandriol, methasterone (Superdrol), methenolone, methyldienolone, methylnortestosterone, methyltrienolone (metribolone), mibolerone, 17a-methyl-1-dohydrotestosterone, nandrolone, norandrostenediol, norandrostenedione, norbolethone, norclostebol, norethandrolone, oxabolone, oxandrolone, oxymesterone, oxymetholone, prostanozol, quinbolone, selective androgen receptor modulators (SAREMs), stanozolol, stenbolone, testosterone, tetrahydrogestrinone, tibolone, trenbolone, zeranol, zilpaterol, any salt, ester, or ether of any listed above, human growth hormone (hGH), insulin-like growth factor (IGF-1) and all isomers (mechano growth factors), gonadotropins (LH, hCG, etc.), aromatase inhibitors, selective estrogen receptor modulator (SERMs), anti-estrogens (clomiphene, cyclofenil, fulvestrant)
Stimulants	Amphetamine, amphetaminil, armodafinil, benfluorex, benzphetamine, benzylpiperazine, bromantan, carphedon, cathine (norpseudoephedrine), chloroampthetamine, clobenzorex, cropropamide, crotetamide, dimethylamphetamine, etilefrine, famprofazone, fenburazate, fencamfamine, fenethylline, fenfluramine, fenproporex, furfenorex, heptaminol, isometheptene, meclofenoxate, mefenorex, mesocarb, mephentermine, methamphatermine (methylamphetamine), methylenedioxyamphetamine, methylenedioxyamphetamine, methylephedrine, methylhexaneamine (dimethylalamine, DMMA), mondafinil, nikethamide, norfenefrine, norfenfluramine, octopamine, oxilorine, pemoline, pentretrazol, phentermine, phenpromethamine, prenylamine, prolintane, phendimetrazine (phenmetrazine), propylhexedrine, pyrovalerone, sibutramine, tuaminoheptane

TESTING PROGRAMS IN OCCUPATIONAL SETTINGS

Drug testing in the workplace has seen dramatic growth since 1988. Former President Ronald Reagan proclaimed the need for a drug-free workplace in America during his years in office. This initiative resulted in the DFW Act, signed into law in November 1988. This legislation (HR-5210-124 Section 5152) laid the groundwork for the existing regulations (49-CFR-40) for virtually all of the drug-testing policies and protocols currently enforced in the workplace today. Interestingly, the DFW legislation was a significant extension of the preexisting "catastrophe driven" testing, where testing was only done after a catastrophic event, such as a serious work-related accident. This new policy offered a proactive deterrent philosophy. The workgroup that drafted the initial legislations comprised almost exclusively federal bureaucrats and lawyers. The National Institute of Mental Health was represented by a clinical research physician who pushed for education to be a key component of the program. As a result, the final program emphasized education and confidential treatment, in addition to the deterrence and testing aspects of the act.

Each DFW program is mandated to include five elements. These include (1) a formal written policy, (2) an employee assistance program, (3) formal training for supervisors, (4) formal employee education, and (5) a drug-testing protocol. There are five participants involved with every DFW drug test: (1) the employer, (2) the donor/employee, (3) the specimen collection site, (4) the laboratory analyzing the sample, and (5) the MRO. The employer is responsible for informing the employee in writing of the Drug Testing Policy, including all policies and procedures of the test, circumstances warranting testing in addition to preemployment, and consequences of a positive test. The employee must sign a form acknowledging that he or she is aware of the Program and the existence of an employee assistance program, and participate in a DFW educational presentation. The employee must also sign an informed consent document agreeing to be tested under the circumstances described in the Policy handbook. The collection site must also conform to specifications described in the Policy handbook. The laboratory used must be certified by the Department of Health and Human Services (DHHS). There are over 80 certified laboratories throughout the United States. An up-to-date list is published regularly in the *Federal Register*. The laboratory is responsible for verifying appropriate chain-of-custody of the sample (Universal Chain of Custody forms became effective in January 1995) and conducting a valid and reliable analysis of the specimen. The laboratory must report any breach in protocol it discovers, including any suspicion of tampering with the sample.

The MRO plays a unique and important role in the drug-testing process. Positive tests are reported to the MRO, who then evaluates the facts in the test. For instance, if a worker was taking a prescribed stimulant for a medical condition with appropriate preauthorized permission, the MRO can reverse a positive test. The MRO is an "independent agent" in the testing process and is responsible for investigating all positive tests before reporting to the employer.

The five substances routinely tested for in the NIDA-5 are marijuana, cocaine, amphetamines, opiates, and PCP. Other drugs, such as alcohol, buprenorphine, and antidepressants, to name a few, may be added to the panel if suspected by the employer from objective evidence (e.g., slurred speech, alcohol on the breath). In keeping with the "rule of fives," there are five situations in which drug testing is conducted: (1)

preemployment, (2) random, (3) postaccident, (4) probable cause, and (5) return to work/follow-up. The employer may request that additional substances be tested for in the case of postaccident, reasonable suspicion, and return-to-work conditions. In order to request this additional testing, the employee must be notified via an official Employee Drug Policy document. Recognizing the high prevalence of alcohol abuse, ethanol testing was mandated in a 1994 amendment. There are separate regulations for alcohol testing, including those not requiring MRO participation.

The program is always designed to give the employee the benefit of the doubt and the benefit of the MRO's advocacy. In workplace testing, the safety of both the public and the individual is at stake. Impaired judgment and hand–eye coordination resulting from intoxication has potentially devastating consequences for professional drivers, pilots, and operators of heavy equipment. Virtually everyone's job performance, with the *possible exception* of rock stars, is adversely affected by drug use in the workplace. The highest rates of current and past-year drug use were reported in construction workers, food preparation workers, waiters, and waitresses. Excessive alcohol consumption was observed in these groups and in auto mechanics, vehicle repairmen, light truck drivers, and laborers (Larson, Eyerman, Foster, & Gfroerer, 2007). According to a National Institue on Drug Abuse (NIDA) (1989) estimate, if every employee/worker between ages 18 and 40 were drug-tested randomly on any given day, between 14 and 25% would test positive.

TYPES OF WORKPLACE TESTING

There are two types of workplace testing: regulated and nonregulated. "Regulated testing" refers to programs conducted under the Federal Testing Guidelines and includes industries working with the DOT, Federal employees, and companies with Federal contracts over $25,000.00 per year. "Nonregulated programs" are typically private sector employers who are not federally required to have a DFW program but voluntarily choose to drug-test employees. These programs are not required to have an MRO, and they are not federally regulated; however, to protect companies from financial losses, they are increasing in popularity.

CONCLUSION

Despite the legitimate concern with false-positive and false-negative test results, the weakest link in the "chain" of drug testing is chain-of-custody violations. Regardless of the sophistication of laboratory technology, human error in completing the requisite paperwork at the drug-testing site remains the single most important inconsistent aspect of the testing process. Given the variety of available methods to cheat, it is likely drug testing will not catch all drug users.

An accurate diagnosis of substance abuse is based on a comprehensive clinical workup; drug testing is only one component of the process. Workplace drug testing serves to deter drug use by employees while on the job (eliminating costly accidents and errors), and to assist in initially identifying individuals with drug use disorders. In the sports world, drug testing aims to create a level playing field for all competitors, while promoting the health of athletes by deterring the use of potentially harmful agents. The role of education, particularly individuals at high risk for drug use, should be the keystone of any DFW program.

As the detriments of substance abuse and associated costs become increasingly known by the general public, education and prevention are vital. Today, opiates, THC, and synthetics are routinely available and abused by an increasingly larger and younger population. Education is paramount in reducing expenses related to drug abuse and addiction. In DSM-5, the category of substance abuse and dependence has been changed to addiction-related disorders. While this is a small step in an ever-lengthening path, we must continue to be vigilant about the nature of these chemicals, to develop new methods to detect them in order to prevent declining workplace and personal performance, and to inform the public of the socioeconomic disasters that could occur if this epidemic is not held in check. The groundwork that President Reagan laid down with the DFW Act continues to evolve and keep pace with the growing problem of drug abuse.

REFERENCES

Buechler, K. F., Moi, S., Noar, B., McGrath, D., Villela, J., Clancy, M., et al. (1992). Simultaneous detection of seven drugs of abuse by the Triage panel for drugs of abuse. *Clin Chem, 38,* 1678–1684.

Center for Substance Abuse Research. (2012a, April 2). Buprenorphine now more likely than methadone to be found in U.S. law enforcement drug seizures. *CESAR FAX, 21*(13).

Center for Substance Abuse Research. (2012b, May 29). Nearly one in ten U.S. high school students report heavy marijuana use in the past month: One-third or more of heavy users also used cocaine, Ectsasy, or other drugs. *CESAR FAX, 21*(21).

Center for Substance Abuse Research. (2012c). The role of biomarkers in the treatment of alcohol use disorders. *SAMHSA Advisory, 11*(2).

Chappell, J. S., Meyn, A. W., & Ngim, K. K. (2004). The extraction and infared identification of gamma-hydroxybutyric acid (GHB) from aqueous solutions. *J Forensic Sci, 49,* 52–59.

Cody, J., & Valtier, S. (2001). Effects of Stealth Adulterant on immunoassay testing for drugs of abuse. *J Anal Toxicol, 25*(6), 466–470.

Cone, E. J. (2001). Legal, workplace and treatment drug testing with alternate biological matrices on a global scale. *Forensic Sci Int, 121*(1–2), 7–15.

Dahl, H., Voltaire Carlsson, A. V., Hillgren, K., & Helander, A. (2011). Urinary ethyl glucuronide and ethly sulfate testing for detection of recent drinking in an outpatient treatment program for alcohol and drug dependence. *Alcohol Alcohol, 46*(3), 278–282.

Hansen, H. J., Caudill, S. P., & Boone, D. J. (1985). Crisis in drug testing: Results of CDC blind study. *JAMA, 253,* 2382–2387.

Larson, S. L., Eyerman, J., Foster, M. S., & Gfroerer, J. C. (2007). *Worker substance use and workplace policies and programs* (DHHS Publication No. SMA 07-4273, Analytic Series A-29). Rockville, MD: Substance Abuse and Mental Health Services Administration, Office of Applied Studies.

National Institute on Drug Abuse (NIDA). (1989). *Drug abuse curriculum for employee assistance program professionals* (DHHS Publication No. ADM 89-1587, pp. i–vi, 98). Washington, DC: U.S. Government Printing Office.

OnTrak TesTcup (1998). [Package insert.] Indianapolis, IN: Roche Applied Science Industrial Business.

Sgan, S. L., & Hanzlick, R. (2003). The medical review officer: A potential role for the medical examiner. *Am J Forensic Med Pathol, 24*(4), 346–350.

Smith, D. E., Glatt, W., Tucker, D. E., et al. (2002). Drug testing in the workplace: Integrating medical review officer duties into occupational medicine. *Occup Med, 17*(1), 79–90.

Willette, R. E. (1986). Drug testing programs. In R. L. Hawks & C. N. Chiang (Eds.), *Urine testing for drugs of abuse* (Vol. 73, pp. 5–12). Rockville, MD: National Institute on Drug Abuse.

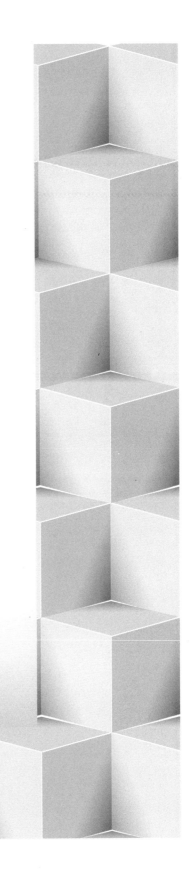

PART III

Substances
of Abuse

CHAPTER 5

Alcohol

ED NACE

Ethyl alcohol (ethanol) is the psychoactive ingredient found in alcoholic beverages. A drink of alcohol in the United States contains 18 ml (12 grams) of alcohol, which is found in a 12-ounce bottle of beer, a 5-ounce glass of wine, and 1½ ounces of liquor (80 proof). Beer contains 4–6% alcohol by volume and is made through fermentation of cereal grains. After water and tea, beer is estimated to be the third most consumed beverage in the world (Nelson, 2005). Wine contains about 10–12% alcohol and is fermented from grapes or occasionally other fruits. If a fermented product is then distilled, then the alcohol content is increased to 40% (80 proof) or more. After one drink, alcohol reaches its peak blood level in 30 minutes and is metabolized primarily by the liver at a rate of one drink per hour (approximately 12 grams of alcohol).

This remarkably simple molecule may be the mostly widely used and most ancient psychoactive substance. Its value for the human race has been its overall improvement in mood, mild euphoria, increased confidence, and increased sociability. For some, it is a sedative enabling sleep and in the past was used as an anesthetic. It seems to blunt the "superego" and provide a time-out from daily cares. The reverse of these benefits is my major purpose in writing this chapter, and I begin with data on alcohol's use, abuse, and dependence, followed by a description of its pharmacology and an outline of psychiatric and other medical complications resulting from its use.

PHARMACOLOGY

Alcohols are compounds with a hydroxyl group; that is oxygen and hydrogen (–OH) bonded to a carbon atom. Ethyl alcohol occurs naturally as a fermentation product of fruits and grains. Its molecular formula is CH_3CH_2OH. It is highly miscible in water and is therefore distributed throughout body water (nonfatty tissue). Since males have more body water by virtue of more muscle mass and proportionally less body fat than females, women achieve a higher blood alcohol concentration (BAC) faster than men, because there is less space for distribution of the alcohol.

Alcohol is primarily metabolized by the enzyme alcohol dehydrogenase (ADH). Metabolism begins in the stomach, where ADH is present. Women have less ADH in the stomach, and this is another reason they may reach a higher BAC faster than men (Frezza et al., 1990). Alcohol is absorbed from the stomach and proximal small intestine up to three times slower if one has consumed a meal with fat, carbohydrate, or protein compared to drinking on an empty stomach (Jones & Jönsson, 1994). Alcohol is absorbed more quickly than it is metabolized. ADH is the enzyme largely responsible for ethanol metabolism, but the enzyme cytochrome P450 2E1 (CYP2E1), which is increased with chronic drinking (Lieber, 1994), accounts for some metabolic activity. One standard drink (12 grams of alcohol) is metabolized to acetaldehyde at the rate of about one drink per hour. Acetaldehyde is then converted to acetic acid, which in turn is metabolized to carbon dioxide and water. A small quantity of alcohol remains unmetabolized and can be detected in urine, breath, and blood for 1–3 days. However a metabolite of alcohol, ethyl glucuronide (EtG) can be detected in the urine for 3–5 days following ingestion. It is not a quantitative test and may be positive as a result of nonbeverage alcohol such as mouthwashes or hand sanitizers (Skipper et al., 2004).

DIAGNOSIS AND DEFINITIONS OF ALCOHOL USE

Over the course of a lifetime, 92% of Americans will have consumed an alcoholic beverage. Of these, 65% are current drinkers, averaging 88 drinking days a year (Greenfield, 2000). The term "at-risk drinking" refers to consumption of more than 14 drinks a week, and "heavy drinking" is often defined as consumption of greater than 60 grams of alcohol (5 drinks) per occasion. The latter measure is associated with increased risk for alcohol-related injury and disease (Rehm et al., 2010) and with psychomotor and cognitive impairment in experimental studies (Lane, Cherek, Pietras, & Tcheremissine, 2004).

As with the other substances of abuse, the current diagnostic classification (DSM-5) utilizes one disorder of use, as opposed to the DSM-IV's previous diagnoses of abuse and dependence. "Alcohol use disorder" can be diagnosed as mild, moderate, or severe, depending on the number of criteria met.

The 11 criteria in DSM-5 are the same as those in DSM-IV—abuse and dependence—except the criterion for legal problems has been dropped and "craving" has been added as a criterion.

Clinically, it was generally assumed that a person who had alcohol abuse could, with proper treatment and motivation, resume a pattern of nonharmful alcohol use. Of course, this is not always the case, and progression to dependence (or "moderate" or "severe" alcohol use disorder) still may occur. In a U.S. representative sample of over 43,000 adults—the National Epidemiologic Survey on Alcohol and Related Conditions (NESARC)—conducted in this century, alcohol abuse has a 12-month prevalence of 4.7% and a lifetime prevalence of 17.8% (Hasin, Stinson, Ogburn, & Grant, 2007). The odds of alcohol abuse within the past 12 months are higher for men, whites, and Native Americans compared to blacks, Hispanics, and Asians, and higher among younger and unmarried people (Hasin et al., 2007). Having alcohol abuse at some point in a lifetime is more likely again in men, whites, and Native Americans. Those ages 30–64 years are more likely to have a history of abuse, while those with a high school education, an income under $20,000/year, or who have never married have lower odds ratios for alcohol abuse. The mean age of onset of an alcohol use disorder is nearly identical for abuse (22.5 years) and dependence (21.9 years) (Hasin et al., 2007).

Referring to the previous DSM-IV terminology, finally, alcohol abuse was not equivalent to "alcoholism" (instead, "alcoholism has been synonymous with alcohol dependence"), and may be reversible if acute situations have precipitated a pathological pattern of use or if the person were motivated to reverse a pattern of harmful drinking. For example, a successful investor was having severe marital conflict. He and his wife had over the past 5 years seen numerous marital therapists without lasting benefit. Alcohol was increasingly used over longer periods of time at home to blunt the tension. As business travel was common for this man, he frequently was away and had no history of excessive drinking on these prolonged trips. His wife would become angry at his absenting himself when at home. He would hide the alcohol, not because he was intending to disguise his drinking, but to minimize his spouse's reaction if she saw an open bottle. Abuse criteria were met because of the continuing personal conflicts over his use of alcohol around his wife. When she filed for divorce, he moved out and quickly stopped drinking—not to assuage his wife but to counter accusations about his drinking as custody arrangements for the children were being processed. Cessation of alcohol use was easily accomplished and has remained in place. No criteria of dependence had been manifest other than an expectable degree of tolerance.

Alcohol dependence has a 12-month prevalence of 3.8% and a lifetime prevalence of 12.5% (Hasin et al., 2007). The odds for lifetime dependence were greater for those with lower incomes, unmarried respondents, the youngest age group, and Native Americans. As in earlier studies (Grant, 1997), the NESARC study indicated that African Americans and Asians are at lower risk for abuse and dependence than whites, and in the NESARC study (Hasin et al., 2007), Hispanics had lower rates of abuse and dependence than whites.

A "severe" alcohol use disorder (or alcohol dependence) is illustrated by a 26-year-old white male who had recently completed his college degree and was found in his apartment after having a seizure. He had been consuming a quart of vodka or other liquors daily for several months. He recognized his dependence on alcohol and agreed to inpatient rehabilitation. Upon discharge he declined follow-up with an addiction psychiatrist and did not attend Alcoholics Anonymous meetings. He soon was drinking again and unable to cut down in spite of repeated efforts and his fear of another seizure. Each drinking episode resulted in drinking more than he intended, and his use of alcohol interfered with applying for either graduate school or employment. A withdrawal seizure occurred again and he agreed to intensive outpatient treatment. This young man illustrates tolerance to alcohol (a quart of liquor per day), withdrawal, use in spite of a known medical complication (seizures), inability to regulate his intake, unsuccessful efforts to cut down or abstain, and failure to pursue occupational or educational goals.

SCREENING AND DIAGNOSIS

Should clinicians, whether they be primary care physicians, emergency department physicians, or mental health professionals, be expected to screen for alcohol use disorders? A medical disorder should have the following criteria if screening is to be recommended: (1) Substantial morbidity and mortality results from the disorder; (2) the disorder should be relatively common; (3) effective treatment is available that can decrease morbidity and mortality; and (4) early treatment should lead to a better outcome than that initiated later in the disease process (Stewart & Connors, 2004–2005). Alcohol use disorders clearly meet these criteria. Fortunately, there are several screening tests available to clinicians. Two of these screening tests ask the patient a brief series of questions. One is the CAGE (Ewing, 1984):

- C: Have you ever felt you should CUT DOWN on your drinking?
- A: Have people ANNOYED you by criticizing your drinking?
- G: Have you ever felt bad or GUILTY about your drinking?
- E—EYE opener: Have you ever had a drink first thing in the morning to steady your nerves or to get rid of a hangover?

Two positive answers are considered a positive test that warrants further assessment.

The TWEAK (Russell et al., 1994) is similar but considered more useful for women:

- T—TOLERANCE: How many drinks can you hold or how many drinks does it take for you to get high? (If it takes more than two drinks to feel "high" or six drinks to feel drunk, tolerance can be assumed.)
- W: Have close friends or relatives WORRIED about your drinking?
- E—EYE opener: Have you ever used alcohol to help you get started in the morning or to steady your nerves?
- A—AMNESIA: Has a friend or family member ever told you of things you said or did while you were drinking that you could not remember?
- K (cut): Do you sometimes feel the need to cut down on your drinking?

Three positive answers warrant further assessment.

Written self-report instruments include the Michigan Alcoholism Screening Test (MAST; Selzer, 1971) and the Alcohol Use Disorders Identification Test (AUDIT; Volk, Steinbauer, Cantor, & Holzer, 1997). The MAST assesses lifetime drinking results, and the AUDIT assesses alcohol use over the previous 12 months.

Several available laboratory tests are useful state biomarkers for detection of alcohol use. Gamma-glutamyl transferase (GGT) is a liver enzyme with a sensitivity of 50% and a specificity of 80% (Bean, 1996). Thus, 50% of problem drinkers will be missed by the GGT, but 80% with an elevation will have a history of heavy alcohol use (excluding other possible causes of an elevated GGT such as prostatitis, pancreatitis, or the effect of other drugs). Alanine aminotransferase (ALT) and aspartate aminotransferase (AST) are two other liver enzymes that may be elevated by heavy drinking. ALT is more specific to alcohol use than AST, and both are indicators primarily of liver disease apart from alcohol use (Halvorson et al., 1993). The volume of red blood cells (mean corpuscular volume [MCV]) when increased may reflect heavy drinking and the combination of an elevated MCV and elevated GGT is found in a high percentage of patients with alcoholism (Holt, Skinner, & Israel, 1981). Carbohydrate-deficient transferrin (CDT) is useful to assess heavy drinking, because five drinks or more per day for 8 weeks or more is likely to elevate this enzyme (Anttila, Jarvi, Latvala, & Niemela, 2004). Finally, EtG is a minor metabolite of ethyl alcohol that can be detected in blood up to 36 hours after the last drink and up to 80 hours in the urine (Wurst, Skipper, & Weinmann, 2003). It is not a satisfactory quantitative test, but it is useful in detecting relapse.

The physician or other clinician qualified to make diagnoses best serves the patient by using established criteria—currently DSM-5. DSM criteria may not be a perfect fit in many cases, but referring to and relying on validated criteria ensure that the clinician is thinking through the presenting history, signs, and symptoms. Careful consideration of a diagnosis is a "defense" against labeling and a buffer against pressure from others who insist that their relative or colleague is an "alcoholic." If the diagnosis is apparent, it becomes a road map for reversing a potentially destructive process. The patient can be tactfully counseled on why abuse or dependence applies. This may involve a review of the patient's experience with alcohol, because it may have compromised his or her health or occupational and social functioning. The effect of his or her drinking on relationships is also an important consideration. An optimistic outlook on how to reverse or alter pathological drinking should be discussed with the patient and his or her family. A professional, thoughtful presentation of a diagnosis helps to overcome resistance and demoralization.

By the same token, a diagnosis may not be clear. There can be a "gray zone" in which it is uncertain whether a substance use disorder (SUD) is present. The process of making a diagnosis does not have to be rushed if the data are not available. Developing a trusting therapeutic relationship with the patient, as well as being sensitive to the concerns of family members while seeking additional history or medical data, is often necessary for an accurate assessment to take place and an appropriate treatment plan to be formulated. For example, a high-achieving physician was experiencing considerable stress over a personal loss that occurred as he took a new and demanding administrative position. Years earlier, he had drunk briefly but heavily during a period of marital discord. His current stressors provoked a similar pattern of "self-medication" and understandingly alarmed his wife. He was highly defensive about being considered the "sick" one and felt unappreciated by and resentful over his spouse's confrontations. The addiction psychiatrist who was consulted on this case had to walk a line between giving the patient "a pass," as the wife saw it, and alienating the physician, who was struggling with anxiety, sleep disturbance and, at the least, overuse of alcohol. The physician-patient formed a trusting relationship with the psychiatrist and spontaneously, without pressure from any party, decided to seek an inpatient rehabilitation program. This was quickly arranged and a successful outcome resulted.

The key to this case was to not rush to a diagnosis but to support the patient and his spouse in reflecting on their experiences and respect their different concerns. A confrontation/intervention or a joining of sides with one partner versus the other would likely have broken a process that was serving the patient's acceptance of help.

COMORBIDITY

A significant advance in the study of addictions over the past 25 years has been the recognition that SUDs commonly co-occur with other psychiatric disorders. The most common form of comorbidity is that between alcohol use disorders and other drug use disorders. When controlled for sociodemographic characteristics and other psychiatric comorbidities, the alcohol-dependent individual is nearly five times more likely than members of the general population to have either drug abuse or drug dependence, and over three times more likely to be nicotine dependent (Hasin et al., 2007). This strong overlap justifies the usual practice of using treatment programs to treat any form of SUD rather than "specialize" in alcohol or in some other drug.

Mood disorders commonly co-occur. Bipolar I and bipolar II disorders are two times more common in alcohol-dependent individuals, and major depression and dysthymia about one and a half times more likely in the person with a lifetime prevalence of alcohol dependence. Fifty-four percent of patients with bipolar disorder also meet criteria for either alcohol abuse or dependence. Bipolar individuals with an alcohol use disorder are at significantly greater risk for making suicide attempts (odds ratio of 2.25) than bipolar patients without an alcohol use disorder (Oquendo et al., 2010). Comorbidity is also common with anxiety disorders; "any anxiety disorder" is nearly twice as likely in the alcohol-dependent person (Hasin et al., 2007).

The NESARC study (Hasin et al., 2007), because it controlled for sociodemographic and other psychiatric comorbidity, found a lesser association with personality disorders and alcohol use disorders than earlier epidemiological studies (e.g., the Epidemiologic Catchment Area study; Helzer & Pryzbeck, 1988). Nevertheless, personality disorders are overrepresented in those with alcohol dependence at a rate nearly twice that of the general population (Hasin et al., 2007).

Alcohol use disorders and comorbid psychiatric disorders should be treated in synchrony, that is, in an integrated program capable of addressing each disorder (Nace & Tinsley, 2007).

ALCOHOL-INDUCED DISORDERS

Alcohol-Induced Brain Damage

Alcohol-related brain damage can be divided between those whose brain damage is associated with nutritional deficiencies or liver disease (complicated alcoholics) and those in whom the latter conditions are not present (uncomplicated alcoholics) (Harper, 2009).

Whether "moderate" drinkers develop brain damage is uncertain, partly because of the different definitions of "moderate." An increase in cerebrospinal-fluid-filled space around the brain was found in studies of drinkers who consumed more than eight drinks a day (Ding et al., 2004), and similar findings in those who drank five to eight drinks a day (Harper, Kril, & Daly, 1988). de Bruin et al. (2005) found that neither current nor lifetime moderate drinking in males or females led to decreases in brain volume. However, their definition of "moderate" was no more than three drinks a week.

The liver damaged by ethanol is not able to remove neurotoxic substances from blood (e.g., acetaldehyde and manganese; Butterworth, 2003). Furthermore, the accumulation of ammonia compromises cerebral blood flow and astrocyte functioning (Felipo & Butterworth, 2002). The hippocampus is especially effected (Matsumoto, 2009). The result is memory deficits, decreased attention span, poor judgment, and compromised capacity for planning.

Thiamine deficiency is the leading nutritional cause of brain damage in "complicated alcoholics" and results in Wernicke's encephalopathy, Korsakoff's psychosis (alcohol-induced persisting amnestic disorder), and cerebellar damage. Current operational criteria for Wernicke's encephalopathy require two of the following: dietary deficiency, occulomotor abnormalities, cerebellar dysfunction, and either altered mental state or mild memory impairment (Caine et al., 1997). Patients with Korsakoff's psychosis have a severe amnestic syndrome characterized by an inability to form new memories. Wernicke's encephalopathy involves damage in the periventricular areas around the third and fourth ventricles; Korsakoff's psychosis damages the anterior nucleus of the thalamus (Harding et al., 2000). Thiamine deficiency also accounts for the cerebellar damage that has been found in at least 25% of alcoholics with Wernicke's encephalopathy or Korsakoff's psychosis (Torvik & Torp, 1986).

So-called "uncomplicated" alcoholics are those whose alcohol-related brain damage is ethanol-specific and referred to as alcohol-induced persisting dementia. Memory loss, apraxia, aphasia, agnosia, and poor executive functioning (planning, initiating, correcting sequencing, and completing a plan of action) are characteristic symptoms. This syndrome occurs in about 9% of alcoholics (Evert & Oscar-Berman, 1995), and unlike Wernicke's encephalopathy or Korsakoff's psychosis, in which recovery occurs in some, the damage is generally irreversible. Loss of both gray- and white-matter volumes has been reported (Harper, 2009). The mechanisms involved include accumulation of acetaldehyde and fatty acid ethyl esters that interrupt mitochondrial function and disrupt neural membranes; generate reactive oxygen species that damage DNA and inhibit gene expression; and inhibit brain-derived neurotrophic factor, which is involved in cell survival and growth (Zahr et al., 2011).

Alcohol Intoxication/Alcohol Intoxication Delirium

Alcohol intoxication is likely to be the most commonly occurring clinical syndrome and is no doubt the one most recognized by the public. In legal settings there is a clear demarcation between intoxication (drunkenness) and not being "drunk." For most states in the United States, a BAC of 80 mg% or above is intoxication. Clinically, such a clear demarcation does not exist. The onset of intoxication from alcohol, in contrast to the commonly sought mild euphoric/sedative effects, is dependent on how tolerant one is to alcohol, individual differences such as body weight, as well as the setting in which dinking occurs. At a blood alcohol level of 50 mg%, the common signs of intoxication in a nontolerant person are expected to appear and to increase with a rising blood alcohol level. These signs include increased talkativeness, decreased attention, euphoria, emotional liability, slurred speech, impulsiveness, impaired reaction time, nystagmus, incoordination, and stupor or coma.

Alcohol intoxication delirium is far less common and, unlike delirium associated with stimulants or cannabis, has a slower onset, typically after days of heavy drinking. Consciousness is disturbed because disorientation may occur, as well as reduced ability to focus, sustain, or shift attention. Memory deficits, as well as hallucinations, may be noted. The symptoms may fluctuate over the course of a day and resolve as the intoxication ends (American Psychiatric Association, 2000).

Alcohol Withdrawal and Alcohol Withdrawal Delirium

Because alcohol's action is primarily through stimulation of gamma-aminobutyric acid (GABA-A) receptors, prolonged stimulation will lead to down-regulation of these receptors. Alcohol also inhibits excitatory N-methyl-D-aspartate (NMDA) glutamate receptors and with prolonged exposure to alcohol these receptors increase in number (i.e., up-regulate). Thus, when alcohol is not present, the brain has a relative deficiency in GABA-A receptors and an excess of NMDA receptors. These changes account for the alcohol withdrawal (AW) syndrome.

AW will begin 6–8 hours after the last drink and when mild to moderate produces nausea, vomiting, insomnia, decreased appetite, tremors, and increased heart rate. If severe, visual and auditory hallucinations ("alcohol hallucinosis") may occur as well. AW may intensify and in the next 48 hours and lead to anxiety, irritability, agitation, headache, sensitivity to light and sound, decreased concentration, and possibly disorientation. AW seizures may develop between 24 and 48 hours after the last drink.

If seizures do occur, there is an increased risk for the development of alcohol withdrawal delirium tremens (DTs). DTs also are more likely to develop if the person has a concomitant medical problem (e.g., pneumonia, fracture, subdural hematoma) and usually develops between 48 and 96 hours after the last drink. This severe and potentially life-threatening syndrome is characterized by disorientation; agitation; gross tremulousness; increased pulse, blood pressure, and respiratory rates; fever; and visual and/or auditory hallucinations (Myrick & Anton, 2000).

Alcohol-Induced Psychotic, Affective, or Anxiety Disorder

Alcohol-induced psychotic disorder is relatively rare, occurring in approximately 0.5% of hospitalized alcoholics. It is characterized by auditory hallucinations, although visual hallucinations may occur; persecutory delusions may be present. These symptoms are present in a clear sensorium and with no more than mild withdrawal symptoms. The prognosis is generally good with only 10 to 20% of individuals developing a chronic schizophrenic-like syndrome. In a German study, the mean age of onset was 47 years (Soyka, 2008).

Major depression and alcohol use disorders commonly co-occur, and having either one doubles the risk of having the other. The alcohol use disorder is most likely the causal agent. When consequences of alcohol dependence, such as job loss and relationship problems, are controlled, the causality remains in favor of the alcohol use disorder leading to major depression. Thus, neurophysiological and metabolic effects from alcohol are likely the causal link. Overall, about 10% of the burden of major depression can be attributed to alcohol (Boden & Fergusson, 2011).

Anxiety disorders are highly comorbid with alcohol use disorders, with 44% of patients presenting for alcoholism treatment meeting criteria for an anxiety disorder

(Kushner et al., 2005). This, of course, does not determine whether the anxiety disorder is alcohol-induced. In a recent study, about one-half of patients entering alcoholism treatment had an anxiety disorder. Of those who had an anxiety disorder at start of treatment and did not relapse, only 31% continued to have an anxiety disorder 4 months later. Of the total sample (those who had an anxiety disorder at baseline and those who did not), 17% had an anxiety disorder at follow-up, which may translate into a conservative estimate of independent (not alcohol-induced) anxiety disorders in a clinical population (Kushner et al., 2005).

An extensive review (Falk, Yi, & Hilton, 2008) found that alcohol use disorders tend to precede generalized anxiety disorder, panic, and panic with agoraphobia, as well as major depression and dysthymia. Alcohol use disorders were more often secondary in comorbid cases of social and specific phobia. Phobias are five times more likely to occur before onset of an alcohol use disorder, and generalized anxiety disorder is five times more likely to occur after onset of an alcohol use disorder. The lag times between comorbid disorders, regardless of which was primary, is quite long, ranging from 7 to 16 years. If the primary disorder has a causative role in the secondary disorder, then it obviously is temporally distant. However, the more severe alcohol use disorder—alcohol dependence—results in a shorter lag time to a secondary anxiety or mood disorder than does alcohol abuse.

According to DSM, in order to diagnose a symptom cluster (e.g., as alcohol-induced), the symptoms must develop during intoxication or within 1 month of withdrawal. And they must be more severe than the usual presentation of such symptoms as they usually occur in intoxicated or withdrawal states. Alcohol-induced disorders would not be expected to be present during prolonged periods of abstinence.

Alcohol-Induced Sexual Dysfunction

Men with alcoholism often have erectile dysfunction and infertility. Alcohol has been recognized as a testicular toxin for decades. Women with a history of chronic, heavy alcohol use are likely to have inhibition of ovulation, decreased gonadal mass, and infertility (Adler, 1992). More recent studies confirm that although acute alcohol intoxication decreases testosterone levels in males, it has an opposite effect in females, raising testosterone levels (Frias, Torres, Miranda, Ruiz, & Orgega, 2002).

Both sexes demonstrate an increase in beta-endorphins, prolactin, adrenocorticotropic hormone (ACTH), and cortisol (Frias et al., 2002). Healthy males, however, who have two or three standard drinks may experience a transient increase in testosterone (Sarkola & Eriksson, 2003). Sexual dysfunction induced by alcohol refers to impairment of desire, arousal, orgasm, or pain associated with intercourse. In contrast to sexual dysfunction from other causes, improvement would be expected with abstinence from alcohol.

Alcohol-Induced Sleep Disorder

Alcohol effects on sleep have been extensively studied. Alcohol before bedtime decreases body temperature and mobility in the first half of the night but increases temperature and motility in the second half. In the first half of the night, the percentage of slow-wave sleep is increased and rapid eye movement (REM) sleep is decreased and delayed. The second half of the night results in increased wakefulness, light Stage 1 sleep and increased REM sleep. The reversal seen between the first and second half of the night reflects a rebound effect as alcohol is metabolized (Arnedt et al., 2011).

People with alcoholism in the general population report higher rates of recent insomnia (18%) than do people without alcoholism (10%). Alcoholics admitted for treatment report even higher rates, ranging from 36 to 72% (Brower, Robinson, & Zucker, 2000). Alcoholics during both drinking times and withdrawal have decreased sleep time. Sleep apnea and periodic limb movements occur at an increased rate in the alcoholic population. Sleep abnormalities in alcoholics may persist after abstinence for up to 1 to 3 years (Brower, 2001).

MEDICAL COMPLICATIONS

Alcohol use is related causally to many major diseases and "causes a considerable part of the global burden of disease" (Rehm et al., 2009). Alcohol consumption has been found to have a causal impact in a dose-related manner on the following major disease categories: cancer (female breast, liver, colon and rectal, esophageal, mouth, and oro- and nasopharynx), tuberculosis, diabetes mellitus, hypertension, epilepsy, stroke, ischemic heart disease, arrhythmias, pneumonia, cirrhosis, unipolar depression, fetal alcohol syndrome, and preterm birth complications. However, beneficial effects are found for ischemic heart disease, stroke, and diabetes mellitus if consumption is light to moderate and free of heavy drinking (defined as 60 grams or five drinks) on any given occasion (Rehm et al., 2010).

Liver

In developed countries, 66% of all chronic liver disease is alcohol-related. Alcohol accounts for 50% of the deaths attributed to cirrhosis. Ninety percent of heavy drinkers (> 60 grams of alcohol per day) will have fatty liver, whereas 10–35% develop alcoholic hepatitis and 5–15% develop cirrhosis (McCullough, O'Shea, & Dasarathy, 2011). Liver disease from alcohol develops at lower doses in women, Hispanics, the obese, and those with hepatitis C. Although fatty liver (hepatic steatosis) is common and reversible, it does lead to cirrhosis in 7% of cases (Gish, 1996). Hepatic inflammation is the hallmark of alcoholic hepatitis, which may be confirmed histologically by infiltration of polymorphonuclear cells, necrosis, and Mallory bodies. Hepatitis per se is not an indication for a transplant, but it may be necessary in those who have liver failure and do not respond to medical treatment—typically a course of steroids (Lucey, 2011).

The consequences of cirrhosis ("scarring") include ascites, kidney failure, esophageal variceal hemorrhage, hepatic encephalopathy, and clotting difficulties. In 2005, the age-adjusted death rate from cirrhosis was 9.2 deaths per 1,000, which is 27,000 deaths a year (Lucey, 2011). Alcoholic liver disease, either alone or in combination with a hepatitis C infection, accounted for 20% of liver transplants between 1988 and 2009 (Lucey, 2011). These figures contradict 1980s predictions, which stated that patients with alcoholic liver disease were unlikely to be selected for liver transplants

(No Author, 1984). Furthermore, the results of liver transplantation for patients with alcoholic liver disease are as good as those for patients with other liver diseases and better than those with hepatitis C (Lucey, Schaubel, Guidinger, Tome, & Merion, 2009).

Gastrointestinal Tract and Pancreas

Abuse of alcohol is associated with acute pancreatitis in 35% of cases and in 70% of cases of chronic pancreatitis. The latter is the result of repeated bouts of acute pancreatitis. Excessive intracellular activation of trypsinogen leads to inflammation and destruction of parenchymal pancreatic cells. Alcohol abuse alone is not likely to cause acute pancreatitis, but it sensitizes the pancreas to injury when factors such as high lipid diet, smoking, infection, or genetic predisposition are present. The pancreas contains stellate cells similar to those found in the liver. Damage to the stellate cells in the pancreas is associated with the fibrotic changes found in pancreatitis (Clemens & Mahan, 2010). Acute pancreatitis is associated with severe pain in the abdomen and the middle of the back. Nausea and vomiting are common and the condition is potentially life-threatening. Chronic pancreatitis can lead to lack of digestive enzymes and lack of insulin, leading to diabetes. Pseudocysts of the pancreas are common and may cause abdominal pressure and infection (Torpy, Lymn, & Golub, 2012).

The relationship between heavy alcohol use and pancreatic cancer remains unclear. Most studies have found no relationship, but a slight increase in risk for male heavy drinkers (> 45 grams of alcohol a day), but not female heavy drinkers, has been established (Michaud et al., 2010).

The inflammatory capacity of alcohol relative to the gastrointestinal tract involves its direct damage of cells and its effect on gut flora. Microorganisms in the gut are affected by alcohol and release lipopolysaccharide (LPS), an inflammation inducer, from the bacterial wall. Gut integrity and permeability are affected by LPS. Zinc deficiency, common to alcoholics, may result (Wang, Lee, Manson, Buring, & Sesso, 2010). Decreased absorption of folate, vitamin B12, thiamine, and vitamin A, as well as some amino acids and lipids, is a well-known effect of alcohol (Hauge, Nilsson, Persson, & Hultberg, 1998). Glossitis, stomatitis, gastritis, and parotid gland enlargement are associated with heavy alcohol use. Acute gastritis is a function of lowered gastric emptying time associated with alcohol, combined with alcohol's disruption of the mucosal barrier that allows hydrogen ions to seep into the mucosa and release histamine. Anorexia, vomiting, epigastric pain, and bleeding are common symptoms. Vomiting may produce a tear at the esophageal–gastric junction (Mallory–Weiss syndrome) and be an additional source of bleeding (Bor et al., 1998).

Cardiovascular System

Moderate, regular consumption of alcohol in generally healthy people is associated with a significantly lower cardiovascular and all-cause mortality compared to abstainers (Costanzo, Di Castelnuovo, Donati, Iacoviello, & de Gaetano, 2010). One drink per day for women and two drinks per day for men reduced total mortality by 18%. Similar findings are found even in patients with known cardiovascular disease.

Mortality is significantly reduced with light to moderate alcohol consumption—5–25 grams per day (i.e., about half a drink to two drinks per day) (Costanzo et al., 2010).

Cardiovascular protection is conferred though improved insulin sensitivity, increased high-density lipoprotein cholesterol, decreased platelet aggregation, beneficial effects on endothelium, and decreased inflammatory responses (O'Keefe, Bybee, & Lavie, 2007). The protective effect is conferred by ethyl alcohol and not the congeners within alcoholic beverages. More than two drinks a day for women or more than three drinks a day for men was associated with increased mortality in a dose-dependent manner (DiCastelnuovo et al., 2006).

Drinking in excess of the amounts referred to earlier is associated with increased risk of the following cardiovascular-related conditions: coronary artery disease, hypertension, congestive heart failure, stroke, dementia, diabetes, and Raynaud's phenomenon (O'Keefe et al., 2007).

Cancer

The American Institute for Cancer Research and the World Cancer Research Fund jointly published reviews indicating that alcohol is a cause of cancer of the mouth, pharynx, larynx, esophagus, breast, and colorecum (in men). Furthermore, alcohol is "probably" a cause of colorectal cancer and liver cancer in women (Latino-Martel et al., 2011). Liver cancer predominately develops in those with cirrhosis. The highest cancer risk is for cancers of the oral cavity, pharynx, larynx, and esophagus, and these are more likely with consumption of greater than 80 grams of alcohol a day and more so in those who also smoke (Pöschl & Seitz, 2004).

Biological mechanisms include the carcinogenic effect of ethanol and its major metabolite acetaldehyde; the formation of DNA adducts (the covalent bonding of a small molecule to DNA); inflammatory processes such as those that occur with cirrhosis; interference with folate metabolism (implicated in colorectal cancer); and increased estrogen levels associated with drinking (breast cancer) (Latino-Martel et al., 2011).

Breast cancer has consistently been associated with a modest (30–50%) increase in women who are moderate drinkers (one to two drinks per day). This association is strongest for those who were premenopausal at time of diagnosis. Polymorphisms of alcohol dehydrogenase have not been found to account for the alcohol–breast cancer association (Terry et al., 2007; Visnanathan et al., 2007). The latter association is limited to women with estrogen-sensitive tumors (Latino-Martel et al., 2011).

Hematology

Alcohol's toxic effect on hematopoiesis usually occurs only in severe alcoholism. Up to 80% of men and 46% of women with macrocytosis (increased MCV) have been found to be alcoholic (Ballard, 1997). Normalization of MCV occurs with abstinence and takes 2–4 months (Latvala, Parkkila, & Niemelä, 2004). Chronic excessive alcohol use decreases red blood cell precursors in the bone marrow, reduces neutrophils, and reduces platelets. Thrombocytopenia from alcoholism can be expected to normalize within 7 days, and neutropenia is transient.

Iron metabolism may be affected, with iron deficiency resulting from gastrointestinal bleeding. Conversely, iron absorption is increased with heavy use of alcohol and can lead to iron deposits in the liver, pancreas, heart, and joints (hemochromatosis) (Lieb et al., 2011).

Blood clotting may be impaired by thrombocytopenia as well as by impairment in the functioning of vitamin K-dependent clotting factors. The clotting mechanism may also be impaired by diminished fibrinolysis secondary to alcohol use. The latter may result in excessive formation of blood clots, with increased risk of stroke (Ballard, 1997).

The effects of alcohol on the blood system are further complicated by the well-known interference of absorption of folate and other B vitamins, all of which are necessary for blood cell precursors to produce red blood cells.

Immune System

Use of alcohol in quantities that exceed two drinks a day for women and three drinks a day for men is likely to compromise the immune system (Szabo & Mandrekar, 2009). Alcohol abuse increases infections of the respiratory tract such as pneumonia and tuberculosis (Zhang, Bagby, happel, Raasch, & Nelson, 2008), and increases the risk for hepatitis C and HIV.

The mechanisms of alcohol's impact on the immune system include damage to the epithelial linings of the gastrointestinal and respiratory tracts. Damage to epithelial cells leads to "leakage" and sets up conditions of chronic inflammation. Polymorphonuclear leukocytes act as phagocytes and engulf invading pathogens. Alcohol suppresses the ability of these cells to act on pathogens and interferes with production of new granulocytes. The immune response includes, in addition to the cellular response of phagocytic cells, humoral responses such as production of cytokines and chemokines. Chronic alcohol exposure increases proinflammatory cytokines, which leads to tissue damage from inflammation. Acute alcohol use such as binge drinking suppresses cytokine production and therefore interferes with this aspect of the host defense response. Thus, the innate immunity system (e.g., the epithelial barrier) and the adaptive immunity system (e. g., production of antigens) are both compromised by chronic alcohol exposure, leading to greater risk of infection in the alcohol-abusing population (Molina, Happel, Zhang, Kolls, & Nelson, 2010).

Musculoskeletal System

The consumption of one drink or less a day is associated with lower risk of hip fracture; whereas abstinence or more than two drinks a day increased the risk of hip fracture. Alcohol use is associated with increased bone density in both men and women if they drink less than two drinks a day. Abstainers and heavier drinkers have increased rates of bone loss. Increased levels of estradiol in moderate drinkers may be a mechanism that supports favorable bone density (Berg et al., 2008). No doubt, it is obvious that falls associated with drinking account for the increased fractures in an alcoholic population. A hospital emergency room study indicated that people with a BAC of 0.1 to 0.15 had triple the rate of falls compared to a control group (Honkanen et al., 1983).

Alcoholic myopathy is an underrecognized complication of drinking and occurs more commonly than do genetically based muscle diseases. The myopathy is not based on cirrhosis, neuropathy, or malnutrition. The myopathy is related to total lifetime alcohol use and can reduce muscle mass by up to 30%. The usual symptoms are muscle weakness and muscle cramps. Serum creatinine kinase is not likely to be elevated. The myopathy is at least partially reversible with abstinence and good nutrition (Preedy et al., 2003).

Skin

Flushing is a common transient reaction to acute alcohol ingestion. A chronic facial erythema due to loss of vasoregulatory control may result from long-term use of alcohol.

Both psoriasis and rosacea may be aggravated by alcohol use. Rosacea may develop pustular eruptions and more pronounced facial telangiectasias. Psoriasis may become more severe, especially in those who drink more than 80 grams of alcohol per day. Treatment resistance develops and plaques are distinctively distributed on acral surfaces (distal aspects of arms and legs and head [ears and nose]; Farber & Nall, 1994).

Nutritional deficiencies contribute to the effect of alcohol on the skin; seborrheic dermatitis is twice as likely in alcoholics, but especially in those whose nutrition is compromised. A thick red tongue and waxy skin may be found in those with thiamine deficiency, which may accompany alcoholism.

Alcoholic liver disease has many cutaneous findings: pruritus, spider angioma, caput medusa (enlarged veins around the umbilicus), nummular dermatitis (coin-shaped lesions of eczema), and palmar erythema (Lui, Lien, & Fenske, 2010).

Fetal Alcohol Effects

Fetal alcohol spectrum disorder (FASD) is a term that includes fetal alcohol syndrome (FAS) and the spectrum of alcohol effects on the fetus that do not meet FAS criteria.

FAS requires prenatal and/or postnatal growth retardation; a distinct facial appearance (short palpebral fissures, smooth philtrum, indistinct fold above the lip), and thin vermillion (thin upper lip); and some central nervous system dysfunction (Riley & Magee, 2005). Prevalence of FAS in the United States is 0.5–2.0 per 1,000 births, but it is considerably higher in some Native American tribes (May & Gossage, 2001). About 13% of women in the United States drink during pregnancy, with 3% of these drinking heavily or binge drinking (Riley & Magee, 2005). Whether or not the facial characteristics of FAS are present, heavy drinking during pregnancy is associated with neuropsychological impairments in memory, language, attention, reaction time, visuospatial abilities, fine and gross motor skills, executive functioning, and lower IQ.

Risk factors for FASD include dose of alcohol, pattern of alcohol (binge or continuous is most harmful), lower socioeconomic status, poor nutritional status, presence of other drugs, and developmental timing of exposure. Animal models indicate that facial characteristics are impacted by the equivalent of first- and third-trimester exposure that impacts prefrontal cortex, cerebellum, and hippocampus development (Riley & Magee, 2005).

TREATMENT PRINCIPLES

There are several principles to consider in the treatment of a patient with an SUD, including specific treatments of pharmacotherapy, individual and group therapies, and 12-step programs.

First, a diagnosis must be made, then presented to the patient. The presentation is done tactfully, optimistically, and professionally. "Tactfully" means that one is sensitive to the potential for stigma or blame; "optimistically" means that a good outcome can be reasonably expected and a variety of treatment options are available; and "professionally" refers to providing the basis for the diagnosis and communicating how the disease may influence one's behavior, thinking, and priorities (Nace & Tinsley, 2007).

Second, the beginning stages of treatment should emphasize abstinence, education about alcoholism, and ego-strengthening (learning to identify affect and to regulate and tolerate affect rather than drinking).

Third, as abstinence is acquired, the specific dynamics or developmental pathway of the patient's addiction may be explored. Coincident with this therapeutic effort, encouragement of spiritual development is undertaken, including gratitude for gains made, humility, and tolerance for one's own shortcomings and the limitations of others, and appreciation of the gradual release from the desire to drink.

Participating in the struggle with the man or woman who has an addiction, tolerating regression, and helping the patient start over as necessary more often than not leads to a good outcome and a grateful patient.

REFERENCES

Adler, R. A. (1992). Clinical Review 33: Clinically important effects of alcohol on endocrine function. *J Clin Endocrinol Metab, 74*(5), 957–960.

American Psychiatric Association. (2000). *Diagnostic and statistical manual of mental disorders* (4th ed., text rev.). Washington, DC: Author.

American Psychiatric Association. (2013). *Diagnostic and statistical manual of mental disorders* (5th ed.). Arlington, VA: Author.

Anttila, P., Jarvi, K., Latvala, J., & Niemela, O. (2004). Method-dependent characteristics of carbohydrate-deficient transferrin measurements in the follow-up of alcoholics. *Alcohol Alcohol, 39*(1), 59–63.

Arnedt, J. T., Rohsenow, D. J., Almeida, A. B., et al. (2011). Sleep following alcohol intoxication in healthy, young adults: Effects of sex and family history of alcoholism. *Alcohol Clin Exp Res, 35*(5), 870–878.

Ballard, H. S. (1997). The hematological complications of alcoholism. *Alcohol Health Res World, 21*(1), 42–52.

Boden, J. M., & Fergusson, D. M. (2011). Alcohol and depression. *Addiction, 106*(5), 906–114.

Bor, S., Caymaz-Bor, C., Tobey, N. A., et al. (1998). The effect of ethanol on the structure and function of rabbit esophageal epithelium. *Am J Physiol, 274*, G819–G826.

Brower, K. J. (2001). Alcohol's effects on sleep in alcoholics. *Alcohol Res Health, 25*(2), 110–125.

Brower, K. J., Robinson, E. A. R., & Zucker, R. A. (2000). Epidemiology of insomnia and alcoholism in the general population. *Alcohol Clinical Exp Res, 25*(Suppl. 5), 43A.

Butterworth, R. F. (2003). Hepatic encephalopathy—a serious complication of alcoholic liver disease. *Alcohol Res Health, 27*, 143–145.

Caine, D., Halliday, G. M., Kril, J. J., et al. (1997). Operational criteria for classification of chronic alcoholics: Identification of Wernicke's encephalopathy. *J Neurol Neurosurg Psychiatry, 62*, 51–60.

Clemens, D. L., & Mahan, K. J. (2010). Alcoholic pancreatitis: Lessons from the liver. *World J Gastroenterol, 16*(11), 1314–1320.

Costanzo, S., Di Castelnuovo, A., Donati, M. B., Iacoviello, L., & de Gaetano, G. (2010). Alcohol consumption and mortality in patients with cardiovascular disease: A meta-analysis. *J Am Coll Cardiol, 55*(13), 1339–1347.

de Bruin, E. A., Hulshoff Pol, H. E., Bijl, S., et al. (2005). Associations between alcohol intake and brain volumes in male and female moderate drinkers. *Alcohol Clin Exp Res, 29*, 656–663.

DiCastelnuovo, A., Castanzo, S., Bagnardi, V., et al. (2006). Alcohol dosing and total mortality in men and women. *Arch Intern Med, 166*, 2437–2445.

Ding, J., Eigenbrodt, M. L., Mosley, T. H., Jr., et al. (2004). Alcohol intake and cerebral abnormalities on magnetic resonance imaging in a community-based population of middle-aged adults: The Atherosclerosis Risk in Communities (ARIC) study. *Stroke, 35*, 16–21.

Evert, D. L., & Oscar-Berman, M. (1995). Alcohol-related cognitive impairments: An overview of how alcohol may effect the workings of the brain. *Alcohol Health Res World, 19*(2), 189–196.

Ewing, J. (1984). Detecting alcoholism: The CAGE questionnaire. *JAMA, 252*(14), 1905–1907.

Falk, D. E., Yi, H. Y., & Hilton, M. E. (2008). Age of onset and temporal sequencing of lifetime DSM-IV alcohol use disorders relative to comorbid mood and anxiety disorders. *Drug Alcohol Depend, 94*(1–3), 234–245.

Farber, E. M., & Nall, L. (1994). Psoriasis and alcoholism. *Cutis, 53*(1), 21–27.

Frezza, M., di Padova, C., Pozzato, G., et al. (1990). High blood alcohol levels in women: The role of decreased gastric alcohol dehydrogenase activity and first-pass metabolism. *N Engl J Med, 322*(2), 95–99. Errata 1990: *322*(21), 1540 and *323*(8), 553.

Frias, J., Torres, J. M., Miranda, M. T., Ruiz, E., & Ortega, E. (2002). Effects of acute alcohol intoxication on pituitary-gonadal axis hormones, pituitary–adrenal axis hormones, beta-endorphin and prolactin in human adults of both sexes. *Alcohol Alcohol, 37*(2), 169–173.

Gish, R. (1996, November 30). *Rational evaluation of liver dysfunction of the chemically dependent patient and diagnosis and treatment of hepatitis C.* Audiotape presentation at the 7th annual meeting and symposium of the American Academy of Addiction Psychiaty, San Francisco, CA.

Grant, B. F. (1997). Prevalence and correlates of alcohol use and DSM-IV alcohol dependence in the United States: Results of the National Longitudinal Alcohol Epidemiologic Survey. *J Stud Alcohol, 58*(5), 464–473.

Greenfield, T. K. (2000). Ways of measuring drinking patterns and the difference they make: Experience with graduated frequencies. *J Subst Abuse, 12*(1–2), 33–49.

Halvorson, M. R., Campbell, J. L., Sprague, G., et al. (1993). Comparative evaluation of the clinical utility of three markers of ethanol intake: The effect of gender. *Alcohol Clin Exp Res, 17*(2), 225–229.

Harding, A., Halliday, G., Caine, D., et al. (2000). Degeneration of anterior thalamic nuclei differentiates alcoholics with amnesia. *Brain, 123*, 141–154.

Harper, C. (2009). The neuropathology of alcohol-related brain damage. *Alcohol Alcohol, 44*(2), 136–140.

Harper, C., Kril, J., & Daly, J. (1988). Does a "moderate" alcohol intake damage the brain? *J Neurol Neurosurg Psychiatry, 51*, 909–913.

Hasin, D. S., Stinson, F. S., Ogburn, E., & Grant, B. F. (2007). Prevalence, correlates, disability, and comorbidity of DSM-IV alcohol abuse and dependence in the United States: Results from the National Epidemiologic Survey on Alcohol and Related Conditions. *Arch Gen Psychiatry, 64*(7), 830–842.

Hauge, T., Nilsson, A., Persson, J., & Hultberg, B. (1998). Gamma-glutamyl transferase, intestinal alkaline phosphatase and beta-hexoaminidase activity in duodenal biopsies of chronic alcoholics. *Hepatogastroenterology, 45,* 985–989.

Helzer, J. E., & Pryzbeck, T. R. (1988). The co-occurrence of alcoholism with other psychiatric disorders in the general population and its impact on treatment. *J Stud Alcohol, 49*(3), 219–224.

Honkanen, R., Ertama, L., Kuosmanen, P., et al. (1983). The role of alcohol in accidental falls. *J Stud Alcohol, 44,* 231–245.

Holt, S., Skinner, H. A., & Israel, Y. (1981). Early identification of alcohol abuse. *CMAJ, 124*(10), 1279–1295.

Jones, A. W., & Jönsson, K. A. (1994). Food-induced lowering of blood-ethanol profiles and increased rate of elimination immediately after a meal. *J Forensic Sci, 39*(4), 1084–1093.

Kushner, M. G., Abrams, K., Thuras, P., et al. (2005). Follow-up study of anxiety disorder and alcohol dependence in comorbid alcoholism treatment patients. *Alcohol Clin Exp Res, 29*(8), 1432–1443.

Lane, S. D., Cherek, D. R., Pietras, C. J., & Tcheremissine, O. V. (2004). Alcohol effects on human risk taking. *Psychopharmacology, 172,* 68–77.

Latino-Martel, P., Arwidson, P., Ancellin, R., et al. (2011). Alcohol consumption and cancer risk: Revisiting guidelines for sensible drinking. *CMAJ, 183*(16), 1861–1865.

Lieb, M., Palm, U., Hock, B., et al. (2011). Effects of alcohol consumption on iron metabolism. *Am J Drug Alcohol Abuse, 37*(1), 68–73.

Lieber, C. S. (1994). Relationships between nutrition, alcohol use, and liver disease. *Alcohol Res Health, 27*(3), 220–231.

Liu, S. W., Lien, M. H., & Fenske, N. A. (2010). The effects of alcohol and drug abuse on the skin. *Clin Dermatol, 28*(4), 391–399.

Lucey, M. R. (2011). Liver transplantation in patients with alcoholic liver disease. *Liver Transpl, 17*(7), 751–759.

Lucey, M. R., Schaubel, D. E., Guidinger, M. K., Tome, S., & Merion, R. M. (2009). Effects of alcoholic liver disease and hepatitis C infection on waiting list and posttransplant mortality and transplant survival benefit. *Hepatology, 50,* 400–406.

Matsumoto, I. (2009). Proteomics approach in the study of the pathophysiology of alcohol-related brain damage. *Alcohol Alcohol, 44*(2), 171–176.

May, P. A., & Gossage, J. P. (2001). Estimating the prevalence of fetal alcohol syndrome: A summary. *Alcohol Res Health, 25*(3), 159–167.

McCullough, A. J., O'Shea, R. S., & Dasarathy, S. (2011). Diagnosis and management of alcoholic liver disease. *Journal of Digestive Diseases, 12,* 257–262.

Michaud, D. S., Vrieling, A., Jiao, L., et al. (2010). Alcohol intake and pancreatic cancer: A pooled analysis from the pancreatic cancer cohort consortium (PanScan). *Cancer Causes Control, 21*(8), 1213–1225.

Molina, P. E., Happel, K. I., Zhang, P., Kolls, J. K., & Nelson, S. (2010). Alcohol and Health—Focus On: Alcohol and the immune system. *Alcohol Res Health, 33,* 97–108.

Myrick, H., & Anton, R. F. (2000). Clinical management of alcohol withdrawal. *CNS Spectr, 5*(2), 22–32.

Nace, E. P., & Tinsley, J. A. (2007). *Patients with substance abuse problems: Effective identification, diagnosis, and treatment.* New York: Norton.

No Authors. (1984). National Institutes of Health Consensus Development Conference on Liver Transplantation (Sponsored by the National Institute of Arthritis, Diabetes, and Digestive and Kidney Diseases and the National Institutes of Health Office of Medical Applications of Research). *Hepatology, 4*(Suppl. 1), 1S–110S.

O'Keefe, J. H., Bybee, K. A., & Lavie, C. J. (2007). Alcohol and cardiovascular health: The razor-sharp double-edged sword. *J Am Coll Cardiol, 50*(11), 1009–1014.

Oquendo, M. A., Currier, D., Liu, S., Hasin, D., Grant, B., & Blanco, C. (2010). Increased risk for suicidal behavior in comorbid bipolar disorder and alcohol use disorders. *J Clin Psychiatry, 71*(7), 902–909.

Pöschl, G., & Seitz, H. K. (2004). Alcohol and cancer. *Alcohol Alcohol, 39,* 155–165.

Preedy, V. R., Ohlendieck, K., Adachi, J., et al. (2003). The importance of alcohol-induced muscle disease. *J Muscle Res Cell Motil, 24*(1), 55–63.

Rehm, J., Baliunas, D., Borges, G. L., et al. (2010). The relation between different dimensions of alcohol consumption and burden of disease: An overview. *Addiction, 105*(5), 817–843.

Rehm, J., Mathers, C., Popova, S., et al. (2009). Global burden of disease and injury and economic cost attributable to alcohol use and alcohol-use disorders. *Lancet, 373*(9862), 2223–2233.

Riley, E. P., & McGee, C. L. (2005). Fetal alcohol spectrum disorders: An overview with emphasis on changes in brain and behavior. *Exp Biol Med (Maywood), 230*(6), 357–365.

Russell, M., Martier, S. S., Sokol, R. J., et al. (1994). Screening for pregnancy risk-drinking. *Alcohol Clin Exp Res, 18*(5), 1156–1161.

Sarkola, T., & Eriksson, C. J. (2003). Testosterone increases in men after a low dose of alcohol. *Alcohol Clin Exp Res, 27*(4), 682–685.

Selzer, M. L. (1971). The Michigan Alcoholism Screening Test: The quest for a new diagnostic instrument. *Am J Psychiatry, 127*(12), 1653–1638.

Skipper, G. E., Weinmann, W., Theirauf, A., et al. (2004). Ethyl glucuronide: A biomarker to identify alcohol use by health professionals recovering from substance use disorders. *Alcohol Alcohol, 39,* 445–449.

Soyka, M. (2008). Prevalence of alcohol-induced psychotic disorders. *Eur Arch Psychiatry Clin Neurosci, 258*(5), 317–318.

Stewart, S. H., & Connors, G. J. (2004–2005). Screening for alcohol problems: What makes a test effective? *Alcohol Res Health, 28*(1), 5–16.

Szabo, G., & Mandrekar, P. (2009). A recent perspective on alcohol, immunity, and host defense. *Alcohol Clin Exp Res, 33*(2), 220–232.

Terry, M. B., Knight, J. A., Zablotska, L., et al. (2007). Alcohol metabolism, alcohol intake, and breast cancer risk: A sister-set analysis using the Breast Cancer Family Registry. *Breast Cancer Res Treat, 106*(2), 281–288.

Torpy, J. M., Lynm, C., & Golub, R. M. (2012). Pancreatitis. *JAMA, 307*(14), 1542.

Torvik, A., & Torp, S. (1986). The prevalence of alcoholic cerebellar atrophy: A morphometric and histological study of autopsy material. *J Neurol Sci, 75,* 43–51.

Visvanathan, K., Crum, R. M., Strickland, P. T., et al. (2007). Alcohol dehydrogenase genetic polymorphisms, low-to-moderate alcohol consumption, and risk of breast cancer. *Alcohol Clin Exp Res, 31*(3), 467–476.

Volk, R. J., Steinbauer, J. R., Cantor, S. B., & Holzer, C. E., III. (1997). The Alcohol Use Disorders Identification Test (AUDIT) as a screen for at-risk drinking in primary care patients of different racial/ethnic backgrounds. *Addiction, 92*(2), 197–206.

Wang, L., Lee, I. M., Manson, J. E., Buring, J. E., & Sesso, H. D. (2010). Alcohol consumption, weight gain, and risk of becoming overweight in middle-aged and older women. *Arch Intern Med, 170*(5), 453–461.

Wurst, F. M., Skipper, G. E., & Weinmann, W. (2003). Ethyl glucuronide—the direct ethanol metabolite on the threshold from science to routine use. *Addiction, 98*(Suppl. 2), 51–61.

Zahr, N. M., Kaufman, K. L., & Harper, C. G. (2011). Clinical and pathological features of alcohol-related brain damage. *Nat Rev Neurol, 7*(5), 284–294.

Zhang, P., Bagby, G. J., Happel, K. I., Raasch, C. E., & Nelson, S. (2008). Alcohol abuse, immunosuppression, and pulmonary infection. *Curr Drug Abuse Rev, 1*(1), 56–67.

CHAPTER 6

Nicotine

DAVID KALMAN
AMY HARRINGTON
JOSEPH DiFRANZA
LORI PBERT
DOUGLAS ZIEDONIS

Tobacco use and dependence continue to be major public health problems in the United States and around the globe, resulting in increased morbidity and mortality to the tobacco user and also others exposed to tobacco smoke. Tobacco control prevention and clinical treatment strategies have effectively reduced tobacco usage in the United States. However, 19% of the population continues to use tobacco, with particularly high rates among individuals with mental illness or other substance use disorders (SUDs). There are effective evidence-based treatments that help improve outcomes, including excellent psychosocial treatments and seven U.S. Food and Drug Administration (FDA)-approved medications. Community-based resources are available via the telephone (1-800-QUIT-NOW), the Internet (*www.becomeanex.org*), and Nicotine Anonymous (12-step program meetings in person, online, on the telephone).

This chapter provides an overview of several key topics in tobacco use and the treatment of tobacco dependence, including the unique characteristics of and treatment strategies recommended for subpopulations of smokers including adolescents, pregnant women, smokers with psychiatric comorbidity, as well as smokers in different ethnic groups. We also briefly discuss neurobiological factors in the development and maintenance of nicotine dependence. We begin by discussing the prevalence of tobacco use, its health consequences, and the health benefits of quitting.

PREVALENCE OF TOBACCO USE

Nearly one in every five persons (19%, or 45.3 million) in the United States is a smoker (Centers for Disease Control and Prevention [CDC], 2011). About 5% of middle school students and 17% of high school students report smoking on at least one day in the past month (Substance Abuse and Mental Health Services Administration [SAMHSA], Office of Applied Studies, 2009; for further detail, see the later section, "Youth and Young Adult Smoking"). Among racial/ethnic populations, Native Americans/Alaska Natives have the highest prevalence of cigarette use (31%), followed by African Americans (21%). Hispanics (13%) and Asians (9%) have the lowest prevalence of cigarette use. Smoking is higher among adults living below the poverty level (29%) than in those at or above the poverty level (18%). Among people with psychiatric comorbidity, the prevalence of smoking is about 40%, twice the rate of that in the general population (Ziedonis et al., 2008; for further detail, see the later section, "Tobacco Use and Psychiatric Comorbidity"). Smokeless tobacco use is highest among high school students and young adults (6–7%).

HEALTH CONSEQUENCES OF TOBACCO USE

About one in every two smokers dies of a disease caused by smoking. In the United States, where tobacco smoking causes approximately 450,000 premature deaths per year, one in five deaths is smoking-related. On average, smokers in the United States live to age 68; people who have never smoked live to age 82. Indeed, tobacco smoking causes more premature deaths each year in the United States than alcohol, illegal drugs, AIDS, traffic accidents, homicide, and suicide all added together.

The medical conditions most responsible for these deaths are cardiovascular disease, pulmonary disease, and cancers of the lung, esophagus, mouth and other organs of the aerodigestive system (U.S. Department of Health and Human Services [USDHHS], 2010). Compared to people who have never smoked, smokers are about 14 times more likely to die from a respiratory disease (chronic bronchitis, emphysema) and about 17 times more likely to die from cancer. Finally, smokers between ages 35 and 65 are about three times more likely to die prematurely as a result of cardiovascular disease than people who have never smoked. African American smokers have a disproportionately high rate of cancer and cardiovascular disease.

Smoking also causes or contributes to the development of many nonfatal diseases and conditions, including cataracts, premature aging of the skin, gum disease, acute respiratory infections in people with chronic obstructive pulmonary disease (COPD), acute respiratory symptoms (e.g., coughing and wheezing), postoperative infections, hip fractures, and peptic ulcers in persons who are *Helicobacter pylori* positive. There is also strong but not conclusive evidence implicating tobacco smoking in colorectal cancer, ectopic pregnancy, spontaneous abortion, sudden infant death syndrome, oral clefts in children whose mothers smoked during pregnancy, childhood asthma, low bone density, dental disease, erectile dysfunction/infertility, and age-related macular degeneration.

People who smoke less often than daily have nearly the same risk for early development of cardiovascular disease as daily smokers. Compared to nonsmokers, they also have a higher risk for developing lung cancer. Similarly, the risk of premature mortality is significantly higher in people who smoke as few as one to four cigarettes per day compared to nonsmokers.

Smokeless tobacco has been linked to tooth decay and tooth loss, gum disease, high blood pressure, lesions of the mouth, and possibly cardiovascular disease. Also, dry snuff, which contains much higher levels of nitrosamines, a potent class of cancer-causing chemicals, than moist snuff and chewing tobacco, has been linked to cancers of the mouth, larynx, and pharynx.

HEALTH BENEFITS OF SMOKING CESSATION

Smokers who quit sharply reduce their chances of premature death (USDHHS, 2010). In general, after 15 years of abstinence, the risk of mortality at any given age for former smokers is the same as it is for those who have never smoked. The benefits of cessation on mortality rates are greatest for smokers who quit at a younger age. Those who quit before age 40 avoid most of the excess risk of premature death due to smoking. However, the benefit also extends to older smokers who quit, including those age 80 and older.

In addition to the effect of quitting smoking on mortality, smoking cessation also leads to improvements in health-related quality of life, including a feeling of vitality, perceptions about one's overall health, and the ability to perform the tasks of daily living. Indeed, the health benefits of quitting are felt almost immediately. Within 2–3 days after cessation, breathing becomes easier as bronchial tubes start to relax and carbon monoxide levels in the blood return to normal. The senses of taste and smell also improve as damaged nerve endings begin to regrow. Within 2–3 months, blood circulation greatly improves, and any chronic coughing disappears. Over the course of the next several months, cilia in the lungs regrow, thereby increasing their ability to keep the lungs clean and reduce infections, and within a year, the excess risk of coronary heart disease, heart attack, and stroke drops to less than half that of a continuing smoker. The risk of pulmonary and cardiovascular disease and cancer continue to drop with increasing abstinence from smoking.

YOUTH AND YOUNG ADULT SMOKING

Most smokers (82%) try their first cigarette before the age of 19 and almost all (98%) try their first cigarette before the age of 26 (SAMHSA, 2011). Current tobacco use ranges from 5.2% among middle school students to 17.2% among high school students. By the senior year, one in four students has used tobacco in the past 30 days. Among high school students, African American youth have a much lower smoking rate (7.5%) than European American and Hispanic youth (both 19.2%). Among young adults ages 18–25, the rate of tobacco use is 34.2% (SAMHSA, 2011). There was a dramatic decline in the prevalence of smoking in this population in 1998, when new initiatives to reduce youth tobacco use became widespread. However, more recently, this decline has slowed, and for some subgroups, may have stopped (USDHHS, 2012).

HEALTH CONSEQUENCES FOR YOUTH

As described earlier, smoking has many serious health consequences for adults. In addition, smoking has widespread negative effects on the developing bodies of youth and young adults (USDHHS, 2012). For adolescents who smoke, the growth of lung function stops at an earlier age, peak lung function is lower, and decline in lung function starts at an earlier age. In addition, they may experience chronic airway inflammation with respiratory symptoms (wheezing, coughing, excess phlegm production). All of these problems can contribute to the development of COPD later in life. In addition, where there is underlying susceptibility, smoking can also lead to the development of asthma in adolescents and, among smokers with asthma, more frequent and severe attacks. Very importantly, adolescents who have stopped smoking show normal lung function.

Cardiovascular disease is the leading cause of death among smokers. Atherosclerosis underlies much of adult cardiovascular disease, and early manifestations of atherosclerosis can be traced to the effects of smoking in adolescence, especially inflammation of the lining of arteries and veins, and the resulting damage to cells and cell functioning. The effect of smoking on early markers of atherosclerosis is evident shortly after youth start to smoke and, over time, leads to rapid acceleration of atherosclerotic disease processes, particularly in the abdominal aorta and coronary artery. As with the effects of smoking on the pulmonary system, the early effects of smoking on the cardiovascular system are reversible, and adolescents who stop smoking show normal cardiovascular function (see USDHHS, 2012).

Finally, nicotine exposure during adolescence negatively affects cognitive functioning in higher brain regions (e.g., prefrontal cortical function), and these effects can last into adulthood. Magnetic resonance imaging (MRI) studies show that during memory and attention tasks, adolescent smokers have reduced prefrontal cortical activation relative to nonsmoking adolescents. This effect is more pronounced in adolescents with longer smoking histories. These nicotine-induced impairments, which begin in adolescence, can persist into later life.

RISK FACTORS FOR INITIATION AND ESCALATION OF TOBACCO USE

Adolescents with high levels of negative affect and problems with behavioral disinhibition are at risk for smoking initiation and progressing to regular smoking. Adolescents with hyperactivity are twice as likely to begin smoking and three times as likely to become regular smokers. At the same time, smoking is also a risk factor for the subsequent development of mood, anxiety, SUDs, and impulse disorders. Studies also suggest that genetic loading predisposes some adolescents to both negative affect and smoking.

TOBACCO USE AND PSYCHIATRIC COMORBIDITY

Overall, about 40–50% of people with a psychiatric disorder—about two times the rate in the general population—are current smokers. The rates of tobacco addiction for particular subtypes of psychiatric disorders are even higher (65–95%), including individuals with bipolar disorder, schizophrenia, and alcoholism, and those with opioid addiction in methadone maintenance treatment. People with a psychiatric disorder are also more likely than smokers without a disorder to be heavy smokers (smokers who consume more than 25 cigarettes/day). Nicotine-dependent smokers with at least one additional psychiatric diagnosis comprise 7% of the population but smoke 34% of all the cigarettes consumed in the United States (Grant, Hasin, Chou, Stinson, & Dawson, 2004). The high rate of smoking in psychiatric populations is most likely the result of genetic and psychosocial factors (Ziedonis et al., 2008).

EFFECTS OF TOBACCO SMOKE ON MEDICATION BLOOD LEVELS

Tobacco smoke accelerates the metabolism of many psychiatric and other medications, which can result in up to a 40% reduction in serum levels of the prescribed medication. Medications that are metabolized by the CYP1A2 enzyme in the liver are most affected. Of note, caffeine is also metabolized by this enzyme and is similarly affected by tobacco use. One of the chemicals in tobacco smoke, polycyclic aromatic hydrocarbons, accelerates activity of this enzyme. Since nicotine is not responsible for these effects, nicotine-based medications do not interact with these medications. See the table "Drug Interactions with Tobacco Smoke" (Smoking Cessation Leadership Center, 2015) for a summary of pharmacokinetic and pharmacodynamic interactions of tobacco smoke and specific medications. As can be seen in this table, several antipsychotic and antidepressant medications as well as mood stabilizers are affected. Therefore, smokers are likely to require higher doses of these medications than nonsmokers and dose adjustments are often needed when patients on these medications quit smoking. Clinicians should also monitor for increased medication side effects during smoking cessation.

NEUROBIOLOGY OF NICOTINE DEPENDENCE

Nicotine binds to receptors in the brain that stimulate the release of hormones and neurotransmitters, including acetylcholine, dopamine, vasopressin, serotonin, and beta-endorphin (Benowitz, 2008). Like most drugs of abuse, nicotine intake stimulates release of dopamine in the mesolimbic or "reward" pathway in the brain, and this phenomenon is associated with reward or reinforcement. However, tolerance to these reinforcing effects develops with chronic nicotine intake and helps sets the stage for the development of nicotine dependence. Nicotine withdrawal symptoms can be divided into two classes: somatic symptoms and affective symptoms. Somatic symptoms likely involve both the central nervous system and parasympathetic nervous system. Affective symptoms are associated with low dopamine activity in the reward circuit of the central nervous system, a condition that arises in nicotine-dependent animals (and presumably humans) when nicotine administration is stopped. Whereas nicotine, as well as other drugs of abuse, such as cocaine and alcohol, initially stimulates the reward circuitry of the brain, *chronic* nicotine exposure may lower stress tolerance by sensitizing brain structures and pathways (e.g., the amygdala and the hypothalamic–pituitary–adrenal pathway) involved in stress reactivity. Thus, chronic exposure to nicotine may increase susceptibility to psychosocial stressors.

DEVELOPMENT OF NICOTINE DEPENDENCE

The first symptoms of dependence begin at a very early point for most smokers. About 25% of adolescents experience at least one symptom of dependence within 1 month of their first smoking occasion. About two-thirds experience their first symptom before onset of daily smoking. Adolescents who smoke as few as two cigarettes per week are at risk for onset of at least one symptoms of dependence. In addition, about 25% of adolescent smokers are nicotine dependent within 2 years and, unlike use of other drugs, there are no significant declines in rates of cigarette smoking from adolescence to young adulthood.

When physical dependence begins, the time it takes before a smoker experiences any withdrawal symptoms (called "latency to withdrawal") may exceed a week. With continued tobacco use, the latency to withdrawal becomes shorter and shorter (DiFranza, Sweet, Savageau, & Ursprung, 2011). This shortening of the latency to withdrawal is a measure of the severity of the addiction. In practical terms, the shortening of the latency to withdrawal means that a smoker will discover that the duration of relief from withdrawal that is provided by each cigarette becomes shorter over time. When the latency to withdrawal shortens to 1 day, daily smoking ensues. Further shortening of the latency to withdrawal prompts a gradual increase in the number of cigarettes smoked per day. This trajectory of gradually increasing frequency of smoking in terms of days per month followed, after the onset of daily smoking, by an increase in the number of cigarettes smoked per day, is well documented (DiFranza et al., 2011). The shortening of the latency to withdrawal is so relentless that smoking an average of two cigarettes per week at age 12 leads to a 174-fold increase in the risk of proceeding to heavy daily smoking by age 24.

PHARMACOKINETICS OF NICOTINE

When a cigarette is smoked, about 80% of the inhaled nicotine is absorbed by the lungs. Absorption is both efficient and extremely rapid because of the large volume of surface area of the lungs and the quick absorption into the pulmonary blood stream.

After absorption in the lungs, nicotine is transported to the brain via arterial blood flow prior to its passing through the liver or being distributed more widely in venous circulation. Thus, after smoking, nicotine levels may be about six to 10 times higher in arterial versus venous blood. Nicotine reaches the brain within 15 seconds after inhalation, where its absorption is also rapid, because of the high affinity of brain tissue for nicotine. Nicotine levels in the brain decline rapidly, however, as the drug is distributed to other body tissues.

The rapid rise and fall of nicotine levels in the brain has important psychobiological effects. The rapid rise releases dopamine in the mesolimbic system that drives the rewarding effects of nicotine. The rapid fall releases norepinephrine in the habenular–peduncular pathway that produces withdrawal symptoms. These symptoms include restlessness, irritability, anxiety, drowsiness, and impaired concentration. A nicotine-dependent smoker can begin to experience low-grade symptoms in as little as 20–30 minutes after smoking a cigarette. These symptoms produce an urge to smoke another cigarette in order to gain symptomatic relief. Since smoking achieves this result, the vicious cycle that is created then leads to and maintains dependence on nicotine.

Nicotine, which is metabolized primarily in the liver, is first metabolized to cotinine, then to trans-3-hydroxycotinine. The rate of metabolism is not constant across people. It also varies across ethnic and racial groups. For example, European Americans and Hispanics metabolize nicotine more rapidly than Asians and African Americans. In addition, the rate of nicotine metabolism is faster in women than in men. Importantly, smokers who metabolize nicotine more rapidly are at higher risk for developing nicotine dependence, may have more difficulty quitting, and may also have a heightened risk for certain cancers (Perez-Stable & Benowitz, 2011).

TREATMENT INTERVENTIONS

Almost 70% of smokers want to stop smoking, and about 50% of smokers make a quit attempt each year (CDC, 2011). The majority of smokers (about 70%) attempt to quit "cold turkey" (without the use of a cessation medication or counseling), although success rates for these smokers are very low—only 5–10% who quit cold turkey achieves long-term abstinence. By contrast, the long-term abstinence rate for smokers who use a medication and/or counseling is typically 25–30% (Fiore et al., 2008). These statistics support the use of evidence-based interventions to achieve long-term cessation.

The Clinical Practice Guideline for Treating Tobacco Dependence (CPG; Fiore et al., 2008) and the *Cochrane Reviews* (e.g., Lai et al., 2008) provide the most authoritative and up-to-date evidence-based recommendations for the treatment of tobacco dependence. These sources recommend treatment that combines medication and behavioral counseling.

There are currently five nicotine-based cessation medications and two non-nicotine-based medications that have received approval by the FDA based on strong support for their ability to help smokers quit (Fiore et al., 2008). In general, placebo-controlled studies have shown that use of a quit-smoking medication can increase the likelihood of quitting and maintaining long-term tobacco abstinence by 50 to 100%. In other words, for every 10 smokers who quit without using a cessation medication, between 15 and 20 are likely to succeed with a medication. Recent studies have also provided strong support for the simultaneous use of a combination of medications for quitting. Regarding behavioral interventions, for smokers not ready to quit, the CPG recommend utilizing advice to quit coupled with a brief motivational intervention. For smokers who are ready to quit, they recommend behavioral counseling and medication. Medication alone is somewhat more effective than counseling alone. However, consistent with the evidence from numerous studies involving thousands of smokers, as noted, the guidelines recommend a combination of behavioral counseling and medication (Fiore et al., 2008).

Nicotine Dependence Treatment Medications

Nicotine Replacement Therapy

Nicotine replacement therapy (NRT) medications come in five forms: transdermal patch, gum, lozenge, nasal spray, and inhaler. The nicotine patch is a passive NRT; once the patch is applied to the skin, a constant stream of nicotine slowly diffuses into the bloodstream without the user having to do anything further. The other forms of NRT permit *ad libitum* nicotine delivery in which the patient can take an additional lozenge, a piece of gum, or other dose form of nicotine when a craving develops. NRT medications primarily improve a smoker's ability to quit by reducing cravings and the intensity of nicotine withdrawal symptoms such as headache, fatigue, irritability, depressed mood, trouble concentrating, and increased appetite. In addition, some of the preparations may help by approximating some of the nonpharmacological effects of using tobacco. For example, the gum and the lozenge provide oral stimulation, and the inhaler is puffed somewhat like a cigarette.

NRT medications are also safe to use and contain only one chemical (nicotine) compared to 4,000 chemicals in smoked tobacco. This is important, because nicotine is not responsible for the multitude of adverse health effects caused by smoking. Rather, these effects are caused by many of these other chemicals, including the approximately 70 carcinogenic chemicals in tobacco smoke. In addition, NRT medications have low abuse liability; the likelihood of becoming addicted to the medication is essentially zero for the nicotine patch and extremely low for all the others NRTs. This is because of the way NRT medications versus smoked tobacco deliver nicotine to the body. As described earlier, nicotine via smoked tobacco quickly enters the arterial vascular system and is delivered very rapidly to the brain, where it reaches peak levels within 15 seconds. These characteristics are responsible for the very high abuse liability of nicotine when it is smoked. By contrast, because they enter the venous system, NRTs cross the blood–brain barrier and reach peak levels more slowly. These characteristics are responsible for the very low abuse liability of NRT medications. According to current guidelines, NRT medications should be used for 8–12 weeks. However, studies have not demonstrated safety concerns for people who use NRT longer than 12 weeks and, as discussed below, some studies indicate that longer-term use results in higher sustained quit rates. The FDA is considering a change in the guidelines on NRT products to include longer-term use (Food and Drug Administration, 2013).

The nicotine patch is available in 7-, 14-, and 21-mg doses. The 21-mg dose is recommended for people who smoke more than 10 cigarettes per day and should be used for at least 6–8 weeks, followed by use of the 14-mg patch for 2 weeks, then the 7-mg patch for 2 weeks. The nicotine patch provides continuous release of nicotine. It is applied upon waking and may be worn overnight or removed at bedtime. Peak nicotine levels are achieved 4–6 hours after application, then gradually decline over the course of the rest of the day. Side effects include tingling where the patch is applied, local skin irritation, and itching. These effects can be minimized by applying the patch to a different site for 3–4 days before returning to the original site of application. Some smokers report vivid and sometimes unpleasant dreams and/or insomnia with overnight use of the patch. Removing the patch at bedtime often alleviates this.

The nicotine gum is available in 2- and 4-mg doses. The 4-mg dose is recommended for people who are more heavily addicted (i.e., those who smoke their first cigarette of the day within 30 minutes of waking); the 2-mg dose is recommended for people who smoke their first cigarette of the day more than 30 minutes after waking. One piece of gum should be used every 1–2 hours for at least 6 weeks, followed by one piece every 2–4 hours for 2 weeks, then one every 4–8 hours for 2 weeks. Smokers who begin with the 4-mg gum may also titrate to the 2-mg medication. The gum should be chewed slowly until a peppery taste is detected, usually after two or three chews; at this point, it should be placed between the teeth and cheek for a few minutes. This procedure should be repeated every few minutes until the taste dissipates or after 30 minutes, at which point the gum should be discarded. In order to be effective, the nicotine in the gum must be absorbed by the oral mucosa; therefore, it should not be swallowed. It is also important to avoid acidic beverages (e.g., coffee, soft drinks) for 30 minutes before and after each use, because the acidity of these beverages prevents absorption of the nicotine. Side effects from the gum include irritation in the mouth and throat, mouth ulcers, hiccups, and jaw ache from chewing. Side effects may also include gastrointestinal symptoms (flatulence, indigestion) and heartburn, symptoms that are most commonly related to improper use (i.e., swallowing the nicotine released from the gum).

The nicotine lozenge shares many of the characteristics of the gum. It is also available in 2- and 4-mg doses; the 4-mg dose is recommended for people who are more heavily addicted. As with nicotine gum, one lozenge should be used every 1–2 hours for the first 6 weeks, followed by one lozenge every 2–4 hours for 2 weeks, then one lozenge every 4–8 hours for 2 weeks. In order to be effective, the nicotine in the lozenge must be absorbed by the oral mucosa; acidic beverages should be avoided. The lozenge is often preferred over the gum because it is easier to use. Lozenges should be sucked slowly and not chewed or swallowed. Side effects include mouth and throat irritation, indigestion, hiccups, and gastrointestinal symptoms.

The nasal spray comes in a 10-ml spray bottle. Each spray delivers approximately 0.5 mg of nicotine. One dose consists of two sprays, one to each nostril. Initial treatment should be one to two doses every hour, and usage should not exceed 40 doses per day. Nicotine from the nasal spray is absorbed by the nasal mucosa. There is some evidence that the nicotine nasal spray may be a good choice for highly dependent smokers because of the relatively more rapid rise to peak levels (compared with other NRTs), which smokers more strongly experience as a "hit" of nicotine. However, discomfort due to side effects is more common with the nasal spray. Side effects include nose and throat irritation, including coughing, runny nose, and watery eyes, although these side effects usually subside with a couple of days of use. Other side effects include dizziness and nausea, chest tightness, gastrointestinal symptoms, paraesthesia (tingling) in limbs, and constipation.

The nicotine inhaler consists of a mouthpiece and a plastic cartridge. The inhaler is "puffed" and therefore partially imitates the sensation of smoking. Peak nicotine levels are achieved within 15 minutes. However, as with the gum and the lozenge, absorption of the nicotine is through the oral mucosa. Therefore, acidic beverages should be avoided for 30 minutes before and after use. Each cartridge provides about 80 inhalations, and smokers should use between six and 16 cartridges per day. Side effects of the inhaler include irritation of the mouth and throat, cough, headache, nausea, runny nose, and gastrointestinal symptoms.

Very importantly, the efficacy of gum, lozenge, nasal spray, and inhaler depends on frequency of dosing as prescribed. While a user can take an additional lozenge, piece of gum, and so forth, when a craving develops, these medications have little efficacy when they are used only when a smoker feels the "need" to use. The only exception is when they are used in combination with another cessation medication (see below).

Bupropion Slow Release

Bupropion slow release (SR) was the first non-nicotine medication approved by the FDA for smoking cessation. It was originally developed as an antidepressant and subsequent study established its efficacy as a smoking cessation aid. Bupropion is available by prescription only, in part because it can lower the seizure threshold. Seizure risk is greatly reduced, however, in the slow-release formulation in which dosing is twice per day and the extended-release (XL) formulation in which dosing is once per day. Bupropion's mechanism of action is not fully understood, but it appears to be unrelated to its efficacy as an antidepressant. Its efficacy as a cessation medication appears to be related to its effect on dopamine and/or norepinephrine. The recommended dose is 300 mg/day, although 150 mg can be used for smokers who experience side effects (e.g., difficulty sleeping) at the higher dose. Bupropion dosing should begin 7 days before cessation, with a 150-mg/day dose for 3 days. The dose should be increased to 150 mg, twice per day, for 8–12 weeks. Although the risk of seizure is small, bupropion SR is contraindicated for smokers with a history of seizures or head injury, or for smokers using other medications that lower the seizure threshold. It is also contraindicated in people with an eating disorder and in those who have used a monoamine oxidase inhibitor (MAOI) in the past 2 weeks. The most common side effects are dry mouth, nausea, and insomnia. Less common side effects include agitation, depressed mood, and suicidal thoughts and behavior. Because of the severe psychiatric side effects, the FDA requires a "black box" warning about these effects and recommends monitoring of patients who are taking bupropion.

Varenicline

Varenicline, which is the only other approved non-nicotine-based medication for smoking cessation, reduces cravings, decreases the rewarding effects of smoking, and attenuates withdrawal symptoms. Its mechanism of action appears to be its ability to bind to and partially block nicotinic receptors, thus blocking nicotine's ability to bind to and stimulate these receptors. It is available by prescription only. Clinical trials have demonstrated that varenicline is somewhat more effective than bupropion SR alone, although the difference is modest and results vary from smoker to smoker. Studies comparing varenicline and any of the NRTs have not been conducted. In addition, varenicline is the only cessation medication that may help to prevent relapse once smoking abstinence is achieved; that is, long-term use (up to 12 months) of varenicline appears to help people who quit maintain tobacco abstinence.

Varenicline is generally well tolerated by people, including psychiatric patients whose symptoms are stable. Nausea is the most common side effect. In recent years, there have been reports of neuropsychiatric symptoms associated with its use (including agitation, depressed mood, and suicidal ideation) and also severe cardiac symptoms risk. The FDA has applied a "black box" warning to varenicline about these two issues and recommends close monitoring of patients taking varenicline. Until more research clarifies the causal relationship between varenicline and these more serious symptoms, caution should also be exercised in prescribing varenicline to smokers with positive histories of these symptoms, especially suicidal ideation and serious cardiac disorders. Its use should be avoided in smokers who are psychiatrically unstable.

Multiple Medication Combinations Therapy

A common clinical practice has been to combine the nicotine patch (a long-acting, passive NRT medication) with a shorter-acting NRT form that requires active dosing (gum, lozenge, spray, inhaler). The rationale for combining NRT medications is that smokers may need a slow delivery system to achieve a constant concentration of nicotine in their blood to relieve withdrawal symptoms and a faster-acting preparation that can be administered on demand for immediate relief of breakthrough cravings. In a recent clinical trial comparing the efficacy of the nicotine patch, nicotine lozenge, bupropion, and a combination of lozenge with either the patch or bupropion, the nicotine patch plus the nicotine lozenge had the greatest benefit for patients. In most smokers with low nicotine dependence, monotherapy is probably sufficient, however.

The Effect of Tobacco Cessation on Psychiatric Symptoms

Clinicians should always carefully monitor their clients for a reemergence or worsening of psychiatric symptoms following a quit attempt. Smokers with a history of recurrent depression may have a somewhat higher risk for a new episode of major depressive disorder when they quit smoking. However, quitting smoking usually leads to either a long-term improvement or no effect on symptoms of depression and anxiety or positive and negative symptoms of schizophrenia (Hitsman, Moss, Montoya, & George, 2009). Among alcoholics and people addicted to other drugs, quitting smoking in early recovery does not jeopardize alcohol and other drug abstinence (Kalman, Kim, DiGirolamo, Smelson, & Ziedonis, 2010). It is also important to realize that several nicotine withdrawal symptoms are indistinguishable from symptoms of other disorders.

Assessment and Psychosocial Interventions

Assessment

Health care providers should ask all patients whether they smoke, advise them to quit if they do, assess their motivation, assist them to quit, and arrange follow-up to more intensive resources within the clinic to review progress. This approach is called the "five A's model" (ask, advise, assess, assist, arrange). Regarding advice, studies indicate that health care providers can influence their patients who smoke simply by advising them to quit (Fiore et al., 2008). The advice should be strong and unequivocal. For example, "Quitting smoking is the most important step you can take to improve your health," is better than "I think it would be a good idea for you to consider quitting smoking." Clinicians should also assess a patient's interest in quitting by asking, "Are you willing to make a quit attempt at this time?"

An assessment should also include information pertaining to a smoker's frequency of smoking and present level of dependence, quit history, psychiatric status, and history of treatment for tobacco dependence. The six-question Fagerstrom Test for Nicotine Dependence (FTND), which assesses time to first cigarette of the day, the number of cigarettes smoked per day, and other smoking character characteristics, is useful for determining severity of nicotine dependence (Heatherton, Kozlowski, Frecker, & Fagerstrom, 1991). Alternatively, two items from the scale (time to first cigarette of the day and number of cigarettes smoked per day), may be used. Smokers who smoke their first cigarette of the day within 5 minutes of waking are considered highly dependent; those who smoke their first cigarette within 30 minutes of waking are considered moderately dependent. Most smokers fall into one of these two categories and are likely to benefit from medication and psychosocial treatment. Assessment for history of prior quit attempts should include treatments used, if any, the length of abstinence, and the full context of relapse. Length of prior abstinence is a good predictor of success. Smokers who have quit for a year or more at some point and whose most recent quit attempt lasted at least 5 days are more likely to succeed on a subsequent quit attempt. The total number of prior quit attempts does not seem to be as important for predicting success. If the patient used a medication, the clinician should review the dose and schedule of treatment to determine whether the medication was used properly and whether the patient experienced any side effect related to its use. If the patient reports having experienced side effects, it is important to determine whether they were due to improper use.

Brief Interventions for Smokers Not Ready to Quit

Only about 30% of smokers are ready to quit at any point in time. To enhance motivation to quit for the remaining 70% of smokers, a 5–10 minute intervention should focus on the "five R's": risks, relevance, reward, roadblocks, repetition. A discussion of the risks of smoking will have the greatest impact if it emphasizes information that is personally relevant to the user. For example, if a client has a positive family history for emphysema, the clinician might say, "Smoking causes emphysema, and because of your family history of the disease, if you continue to smoke, you also run the risk of developing emphysema. Quitting is by far the most important thing you can do to minimize this risk." More generally, clinicians should be prepared to discuss the short- and long-term risks to the smoker's health, as well as the risks of secondhand smoke to others, especially children and older adults. A discussion about rewards should highlight the benefits of quitting, and a discussion about roadblocks (the perceived costs of quitting) should attempt to address a client's concerns about quitting. For example, clients who are concerned about withdrawal symptoms should be given information about the relatively short time course of most withdrawal symptoms and how medications help to alleviate them.

Rollnick, Butler, and Stott (1997) developed an easy-to-use, structured approach to intervention that derives from the principles of motivational interviewing. In motivational interviewing, the clinician asks questions that are designed to elicit the client's own motivation for behavior change (e.g., to quit smoking) rather than provide direct information for this purpose. In the brief intervention developed for smokers by Rollnick and colleagues, the clinician begins by asking, "If, on a scale of 1 to 10, 1 is *not at all important to give up smoking* and 10 is *extremely important*, what number would you give yourself at the moment?" Self-motivational statements are elicited by the follow-up questions. For example, if a client were to say "5," the clinician asks, "Why are you a 5 and not a 2?" This prompts the client for reasons why he or she wants to quit—a self-motivational statement that involves having the client identify personally relevant risks of smoking and rewards of quitting. Following a brief discussion based on the client's responses, the clinician asks the client, "What would it take for you to move from a 5 to an 8 or 9?" This question is designed to identify roadblocks to quitting. For example, a client might say that when he tried to quit in the past, the withdrawal symptoms were severe. If he then reveals that he quit "cold turkey," the clinician would then have an opportunity to inform the client about the potential benefits of a cessation medication. Following this discussion, while being careful not to push too hard, the clinician might then ask the client for one thing he or she might do to move higher on the 1- to 10-point scale. The clinician then moves on to the second (and final) step of the intervention, which focuses on assessing the client's confidence in quitting. The clinician asks, "If, on a scale of 1 to 10, 1 means that you are *not at all confident* and 10 means that you are 100% confident you could *give up smoking and remain a nonsmoker*, what number would you give yourself now?" The clinician then follows the same procedure as described for assessing importance, eliciting the client's reasons for confidence and roadblocks to greater confidence. Smokers who receive this intervention (which takes about 5–10 minutes to deliver) are more likely to quit in the following few months than those who only receive brief advice.

A study of smokers with schizophrenia showed that carbon monoxide testing, when combined with personalized feedback, increased motivation to seek treatment for quitting (Steinberg, Ziedonis, Krejci, & Brandon, 2004). However, more studies are needed to evaluate this approach with smokers with and without psychiatric comorbidity. In addition, there is little evidence that biochemical risk assessment (carbon monoxide testing, spirometric assessment of lung function) by itself promotes quitting. A practice quit attempt combined with a cessation medication during the attempt may promote long-term quitting in smokers who say they do not intend to quit in the near future (Carpenter et al., 2010). However, this finding is preliminary and requires further study.

Interventions for Smokers Who Are Ready to Quit

As noted earlier, counseling interventions are effective in helping people to quit. Interventions delivered by means of individual, group, and proactive telephone counseling all increase quit rates relative to no intervention (Fiore et al., 2008). The intensity of the intervention is also related to its effectiveness. For example, two sessions are more effective than one; four sessions are more effective than two; and eight are more effective than four. Similarly, longer counseling sessions (e.g., more than 10 minutes) generally produce higher quit rates. However, even a single counseling session that is limited to only a few minutes is more effective than none.

There is good support from high-quality studies for the effectiveness of counseling that includes supportive interventions, provision of basic information about quitting, and problem-solving skills related to smoking cessation. Miller and Rollnick (2002) provide excellent guidance on the use of supportive interventions in their book on motivational interviewing, in which they discuss the importance of counselor empathy, the use of reflective listening, exploration of a smoker's ambivalence about quitting, rolling with resistance, and supporting self-efficacy. Importantly, clinicians sometimes believe that ambivalence is no longer an issue for smokers who have decided to quit. However, a smoker's commitment to quitting often vacillates even once the "decision" to quit is made, and these motivational techniques are especially useful for clinicians to empathically help clients work through their ambivalence without losing their commitment to quit. Key information that counselors should provide to all smokers includes the consequences of smoking and the benefits of quitting, the advantages and possible side effects of the different quit smoking medications, combination medication approaches, and the symptoms and typical course of nicotine withdrawal.

Problem-solving interventions focus primarily on identifying smoking triggers, and developing and strengthening clients' skills for coping with them. Usually, clients are easily able to identify their smoking triggers (e.g., activities associated with smoking such as drinking coffee and driving, stress, and being around other smokers). The process of building coping skills should begin prior to quitting. For clients who smoke soon after waking in the morning, it can be helpful to increase gradually the amount of time the client is awake before smoking the first cigarette of the day. These and similar strategies regarding other smoking triggers can help build self-efficacy. Clients might also be encouraged not to carry their cigarettes around all of the time prior to quitting, and each time they light up, they can remind themselves of their reasons for quitting. Furthermore, while the evidence does not support the use of relaxation training as a stand-alone treatment for smoking cessation, relaxation techniques may prepare clients to cope more effectively with negative affect during a quit attempt. More recently, studies have supported the use of mindfulness skills in promoting successful quitting (Brewer et al., 2011). Mindfulness skills (which include the ability to "step back" psychologically from a difficult situation rather than being swept up by it) can help smokers cope with urges to smoke associated with negative affect and other smoking triggers. Finally, many clients express an interest in gradually reducing the number of cigarettes they smoke each day for some period of time before quitting. Studies indicate that success in quitting is unrelated to whether or not smokers reduce their smoking before quitting; thus, clinicians can simply support client preference.

A typical counseling protocol comprises between four and eight sessions. However, since the majority of smokers will relapse during or shortly after a treatment episode, there is growing interest in studying the effects of a long-term "continuity of care" treatment model that helps successful quitters to maintain abstinence and those who relapse to recommit to quitting. For example, in one recent study, smokers received either 8 or 52 weeks of treatment (Joseph et al., 2011). Participants in both conditions received weekly telephone sessions in the first month of treatment. Participants in the yearlong treatment condition then received between one and two telephone sessions per month. For these participants, relapse prevention strategies (e.g., making lifestyle changes that support abstinence) were provided to those who were abstinent; counselors urged participants who relapsed to make a new quit attempt as soon as they were willing; and counselors explained to participants who were not interested in making another quit attempt that smoking reduction was an option and a step toward quitting. The long-term intervention increased both quit rates and quit attempts compared to the 8-week treatment. Importantly, while abstinence rates were similar in the two groups for the first 6 months, in the following 12 months, abstinence rates continued to increase only in the long-term care condition. It is unclear, however, whether the advantage was due to benefits to abstainers, relapsers, or both. A few additional studies of long-term counseling treatment have also supported this approach. Studies of extended treatment of medication have been more mixed. Studies with bupropion and NRT have not shown a benefit for extended treatment. Benefit was seen, however, in the only study to date of extended varenicline treatment (Tonstad et al., 2006). As is typical in these medication studies, only smokers who are tobacco abstinent at the end of an 8- to 12-week course of medication are eligible for extended treatment. Thus, these studies focus on the use of medication for relapse prevention only.

Importantly, studies have demonstrated the efficacy of telephone quit lines and Internet-based interventions (Myung, McDonell, Kazinets, Seo, & Moskowitz, 2009). The telephone counseling protocols showing clearest effects included at least one pre-counseling session and additional calls scheduled close to the quit date. Following an initial contact by a smoker, the evidence supports the use of proactive calls by the counselor (i.e., the counselor calls the smoker). The evidence does not support the use of reactive telephone counseling (counseling that is provided only if the smoker calls).

Some quit lines also offer free or low-cost nicotine patches or other nicotine replacement medication. Quit line and Web-based interventions are about equally effective as face-to-face counseling in helping smokers achieve long-term abstinence.

Finally, the evidence does not support the use of relaxation training alone, hypnosis, acupuncture, acupressure, laser therapy, and electrostimulation, although the lack of support for all but relaxation training derives from a paucity of high-quality studies. Additional research is needed before any definitive conclusions about their effectiveness can be drawn.

Treatment for Special Populations

Youth and Young Adults

Most youth and young adult smokers want to quit. About 68% have made a serious quit attempt in the past year. However, relapse rates are high: About 90% will return to smoking within 6 months. A review of studies of tobacco treatment for adolescents found little support for the use of pharmacotherapy in this population (Grimshaw & Stanton, 2006). However, there is good support for multicomponent behavioral interventions. Effective programs were found to include motivational enhancement techniques to decrease ambivalence about quitting and cognitive-behavioral strategies, such as skills for refusing cigarettes when they are offered (Grimshaw & Stanton, 2006).

Given that youth and young adult smokers do not typically attend traditional smoking cessation treatments, there is a need to test innovative approaches to reach these smokers. Mobile phone-based smoking cessation interventions show promise with short-term abstinence but have not yet demonstrated long-term benefits. In one study, a program of personalized cognitive-behaviorally oriented cell phone text messaging appeared promising compared to a control group of general text messages (29 vs. 19% at 12 weeks). The National Cancer Institute has developed the Smokefree TXT program, a free text message cessation service designed to provide 24/7 encouragement, advice, and tips to teens trying to quit smoking (texting the word "QUIT" to IQUIT.

Smokers with Other Psychiatric Disorders

Most smokers with a psychiatric illness recognize the health benefits of quitting. In addition, few smokers with a psychiatric illness believe quitting would have a long-term negative effect on their psychiatric symptoms, and importantly, research supports this perception. However, as in the general population, only a minority (about 20–30%) are ready to quit.

Because the benefits of quitting smoking far outweigh the risks, smokers with other psychiatric disorders should always be advised to quit unless they are in crisis. Steinberg et al. (2004) tested a 40-minute motivational intervention for smokers with schizophrenia. Of those who received the intervention, 31% sought treatment to quit within a month, compared to only 11% of those who received psychoeducation only, and 0% who received only brief advice. Given the present state of knowledge for this population, we recommend the use of the previously described motivational intervention, which is relatively brief and easy to administer (see the section "Brief Interventions for Smokers Not Ready to Quit"). There is clearly a need for more research into strategies that can enhance motivation to quit in this population.

For those who want to quit, a combination of counseling and medication, including a combination of medications, is recommended. For example, Evins et al. (2007) randomly assigned 51 smokers with schizophrenia to a 12-week trial of bupropion or placebo. All smokers received transdermal nicotine patch, nicotine polacrilex gum, and cognitive-behavioral therapy (CBT). At the end of 8 weeks of treatment, smoking abstinence rates in the bupropion and placebo conditions were 36 and 19%, respectively; at the end of 1 year, the rates were 12 and 8%, respectively. A study that tested a combination of medications (nicotine patch and gum) produced the best results to date for smokers in early alcohol recovery (Cooney et al., 2009). Among smokers with a history of recurrent major depression, a smoking cessation treatment that specifically addresses mood regulation can significantly increase the long-term abstinence rate compared to standard smoking cessation counseling (Haas, Munoz, Humfleet, Royce, & Hall, 2004). Finally, studies of smoking cessation treatment for smokers with anxiety disorders have been limited to smokers with posttraumatic stress disorder (PTSD). One study demonstrated that mental health clinicians can effectively deliver smoking cessation treatment to their patients with PTSD when proper training is provided (McFall et al., 2010).

Ethnic and Racial Groups

Only a few studies have investigated the efficacy of cessation interventions among ethnic and racial minorities (Cox, Okuyemi, Choi, & Ahluwalia, 2011). Quit rates were similar for nonwhite and white smokers in the only study designed to compare these groups directly.

Pregnant Women

Smoking in pregnancy leads to adverse outcomes for fetal, neonatal, and long-term development (e.g., risk of attention-deficit/hyperactive disorder [ADHD]). Nicotine and many other chemicals in cigarettes restrict the supply of oxygen and other essential nutrients, which retards fetal growth and neurodevelopment (Herrmann, King, & Weitzman, 2008). Smoking-related adverse pregnancy and birth outcomes include placental abruption, miscarriage, premature birth, low birthweight, congenital abnormalities, and sudden infant death. Importantly, these adverse outcomes are less likely in women who quit smoking during pregnancy.

In the United States, the prevalence of smoking during pregnancy is 9.3%, down from 18.4% in 1990. African American, Hispanic, and Pacific Islander women have a lower prevalence of smoking in pregnancy than do European American women. Low socioeconomic status and psychiatric illness are strongly associated with smoking during pregnancy. For example, depressed women are up to four times more likely than nondepressed women to smoke during pregnancy. On the other hand, more women stop smoking during pregnancy (up to 45%) than at any other time in their lives. Only one-third of these women are still abstinent 1 year later, however.

Smoking cessation interventions with this population are more effective than brief advice to quit. Interventions have generally included the strategies describe earlier to motivate smokers to quit and help them succeed, as well as information related to the health effects of smoking on the fetus. For example, Pbert et al. (2004) compared a no-intervention condition ("usual care") with a cognitive-behavioral intervention that comprised advice to quit, elicitation of a commitment to quit, and provision of support and skills-based counseling. The intervention was delivered by health care providers during routine prenatal care. Abstinence rates at the end of pregnancy were 26 and 12% in the intervention and usual care conditions, respectively; at 3 months postpartum, abstinence rates by condition were 10 and 5%, respectively. Finally, NRT for cessation is less efficacious in this population, and the safety of NRT on fetal development and birth outcomes remain unclear. The reduced efficacy of NRT for this population may be the result of inadequate dosing due to safety concerns and low compliance with its use.

Electronic Cigarettes and New Products

Electronic cigarettes (e-cigarettes) consist of a metal tube that resembles a cigarette and a battery-powered vaporizer that delivers nicotine via inhalation of a vapor into the lungs, in a manner similar to smoking a cigarette. Electronic cigarettes contain some carcinogens and other toxins; therefore, use of this product poses some health risks. These risks are somewhat lower than they are with conventional cigarettes, however, although the degree of risk varies due to differences in levels of toxic chemicals between brands. As a cessation aid, limited data suggest that the efficacy of electronic cigarettes is somewhat similar to that of nicotine replacement products (World Health Organization, 2014).

There is a need to be aware of the new ways tobacco and nicotine products are being sold and used. Hookah bars have become popular and offer a way to smoke tobacco through a water pipe. These have become popular among college students, yet the smoke poses the same health risks and individuals often smoke more than they would if smoking cigarettes. As the cost of cigarettes rises, individuals on fixed incomes are also switching to little cigars that are sold in packs that look like cigarettes. In addition, more individuals are rolling their own cigarettes to avoid the tobacco tax.

CONCLUSION

Tobacco addiction continues to be the most prevalent addiction and the leading cause of increased morbidity and mortality. There are a range of tobacco users, with different comorbidities, ages of onset, and use of a wide range of products. Integrated psychosocial and medication treatment achieves the best outcomes; however, most individuals quit on their own or receive medication treatment. There is a need to help more smokers learn about their community treatment resources, including the

1-800-QUIT-NOW quit line, numerous Internet counseling options, and even face-to-face treatment and support groups such as Nicotine Anonymous. There are seven FDA-approved medications to consider. Strategies to help less-motivated individuals can increase the odds that they will seek treatment, and each treatment attempt increases the odds that treatment will be successful.

ACKNOWLEDGMENTS

We thank Sun Kim, PhD, RN, Andrew Tapper, PhD, Rashelle Hayes, PhD, and Norman Hymowitz, PhD, for their comments in the preparation of this chapter.

REFERENCES

Benowitz, N. L. (2008). Neurobiology of nicotine addiction: Implications for smoking cessation treatment. *Am J Med, 121*(4), S3–S10.

Brewer, J. A., Mallik, S., Babuscio, T. A., Nich, C., Johnson, H. E., Deleone, C. M., et al. (2011). Mindfulness training for smoking cessation: Results from a randomized controlled trial. *Drug Alcohol Depend*, 119(1–2), 72–80.

Carpenter, M. J., Hughes, J. R., Gray, K. M., Wahlquist, A. E., Saladin, M. E., & Alberg, A. J. (2010). Nicotine therapy sampling to induce quit attempts among smokers unmotivated to quit: A randomized clinical trial. *Arch Int Med, 171*(21), 1901–1907.

Castellsague, X., Munoz, N., De Stefani, E., Victora, C. G., Castelletto, R., Rolon, P. A., et al. (1999). Independent and joint effects of tobacco smoking and alcohol drinking on the risk of esophageal cancer in men and women. *Intl J Cancer, 82*(5), 657–664.

Centers for Disease Control and Prevention (CDC). (2011). Quitting Smoking Among Adults—United States, 2001–2010. *Morbid Mortal Weekly Rep, 60*(44), 1513–1519. Retrieved from *www.cdc.gov/mmwr/preview/mmwrhtml/mm6044a2.htm*.

Cooney, N. L., Cooney, J. L., Perry, B. L., Carbone, M., Cohen, E. H., Steinberg, H. R., et al. (2009). Smoking cessation during alcohol treatment: A randomized trial of combination nicotine patch plus nicotine gum. *Addiction, 104*(9), 1588–1596.

Cox, L. S., Okuyemi, K., Choi, W. S., & Ahluwalia, J. S. (2011). A review of tobacco use treatments in U.S. ethnic minority populations. *Am J Health Promot, 25*(Suppl. 5), S11–S30.

DiFranza, J. R., Sweet, M., Savageau, J., & Ursprung, W. W. (2011). An evaluation of a clinical approach to staging tobacco addiction. *J Pediatr, 159*(6), 999–1003.

Evins, A. E., Cather, C., Culhane, M. A., Birnbaum, A., Horowitz, J., Hsieh, E., et al. (2007). A 12-week double-blind, placebo-controlled study of bupropion SR added to high-dose dual nicotine replacement therapy for smoking cessation or reduction in schizophrenia. *J Clin Psychopharmacol, 27*, 380–386.

Fiore, M. C., Jaen, C. R., Baker, T. B., Bailey, W. C., Benowitz, N. L., Curry, S. J., et al. (2008). *Treating tobacco use and dependence: 2008 update: Clinical practice guideline*. Rockville, MD: USDHHS, Public Health Service. Retrieved from *www.surgeongeneral.gov/tobacco/treating tobacco use08.pdf*.

Food and Drug Administration (FDA). (2013). Modifications to labeling of nicotine replacement therapy products for over-the-counter human use. Retrieved from *https://www.federalregister.gov/articles/2013/04/02/2013-07528/modifications-to-labeling-of-nicotine-replacement-therapy-products-for-over-the-counter-human-use*.

Grant, B. F., Hasin, D. S., Chou, S. P., Stinson, F. S., & Dawson, D. A. (2004). Nicotine dependence and psychiatric disorders in the United States: Results from the National Epidemiologic Survey on Alcohol and Related Conditions. *Arch Gen Psychiatry, 61*(11), 1107–1115.

Grimshaw, G. M., & Stanton, A. (2006). Tobacco cessation interventions for young people. *Cochrane Database Syst Rev, 4*, CD003289.

Haas, A. L., Munoz, R. F., Humfleet, G. L., Royce, G. I., & Hall, S. M. (2004). Influences of mood, depression history and treatment modality on outcomes in smoking cessation. *J Consult Clin Psychol, 72*, 563–570.

Heatherton, T. F., Kozlowski, L. T., Frecker, R. C., & Fagerstrom, K. O. (1991). The Fagerstrom Test for Nicotine Dependence: A revision of the Fagerstrom Tolerance Questionnaire. *Brit J Addict, 86*, 1119–1127.

Herrmann, M., King, K., & Weitzman, M. (2008). Prenatal tobacco smoke and postnatal second-hand smoke exposure and child neurodevelopment. *Curr Opin Pediatr, 20*, 184–190.

Hitsman, B., Moss, T. G., Montoya, I. D., & George, T. P. (2009). Treatment of tobacco dependence in mental health and addictive disorders. *Can J Psychiatry, 54*(6), 368–378.

Joseph, A. M., Fu, S. S., Lindgren, B., Rothman, A. J., Kodl, M., Lando, H., et al. (2011). Chronic disease management for tobacco dependence: A randomized, controlled trial. *Arch Int Med, 171*(21), 1894–1900.

Kalman, D., Kim, S., DiGirolamo, G., Smelson, D., & Ziedonis, D. (2010). Addressing tobacco use disorder in smokers in early remission from alcohol dependence: The case for integrating smoking cessation services in substance use disorder treatment programs. *Clin Psychol Rev, 30*, 12–24.

Lai, D. T. C., Qin, Y., & Tang, J. L. (2008). Motivational interviewing for smoking cessation. *Cochrane Database of Systematic Reviews*, Issue 1. Art. No. CD006936.

McFall, M., Saxon, A. J., Malte, C. A., Chow, B., Bailey, S., Baker, D. G., et al. (2010). Integrating tobacco cessation into mental health care for posttraumatic stress disorder: A randomized controlled trial. *JAMA, 304*(22), 2485–2493.

Miller, W. R., & Rollnick, S. (2002). *Motivational interviewing: Preparing people for change* (2nd ed.). New York: Guilford Press.

Myung, S. K., McDonell, Y. J., Kazinets, G., Seo, H. G., & Moskowitz, J. M. (2009). Effects of web- and computer-based smoking cessation programs: Meta-analysis of randomized controlled trials. *Arch Intern Med, 169*, 929–937.

Pbert, L., Ockene, J. K., Zapka, J., Ma, Y., Goins, K. V., Oncken, C., et al. (2004). A community health center smoking-cessation intervention for pregnant and postpartum women. *Am J Prev Med, 26*(5), 377–385.

Perez-Stable, E., & Benowitz, N. L. (2011). Do biological differences help explain tobacco-related disparities? *Am J Health Promot, 25*(5), S8–S11.

Rollnick, S., Butler, C. C., & Stott, N. (1997). Helping smokers make decisions: The enhancement of brief intervention for general medical practice. *Patient Educ Couns, 31*, 191–203.

Smoking Cessation Leadership Center. (2015). Drug interactions with tobacco smoke. Retrieved February 2016, from *smokingcessationleadership.ucsf.edu/sites/smokingcessationleadership.ucsf.edu/files/Drug-Interactions-with-Tobacco-Smoke.pdf*.

Steinberg, M. L., Ziedonis, D. M., Krejci, J. A., & Brandon, T. H. (2004). Motivational interviewing with personalized feedback: A brief intervention for motivating smokers with schizophrenia to seek treatment for tobacco dependence. *J Consult Clin Psychol, 72*(4), 723–728.

Substance Abuse and Mental Health Services Administration (SAMHSA). (2011). Results from the 2010 National Survey on Drug Use and Health: Summary of national findings (NSDUH Series H-41, HHS Publication No. [SMA] 11-4658). Retrieved from *www.samhsa.gov/data/nsduh/2k10nsduh/2k10results.htm*.

Substance Abuse and Mental Health Services Administration (SAMHSA), Office of Applied Studies. (2009, February). The NSDUH report: Smokeless tobacco use, initiation, and relationship to cigarette smoking: 2002 to 2007. Retrieved from *www.samhsa.gov/data/2k9/smokelesstobacco/smokelesstobacco.htm*.

Tonstad, S., Tonnesen, P., Hajek, P., Williams, K. E., Billing, C. B., & Reeves, K. R. (2006). Effect of maintenance therapy with varenicline on smoking cessation: A randomized controlled trial. *JAMA, 296*, 64–71.

U.S. Department of Health and Human Services (USDHHS), Centers for Disease Control and Prevention, National Center for Chronic Disease Prevention and Health Promotion, Office on Smoking and Health. (2010). How tobacco smoke causes disease: The biology and behavioral basis for smoking-attributable disease: A report of the Surgeon General. Retrieved from *www.surgeongeneral.gov/library/reports/tobaccosmoke/full_report.pdf.*

U.S. Department of Health and Human Services (USDHHS), Centers for Disease Control and Prevention, National Center for Chronic Disease Prevention and Health Promotion, Office on Smoking and Health. (2012). Preventing tobacco use among youth and young adults. Retrieved from *www.surgeongeneral.gov/library/reports/tobaccosmoke/full_report.pdf.*

World Health Organization, Conference of the Parties to the WHO Framework Convention on Tobacco Control. (2014). Retrieved from *http://apps.who.int/gb/fctc/PDF/cop6/FCTC_COP6_10-en.pdf?ua=1.*

Ziedonis, D., Hitsman, B., Beckham, J. C., Zvolensky, M., Adler, L. E., Audrain-McGovern, J., et al. (2008). Tobacco use and cessation in psychiatric disorders: National Institute of Mental Health report. *Nicotine Tob Res, 10*(12), 1691–1715.

CHAPTER 7

Opioids

SUDIE E. BACK
JENNA L. McCAULEY
KELLY S. BARTH
KATHLEEN T. BRADY

Since the early 19th century, when Sertürner (1817) isolated morphine from opium, opioids have been a mainstay in the implementation of surgical procedures and in the management of acute and chronic pain. Opioids exert their effects primarily through their action at the opioid mu, kappa, and sigma receptors. Mu opioid receptors are involved in the perception of pain and in reward. Opioid receptors located in the brainstem are involved in control of critical automatic processes, such as blood pressure, arousal, and respiration.

Opioids may be categorized as (1) naturally occurring, (2) semisynthetic, or (3) synthetic. Morphine, codeine, and thebaine are phenanthrene alkaloids that occur naturally in the opium plant. Thebaine is converted into medically useful compounds such as codeine, hydrocodone (Vicodin), oxycodone (OxyContin, Percodan, Percocet, Tylox), oxymorphone (Numorphan), nalbuphine (Nubain) and diacetylmorphine (heroin). Thus, raw opium, morphine, codeine, and thebaine are referred to as "naturally occurring opioids." In contrast, compounds such as hydrocodone and oxycodone, which are produced from naturally occurring compounds, are referred to as "semisynthetic opioids."

Attempts to synthesize compounds have produced a variety of agents, referred to as the "synthetic opioids," which are chemically distinct from morphine yet exert their effects via similar mechanisms and demonstrate cross-tolerance. These include, for example, methadone (Dolophine), meperidine (Demerol), propoxyphene (Darvon), and levo-alpha-acetylmethadol (LAAM). Fentanyl (Sublimaze) and sufentanil (Sufenta) are potent and short-acting opioids that are used mainly in anesthesia. Buprenorphine is a partial mu agonist that is used in the treatment of opioid dependence and has recently received approval for pain management. Most opioids, with the exception of methadone and LAAM, have short half-lives. However, extended release preparations of morphine (MS Contin), oxycodone (OxyContin), and buprenorphine have become more widely used in pain management because they result in fewer peaks and troughs over a 24-hour period.

The majority of prescription opioids are used legitimately for pain management or to treat physical ailments. However, prescription opioids are increasingly being used nonmedically for alternative reasons (e.g., euphoric effects). In this chapter, we review the scope of the problem of nonmedical prescription and nonprescription (i.e., heroin) opioid use, important issues concerning assessment and diagnosis, clinical features and pharmacology, as well the treatment of opioid use disorders. Table 7.1

TABLE 7.1. Commonly Used Oral Opioid Analgesics

Medication	Brand name examples	Onset of action	Duration of action	Equianalgesic dosing
Hydrocodone	Lortab, Vicodin, various	30 to 60 min	4 to 6 hr	30 mg
Oxycodone, immediate release	Roxicodone, OxyIR, Percocet, various	10 to 15 min	4 to 6 hr	20 mg
Oxycodone, controlled release	OxyContin, various	1 hr	12 hr	20 mg
Codeine	Tylenol with codeine No. 2, various	30 to 60 min	4 to 6 hr	200 mg
Hydromorphone	Dilaudid	15 to 30 min	4 to 6 hr	7.5 mg
Morphine, immediate release	MSIR, Roxanol, various	30 to 60 min	3 to 6 hr	30 mg
Morphine, extended release	MS Contin	30 to 90 min	8 to 12 hr	30 mg
	Kadian, Avinza	30 to 90 min	12 to 24 hr (Kadian) 24 hr (Avinza)	30 min
Methadone	Dolophine, various	30 to 60 min	>8 hr (chronic use)	Variable with chronic dosing
Oxymorphone, immediate release	Opana, various	30 to 60 min	3 to 6 hr	10 mg
Oxymorphone, extended release	Opana ER, various	30 to 60 min	8 to 12 hr	10 mg

Note. Adapted from the Medical University of South Carolina's Opioid Analgesic Comparison Chart, updated June 2013. Equianalgesic dosing is based on morphine 10 mg administered parenterally (i.e., intravenously/subcutaneously) in opioid-naive persons. For our purposes in this chapter, this information is meant to be general and not as a guide to patient care or as an opioid conversion chart. For clinical information, it is the user's responsibility to examine all available information on opioid conversions and to integrate this with knowledge about the patient (i.e., tolerance, cross-tolerance, medical issues, and other medications). The clinician should always use good clinical judgment when making decisions for an individual patient.

provides examples of commonly used oral opioid analgesics, including their onset and duration of action and equianalgesic dosing.

NONMEDICAL USE OF PRESCRIPTION OPIOIDS

The nonmedical use of prescription opioids is a serious public health concern. As the number of legitimate prescriptions for opioids has increased, so has the incidence of nonmedical use and adverse events. Over the past two decades, the number of opioid prescriptions has increased significantly, from approximately 76 million in 1991 to over 210 million in 2010, making opioid analgesics the most commonly prescribed medication category in the United States (Volkow, McLellan, Cotto, Karithanom, & Weiss, 2011). Prescription opioids are now one of the most commonly initiated drugs, second only to marijuana (Substance Abuse and Mental Health Services Administration [SAMHSA], 2012). Epidemiological data from the National Survey on Drug Use and Health (NSDUH; N = 55,279) demonstrate that 14% of individuals in the general population endorse lifetime nonmedical use of prescription opioids (i.e., using a prescription opioid that was not prescribed to that individual or using it only for the experience or feeling it caused; Back, Payne, Simpson, & Brady, 2010). Similarly, in a nationally representative sample of college students (N = 10,904), McCabe, Teter, and Boyd (2005) observed a 12% lifetime prevalence rate of prescription opioid nonmedical use. Among 18- to 25-year-old young adults in the general population (N = 22,931), 18.2% endorsed lifetime nonmedical use of prescription opioids (SAMHSA, 2003). Among users for nonmedical reasons, a substantial percentage (13%) met DSM-IV diagnostic criteria for an opioid use disorder (Back et al., 2010).

Serious adverse consequences are associated with nonmedical use of prescription opiates (Bohnert et al., 2011; Cicero, Surrat, Inciardi, & Munoz, 2007; Manchikanti et al., 2012). For example, rates of opioid-related emergency department visits increased 219% over a 5-year period (SAMHSA, 2010). In addition, prescription opioids are implicated in more overdose fatalities than heroin and cocaine combined (Warner, Chen, Makuc, Anderson, & Minino, 2011). Although more men die from prescription opioid overdose than women, the death rate from prescription opioid overdose increased more than fivefold among women from 1999 to 2010 (Centers for Disease Control and Prevention [CDC], 2013). Finally, prescription opioids are the most commonly implicated drug in unintentional overdose fatalities, usually in combination with other substances. In one study of unintentional pharmaceutical overdoses (N = 295), Hall and colleagues (2008) found that 93% of decedents had consumed prescription opioids, and only 44% had ever been prescribed the medication. In 80% of the decedents, multiple substances in addition to opioids contributed to their fatal overdoses, the most common being benzodiazepines (38%).

The most common types of opioids used nonmedically include oxycodone and hydrocodone compounds, and the most common sources are physicians and family/friends (Back, Lawson, Singleton, & Brady, 2011; Barth et al., 2013; Osgood, Eaton, Trudeau, & Katz, 2012). When queried about motives for engaging in nonmedical opioid use, individuals typically report using to reduce pain, to experience a "high," to increase energy, and to improve sleep (Barth et al., 2013; Rigg & Ibañez, 2010).

Gender differences have been noted, with men being more likely to use prescription opioids via alternative routes (e.g., crushing and snorting pills), and women being more likely to use in response to negative emotions or interpersonal stress (Back et al., 2010, 2011).

HEROIN USE

Heroin is an opioid drug that is synthesized from morphine and usually appears as a white or brown powder or as a black sticky substance, known as "black tar heroin." It can be injected, inhaled by snorting or sniffing, or smoked, and it is rapidly delivered to the brain by all routes of administration. When heroin enters the brain, it is converted back into morphine, which binds to mu opioid receptors. After an intravenous injection of heroin, users feel a surge of euphoria ("rush") accompanied by dry mouth, flushing of the skin, heaviness of the extremities, and clouded mental functioning. Following this initial euphoria, the user generally goes "on the nod," an alternately wakeful and drowsy state. Users who do not inject the drug may not experience the initial rush, but other effects are the same.

Heroin abuse is associated with a number of serious health conditions, including fatal overdose, spontaneous abortion, and infectious diseases such as hepatitis and HIV. Chronic users may develop collapsed veins, endocarditis, abscesses, constipation and gastrointestinal cramping, and liver or kidney disease. Pulmonary complications, including various types of pneumonia, may result from the poor health of the user, as well as heroin's effects on pulmonary function. In addition, street heroin often contains contaminants or additives that can damage blood vessels and vital organs.

In 2011, 4.2 million Americans age 12 or older (or 1.6%) had used heroin at least once in their lives (SAMHSA, 2012). It is estimated that about 23% of individuals who use heroin become dependent. While the percentage of individuals with heroin dependence in the United States has been fairly consistent over the last 20 years, research suggests that abuse of prescription opiate drugs may provide a pathway to heroin abuse. Some individuals reported taking up heroin because it is cheaper and easier to obtain than prescription opioids (Peavy et al., 2012). As such, an increase in heroin use may be yet another consequence of the recent increases in prescription opiate misuse.

ASSESSMENT AND DIAGNOSIS

The fifth edition of the *Diagnostic and Statistical Manual of Mental Disorders* (DSM-5; American Psychiatric Association, 2013) defines a substance use disorder (SUD) as a problematic pattern of use resulting in significant distress or impairment of major role functioning in social, occupational, and/or recreational areas of life. Whereas the previous DSM edition (DSM-IV) divided SUDs into two discrete categories, abuse and dependence, DSM-5 rates severity of an SUD on a dimensional scale based on the number of criteria individuals have experienced in the previous 12 months: mild (two to three criteria), moderate (four to five criteria), or severe (six or more criteria). DSM-5 diagnostic criteria include a newly added *craving* criterion, in addition to all previous DSM-IV criteria for abuse and dependence, and it removes legal problems. Empirical evidence, albeit a limited amount, suggests a high correspondence between DSM-IV opioid dependence and DSM-5 moderate or severe (four or more criteria) opioid use disorder (Compton, Dawson, Goldstein, & Grant, 2013; Peer et al., 2013).

Thorough assessment facilitates identification and diagnosis of individuals presenting with opioid use disorder and can result in links with appropriate treatment resources. Initial assessment strategies that are helpful in diagnosing opioid use disorders, including history and physical, laboratory, and standardized assessments (self-report and clinician administered) are reviewed subsequently. In addition, attention is given to strategies for ongoing assessment and monitoring of abuse risk among individuals receiving opioid therapy under the care of a physician.

Initial assessment includes a thorough history of the individual's major medical conditions, onset and course of opioid use, and the interaction between significant medical history and use over the lifespan. Particular attention should be given to the progression of opioid use over time and the impact that opioid use has had on the individual's ability to function across multiple life domains (e.g., social, occupational, leisure, family). Determination of the most recent use or time since the last use, and type and amount of opiate (and potentially other substances) used is critical in determining the impact of intoxication or withdrawal on the immediate clinical presentation. Assessing for additional substances of abuse, including the use and misuse of prescription medications, is warranted given documented high rates of multiple substance dependences among this population (Conway et al., 2013), as well as the increased risks of overdose and death associated with concomitant substance use (Calcaterra, Glanz, & Binswanger, 2013). In addition, collecting information regarding the individual's family history, social support, legal problems, and involvement in activities unrelated to substance abuse may be useful in determining treatment readiness and selecting appropriate levels of intervention. A standard medical review of systems, including a neurological examination, mental status examination, and physical examination, is also recommended. Physical examination of the individual may reveal indications of opioid use disorder such as needle marks from injection (i.e., tracks), skin abscesses, thrombosis of the veins, and weight loss, as well as medical conditions, such as enlarged or tender liver, bowel disruptions (hypoactive or hyperactive), and endocarditis.

As with other substance-abusing populations, it is important to corroborate the individual's self-reported history via collateral reports or the use of laboratory studies when possible. Useful laboratory studies include serum liver function studies (e.g., serum aspartate aminotransferase, serum alanine aminotransferase, alkaline phosphatase, bilirubin, clotting factors, immunoglobulin, and reduction in total protein), as well as testing for conditions commonly associated with injection drug use, including Hepatitis A, B, and/or C, and human immunodeficiency virus (HIV). Urine drug screening (UDS), or urinalysis, is the most common and preferred method for detecting illicit drug use (Richter & Johnson, 2001). UDS is minimally invasive and cost-effective, and it facilitates measurement of an individual's pattern, frequency, and amount of use (Preston, Silverman, Schuster, & Cone, 1997). However, limitations of UDS testing include its relatively narrow window of detection (usually 3 days or less for most substances), susceptibility to false positives, and easy alteration with chemicals or clean urine samples (Jaffe, 1998), making observed UDS testing preferable.

Initial assessment of symptoms and subsequent diagnosis of opioid dependence may also be aided by the use of standardized assessments. These assessments vary with respect to degree of clinician involvement and time for completion. Screening instruments such as the Drug Use Disorder Identification Test (DUDIT; Berman, Bergman, Palmsteirna, & Schlyter, 2005), the Drug Abuse Screening Test (DAST; Gavin, Ross, & Skinner, 1989), and the Alcohol, Smoking, and Substance Involvement Screening Test (ASSIST; Humeniuk et al., 2008), offer low-cost, quick options for identifying a range of potential SUDs, including opioid use, and are commonly used. In addition, screening instruments have been designed to assist in medical settings with identification of patients presenting for treatment of chronic pain who are at risk for abuse of prescription opioids. Examples of screeners for prescription opioid misuse include the Screener and Opioid Assessment for Patients with Pain—Revised (SOAPP-R; Passik, Kirsh, & Casper, 2008) and the Opioid Risk Tool (ORT; Webster, 2005). Structured diagnostic assessments include the Structured Clinical Interview for DSM-IV Axis I Disorders (SCID; First, Spitzer, Gibbon, & Williams, 1996); the Mini-International Neuropsychiatric Interview (MINI; Sheehan et al., 1998); and the Composite International Diagnostic Interview–2 (CIDI-2; Robins et al., 1989), which serves the criteria of both DSM-IV and the ICD-10. Finally, several standardized assessments exist to monitor the characteristics, motives, and impact associated with opioid use. These include the Timeline Followback (TLFB; Sobell & Sobell, 1995), an assessment that uses a calendar to record estimates of daily drug use over long periods of time, and the Addiction Severity Index (ASI; McLellan et al., 1992), a semistructured interview that assesses the severity of use and consequences on psychological and health functioning. Self-report forms specific to prescription opioid misuse include the Current Opioid Misuse Measure (COMM; Butler et al., 2007), a 17-item self-report measure to monitor pain patients on opioid therapy and identify potential misuse, and the Nonmedical Use Questionnaire (McCabe, Cranford, Boyd, & Teter, 2007), a six-item instrument that evaluates motives for opioid analgesic misuse, sources, and routes of administration. Use of standardized assessment measures, such as those mentioned in this chapter, have been found useful across varying levels of opioid use disorder severity and can be informative in treatment planning; however, it should be noted that to date, these measures have not been updated to reflect altered DSM-5 criteria.

PHYSICAL DEPENDENCE AND THE TREATMENT OF WITHDRAWAL

Regular opiate use is associated with tolerance, which means more of the drug is needed to achieve the same intensity of effect, and physical dependence, which is manifested by a characteristic set of signs and symptoms when drug taking is abruptly stopped. The amount and duration of use associated with physical dependence is variable, but daily use for more than 2–3 weeks is often accompanied by some signs/symptoms of withdrawal. Early symptoms of opioid withdrawal include yawning, agitation, anxiety, muscle aches, lacrimation, insomnia, rhinorrhea, and sweating. Late symptoms include abdominal cramping, diarrhea, dilated pupils, piloerection, nausea, and vomiting. Opioid withdrawal is very uncomfortable but generally not life threatening. The course of the symptoms depends on the half-life of the drug from which the individual is withdrawing. In heroin withdrawal, symptoms usually begin within 12 hours of last use. Methadone withdrawal symptoms generally begin within 30 hours of last use.

The goal of medically supervised detoxification is to limit patient discomfort by decreasing or ameliorating withdrawal symptoms. Medications commonly used to treat acute opioid withdrawal include the alpha$_2$-adrenergic agonist clonidine (Catapres), cyclobenzaprine (Flexeril) or benzodiazepines for muscle cramps, the antispasmodic dicyclomine (Bentyl) for abdominal cramping, antidiarrheals such as loperamide, antiemetics such as prochlorperazine (Compazine), and sedatives such as benzodiazepines. If an individual is using heroin or another form of opiate, another option is to convert the patient to an equivalent dose of either methadone or buprenorphine, then gradually reduce the dose to minimize withdrawal (described below). If the goal is to expedite the withdrawal process, particularly in the case of a long-acting opioid, administration of an opioid antagonist, such as naloxone (Narcan) or naltrexone (Revia), hastens the onset of the withdrawal syndrome. However, caution must be taken when using this approach because of the discomfort associated with the abrupt onset of withdrawal symptoms that can appear in precipitated withdrawal. As mentioned earlier, adjunctive medications may also be used for symptomatic treatment of withdrawal.

The use of *ultrarapid opioid detoxification* involving the administration of general anesthesia or heavy sedation in individuals undergoing withdrawal, while effective in reducing physiological dependence, has been demonstrated to lead to a greater number of serious adverse events compared to approaches without superior outcomes, so it is not recommended (Laheij, Krabbe, & de Jong, 2000).

Methadone

Methadone is an opiate agonist that was originally developed for the treatment of opioid dependence in the mid-1960s (Dole, Nyswander, & Kreek, 1966). Methadone's dramatic efficacy in reducing heroin use, decreasing crime, and improving mortality rates made it a prosocial and lifesaving intervention for countless opioid-dependent persons. Methadone continues to be used worldwide in the treatment of opiate dependence.

Methadone's primary therapeutic effect is through the mu opioid receptor. It is 70–80% bioavailable when swallowed, but it can also be administered rectally or by injection (Walsh & Strain, 2006). Peak effects with oral administration vary; in a nondependent person, the peak generally occurs in about 2–3 hours, while in an opioid-dependent person, the peak may last longer. The half-life can vary considerably as a function of genetic differences in enzymatic activity, duration of treatment, and urinary pH (Eap, Buclin, & Baumann, 2002). In addition, as a person stabilizes on methadone, metabolism increases with a resultant half-life decrease. In general, half-life is 15–36 hours (average is 24 hours), permitting once per day dosing. Methadone is primarily metabolized in the liver, with a small percentage excreted unchanged in the urine.

Methadone was initially developed as an analgesic. The duration of its analgesic effects is shorter than the half-life would suggest, necessitating dosing 2–3 times per day for pain control. Methadone is also a respiratory depressant, reflecting its mu agonist function. Such effects are more likely to be seen in nondependent persons receiving a relatively high dose. Other acute effects include miosis, nausea, and vomiting (especially in a nondependent person), histaminic effects (itching, flushing, sweating), and constipation.

TREATMENT OF OPIATE DEPENDENCE

Most of the studies investigating the treatment of opiate dependence were conducted with individuals who were primarily heroin users. As such, the treatment of prescription opiate dependence is relatively underexplored. However, the principles of opiate agonist and antagonist treatment as described below should apply across both heroin and prescription opiate dependence.

Methadone Maintenance Treatment

Methadone maintenance treatment (MMT) for opioid dependence in the United States is provided at clinics that are regulated by the Drug Enforcement Agency and the Center for Substance Abuse Treatment. The clinics provide medications and other services such as counseling, urine testing, and vocational assistance. MMT clinics have a medical director, counseling staff (with the patient: counselor ratio determined by local regulations), nursing staff, and other support staff. Federal eligibility requirements for MMT stipulate that individuals entering treatment have a minimum 1-year history of opioid dependence. While the minimum age requirement for MMT is 18 years of age, under certain conditions, individuals between 16 and 18 years of age may receive MMT. Individuals with major medical conditions and polydrug abusers are eligible for MMT. Patients initially attend the clinic 6 or 7 days per week (some clinics are routinely closed on Sundays) to receive a supervised dose of methadone, typically delivered in a flavored liquid form. While in clinic, the patient may be asked to provide a urine sample for drug testing, have minor medical problems addressed, and/or attend an individual or group counseling session. For days on which the patient is not required to attend the clinic, a "take-home" dose of medication is provided. The maximum number of take-home doses allowed per week is tied to the patient's response and time in treatment.

Counseling in MMT clinics can vary depending on clinical stability indicators such as drug and alcohol use, level of social needs, effectiveness of coping skills, and vocational/legal status. Early in treatment there is usually an emphasis on drug use, education regarding risk behaviors, and assistance in obtaining other needed services (e.g., medical care, social services, other psychiatric services). As the patient stabilizes in treatment, counseling may decrease in frequency and intensity, and shift in focus (e.g., familial relationships, work and education needs). The approaches used in counseling (e.g., motivational enhancement) are addressed in other chapters. Contingency management is particularly useful in the context of methadone treatment, where the availability of methadone take-home doses can serve as a powerful reward for behavior change (Brooner & Kidorf, 2002).

Outcomes in MMT are dose related, and there is great individual variability in the effective dose. Lower doses (20–40 mg per day) that are effective at suppressing opioid withdrawal may not suffice in decreasing craving or blocking the effects of other opioids (Strain, Stitzer, Liebson, & Bigelow, 1993). Maintenance doses are generally in the range of 70–120 mg/day, although some patients may require more than 120 mg/day for optimal therapeutic response. The blood level of methadone does not correspond well to dose, however; there is value in checking a 24-hour blood level in patients on a dose of 120 mg/day or higher, or in those taking medications known to alter serum methadone levels. There do not appear to be problems with performance or clinically significant cognitive impairment in individuals maintained on a steady dose of methadone. There is some controversy as to whether methadone can produce prolongation of the QTc interval, but studies to date have been quite variable in their electrocardiographic (EKG) findings on this matter. For patients who have other risk factors for QTc prolongation (e.g., other medications that can prolong the QTc, preexisting cardiac conditions, electrolyte abnormalities), closer monitoring of the EKG may be warranted (Cruciani et al., 2005).

While methadone can be very useful for suppressing withdrawal and blocking the effects of other opioids, MMT provides a context in which a number of prosocial activities and health issues can be addressed. Studies using outcomes of treatment retention and rates of illicit opioid use (e.g., as measured by urine testing) have clearly demonstrated that MMT can be highly effective (Strain et al., 1993; Ling, Wesson, Charuvastra, & Klett, 1996; Sees et al., 2000). In addition, MMT is associated with decreases in criminal activity, illicitly obtained income, and nonopioid illicit drug use.

Buprenorphine

Buprenorphine was initially developed and marketed as an analgesic in the 1970s. In 2002, the U.S. Food and Drug Administration (FDA) approved it for the treatment of opioid dependence. Buprenorphine has become a widely used medication for treatment of opioid dependence worldwide, and its availability outside the traditional methadone clinic system has transformed the treatment of opioid dependence in the United States.

Buprenorphine is classified among "mixed agonist–antagonist opioids" (others include butorphanol, nalbuphine, and pentazocine) and has a high affinity for and slow dissociation from the mu opioid receptor. Buprenorphine has a bell-shaped dose–response curve, such that initially as the dose of buprenorphine is increased, the effects increase (i.e., analgesia, decreased gastrointestinal [GI] motility, or respiratory depression); however, with increases beyond a certain dose of drug, the response curve begins to descend, so that increasing the dose produces less of an effect. While this profile has been shown in a number of animal models (Lizasoain, Leza, & Lorenzo,

1991), it has not been clearly demonstrated in a human study. However, pharmacological profile suggests that there should be relative safety with buprenorphine, in comparison to a full mu agonist opioid such as methadone (i.e., that there would be less respiratory depression with very high doses of the medication).

While initially approved in the United States as a parenteral analgesic in the treatment of opioid dependence, buprenorphine is taken by the sublingual route, providing slightly better bioavailability than oral administration. Buprenorphine has a long duration of action, which allows once-daily dosing. A number of studies have shown that it can be dosed less than daily (e.g., every 48–72 hours, and perhaps even less frequently), although the most common practice appears to have patients take it daily. It is metabolized by cytochrome P450 3A4, with a primary metabolite (norbuprenorphine) that has some bioactivity. As with methadone, there can be wide variability between patients in the blood level for a given dose (Strain, Moody, Stoller, Walsh, & Bigelow, 2002), although it is not common in clinical practice to check buprenorphine blood levels. A formulation of buprenorphine containing naloxone (initially marketed under the trade name Suboxone and marketed as a tablet, and now available as a soluble film) is commonly used. Naloxone is an opioid antagonist that will precipitate opioid withdrawal if injected by a person who is physically dependent on typical mu agonist opioids (e.g., heroin, oxycodone). The inclusion of naloxone in buprenorphine tablets and soluble film is a pharmacological strategy to decrease parenteral misuse of buprenorphine. While sublingual naloxone has poor bioavailability (Preston, Bigelow, & Liebson, 1990), injected naloxone has good bioavailability. As such, there is no naloxone effect if the buprenorphine–naloxone is taken as indicated (sublingually), but if the combination is dissolved and injected by an opioid-dependent person, the person will experience precipitated opioid withdrawal (Stoller, Bigelow, Walsh, & Strain, 2001). Buprenorphine–naloxone tablets and soluble film are marketed in a dose ratio of 4:1 (i.e., 12/3 mg, 8/2 mg, 4/1 mg, and 2/0.5 mg), and buprenorphine tablets without naloxone are marketed in 8- and 2-mg doses. Trials have established the safety and efficacy of buprenorphine in opioid dependence maintenance treatment in doses ranging from 2–32 mg per day.

Because buprenorphine is a partial agonist, a dose of buprenorphine administered to a person who is physically dependent on a full agonist opioid, such as heroin, could result in opioid withdrawal (Rosado, Walsh, Bigelow, & Strain, 2007). In order to minimize the risk of buprenorphine-precipitated withdrawal, it is best to begin with a low dose (e.g., 2–4 mg) that is given well after the last dose of opioid agonist (early opioid withdrawal). The first dose is generally monitored in an office setting.

In contrast to methadone, a physician in an office-based setting in the United States can prescribe buprenorphine for the treatment of opioid dependence. In 2000, the Drug Addiction Treatment Act (DATA 2000) marked the beginning of a process designed to allow qualified physicians to prescribe approved narcotic drugs for the treatment of opioid dependence in office-based settings. There are a number of approved training programs in place to teach physicians about the use of buprenorphine. There is a limit in the number of patients a physician can concurrently treat with buprenorphine (30 in the first year, then up to 100 in subsequent years after requesting this increase). This is the first time in modern medicine that physicians in the United States practicing in a variety of clinical settings, including office-based practice, are able to treat opioid dependence adequately with pharmacotherapy. It is our hope that this will greatly increase access to treatment for opioid-dependent individuals.

As noted earlier, patients started on buprenorphine should begin with a relatively low dose (either 2 or 4 mg), and ideally should be experiencing slight opioid withdrawal. A second dose can be given the same day, after 1–2 hours, if the first dose is tolerated without problems. The individual should be monitored during initial dosing. If the person is not physically dependent on opioids (e.g., a person who was on buprenorphine previously, then incarcerated, and now returns to restart buprenorphine), low doses (2 mg) should be started and stabilization should be slowed. Typical maintenance doses of buprenorphine are in the range of 8–16 mg/day, although some patients have required higher doses (e.g., 24 mg/day). If a patient seems to require high doses (e.g., 24–32 mg/day), risk of diversion or misuse of the medication must be assessed.

As with methadone, buprenorphine can be used for medically supervised withdrawal, as well as maintenance treatment. When tapering buprenorphine, 2 mg increments are typically used. The tablets are not made to be broken, and the soluble films are not designed to be cut (although some clinicians cut them, and it is a convenient mechanism to produce doses that contain less than 2 mg of buprenorphine). While there is limited research on buprenorphine tapering schedules, gradual rather than rapid withdrawal is likely to be more effective. Maintenance on buprenorphine can occur for years (similar to methadone), and physicians can prescribe a month's worth of the medication at a time, with up to five refills. Providing nonpharmacological treatment along with buprenorphine is recommended for most patients (especially early in treatment), but DATA 2000 only requires that the physician have access to such services and does not require that on-site services be provided.

In general, studies show that buprenorphine outcomes in opioid dependence (treatment retention, illicit opiate use) are superior to placebo or placebo-like doses of medication (Johnson et al., 1995) and are similar to daily methadone doses of about 50–60 mg/day. However, responses seen with higher doses of methadone (80 mg/day or greater) have generally not been seen with daily buprenorphine in controlled trials (Ling et al., 1996). Clinical trials suggest that a dose of about 12–16 mg/day of sublingual buprenorphine produces outcomes similar to a dose of about 50–60 mg/day of methadone (Strain, Stitzer, Liebson, & Bigelow, 1994). Despite initial concerns that buprenorphine may cause a slight increase in liver function tests (LFTs) in persons with a history of hepatitis (Petry, Bickel, Piasecki, Marsch, & Badger, 2000), a large, multicenter trial did not find any problems with LFTs in individuals being treated with buprenorphine or methadone over the first 6 months of treatment (Saxon et al., 2013). There are not significant cognitive or performance-impairing effects associated with buprenorphine treatment of opioid dependence.

A recent multisite trial compared a short versus extended taper of buprenorphine–naltrexone combination in a group of prescription-opiate-dependent individuals (Weiss et al., 2011). They found that both groups reduced opiate use during treatment; however, when tapered off buprenorphine–naloxone, even after 12 weeks of treatment (extended taper group), the likelihood of an unsuccessful outcome was high, even in patients receiving counseling in addition to standard medical management. This study suggests that buprenorphine is an effective treatment for prescription opiate dependence, but the necessary duration of treatment and best strategy for transition to medication-free treatment remains an open question.

Buprenorphine has expanded the capacity for opioid dependence treatment into mainstream medical practice in the United States. Despite this, only a small number of physicians prescribe buprenorphine (less than 2% of U.S. physicians). Despite this relatively small number, a substantial number of patients are currently receiving buprenorphine.

Treatment of Opioid Dependence in Pregnancy

MMT is the recommended treatment for opioid dependence during pregnancy. However, prenatal exposure to methadone is associated with a neonatal abstinence syndrome, which is characterized by central nervous system hyperirritability and autonomic nervous system dysfunction that often require medication and extended hospitalization. A study comparing methadone and buprenorphine treatment during pregnancy found a slightly higher dropout rate but better neonatal outcomes in the buprenorphine-treated group (Jones et al., 2010). There were no significant differences between groups in other primary or secondary outcomes, or in rates of maternal or neonatal adverse events. As such, it is likely that either methadone or buprenorphine (Subutex) can safely be used in the treatment of opiate dependence during pregnancy.

Naltrexone Treatment

Naltrexone is an opioid antagonist that has no euphoric effects and may provide a nonaddicting treatment for opioid users. In a recent Cochrane review of 10 controlled studies of oral naltrexone compared with placebo (Minozzi et al., 2011), naltrexone was clearly associated with superior results. Despite the strong theoretical potential of naltrexone for treating opioid dependence, clinical experience has been disappointing because of high dropout rates and poor compliance. People such as health professionals, business executives, and those who are under probation in the legal system have strong incentives to complete treatment and may be good candidates for naltrexone treatment. Prior to starting naltrexone, a naloxone challenge test should be performed to ensure that no residual physiological dependence remains, or naltrexone could cause a prolonged, precipitated withdrawal episode. Naltrexone may be dosed at 50 mg/day or 100–150 mg two to three times a week.

A long-acting (4 weeks) injectable form of naltrexone was tested in 60 heroin-dependent adults. There was a dose-dependent increase in retention in the naltrexone-treated group, and individuals who attended treatment in all groups had high rates of urine drug screens that were negative for opioids (75–80%) (Comer et al., 2006). Other studies exploring the use of this promising agent in the treatment of opiate dependence are in progress.

Treatment of Prescription Opioid Overdose

As discussed previously, prescription opioid overdose deaths have increased steadily over the past decade. While improvements are being made in treatment for prescription opioid dependence and in access to care, many communities are faced with overdose fatalities that occur prior to access to treatment. Since the 1990s, community-based programs that have developed in response to this growing issue have provided opioid overdose prevention services and education to opioid-dependent individuals, their families and friends, and service providers. There are now over 180 local programs across the Unites States that provide training in the use of the opioid antagonist naloxone hydrochloride to reverse the fatal respiratory depression that occurs during an opioid overdose. These community-based programs have provided naloxone to over 50,000 persons, resulting in approximately 10,000 drug overdose reversals using naloxone (intranasal or intramuscular) (CDC, 2012). Preliminary evidence supports a reduction in opioid overdose death rates in communities that implement overdose education and naloxone distribution compared to those with low rates of implementation (Walley et al., 2013). This suggests that training family, friends, and care providers to recognize, prevent, and respond to opioid overdoses can be effective in reducing opioid overdose mortality.

CONCLUSIONS

In conclusion, the public health importance of opiate dependence has taken on increasing significance with the increase in prescription opiate misuse over the past 10 years. Fortunately, treatment options have also increased with the introduction of buprenorphine and a long-acting formulation of the opiate antagonist, naltrexone. In the treatment of opiate dependence, medication therapy must be coupled with psychosocial rehabilitation for optimal results.

ACKNOWLEDGMENTS

This work was supported by National Institute on Drug Abuse Grant No. K12 DA031794 to Kathleen T. Brady.

REFERENCES

American Psychiatric Association. (2013). *Diagnostic and statistical manual of mental disorders* (5th ed.). Arlington, VA: Author.

Back, S. E., Lawson, K. M., Singleton, L. M., & Brady, K. T. (2011). Characteristics and correlates of men and women with prescription opioid dependence. *Addict Behav, 36*, 829–834.

Back, S. E., Payne, R. A., Simpson, A. N., & Brady, K. T. (2010). Gender and prescription opioids: Findings from the National Survey on Drug Use and Health. *Addict Behav, 35*, 1001–1007.

Barth, K. S., Back, S. E., Maria, M. M., Lawson, K., Shaftman, S., Brady, K. T., et al. (2013). Pain and motives for use among non-treatment seeking individuals with prescription opioid dependence. *Am J Addict, 22*(5), 486–491.

Berman, A. H., Bergman, H., Palmstierna, T., & Schlyter, F. (2005). Evaluation of the Drug Use Disorders Identification Test (DUDIT) in criminal justice and detoxification settings and in a Swedish population sample. *Euro Addict J, 11*, 22–31.

Bohnert, A. S., Valenstein, M., Bair, M. J., Ganoczy, D., McCarthy, J. F., Ilgen, M. A., et al. (2011). Association between opioid prescribing patterns and opioid overdose-related deaths. *JAMA, 305*(13), 1315–1321.

Brooner, R. K., & Kidorf, M. (2002). Using behavioral reinforcement to improve methadone treatment participation. *Sci Pract Perspect, 1*(1), 38–47.

Butler, S. F., Budman, S. H., Fernandez, K. C., Houle, B., Benoit, C., Katz, N., et al. (2007). Development and validation of the Current Opioid Misuse Measure. *Pain, 130*(1–2), 144–156.

Calcaterra, S., Glanz, J., & Binswanger, I. A. (2013). National trends in pharmaceutical opioid related deaths compared to other substance related overdose deaths: 1999–2009. *Drug Alcohol Depend, 131*(3), 263–270.

Centers for Disease Control and Prevention (CDC). (2012). Community-based opioid overdose prevention programs providing naloxone—United States, 2010. *MMWR Morb Mortal Wkly Rep, 61*(6), 101–105.

Centers for Disease Control and Prevention (CDC). (2013). Vital signs: Overdoses of prescription opioid pain relievers and other drugs among women—United States, 1999–2010. *MMWR Morb Mortal Wkly Rep, 62*(26), 537–542.

Cicero, T. J., Surratt, H., Inciardi, J. A., & Muñoz, A. (2007). Relationship between therapeutic use and abuse of opioid analgesics in rural, suburban, and urban locations in the United States. *Pharmacoepidem Dr S, 16*(8), S27–S40.

Comer, S. D., Sullivan, M. A., Yu, E., Rothenberg, J. L., Kleber, H. D., Kampman, K., et al. (2006). Injectable sustained released naltrexone for the treatment of opioid dependence: A randomized placebo controlled trial. *Arch Gen Psychiatry, 63*(2), 210–218.

Compton, W. M., Dawson, D. A., Goldstein, R. B., & Grant, B. F. (2013). Crosswalk between DSM-IV dependence and DSM-5 substance use disorders for opioids, cannabis, and alcohol. *Drug Alcohol Depend, 132*(1–2), 387–390.

Conway, K. P., Vullo, G. C., Nichter, B., Wang, J., Compton, W. M., Iannotti, R. J., et al. (2013). Prevalence and pattern of polysubstance use in a nationally representative sample of 10th graders in the United States. *J Adolesc Health, 52*(6), 716–723.

Cruciani, R. A., Sekine, R., Homel, P., Lussier, D., Yap, Y., Suzuki, Y., et al. (2005). Measurement of QTc in patients receiving chronic methadone therapy. *J Pain Symptom Manage, 29*(4), 385–391.

Dole, V. P., Nyswander, M. E., & Kreek, M. J. (1966). Narcotic blockade. *Arch Intern Med, 118*(4), 304–309.

Eap, C. B., Buclin, T., & Baumann, P. (2002). Interindividual variability of the clinical pharmacokinetics of methadone: Implications for the treatment of opioid dependence. *Clin Pharmacokinet, 41*(14), 1153–1193.

First, M. B., Spitzer, R. L., Gibbon, M., & Williams, J. B. W. (1996). *Structured Clinical Interview for DSM-IV Axis I Disorders (SCID)*. Washington, DC: American Psychiatric Press.

Gavin, D. R., Ross, H. E., & Skinner, H. (1989). Diagnostic validity of the Drug Abuse Screening Test in the assessment of DSM-III drug disorders. *British J Addict, 84*, 301–307.

Hall, A. J., Logan, J. E., Toblin, R. L., Kaplan, J. A., Kraner, J. C., Bixler, D., et al. (2008). Patterns of abuse among unintentional pharmaceutical overdose fatalities. *JAMA, 300*(22), 2613–2620.

Humeniuk, R. E., Ali, R. L., Babor, F., Farrell, M., Formigoni, K. L., Jittiwutikarn, J., et al. (2008). Validation of the alcohol, smoking and substance involvement screening test (ASSIST). *Addiction, 103*(6), 1039–1047.

Jaffe, S. L. (1998). Adolescent substance abuse: Assessment and treatment. In A. H. Esman, L. T. Flaherty, & H. A. Horowitz (Eds.), *Adolescent psychiatry: Developmental and clinical studies* (Vol. 23, pp. 61–71). Mahwah, NJ: Analytic Press.

Johnson, R. E., Eissenberg, T., Stitzer, M. L., Strain, E. C., Liebson, I. A., & Bigelow, G. E. (1995).

Buprenorphine treatment of opioid dependence: Clinical trial of daily versus alternate-day dosing. *Drug Alcohol Depend, 40,* 27–35.

Jones, H. E., Kaltenbach, K., Heil, S. H., Stine, S. M., Coyle, M. G., Arria, A. M., et al. (2010). Neonatal abstinence syndrome after methadone or buprenorphine exposure. *N Engl J Med, 363,* 2320–2331.

Laheij, R. J. F., Krabbe, P. F. M., & de Jong, C. A. J. (2000). Rapid heroin detoxification under general anesthesia. *JAMA, 283*(9), 1143.

Ling, W., Wesson, D. R., Charuvastra, C., & Klett, C. J. (1996). A controlled trial comparing buprenorphine and methadone maintenance in opioid dependence. *Arch Gen Psychiatry, 53,* 401–407.

Lizasoain, I., Leza, J. C., & Lorenzo, P. (1991). Buprenorphine: Bell-shaped dose–response curve for its antagonist effects. *Gen Pharmacol, 22*(2), 297–300.

Manchikanti, L., Helm, S., Fellows, B., Janata, J. W., Pampati, V., Grider, J. S., et al. (2012). Opioid epidemic in the United States. *Pain Physician, 15,* ES9–ES38.

McCabe, S. E., Cranford, J. A., Boyd, C. J., & Teter, C. J. (2007). Motives, diversion, and routes of administration associated with nonmedical use of prescription opioids. *Addict Behav, 32*(3), 562–575.

McCabe, S. E., Teter, C. J., & Boyd, C. J. (2005). Illicit use of prescription pain medication among college students. *Drug Alcohol Depend, 77,* 37–47.

McLellan, A. T., Kushner, H., Metzger, D., Peters, R., Grisson, G., Pettinati, H., et al. (1992). The fifth edition of the Addiction Severity Index. *J Subst Abuse Treat, 9*(3), 199–213.

Minozzi, S., Amato, L, Vecchi, S., Davoli, M., Kirchmayer, U., & Verster, A. (2011). Oral naltrexone maintenance treatment for opiate dependence. *Cochrane Database Syst Rev, 13*(4), CD001333.

Osgood, E. D., Eaton, T. A., Trudeau, J. J., & Katz, N. P. (2012). A brief survey to characterize oxycodone abuse patterns in adolescents enrolled in two substance abuse recovery high schools. *Am J Drug Alcohol Abuse, 38*(2), 166–170.

Passik, S. D., Kirsh, K. L., & Casper, D. (2008). Addiction-related assessment tools and pain management: Instruments for screening, treatment planning and monitoring compliance. *Pain Med, 9,* S145–S166.

Peavy, K. M., Banta-Green, C. J., Kingston, S., Hanrahan, M., Merrill, J. O., & Coffin, P. O. (2012). Hooked on prescription-type opiates prior to using heroin: Results from a survey of syringe exchange clients. *J Psychoactive Drugs, 44*(3), 259–265.

Peer, K., Rennert, L., Lynch, K. G., Farrer, L., Gelernter, J., & Kranzler, H. R. (2013). Prevalence of DSM-IV and DSM-5 alcohol, cocaine, opioid, and cannabis use disorders in a largely substance dependent sample. *Drug Alcohol Depend, 127,* 215–219.

Petry, N. M., Bickel, W. K., Piasecki, D., Marsch, L. A., & Badger, G. J. (2000). Elevated liver enzyme levels in opioid-dependent patients with hepatitis treated with buprenorphine. *Am J Addict, 9*(3), 265–269.

Preston, K. L., Bigelow, G. E., & Liebson, I. A. (1990). Effects of sublingually given naloxone in opioid-dependent human volunteers. *Drug Alcohol Depend, 25*(1), 27–34.

Preston, K. L., Silverman, K., Schuster, C. R., & Cone, E. J. (1997). Assessment of cocaine use with quantitative urinalysis and estimation of new uses. *Addiction, 92*(6), 717–727.

Richter, L., & Johnson, P. B. (2001). Current methods of assessing substance use: A review of strengths, problems, and developments. *J Drug Issues, 31*(4), 809–832.

Rigg, K. K., & Ibañez, G. E. (2010). Motivations for non-medical prescription drug use: A mixed methods analysis. *J Subst Abuse Treat, 39*(3), 236–247.

Robins, L. N., Wing, J., Wittchen, H. U., Leltzer, J. E., Babor, T. F., Burke, J., et al. (1989). The Composite International Diagnostic Interview: An epidemiologic instrument suitable for use in conjunction with different diagnostic systems and in different cultures. *Arch Gen Psychiatry, 45,* 1069–1077.

Rosado, J., Walsh, S. L., Bigelow, G. E., & Strain, E. C. (2007). Sublingual buprenorphine/naloxone precipitated withdrawal in subjects maintained on 100 mg of daily methadone. *Drug Alcohol Depend, 90*(2–3), 261–269.

Saxon, A. J., Ling, W., Hillhouse, M., Thomas, C., Hasson, A., Ang, A., et al. (2013). Buprenor-phine/naloxone and methadone effects on laboratory indices of liver health: A randomized trial. *Drug Alcohol Depend 128*(1–2), 71–76.

Sees, K. L., Delucchi, K. L., Masson, C., Rosen, A., Clark, H. W., Robillard, H., et al. (2000). Methadone maintenance vs. 180-day psychosocially enriched detoxification for treatment of opioid dependence: A randomized controlled trial. *JAMA, 283*(10), 1303–1310.

Sertürner, F. W. (1817). Ueber das Morphium, eine neue salzfähige Grundlage, und die Mekon-säure, als Hauptbestandtheile des Opiums. *Ann Phys-Berlin, 55*, 56–89.

Sheehan, D. V., Lecrubier, Y., Sheehan, K. H., Amorim, P., Janavs, J., Weiller, E., et al. (1998). The Mini-International Neuropsychiatric Interview (MINI): The development and validation of a structured diagnostic psychiatric interview for DSM-IV and ICD-10. *J Clin Psychiatry, 59*, 22–33.

Sobell, L. C., & Sobell, M. B. (1995). *Alcohol Timeline Follow-back user's manual.* Toronto: Addictions Research Foundation.

Stoller, K. B., Bigelow, G. E., Walsh, S. L., & Strain, E. C. (2001). Effects of buprenorphine/nalox-one in opioid-dependent humans. *Psychopharmacol (Berl), 154*(3), 230–242.

Strain E. C., Bigelow, G. E., Liebson, I. A., & Stitzer, M. L. (1999). Moderate- vs. high-dose meth-adone in the treatment of opioid dependence: A randomized trial. *JAMA, 281*, 1000–1005.

Strain, E. C., Moody, D. E., Stoller, K., Walsh, S. L., & Bigelow, G. E. (2002). Bioavailability of buprenorphine solution versus tablets during chronic dosing in opioid-dependent subjects. *Drug Alcohol Depend, 66*(Suppl. 1), S176.

Strain, E. C., Stitzer, M. L., Liebson, I. A., & Bigelow, G. E. (1993). Methadone dose and treat-ment outcome. *Drug Alcohol Depend, 33*(2), 105–117.

Strain, E. C., Stitzer, M. L., Liebson, I. A., & Bigelow, G. E. (1994). Comparison of buprenorphine and methadone in the treatment of opioid dependence. *Am J Psychiatry, 151*(7), 1025–1030.

Substance Abuse and Mental Health Services Administration (SAMHSA). (2003). *Results from the 2002 National Survey on Drug Use and Health: National findings.* Washington, DC: National Institute on Drug Abuse.

Substance Abuse and Mental Health Services Administration (SAMHSA). (2010). National Sur-vey on Drug Use and Health: National findings. Retrieved from *http://oas.samhsa.gov/nsduh/2k20nsduh/tabs/sect7petabs1to21.pdf.*

Substance Abuse and Mental Health Services Administration (SAMHSA). (2012). *Results from the 2011 National Survey on Drug Use and Health: Summary of national findings* (Office of Applied Studies, NSDUH Series H-44, DHHS Publication No. SMA 12-4713). Rockville, MD: Author.

Volkow, N. D., McLellan, T. A., Cotto, J. H., Karithanom, M., & Weiss, S. R. B. (2011). Charac-teristics of opioid prescriptions in 2009. *JAMA, 305*(13), 1299–1301.

Walley, A. Y., Xuan, Z., Hackmann, H. H., Quinn, E., Doe-Simkins, M., Sorensen-Alawad, A., et al. (2013). Opioid overdose rates and implementation of overdose education and nasal nalox-one distribution in Massachusetts: Interrupted time series analysis. *BMJ, 346*, f174.

Walsh, S. L., & Strain, E. C. (2006). Pharmacology of methadone. In E. C. Strain & M. L. Stitzer (Eds.), *The treatment of opioid dependence* (pp. 60–76). Baltimore, MD: Johns Hopkins University Press.

Warner, M., Chen, L. H., Makuc, D. M., Anderson, R. N., & Minino, A. M. (2011). *Drug poi-soning deaths in the United States, 1980–2008* (NCHS Data Brief No. 81). Hyattsville, MD: National Center for Health Statistics.

Webster, L. R. (2005). Predicting aberrant behaviors in opioid-treated patients: Preliminary vali-dation of the opioid risk tool. *Pain Med, 6*(6), 432–442.

Weiss R. D., Potter, J. S., Feilin, D. A., Byrne, M., Connery H. S., Dickinson, W., et al. (2011). Adjunctive counseling during brief and extended buprenorphine–naloxone treatment for pre-scription opioid dependence: A 2-phase randomized controlled trial. *Arch Gen Psychiatry, 68*(12), 1238–1246.

CHAPTER 8

Cannabis

ALICIA R. MURRAY
FRANCES R. LEVIN

Cannabis has been used since ancient times. The cannabis plant has a long history of use as medicine, with historical evidence dating back to 2737 B.C.E. (Ben Amar, 2006). The cultivation and sale of cannabis continued unfettered until the Marijuana Tax Act of 1937 legislated a tax on the sale of cannabis. It was drafted by Harry Anslinger and levied a tax on anyone who commercially sold cannabis, hemp, or marijuana, and included a penalty and enforcement provisions to which marijuana, cannabis, or hemp handlers were subject. Violation could result in a fine of up to $2,000 and up to 5 years imprisonment. Some have suggested the Act was implemented because of increased reports of smoked cannabis (Bonnie & Whitebread, 1974), although others have argued that the aim of the Act was to reduce the size of the hemp industry. This act was overturned in 1969 in *Leary v. United States,* and was repealed by Congress the next year. Subsequently, the Controlled Substances Act of 1970 classified cannabis along with heroin and D-lysergic acid diethylamide (LSD) as a Schedule I drug (i.e., having the relatively highest abuse potential and no accepted medical use (Erowid Vaults, 2010). Marijuana's peak use was in 1979, when approximately 51% of high schools seniors admitted to trying it. Cannabis use declined in the 1980s, possibly due to newly emerging laws on drugs and increased perceived risk (Bachman, Johnston, & O'Malley, 1998; Johnston, O'Malley, Bachman, & Schulenberg, 2009). Its use then increased again in the mid-1990s, especially among young adults, which may have been due to the public perception that cannabis is a benign drug and view it as relatively safe compared to alcohol, cocaine, or heroin (Raphael, Wooding, Stevens, & Connor, 2005). Despite this perception, early and heavy use of cannabis has been associated with a greater likelihood of developing certain mental health problems, such as psychosis and depression. Additionally, poorer treatment outcomes have been noted among those with co-occurring mental disorders (Agosti, Nunes, & Levin, 2002). We review in this chapter the neuropharmacology of cannabis, prevalence of use, cannabis's role as a possible "gateway" drug, its relationship to mental health disorders, treatment strategies, and future areas of research.

OVERVIEW OF CANNABIS AND EPIDEMIOLOGY OF USE

Marijuana consists of the dried leaves, stems, and seeds of the hemp plant and has been used for religious and medicinal purposes for more than 1,000 years. It is most commonly smoked but may be ingested via multiple routes. Cannabis cigarettes have a variety of names, including joints, nails, herb, pot, and reefers; pipes for smoking are also known as bongs and bowls (Neuspiel, 2007). Cannabis may also be incorporated into food items or brewed as tea. A powerful resin of marijuana (hashish) is usually smoked in pipes or in cigarette form; its potency may vary due to its cultivation. Marijuana's active ingredient is THC (delta-9-tetrahydrocannabinol) and because of creative agriculture, the THC content of cannabis has more than quadrupled, from 0.5 to 2.0% in the 1970s to 6 to 10% in 2000 (Neuspiel, 2007). This increase in THC potency and increase in availability of cannabis may contribute to recent increases in dependence on cannabis.

Cannabis is the most widely used illicit drug in United States, as well as throughout the world. Globally, its use appears to be increasing, with an estimated 162 million (4%) of the world's adults using it in 2004, and approximately 0.6% (22.5 million) people using cannabis daily (United Nations Office on Drugs and Crime, 2006), a 10% increase in use from the mid-1990s (Hall & Degenhardt, 2007). In 2009, more than 28 million Americans (11.3%) age 12 or older reported abusing cannabis, and 4.3 million met DSM-IV criteria for abuse or dependence (National Institute on Drug Abuse, 2011).

In the 2013 National Survey on Drug Use and Health (NSDUH), 5.7 million persons ages 12 or older used marijuana on a daily or almost daily basis in the past 12 months (i.e., on 300 or more days in that period), which was an increase from the 3.1 million daily or almost daily users in 2006. In addition, 8.1 million persons ages 12 or older used marijuana on 20 or more days in the past month, which was an increase from the 5.1 million daily or almost daily past month users in 2005 to 2007. (National Center for Health Statistics, 2013) The number of daily or almost daily users in 2013 represented 41.1 percent of past month marijuana users.

The 2009 the NSDHU reported that of the more than 16 million Americans who use cannabis on a regular basis, most started using cannabis and other drugs during their teenage years. The NSUDH recently reported that 78% of the 2.4 million people who began using in the last year were ages 12 to 20 (National Center for Health Statistics, 2013). According to the Monitoring the Future study (Terry-McElrath, O'Malley, & Johnston, 2014), over a 1-month period, 6.5% of eighth graders, 16.6% of sophomores, and 21.2% of high school seniors reported using marijuana, with 6% of high school seniors smoking marijuana daily; this number has increased slightly since 2000. The only substance that was found to be reduced among teens during this period was nicotine. Reported lifetime use among 10th and 12th graders is 34.1 and 44.8%, respectively, and daily use of cannabis is 3.1 and 5%, respectively (Harvey, Sellman, Porter, & Frampton, 2007; Wallace et al., 2009).

According to the Drug Abuse Warning Network (DAWN) for 2009, 973,591 emergency room visits involved an illicit drug. Cannabis was involved in 376,467 visits, or 38.7%, and cannabis-related visits were highest for those ages 18–20 (Owens, Mutter, & Stocks, 2007).

Many tend to think of cannabis use as an "adolescent problem." But, in fact, a substantial subset of individuals continue to have problems into adulthood. Of note, the prevalence of cannabis use among 45- to 64-year-olds has also increased in the last 10 years. Perhaps of greater concern is the increased rate of cannabis abuse/dependence. The National Comorbidity Survey observed a 4.2% lifetime prevalence rate for cannabis dependence, and among those treated for substance abuse, 13% of admissions were for cannabis dependence (Agosti et al., 2002). Consistent with this, a recent Substance Abuse and Mental Health Services Administration (SAMSHA) survey found that 16% of all patients admitted to public-sponsored treatment facilities reported cannabis as their primary drug of abuse, more than a twofold increase over a similar survey conducted more than 10 years earlier (National Survey on Drug Use and Health [NSDUH], 2009).

Compton, Grant, Colliver, Glantz, and Stinson (2004) found that more adults in the United States had a cannabis use disorder in 2001–2002 than in 1991–1992. They found that increased prevalence rates of cannabis use disorders were most notable among young black men and women, and young Hispanic men. The rates among young white men and women also remained high (Compton et al., 2004).

EFFECTS OF CANNABIS ON THE CENTRAL NERVOUS SYSTEM

When smoked, THC passes quickly from the respiratory tract to the bloodstream and binds to cannabinoid receptors in the brain. Within minutes, the active component of the drug changes brain chemistry and peaks 15–30 minutes later. The effect lasts 2–3 hours, and THC has a serum half-life of approximately 19 hours (Ameri, 1999).

THC passes readily across the blood–brain barrier, because it is lipid soluble (Iversen, 2003). The acute psychoactive effects of cannabis can produce pleasant and unpleasant reactions that include euphoria; perceptual disturbances; the subjective effect of time being slowed down; and a sense of calm and relaxation, but also depression, paranoia, anxiety or panic attacks. Studies have shown that high-dose intravenous THC given acutely produces transient symptoms such as perceptual alterations, anxiety, deficits in working memory and recall, and impairment of executive functioning that resembles symptoms of psychosis (D'Souza et al., 2004). Yucel et al. (2008) found significant reductions in brain volume in both the hippocampus and amygdala in chronic heavy cannabis users likely related to cumulative cannabis exposure. Yucel found these reductions to also be associated with psychosis and related cognitive deficits (Yucel et al., 2008).

There are more than 60 different cannabinoids found within *Cannabis sativa*. The two most abundant naturally occurring cannabinoids are THC and cannabidiol (CBD), which have different effects. THC is psychotomimetic and accounts for the "high" associated with cannabis use; CBD has been found to be anxiolytic and to have antipsychotic properties (Zuardi, Crippa, et al., 2006a; Zuardi, Hallak, et al.,

2006b; Ameri, 1999). Cannabis cultivated with variations in the ratio of these two cannabinoids, as well as numerous others, likely impacts the intensity and quality of the associated experience. A recent study examining levels of THC and CBD in hair samples of cannabis users and nonusers found that users with THC alone reported higher levels of positive schizophrenia-like symptoms, while the THC and CBD group reported less anhedonia (Morgan & Curran, 2008).

Of the cannabinoid receptors throughout the brain, two types of cannabinoid receptors (CB_1 and CB_2) have been characterized. The CB_1 receptor is most abundant in the nerve terminals of the frontal regions of the cerebral cortex, hippocampus, and basal ganglia. CB_2 receptors are found mainly on cells of the immune system. When CB_1 receptors are activated presynaptically, they modulate the release of other neurotransmitters such as gamma-aminobutyric acid (GABA), glutamate, and serotonin in these brain regions. THC is reinforcing because of its ability to indirectly release dopamine within the brain's reward system by switching off GABA interneurons that normally inhibit these dopaminergic pathways (Ameri, 1999). There are three different groups of cannabinoids: the phytocannabinoids, the endocannabinoids, and the synthetic cannabinoids. The phytocannabinoids are produced within the cannabis plant. There are several dozen different phytocannabinoids that have not been detected in any other plant, and new phytocannabinoids continue to be isolated (Radwan et al., 2009). The endocannabinoid neurotransmitter system consists of two known cannabinoid receptor types (CB_1 and CB_2) and endogenous ligands (endocannabinoids), the best known being 2-arachindonoylglycerol (2-AG) and anandamide. The endocannabinoids are ligands targeted to interact with cannabinoid receptors. The most well-known cannabinoids include (1) cannabidiol, a CB_1 and CB_2 antagonist; (2) delta-9-tetrahydrocannabivarin (THCV), which acts as a partial agonist *in vitro*, and an antagonist *in vivo*; and (3) THC, which is a CB_1 and CB_2 receptor partial agonist (Pertwee, 2008).

The synthetic cannabinoids do not occur naturally, but they interact with cannabinoid receptors (Sun & Bennett, 2007). There are currently two cannabinoids available by prescription in the United States: dronabinol and nabilone. Dronabinol is synthetically made and chemically identical to THC in the cannabis plant. It is a Schedule III drug and is approved for refractory treatment of anorexia associated with AIDS and nausea associated with chemotherapy and cancer. Nabilone acts as a partial agonist at cannabinoid receptors and is also approved to treat nausea and vomiting due to chemotherapy not responsive to standard treatments. Nabilone is controlled as a Schedule II drug in the United States, although reports of abuse of nabilone are extremely rare (Ware & St. Arnaud-Trempe, 2010). Rimonabant is also a synthetic compound with cannabinoid antagonist activity that acts as an inverse agonist at CB_1 receptors. It was evaluated as an antiobesity drug in Europe, but it was rejected by the U.S. Food and Drug Administration (FDA) because of an adverse psychiatric symptom profile (Butler & Korbonits, 2009).

K2 or "Spice" refers to a series of synthetic cannabinoid products that are advertised and sold legally as herbal blend incense. They produce similar effects to those of marijuana when smoked. They are intentionally sprayed on dried herbs before packaged and sold as K2. They mimic intoxication with marijuana, with longer duration and poor detection on typical urine screens (Hu, Primack, Barnett, & Cook, 2011).

These herbs have emerged as popular legal alternatives to marijuana among adolescents and young adults. In response to the dangers of these products, on March 1, 2011, the Drug Enforcement Agency (DEA, 2011) issued the final order to temporarily ban five synthetic cannabinoids (JWH-018, JWH-073, JWH-200, CP 47,497 and CP 47,497 C8), following 18 states that had already implemented their own law or policy of controlling one or more of these five synthetic cannabinoids. According to the American Association of Poison Control Centers (AAPCC), more than 2,500 calls related to K2 were reported in 2010, compared with only 53 in 2009 (Muller et al., 2010). In 2011 this number jumped to 2,906 calls (*www.WhiteHouse.gov/ ONDCP*).

Smoking K2 may produce several adverse health events, such as hallucinations, severe agitation, extremely elevated heart rate and blood pressure, coma, suicide attempts, and drug dependence (Schneir, Cullen, & Ly, 2011). Synthetic cannabinoids have been associated with both seizures (Schneir et al., 2011) and heart attacks (Mir, Obafemi, Young, & Kane, 2011). Greater awareness of the adverse effects of these synthetic cannabinoids is needed to stem the tide of growing use. Governments around the world are taking actions to ban or control synthetic cannabinoids. At present, standard toxicology testing does not detect the most commonly available synthetic cannabinoids.

DIAGNOSIS OF CANNABIS DEPENDENCE

The classifications of cannabis dependence in the DSM-IV-TR and ICD-10 are very similar. The DSM-5 (American Psychiatric Association, 2013) cannabis use disorder criteria are nearly identical to the DSM-IV cannabis abuse and dependence criteria combined into a single list, but with the deletion of recurrent legal problems and the addition of craving/urge or strong desire to use cannabis.

The most pertinent diagnostic change in DSM-5 is the addition of the diagnosis of cannabis withdrawal, which reflects ongoing recognition of such a condition. Its diagnosis requires cessation of cannabis use, a resulting period of clinical significance, and at least three other symptoms within 1 week of cessation (Wiesbeck et al., 1996; Kouri, Pope, & Lukas, 1999; Kouri & Pope, 2000; Pope, Gruber, & Yurgellun-Todd, 2001; Budney & Moore, 2002; American Psychiatric Association, 2013). The National Comorbidity Study (NCS) conducted in the United States reported that for those meeting criteria for cannabis dependence at some time in their lives, withdrawal symptoms and a persistent desire or attempts to control use were among the most commonly reported symptoms (Swendsen et al., 2010).

CANNABIS AS A GATEWAY DRUG

Many studies have indicated that adolescent cannabis use is often related to the subsequent use of other illicit substances. As the data indicate, there is the widespread use of cannabis among young people. The "gateway hypothesis" suggests that adolescent cannabis use increases risk for later use and abuse of other illicit substances, and public health research appears to support this idea (Kandel & Davies, 1986). What is unclear is the degree to which the link between early cannabis use causes the later use of other drugs (Morral, McCaffrey, & Paddock, 2002).

Research suggests that cannabis's gateway effect remains significant when researchers control for stress exposure, age, and age-linked social roles. This provides some supporting evidence for the hypothesis that the use of cannabis, independent of other factors, increases the use of other illicit substances (Van Gundy & Rebellon, 2010).

Research focused on the initiation and continuation of cannabis use in young people has indicated that use usually begins in high school, with the possibility of occasional use progressing into dependence. However, other factors may need to be taken into account, such as access to drugs, supply, and cost, which may have greater influence on patterns of subsequent drug use and continuation (Raphael et al., 2005).

Males have a greater likelihood of becoming regular users due to availability and peer use (Coffey, Lynskey, Wolfe, & Patton, 2000).

In support of the "gateway hypothesis" in a recent Australian study of over 30,000 students, 38.75% of regular cannabis users also reported use of other illicit substances, compared with 4.7% of nonregular cannabis users (Lynskey, White, Hill, Letcher, & Hall, 1999). In a large-scale birth cohort study in New Zealand, researchers observed that 70% of subjects had used cannabis and 26% had used other illicit substances. With the exception of three subjects (i.e., in more than 99% of cases), cannabis use had preceded the use of other illicit drugs (Fergusson & Horwood, 2000).

On the other hand, when researchers examine initiation of drug use across other countries and cohorts, the strength of associations between substance use progression may be due more to background prevalence or cultural factors than to causal mechanisms (Hall & Degenhardt, 2007). Differences in patterns of gateway drug use seen across countries in the World Mental Health Survey (WMHS) support the likely influence of attitudes toward substance use in influencing order of initiation. For example, higher levels of other illicit drug use before cannabis were related to lower levels of cannabis use in Japan and Nigeria. Similarly, first use of other illicit drugs before alcohol and tobacco was found to be most prevalent in Japan and Nigeria, countries with relatively low rates of alcohol and tobacco use compared to other WMHS countries (Degenhardt et al., 2010). Notably, cannabis use before alcohol and tobacco use was extremely rare in countries with some of the highest rates of cannabis use, such as the United States and New Zealand. Moreover, cannabis users in the United States were also much more likely to progress to other illicit drug use than those in the Netherlands.

Studies also indicate that early-onset drug use and mental health problems are risk factors for later dependent drug use (Lubman, Allen, Rogers, Cementon, & Bonomo, 2007), and that comorbid mental health problems escalate risk of developing dependence once drug use begins.

This suggests that prevention efforts are probably better targeted at all types of drug use, particularly among young people who are already dealing with other challenges such as comorbid psychiatric issues, deviance (Osgood, Johnston, O'Malley, & Bachman, 1988), and other unmeasured developmental factors, since it may be this group that is most at risk of developing problems later on (Degenhardt et al., 2010).

COMORBID DISORDERS

Cannabis Use and Affective Disorders

Anxiety and mood disorders are among the most common psychiatric disorders. About 10% of the U.S. adult population experiences these disorders over a 1-year period (Merikangas et al., 1998; Kessler, Chiu, Demler, & Walters, 2005). The possible relationship between cannabis use and the development of anxiety and mood disorders, such as depression, has received less attention than the relationship between cannabis and psychosis. Some studies suggest that as cannabis use increases, episodes of depression and mood or anxiety problems increase (Troisi, Vicario, Nuccetelli, Ciani, & Pasini, 1995; Alpert, Maddocks, Rosenbaum, & Fava, 1994), although not all studies support this relationship (Kouri, Pope, Yurgelun-Todd, & Gruber, 1995).

Cheung et al. (2010) found that regular cannabis users have increased levels of anxiety and mood disorders in comparison with 12-month abstainers. This finding is consistent with results from the NCS, which indicate that increased cannabis use is associated with a higher risk of having experienced a major depressive episode (Hao et al., 2002). Patton et al. (2002) found that early-onset weekly cannabis use in adolescent women predicts a twofold increase in rates of depression later on, with daily use increasing the risk fourfold.

Several other epidemiological studies have also reported higher levels of depression among those who chronically use marijuana, although a recent systematic review highlighted that the association is modest, and noncausal explanations often remain unaddressed in these studies. Others have suggested that these inconsistencies in the literature may be due to several factors: small sample sizes; inconsistencies in the measurement of marijuana use, including failure to differentiate different levels of use; and divergence in measures of mood and anxiety disorders (Degenhardt, Hall, & Lynskey, 2003). Despite these limitations, evidence from longitudinal studies suggests that heavy cannabis use may increase depressive symptoms in some users, and that using cannabis to cope with negative affect is commonly reported by young people seeking mental health services for mood or anxiety disorders (Degenhardt et al., 2003). This highlights the importance of targeting coping skills during treatment. Adolescents and young adults with co-occurring affective and substance use disorders (SUDs) continue to experience significant problems with their symptoms and their functioning 6 months after presentation to mental health services, which suggests that integrated approaches addressing both mental health and cannabis use simultaneously should be considered (Hall, 2006b).

Although the role of anxiety in cannabis treatment is largely unexplored, patients seeking treatment for cannabis problems report significantly more elevated anxiety than do nonpatient samples (Copeland, Swift, Roffman, & Stephens, 2001). A high level of anxiety in individuals with SUDs is noteworthy, because the co-occurrence of elevated anxiety and cannabis dependence may result in greater impairment than that in either condition independently (Buckner & Carroll, 2010). Anxiety may also increase the risk of relapse. Among patients receiving treatment for cannabis dependence, history of being treated for an anxiety disorder is associated with reentry into cannabis treatment following cannabis treatment completion (Arendt, Rosenberg, Foldager, Perto, & Munk-Moffitt, 2007).

Individuals often report using cannabis to cope with stress and anxiety, and to help them relax or relieve tension (Reilly, Didcott, Swift, & Hall, 1998). Moreover, cannabis users with elevated anxiety (e.g., social anxiety, anxiety sensitivity, or fear of anxiety-related sensations) report using cannabis to cope with negative affect (Buckner, Bonn-Miller, Zvolensky, & Schmidt, 2007). These data suggest that the elevated anxiety associated with withdrawal may increase the risk of using cannabis to manage anxiety, thereby increasing relapse vulnerability. Buckner et al. used data from a large, multisite, randomized trial of 450 cannabis users who entered treatment and were randomly assigned to one of three psychosocial treatment conditions: motivational enhancement therapy (MET) alone, combined cognitive-behavioral therapy (CBT) and MET, and delayed treatment. At baseline, anxiety was linked to more cannabis-related problems. At follow-up, reduction in anxiety was related to less cannabis use (Buckner et al., 2007). Thus, anxiety may be an important characteristic that deserves further attention in cannabis dependence treatment.

Cannabis Use and Panic Disorder

The lifetime rates of panic disorder among the general population are approximately 5–8% (Katerndahl & Realini, 1993). Studies suggest that more frequent cannabis use and/or more severe cannabis problems may be related to an increased risk of panic attacks (Realini & Katerndahl, 1993). MacDonald et al. (2003) found that among weekly users of cannabis, approximately 40% reported having had at least one panic attack related to such use. Other investigations show that daily or weekly users of cannabis report a greater level of somatic tension and arousal symptoms, such as feeling dizzy and cognitive dyscontrol symptoms (e.g., depersonalization) compared to nonusers (Buckner & Schmidt, 2008). Zvolensky and colleagues (2006) report that cannabis dependence, but not use, was associated with an increased risk of panic attacks. A substantial percentage (30.1%) of cannabis-related visits to emergency rooms results from unexpected reactions to the drug. These findings collectively suggest that either cannabis use and/or dependence may be a risk factor for panic psychopathology. Alternatively, some individuals with panic disorder may be more likely to abuse cannabis. It is important for future research to understand the mechanisms linking cannabis use and dependence and panic psychopathology.

Cannabis Use and Posttraumatic Stress Disorder

The NCS demonstrated that those with posttraumatic stress disorder (PTSD) are three times more likely to have cannabis dependence as those without PTSD (Kilpatrick et al., 2003). In a recent study by Tepe, Dalrymple, and Zimmerman (2012), patients with comorbid social anxiety disorder and cannabis use disorder were more likely to have a lifetime diagnosis of PTSD and specific phobia than patients without cannabis use disorders. Cougle, Bonn-Miller, Vujanovic, Zvolensky, and Hawkins (2011) found that lifetime and current PTSD diagnoses were associated with increased odds of a lifetime history of cannabis use, as well as past-year daily cannabis use. Lifetime diagnosis of PTSD also was associated with increased risk for past-year cannabis use. These relationships remained statistically significant after Cougle et al. adjusted for co-occurring other anxiety and mood disorders and trauma type frequency. Agosti et al. (2002) found that PTSD was the second most common anxiety disorder, following generalized anxiety disorder, in those with cannabis dependence. Studies evaluating the relationship between PTSD and cannabis use disorders are particularly scarce among adolescent populations, despite the fact that cannabis use typically has its onset during adolescence. PTSD is often neglected in clinical evaluations of adolescents with SUDs (Clark & Power, 2005; Driessen et al., 2008).

Cornelius et al. (2010) evaluated the effect of PTSD on the rates of development of cannabis use disorders among teenagers transitioning to young adulthood. They controlled for variables associated with cannabis use (e.g., affiliation with deviant peers, gender, race), and found that PTSD contributes to the etiology of cannabis use disorders among teenagers making the transition to young adulthood, regardless of deviant peers or other demographic factors. These findings emphasize the importance of adequately assessing for PTSD among those at risk for cannabis dependence.

Cannabis Use and Attention-Deficit/Hyperactivity Disorder

Recent literature suggest that there is overrepresentation of attention-deficit/hyperactivity disorder (ADHD) in cannabis-abusing populations (Riggs et al., 2011), with ADHD rates of up to 35%. Perhaps because of the availability and social acceptability of cannabis use (Biederman et al., 1995), cannabis seems to be the preferred drug of abuse in participants with ADHD (Biederman et al., 1995). Anecdotally, cannabis users with ADHD report that cannabis helps to reduce emotional dysregulation, inner restlessness, and excessive arousal (Sobanski, 2006). While some studies have found that chronic cannabis use exacerbates signs and symptoms of ADHD, other studies have not found differences between participants with and without ADHD, and adolescents and adults without ADHD who abuse cannabis (Clure et al., 1999; Biederman et al., 1997; Thompson, Riggs, Mikulich, & Crowley, 1996).

Several studies that have considered the impact of stimulant treatment on subsequent substance abuse (often cannabis) found that stimulant treatment prior to the initiation of substance use is associated with a significant reduction in the likelihood of substance abuse/dependence in adolescence and adulthood (Biederman, 2003; Wilens, 2004). While ADHD may occur in a minority of cannabis-dependent individuals, most cannabis users do not have ADHD. However, even in the absence of a diagnosis, some cannabis users have impairment of attention, even when they are not intoxicated (Fergusson & Boden, 2008; Lundqvist, 2005; Pope et al., 2001). Harvey et al. (2007) found that adolescents who used cannabis at least once a week performed more poorly on cognitive tasks requiring attention and spatial working memory. Another study indicated that long-term cannabis users have attention and processing speed impairments when using a battery of neuropsychological tests (Messinis, Kyprianidou, Malefaki, & Papathanasopoulos, 2006). Similarly, Solowij, Stephens, Roffman, and Babor (2002) reported that heavy cannabis users showed impaired attention and executive functioning across several neuropsychological tests, and that the degree of impairment of attention was associated with increasing years of heavy cannabis use. Notably, Ehrenrich et al. (1999) found that impairments in attention were more persistent and significant for those individuals who began using cannabis prior to age 16 years. Other studies indicate that these effects are short-lived. Pope et al. (2001) found that about 1 month after cessation of use, neuropsychiatric deficits diminished. Although several studies have indicated an association between cannabis use and attention problems, a number of the studies were cross-sectional or retrospective, making it difficult to determine whether cannabis use or underlying ADHD were causal factors. More research is needed to determine if these neuropsychiatric effects are long-lasting if the individual stops using cannabis.

Cannabis Use and Psychosis

Various hypotheses have been developed concerning the association between cannabis use and psychosis (Swift, Hall, Didcott, & Reilly, 1998; Hall & Degenhardt, 2000; Degenhardt et al., 2007). First is that cannabis use precipitates psychosis among those vulnerable to developing the disorder; second, cannabis use exacerbates symptoms or prolongs the illness; third, those with schizophrenia, or a vulnerability to it, use cannabis to self-medicate premorbid psychiatric symptoms or medication side effects; and, finally, the association results from either common risk factors such as family history of schizophrenia, drug use, or poor adherence to antipsychotic medication.

Because cannabis use may increase the risk of psychotic disorders and result in a poorer prognosis for those with a vulnerability to psychosis, it has been suggested that some cases of psychosis may be prevented by discouraging cannabis use, particularly among those who are vulnerable (Arseneault, Cannon, Witton, & Murray, 2004). Epidemiological studies indicate that cannabis use among adolescents increases the relative risk of developing schizophrenia by 2.4 times and up to 6.0 times in heavy users (Arseneault et al., 2002). The hypothesis that cannabis use is a risk factor for psychosis has received support from a number of recent longitudinal cohort and population-based studies. Moore et al. (2007) reported that regular cannabis use may be associated with an approximate twofold increase in the relative risk of developing schizophrenia or other psychoses, with greater risk among those who use cannabis more frequently. Many of the existing longitudinal studies indicate a significant association between cannabis use and a higher risk of developing schizophrenia or relapse of psychotic symptoms (Andreasson, Allebeck, Engstrom, & Rydberg, 1988; Linszen, Dingemans, & Lenior, 1994). A longer term follow-up of the cohort in the study by Andreassonet al. (1988) confirmed the earlier findings that cannabis is associated with later schizophrenia and that this is not explained by prodromal symptoms (Andreasson & Allebeck, 1990). Other researchers have reported that cannabis use increased both the risk of psychosis in individuals without psychosis and a poorer prognosis in those with an established vulnerability to psychotic disorders. In this study, duration of cannabis use predicted the severity of the psychosis, which was not explained by other drugs. Those with psychotic symptoms who smoked cannabis at baseline had a worse outcome (van Os et al., 2002).

There is also evidence to suggest that individuals use cannabis to treat their positive and negative symptoms and also the side effects of antipsychotic medication. As discussed earlier, THC increases dopamine in the nucleus accumbens and has therefore been considered a potential cause of psychosis or relapse. However, increased dopamine in this area also has an arousing, anti-anhedonic effect that individuals with schizophrenia or other psychotic illnesses may actively seek (Negrete, 2003).

For those who have already developed psychosis, chronic cannabis use may negatively impact the course of the illness and treatment outcome. These individuals are likely to have poor medication compliance, more severe psychotic symptoms, more hospitalizations, and earlier relapses (Hall, 2006a). Most research and clinic data suggest that cannabis intoxication can lead to acute transient psychotic episodes in some individuals (Lambert et al., 2005) and that it can produce short-term exacerbation or recurrences of preexisting psychotic symptoms (Mathers & Ghodse, 1992; Kilpatrick et al., 2000). Although, it remains controversial whether cannabis use causes psychotic illness over the long term, some review articles reach no solid conclusions about causality and stress the importance of prospective longitudinal, population-based cohort studies to elucidate a possible causal association (Thornicroft, 1990). A recent study by Frischer, Crome, Martino, and Croft (2009) suggests that while early onset of heavy cannabis use is a risk factor for later psychosis, the incidence of schizophrenia (in the United Kingdom) does not appear to be increasing despite elevated rates of cannabis use in the general community. Conversely, Large, Sharma, Compton, Slade, and Nielssen (2011) published a meta-analysis providing evidence to support the hypothesis that cannabis use plays a causal role in the development of psychosis in some patients and suggested the need for renewed warnings about the potentially harmful effects of cannabis. Other data indicate that the vulnerability to develop psychosis can come from common risk factors, such as family history of schizophrenia, drug use, or poor adherence to psychotropic medication (Stowkowy, Addington, Liu, Hollowell, & Addington, 2012). This suggests that the relationship between cannabis use and psychosis is complex, and it highlights the need for future research to develop longitudinal studies with larger cohorts and prospective studies that examine cannabis use during adolescence and young adulthood.

TREATMENT OF CANNABIS USE DISORDERS

The mainstay of cannabis treatment is psychotherapy. Most of the clinical trials targeting cannabis dependence have evaluated the efficacy of psychotherapeutic interventions rather than pharmacotherapies. Unlike alcohol or opiate dependence, there are no FDA-approved medications for cannabis dependence. Although the finding are not exhaustive, we present in this section the major critical findings from some of the larger, well-controlled psychotherapeutic treatment trials, as well as the laboratory and outpatient treatment trials assessing emerging pharmacotherapies for cannabis dependence.

Psychotherapeutic Approaches

Data indicate that various psychotherapeutic approaches are effective in reducing cannabis use. The most common approaches have been motivational interviewing, 12-step facilitation counseling, CBT, and contingency management strategies. Most studies looking at psychotherapeutic approaches for the treatment of cannabis abuse and dependence have focused on reduction of use, not necessarily abstinence.

MET and CBT have been evaluated in several clinical trials. One of the largest trials compared a nine-session MET/CBT intervention, a two-session MET intervention, and a delayed treatment condition in 450 adult cannabis abusers. The MET/CBT and MET interventions exhibited greater cannabis use reduction and abstinence than the control condition. Additionally, the nine-session MET/CBT treatment was superior to the brief MET-only intervention in reducing cannabis use (Marijuana Treatment Project Research Group, 2004). Several research groups have found that contingency management strategies that provide vouchers for THC-negative urines are most effective either alone or in combination with MET/CBT in promoting abstinence. However, the reduction of cannabis use with contingency management is often not maintained unless there is concurrent CBT (Carroll & Rounsaville, 2007; Budney & Hughes, 2006; Budney, Vandrey, & Stanger, 2010).

For adolescents, most of the available treatment studies include youth who use multiple substances, most commonly cannabis and alcohol. Combined MET/CBT interventions studied have been found to be beneficial in reducing cannabis use, although, similar to adults, their abstinence rates are relatively low (Waldron & Turner, 2008). Several randomized trials have found family-based treatments to be efficacious. This included brief strategic family therapy (Szapocznik, Kurtines, Foote, Perez-Vidal, & Hervis, 1983), family behavior therapy (Azrin et al., 1994), family support network intervention and community reinforcement approach counseling (Dennis et al., 2004). These family interventions attempt to unite parents, schools, and other social agencies to help motivate change and recognize the problem areas and maladaptive coping patterns in both the child and parents. It has been suggested that family approaches may produce more effective outcomes than those without family involvement (Budney et al., 2010).

Contingency management (CM) has also been studied in young adults with hopes of improving outcomes of already established treatments. Although, the addition of abstinence-based incentive CM programs to Drug Court did not improve outcomes (Henggeler et al., 2006). However, when integrated with MET/CBT, CM was found to be superior to MET/CBT alone in promoting abstinence, but it was not as robust during posttreatment assessments (Kamon, Budney, & Stanger, 2005; Stanger, Budney, Kamon, & Thostensen, 2009). Similar to the adult studies, CM strategies used alone or in combination with MET/CBT in youth seem to be most effective in promoting abstinence. Unfortunately, the reduction or cessation of cannabis use elicited by CM is often not maintained after active treatment is ended. Several studies indicate that CM helps promote abstinence initially and CBT maintains it, leading to greater improvement after CM (Carroll & Rounsaville, 2007). In both adults and young adults, abstinence is difficult to achieve with psychotherapy alone. Thus, the combination of both psychotherapy and medications might enhance this goal. The overall conclusion in most adolescent studies is that psychotherapies are helpful, but superior when CM is implemented with the psychotherapy.

Pharmacotherapies

There is a growing interest in developing pharmacological treatments for cannabis dependence. Several laboratory and clinical studies have been conducted to date evaluating various pharmacological agents for treatment of cannabis dependence. We discuss in this section the different pharmacological agents studied by class.

Mood Stabilizers

Both lithium and valproate have been studied as treatments for cannabis dependence and have produced mixed results. In a small (*n* = 9) community-based, open-label study of the effects of lithium on non-treatment-seeking individuals meeting DSM-IV criteria for cannabis dependence, a variable response was reported (Bowen, McIlwrick, Baetz, & Zhang, 2005). In a subsequent open trial Winstock, Lea, and Copeland (2009) provided evidence that lithium has potential as a safe, acceptable, and clinically useful treatment modality for the alleviation of many commonly experienced symptoms of cannabis withdrawal. Follow-up of study participants showed a high rate of abstinence from cannabis use and also reductions in symptoms of depression and anxiety, and cannabis-related problems. However, placebo-controlled trials are needed to determine lithium's clinical efficacy.

Alternatively, valproate has not been found to be useful in reducing cannabis withdrawal symptoms. In a randomized, double-blind, placebo-controlled crossover laboratory trial of depakote in seven non-treatment-seeking cannabis users, the investigators found decreased ratings of cannabis craving during withdrawal but increased ratings of anxiety, irritability, and tiredness (Haney et al., 2004). When Levin et al. (2004) conducted a small (*n* = 25), double-blind treatment trial comparing depakote sodium to placebo, both groups reduced their cannabis use, but there was no difference between the groups, and medication adherence was poor.

Gabapentin was studied in a 12-week, randomized, double-blind, placebo-controlled clinical trial of 50 treatment-seeking outpatients diagnosed with current cannabis dependence. Subjects received either gabapentin (1,200 mg/day) or matched placebo. Although study completion was low (36%), gabapentin was found to significantly reduce cannabis use, decrease withdrawal symptoms, and improve overall performance on tests of executive function (Mason et al., 2012). While this is promising, larger controlled trials are needed to determine whether gabapentin is an effective treatment for cannabis dependence.

Antidepressants and Anxiolytics

Several antidepressants have been studied to assess their effectiveness in treating both withdrawal and relapse. Laboratory studies have been conducted in non-treatment-seeking heavy cannabis users, whereas outpatient trials have been primarily conducted in cannabis-dependent treatment seekers. Bupropion is an effective treatment for nicotine dependence, and it was hypothesized that bupropion might be effective in treating cannabis dependence. Using a randomized, double-blind, placebo-controlled, crossover design, bupropion SR was found to worsen irritability, restlessness, depression, and sleeping difficulties associated with withdrawal (Haney et al., 2001).

In another trial, Haney (2002) evaluated nefazodone and found that it reduced anxiety but not other withdrawal symptoms, and it did not change subjective effects of smoked cannabis. A subsequent treatment study compared nefazodone and bupropion to placebo in a randomized controlled trial of 106 cannabis-abusing adults. While all three treatment arms demonstrated improvement, none was superior (Carpenter, McDowell, Brooks, Cheng, & Levin, 2009). Haney et al. (2010) evaluated the effects of mirtazapine in the laboratory and found that it improved sleep during abstinence and increased food intake but had no effect on other withdrawal symptoms; moreover, it did not decrease self-administration after a period of cannabis abstinence.

Finally, McRae, Brady, and Carter (2006) conducted a double-blind treatment trial in 50 cannabis-dependent adults, comparing buspirone to placebo, and found that the active treatment group had greater reductions in craving and irritability, and a trend toward a greater percentage of negative urinalyses. However, the high dropout rate makes it difficult to draw conclusions regarding the medication's utility. Taken together, antidepressants might have clinical utility, particularly those with sedative properties, and anxiolytic agents might reduce cannabis use, but further investigation is needed.

ADHD Medications/Stimulant-Like Drugs

Individuals with cannabis dependence often have difficulties with concentration and executive functioning (Solowij et al., 2002), and some individuals are likely to have ADHD. Atomoxetine, approved for the treatment of adult ADHD, was shown to reduce cannabis use in an open clinical trial of cannabis-dependent individuals without ADHD, but it was poorly tolerated and produced marked gastrointestinal side effects (Tirado, Goldman, Lynch, Kampman, & O'Brien, 2008). In a double-blind, placebo-controlled outpatient study, modafinil has also been found to reduce the euphoria associated with oral THC (Sugarman, Poling, & Sofuoglu, 2011) but more investigation is needed.

Antagonists

Antagonist medications have been extensively studied for other drug classes and have been found to be effective as long as adherence is ensured (Garbutt, West, Carey, Lohr, & Crews, 1999). While naltrexone is not necessarily considered an antagonist for cannabis dependence, there is evidence that some of cannabis's subjective and potential amelioration of pain is mediated through the opiate system (Haney, 2007). Notably, naltrexone was found to reduce the discriminative effects of THC in animals (Solinas & Goldberg, 2005) and also self-administration (Justinova, Tanda, Munzar, & Goldberg, 2004). Contrasting this, in human laboratory studies, naltrexone did not reduce the effects of oral THC in participants pretreated with naltrexone (Wachtel & de Wit, 2000). Similarly, at both low and high doses, pretreatment with naltrexone in non-treatment-seeking cannabis users did not reduce the subjective effects of oral THC (Haney, 2007) and actually enhanced THC's pleasurable effects (Cooper & Haney, 2010). However, a recent study indicated that when naltrexone was given a couple hours prior to smoking cannabis, it did not change the subjective effects of THC (Ranganathan et al., 2012). While naltrexone may indirectly act as a cannabinoid antagonist, rimonabant, a partial CB_1 receptor antagonist, has been evaluated in heavy cannabis users under laboratory conditions. An initial study indicated that rimonabant significantly reduced the subjective and physiological effects of smoked cannabis (Huestis et al., 2001). However, a subsequent study showed inconsistent effects (Huestis et al., 2007). Rimonabant is unlikely to be available for future use, because it was not approved for treatment of obesity, due to its to its propensity to produce depressive symptoms and suicidal ideation.

Agonists

The primary psychoactive cannabinoid in cannabis is THC. Therefore, using oral THC (dronabinol), a partial agonist, may be an effective substitution agent to treat cannabis withdrawal and facilitate abstinence. Laboratory studies have shown that oral THC reduces the positive subjective effects of smoked cannabis (Hart et al., 2002) and also decreased rates of cannabis withdrawal and craving (Haney et al., 2004). In an outpatient study of non-treatment-seeking heavy cannabis users, Budney, Vandrey, Hughes, Moore, and Bahrenburg (2007) found that high-dose oral THC significantly alleviated withdrawal symptoms. However, oral THC has not been found to reduce self-administration (Hart et al., 2002), even after a period of abstinence (Haney et al., 2008). Two case reports of outpatients suggest that oral THC may be effective in reducing cannabis use and facilitating abstinence (Levin & Kleber, 2008). In the largest randomized controlled pharmacological trial to date, oral THC was compared to placebo in cannabis-dependent adults (Levin et al., 2011). Those receiving oral THC had greater treatment retention and reduction in withdrawal symptoms. However, there were no group differences in reductions in cannabis use or abstinence rates.

Combination

Since oral THC has shown some promise, and lofexidine, an alpha$_2$ receptor agonist, has been useful for opiate withdrawal, these medications were evaluated alone and in combination in a laboratory setting with eight heavy users of cannabis. The combination was superior to the other conditions in alleviating withdrawal symptoms. Moreover, both the combination and lofexidine alone were superior to placebo in reducing self-administration after a period of abstinence (Haney et al., 2008). This promising combination is currently being investigated among treatment seekers in an outpatient setting.

Other

N-acetylcysteine (NAC) has also been investigated for the treatment of cannabis dependence. NAC has been shown to reduce reinstatement of drug-seeking behavior in animals, possibly through modification of glutaminergic transmission via the cystine–glutamate exchanger (LaRowe et al., 2006; Kau et al., 2008). An open trial in adolescents found that the agent was well-tolerated, with a reduction in self-reported use, although urinalysis results did not change. A larger trial in adolescents found that those on NAC, along with contingency reinforcement for negative urinalyses, were more likely to provide negative urine results than the placebo arm that also received contingency reinforcement (Gray, Watson, Carpenter, & LaRowe, 2010). Because CM was the behavioral platform, it is unclear whether these findings will apply to cannabis-dependent individuals who are administered NAC without CM interventions. Baclofen, a GABA-B receptor agonist and antispasmodic medication, has sedating properties and has been hypothesized to improve agitation and sleep disruption. In a placebo-controlled laboratory study, baclofen was found to reduce craving, but mood symptoms were not affected, and it did not reduce self-administration after cannabis abstinence (Haney et al., 2010). Thus, the data supporting the potential benefit of baclofen as a treatment for cannabis dependence are limited.

Dual Diagnosis

There is a strong association between cannabis dependence and psychiatric disorders. This may be due to attempts at self-medication (Cornelius et al., 1999), or psychiatric symptoms may be a direct effect of the cannabis use. Although few clinical treatment trials have looked directly at cannabis dependence and psychiatric comorbidity, some studies have indicated that medications are effective in reducing cannabis use and craving. For example, in a small, open trial of cannabis-dependent individuals with bipolar illness or schizophrenia, quetiapine reduced their cannabis use (Potvin, Stip, & Roy, 2004). In a secondary analysis of adult cannabis users entering a double-blind, randomized, placebo-controlled trial for depressed alcoholics, those receiving fluoxetine were more likely than the placebo group to reduce their amount and frequency of cannabis use (Cornelius et al., 1999).

However, another study that evaluated depressed adolescents seeking treatment for their problematic cannabis use indicated that fluoxetine was not superior in reducing depressive symptoms compared to placebo, and there was no reduction in cannabis use. A recent double-blind trial of cannabis-dependent adults with depressive disorders found that venlafaxine extended release was not superior to placebo in reducing depressive symptoms (Levin et al., 2012). Strikingly, the venlafaxine group had greater severity of withdrawal symptoms than the placebo group and were less likely to achieve abstinence. To date, there has been little research evaluating treatment options for patients with ADHD and cannabis use disorders. In a small, double-blind, randomized trial of cannabis-dependent adolescents with ADHD, atomoxetine was not superior to placebo in reducing ADHD symptoms or cannabis use (Thurstone, Riggs, Salomonsen-Sautel, & Mikulich-Gilbertson, 2010). The small sample size and high dropout rate may have precluded finding significant differences. Non-stimulants, which usually have smaller effect sizes compared to stimulant ADHD medications, may be less effective in drug-abusing populations.

Furthermore, in another study of adult cannabis abusers with ADHD, atomoxetine was not superior to placebo in reducing ADHD symptoms or cannabis use (McRae-Clark et al., 2010); suggesting that atomoxetine may not be useful in this dually disordered population.

Riggs et al. (2011) studied the effects of osmotic-release oral system (OROS) methylphenidate treatment in adolescent substance abusers with ADHD and found that the active treatment was superior to placebo on secondary outcome measures of ADHD but not on primary outcome measures. While there were no differences in drug use for the OROS methylphenidate or placebo arms, there was significantly greater improvement in the Clinician Global Improvement Scale and less positive urinalyses for those receiving OROS methylphenidate (Riggs et al., 2011). Although the findings are not wholly positive, the data suggest that improvement of ADHD symptoms may lead to reduction in use among those receiving active medication.

CONCLUSION

Cannabis use is a public health concern that is steadily worsening in terms of the extent of use, the perception of risk, and the costs associated with it. With the widespread availability of cannabis, it is important to note the added risks that chronic cannabis use may pose in those with comorbid psychiatric disorders.

There is growing evidence of an association between chronic cannabis use and the onset or exacerbation of mental illness. Discouraging cannabis use in vulnerable populations may improve overall functionality. As described earlier in the treatment section, several controlled cannabis treatment trials have reported results supporting the use of cognitive-behavioral interventions, MET, and CM. While there are no definitve pharmacological treatments for cannabis dependence, several pharmacotherapies appear to be helpful in alleviating withdrawal symptoms and reduce use. Due to the high prevalence of regular cannabis use in the United States, particularly among young people with comorbid mental illness, it is important to focus on both prevention and treatment.

More research is needed to clarify the most effective way to treat cannabis-dependent individuals.

REFERENCES

Agosti, V., Nunes, E., & Levin, F. (2002). Rates of psychiatric comorbidity among U.S. residents with lifetime cannabis dependence. *Am J Drug Alcohol Abuse, 28*, 643–652.

Alpert, J. E., Maddocks, A., Rosenbaum, J. F., & Fava, M. (1994). Childhood psychopathology retrospectively assessed among adults with early onset major depression. *J Affect Disord, 31*, 165–171.

Ameri, A. (1999). The effects of cannabinoids on the brain. *Prog Neurobiol, 58*, 315–348.

American Psychiatric Association. (2000). *Diagnostic and statistical manual of mental disorders* (4th ed., text rev.). Washington, DC, Author.

American Psychiatric Association. (2013). *Diagnostic and statistical manual of mental disorders* (5th ed.). Arlington, VA: Author.

Andreasson, S., & Allebeck, P. (1990). Cannabis and mortality among young men: A longitudinal study of Swedish conscripts. *Scand J Soc Med, 18*, 9–15.

Andreasson, S., Allebeck, P., Engstrom, A., & Rydberg, U. (1988). Cannabis and schizophrenia. *Lancet, 1*, 1000–1001.

Arendt, M., Rosenberg, R., Foldager, L., Perto, G., & Munk-Jorgensen, P. (2007). Psychopathology among cannabis-dependent treatment seekers and association with later substance abuse treatment. *J Subst Abuse Treat, 32*, 113–119.

Arseneault, L., Cannon, M., Poulton, R., Murray, R., Caspi, A., & Moffitt, T. E. (2002). Cannabis use in adolescence and risk for adult psychosis: Longitudinal prospective study. *BMJ, 325*, 1212–1213.

Arseneault, L., Cannon, M., Witton, J., & Murray, R. M. (2004). Causal association between cannabis and psychosis: Examination of the evidence. *Br J Psychiatry, 184*, 110–117.

Azrin, N. H., McMahon, P. T., Donohue, B., Besalel, V. A., Lapinski, K. J., Kogan, E. S., et al. (1994). Behavior therapy for drug abuse: A controlled treatment outcome study. *Behav Res Ther, 32*, 857–866.

Bachman, J. G., Johnson, L. D., & O'Malley, P. M. (1998). Explaining recent increases in students' marijuana use: Impacts of perceived risks and disapproval, 1976 through 1996. *Am J Public Health, 88*, 887–892.

Ben Amar, M. (2006). Cannabinoids in medicine: A review of their therapeutic potential. *J Ethnopharmacol, 105*, 1–25.

Biederman, J. (2003). Pharmacotherapy for attention-deficit/hyperactivity disorder (ADHD) decreases the risk for substance abuse: Findings from a longitudinal follow-up of youths with and without ADHD. *J Clin Psychiatry, 64*(Suppl. 11), 3–8.

Biederman, J., Wilens, T., Mick, E., Faraone, S. V., Weber, W., Curtis, S., et al. (1997). Is ADHD a risk factor for psychoactive substance use disorders?: Findings from a four-year prospective follow-up study. *J Am Acad Child Adolesc Psychiatry, 36*, 21–29.

Biederman, J., Wilens, T., Mick, E., Milberger, S., Spencer, T. J., & Faraone, S. V. (1995). Psychoactive substance use disorders in adults with attention deficit hyperactivity disorder (ADHD): Effects of ADHD and psychiatric comorbidity. *Am J Psychiatry, 152*, 1652–1658.

Bonnie, R. J., & Whitebread, C. H., II. (1974). *The Marijuana conviction: A history of marijuana prohibition in the United States.* Charlottesville: University of Virginia Press.

Bowen, R., McIlwrick, J., Baetz, M., & Zhang, X. (2005). Lithium and marijuana withdrawal. *Can J Psychiatry, 50*, 240–241.

Buckner, J. D., Bonn-Miller, M. O., Zvolensky, M. J., & Schmidt, N. B. (2007). Marijuana use motives and social anxiety among marijuana-using young adults. *Addict Behav, 32*, 2238–2252.

Buckner, J. D., & Carroll, K. M. (2010). Effect of anxiety on treatment presentation and outcome: results from the Marijuana Treatment Project. *Psychiatry Res, 178*, 493–500.

Buckner, J. D., & Schmidt, N. B. (2008). Marijuana effect expectancies: relations to social anxiety and marijuana use problems. *Addict Behav, 33*, 1477–1483.

Budney, A. J., & Hughes, J. R. (2006). The cannabis withdrawal syndrome. *Curr Opin Psychiatry, 19*, 233–238.

Budney, A. J., & Moore, B. A. (2002). Development and consequences of cannabis dependence. *J Clin Pharmacol, 42*, 28S–33S.

Budney, A. J., Vandrey, R. G., Hughes, J. R., Moore, B. A., & Bahrenburg, B. (2007). Oral delta-9-tetrahydrocannabinol suppresses cannabis withdrawal symptoms. *Drug Alcohol Depend, 86*, 22–29.

Budney, A. J., Vandrey, R. G., & Stanger, C. (2010). [Pharmacological and psychosocial interventions for cannabis use disorders]. *Rev Bras Psiquiatr, 32*(Suppl. 1), S46–S55.

Butler, H., & Korbonits, M. (2009). Cannabinoids for clinicians: The rise and fall of the cannabinoid antagonists. *Eur J Endocrinol, 161*, 655–662.

Carpenter, K. M., McDowell, D., Brooks, D. J., Cheng, W. Y., & Levin, F. R. (2009). A preliminary trial: double-blind comparison of nefazodone, bupropion-SR, and placebo in the treatment of cannabis dependence. *Am J Addict, 18*, 53–64.

Carroll, K. M., & Rounsaville, B. J. (2007). A perfect platform: Combining contingency management with medications for drug abuse. *Am J Drug Alcohol Abuse, 33*, 343–365.

Cheung, J. T., Mann, R. E., Ialomiteanu, A., Stoduto, G., Chan, V., Ala-Leppilampi, K., et al. (2010). Anxiety and mood disorders and cannabis use. *Am J Drug Alcohol Abuse, 36*, 118–122.

Clark, H. W., & Power, A. K. (2005). Women, Co-occurring Disorders, and Violence Study: A case for trauma-informed care. *J Subst Abuse Treat, 28*, 145–146.

Clure, C., Brady, K. T., Saladin, M. E., Johnson, D., Waid, R., & Rittenbury, M. (1999). Attention-deficit/hyperactivity disorder and substance use: Symptom pattern and drug choice. *Am J Drug Alcohol Abuse, 25*, 441–448.

Coffey, C., Lynskey, M., Wolfe, R., & Patton, G. C. (2000). Initiation and progression of cannabis use in a population-based Australian adolescent longitudinal study. *Addiction, 95,* 1679–1690.

Compton, W. M., Grant, B. F., Colliver, J. D., Glantz, M. D., & Stinson, F. S. (2004). Prevalence of marijuana use disorders in the United States: 1991–1992 and 2001–2002. *JAMA, 291,* 2114–2121.

Cooper, Z. D., & Haney, M. (2010). Opioid antagonism enhances marijuana's effects in heavy marijuana smokers. *Psychopharmacology (Berl), 211,* 141–148.

Copeland, J., Swift, W., Roffman, R., & Stephens, R. (2001). A randomized controlled trial of brief cognitive-behavioral interventions for cannabis use disorder. *J Subst Abuse Treat, 21,* 55–64; discussion 65–66.

Cornelius, J. R., Kirisci, L., Reynolds, M., Clark, D. B., Hayes, J., & Tarter, R. (2010). PTSD contributes to teen and young adult cannabis use disorders. *Addict Behav, 35,* 91–94.

Cornelius, J. R., Salloum, I. M., Haskett, R. F., Ehler, J. G., Jarrett, P. J., Thase, M. E., et al. (1999). Fluoxetine versus placebo for the marijuana use of depressed alcoholics. *Addict Behav, 24,* 111–114.

Cougle, J. R., Bonn-Miller, M. O., Vujanovic, A. A., Zvolensky, M. J., & Hawkins, K. A. (2011). Posttraumatic stress disorder and cannabis use in a nationally representative sample. *Psychol Addict Behav, 25,* 554–558.

Degenhardt, L., Dierker, L., Chiu, W. T., Medina-Mora, M. E., Neumark, Y., Sampson, N., et al. (2010). Evaluating the drug use "gateway" theory using cross-national data: Consistency and associations of the order of initiation of drug use among participants in the WHO World Mental Health Surveys. *Drug Alcohol Depend, 108,* 84–97.

Degenhardt, L., Hall, W., & Lynskey, M. (2003). Exploring the association between cannabis use and depression. *Addiction, 98,* 1493–1504.

Degenhardt, L., Tennant, C., Gilmour, S., Schofield, D., Nash, L., Hall, W., et al. (2007). The temporal dynamics of relationships between cannabis, psychosis and depression among young adults with psychotic disorders: Findings from a 10-month prospective study. *Psychol Med, 37,* 927–934.

Dennis, M., Godley, S. H., Diamond, G., Tims, F. M., Babor, T., Donaldson, J., et al. (2004). The Cannabis Youth Treatment (CYT) Study: Main findings from two randomized trials. *J Subst Abuse Treat, 27,* 197–213.

Driessen, M., Schulte, S., Luedecke, C., Schaefer, I., Sutmann, F., Ohlmeier, M., et al. (2008). Trauma and PTSD in patients with alcohol, drug, or dual dependence: A multi-center study. *Alcohol Clin Exp Res, 32,* 481–488.

Drug Enforcement Agency. (2011). Schedules of controlled substances: Temporary placement of five synthetic cannabinoids into Schedule I. *Fed Regist, 76*(40), 11075–11078.

D'Souza, D. C., Perry, E., MacDougall, L., Ammerman, Y., Cooper, T., Wu, Y. T., et al. (2004). The psychotomimetic effects of intravenous delta-9-tetrahydrocannabinol in healthy individuals: Implications for psychosis. *Neuropsychopharmacology, 29,* 1558–1572.

Ehrenreich, H., Rinn, T., Kunert, H. J., Moeller, M. R., Poser, W., Schilling, L., et al. (1999). Specific attentional dysfunction in adults following early start of cannabis use. *Psychopharmacology (Berl), 142,* 295–301.

Erowid Vaults. (2010). Cannabis: Legal status. Retrieved from *erowid.org.*

Fergusson, D. M., & Boden, J. M. (2008). Cannabis use and adult ADHD symptoms. *Drug Alcohol Depend, 95,* 90–96.

Fergusson, D. M., & Horwood, L. J. (2000). Does cannabis use encourage other forms of illicit drug use? *Addiction, 95,* 505–520.

Frisher, M., Crome, I., Martino, O., & Croft, P. (2009). Assessing the impact of cannabis use on trends in diagnosed schizophrenia in the United Kingdom from 1996 to 2005. *Schizophr Res, 113,* 123–128.

Garbutt, J. C., West, S. L., Carey, T. S., Lohr, K. N., & Crews, F. T. (1999). Pharmacological treatment of alcohol dependence: A review of the evidence. *JAMA, 281,* 1318–1325.

Gray, K. M., Watson, N. L., Carpenter, M. J., & Larowe, S. D. (2010). *N*-Acetylcysteine (NAC) in young marijuana users: An open-label pilot study. *Am J Addict, 19,* 187–189.

Hall, W. (2006a). Is cannabis use psychotogenic? *Lancet, 367,* 193–195.

Hall, W. D. (2006b). Cannabis use and the mental health of young people. *Aust N Z J Psychiatry, 40,* 105–113.

Hall, W., & Degenhardt, L. (2000). Cannabis use and psychosis: A review of clinical and epidemiological evidence. *Aust N Z J Psychiatry, 34,* 26–34.

Hall, W., & Degenhardt, L. (2007). Prevalence and correlates of cannabis use in developed and developing countries. *Curr Opin Psychiatry, 20,* 393–397.

Haney, M. (2002). Effects of smoked marijuana in healthy and HIV + marijuana smokers. *J Clin Pharmacol, 42,* 34S–40S.

Haney, M. (2007). Opioid antagonism of cannabinoid effects: Differences between marijuana smokers and nonmarijuana smokers. *Neuropsychopharmacology, 32,* 1391–1403.

Haney, M., Hart, C. L., Vosburg, S. K., Comer, S. D., Reed, S. C., Cooper, Z. D., et al. (2010). Effects of baclofen and mirtazapine on a laboratory model of marijuana withdrawal and relapse. *Psychopharmacology (Berl), 211,* 233–244.

Haney, M., Hart, C. L., Vosburg, S. K., Comer, S. D., Reed, S. C., & Foltin, R. W. (2008). Effects of THC and lofexidine in a human laboratory model of marijuana withdrawal and relapse. *Psychopharmacology (Berl), 197,* 157–168.

Haney, M., Hart, C. L., Vosburg, S. K., Nasser, J., Bennett, A., Zubaran, C., et al. (2004). Marijuana withdrawal in humans: Effects of oral THC or divalproex. *Neuropsychopharmacology, 29,* 158–170.

Haney, M., Ward, A. S., Comer, S. D., Hart, C. L., Foltin, R. W., & Fischman, M. W. (2001). Bupropion SR worsens mood during marijuana withdrawal in humans. *Psychopharmacology (Berl), 155,* 171–179.

Hao, W., Xiao, S., Liu, T., Young, D., Chen, S., Zhang, D., et al. (2002). The second National Epidemiological Survey on illicit drug use at six high-prevalence areas in China: Prevalence rates and use patterns. *Addiction, 97,* 1305–1315.

Hart, C. L., Ward, A. S., Haney, M., Comer, S. D., Foltin, R. W., & Fischman, M. W. (2002). Comparison of smoked marijuana and oral Delta(9)-tetrahydrocannabinol in humans. *Psychopharmacology (Berl), 164,* 407–415.

Harvey, M. A., Sellman, J. D., Porter, R. J., & Frampton, C. M. (2007). The relationship between non-acute adolescent cannabis use and cognition. *Drug Alcohol Rev, 26,* 309–319.

Henggeler, S. W., Halliday-Boykins, C. A., Cunningham, P. B., Randall, J., Shapiro, S. B., & Chapman, J. E. (2006). Juvenile drug court: Enhancing outcomes by integrating evidence-based treatments. *J Consult Clin Psychol, 74,* 42–54.

Hu, X., Primack, B. A., Barnett, T. E., & Cook, R. L. (2011). College students and use of K2: An emerging drug of abuse in young persons. *Subst Abuse Treat Prev Policy, 6,* 16.

Huestis, M. A., Boyd, S. J., Heishman, S. J., Preston, K. L., Bonnet, D., Le Fur, G., et al. (2007). Single and multiple doses of rimonabant antagonize acute effects of smoked cannabis in male cannabis users. *Psychopharmacology (Berl), 194,* 505–515.

Huestis, M. A., Gorelick, D. A., Heishman, S. J., Preston, K. L., Nelson, R. A., Moolchan, E. T., et al. (2001). Blockade of effects of smoked marijuana by the CB$_1$-selective cannabinoid receptor antagonist SR141716. *Arch Gen Psychiatry, 58,* 322–328.

Iversen, L. (2003). Cannabis and the brain. *Brain, 126,* 1252–1270.

Johnston, L., O'Malley, P. M., Bachman, J. G., & Schulenberg, J. E. (2009). *Monitoring the Future national survey results on drug use, 1975–2008: Vol. I. Secondary school students* (NIH Publication No. 09-7402). Bethesda, MD: NIDA.

Justinova, Z., Tanda, G., Munzar, P., & Goldberg, S. R. (2004). The opioid antagonist naltrexone reduces the reinforcing effects of delta 9 tetrahydrocannabinol (THC) in squirrel monkeys. *Psychopharmacology (Berl), 173,* 186–194.

Kamon, J., Budney, A., & Stanger, C. (2005). A contingency management intervention for adolescent marijuana abuse and conduct problems. *J Am Acad Child Adolesc Psychiatry, 44,* 513–521.

Kandel, D. B., & Davies, M. (1986). Adult sequelae of adolescent depressive symptoms. *Arch Gen Psychiatry, 43,* 255–262.

Katerndahl, D. A., & Realini, J. P. (1993). Lifetime prevalence of panic states. *Am J Psychiatry, 150,* 246–249.

Kau, K. S., Madayag, A., Mantsch, J. R., Grier, M. D., Abdulhameed, O., & Baker, D. A. (2008). Blunted cystine–glutamate antiporter function in the nucleus accumbens promotes cocaine-induced drug seeking. *Neuroscience, 155,* 530–537.

Kessler, R. C., Chiu, W. T., Demler, O., & Walters, E. E. (2005). Prevalence, severity, and comorbidity of twelve-month DSM-IV disorders in the National Comorbidity Survey Replication (NCS-R). *Arch Gen Psychiatry, 62,* 617–627.

Kilpatrick, D. G., Acierno, R., Saunders, B., Resnick, H. S., Best, C. L., & Schnurr, P. P. (2000). Risk factors for adolescent substance abuse and dependence: Data from a national sample. *J Consult Clin Psychol, 68,* 19–30.

Kilpatrick, D. G., Ruggiero, K. J., Acierno, R., Saunders, B. E., Resnick, H. S., & Best, C. L. (2003). Violence and risk of PTSD, major depression, substance abuse/dependence, and comorbidity: results from the National Survey of Adolescents. *J Consult Clin Psychol, 71,* 692–700.

Kouri, E. M., & Pope, H. G., Jr. (2000). Abstinence symptoms during withdrawal from chronic marijuana use. *Exp Clin Psychopharmacol, 8,* 483–492.

Kouri, E. M., Pope, H. G., Jr., & Lukas, S. E. (1999). Changes in aggressive behavior during withdrawal from long-term marijuana use. *Psychopharmacology (Berl), 143,* 302–308.

Kouri, E., Pope, H. G., Jr., Yurgelun-Todd, D., & Gruber, S. (1995). Attributes of heavy vs. occasional marijuana smokers in a college population. *Biol Psychiatry, 38,* 475–481.

Lambert, M., Conus, P., Lubman, D. I., Wade, D., Yuen, H., Moritz, S., et al. (2005). The impact of substance use disorders on clinical outcome in 643 patients with first-episode psychosis. *Acta Psychiatr Scand, 112,* 141–148.

Large, M., Sharma, S., Compton, M. T., Slade, T., & Nielssen, O. (2011). Cannabis use and earlier onset of psychosis: A systematic meta-analysis. *Arch Gen Psychiatry, 68,* 555–561.

LaRowe, S. D., Mardikian, P., Malcolm, R., Myrick, H., Kalivas, P., McFarland, K., et al. (2006). Safety and tolerability of *N*-acetylcysteine in cocaine-dependent individuals. *Am J Addict, 15,* 105–110.

Levin, F. R., & Kleber, H. D. (2008). Use of dronabinol for cannabis dependence: Two case reports and review. *Am J Addict, 17,* 161–164.

Levin, F. R., Mariani, J. J., Brooks, D. J., Pavlicova, M., Cheng, W., & Nunes, E. V. (2011). Dronabinol for the treatment of cannabis dependence: A randomized, double-blind, placebo-controlled trial. *Drug Alcohol Depend, 116,* 142–150.

Levin, F. R., Mariani, J. J., Paulicova, M., Brooks, D. J., Nunes, E. V., Agosti, V., et al. (2012, June 9–14). *Venlaxafine treatment lowers abstinence rates in marijuana-dependent adults with depression.* Presented at the College on Problems of Drug Dependence 74th Annual Scientific Meeting, Palm Springs, CA.

Levin, F. R., McDowell, D., Evans, S. M., Nunes, E., Akerele, E., Donovan, S., et al. (2004). Pharmacotherapy for marijuana dependence: A double-blind, placebo-controlled pilot study of divalproex sodium. *Am J Addict, 13,* 21–32.

Linszen, D. H., Dingemans, P. M., & Lenior, M. E. (1994). Cannabis abuse and the course of recent-onset schizophrenic disorders. *Arch Gen Psychiatry, 51,* 273–279.

Lubman, D. I., Allen, N. B., Rogers, N., Cementon, E., & Bonomo, Y. (2007). The impact of co-occurring mood and anxiety disorders among substance-abusing youth. *J Affect Disord, 103,* 105–112.

Lundqvist, T. (2005). Cognitive consequences of cannabis use: Comparison with abuse of stimulants and heroin with regard to attention, memory and executive functions. *Pharmacol Biochem Behav, 81,* 319–330.

Lynskey, M., White, V., Hill, D., Letcher, T., & Hall, W. (1999). Prevalence of illicit drug use among youth: Results from the Australian School Students' Alcohol and Drugs Survey. *Aust N Z J Public Health, 23,* 519–524.

MacDonald, S., Anglin-Bodrug, K., Mann, R. E., Erickson, P., Hathaway, A., Chipman, M., et al. (2003). Injury risk associated with cannabis and cocaine use. *Drug Alcohol Depend, 72,* 99–115.

Marijuana Treatment Project Research Group. (2004). Brief treatments for cannabis dependence: Findings from a randomized multisite trial. *J Consult Clin Psychol, 72,* 455–466.

Mason, B. J., Crean, R., Goodell, V., Light, J. M., Quello, S., Shadan, F., et al. (2012). A proof-of-concept randomized controlled study of gabapentin: Effects on cannabis use, withdrawal and executive function deficits in cannabis-dependent adults. *Neuropsychopharmacology, 37,* 1689–1698.

Mathers, D. C., & Ghodse, A. H. (1992). Cannabis and psychotic illness. *Br J Psychiatry, 161,* 648–653.

McRae, A. L., Brady, K. T., & Carter, R. E. (2006). Buspirone for treatment of marijuana dependence: A pilot study. *Am J Addict, 15,* 404.

McRae-Clark, A. L., Carter, R. E., Killeen, T. K., Carpenter, M. J., White, K. G., & Brady, K. T. (2010). A placebo-controlled trial of atomoxetine in marijuana-dependent individuals with attention deficit hyperactivity disorder. *Am J Addict, 19,* 481–489.

Merikangas, K. R., Mehta, R. L., Molnar, B. E., Walters, E. E., Swendsen, J. D., Aguilar-Gaziola, S., et al. (1998). Comorbidity of substance use disorders with mood and anxiety disorders: Results of the International Consortium in Psychiatric Epidemiology. *Addict Behav, 23,* 893–907.

Messinis, L., Kyprianidou, A., Malefaki, S., & Papathanasopoulos, P. (2006). Neuropsychological deficits in long-term frequent cannabis users. *Neurology, 66,* 737–739.

Mir, A., Obafemi, A., Young, A., & Kane, C. (2011). Myocardial infarction associated with use of the synthetic cannabinoid K2. *Pediatrics, 128,* e1622–e1627.

Moore, T. H., Zammit, S., Lingford-Hughes, A., Barnes, T. R., Jones, P. B., Burke, M., et al. (2007). Cannabis use and risk of psychotic or affective mental health outcomes: A systematic review. *Lancet, 370,* 319–328.

Morgan, C. J., & Curran, H. V. (2008). Effects of cannabidiol on schizophrenia-like symptoms in people who use cannabis. *Br J Psychiatry, 192,* 306–307.

Morral, A. R., Mccaffrey, D. F., & Paddock, S. M. (2002). Reassessing the marijuana gateway effect. *Addiction, 97,* 1493–1504.

Muller, H., Sperling, W., Kohrmann, M., Huttner, H. B., Kornhuber, J., & Maler, J. M. (2010). The synthetic cannabinoid Spice as a trigger for an acute exacerbation of cannabis induced recurrent psychotic episodes. *Schizophr Res, 118,* 309–310.

National Center for Health Statistics, Office of Information Services. (2013, August). *National Health Interview Survey (NHIS): 2012 data release.* Retrieved from *http://www.cdc.gov/nchs/nhis/nhis_2012_data_release.htm.*

National Institute on Drug Abuse. (2011). *Topics in brief: Marijuana.* Washington, DC: U.S. Department of Health and Human Services.

National Survey on Drug Use and Health (NSDUH). (2009). *Results from the 2008 National Survey on Drug Use and Health: National findings.* Rockville, MD: Substance Abuse and Mental Health Services Administration.

Negrete, J. C. (2003). Clinical aspects of substance abuse in persons with schizophrenia. *Can J Psychiatry, 48,* 14–21.

Neuspiel, D. R. (2007). Marijuana. *Pediatr Rev, 28,* 156–157.

Osgood, D. W., Johnston, L. D., O'Malley, P. M., & Bachman, J. G. (1988). The generality of deviance in late adolescence and early adulthood. *Am Sociol Rev, 53,* 81–93.

Owens, P. L., Mutter, R., & Stocks, C. (2007). *Mental health and substance abuse-related emergency department visits among adults, 2007* (Statistical Brief #92). Rockville, MD: Agency for Healthcare Research and Quality.

Patton, G. C., Coffey, C., Carlin, J. B., Degenhardt, L., Lynskey, M., & Hall, W. (2002). Cannabis use and mental health in young people: Cohort study. *BMJ, 325,* 1195–1198.

Pertwee, R. G. (2008). Ligands that target cannabinoid receptors in the brain: From THC to anandamide and beyond. *Addict Biol, 13,* 147–159.

Pope, H. G., Jr., Gruber, A. J., & Yurgelun-Todd, D. (2001). Residual neuropsychologic effects of cannabis. *Curr Psychiatry Rep, 3,* 507–512.

Potvin, S., Stip, E., & Roy, J. Y. (2004). The effect of quetiapine on cannabis use in 8 psychosis patients with drug dependency. *Can J Psychiatry, 49,* 711.

Radwan, M. M., Elsohly, M. A., Slade, D., Ahmed, S. A., Khan, I. A., & Ross, S. A. (2009). Biologically active cannabinoids from high-potency *Cannabis sativa. J Nat Prod, 72,* 906–911.

Ranganathan, M., Carbuto, M., Braley, G., Elander, J., Perry, E., Pittman, B., et al. (2012). Naltrexone does not attenuate the effects of intravenous delta-9-tetrahydrocannabinol in healthy humans. *Int J Neuropsychopharmacol, 15*(9), 1251–1264.

Raphael, B., Wooding, S., Stevens, G., & Connor, J. (2005). Comorbidity: Cannabis and complexity. *J Psychiatr Pract, 11,* 161–176.

Realini, J. P., & Katerndahl, D. A. (1993). Factors affecting the threshold for seeking care: The Panic Attack Care-Seeking Threshold (PACT) Study. *J Am Board Fam Pract, 6,* 215–223.

Reilly, D., Didcott, P., Swift, W., & Hall, W. (1998). Long-term cannabis use: Characteristics of users in an Australian rural area. *Addiction, 93,* 837–846.

Riggs, P. D., Winhusen, T., Davies, R. D., Leimberger, J. D., Mikulich-Gilbertson, S., Klein, C., et al. (2011). Randomized controlled trial of osmotic-release methylphenidate with cognitive-behavioral therapy in adolescents with attention-deficit/hyperactivity disorder and substance use disorders. *J Am Acad Child Adolesc Psychiatry, 50,* 903–914.

Schneir, A. B., Cullen, J., & Ly, B. T. (2011). "Spice" girls: Synthetic cannabinoid intoxication. *J Emerg Med, 40,* 296–299.

Sobanski, E. (2006). Psychiatric comorbidity in adults with attention-deficit/hyperactivity disorder (ADHD). *Eur Arch Psychiatry Clin Neurosci, 256*(Suppl. 1), i26–i31.

Solinas, M., & Goldberg, S. R. (2005). Involvement of mu-, delta- and kappa-opioid receptor subtypes in the discriminative-stimulus effects of delta-9-tetrahydrocannabinol (THC) in rats. *Psychopharmacology (Berl), 179,* 804–812.

Solowij, N., Stephens, R., Roffman, R. A., & Babor, T. (2002). Does marijuana use cause long-term cognitive deficits? *JAMA, 287,* 2653–2654.

Stanger, C., Budney, A. J., Kamon, J. L., & Thostensen, J. (2009). A randomized trial of contingency management for adolescent marijuana abuse and dependence. *Drug Alcohol Depend, 105,* 240–247.

Stowkowy, J., Addington, D., Liu, L., Hollowell, B., & Addington, J. (2012). Predictors of disengagement from treatment in an early psychosis program. *Schizophr Res, 136,* 7–12.

Sugarman, D. E., Poling, J., & Sofuoglu, M. (2011). The safety of modafinil in combination with oral 9-tetrahydrocannabinol in humans. *Pharmacol Biochem Behav, 98,* 94–100.

Sun, Y., & Bennett, A. (2007). Cannabinoids: A new group of agonists of PPARs. *PPAR Res, 2007,* 23513.

Swendsen, J. C. K., Degenhardt, L., Glantz, M., Jin, R., Merikangas, K. R., Sampson, N., et al. (2010). Mental disorders as risk factors for substance use, abuse and dependence: Results from the 10-year follow-up of the National Comorbidity Survey. *Addiction, 105*(6), 1117–1128.

Swift, W., Hall, W., Didcott, P., & Reilly, D. (1998). Patterns and correlates of cannabis dependence among long-term users in an Australian rural area. *Addiction, 93,* 1149–1160.

Szapocznik, J., Kurtines, W. M., Foote, F. H., Perez-Vidal, A., & Hervis, O. (1983). Conjoint versus one-person family therapy: Some evidence for the effectiveness of conducting family therapy through one person. *J Consult Clin Psychol, 51,* 889–899.

Tepe, E., Dalrymple, K., & Zimmerman, M. (2012). The impact of comorbid cannabis use disorders on the clinical presentation of social anxiety disorder. *J Psychiatr Res, 46,* 50–56.

Terry-McElrath, Y. M., O'Malley, P. M., & Johnston, L. D. (2014). Reasons for drug use among

American youth by consumption level, gender, and race/ethnicity: 1976–2005. *J Drug Issues, 39,* 677–714.

Thompson, L. L., Riggs, P. D., Mikulich, S. K., & Crowley, T. J. (1996). Contribution of ADHD symptoms to substance problems and delinquency in conduct-disordered adolescents. *J Abnorm Child Psychol, 24,* 325–347.

Thornicroft, G. (1990). Cannabis and psychosis: Is there epidemiological evidence for an association? *Br J Psychiatry, 157,* 25–33.

Thurstone, C., Riggs, P. D., Salomonsen-Sautel, S., & Mikulich-Gilbertson, S. K. (2010). Randomized, controlled trial of atomoxetine for attention-deficit/hyperactivity disorder in adolescents with substance use disorder. *J Am Acad Child Adolesc Psychiatry, 49,* 573–582.

Tirado, C. F., Goldman, M., Lynch, K., Kampman, K. M., & O'Brien, C. P. (2008). Atomoxetine for treatment of marijuana dependence: A report on the efficacy and high incidence of gastrointestinal adverse events in a pilot study. *Drug Alcohol Depend, 94,* 254–257.

Troisi, A., Vicario, E., Nuccetelli, F., Ciani, N., & Pasini, A. (1995). Effects of fluoxetine on aggressive behavior of adult inpatients with mental retardation and epilepsy. *Pharmacopsychiatry, 28,* 73–76.

United Nations Office on Drugs and Crime. (2006). World drug report 2006: Vol. 1. Analysis. Vienna: Author. Retrieved March 26, 2007, from *www.unodc.org/pdf/wdr_2006/wdr2006_volume1.pdf.*

Van Gundy, K., & Rebellon, C. J. (2010). A life-course perspective on the "gateway hypothesis." *J Health Soc Behav, 51,* 244–259.

Van Os, J., Bak, M., Hanssen, M., Bijl, R. V., De Graaf, R., & Verdoux, H. (2002). Cannabis use and psychosis: A longitudinal population-based study. *Am J Epidemiol, 156,* 319–327.

Wachtel, S. R., & de Wit, H. (2000). Naltrexone does not block the subjective effects of oral delta(9)-tetrahydrocannabinol in humans. *Drug Alcohol Depend, 59,* 251–260.

Waldron, H. B., & Turner, C. W. (2008). Evidence-based psychosocial treatment for adolescent substance abuse disorder. *J Clin Child Adolesc Psychol, 37*(1), 238–261.

Wallace, J. M., Jr., Vaughn, M. G., Bachman, J. G., O'malley, P. M., Johnston, L. D., & Schulenberg, J. E. (2009). Race/ethnicity, socioeconomic factors, and smoking among early adolescent girls in the United States. *Drug Alcohol Depend, 104*(Suppl. 1), S42–S49.

Ware, M. A., & St. Arnaud-Trempe, E. (2010). The abuse potential of the synthetic cannabinoid nabilone. *Addiction, 105,* 494–503.

Wiesbeck, G. A., Schuckit, M. A., Kalmijn, J. A., Tipp, J. E., Bucholz, K. K., & Smith, T. L. (1996). An evaluation of the history of a marijuana withdrawal syndrome in a large population. *Addiction, 91,* 1469–1478.

Wilens, T. E. (2004). Impact of ADHD and its treatment on substance abuse in adults. *J Clin Psychiatry, 65*(Suppl. 3), 38–45.

Winstock, A. R., Lea, T., & Copeland, J. (2009). Lithium carbonate in the management of cannabis withdrawal in humans: An open-label study. *J Psychopharmacol, 23,* 84–93.

Yucel, M., Solowij, N., Respondek, C., Whittle, S., Fornito, A., Pantelis, C., et al. (2008). Regional brain abnormalities associated with long-term heavy cannabis use. *Arch Gen Psychiatry, 65,* 694–701.

Zuardi, A. W., Crippa, J. A., Hallak, J. E., Moreira, F. A., & Guimaraes, F. S. (2006). Cannabidiol, a *Cannabis sativa* constituent, as an antipsychotic drug. *Braz J Med Biol Res, 39,* 421–429.

Zuardi, A. W., Hallak, J. E., Dursun, S. M., Morais, S. L., Sanches, R. F., Musty, R. E., et al. (2006b). Cannabidiol monotherapy for treatment-resistant schizophrenia. *J Psychopharmacol, 20,* 683–686.

Zvolensky, M. J., Bernstein, A., Sachs-Ericsson, N., Schmidt, N. B., Buckner, J. D., & Bonn-Miller, M. O. (2006). Lifetime associations between cannabis, use, abuse, and dependence and panic attacks in a representative sample. *J Psychiatr Res, 40,* 477–486.

CHAPTER 9

Hallucinogens and Inhalants

STEPHEN ROSS
AVRAM H. MACK

This chapter covers two classes of substances (hallucinogens and inhalants) that have not only differing pharmacological and behavioral effects but also overlapping features. Both classes include their tendency be used by youth and their lesser epidemiological magnitude than other substances, such as alcohol or nicotine. In addition, while for each class there are "core" substances, each is a dynamic category in which new substances are constantly being developed and utilized in the community. Another common feature is that besides immediate supportive care and the prevention of violence or injury during intoxication, there are few specific treatments for long-term problem use of these substances. Short-term therapies include attention to general supportive care, as well as medical conditions induced by the substance.

HALLUCINOGENS

Hallucinogens are a diverse group of substances that vary in source (plant derived or synthetic), chemical and molecular structure, pharmacodynamic effects, and addictive liability versus potential for anti-addictive effects and toxic effects (medical, neurological, psychiatric) versus therapeutic applicability. DSM-5, like DSM-IV, does not include the cannabinoids in the hallucinogen category, even though they produce subjective states along the "hallucinogenic" spectrum but are considered sufficiently different in their psychological and behavioral effects to merit their own category (DSM-5). In recognition of the need to expand the hallucinogen drug category, DSM-5 now includes the following subtypes: the N-methyl-D-aspartate (NMDA) antagonist hallucinogens such as phencyclidine (PCP), ketamine, and dextromethorphan (DXM); serotonergic hallucinogens such as D-lysergic acid diethylamide (LSD), psilocybin, ayahuasca, ibogaine, and mescaline; the 3,4-methylenedioxymethamphetamine (MDMA) subtype; and another (single-substance) subtype (i.e., *Salvia divinorum*, jimsom weed).

The desired drug effect of the "hallucinogens" falls along a phenomenological spectrum of varying intensity of consciousness alteration, with unique changes in perception, cognition, affect, and spiritual states (i.e., mystical states of consciousness). Most hallucinogens are included in the Schedule I category as originally defined by the Controlled Substances Act of 1970. As such, by definition, they are classified as having no currently accepted medical use in the United States, as lacking in safety for use under medical supervision, and as having a high addictive liability. From an addiction perspective, it is worth examining the evidence base for this classification to understand the true addictive liability of this class of agents and how it differs depending on the type of hallucinogen. Moreover, given the history of research suggesting a role for certain hallucinogen treatment models to treat psychiatric and addictive disorders, it is further worth exploring how some of these agents may confer their therapeutic effects and to weigh this against potential toxic effects depending on the particular hallucinogen. Given the breadth of this topic, the focus will be on the NMDA antagonist hallucinogens, serotonergic hallucinogens, and MDMA.

NMDA Antagonist Hallucinogens: PCP and Related Substances

Classification

The NMDA antagonist hallucinogens (NAHs) are hallucinogens known as *dissociative anesthetics* because of their ability to disconnect mental from somatic processes (Domino & Miller, 2009). However, they are more psychotogenic than the serotonergic hallucinogens (SHs) and can indeed produce frank hallucinations. The NAHs include the arylcyclohexylamines (i.e., PCP; ketamine; DXM and its active metabolic dextrorphan [DXO]; dizocilpine (MK-801); and cyclohexamine). There are other agents that are known to potently antagonize the NMDA receptor with associated psychedelic properties (i.e., nitrous oxide, ethanol, propofol), but they are not included in this category.

Administration and Pharmacokinetics

PCP, a Schedule I drug, is prepared illicitly in tablet, powder, and liquid form, with the liquid sprayed onto leafy plant material, such as tobacco and cannabis, and smoked. PCP tends to have a wide range in plasma half-life (7–46 hours), and even with normal doses it is not unusual for effects to persist for days after a period of diagnosable intoxication (as defined in DSM-5) has passed. The desired and toxic behavioral effects of PCP are related to serum level, with psychotomimetic effects seen at approximately 0.05–0.2 micromoles (μM) serum concentration, anesthetic doses at approximately 0.2–1.0 μM, and lethal doses at 1.0 μM and above (Domino & Miller, 2009).

Ketamine, a Schedule III drug, was synthesized in 1962 for use as a novel anesthetic agent, and it has a well-established safety profile based on greater than 7,000 published reports (Krupitsky, 2007). Available in powder and liquid form, it can be snorted or injected intramuscularly or intravenously. Ketamine's plasma half-life (alpha T1/2 approximately 7 minutes; beta T1/2 of 3–4 hours) is much shorter than that of PCP, accounting for its diminished psychiatric and medical toxicity relative to PCP (Domino & Miller, 2009).

DXM was patented in 1954 and designed as a substitute for codeine as a cough suppressant. It was excluded from the 1970 Controlled Substance Act; over the years, DXM has been made increasingly available as a part of over-the-counter cold medicine preparations, which provided a surge of abuse starting in the early 1990s. DXM gets converted to DXO, a potent NMDA antagonist that produces effects similar to ketamine and PCP. To produce its psychoactive effects, large doses of DXM are needed (typically 300–1,800 mg, and well above the recommended antitussive dose of 15–30 mg) to produce a sufficient amount of the psychoactive DXO. The time course of DXOs effects depend on a genetic polymorphism for the catabolism of DXM in which rapid metabolizers (representing approximately 90% of the population) have a T1/2 of approximately 3 hours and slow metabolizers have a T1/2 of approximately 24 hours or more (Zawertailo et al., 1998).

Epidemiology

The peak use of PCP in the United States occurred during the 1970s and has decreased considerably since then. For instance, the recreational use of PCP in the prior year by high school seniors in the United States decreased from 7% in 1979 to 1% in 2008 (Johnston, O'Malley, Bachman, & Schulenberg, 2013). PCP abuse appears to be limited to major cities in the United States and is particularly prevalent in Philadelphia, Washington, DC, Los Angeles, and Houston. Since 1999, according to the Drug Abuse Warning Network, there has been a marked increase in emergency department visits associated with PCP, with a 400% increase from 2005 to 2011 (which was in addition to earlier increases; Substance Abuse and Mental Health Services Administration [SAMHSA], 2013). The reason behind this is unclear, but it may represent an increase in use among people not typically covered in community surveys.

It is difficult to establish the true prevalence of ketamine use disorders, because the users remain a mostly hidden group. One study in Britain reported that close to 30% of surveyed club-goers reported a lifetime use of ketamine (Wolff & Winstock, 2006).

Starting in the early 1990s, DXM began to emerge as a drug of abuse especially among teenagers and young adults. This is consistent with data from the National Poison Data System, which indicated that between 2000 and 2010, the peak in calls related to DXM nationally occurred in 2006, with concerted legislative and educational initiatives likely accounting for the drop-off in use and adverse medical events (Wilson, Ferguson, Mazer, et al., 2011).

Neurobiology

The NAHs primarily exert their psychoactive effects via noncompetitive blockade at the ionotropic NMDA glutamate receptor at the PCP binding site (located inside the calcium channel and leading to blockade of calcium influx through the channel), with psychoactivity directly correlating with receptor affinity (Oye, Paulsen, & Maurset, 1992). NAHs increase glutamate release and the firing rate of pyramidal neurons in the medial prefrontal cortex (mPFC), an effect likely due to blockade of NMDA receptors on gamma-aminobutyric acid (GABA)-ergic interneurons in cortical and subcortical structures, which normally antagonize cortical glutamate neurons, leading to a reduction of inhibitory control over PFC glutamatergic neurons (Homayoun & Moghaddam, 2007; Jodo et al., 2005). In turn, cortical glutamatergic activation stimulates monoaminergic terminals within the cortex, limbic system, midbrain, and brainstem (Krystal et al., 2003). As part of this, extracellular dopamine (DA) levels are increased in reward-related areas (i.e., ventral tegmental area [VTA] and nucleus accumbens [NA]) in the mesolimbic system and account for the addictive liability of this class of drugs (see below).

Regional Brain Activity

See below in the section "Classical or Serotonergic Hallucinogens."

Addictive Liability

Several converging pieces of data point to NAHs having real addictive liability. These include positron emission tomographic (PET) studies demonstrating increases in DA in the VTA in humans correlating with elevated mood (Vollenweider, Liechti, Gamma, Greer, & Geyer, 2000); increases in DA in the NA of humans (Smith et al., 1998); induction of self-administration in animal models (Newman, Perry, & Carroll, 2007); repeated administration leading to tolerance in animals (Benthuysen, Hance, Quam, & Winters, 1989) and humans (Wolff & Winstock, 2006); and heavy, habitual use and dependence syndromes in humans (Moore & Bostwick, 1999). Despite having known addictive liability, the NAHs are one of the least "addictive" classes of abusable substances. Only about 5% of individuals who try these drugs will go on to develop dependence syndromes (Anthony, Warner, & Kessler, 1994).

Intoxication/Phenomenology

The NAHs produce a range of psychic and toxic states that can be grouped into three stages. Stage I is the desired rewarding state characterized by euphoria, anxiolysis, dissociation, and psychedelic effects. The spiritual or mystical type experiences induced by the NAHs, separate from their dissociative properties (i.e., out-of-body experiences) and perhaps overlapping with what is traditionally understood as psychotic phenomenon, may include feelings of ego dissolution and loss of identity; experience of psychological death and rebirth; emotionally intense visions and dream-like states; enhanced insight/self-reflection and meaning in life; and feelings of unity with humanity, nature, the universe, and deity (Krupitsky & Kolp, 2007). With respect to the NAHs, it has been postulated that the NMDA blockade accounts for their negative and cognitive dysfunction potential, while the increased glutamate transmission accounts for the positive symptoms of psychosis (Domino & Miller, 2009).

There is a narrow difference between the desired effects of the NAHs and psychological toxicity, which includes psychosis (i.e., positive, negative, cognitive symptoms), delirium, catatonia, depression, mania, agitation, and violence toward self and others. The latter stages of intoxication (i.e., Stages II and III), especially with PCP, are marked by increasingly serious medical complications, including death. Intoxication due to a NAH may include many different symptoms and signs, but formal diagnosis requires several specific findings of cardiac, somatic, pain, or neuro/neuromuscular systems as noted in DSM-5 (American Psychiatric Association, 2013).

Adverse Psychiatric Effects

Psychiatric conditions recognized as being exacerbated by the NAHs include psychotic, bipolar, and depressive spectrum disorders. In addition, hallucinogen persisting perceptual disorder (HPPD) may result from exposure to an NAH. Beyond the acute stage of intoxication, heavy chronic PCP use (with its potentially long half-life), can engender enduring psychotic symptoms lasting weeks to months even in the absence of underlying psychotic spectrum illness and as such, schizophrenia should not be ruled in unless the psychosis continues chronically and there is other evidence to suggest schizophrenia (i.e., history of psychotic symptoms predating any drug use, [+] family history of schizophrenia) (Ross, 2012). Psychiatric treatment of NAH intoxication depends on the clinical findings. Many individuals, especially those intoxicated with PCP, come to clinical attention due to extremely violent or agitated behavior; others are referred in severe conditions that affect consciousness, such as delirium. Behavioral management usually requires supportive care in a manner that protects the individual from self and others. This can include not only placing patients in a quiet environment with little environmental stimuli but may also necessitate physical restraints to manage violent behavior. Benzodiazepines or antipsychotics are often necessary to treat symptoms such as violence, agitation, and psychosis. It is important to avoid low-potency typical neuroleptics (i.e., chlorpromazine) due to additive increased risks of seizures and cardiovascular effects. While it is important to continue antipsychotic medication in individuals with subacute (days to several months) psychosis due to PCP use, unless there is other evidence to suggest an independent psychotic spectrum illness, it would be reasonable to taper off antipsychotic pharmacotherapy once the psychotic symptoms resolve.

Adverse Medical Effects

The serious medical toxicity of the NAHs is mostly associated with PCP due to its relatively long half-life. The potential medical toxicities due to PCP are wide ranging and may include severe and permanent problems. As noted earlier, Stage I intoxication is associated with few serious physiological or medical sequelae, but it is characterized by ataxia, dysarthria, tachycardia, hypertension, increased salivation, hyperreflexia, and nystagmus (horizontal, vertical, rotary), with both rotary and vertical nystagmus being pathognomonic for NAH intoxication. In Stage II, patients range from a stuporous state to mild coma, are responsive to pain, and have pupils in the midposition and responsive to light. In Stage III, patients are comatose and unresponsive to painful stimuli. Stages II and III are associated with serious adverse medical outcomes, including malignant hypertension and hyperthermia, seizures, rhabdomyolysis and acute renal failure, stroke, heart failure, coma, and death. Supportive medical treatment should be provided especially for Stages II and III of intoxication.

The medical toxicity associated with DXM use includes serotonin syndrome (when combined with monoamine oxidase inhibitors [MAOIs], selective serotonin reuptake inhibitors [SSRIs], or other serotonergically active medications, because DXM increases the synthesis and release of the serotonin transporter 5-HT and blocks the 5-HT reuptake transporter) and toxicity related to the other substances contained in cold preparations (i.e., pseudophedrine, phenylephrine, antihistamines, acetaminophen).

Therapeutic Applicability: Addiction, Mood Disorders, and Pain Syndromes

Despite the known addictive liability of NAHs, it is interesting that there is experimental evidence to suggest antiaddictive or antidepressant effects of ketamine. For example, ketamine's antiaddictive properties have been studied in hundreds of participants in Russia as part of ketamine psychedelic therapy (KPT; Krupitsky & Kolp, 2007). An emerging body of scientific literature has demonstrated the ability of single or repeated subanesthetic doses of IV ketamine to rapidly and reproducibly reduce depressive symptoms (including reductions in suicidal ideation) in patients with treatment-resistant major depression or bipolar depression, with antidepressant responses detected within 1–2 hours postinfusion, maintained in a majority of patients for at least 24 hours, and enduring for up to several days to several weeks (Murrough et al., 2013; Lee, Della Selva, Liu, & Himelhoch, 2015).

Research with ketamine has also strongly supported a role in treating refractory pain syndromes such as complex regional pain syndrome (CRPS; Goldberg et al., 2005) and breakthrough pain in chronic pain syndromes such as that related to advanced cancer (Carr et al., 2004).

Classical or Serotonergic Hallucinogens: LSD and Related Substances

Classification

SH plant-derived compounds occur in nature, including psilocybin mushrooms, peyote cacti, iboga alkaloids, and ayahuasca. SHs consist of an arylalkylamine skeleton and are divided into two main categories: the *indolealkylamines* and the *phenylalkylamines*.

The indolealkylamines have a core structure similar to serotonin and include:

- Tryptamines, such as N,N-dimethyltryptamine (DMT, found in ayahuasca), psilocybin, and its psychoactive metabolite psilocin.
- Semisynthetic ergolines or lysergamides (the ergot LSD).
- Iboga alkaloids (ibogaine).

The phenylalkylamines have a core structure more similar to norepinephrine (NE) and include

- Phenylethylamines, such as "STP" (2,5-dimethoxy-4-methylamphetamine), mescaline (from the peyote cactus *Lophophora williamsii*), and the 2C series of compounds (i.e., 2CB, 2CI).
- Phenylisopropylamines, which are amphetamine derivatives such as DOM (2,5-dimethoxy-4-methylamphetamine). This group also includes "Ecstasy" MDMA (3,4-methylenedioxymethamphetamine). Note that MDMA, which is discussed in more detail below, is not a "classical" hallucinogen, because it does not appreciably agonize the serotonin 2A receptor and does not typically induce mystical states or psychosis.

Administration and Pharmacokinetics

One of the simple tryptamine indolealkylamines, DMT, is produced in the pineal gland (Barker, McIlhenny, & Strassman, 2012) and its endogenous function remains a mystery. Synthetic DMT, typically smoked or, much less commonly, injected by the user, leads to a rapid onset of action within seconds to minutes and has a short duration of action lasting approximately 10–20 minutes. The major route of catabolism of DMT is via oxidative deamination by MAO, and because of the significant present of MAO in the gastrointenstinal system, orally ingested DMT is degraded in the gut and is therefore not psychoactive. The South American hallucinogen aqueous decoction ayahuasca was designed to account for this process by containing two plant-derived components: *Psychotria viridis* (which contains DMT) and *Banisteriopsis capii*, containing several beta-carbolines (harmine, harmaline, and tetrahydroharmine) that have MAO inhibitory properties that prevent gastrointestinal degradation of DMT and allow for its entry into the central nervous system (CNS) (Dos Santos et al., 2011). Unlike smoked or injected DMTs rapid on–off effects, ayahuasca has a delayed onset of psychedelic effects (20–60 minutes), a plateau of 1–2 hours, DMT half-life of approximately 1 hour, and a gradual return to baseline around 6 hours postingestion (Riba et al., 2003).

Psilocybin, a ring-substituted tryptamine indolealkylamine, is considered a prodrug. It is dephosphorylated to psilocin, which is considered its major psychoactive metabolite, with a mean elimination half-life of 50 minutes (Passie, Seifert, Schneider, & Emrich, 2002). Typical hallucinogenic doses of psilocybin range from 8–30 mg in humans, with onset of action at approximately 30–60 minutes, which coincides with when psilocin first appears in plasma; peak effects occur at approximately 60–90 minutes postingestion, plateau for approximately 50 minutes (corresponding to a plateau of plasma psilocin over the same time period), followed by a gradual decline of psychoactive effects until about 360 minutes postingestion (Passie et al., 2002).

LSD is among the most potent SHs, with pronounced alterations in consciousness at doses as low as 50–75 µg, with a typical dose of 100–200 µg (Passie et al., 2008). It is synthetically derived, available as a liquid, and typically ingested on "blotter paper," microdots, or other material (i.e., sugar cubes) impregnated with LSD solution. Following oral intake and complete absorption of LSD in the gastrointestinal tract, psychological effects begin approximately 30–45 minutes postingestion, peak at approximately 1.5–2.5 hours, with the total duration of the experience lasting 6–10 hours. In humans, LSD's elimination half-life is approximately 4 hours, and it is extensively metabolized, with less than 1% of LSD appearing in urine. It is metabolized by NADH-dependent microsomal liver enzymes to several inactive metabolites, including 2-oxy-LSD, 2-oxy-3-hydroxy-LSD, and nor-LSD; the latter two are the most abundant in urine and detectable for 2–5 days postuse (Canezin et al., 2001)

Ibogaine is one of the longest acting hallucinogens. With dose-dependent bioavailability, the onset and peak of the hallucinogenic effects occur 1–3 hours after ingestion, with a plateau phase of approximately 4–8 hours, and residual alterations of consciousness that can last another 12–24 hours (Alper, 2001). The major metabolite of ibogaine, nor-ibogaine (produced by cytochrome P450 2D6 [CYP2D6] demethylation) has a longer half-life and greater binding at the mu opioid receptor than ibogaine (Mash et al., 2000). Ibogaine's estimated half-life in humans is 7.5 hours, and both ibogaine and nor-ibogaine are excreted by the kidneys and gastrointestinal tract (Alper, 2001).

The metabolism of most of the phenylalkylamines has not been well researched and documented in humans, but most are thought to be substrates for cytochrome P450 and MAO (Glennon, 2009). Mescaline is the active ingredient in the peyote cactus, with documented ceremonial and sacramental use by Native Americans for hundreds of years. Mescaline possesses psychoactivity at oral doses of 200–400 mg/kg, has a relatively slow onset (1–3 hours) and a long duration of action up to 10 hours (Glennon, 2009). Mescaline is approximately one-tenth as potent as psilocybin and one-thousandth as potent as LSD. The approximate half-life of mescaline is 6 hours, and it appears not to be metabolized by the cytochrome P450 system, with 20–50% of mescaline excreted unchanged in urine and the remainder excreted as the carboxylic acid form of the drug, likely due to MAO degradation (Cochin, Woods, & Seevers, 1951).

Epidemiology

There is a relative lack of epidemiological data detailing the course of hallucinogen use disorders specific to the SHs, but they are among the most rare of all use disorders and the least likely to be associated with frank addiction, if any addiction at all, and are associated with high rates of recovery (Ross, 2012). They typically begin in adolescence, peak at 18–29 years (0.6%) and decrease to 0% among those 45 and older. Regarding the DSM-IV hallucinogen use disorders, past 12-month prevalence among age groups has included adults (0.14%), 12- to 17-year-olds (0.5%), and 18-year-olds and older (0.1%) (SAMHSA, 2011). Adolescents have the greatest rates of use, with approximately 8% of adolescents ages 16–23 using one or more SHs in a prior 12-month period, with MDMA by far being the most commonly used SH (despite its inaccurate characterization as an SH) (Wu, Schlenger, & Galvin, 2006). Adult men are twice as likely to meet criteria, although girls are more likely to use than boys ages 12–17 (SAMHSA, 2011).

Neurobiology

All of the SHs have marked affinity as agonists for the 2AR but also interact to some degree with 5-HT$_1$, 5-HT$_4$, 5-HT$_5$, 5-HT$_6$, and 5-HT$_7$ receptors. In addition, the semisynthetic ergolines (i.e., LSD) display high intrinsic activity at D$_2$ and alpha-adrenergic receptors (Marona-Lewicka, Thisted, & Nichols, 2005). Ibogaine has the most complicated pharmacodynamic profile of the SHs, and in addition to its agonist effects at the serotonin receptors (2ARs), it also interacts with the glutamatergic, opioidergic, and cholinergic neurotransmitter systems (Alper, 2001). Converging lines of evidence from pharmacological, electrophysiological, and behavioral research in animals strongly suggest that activation of cortical 2ARs is the most critical step in initiating a cascade of biological events that accounts for their hallucinogenic properties (Vollenweider & Kometer, 2010). In humans, preadministration of ketanserin (a 2AR antagonist) abolishes almost all of the psilocybin-induced psychoactive effects (Vollenweider, Vollenweider-Scherpenhuyzen, et al., 1998).

There is also evidence that 2AR agonists activate differing intracellular signaling pathways depending on whether they have hallucinogenic properties (i.e., lisuride; Nichols, 2004). The 2AR is a Gq-coupled G protein-coupled receptor (GPCR) that responds to the endogenous neurotransmitter, serotonin, whereas the metabotropic glutamate receptor (mGluR2) is a Gi-coupled, pertussis toxic-sensitive GPCR that responds to glutamate. It has been demonstrated that 2AR and mGluR2 receptors form a functional heteromeric complex through which classical hallucinogens cross-signal to the Gi-coupled receptor (Gonzalez-Maeso et al., 2008). Furthermore, formation of the mGluR2–2AR complex establishes an optimal Gi–Gq balance in response to glutamate and serotonin (increase in Gi and decrease in Gq) and the classical hallucinogens may produce their propsychotic states by effecting decreases in Gi and increases in Gq (Fribourg et al., 2011).

2AR activation by classical hallucinogens modulates prefrontal network activity by causing marked increases in extracellular glutamate levels that account for increased activity of pyramidal neurons, most pronounced in layer V of the PFC (Béïque et al., 2007). Also, activation of 2AR receptors in the mPFC affects subcortical transmission by increasing the activity of serotonin neurons in the dorsal raphe and DA neurons in the VTA, the latter resulting in increased DA transmission in mesocortical and mesostriatal areas (Puig et al., 2003). In a human study, psilocybin induced increase in striatal DA was correlated with euphoria and depersonalization (Vollenweider et al., 1999). This is interesting to note in light of the lack of psilocybin's ability to produce dependence or addiction (Ross, 2012).

Regional Brain Activity

SHs and NAHs both produce similar altered states of consciousness in human studies (Vollenweider & Kometer, 2010). Both are capable of producing mystical states of consciousness. Consistent with similar phenomenological states, human brain imaging studies have demonstrated that both psilocybin and ketamine produce similar patterns of prefrontal–limbic activation. They showed marked prefrontal activation (hyperfrontality): frontomedial, dorsolateral cortices, anterior cingulate, insula and temporal poles; decreased activation of areas important for gating or integrating cortical information processing, such as the bilateral thalamus, right globus pallidus, bilateral pons, and cerebellum; and decreased activity in the somatosensory cortical areas, occipital cortex, and visual pathways (Geyer & Vollenweider, 2008). Taken together, psilocybin and ketamine both produce hyperfrontality with divergent prefrontal–subcortical activation in such a way as to increase cognitive and affective processing in the context of reduced gating and reduced focus on external stimulus processing. Interestingly, the dimension of "oceanic boundlessness" on the Swiss APZ Scale (translated as Altered States of Consciousness Scale, correlating with mystical states of consciousness) was correlated with ketamine and psilocybin activation of a prefrontal–parietal network and the deactivation of a striatolimbic amygdalocentric network (Vollenweider & Kometer, 2010). Other similarities between psilocybin and ketamine are that both stimulate cortical glutamate transmission, with increased activation of alpha-amino-3-hydroxy-5-methyl-4-isoxazolepropionic acid (AMPA) receptors relative to NMDA ones, and that both increase brain-derived neurotrophic factor (BDNF) levels in prefrontal and limbic brain areas in rats (Vaidya et al., 1997; Cavus & Duman, 2003; Garcia et al., 2009).

Addictive Liability

In contrast to all other drugs of abuse, SHs are not considered to be capable of producing sufficient reinforcing effects to cause dependence (addiction) syndromes associated with compulsive use (O'Brien, 2006; Ross, 2012). Animal models have failed to reliably demonstrate addictive liability of the SHs, suggesting that they do not possess sufficient pharmacological properties to initiate or maintain dependence (Fantegrossi, Woods, & Winger, 2004; Nichols, 2004; Poling & Bryceland, 1979). All of the SHs (except LSD; Watts et al., 1995; Giacomelli et al., 1998) lack affinity for DA receptors or dopamine transporters (DATs) and do not directly affect dopaminergic transmission. Interestingly, despite evidence that SHs have been shown to increase DA transmission in striatal areas in humans, they fail to activate the nucleus accumbens significantly in PET imaging studies. This is consistent with the lack of evidence linking classical hallucinogens with addiction syndromes (Vollenweider et al., 1999; Geyer & Vollenweider, 2008). In fact, in animals, ibogaine (as well as nor-ibogaine and 18-methoxycoronaridine [18-MC]) has been shown to decrease dopamine efflux in the nucleus accumbens in response to opioids (Maisonneuve et al., 1991; Glick, Maissonneuve, & Dickinson, 2000; Taraschenko et al., 2007) and nicotine (Benwell et al., 1996; Maisonneuve et al., 1997). Furthermore, rapid tachyphylaxis occurs with repeated administration of the SHs (with the exception of DMT) and with repeated daily dosing, psychological effects disappear within several days, an effect correlated with and likely mediated by 5-HT_{2A} downregulation (Buckholtz et al., 1990). The lack of a withdrawal syndrome eliminates another avenue toward addiction, that of negative reinforcement to avoid painful withdrawal states (i.e., opioids, alcohol). In addition to the lack of biological evidence, epidemiological studies have also failed to reliably demonstrate a link between SHs and their ability to engender enduring dependence syndromes, and the National Institute on Drug Abuse (NIDA; 2001,

2005) does not consider the SHs drugs of "addiction" because they do not produce compulsive drug-seeking behavior, and most recreational users decrease or stop their use over time.

Intoxication/Phenomenology

The acute psychological and behavioral effects of the SHs are greatly influenced by set (personality and expectations of the individual), setting (environmental conditions and context of use) and dose, with the factors combining to influence the valence (positive or negative) of the experience (Ross, 2012). Affective changes can range from euphoric or ecstatic spiritual states to anxiety, terror, and panic. Perception is intensified and amplified, with alterations in time, space, and boundaries between self and others. Synesthesia is common, with mixing of various sensory stimuli (i.e., hearing colors). Sensory illusions (i.e., walls breathing) are common and frank hallucinations occur but less frequently. Thought processes are loosened, with effects ranging from increased creativity to thought disorder. Cognition is altered and can range from increased and sudden insight ("noetic" effect) to confusion and disorientation (Wilkins, Danovitch, & Gorelick, 2009). The sum total of the experience can range from positive mystical-type experiences associated with enduring positive changes in affect–cognition–behavior to "bad trips" or hallucinogen persisting perceptual disorder (HPPD) (see below) (Griffiths, Richards, McCann, & Jesse, 2006; Griffiths, Richards, Johnson, McCann, & Jesse, 2008; Griffiths et al., 2011; Johnson, Richards, & Griffiths, 2008).

When LSD was first discovered in 1943, its effects were thought to be similar to endogenous psychotic states and the term "psychotomimetic" was coined. The SHs cause states that resemble acute positive symptoms of psychosis (i.e., illusions, hallucinations, thought disorder); however, reality testing tends to remain intact during intoxication with these agents, and they rarely cause frank hallucinations, delusions, or prominent negative or cognitive symptoms in individuals without underlying psychotic spectrum illness or major affective psychoses (Ross & Peselow, 2012). The vague term "psychedelic," meaning mind manifesting, has remained as the most commonly used term in popular culture (Osmond, 1957). The term "hallucinogen" is a misnomer, because the SHs are less likely to cause frank hallucinations than to cause illusions. Perhaps a more precise phenomenological descriptor, "mysticomimetic," comes from the psychology of religion literature.

Adverse Psychiatric Effects

ACUTE EFFECTS

Severe adverse psychological experiences ("bad trips") tend to occur in poorly prepared individuals who use the particular SH in an uncontrolled setting and who have psychological risk factors (i.e., severe mental illness, recent trauma) (Johnson et al., 2008). These experiences typically include anxiety, panic, dysphoria, depersonalization, paranoid ideation, and fear that the experience will never end or that one will lose one's mind. Despite such adverse reactions, users usually retain insight into the fact that their symptoms are related to drug ingestion and usually respond to verbal reassurance. SHs can acutely engender frank psychosis marked by hallucinations, thought disorder, and delusions, although this is rare in individuals without underlying psychotic spectrum illnesss (Ross, 2012). Such adverse psychological experiences can potentially lead to dangerous behavior toward self or others (Strassman, 1984). First-line treatment of acute panic reactions and psychotic phenomena (i.e., paranoid ideation, hallucinations), engendered by SHs, should include placement in a quiet setting and "talking down" the patient with verbal reassurance about the time-limited nature of the experience. Pharmacological interventions can also be used, if necessary, including fast-acting oral or parenteral benzodiazepines (i.e., diazepam, lorazepam) and antipsychotics. The atypical antipsychotics may be especially helpful because of their antagonist effects at the 5-HT_{2A} receptor.

PROLONGED EFFECTS

Psychosis. It is well-established that SHs use can provoke sustained psychosis in vulnerable people with psychotic spectrum illnesses (i.e., schizophrenia, schizoaffective disorder, bipolar disorder with psychotic features). However there is little to no evidence linking SH use to prolonged psychosis in individuals without a psychotic diathesis (Ross & Peselow, 2012). Estimates of the prevalence of LSD-induced psychosis as assessed by early psychedelic researchers and clinicians (many working with and administering LSD to psychiatric inpatients) were as follows from two reports: 0.8/1000 research volunteers and 1.8/1000 psychiatric patients (Cohen, 1960); and 0/170 research volunteers and 9/1000 psychiatric patients (Malleson, 1971). A recent cross-sectional study evaluating data taken from years 2001–2004 of the National Survey on Drug Use and Health with a sample of 130,152 (representing a random sample of the U.S. population living in households) did not find any significant associations between lifetime use of any psychedelic or past year use of LSD and increased rates of any psychiatric symptoms (including psychosis) or mental health outcomes (Krebs & Johansen, 2013).

Hallucinogen Persisting Perception Disorder. In HPPD, users experience perceptual effects ("flashbacks") similar to those experienced during previous hallucinogen use; these flashbacks must cause distress and impair functioning (DSM-5). Flashbacks can occur spontaneously or be triggered by stress, exercise, or use of another drug (i.e., cannabis). Although the exact prevalence of HPPD is unknown, it is thought to be a rare condition and less common in research settings with careful screening and preparation (Johnson et al., 2008; Halpern & Pope 2003). The longitudinal course tends to be brief, and the condition usually remits on its own over time (Strassman, 1984). Supportive psychotherapy is warranted to reassure individuals. There is no established evidence-based pharmacologic algorithm to treat HPPD with most of the trials coming from case reports, case series, and open label trials with little in the way of randomized controlled trials. Benzodiazepines (e.g., alprazolam, clonazepam), naltrexone, and typical antipsychotics (haloperidol, trifluoperazine, perphenazine) have been shown to reduce some symptoms of HPPD without leading to disease remission; data on the utility of SSRIs to ameliorate symptoms of HPPD is mixed, with some data supporting their efficacy and some suggesting a worsening of symptoms; risperidone (and possibly the atypical antipsychotics in general) should be avoided as a treatment option in HPPD as there is evidence that risperidone worsens HPPD symptoms (Wilkins et al., 2009). More controlled trials are needed to establish better pharmacologic treatments for HPPD, which could help further elucidate the pathophysiology of the illness.

Adverse Medical Effects

In general, SHs possess low physiological toxicity and are not typically associated with end organ damage, carcinogenicity, teratogenicity, lasting neuropsychological deficits, or overdose fatalities (Johnson et al., 2008; Halpern et al., 2005, 2008). An exception to this is ibogaine which has been associated with fatalities and is known to induce cardiac arrhythmias: bradyarrhythmias, QT prolongation possibly leading to Torsade de points (Alper, Stajić, & Gill, 2012). Also some relatively new designer phenethylamine SHs (Bromo-DragonFLY and 2,5-dimethoxy-N-[2-methoxybenzyl] phenylethylamine—referred to as NBOMe), with very high potency at the serotonin 2AR, have been associated with fatalities (Baumann et al., 2012). The SHs produce sympathomimetic effects and can moderately increase pulse, as well as diastolic and systolic blood pressure, but this has not been associated with cardiac, neurological, or other organ damage (Griffths & Grob, 2010). Common physiological side effects of the SHs include mydriasis, blurry vision, dizziness, tremors, weakness, paresthesias, and increased deep tendon reflexes (Johnson et al., 2008).

Therapeutic Applicability

Although often forgotten and not part of modern psychiatric training, from approximately the late 1950s to the mid-1970s, there was extensive research on the therapeutic applicability of hallucinogen treatment models. Much of the research centered in the United States and Europe. Two treatment models emerged: *psycholytic* and *psychedelic* (Ross, 2012). The psycholytic model predominated in Europe, where lower doses of LSD (30–200 µg) and psilocybin (3–15 mg) were used as tools to activate and enhance the psychoanalytic process by allowing greater access to unconscious material to effect personality changes in disease states such as personality disorders, neurotic spectrum disorders, and psychosomatic illness. The psychedelic model utilized high doses of LSD (400–1,500 mcg) and psilocybin (20–40 mg) to access novel dimensions of consciousness remarkably similar to mystical states of consciousness, with oneness, illuminative insight, a sense of the sacred, and ecstatic joy as core parts of the experience. This new therapeutic model with no previous basis within the field of mental health research had more parallels toward religion and mysticism. By the end of nearly three decades of research, over 1,000 articles were published in the literature and over 40,000 participants were included in basic or therapeutic clinical hallucinogen research (Malleson, 1971). A treatment model that established the parameters of set (psychological frame of mind, intention, excluding participants with major mental illness or family history of such illness), setting (environment/

room on dosing days), dose, preparation with therapeutic dyad teams, and integration of the experience was established.

LSD/PSILOCYBIN AND ADDICTION TREATMENT STUDIES

Overall, the studies of LSD's effect in alcoholism during the 1950s and 1960s varied widely, from astonishingly positive results to worsening of the alcoholism, depending on the design of the study, set, and setting of the dosing sessions and the degree to which preparatory and integrative psychotherapy was used. While a 1971 meta-analysis reduced enthusiasm for this line of investigation (Abuzzahab & Anderson, 1971), a 2012 review (Krebs & Johansen, 2012) found new evidence supporting this as a potential therapy. Recently, a re-emergence of research has occurred utilizing psilocybin-assisted psychotherapy to treat addiction with two recently published open label trials suggesting efficacy of psilocybin treatment for alcoholism (Bogenschutz et al., 2015) and tobacco addiction (Johnson et al., 2014). Randomized controlled trials utilizing a similar model to treat alcoholism, tobacco addiction, and cocaine addiction are underway at several academic medical centers in the United States.

IBOGAINE, IBOGA CONGENERS, AND OPIOID WITHDRAWAL

Ibogaine, a psychoactive indole alkaloid that is the most abundant alkaloid found in the root bark of the apocynaceous shrub *Tabernathe iboga* in West Central Africa, has been studied as a substance that may attenuate opioid withdrawal in nonhumans (Maisonneuve & Glick, 2003). Anecdotal reports and several case series have indicated that ibogaine diminishes or eliminates opioid withdrawal symptoms in humans and may be associated with longer term abstinence even after a single dose (Alper, 2001). The ability of ibogaine and related congeners to attenuate or suppress opioid withdrawal is unique among the SHs, and there is no evidence of other, similar agents (i.e., LSD, psilocybin, DMT, mescaline) having any efficacy in diminishing opioid withdrawal. Agonism at the mu opioid receptor has been considered a potential mechanism (Maciulaitis et al., 2008).

Ibogaine remains unavailable for use in the United States because of concerns regarding its safety, specifically, cardiotoxic and neurotoxic issues, which is consistent with anthropological reports of fatalities during initiation rites of the Fang people of West Africa; there have been at least a dozen deaths reported within 72 hours of ibogaine use since 1990 (Alper et al., 2012).

MDMA

Classification

MDMA is a ring-substituted analog of methamphetamine in the phenylisopropylamine category of substances, which includes a variety of SH with amphetamine-like effects. However, MDMA is not considered a "classical" SH, because it does not appreciably agonize the 5-HT_{2A} receptor to the same extent as the SHs and does not typically induce mystical states or psychosis (Vollenweider et al., 2002). It exists in a unique category, described as an "entactogen" (Nichols, 2004), producing a diverse set of effects (amphetamine, prosocial/empathogen, anxiolytic, mild psychedelic). "Bath Salts" should not be unduly confused with MDMA. "Bath Salts," a group of synthetic derivatives of the CNS stimulant cathinone, have rewarding effects somewhere between MDMA and methamphetamine and are associated with adverse psychological (i.e., mania, psychosis) and medical (i.e., seizures, arrhythmias, deaths) effects (Spiller, Ryan, Weston, & Jansen, 2011).

Administration and Pharmacokinetics

MDMA is almost exclusively available in pill form, is usually taken orally but it can be snorted and rarely is injected intravenously. The usual single recreational dose is 50–150 mg. MDMA possesses good oral bioavailability, easily crosses the blood–brain barrier, has an onset of action 20–40 minutes after ingestion, which is often experienced with immediacy or a "rush" that lasts approximately 30–45 minutes, and is associated with peak plasma concentrations achieved in 1–3 hours postingestion; the next phase (plateau) typically lasts several hours, is somewhat less pleasurable than the initial phase, and is usually accompanied by heightened motor activity (i.e., dancing); the elimination half-life of MDMA is 7–8 hours, and most users experience a "coming down" 3–6 hours after drug intake (Wilkins et al., 2009).

MDMA's major metabolic pathway in humans involves O-demethylenation by CYP2D6 to 3,4-dihydroxymethamphetamine (HHMA) and subsequent methylation of HHMA by catechol-O-methyltransferase (COMT) to 4-hydroxy-3-methoxymethamphetamine (HMMA) (de la Torre et al., 2004). A minor pathway involves N-demethylation of MDMA by CYP3A4 to 3,4-methylenedioxyamphetamine (MDA), which possesses psychoactive effects similar to MDMA and has a longer half-life of 16–40 hours (Monks et al., 2004). MDMA displays nonlinear kinetics in humans whereby increasing doses, or multiple doses taken in a single-use episode, leads to unpredicatbly high plasma levels of the drug, which could account for the serious adverse medical and psychiatric toxicity reported with multiple-dose usage (Baumann, Wang, & Rothman, 2007).

Epidemiology

Adolescents are frequent users of MDMA and the population most likely to present with this as the drug causing the most problems for them. Furthermore, they are more likely to be involved with the subculture (i.e., clubs, raves, circuit parties) that is enmeshed with MDMA, and more likely to have a decreased perception of harm of the drug that is associated with a greater likelihood of using MDMA (Pentney, 2001). According to Monitoring the Future (Johnston, O'Malley, Bachman, & Schulenberg, 2013) data, MDMA use peaked among adolescents in 2001, with annual prevalence of use as follows: eighth graders 3.5%, 10th graders 6.2%, and 12th graders 9.2%. A marked reduction of use in all grades occurred from 2001 until approximately 2005–2006, with a rebound in use among 8th and 10th graders occurring over the next 2 years; after 2007, usage became flat in all grades; annual use increased significantly from 2009–2010 in 8th graders (1.3 → 2.4%) and 10th graders (3.7 → 4.7%)

but then declined over the next 2 years, and annual use among 12th graders increased from 2010 to 2011 (7.3 → 8%) but then significantly decreased back to 7.2% in 2012 (Johnston et al., 2013). It is of concern that from 2004 to 2011, the perceived risk of MDMA use declined in all grades and likely accounted for some of the previously mentioned rebound in usage patterns (Johnston et al., 2013). The most recent National Survey on Drug Use and Health (SAMHSA, 2011) data indicate that in 2011, an estimated 555,000 individuals (0.2% of the population) in the United States over the age of 12 had used MDMA in the month prior to the survey. Lifetime use in this same demographic group was significantly increased from 4.3% in 2002 to 5.7% in 2011. The 18–25 age range represents the highest lifetime use rates, with rates at approximately 12% in the last several years. Regarding past year initiates of MDMA in those 12 and older, the peak in 2002 (1.2 million new users) decreased to 607,000 in 2004, and has significantly increased from 2005 (615,000) to 2011 (922,000); the majority (61%) of new users in 2011 were 18 or older (NSDUH, 2011).

Regarding MDMA use and use syndromes, there appear to be two main groups of individuals who ingest MDMA. The vast majority of humans who try MDMA will not progress to compulsive, addictive use. In one of the few epidemiological studies that analyzed the rates of MDMA use disorders in a general population sample in the United States (analyzed from the 2005 NSDUH), among past-year Ecstasy users, only 3.6% met criteria for DSM-IV hallucinogen dependence (Wu, Howard, & Pilowsky, 2008). This may be explained by attenuation of mesolimbic dopaminergic release by antagonist MDMA-induced increased serotonergic activity (Bankson & Yamamoto, 2004) or due to the phenomenon of chronic tolerance, whereby most people who continue to use MDMA report a precipitous decline in the pleasurable effects of the drug and an increase in the undesirable effects such as psychomotor agitation (Parrott, 2005). First-time users are often instant advocates of MDMA only to have their enthusiasm dampen with time. However, there does appear to be a small but significant group of chronic MDMA users that develop frank addiction to the drug. For example, in an epidemiological study looking examining use syndromes among 600 MDMA users in 2 U.S. cities and one city in Australia, MDMA dependence was found in 83% of moderate (100–499 doses per lifetime) or heavy (greater than 500 doses per lifetime) users and in 48% of light users (1–99 doses per lifetime) (Cottler et al., 2006; Leung & Cottler, 2008). Furthermore, an MDMA withdrawal phenomenon has been described. In another epidemiological study of 52 club drug users in St Louis, 34% met criteria for MDMA abuse, 43% met criteria for dependence, and 59% met criteria for withdrawal-related symptoms (Cottler et al., 2001).

Neurobiology

MDMA has a variety of effects on several neurotransmitter systems: MDMA increases monoaminergic signaling by interacting with monoamine transporters to stimulate nonexocytotic release of DA, NE, and 5-HT, as well as inhibit the DAT, 5-HT transporter (SERT), and NE transporter (NET) (Baumann et al., 2007); MDMA has especially pronounced effects on the 5-HT system in addition to stimulating presynaptic release of 5-HT; it also increases 5-HT transmission by inhibiting SERT, reversibly inhibiting monoamine oxidase A (MAO-A) and slowing down the degradation of

5-HT, and inhibiting tryptophan hydroxylase, which slows down the production of 5-HT (Hasler, Studerus, Lindner, Ludewig, & Vollenweider, 2009), with increases in extracelluar 5-HT that are greater in magnitude those that for DA (Baumann et al., 2007) but less so than its effects on NE (Verrico, Miller, & Madras, 2007). Some conclusions can be drawn from these varying effects:

1. Some of the psychological and physical effects of MDMA are due to SERT-mediated increases in presynaptic release of 5-HT (Vollenweider et al., 2002). In animal studies, SSRIs inhibit MDMA-induced 5-HT release and block the behavioral effects of MDMA (Gudelsky & Nash, 1996; Geyer & Callaway, 1994). In a human laboratory study, pretreatment with citalopram significantly reduced the spectrum of psychological effects (i.e., positive mood, self-confidence, extraversion, derealization, depersonalization, and thought disorder), as well as cardiovascular and side effects associated with MDMA administration (Liechti, Baumann, Gamma, & Vollenweider, 2000).

2. The NET plays a key role in stimulant and cardiovascular effects (i.e., sympathomimetic) of MDMA. In a human study, reboxetine (a NET) pretreatment reduced the effects of MDMA on increases in plasma levels of NE, increases in blood pressure (BP) and heart rate (HR), subjective drug high, and emotional excitation (Hysek et al., 2011). In a recent study that further confirms the role of the SERT and NET in mediating MDMA effects, duloxetine (a dual SERT and NET inhibitor) markedly decreased the psychological and cardiovascular responses to MDMA in human participants (Hysek, Simmler, et al., 2012).

3. $5-HT_{2A}$ activation is responsible for the mild perceptual and hallucinogen-like properties of MDMA. MDMA has relatively mild to moderate affinity for the $5-HT_{2A}$ receptor in animal studies (Vollenweider et al., 2002) and although not considered a classical hallucinogen, it does possess mild hallucinogenic properties along the spectrum with the SHs, with increased hallucinogenic and psychotic experiences reported at higher doses (Solowij, Hall, & Lee, 1992). Furthermore, in a human laboratory study, pretreatment with ketanserin (a $5-HT_{2A}$ antagonist) led to a significant reduction in hallucinogenic perceptual phenomenon associated with MDMA administration (Liechti, Saur, Gamma, Hell, & Vollenweider, 2000).

4. Dopamine activation is responsible for the addictive liability and some of the mood-elevating effects of MDMA (Kehr et al., 2011). In a human laboratory study, pretreatment with haloperidol selectively reduced the euphoric effects of MDMA while increasing certain negative psychological effects (i.e., anxiety and derealization), and having no effect on physiological responses (Liechti & Vollenweider, 2000).

5. With regard to neurohormonal effects, MDMA increases prolactin and cortisol levels acutely (Harris, 2002) and can diminish cortisol reactivity in chronic users (Parrott et al., 2014); MDMA increases levels of oxytocin in animals and humans. Serotonin release, directly or indirectly, causes an increase in oxytoxin transmission, possibly due to $5-HT_{1A}$ stimulation (Thompson et al., 2007; Dumont et al., 2009; Wolff & Winstock, 2006). MDMA-induced increases in oxytocin signaling likely mediate the prosocial and empathic properties of MDMA in humans (Thompson et

al., 2007; Hysek, Domes, & Liechti, 2012). In human Ecstasy users, MDMA administration diminishes the accuracy of facial fear recognition (Bedi, Hyman, & de Wit, 2010) and attenuates amygdaloid activity in response to threatening faces, while increasing ventral striatal activity in response to happy facial expressions (Bedi et al., 2009). Together, MDMA may increase prosocial or approach behavior by enhancing responsivity to positive social stimuli and decreasing reactivity to negative social stimuli leading to higher social risk behavior (Hysek, Domes, et al., 2012). It is plausible that MDMA's ability to reduce fear acutely and increase interpersonal trust and bonding may make it a useful adjunct to psychotherapy and might particularly be helpful for certain conditions such as posttraumatic stress disorder (PTSD) and attachment disorders (i.e., Asperger's syndrome; see below).

Regional Brain Activity

Imaging studies (i.e., PET) in human participants who ingest MDMA have demonstrated the following in differential regional brain activity: (1) cerebral blood flow (CBF) increases bilaterally in the ventromedial PFC, the anterior cingulate cortex (ACC), and the cerebellum; (2) CBF decreases bilaterally in motor and somatosensory cortices, superior temporal lobe, posterior cingulate cortex, insula, and thalamus; and (3) unilateral CBF decreases in the left amygdala, right parahippocampal formation, and uncus (Vollenweider et al., 2002). In one study, lower activity in the left amygdala was correlated with lower scores in anxiety-related measures (Gamma, Buck, Berthold, Liechti, & Vollenweider, 2000). This is interesting because MDMA, at typical recreational doses, is known to have anxiolytic-type properties despite having stimulant effects. In the same imaging study by Gamma et al., activity in the temporal cortex, amygdala, and orbitofrontal cortex was correlated with "extraversion" ratings, which is interesting given MDMA's known effects at increasing prosocial behavior and evidence that these brain regions are involved in aspects of social communication (Vollenweider et al., 2002).

Addictive Liability

MDMA's addictive liability appears to be lower than that of other drugs of abuse, as demonstrated in both animal models (Degenhardt, Bruno, & Topp, 2010) and human epidemiological studies (Parrott, 2012). For example, a significant number of rats fail repeatedly to self-administer MDMA even after extended periods of training (Schenk et al., 2007), and unlike cocaine and methamphetamine, low fixed-ratio operant paradigms fail to sustain MDMA self-administration (Fantegrossi, 2007). (One possible explanation for MDMA's relative lack of addictive liability, especially compared to other stimulants (i.e., cocaine, methamphetamine), is likely related to its serotonergic effects; it has been demonstrated in animals that mesoaccumbens dopaminergic release is attenuated by antagonistic MDMA-occasioned serotonergic signaling (Bankson & Yamamoto, 2004) and further evidenced by studies demonstrating that coadministration of MDMA attenuates the reinforcing effects of methamphetamine (Clemens et al., 2007), and cocaine (Diller et al., 2007) in rats.

Intoxication/Phenomenology

MDMA produces a diverse and unique profile of psychological and behavioral effects at typical recreational doses that includes an affective state marked by mood elevation, sense of well-being, low anxiety, increased emotional sensitivity, heightened openness, a sense of being close and connected to others, increased sociability, increased sexual desire, stimulant effects (e.g., increased heart rate and blood pressure, increased core body temperature, decreased appetite, increased alertness, decreased speech fluency, jaw clenching, and an increase in sleep latency), mild hallucinogenic effects that include mild perceptual changes (i.e., heightened sensory perception), depersonalization, derealization, and a loosening of ego boundaries (Vollenweider, Gamma, et al., 1998; Baylen & Rosenberg, 2006; Burgess, O'Donohoe, & Gill, 2000). In summary, MDMA could be uniquely classified across drug categories as an anxiolytic, amphetaminergic stimulant with mild psychedelic properties that enhance sociability and empathy. Its previously described diverse pharmacological effects (increased monoaminergic signaling, 5-HT–DA–NE; increased oxytocin signaling) account for its spectrum of subjective effects.

Adverse Psychiatric/Neurological Effects

ACUTE/SUBACUTE EFFECTS

Acute adverse psychological effects from MDMA that can occur with single doses but are more likely seen with repeated dosing or use at higher doses may include anxiety, agitation, dysphoria, hyperactivity, mental fatigue, depersonalization, derealization, confused thinking, decreased appetite, and insomnia (Baylen & Rosenberg, 2006). High-dose MDMA can rarely cause transient panic attacks, brief psychotic episodes, and delirium even in individuals without underlying psychiatric illness (Vecellio, Schopper, & Modestin, 2003). MDMA can acutely exacerbate or precipitate relapse in vulnerable individuals, especially those with psychotic or bipolar spectrum disorders. Although typical recreational doses are associated with an anxiolytic state, associated with decreased amygdaloid activity, and there is some evidence to suggest the efficacy of MDMA-assisted psychotherapy for PTSD (Mithoefer et al., 2011, 2013), higher doses of MDMA can be anxiogenic and exacerbate underlying anxiety spectrum disorders (i.e., panic disorder).

   Following the acute effects of MDMA intoxication (typically 3–6 hours), subacute persisting psychological symptoms in the 24- to 48-hour period postingestion include depression, irritability, anxiety, difficulty concentrating, headache, fatigue, and muscle aches (Peroutka, Newman, & Harris, 1988; Verheyden, Henry, & Curran, 2003). These symptoms usually subside with support and reassurance, which often are all that is needed. If the symptoms are severe, brief pharmacotherapy to alleviate symptoms is recommended. A minority of MDMA users continue to experience these symptoms for more than 3 days after a single ingestion of MDMA (Liechti, Baumann, et al., 2000; Liechti, Saur, et al., 2000; Liechti & Vollenweider, 2000; Huxster, Pirona, & Morgan, 2006). However, individuals who are heavy/chronic users of MDMA are at higher risk of experiencing such adverse psychological symptoms over a longer period of time, especially if they have underlying psychiatric illness. This group is also likely to be at higher risk of experiencing sustained cognitive impairment (see below).

As mentioned, a small group of patients chronically and compulsively use MDMA and develop addiction to it. For these people, the standard psychosocial treatments for addictive disorders should be employed. There are no known pharmacological treatments for MDMA addiction.

PROLONGED EFFECTS

In animal studies, single high doses or repeated dosing of MDMA is usually assessed 1–2 weeks after final drug administration; these studies have consistently revealed major reductions in 5-HT, 5-HIAA, 5-HT uptake, and SERT binding, with the most pronounced effects in certain brain regions such as the cortex, hippocampus, and striatum (Battaglia et al., 1991). Whether these serotonergic changes reflect neurodegenerative neurotoxicity or simply neuroadaptations is a matter of debate. One hypothesis is that these changes reflect neurodegenerative distal axotomy in the long ascending 5-HT axons and their synaptic terminals in higher brain regions. Early studies demonstrated MDMA-induced swelling and fragmentation of 5-HT fibers in rat forebrain followed by loss of these fibers (O'Hearn et al., 1988; Molliver et al., 1990) and while some long-term studies (i.e., 8 weeks to over a year) showed recovery of these serotonergic changes (Battaglia, Yey, & De Souza, 1988; Battaglia et al., 1991), other ones showed an incomplete recovery (Fischer et al., 1995; Scanzello et al., 1993). Some have interpreted these findings as reflective of "neurotoxicity" and a neurodegenerative process. Others have challenged these interpretations by looking at whether MDMA causes glial responses that are characteristic of CNS damage. There is now substantial evidence from the animal literature that long-lasting reductions in serotonergic markers are not reliably associated with microglial or astroglial responses, causing some to conclude that MDMA does not necessarily lead to structural damage to the serotonergic system (Biezonski & Meyer, 2011).

In humans, the argument for MDMA-induced serotonergic "neurotoxicity" has been made based on neuroimaging studies and cognitive/psychological assessments in long-term Ecstasy users. Neuroimaging studies have consistently shown that repeated MDMA use in humans is associated with chronic reductions in cortical serotonin signaling, as evidenced by reductions in SERT, up-regulation in 5-HT_{2A} receptors, and increased neocortical excitability; although there is some evidence for SERT recovery in subcortical areas with extended abstinence, the reductions in SERT in the neocortex appear long-lasting (Benningfield & Cowan, 2013). A number of studies have examined functional problems in abstinent individuals with a history of substantial Ecstasy use, and a variety of pathological conditions has been reported, including neurocognitive impairment, especially related to frontal and hippocampal regions (retrospective–prospective–procedural–working memory, simple–complex cognition, and social intelligence); visual and psychomotor deficits; greater pain perception; changes in appetite; and psychopathology (i.e., depression, anxiety, disturbed sleep, impulsivity, increased stress reactivity (Parrott, 2012). It is important to note that none of these studies was designed to conclude definitively that MDMA is the causative agent (such a study would be unethical to conduct) and it cannot be ruled out that preexisting differences, polydrug use, or other unknown factors may account for these effects. We cannot conclude at this point that MDMA causes irreversible neurological and psychiatric pathology. However, given the animal and human data, heavy prolonged use of MDMA is highly concerning and should be assumed to cause enduring cognitive impairment, although the functional implications and impact of these deficits are unclear at present.

Adverse Medical Effects

Serious adverse medical sequelae related to MDMA ingestion are uncommon and predominantly relate to its stimulant–sympathomimetic effects and include cardio-vascular toxicity (i.e., tachyarrhythmias, malignant hypertension, myocardial infarc-tion), neurological toxicity (i.e., seizures, ischemic or hemorrhagic strokes, delirium), malignant hyperthermia, hyponatremia, hepatotoxicity, renal failure, and death (Kalant, 2001). Malignant hyperthermia is caused by MDMA-induced sympathetic activation, exacerbated by excessive motoric activity (i.e., dancing) in a warm and crowded club setting, and associated with an array of serious adverse events such as rhabdomyolysis (also exacerbated by excessive motoric activity) leading to myoglo-binuria/acute tubular necrosis/renal failure, disseminated intravascular coagulation, hepatic failure, seizures, and death (Ricaurte & McCann, 2005). Hyponatremia, a serious adverse medical event that can lead to seizures, coma and death, is likely related to MDMA-induced syndrome of inappropriate antidiuretic hormone secre-tion (SIADH; Henry et al., 1998) or is related to the law of unintended consequences. The "harm reduction" admonition of advising MDMA users to adopt the strategy of ingesting copious amounts of water prior to, and while taking MDMA to pre-vent dehydration likely contributes to development of this potentially fatal condition (Hartung et al., 2002).

MDMA intoxication or overdose may be suspected in any individual with altera-tions of sensorium, hyperthermia, muscle rigidity, and/or fever. Because the drug is used in specific settings and by specific subgroups, the level of suspicion should be proportional to the user and the circumstances involved. If an individual patient has been to a rave, or some club event, this should raise the clinician's suspicion that MDMA was ingested. In addition, the clinician should have a high degree of suspi-cion that the patient may have taken multiple drugs. Ecstasy overdose would most likely involve the ingestion of multiple doses and would also most likely occur in an environment that induced dehydration. Supportive measures, such as effective hydra-tion using intravenous fluids and lowering the temperature of the patient with cooling blankets or an ice bath, are often necessary. Physical restraint, which may be neces-sary for agitated patients, should be used sparingly so as not to potentially exacerbate rhabdomyolysis. Benzodiazepines are the preferred choice for a sedating agent (Shan-non, 2000). Hypertension often resolves with sedation. If it persists, nitroprusside, or a calcium-channel blocker, is preferred over a beta-blocker, which may worsen vasospasm and hypertension (Albertson & Marelich, 1998).

Therapeutic Applicability

MDMA was used as an adjunct to psychotherapy for certain conditions (i.e., PTSD, couple therapy) by over 1,000 U.S. clinicians from the mid-70s to 1985, when it was placed in the Schedule I category after gaining popularity as a club drug (Pentney, 2001). Given MDMA's unique profile of psychic effects (especially its prosocial and empathogenic properties), it could theoretically be used therapeutically as an adjunct to psychotherapy for an array of psychiatric conditions, such as anxiety spectrum disorders (i.e., PTSD), attachment disorders (i.e., autism spectrum disorders), personality disorders (i.e., narcissistic and antisocial personality disorders), and couple therapy. A recent reemergence of controlled therapeutic trials for MDMA to treat PTSD has occurred in the United States and several other countries (Doblin, 2002) with evidence so far from a randomized controlled trial (RCT) of 20 participants pointing to a therapeutic effect of MDMA versus placebo in treating core symptoms of PTSD with enduring benefits and without evidence of medical or psychiatric harm to participants (Mithoefer et al., 2011, 2013). Notwithstanding these studies, MDMA is a potentially dangerous substance and its risks need to be weighed against any experimental or clinical use.

INHALANTS

Inhalants, a heterogeneous group of substances, are recognized as a category in DSM. One might subclassify them as volatile solvents, aerosols, gases, and nitrates, although that grouping is imperfect given the range of other substances that are used to provide a psychoactive effect. With the exception of nitrates, these substances act directly on the CNS. Volatile solvents are found within household and industrial items such as paint thinners, glues, correction fluids, and other products. Aerosols are sprays that contain propellants and solvents. Gases include medical anesthetics and those found in various household or industrial products, including nitrous oxide, which is also found in whipped cream dispensers, as well as refrigerant. Finally, nitrates, which dilate blood vessels and relax muscles, are a special group. They have a reputation as being "sexual enhancers," and amyl nitrate is particularly used for that purpose.

Many individuals have used inhalants, and some subgroups utilize certain inhalants more than others. According to the 2010 NSDUH, there were 793,000 adults who had ever used such a substance; they are clearly used mostly by youth ages 12–17 (and more among females), likely owing to their ease of access. The rate of cases reported to U.S. poison control centers declined from 1993 to 2008 by around 33%. Also, use among adolescents has declined over time: Overall rates decreased from 3.3% in 2011 to 2.6% in 2012 (SAMHSA, 2014). Use is higher among Hispanics than among other ethnic groups. Often a particular substance is favored in one geographic area over another. Toluene, which is a solvent found in many commonly abused inhalants, activates the brain's dopamine system, suggesting a link to its role in the reward system.

The pharmacological effects of inhalants vary by substance, but in general these substances produce an anesthetic, intoxicating, and reinforcing effect through CNS depression, except in the case of the nitrites, which act as dilators and relaxers of blood vessels rather than as anesthetics. They disseminate quickly to the CNS and lead to a rapid "high" that is akin to alcohol intoxication and lasts a few minutes, leading to frequent reexposure. Like alcohol intoxication, symptoms include dizziness, euphoria, and inability to coordinate movements. Users may experience disinhibition, lightheadedness, or even psychotic features. In high amounts, the solvents and gases produce anesthesia and possibly unconsciousness. During intoxication there may be other effects: belligerence, apathy, and impaired judgment and functioning. Further doses may lead to confusion or delirium.

Toxicity from inhalants may affect other organs or lead to permanent brain injury. This may include cardiac conduction abnormalities, a manner in which an otherwise healthy individual may die after a single dose. Other morbidity and mortality may arise due to asphyxiation, suffocation, convulsions, coma, choking, or injuries that occur while intoxicated. Over long-term exposure, damage to the CNS, bone marrow, immune system, hepatic, renal, and sensory damage are all possible. Finally, both unsafe sexual practices (Mimiaga et al., 2008) and disordered eating have been associated with inhalant use (Pisetsky & Chao, 2008). Individuals with inhalant use disorder receiving clinical care often have numerous other substance use disorders (SUDs; Wu et al., 2008). Inhalant use disorder commonly co-occurs with adolescent conduct disorder and adult antisocial personality disorder. Adult inhalant use and inhalant use disorder also are strongly associated with suicidal ideation and suicide attempts (Howard et al., 2010).

In DSM-IV, the disorders inhalant abuse and inhalant dependence were recognized. There were no specific criteria sets for either one. Inhalant intoxication was delineated specifically. Inhalant-induced disorders included inhalant-induced persisting dementia, as well as disorders of mood, psychosis, anxiety, and delirium. DSM-5 made a change and includes only hydrocarbons among the inhalants, with the other inhaled substances moved to the section on "other" substances of abuse. In DSM-5 the various inhalant-induced disorders are like those in DSM-IV.

REFERENCES

Abuzzahab, F. S., Sr., & Anderson, B. J. (1971). A review of LSD treatment in alcoholism. *Int Pharmacopsychiatry, 6*(4), 223–235.
Albertson, T. E., & Marelich, G. P. (1998). Pharmacologic adjuncts to mechanical ventilation in acute respiratory distress syndrome. *Crit Care Clin, 14*(4), 581–610.
Alper, K. R. (2001). Ibogaine: A review. *Alkaloids Chem Biol, 56,* 1–38.
Alper, K. R., Stajić, M., & Gill, J. R. (2012). Fatalities temporally associated with the ingestion of ibogaine. *J Forensic Sci, 57*(2), 398–412.
American Psychiatric Association. (2013). *Diagnostic and statistical manual of mental disorders* (5th ed.). Arlington, VA: Author.
Anthony, J. C., Warner, L. A., & Kessler, R. C. (1994). Comparative epidemiology of dependence on tobacco, alcohol, controlled substances, and inhalants: Basic findings from the National Comorbidity Survey. *Exp Clin Psychopharmacol, 2,* 244–268.
Bankson, M. G., & Yamamoto, B. K. (2004). Serotonin–GABA interactions modulate MDMA-induced mesolimbic dopamine release. *J Neurochem, 91,* 852–859.
Barker, S. A., McIlhenny, E. H., & Strassman, R. (2012). A critical review of reports of endogenous

psychedelic N, N-dimethyltryptamines in humans: 1955–2010. *Drug Test Anal, 4*(7–8), 617–635.

Battaglia, G., Sharkey, J., Kuhar, M. J., et al. (1991). Neuroanatomic specificity and time course of alterations in rat brain serotonergic pathways induced by MDMA (3,4-methylenedioxymethamphetamine): Assessment using quantitative autoradiography. *Synapse, 8,* 249–260.

Battaglia, G., Yeh, S. Y., & De Souza, E. B. (1988). MDMA-induced neurotoxicity: Parameters of degeneration and recovery of brain serotonin neurons. *Pharmacol Biochem Behav, 29,* 269–274.

Baumann, M. H., Ayestas, M. A., Partilla, J. S., et al. (2012). The designer methcathinon analogs, mephedrone and methylone, are substrates for monoamine transporters in brain tissue. *Neuropsychopharmacol, 37*(5), 1192–1203.

Baumann, M. H., Wang, X., & Rothman, R. B. (2007). 3,4-Methylenedioxymethamphetamine (MDMA) neurotoxicity in rates: A reappraisal of past and present findings. *Psychopharmacol, 189,* 407–424.

Baylen, C. A., & Rosenberg, H. (2006). A review of the acute subjective effects of MDMA/ecstasy. *Addiction, 101,* 933–947.

Bedi, G., Hyman, D., & de Wit, H. (2010). Is ecstasy an "empathogen"?: Effects of ±3,4-methylenedioxymethamphetamine on prosocial feelings and identification of emotional states in others. *Biol Psychiatry, 68,* 1134–1140.

Bedi, G., Phan, K. L., Angstadt, M., et al. (2009). Effects of MDMA on sociability and neural response to social threat and social reward. *Psychopharmacol (Berl), 207,* 73–83.

Béïque, J. C., Imad, M., Mladenovic, L., et al. (2007). Mechanism of the 5-hydroxytryptamine 2A receptor-mediated facilitation of synaptic activity in prefrontal cortex. *Proc Natl Acad Sci USA, 104*(23), 9870–9875.

Benningfield, M. M., & Cowan, R. L. (2013). Brain serotonin function in MDMA (Ecstasy) users: Evidence for persisting neurotoxicity. *Neuropsychopharmacol Rev, 28,* 252–253.

Benthuysen, J. L., Hance, A. J., Quam, D. D., & Winters, W. D. (1989). Comparison of isomers of ketamine on catalepsy in the rat and electrical activity of the brain and behavior in the cat. *Neuropharmacol, 28,* 1003–1009.

Benwell, M. E., Holtom, P. E., Moran, R. J., et al. (1996). Neurochemical and behavioural interactions between ibogaine and nicotine in the rat. *Br J Pharmacol, 117*(4), 743–749.

Biezonski, D., & Meyer, J. S. (2011). The nature of 3,4-methylenedioxymethamphetamine (MDMA)-induced serotonergic dysfunction: Evidence for and again the neurodegenerative hypothesis. *Curr Neuropharmacol, 9,* 84–90.

Bogenszhutz, M. P., Forcehimes, A. A., Pommy, J. A., et al. (2015). Psilocybin-assisted treatment for alcohol dependence: A proof-of-concept study. *J Psychopharmacol, 29*(3), 289–299.

Buckholtz, N. S., Zhou, D. F., Freedman, D. X., et al. (1990). Lysergic acid diethylamide (LSD) administration selectively downregulates serotonin$_2$ receptors in rat brain. *Neuropsychopharmacol, 3,* 137–148.

Burgess, C., O'Donohoe, A., & Gill, M. (2000). Agony and ecstasy: A review of MDMA effects and toxicity. *Eur Psychiatry, 15,* 287–294.

Canezin, J., Cailleux, A., Turcant, A., et al. (2001). Determination of LSD and its metabolites in human biological fluids by high-performance liquid chromatography with electrospray tandem mass spectrometry. *J Chromatogr B Biomed Sci Appl, 765*(1), 15–27.

Carr, D. B., Goudas, D. B., Denman, W. T., et al. (2004). Safety and efficacy of intranasal ketamine for the treatment of breakthrough pain in patients with chronic pain: A randomized, double-blind, placebo-controlled, crossover study. *Pain, 108*(1–2), 17–27.

Cavus, I., & Duman, R. S. (2003). Influence of estradiol, stress, and 5-HT$_{2A}$ agonist treatment on brain-derived neurotrophic factor expression in female rats. *Biol Psychiatry, 54,* 59–69.

Clemens, K. J., McGregor, I. S., Hunt, G. E., et al. (2007). MDMA, methamphetamine and their combination: Possible lessons for party drug users from recent preclinical research. *Drug Alcohol Rev, 26,* 9–15.

Cochin, J., Woods, L. A., & Seevers, M. H. (1951). The absorption, distribution and urinary excretion of mescaline in the dog. *J Pharmacol Exp Ther, 101*(2), 205–209.

Cohen, S. (1960). Lysergic acid diethylamide: Side effects and complications. *J Nerv Ment Dis, 130,* 30–40.

Cottler, L. B., Ben Abdallah, A., Inciardi, J., et al. (2006, July 12–16). *Use, abuse, and dependence on club drugs in Sydney, St. Louis and Miami.* Paper presented at the 2006 World Psychiatric Association International Congress, Istanbul, Turkey.

Cottler, L. B., Womack, S. B., Compton, W. M., et al. (2001). Ecstasy abuse and dependence among adolescents and young adults: Applicability and reliability of DSM-IV criteria. *Hum Psychopharmacol, 16,* 599–606.

Degenhardt, L., Bruno, R., & Topp, L. (2010). Is ecstasy a drug of dependence? *Drug Alcohol Depend, 107,* 1–10.

de la Torre, R., Farre, M., Roset, P. N., et al. (2004). Human pharmacology of MDMA: Pharmacokinetics, metabolism, and disposition. *Ther Drug Monit, 26,* 137–144.

Diller, A., Rocha, A., Cardon, A., et al. (2007). The effects of concurrent administration of ±3,4-methylenedioxymethamphetamine and cocaine on conditioned placed preference in the adult male rat. *Pharmacol Biochem Behav, 88,* 165–170.

Doblin, R. (2002). A clinical plan for MDMA (Ecstasy) in the treatment of posttraumatic stress disorder (PTSD): Partnering with the FDA. *J Psychoactive Drugs, 34,* 185–194.

Domino, E. F., & Miller, S. C. (2009). The pharmacology of dissociatives. In R. K. Ries, D. A. Fiellin, S. C. Miller, & R. Saitz (Eds.), *Principles of addiction medicine* (4th ed., pp. 231–240). Philadelphia: Lippincott Williams & Wilkins.

Dos Santos, R. G., Valle, M., Bouso, J. C., et al. (2011). Autonomic, neuroendocrine, and immunological effects of ayahuasca: A comparative study with *d*-amphetamine. *J Clin Psychopharmacol, 31*(6), 717–726.

Dumont, G. J., Sweep, F. C., van der Steen, R., et al. (2009). Increased oxytocin concentrations and prosocial feelings in humans after ecstasy (3,4-methylenedioxymethamphetamine) administration. *Soc Neurosci, 4,* 359–366.

Fantegrossi, W. E. (2007). Reinforcing effects of methylenedioxy amphetamine congeners in rhesus monkeys: Are intravenous self-administration experiments relevant to MDMA neurotoxicity? *Psychopharmacology, 189,* 471–482.

Fantegrossi, W. E., Woods, J. H., & Winger, G. (2004). Transient reinforcing effects of phenylisopropylamine and indolealkylamine hallucinogens in rhesus monkeys. *Behav Pharmacol, 15*(2), 149–157.

Fischer, C., Hatzidimitriou, G., Wlos, J., et al. (1999). Reorganization of ascending 5-HT axon projections in animals previously exposed to the recreational drug (±)3,4-methylenedioxymethamphetamine (MDMA, "ecstasy"). *J Neurosci, 15,* 5476–5485.

Fribourg, M., Moreno, J. L., Holloway, T., et al. (2011). Decoding the signaling of a GPCR heteromeric complex reveals a unifying mechanism of action of antipsychotic drugs. *Cell, 147*(5), 1011–1023.

Gamma, A., Buck, A., Berthold, T., Liechti, M. E., & Vollenweider, F. X. (2000). 3,4-Methylenedioxymethamphetamine (MDMA) modulates cortical and limbic brain activity as measured by [H(2)(15)O]-PET in healthy humans. *Neuropsychopharmacol, 23*(4), 388–395.

Garcia, L. S., Comim, C. M., Valvassori, S. S., et al. (2009). Ketamine treatment reverses behavioral and physiological alterations induced by chronic mild stress in rats. *Prog Neuropsychopharmacol Biol Psychiatry, 33,* 450–455.

Geyer, M. A., & Callaway, C. W. (1994). Behavioral pharmacology of ring-substituted amphetamine analogs. In A. K. Cho & D. S. Segal (Eds.), *Amphetamine and its analogs: Psychopharmacology, toxicology, and abuse.* San Diego, CA: Academic Press.

Geyer, M. A., & Vollenweider, F. X. (2008). Serotonin research: Contributions to understanding psychoses. *Trends Pharmacol Sci, 29*(9), 445–453.

Giacomelli, S., Palmery, M., Romanelli, L., et al. (1998). Lysergic acid diethylamide (LSD) in a partial agonist of D_2 dopaminergic receptors and it potentiates dopamine-mediated prolactin secretion in lactotrophs *in vitro*. *Life Sci, 63,* 215–222.

Glennon, R. A. (2009). The pharmacology of classical hallucinogens and related designer drugs. In R. K. Ries, D. A. Fiellin, S. C. Miller, & R. Saitz (Eds.), *Principles of addiction medicine* (4th ed., pp. 215–240). Philadelphia: Lippincott/Williams & Wilkins.

Glick, S. D., Maisonneuve, I. M., & Dickinson, H. A. (2000). 18-MC reduced methamphetamine and nicotine self-administration in rats. *NeuroReport, 11*(9), 2013–2015.

Goldberg, M. E., Domsky, R., Scaringe, D., et al. (2005). Multi-day low dose ketamine infusion for the treatment of complex regional pain syndrome. *Pain Physician, 8,* 175–179.

Gonzalez-Maeso, J., Ang, R. L., Yuen, T., et al. (2008). Identification of a serotonin/glutamate receptor complex implicated in psychosis. *Nature, 452,* 93–97.

Griffiths, R. R., & Grob, C. S. (2010). Hallucinogens as medicine. *Sci Am, 303*(6), 76–79.

Griffiths, R. R., Johnson, M. W., Richards, W. A., et al. (2011). Psilocybin occasioned mystical-type experiences: Immediate and persisting dose-related effects. *Psychopharmacol (Berl), 218*(4), 649–665.

Griffiths, R., Richards, W., Johnson, M., McCann, U., & Jesse, R. (2008). Mystical-type experiences occasioned by psilocybin mediate the attribution of personal meaning and spiritual significance 14 months later. *J Psychopharmacol, 22*(6), 621–632.

Griffiths, R. R., Richards, W. A., McCann, U., & Jesse, R. (2006). Psilocybin can occasion mystical-type experiences having substantial and sustained personal meaning and spiritual significance. *Psychopharmacol (Berl), 187*(3), 268–283.

Gudelsky, G. A., & Nash, J. F. (1966). Carrier-mediated release of serotonin by 3,4-methylenedioxymethamphetamine: Implications for serotonin–dopamine interactions. *J Neurochem, 66,* 243–249.

Halpern, J. H., & Pope, H. G., Jr. (2003). Hallucinogen persisting perception disorder: What do we know after 50 years? *Drug Alcohol Depend, 69*(2), 109–119.

Halpern, J. H., Sherwood, A. R., Hudson, J. I., et al. (2005). Psychological and cognitive effects of long-term peyote use among Native Americans. *Biol Psychiatry, 58,* 624–631.

Halpern, J. H., Sherwood, A. R., Passie, T., et al. (2008). Evidence of health and safety in American members of a religion who use a hallucinogenic sacrament. *Med Sci Monit, 14*(8), SR15–SR22.

Harris, D. S., Baggott, M., Mendelson, J. H., et al. (2002). Subjective and hormonal effects of 3,4-methylenedioxymethamphetamine (MDMA) in humans. *Psychopharmacol, 162*(4), 396–405.

Hartung, T. K., Schofield, E., Short, A. I., et al. (2002). Hyponatraemic states following 3,4-methylenedioxymethamphetamine (MDMA, "ecstasy") ingestion. *QJM, 95*(7), 431–437.

Hasler, F., Studerus, E., Lindner, K., Ludewig, S., & Vollenweider, F. X. (2009). Investigation of serotonin-1A receptor function in the human psychopharmacology of MDMA. *J Psychopharmacol, 23*(8), 923–935.

Henry, J. A., Fallon, J. K., Kicman, A. T., et al (1998). Low-dose MDMA ("ecstasy") induces vasopressin secretion. *Lancet, 13,* 351(9118), 1784.

Homayoun, H., & Moghaddam, B. (2007). NMDA receptor hypofunction produces opposite effects on prefrontal cortex interneurons and pyramidal neurons. *J Neurosci, 27,* 11496–11500.

Howard, M. O., Perron, B. E., Sacco, P., et al. (2010). Suicide ideation and attempts among inhalant users: Results from the National Epidemiologic Survey on Alcohol and Related Conditions. *Suicide Life Threat Behav, 40*(3), 276–286.

Huxster, J. K., Pirona, A., & Morgan, M. J. (2006). The sub-acute effects of recreational ecstasy (MDMA) use: A controlled study in humans. *J Psychopharmacol, 20*(2), 281–290.

Hysek, C. M., Domes, G., & Liechti, M. E. (2012). MDMA enhances "mind reading" of positive emotions and impairs "mind reading" of negative emotions. *Psychopharmacol, 222,* 293–302.

Hysek, C. M., Simmler, L. D., Nicola, V. G., et al. (2012). Duloxetine inhibits effects of MDMA ("Ecstasy") *in vitro* and in humans in a randomized placebo-controlled laboratory study. *PLoS ONE, 7*(5), e36476.

Hysek, C. M., Simmler, L. D., Ineichen, M., et al. (2011). The norepinephine transporter inhibitor Reboxetine reduces stimulant effects of MDMA ("Ecstasy") in humans. *Clin Pharmacol Therapeut, 90*(2), 246–255.

Jodo, E., Suzuki, Y., Katayama, T., et al. (2005). Activation of medial prefrontal cortex by phencyclidine is mediated via a hippocampo-prefrontal pathway. *Cereb Cortex, 15,* 663–669.

Johnson, M. W., Garcia-Romeu, A., Cosimano, M. P., et al. (2014). Pilot study of the 5-HT2AR agonist psilocybin in the treatment of tobacco addiction. *J Psychopharmacol, 28*(11), 983–992.

Johnson, M. W., Richards, W. A., & Griffiths, R. R. (2008). Human hallucinogen research: Guidelines for safety. *J Psychopharmacol, 22*(6), 603–620.

Johnston, L. D., O'Malley, P. M., Bachman, J. G., & Schulenberg, J. E. (2013). *Monitoring the Future national survey results on drug use, 1975–2012: Vol. I. Secondary school students.* Ann Arbor: Institute for Social Research, University of Michigan.

Kalant, H. (2001). The pharmacology and toxicology of "ecstasy" (MDMA) and related drugs. *CMAJ, 165*(7), 917–928.

Kehr, J., Ichinose, F., Yoshitake, S., et al. (2011). Mephedrone, compared with MDMA (ecstasy) and amphetamine, rapidly increases both dopamine and 5-HT levels in nucleus accumbens in awake rats. *Br J Pharmacol, 164,* 1949–1958.

Krebs, T. S., & Johansen, P. O. (2012). Lysergic acid diethylamide (LSD) for alcoholism: Meta-analysis of randomized controlled trials. *J Psychopharmacol, 26*(7), 994–1002.

Krebs, T. S., & Johansen, P. O. (2013). Psychedelics and mental health: A population study. *PLoS ONE, 8,* e63972.

Krupitsky, E. M. (2007). Single versus repeated sessions of ketamine-assisted psychotherapy for people with heroin dependence. *J Psychoactive Drugs, 39*(1), 13–19.

Krupitsky, E., & Kolp, E. (2007). Ketamine psychedelic psychotherapy. In T. B. Roberts & M. J. Winkelman (Eds.), *Psychedelic medicine: New evidence for hallucinogen substances as treatments.* Portsmouth, NH: Greenwood.

Krystal, J. H., D'Souza, D. C., Mathalon, D., et al. (2003). NMDA receptor antagonist effects, cortical glutamatergic function, and schizophrenia: Toward a paradigm shift in medication development. *Psychopharmacol, 169,* 215–233.

Lee, E. E., Della Selva, M. P., Liu, A., & Himelhoch, S. (2015). Ketamine as a novel treatment for major depressive disorder and bipolar depression: A systematic review and quantitative meta-analysis. *Gen Hosp Psychiatry, 37*(2), 178–184.

Leung, K. S., & Cottler, L. B. (2008). Ecstasy and other club drugs: A review of recent epidemiologic studies. *Curr Opin Psychiatry, 21,* 234–241.

Liechti, M. E., Baumann, C., Gamma, A., & Vollenweider, F. X. (2000). Acute psychological effects of 3,4-methylenedioxymethamphetamine (MDMA, or "Ecstasy") are attenuated by the serotonin uptake inhibitor citalopram. *Neuropsychopharmacol, 22,* 513–521.

Liechti, M. E., Saur, M. R., Gamma, A., Hill, D., & Vollenweider, F. X. (2000). Psychological and physiological effects of MDMA ("Ecstasy") after pretreatment with the 5-HT2 antagonist ketanserin in healthy humans. *Neuropsychopharmacol, 23,* 396–404.

Liechti, M. E., & Vollenweider, F. X. (2000). Acute psychological and physiological effects of MDMA ("Ecstasy") after haloperidol pretreatment in healthy humans. *Eur Neuropsychopharmacol, 10,* 289–295.

Maciulaitis, R., Kontrimaviciute, V., Bressolle, F. M. M., & Briadis, V. (2008). Ibogaine, an anti-addictive drug: pharmacology and time to go further in development: A narrative review. *Hum Exp Toxicol, 27,* 181–194.

Maisonneuve, I. M., & Glick, S. D. (2003). Anti-addictive actions of an iboga alkaloid congener: A novel mechanism for a novel treatment. *Pharmacol Biochem Behav, 75*(3), 607–618.

Maisonneuve, I. M., Keller, R. W., & Glick, S. D. (1991). Interactions of ibogaine, a potential anti-addictive agent, and morphine: An *in vivo* microdialysis study. *Eur J Pharmacol, 199*(1), 35–42.

Maisonneuve, I. M., Mann, G. L., Deibel, C. R., & Glick, S. D. (1997). Ibogaine and the dopaminergic response to nicotine. *Psychopharmacol (Berl), 129*(3), 249–256.

Malleson, N. (1971). Acute adverse reactions to LSD in clinical and experimental use in the United Kingdom. *Br J Psychiatry, 118*(543), 229–230.

Marona-Lewicka, D., Thisted, R. A., & Nichols, D. E. (2005). Distinct temporal phases in the behavioral pharmacology of LSD: Dopamine D2 receptor-mediated effects in the rat and implications for psychosis. *Psychopharmacol (Berl), 180*, 427–435.

Mash, D. C., Kovera, C. A., Pablo, J., et al. (2000). Ibogaine: Complex pharmacokinetics, concerns for safety, and preliminary efficacy measures. *Ann NY Acad Sci, 914*, 394–401.

Mimiaga, M. J., Reisner, S. L., Vanderwarker, R., et al. (2008). Polysubstance use and HIV/STD risk behavior among Massachusetts men who have sex with men accessing Department of Public Health mobile van services: Implications for intervention development. *AIDS Patient Care STDS, 22*(9), 745–751.

Mithoefer, M. C., Wagner, M. T., Mithoefer, A. T., et al. (2011). The safety and efficacy of (±)3,4-methylenedioxymethamphetamine-assisted psychotherapy in subjects with chronic, treatment-resistant posttraumatic stress disorder: The first randomized controlled pilot study. *J Psychopharmacol, 25*(4), 439–452.

Mithoefer, M. C., Wagner, M. T., Mithoefer, A. T., et al. (2013). Durability of improvement in post-traumatic stress disorder symptoms and absence of harmful effects or drug dependency after 3,4-methylenedioxymethamphetamine-assisted psychotherapy: A prospective long-term follow-up study. *J Psychopharmacol, 27*(1), 28–39.

Molliver, M. E., Berger, U. V., Mamounas, L. A., et al. (1990). Neurotoxicity of MDMA and related compounds: Anatomic studies. *Ann NY Acad Sci, 600*, 649–661.

Monks, T. J., Jones, D. C., Bai, F., & Lau, S. S. (2004). The role of metabolism in 3,4-(+)-methylenedioxyamphetamine and 3,4-(+)-methylenedioxymethamphetamine (ecstasy) toxicity. *Ther Drug Monit, 26*(2), 132–136.

Moore, N. N., & Bostwick, J. M. (1999). Ketamine dependence in anesthesia providers. *Psychosomatics, 40*(4), 356–359.

Murrough, J. W., Iosifescu, D. V., Chang, L. C., et al. (2013). Antidepressant efficacy of ketamine in treatment-resistant major depression: A two-site randomized controlled trial. *Am J Psychiatry, 170*(10), 1134–1142.

National Institute on Drug Abuse (NIDA). (2001). *Hallucinogens and dissociative drugs* (NIDA Research Report Series, NIH Publication Vol. 01-4209). Rockville, MD: Author.

National Institute on Drug Abuse (NIDA). (2005). *LSD NIDA infofacts*. Rockville, MD: Author.

Newman, J. L., Perry, J. L., & Carroll, M. E. (2007). Social stimuli enhance phencyclidine (PCP) self-administration in rhesus monkeys. *Pharmacol Biochem Behav, 87*(2), 280–288.

Nichols, D. E. (2004). Hallucinogens. *Pharmacol Therapeut, 101*, 131–181.

O'Brien, C. P. (2006). Drug addiction and drug abuse. In L. L. Brunton, J. S. Lazo, & K. L. Parker (Eds.), *Goodman & Gilman's the pharmacological basis of therapeutics* (11th ed., pp. 607–627). New York: McGraw-Hill.

O'Hearn, E., Battaglia, G., De Souza, E. B., et al. (1988). Methylenedioxyamphetamine (MDA) and methylenedioxymethamphetamine (MDMA) cause selective ablation of serotonergic axon terminals in forebrain: Immunocytochemical evidence for neurotoxicity. *J Neurosci, 8*, 2788–2803.

Osmond, H. (1957). A review of the clinical effects of psychotomimetic agents. *Ann NY Acad Sci, 66*, 418–434.

Oye, I., Paulsen, O., & Maurset, A. (1992). Effects of ketamine on sensory perception: Evidence for a role of N-methyl-D-aspartate receptors. *J Pharmacol Exp Ther, 260*(3), 1209–1213.

Parrott, A. C. (2005). Chronic tolerance to recreational MDMA (3,4-methylenedioxymetham-phetamine) or Ecstasy. *J Psychopharmacol, 19,* 71–83.

Parrott, A. C. (2012). MDMA and 5-HT neurotoxicity: The empirical evidence for its adverse effects in humans. *Br J Pharmacol, 166*(5), 1518–1522.

Parrott, A. C., Sands, H. R., Jones, L., et al. (2014). Increased cortisol levels in hair of recent Ecstasy/MDMA users. *Eur Neuropsychopharmacol, 24*(3), 369–374.

Passie, T., Halpern, J. H., Stichtenoth, D. O., et al. (2008). The pharmacology of lysergic acid diethylamide: A review. *CNS Neurosci Ther, 14*(4), 295–314.

Passie, T., Seifert, J., Schneider, U., & Emrich, H. M. (2002). The pharmacology of psilocybin. *Addict Biol, 7*(4), 357–364.

Pentney, A. R. (2001). An exploration of the history and controversies surrounding MDMA and MDA. *J Psychoactive Drugs, 33*(3), 213–221.

Peroutka, S. J., Newman, H., & Harris, H. (1988). Subjective effects of 3,4-methylenedioxymeth-amphetamine in recreational users. *Neuropsychopharmacol, 1,* 273–277.

Pisetsky, E. M., Chao, Y. M., Dierker, L. C., May, B. A., & Striegel-Moore, R. H. (2008). Disor-dered eating and substance use in high school students: Results from the Youth Risk Surveil-lance System. *Int J Eating Dis, 41*(5), 464–470.

Poling, A., & Bryceland, J. (1979). Voluntary drug self-administration by nonhumans: A review. *J Psychedelic Drugs, 11*(3), 185–190.

Puig, M. V., Celada, P., Diaz-Mataix, L., et al. (2003). *In vivo* modulation of the activity of pyramidal neurons in the rat medial prefrontal cortex by 5-HT$_{2A}$ receptors: Relationship to thalamocortical afferents. *Cereb Cortex, 13*(8), 870–882.

Riba, J., Valle, M., Urbano, G., et al. (2003). Human pharmacology of ayahuasca: Subjective and cardiovascular effects, monoamine metabolite excretion, and pharmacokinetics. *J Pharmacol Exp Ther, 306*(1), 73–83.

Ricaurte, G. A., & McCann, U. D. (2005). Recognition and management of complications of new recreational drug use. *Lancet, 365,* 2137–2145.

Ross, S. (2012). Serotonergic hallucinogens and emerging targets for addiction pharmacothera-pies. *Psychiatric Clin North Am, 35*(2), 357–374.

Ross, S., & Peselow, E. (2012). Co-occurring psychotic and addictive disorders: Neurobiology and diagnosis. *Clin Neuropharmacol, 35*(5), 235–243.

Scanzello, C. R., Hatzidimitriou, G., Martello, A. L., et al. (1993). Serotonergic recovery after (±)3,4-(methylenedioxy) methamphetamine injury: Observations in rats. *J Pharmacol Exp Ther, 264,* 1484–1491.

Schenk, S., Hely, L., Lake, B., et al. (2007). MDMA self-administration in rats: Acquisition, progressive ration responding and serotonin transporter binding. *Eur J Neurosci. 26*(11), 3229–3236.

Shannon, M. (2000). Methylenedioxymethamphetamine (MDMA, "ecstasy"). *Pediatr Emerg Care, 16*(5), 377–380.

Smith, G. S., Schloesser, R., Brodie, J. D., et al. (1998). Glutamate modulation of dopamine mea-sured *in vivo* with positron emission tomography (PET) and 11C-raclopride in normal human subjects. *Neuropsychopharmacol, 18*(1), 18–25.

Solowij, N., Hall, W., & Lee, N. (1992). Recreational MDMA use in Sydney: A profile of "Ecstasy" users and their experiences with the drug. *Br J Addict, 87*(8), 1161–1172.

Spiller, H. A., Ryan, M. L., Weston, R. G., & Jansen, J. (2011). Clinical experience with and ana-lytical conformation of "bath salts" and "legal highs" (synthetic cathinones) in the United States. *Clin Toxicol, 49,* 499–505.

Strassman, R. J. (1984). Adverse reactions to psychedelic drugs. A review of the literature. *J Nerv Mental Dis, 172*(10), 577–595.

Substance Abuse and Mental Health Services Administration (SAMHSA). (2011). *Results from the 2010 National Survey on Drug Use and Health: National findings.* Rockville, MD: Author.

Substance Abuse and Mental Health Services Administration, Center for Behavioral Health Statistics and Quality. (2013, November 12). *The DAWN Report: Emergency department visits involving phencyclidine (PCP)*. Rockville, MD: Author.

Substance Abuse and Mental Health Services Administration, Center for Behavioral Health Statistics and Quality. (2014, March 18). *The NSDUH Report: Recent declines in adolescent inhalant use*. Rockville, MD: Author.

Taraschenko, O. D., Shulan, J. M., Maisonneuve, I. M., et al. (2007). 18-MC acts in the medial habenula and interpeduncular nucleus to attenuate dopamine sensitization to morphine in the nucleus accumbens. *Synapse, 61*(7), 547–560.

Thompson, M. R., Callaghan, P. D., Hunt, G. E., et al. (2007). A role for oxytocin and 5-HT$_{1A}$ receptors in prosocial effects of 3,4-methylenedioxymethamphetamine ("Ecstasy"). *Neurosci, 146*, 509–514.

Vaidya, V. A., Marek, G. J., Aghajanian, G. K., et al. (1997). 5-HT$_{2A}$ receptor-mediated regulation of brain-derived neurotrophic factor mRNA in the hippocampus and the neocortex. *J Neurosci, 17*, 2785–2795.

Vecellio, M., Schopper, C., & Modestin, J. (2003). Neuropsychiatric consequences (atypical psychosis and complex-partial seizures) of ecstasy use: Possible evidence for toxicity-vulnerability predictors and implications for preventative and clinical care. *J Psychopharmacol, 17*(3), 342–345.

Verheyden, S., Henry, J., & Curran, V. (2003). Acute, sub-acute and long-term subjective consequences of "ecstasy" (MDMA) consumption in 430 regular users. *Hum Psychopharmacol, 18*, 507–517.

Verrico, C. D., Miller, G. M., & Madras, B. K. (2007). MDMA (Ecstasy) and human dopamine, norepinephrine, and serotonin transporters: Implications for MDMA-induced neurotoxicity and treatment. *Psychopharmacol (Berl), 189*, 489–503.

Vollenweider, F. X., Gamma, A., Liechti, M. E., et al. (1988). Psychological and cardiovascular effects and short-term sequelae of MDMA ("Ecstasy") on MDMA-naïve healthy volunteers. *Neuropsychopharmacol, 19*, 241–251.

Vollenweider, F. X., & Kometer, M. (2010). The neurobiology of psychedelic drugs: Implications for the treatment of mood disorders. *Nat Rev Neurosci, 11*(9), 642–651.

Vollenweider, F. X., Liechti, M. E., Gamma, A., et al. (2002). Acute psychological and neurophysiological effects of MDMA in humans. *J Psychoactive Drugs, 34*(2), 171–184.

Vollenweider, F. X., Vollenweider-Scherpenhuyzen, M. F., Babler, A., et al. (1998). Psilocybin induces schizophrenia-like psychosis in humans via a serotonin-2 agonist action. *NeuroReport, 9*(17), 3897–3902.

Vollenweider, F. X., Vontobel, P., Hell, D., et al. (1999). 5-HT modulation of dopamine release in basal ganglia in psilocybin-induced psychosis in man: A PET study with [^{11}C] raclopride. *Neuropsychopharmacol, 20*, 424–433.

Vollenweider, F. X., Vontobel, P., Oye, I., Hell, D., & Leenders, K. L. (2000). Effects of (S)-ketamine on striatal dopamine: A [^{11}C] raclopride PET study of a model psychosis in humans. *J Psychiatric Res, 34*, 35–43.

Watts, V. J., Lawler, C. P., Fox, D. R., et al. (1995). LSD and structural analogs: Pharmacological evaluation at D$_1$ dopamine receptors. *Psychopharmacol (Berl), 118*, 401–409.

Wilkins, J. N., Danovitch, I., & Gorelick, M. D. (2009). Management of stimulant, hallucinogen, marijuana, phencyclidine, and club drug intoxication and withdrawal. In R. K. Ries, D. A. Fiellin, S. C. Miller, & R. Saitz (Eds.), *Principles of addiction medicine* (4th ed., pp. 607–628). Philadelphia: Lippincott/Williams & Wilkins.

Wilson, M. D., Ferguson, R. W., Mazer, M. E., & Litovitz, T. L. (2011). Monitoring trends in dextromethorphan abuse using the National Poison Data System: 2000–2010. *Clin Toxicol (Phila), 49*(5), 409–415.

Wolff, K., & Winstock, A. R. (2006). Ketamine: From medicine to misuse. *CNS Drugs, 20*(3), 199–218.

Wu, L. T., Howard, M. O., & Pilowsky, D. J. (2008). Substance use disorders among inhalant users: Results from the National Epidemiologic Survey on Alcohol and Related Conditions. *Addict Behav, 33*(7), 968–973.

Wu, L. T., Schlenger, W. E., & Galvin, D. M. (2006). Concurrent use of methamphetamine, MDMA, LSD, ketamine, GHB, and flunitrazepam among American youths. *Drug Alcohol Depend, 84*(1), 102–113. Erratum in *Drug Alcohol Depend* (2007), *86*(2–3), 301.

Zawertailo, L. A., Kaplan, H. L., Busto, U. E., et al. (1998). Psychotropic effects of dextromethorphan are altered by the CYP2D6 polymorphism: A pilot study. *J Clin Psychopharmacol, 18*(4), 332–337.

CHAPTER 10

Caffeine

LAURA M. JULIANO
GRETA BIELACZYC RAGLAN

Caffeine (1,3,7-trimethylxanthine) has been ingested in one form or another throughout various parts of the world for thousands of years, and any attempts to prohibit its use have repeatedly failed (Pendergrast, 1999). Currently, caffeine is the most widely used psychoactive drug in the world. It is found naturally in more than 60 species of plants (e.g., coffee, tea, kola, guarana, mate) and belongs to the methylxanthine class of alkaloids, which also includes theobromine and theophylline. In the United States, approximately 85% of adults and children regularly ingest caffeine (Mitchell, Knight, Hockenberry, Teplansky, & Hartman, 2014). As a nonselective adenosine antagonist and central nervous system (CNS) stimulant, caffeine produces various physiological and psychological effects (Ferre, 2008). Typical dietary doses (e.g., 20–300 mg) of caffeine are generally consumed without incident and are not associated with any life-threatening illnesses. Moreover, caffeine has some valuable therapeutic effects (e.g., analgesic adjuvant, energy aid) and may possibly offer protective effects against some diseases (e.g., Parkinson's disease; Liu et al., 2012). However, caffeine is not completely innocuous. It can produce clinically significant negative psychological and physiological effects, tolerance and withdrawal, and discrete psychiatric symptoms and disorders (e.g., caffeine intoxication, caffeine-induced anxiety disorder). Like other recreational drugs, some individuals develop caffeine use disorder, characterized in part by an inability to modify caffeine use despite negative psychological and/or physical consequences (American Psychiatric Association, 2013; Juliano, Evatt, Richards, & Griffiths, 2012). In addition, caffeine interacts with some commonly used psychotherapeutic (e.g., benzodiazepines) and recreational drugs (e.g., nicotine). The widespread use of caffeine and its well accepted integration into daily activities and cultural routines (e.g., coffee break) may obscure the recognition of caffeine-associated problems. It is important for clinicians to be familiar with sources of caffeine; the pharmacological effects, psychiatric symptoms, and disorders that can result from its use; and methods to help individuals curtail caffeine use.

SOURCES OF CAFFEINE

Caffeine is found in a variety of beverages, foods, dietary supplements, and over-the-counter and prescription medications (see Table 10.1). It is important to note that caffeine levels can vary significantly across product types and even within the same product type. For example, the amount of caffeine in a 12 oz serving of coffee can range from 108 to 420 mg. Caffeine levels vary more than 10-fold across different brands of energy drinks (i.e., 36–375 mg). In the United States, coffee and soft drinks are the major dietary sources of caffeine. However, since Red Bull became available in the United States in 1997, energy drink consumption has increased every year, and hundreds of brands of energy drinks are now marketed to consumers (Reissig, Strain, & Griffiths, 2009). In the past decade, the practice of mixing alcohol with energy drinks (e.g., Red Bull and vodka) has become increasingly common. This is potentially problematic, because research has shown that the co-ingestion of caffeinated energy drinks and alcohol increases alcohol consumption, and alters its psychological and behavioral effects (e.g., decreases perceived impairment), which may increase harmful effects (Howland & Rohsenow, 2013; Marczinski & Fillmore, 2006). Caffeinated beer, malt beverages, and hard liquors were available to consumers for a short while before the U.S. Food and Drug Administration (FDA) banned the sale of these products in 2010 due to safety concerns. In recent years there has been widespread marketing of highly caffeinated energy shots (e.g., 5-Hour Energy), and certain manufactures have begun to add caffeine to foods that have traditionally not contained caffeine (e.g., oatmeal, jelly beans, peanut butter).

The FDA limits the amount of caffeine that can be added to soft drinks to 0.2 mg per ml or 71.5 mg for a 12 oz serving. This limit does not apply to energy drinks, because they may be considered dietary supplements. Although manufacturers are required to list caffeine as an ingredient when it is added to products, they are not required to disclose how much caffeine the product contains. In recent years, major soft drink manufacturers have voluntarily begun to label actual caffeine content. Some companies readily provide the caffeine content of their products to consumers who inquire. However, other manufacturers refuse to disclose actual caffeine amounts added to their products, stating their caffeine is part of a proprietary blend. In these instances, consumers may have difficulty assessing and regulating their caffeine exposure. In 2013, the FDA launched an investigation into the safety of caffeine in food products.

EPIDEMIOLOGY

Approximately 85% of the U.S. population age 2 years and older regularly consume caffeine (Mitchell et al., 2014). In a recent study, Mitchell et al. reported an average

TABLE 10.1. Caffeine Content of Common Foods and Medications

Product	Serving size (volume or weight)	Caffeine content (mg)
Beverages		
Coffee		
Brewed/drip	6 oz	54–210
Instant	6 oz	20–130
Espresso	1 oz	60–95
Tea		
Decaffeinated	6 oz	0–10
Brewed	6 oz	30–90
Instant	6 oz	10–35
Canned or bottled	12 oz	8–32
Soft drinks		
Pepsi Max/Diet Pepsi Max	12 oz	69
Mountain Dew/Diet Mt Dew	12 oz	55
Pepsi One	12 oz	55
Diet Coke	12 oz	47
Sunkist/Diet Sunkist	12 oz	41
Dr. Pepper/Diet Dr. Pepper	12 oz	41
Pepsi-Cola	12 oz	38
Diet Pepsi	12 oz	36
Coke Classic	12 oz	35
A&W Cream Soda	12 oz	29
Barq's Root Beer	12 oz	23
A&W Diet Cream Soda	12 oz	22
Cocoa/hot chocolate	6 oz	2–10
Chocolate milk	6 oz	2–7
Energy drinks		
Rage Inferno	24 oz	375
Cocaine	8.4 oz	280
Jolt	23.5 oz	278
NOS	16 oz	260
Rockstar	16 oz	160
Monster	16 oz	160
Full Throttle	16 oz	144
AMP Energy Boost	16 oz	142
Red Bull	8.3 oz	80
Lift Plus	8.45 oz	36
5-Hour Energy	2 oz	215
5-Hour Energy Ext. Strength	2 oz	242
Caffeinated water		
Element	16.9 oz	50
Water Joe	16.9 oz	60
Buzzwater	16.9 oz	100 or 200
Mio Energy Water Enhancer	.06 oz	60
Foods		
Chocolate		
Reese's Peanut Butter Cups	1.45 oz	4
Kit Kat Wafer Bar	1.5 oz	6

(continued)

TABLE 10.1. *(continued)*

Product	Serving size (volume or weight)	Caffeine content (mg)
Hershey's Chocolate Bar	1.55 oz	9
Baking Chocolate, Unsweetened	1 block	17
Hershey's Special Dark	1.45 oz	20
Miscellaneous foods		
Penguin Peppermints	1 mint	7
Dannon Coffee Yogurt	6 oz	30
Powerbar Tangerine Powergel	41 g	50
Morning Spark Instant Energy Oatmeal	1 packet	50
Jelly Belly Sport (Jelly) Beans	1 oz	50
Starbucks Classic Coffee Ice Cream	8 oz	60
Military Energy Gum	1 piece	100
Dietary supplements/weight loss products		
Dexatrim Max	1 caplet	50
Metabolife Weight Management	2 tablets	101
Metabolife Ultra	2 caplets	150
Hydroxycut Weight Loss Formula	2 caplets	200
Twinlab Ripped Fuel	2 capsules	220
Leptopril	2 capsules	220
Stacker 2	1 capsule	253
Stacker 3	1 capsule	254
Swarm Extreme Energizer	1 capsule	300
Over-the-counter medications		
Stimulants		
Vivarin	1 tablet	200
Ultra Pep-Back	1 tablet	200
No-Doz/No-Doz Maximum Strength	1 tablet	100 or 200
Analgesics		
Goody's Headache Powder	1 powder packet	32.5
BC Fast Pain Relief	1 powder packet	33.3
Vanquish	1 caplet	33
BC Arthritis Pain and Influenza	1 powder packet	38
Anacin Advanced Headache	2 tablets	130
Excedrin Extra Strength	2 tablets	130
Menstrual pain relief/diuretics		
Diurex Water Pills	1 tablet	50
Midol Menstrual Complete	1 caplet	60
Pamprin Max	1 caplet	65
Prescription medications		
Headache/migraine/pain		
Norgesic	2 tablets	60
Fiorinal	2 capsules	80
Fioricet/Esgic/many others	2 tablets	80
Cafergot	2 tablets	200

Note. Caffeine values for all brand name products were obtained directly from product labels, or the manufacturer's website or customer service department. Other sources: Juliano, Ferre, and Griffiths (2014); McCusker, Fuehrlein, Goldberger, Gold, and Cone (2006); McCusker, Goldberger, and Cone (2003).

daily caffeine intake of 165 mg when including all age groups. Mean daily intake of caffeine among U.S. adult caffeine consumers has been estimated to be 200–300 mg, with higher intakes estimated for individuals in some European countries and Canada (Barone & Roberts, 1996; Frary, Johnson, & Wang, 2005; Somogyi, 2010). The greatest caffeine consumption is generally found among those 35 years and older (Frary et al., 2005; Mitchell et al., 2014). Coffee is the largest source of caffeine, followed by soft drinks and tea (Frary et al., 2005; Mitchell et al., 2014), and more than 50% of the adult U.S. population consume coffee every day. The last century has seen a large increase in soft drink consumption and, more recently, energy drink consumption (Reissig et al., 2009). Smokers, alcoholics, psychiatric patients, prisoners, and those with eating disorders have been identified as heavier users of caffeine than the general population.

GENETICS

Genetic factors account for some of the variability in caffeine use and effects. Relative to dizygotic twins, monozygotic twins have higher concordance rates for total caffeine consumption, heavy caffeine consumption, coffee and tea intake, caffeine intoxication, caffeine withdrawal, caffeine tolerance, and caffeine-related sleep disturbances, with heritability ranging between 30 and 77% (Cornelis, El-Sohemy, & Campos, 2007; Yang, Palmer, & de Wit, 2010). Findings from twin studies also suggest that there may be common genetic factors that underlie the use of caffeine, cigarette smoking, and alcohol, which appear to be distinct from genetic factors associated with illicit drug use (Kendler, Myers, & Prescott, 2007).

The *CYP1A2* gene, which codes for the primary enzyme responsible for caffeine metabolism (P-450 1A2) and the *ADORA2A* gene, which codes for the adenosine A_{2A} receptor, have been shown to be associated with caffeine use, effects of caffeine, and health outcomes. Variability in the *CYP1A2* gene is associated with variability in caffeine consumption (Josse, Da Costa, Campos, & El-Sohemy, 2012; Yang et al., 2010). Furthermore, individuals who carry the slow metabolism variant of the *CYP1A2* gene have been shown to be at increased risk for coffee-associated hypertension and myocardial infarction (Palatini et al., 2009; Cornelis, El-Sohemy, Kabagambe, & Campos, 2006), and decreased risk for Parkinson's Disease (Popat et al., 2011). One study also indicated an association between the *CYP1A2* gene and greater ergogenic effects of caffeine as measured by cycling time (Womack et al., 2012). *ADORA2A* receptor gene polymorphisms have been shown to be associated with caffeine consumption (Cornelis et al., 2007), self-reported caffeine sensitivity, and caffeine's effects on psychomotor vigilance (Bodenmann et al., 2012), anxiety (Childs, Hohoff, Deckert, Xu, Badner, & de Wit, 2008; Rogers et al., 2010), sleep (Byrne et al., 2012; Retey et al. 2007), and blood pressure (Renda et al., 2012). Recent meta-analyses have found genomewide associations between caffeine use and variants of the ACH receptor gene (aryl hydrocarbon receptor, which regulates *CYP12A*) and the *CYP12A* gene (Cornelis et al., 2011; Sulem et al., 2011; Amin et al., 2012).

PHARMACOLOGICAL EFFECTS

Pharmacokinetics

After oral ingestion, caffeine is absorbed quickly from the gastrointestinal tract and distributed throughout all body fluids. Caffeine readily crosses the blood–brain barrier and placental barrier. Peak plasma concentrations typically occur within 45–60 minutes (Mumford et al., 1996). Caffeine is metabolized by the liver primarily via the P450 1A2 system, which also plays an important role in the metabolism of other substances (Furge & Guengerich, 2006). More than 25 metabolites of caffeine have been identified in humans, including the active metabolites paraxanthine, theobromine, and theophylline. In general, the half-life of caffeine is 4–6 hours, but it can vary widely among individuals (Denaro & Benowitz, 1992). Caffeine half-life is much longer among infants (e.g., 80–100 hours) until the liver enzyme system develops more fully around 6 months of age. Cigarette smoking induces *CYP1A2* enzyme activity, which speeds the elimination of caffeine by as much as 50% (Benowitz, Peng, & Jacob, 2003). Oral contraceptives and hormonal changes in the later stages of pregnancy significantly slow caffeine elimination, which may increase the risk of caffeine toxicity in women who maintain very high levels of caffeine use during pregnancy (Anderson, Juliano, & Schulkin, 2009). There are numerous drugs that interact with caffeine, including the sleep medication zolpidem, the antipsychotic clozapine, the stomach acid inhibitor cimetidine, and the bronchodilator theophylline (Carillo & Benitez, 2000). Caffeine is used as a probe drug for *CYP1A2* activity (Perera, Gross, & McLachlan, 2012).

CNS Effects

Caffeine is a stimulant that influences various neurotransmitter systems primarily via antagonism of A_{2A} and A_1 adenosine receptors (Ferre, 2008). Adenosine is formed from the breakdown of adenosine triphosphate (ATP) and modulates a variety of CNS and peripheral nervous system effects. Caffeine is structurally similar to adenosine. As a competitive A_1 and A_{2A} adenosine receptor antagonist, caffeine produces a variety of effects that are opposite to the effects of adenosine (e.g., CNS stimulation, vasoconstriction). Adenosine is a neuromodulator in the brain that produces largely inhibitory effects (e.g., reduces spontaneous neuronal firing, suppresses motor activity, promotes sleep). A_1 receptors are expressed throughout various brain regions, with the highest concentrations in the hippocampus, cerebral cortex, thalamus, and cerebellum. A_{2A} receptors are concentrated in dopamine-rich areas of the brain, including the striatum, nucleus accumbens, and olfactory tubercle. Adenosine receptors functionally interact with each other, as well with other receptors (i.e., receptor heteromers; Ferre et al., 2008). For example, some of the motor stimulant properties of caffeine are likely a result of increased dopamine release resulting from antagonism of adenosine at the A_{2A}–D_2 receptor heteromer. Lazarus et al. (2011) concluded that caffeine-induced wakefulness is dependent on A_{2A} receptors in the nucleus accumbens. There is also evidence that caffeine increases dopamine release in the shell of the nucleus accumbens, a common neuropharmacological mechanism underlying the rewarding effects of all drugs of dependence (Solinas et al., 2002).

Physiological Effects

Caffeine produces various physiological effects. It increases broncodilation and respiration, and is used therapeutically to treat apnea of prematurity. Caffeine increases gastric acid secretion, diuresis, and urinary calcium excretion, but there is not convincing evidence that these effects have clinical implications for gastrointestinal problems, dehydration, or osteoporosis, respectively (Nawrot et al., 2003). Caffeine increases detrusor pressure on the bladder and may have implications for complaints of urinary urgency and detrusor instability (Gleason et al., 2013). Heavy caffeine use during pregnancy is associated with increased risk of spontaneous abortion (Weng, Odouli, & Li, 2008). Caffeine promotes the release of various hormones, including plasma epinephrine, norepinephrine, cortisol, renin, insulin, and adrenocorticotropic hormone. Research has demonstrated that caffeine consumption increases blood glucose levels and may play a role in insulin resistance among diabetics (Lane, Lane, Surwit, Kuhn, & Feinglos, 2012). Caffeine increases blood pressure to an extent that some have proposed is clinically significant (James, 1997), but this has been debated (Uiterwaal et al., 2007). Caffeine constricts cerebral blood vessels, and chronic use results in a compensatory dilation of blood vessels (via adenosine up-regulation) that accounts for the characteristic throbbing and diffuse withdrawal headache that manifests during caffeine abstinence. Caffeine has thermogenic and ergogenic effects, and as a consequence is added to weight loss products and used to enhance exercise performance (Astorino & White, 2012). Caffeine is believed to be an analgesic adjuvant and is added to many common pain medications (e.g., aspirin, ibuprofen). A Cochrane Review concluded that the addition of caffeine to pain medication increases the percentage of people having a significant analgesic effect by 5–10% (Derry, Derry, & Moore, 2012).

Subjective and Performance Effects

Subjective effects of caffeine are dose dependent and may vary depending on individual differences in caffeine sensitivity and tolerance. Low to moderate doses of caffeine (i.e., 20–200 mg) generally produce positive subjective effects, such as increased alertness, wellbeing, energy, sociability, concentration, motivation to work, and decreased sleepiness and fatigue. Doses greater than 200 mg are more likely to produce anxiety, nervousness, jitteriness, negative mood, and upset stomach. Higher caffeine doses (> 400 mg) can trigger panic attacks. Individuals with anxiety tend to be particularly sensitive to the negative effects of caffeine (Telch, Silverman, & Schmidt, 1996). At typical dietary doses people will choose caffeine over placebo and choose caffeine over money, demonstrating its reinforcing qualities (Schuh & Griffiths, 1997). Among regular caffeine users, the reinforcing effects of caffeine appear to be driven primarily by its ability to suppress withdrawal symptoms (i.e., negative reinforcement) (Schuh & Griffiths, 1997).

There is a rich body of research on the cognitive and motor performance enhancing effects of caffeine. Relative to placebo, caffeine reliably leads to greater sustained attention (vigilance), faster tapping speed, and faster reaction time (Adan & Serra-Grabulosa, 2010; Smith, Christopher, & Sutherland, 2013). The effects of caffeine on memory and other cognitive effects are less conclusive. An expanding literature on caffeine and exercise performance has shown that relative to placebo, caffeine can enhance performance during endurance exercise, reduce ratings of perceived exhaustion, and increase speed and power output (Doherty & Smith, 2004; Ganio, Klau, Casa, Armstrong, & Maresh, 2009). Beneficial effects of caffeine on short-term, high-intensity exercise are harder to demonstrate (e.g., Glaister et al., 2012). Studies have shown that sleep deprivation is associated with decrements in performance on a variety of tasks, and caffeine can reduce but not completely reverse these performance decrements (Wyatt, Cajochen, Ritz-De Cecco, Czeisler, & Dijk, 2004).

An important consideration in interpreting subjective and performance effects of caffeine is that studies typically compare caffeine to placebo among habitual caffeine users after requiring overnight abstinence. Thus, differences between caffeine and placebo may reflect withdrawal reversal (i.e., restoration to baseline performance), a net benefit of caffeine, or some combination of the two (Smith et al., 2013; James & Rogers, 2005). Some studies have demonstrated caffeine-related performance enhancements among nondependent caffeine consumers and nonconsumers, suggesting that not all enhancements are explained by withdrawal reversal (Christopher, Sutherland, & Smith, 2005; Childs & de Wit, 2006; Adan & Serra-Grabulosa, 2010). Taken together it seems reasonable to conclude that caffeine can have modest beneficial performance effects, especially under conditions of sleep deprivation, prolonged vigilance or exercise, or when reversing the effects of caffeine withdrawal. Performance effects might be greater among individuals who are not caffeine dependent; however, beneficial effects may be offset by coinciding negative subjective effects (e.g., anxiety) that may emerge in the absence of tolerance (Rogers, Heatherley, Mullings, & Smith, 2013).

CAFFEINE AND ANXIETY

There is a great deal of evidence showing that caffeine has anxiogenic effects. As previously discussed, genetic factors may underlie individual sensitivity to the anxiogenic effects of caffeine (Telch et al., 1996). Acute doses of caffeine, generally greater than 200 mg, increase anxiety ratings among those with anxiety disorders, as well as nonclinical samples, with higher caffeine doses sometimes producing panic attacks (Nardi et al., 2009). Individuals with anxiety disorders generally experience greater anxiety after consuming caffeine than control subjects (Bruce, Scott, Shine, & Lader, 1992). Some may naturally limit their caffeine intake, but others who do not may fail to recognize the role that caffeine plays in their anxiety. One study reported significant improvements in anxiety symptoms of patients seeking treatment at an anxiety disorders clinic, who had been instructed to cease caffeine use for 1 week (Bruce et al., 1992). Notably, some patients required no additional treatment and were able to stop taking anxiolytic medications.

DSM-5 recognizes caffeine-induced anxiety disorder, which is defined as having the symptoms of an anxiety disorder (e.g., panic disorder, generalized anxiety disorder) as a result of caffeine use. According to DSM-5, one does not need to meet the full criteria for any specific anxiety disorder to be diagnosed with caffeine-induced anxiety disorder. The diagnosis depends on linking the use of caffeine to the anxiety symptoms of concern. For a patient with a suspected caffeine-induced anxiety disorder, a trial caffeine abstinence period may aid in clarifying the diagnosis. There are no epidemiological data on caffeine-induced anxiety disorder.

Clinicians should encourage individuals with anxiety symptoms to reduce or eliminate caffeine use, especially if considering anxiolytic therapy. However, clinicians should be aware that some patients may be hesitant about eliminating caffeine and may express skepticism or defensiveness about the role of caffeine in their anxiety symptoms.

CAFFEINE AND SLEEP

There is abundant evidence that caffeine promotes wakefulness and has disruptive effects on planned sleep (Albert, Uhde, Slate, & McCann, 1997). Caffeine antagonizes adenosine, which is believed to promote sleep as levels increase during prolonged wakefulness (Bjorness & Greene, 2009). Research suggests that caffeine-induced wakefulness is a result of antagonism of A_{2A} receptors in the shell of the nucleus accumbens (Lazarus et al., 2011). As previously discussed, genetic factors may underlie individual differences in the sleep-disruptive effects of caffeine.

Greater sleep disruption is observed as doses of caffeine increase, and as the latency between caffeine consumption and the time to planned sleep decreases. Consuming 200 mg of caffeine before bedtime delays sleep onset, and reduces sleep efficiency and total sleep time (Keenan, Tiplady, Priestley, & Rogers, 2015). A morning dose of 200 mg caffeine is sufficient to disrupt that evening's sleep (Landolt, Werth, Borbely, & Dijk, 1995). Caffeine-related sleep disturbances are more likely to occur among people who do not regularly consume caffeine. Habitual caffeine consumers develop some tolerance to the sleep-disrupting effects of caffeine but may be vulnerable to caffeine-related sleep problems, especially when caffeine is taken closer to bedtime.

Caffeine-induced sleep disorder, as defined in DSM-5, is characterized by a sleep disturbance that is etiologically related to caffeine consumption (American Psychiatric Association, 2013). One does not need to meet full criteria for a DSM-5 sleep disorder to qualify for a diagnosis of caffeine-induced sleep disorder. Insomnia is the most common sleep disturbance caused by caffeine. There are no epidemiological data on caffeine-induced sleep disorder.

Caffeine use should be assessed anytime a patient is complaining of sleep difficulties. It is not uncommon for patients to fail to make a connection between the ingestion of caffeinated products (e.g., caffeine-containing analgesics) and difficulty falling asleep. Although some patients show reluctance to eliminate caffeine, especially when they feel sleep deprived, they should be encouraged to attempt a caffeine abstinence trial in order to rule out an etiological role of caffeine in sleep problems. Furthermore, caffeine reduction or elimination should be considered before prescribing sleep medications (e.g., benzodiazepines).

While caffeine can have negative effects on planned sleep, it is important to acknowledge the beneficial effects of caffeine in preventing unwanted sleep, such as when driving long distances or engaging in other activities that require wakefulness (Kamimori et al., 2015).

CAFFEINE INTOXICATION

Caffeine intoxication results from excessive caffeine consumption. It is defined by the presence of five or more specific mental states, or autonomic signs defined in DSM-5. In addition, fever, irritability, sensory disturbances, tachypnea, vomiting, hallucinations, and headaches have also been reported after excessive caffeine use. Caffeine intoxication usually resolves quickly (i.e., within the first day), often with supportive care and no long-term negative effects. However, very high doses of caffeine (5–10 g) can be fatal (Benowitz, 1990; Banerjee, Ali, Levine, & Fowler, 2014), and there are case reports of accidental overdose and suicide by caffeine ingestion.

There are a number of disorders that should be considered in the differential diagnosis of caffeine intoxication. These include intoxication from other drugs (e.g., cocaine) and withdrawal from other drugs (e.g., benzodiazepines). In addition, other psychiatric disorders (e.g., anxiety disorders, mania, sleep disturbances), medical disorders (e.g., arrhythmia, hyperthyroidism), and medication side effects (e.g., akathisia) should be ruled out.

There are no large-scale epidemiological data on the incidence or prevalence of caffeine intoxication. One random-digit telephone survey in Vermont involving 162 caffeine users found that 7% met the DSM criteria for caffeine intoxication in the past year. Another study, which assessed more than 3,600 twins, reported that nearly 30% of subjects indicated having experienced feeling ill or shaky or jittery after consuming caffeine (Kendler, Myers, & Gardner, 2006). Caffeine was implicated in 4,656 reports to poison control centers in the United States in 2005, with half requiring treatment in a health care facility. One study evaluated 265 cases of caffeine intoxication (resulting from products other than coffee or tea) that were reported to a local area poison center between 2001 and 2004. Patients were 21 years old on average (50% female), and 12% received hospital care. In 77% of these cases, caffeine was ingested in the form of a medication, in 14% as a dietary supplement, and in 16% as a caffeine-enhanced beverage. In addition, numerous case reports have been published in recent years describing caffeine intoxication resulting from the use of energy drinks (e.g., Babu, Zuckerman, Cherkes, & Hack, 2011; Trabulo, Marques, & Pedroso, 2011). A report by the Drug Abuse Warning Network (DAWN) indicated that the number of emergency department (ED) visits involving energy drinks doubled from 2007 to 2011. Of the 20,783 energy drink-related ED visits in 2011, 58% involved only energy drinks and 42% involved energy drinks combined with other drugs or alcohol (Substance Abuse and Mental Health Services Administration, 2013).

CAFFEINE WITHDRAWAL

Physical dependence on caffeine is evidenced by the manifestation of a withdrawal syndrome (time-limited biochemical, physical, and behavioral disruptions) in response to a significant reduction or cessation of caffeine after a period of regular use. Symptoms of caffeine withdrawal have been described in medical reports for more than 175 years and the caffeine withdrawal syndrome is currently well characterized. In 2004, a comprehensive review of 66 caffeine withdrawal studies empirically validated 13 caffeine withdrawal symptoms and identified additional symptoms that were likely caffeine withdrawal but warranted further investigation (Juliano & Griffiths, 2004). These symptoms are shown in Table 10.2.

Caffeine withdrawal is currently defined by DSM-5 as the presence of three or more of five specific symptoms that occur after abruptly stopping or reducing caffeine intake. Symptoms must cause clinically significant distress or impairment in social, occupational, or other important areas of functioning.

Headache is a hallmark feature of caffeine withdrawal. About 50% of research volunteers report headache within 24 hours of caffeine abstinence in controlled, double-blind studies, and the incidence is likely higher under naturalistic conditions (Juliano & Griffiths, 2004). Caffeine withdrawal headaches are described as severe, diffuse, throbbing, gradual in development, and sensitive to movement. The mechanism underlying caffeine withdrawal headache is likely rebound cerebral vasodilation and increased cerebral blood flow that occurs during caffeine abstinence (Sigmon, Herning, Better, Cadet, & Griffiths, 2010) subsequent to the upregulation of adenosine receptors due to chronic caffeine use.

Physical dependence on caffeine can develop after chronic exposure to as little as 100 mg per day, the amount of caffeine in a small cup of coffee. Although there is wide variability across individuals, in general, the incidence and severity of caffeine withdrawal increases as usual daily dose of caffeine increases. Caffeine withdrawal can occur after relatively short-term exposure to daily caffeine.

TABLE 10.2. Empirically Validated Caffeine Withdrawal Symptoms

Strong evidence	Suggestive evidence
Increased	Increased
Headache	Yawning
Tiredness/fatigue	Unmotivated for work
Drowsiness/sleepiness	Heavy feelings in arms and legs
Irritability	Analgesic use
Depressed mood	Craving/strong desire to use
Muzzy/foggy/not clearheaded	Nighttime sleep quality/duration
Flu-like symptoms	Cerebral blood flow velocity
Nausea/vomiting	
Muscle pain/stiffness	
Decreased	Decreased
Energy/activeness	Self-confidence
Alertness/attentiveness	Desire to socialize
Contentedness/well-being	Motor activity
Ability to concentrate	Behavioral and cognitive performance

Note. Data from Juliano and Griffiths (2004).

Withdrawal symptoms have been observed after only 3 days' exposure to 300 mg/ day caffeine, with greater severity occurring after a week or two of daily caffeine use (Evans & Griffiths, 1999). Caffeine withdrawal symptoms typically emerge 12–24 hours after the last dose of caffeine, peak within the first 2 days of abstinence, and can persist for more than a week. Caffeine withdrawal can vary in severity from mild to incapacitating, even within the same individual across difference abstinence trials. The incidence of caffeine withdrawal-related impairment or distress to the point of significantly interfering with normal functioning (e.g., missing work, unable to care for children) is about 13%. Doses well below the usual daily dose can suppress caffeine withdrawal. For example, one study found that as little as 25 mg of caffeine was sufficient to prevent headache after daily dosing of 300 mg (Evans & Griffiths, 1999). Thus, clinically significant caffeine withdrawal symptoms may not manifest unless there is a substantial decrease in caffeine consumption.

There is evidence that children and adolescents who use caffeine experience caffeine withdrawal symptoms upon abstinence (Oberstar, Bernstein, & Thuras, 2002). It is possible that children may be particularly vulnerable to caffeine withdrawal as they may have less control over the regular availability of caffeine. Caffeine withdrawal has also been documented in newborns who have had prenatal caffeine exposure (McGowan, Altman, & Kanto, 1988).

Caffeine withdrawal symptoms overlap with various psychological and physical ailments. Caffeine withdrawal should be considered when patients present with headaches, fatigue, mood disturbances, impaired concentration, and flu-like symptoms. Fasting requirements for certain blood tests, surgery, or medical procedures (e.g., colonoscopies, fasting blood sugar tests) may lead to caffeine withdrawal symptoms that could be misattributed to other causes if patients are not aware of their dependence on caffeine. Caffeine withdrawal has been identified as a significant cause of postoperative headaches (Fennely, Galletly, & Purdie, 1991). The more caffeine someone uses, the greater the risk of postoperative headache. Caffeine consumers administered caffeine on the day of the surgical procedure have lower rates of postoperative headache (Weber, Ereth, & Danielson, 1993). In general, caffeine withdrawal symptoms resolve quickly after caffeine reexposure (i.e., 60 minutes or less).

CAFFEINE USE DISORDER

There is growing recognition that caffeine use can be problematic for some individuals. Case reports and research studies have described individuals who have a pattern of symptoms resulting from caffeine use reflective of a drug use disorder. For example, one investigation characterized 94 individuals who were seeking treatment for problematic caffeine use and self-identified as being physically or psychologically dependent on caffeine, or having been unsuccessful at previous attempts to modify caffeine use (Juliano et al., 2012). Participants (mean age 41 years, 55% female) had a clinical interview and completed an assessment battery. Participants consumed 548 mg caffeine per day on average (120–2,667 mg), and half of the participants reported coffee as their primary source of caffeine. Ninety-three percent met criteria for caffeine dependence using generic DSM-IV-TR drug dependence criteria. The most common symptoms were withdrawal (96%), persistent desire or unsuccessful efforts to control use (89%), use despite knowledge of physical or psychological problems caused by caffeine (87%), and tolerance (70%). Only 8% reported having given up or reduced important social, occupational, or recreational activities due to caffeine use, which is not a surprise considering that caffeine is legal, socially accepted, and widely available. Four other clinical studies have also identified individuals who meet criteria for caffeine dependence using DSM criteria (Jones & Lejuez, 2005; Oberstar et al., 2002; Strain, Mumford, Silverman, & Griffiths, 1994; Svikis, Berger, Haug, & Griffiths, 2005).

Caffeine use disorder is recognized by DSM-5 as a condition for further study using a more restrictive set of criteria than the generic DSM-5 substance use disorder criteria that apply to other recreational drugs (American Psychiatric Association, 2013). As is intended with a research diagnosis, additional research is needed to characterize more fully the features and prevalence of caffeine use disorder, as well as effective treatment strategies.

CAFFEINE MODIFICATION AND TREATMENT

There are various reasons why individuals may want to modify their caffeine use, including but not limited to health concerns, undesirable side effects, and not wanting to be dependent on caffeine (Juliano et al., 2012). It should be recognized that reducing or eliminating caffeine may be difficult for some. In fact, a population-based survey in Vermont indicated that 56% of respondents reported having had a strong desire or unsuccessful attempts to stop use (Hughes, Oliveto, Liguori, Carpenter, & Howard, 1998). Health providers often recommend that patients modify caffeine use for various conditions (e.g., anxiety, insomnia, tachycardia, pregnancy). Clinicians should not assume that the simple suggestion to modify caffeine use will be sufficient for successful behavior change. Some studies have identified caffeine-dependent individuals who report being unable to follow their doctors' recommendations to modify caffeine use. For example, in a clinical study involving pregnant women, a diagnosis of caffeine dependence combined with a family history of alcoholism predicted difficulty abstaining from caffeine use during pregnancy despite their doctors' advice to do so (Svikis et al., 2005). In a recent study, among 94 individuals seeking treatment for problematic caffeine use, 43% were advised by a medical professional to reduce or eliminate caffeine, but fewer than 20% were given any advice or assistance (Juliano et al., 2012).

There are only a handful of published reports (mostly case studies) on the treatment of problematic caffeine use (e.g., Bryant, Dowell, & Fairbrother, 2002; Foxx & Rubinoff, 1979; James, Stirling, & Hampton, 1985). In the absence of empirically validated treatments for modifying caffeine use, it seems prudent to draw from effective treatments for other drugs, such as tobacco. Such strategies may include education, self-monitoring, coping response training, social support, rewards for successful behavior change, and follow-up. Validated treatment approaches such as relapse prevention and motivational interviewing might also be readily applied to the treatment of problematic caffeine use. There is some evidence that caffeine withdrawal symptoms may thwart caffeine reduction or cessation. A gradual tapering off of caffeine over time may help to attenuate caffeine withdrawal symptoms. Table 10.3 provides suggestions to help patients modify caffeine use.

TABLE 10.3. Caffeine Treatment Guidelines

1. *Identification of problematic caffeine use.* Caffeine modification should be advised for individuals who are using excessive amounts of caffeine and/or have anxiety, sleep problems, caffeine intoxication, caffeine use disorder, are pregnant, and have cardiovascular complaints, chronic headaches, urinary complaints, or any other medical or psychological conditions that are believed to be aggravated by caffeine use. It should be noted that some individuals simply do not want to be dependent on caffeine and are interested in treatment assistance. Caffeine reduction or elimination should also be advised when patients are taking medications that interact with caffeine.

2. *Assessment, education, and self-monitoring.* The clinician should be familiar with potential sources of caffeine (see Table 10.1) and educate patients about caffeine-containing products. It is important to recognize that caffeine is present in some non-cola soft drinks (e.g., orange soft drinks), foods (e.g., coffee yogurt), and over-the-counter medications, and that there is wide variability in caffeine levels within and across product types. Patients should also be educated about the physiological and psychological effects of caffeine and be informed that relatively small amounts of daily caffeine (e.g., ~100 mg) are associated with physical dependence (i.e., withdrawal symptoms upon abstinence).
   The clinician can estimate caffeine exposure amount based on self-report or have the patient self-monitor caffeine use for 1 to 2 weeks to establish a baseline level.
   For patients who are consuming multiple caffeine containing products, caffeine exposure in milligrams should be calculated, taking into account the caffeine content of specific products, the serving sizes, and the number of servings.
   Patients should continue to self-monitor during the caffeine reduction phase of treatment.

3. *Goal setting and dose reduction schedule.* Some individuals may be interested in eliminating caffeine entirely, whereas others may wish to reduce their caffeine consumption. Patients should be advised to keep caffeine exposure under 50 mg per day or use caffeine only occasionally (e.g., use no more than 2 consecutive days) if they want to avoid physical dependence on caffeine.
   Tapering caffeine exposure over the course of 3 to 4 weeks may help to lessen or prevent caffeine withdrawal symptoms. Caffeinated beverages can either be gradually omitted or mixed with decaffeinated beverages and decreasing the ratio of caffeinated product over time (e.g., gradually transitioning from caffeinated coffee to decaffeinated coffee).
   Individuals who prefer to quit "cold turkey" may expect withdrawal symptoms that peak in the first couple days of acute abstinence, then gradually improve over the course of a week.

4. *Treatment strategies.* At this time there are no empirically validated treatments for problematic caffeine use. However, patients may benefit from behavior modification techniques that are effective in treating dependence on other drugs (e.g., nicotine). These techniques may include psychoeducation, self-monitoring, coping response training, reinforcement for abstinence, identifying barriers to change, social support, and framing withdrawal as a temporary inconvenience.

5. *Follow-up.* Schedule a time to follow-up with patients at a later date to check on their progress. As with other recreational drugs, some amount of treatment failure and relapse is to be expected. Some patients may need to make repeated attempts to modify caffeine use before achieving success.

REFERENCES

Adan, A., & Serra-Grabulosa, J. M. (2010). Effects of caffeine and glucose, alone and combined, on cognitive performance. *Hum Psychopharmacol Clin Exp, 25*(4), 310–317.

Albert, S. L., Uhde, T. W., Slate, S. O., & McCann, U. D. (1997). Effects of intravenous caffeine administered to health males during sleep. *Depress Anxiety, 5*(1), 21–28.

American Psychiatric Association. (2013). *Diagnostic and statistical manual of mental disorders* (5th ed.). Arlington, VA: Author.

Amin, N., Byrne, E., Johnson, J., Chenevix-Trench, G., Walter, S., Nolte, I. M., et al. (2012). Genome-wide association analysis of coffee drinking suggests association with CYP1A1/CYP1A2 and NRCAM. *Mol Psychiatry, 17*(11), 1116–1129.

Anderson, B. L., Juliano, L. M., & Schulkin, J. (2009). Caffeine's implications for women's health and survey of obstetrician-gynecologists' caffeine knowledge and assessment practices. *Journal of Women's Health, 18*(9), 1457–1466.

Astorino, T. A., & White, A. C. (2012). Caffeine and exercise performance. In V. R. Preedy (Ed.), *Caffeine: Chemistry, analysis, function and effects* (pp. 314–336). London: Royal Society of Chemistry.

Babu, K. M., Zuckerman, M. D., Cherkes, J. K., & Hack, J. B. (2011). First-onset seizure after use of 5-hour ENERGY. *Pediatr Emerg Care, 27*(6), 539–540.

Banerjee, P., Ali, Z., Levine, B., & Fowler, D. R. (2014). Fatal caffeine intoxication: A series of eight cases from 1999 to 2009. *J Forensic Sci, 59*(3), 865–868.

Barone, J. J., & Roberts, H. R. (1996). Caffeine consumption. *Food Chem Toxicol, 34*(1), 119–129.

Benowitz, N. L. (1990). Clinical pharmacology of caffeine. *Ann Rev Med, 41*(1), 277–288.

Benowitz, N. L., Peng, M., & Jacob, P., III. (2003). Effects of cigarette smoking and carbon monoxide on chlozoxazone and caffeine metabolism. *Clin Pharmacol Ther, 74*, 468–474.

Bjorness, T. E., & Greene, R. W. (2009). Adenosine and sleep. *Curr Neuropharmacol, 7*(3), 238–245.

Bodenmann, S., Hohoff, C., Freitag, C., Deckert, J., Retey, J. V., Bachmann, V., et al. (2012). Polymorphisms of ADORA2A modulate psychomotor vigilance and the effects of caffeine on neurobehavioral performance and sleep EEG after sleep deprivation. *Br J Pharmacol, 165*(6), 1904–1913.

Bruce, M., Scott, N., Shine, P., & Lader, M. (1992). Anxiogenic effects of caffeine in patients with anxiety disorders. *Arch Gen Psychiatry, 49*, 867–869.

Bryant, C. M., Dowell, C. J., & Fairbrother, G. (2002). Caffeine reduction education to improve urinary symptoms. *Br J Nurs, 11*(8), 560–565.

Byrne, E. M., Johnson, J., McRae, A. F., Nyholt, D. R., Medland, S. E., Gehrman, P. R., et al. (2012). A genome-wide association study of caffeine-related sleep disturbance: Confirmation of a role for a common variant in the adenosine receptor. *Sleep, 35*(7), 967–975.

Carrillo, J. A., & Benitez, J. (2000). Clinically significant pharmacokinetic interactions between dietary caffeine and medications. *Clin Pharmacokinet, 39*(2), 127–153.

Childs, E., & de Wit, H. (2006). Subjective, behavioral, and physiological effects of acute caffeine in light, nondependent caffeine users. *Psychopharmacol, 185*(4), 514–523.

Childs, E., Hohoff, C., Deckert, J., Xu, K., Badner, J., & de Wit, H. (2008). Association between ADORA2A and DRD2 polymorphisms and caffeine-induced anxiety. *Neuropsychopharmacol, 33*, 2791–2800.

Christopher, G., Sutherland, D., & Smith, A. (2005). Effects of caffeine in non-withdrawn volunteers. *Hum Psychopharmacol Clin Exp, 20*(1), 47–53.

Cornelis, M. C., El-Sohemy, A., & Campos, H. (2007). Genetic polymorphism of the adenosine A_{2A} receptor is associated with habitual caffeine consumption. *Am J Clin Nutr, 86*(1), 240–244.

Cornelis, M. C., El-Sohemy, A., Kabagambe, E. K., & Campos, H. (2006). Coffee, CYP1A2 genotype, and the risk of myocardial infarction. *JAMA, 295*(10), 1135–1141.

Cornelis, M. C., Monda, K. L., Yu, K., Paynter, N., Azzato, E. M., Bennett, S. N., et al. (2011). Genome-wide meta-analysis identifies regions on 7p21 (AHR) and 15q24 (CYP1A2) as determinants of habitual caffeine consumption. *PLoS Genet, 7*(4), e1002033.

Denaro, C. P., & Benowitz, N. L. (1992). Caffeine metabolism: Disposition in liver disease and hepatic-functioning testing. *Drug Alcohol Abuse Rev, 2*, 513–539.

Derry, C. J., Derry, S., & Moore, R. A. (2012). Caffeine as an analgesic adjuvant for acute pain in adults (Review). *Cochrane Database Syst Rev, 3*, 1–37.

Doherty, M., & Smith, P. M. (2004). Effects of caffeine ingestion on exercise testing: A meta-analysis. *Int J Sport Nutr Exerc Metab, 14*(6), 626–646.

Evans, S. M., & Griffiths, R. R. (1999). Caffeine withdrawal: A parametric analysis of caffeine dosing conditions. *J Pharmacol Exp Ther, 289*(1), 285–294.

Fennelly, M., Galletly, D. C., & Purdie, G. I. (1991). Is caffeine withdrawal the mechanism of postoperative headache? *Anesth Analg, 72*, 449–453.

Ferre, S. (2008). An update on the mechanisms of the psychostimulant effects of caffeine. *J Neurochem, 105*(4), 1067–1079.

Ferre, S., Ciruela, F., Borycz, J., Solinas, M., Quarta, D., Antoniou, K., et al. (2008). Adenosine A1-A2A receptor heteromers: New targets for caffeine in the brain. *Front Biosci, 13*, 2391–2399.

Foxx, R. M., & Rubinoff, A. (1979). Behavioral treatment of caffeinism: Reducing excessive coffee drinking. *J Appl Behav Anal, 12*(3), 335–344.

Frary, C. D., Johnson, R. K., & Wang, M. Q. (2005). Food sources and intakes of caffeine in the diets of persons in the United States. *J Am Diet Assoc, 105*(1), 110–113.

Furge, L. L., & Guengerich, F. P. (2006). Cytochrome P450 enzymes in drug metabolism and chemical toxicology: An introduction. *Biochem Mol Biol Educ, 34*(2), 66–74.

Ganio, M. S., Klau, J. F., Casa, D. J., Armstrong, L. E., & Maresh, C. M. (2009). Effect of caffeine on sport-specific endurance performance: A systematic review. *J Strength Cond Res, 23*(1), 315–324.

Glaister, M., Patterson, S. D., Foley, P., Pedlar, C. R., Pattison, J. R., & McInnes, G. (2012). Caffeine and sprinting performance: Dose responses and efficacy. *J Strength Cond Res, 26*(4), 1001–1005.

Gleason, J. L., Richter, H. E., Redden, D. T., Goode, P. S., Burgio, K. L., & Markland, A. D. (2013). Caffeine and urinary incontinence in US women. *Int Urogynecol J, 24*(2), 295–302.

Howland, J., & Rohsenow, D. J. (2013). Risks of energy drinks mixed with alcohol. *JAMA, 309*, 245–246.

Hughes, J. R., Oliveto, A. H., Liguori, A., Carpenter, J., & Howard, T. (1998). Endorsement of DSM-IV dependence criteria among caffeine users. *Drug Alcohol Depend, 52*(2), 99–107.

James, J. E. (1997). *Understanding caffeine: A biobehavioral analysis*. Thousand Oaks, CA: Sage.

James, J. E., & Rogers, P. J. (2005). Effects of caffeine on performance and mood: Withdrawal reversal is the most plausible explanation. *Psychopharmacol, 182*(1), 1–8.

James, J. E., Stirling, K. P., & Hampton, B. A. M. (1985). Caffeine fading: Behavioral treatment of caffeine abuse. *Behav Ther, 16*(1), 15–27.

Jones, H. A., & Lejuez, C. W. (2005). Personality correlates of caffeine dependence: The role of sensation seeking, impulsivity, and risk taking. *Exp Clin Psychopharmacol, 13*(3), 259–266.

Josse, A. R., Da Costa, L. A., Campos, H., & El-Sohemy, A. (2012). Associations between polymorphisms in the AHR and CYP1A1–CYP1A2 gene regions and habitual caffeine consumption. *Am J Clin Nutr, 96*(3), 665–671.

Juliano, L. M., Evatt, D. P., Richards, B. D., & Griffiths, R. R. (2012). Characterization of individuals seeking treatment for caffeine dependence. *Psychol Addict Behav, 26*(4), 948–954.

Juliano, L. M., Ferre, S., & Griffiths, R. R. (2014). The pharmacology of caffeine. In R. K. Ries,

D. A. Fiellin, S. C. Miller, & R. Saitz (Eds.), *ASAM principles of addiction medicine* (5th ed., pp. 180–200). Baltimore, MD: Lippincott Williams & Wilkins.

Juliano, L. M., & Griffiths, R. R. (2004). A critical review of caffeine withdrawal: Empirical validation of symptoms and signs, incidence, severity, and associated features. *Psychopharmacol, 176,* 1–29.

Kamimori, G. H., McLellan, T. M., Tate, C. M., Voss, D. M., Niro, P., & Lieberman, H. R. (2015). Caffeine improves reaction time, vigilance and logical reasoning during extended periods with restricted opportunities for sleep. *Psychopharmacol, 232*(12), 2031–2042.

Keenan, E. K., Tiplady, B., Priestley, C. M., & Rogers, P. J. (2014). Naturalistic effects of five days of caffeine use on sleep, next-day cognitive performance, and mood. *J Caffeine Res, 4*(1), 13–20.

Kendler, K. S., Myers, J., & Gardner, C. O. (2006). Caffeine intake, toxicity, and dependence and lifetime risk for psychiatric and substance use disorders: An epidemiologic and co-twin control analysis. *Psychol Med, 36,* 1717–1725.

Kendler, K. S., Myers, J., & Prescott, C. A. (2007). Specificity of genetic and environmental risk factors for symptoms of cannabis, cocaine, alcohol, caffeine, and nicotine dependence. *Arch Gen Psychiatry, 64*(11), 1313–1320.

Landolt, H., Werth, E., Borbely, A. A., & Dijk, D. (1995). Caffeine intake (200 mg) in the morning affects human sleep and EEG power spectra at night. *Brain Res, 675*(1–2), 67–74.

Lane, J. D., Lane, A. L., Surwit, R. S., Kuhn, C. M., & Feinglos, M. N. (2012). Pilot study of caffeine abstinence for control of chronic glucose in Type 2 diabetes. *J Caffeine Res, 2*(1), 45–47.

Lazarus, M., Shen, H. Y., Cherasse, Y., Qu, W. M., Huang, Z. L., Bass, C. E., et al. (2011). Arousal effect of caffeine depends on adenosine A_{2A} receptors in the shell of the nucleus accumbens. *J Neurosci, 31*(27), 10067–10075.

Liu, R., Guo, X., Park, Y., Huang, X., Sinha, R., Freedman, N. D., et al. (2012). Caffeine intake, smoking, and risk of Parkinson disease in men and women. *Am J Epidemiol, 175*(11), 1200–1207.

Marczinski, C. A., & Fillmore, M. T. (2006). Clubgoers and their trendy cocktail: Implications of mixing caffeine into alcohol on information processing and subjective reports of intoxication. *Exp Clin Psychopharmacol, 14*(4), 450–458.

McCusker, R. R., Fuehrlein, B., Goldberger, B. A., Gold, M. S., & Cone, E. J. (2006). Caffeine content of decaffeinated coffee. *J Anal Toxicol, 30*(8), 611–613.

McCusker, R. R., Goldberger, B. A., & Cone, E. J. (2003). Caffeine content of specialty coffees. *J Anal Toxicol, 27*(7), 520–522.

McGowan, J. D., Altman, R. E., & Kanto, W. P., Jr. (1988). Neonatal withdrawal symptoms after chronic maternal ingestion of caffeine. *South Med J, 81*(9), 1092–1094.

Mitchell, D. C., Knight, C. A., Hockenberry, J., Teplansky, R., & Hartman, T. J. (2014). Beverage caffeine intakes in the US. *Food Chem Toxicol, 63,* 136–142.

Mumford, G. K., Benowitz, N. L., Evans, S. M., Kaminski, B. J., Preston, K. L., Sannerud, C. A., et al. (1996). Absorption rate of methylxanthines following capsules, cola and chocolate. *Eur J Clin Psychol, 51*(3–4), 319–325.

Nardi, A. E., Lopes, F. L., Freire, R. C., Veras, A. B., Nascimento, I., Valenca, A. M., et al. (2009). Panic disorder and social anxiety disorder subtypes in a caffeine challenge test. *Psychiatry Res, 169*(2), 149–153.

Nawrot, P., Jordan, S., Eastwood, J., Rotstein, J., Hugenholtz, A., & Feeley, M. (2003). Effects of caffeine on human health. *Food Addit Contam, 20*(1), 1–30.

Oberstar, J. V., Bernstein, G. A., & Thuras, P. D. (2002). Caffeine use and dependence in adolescents: One-year follow-up. *J Child Adolesc Psychopharmacol, 12*(2), 127–135.

Palatini, P., Ceolotto, G., Ragazzo, F., Dorigatti, F., Saladini, F., Papparella, I., et al. (2009). CYP1A2 genotype modifies the association between coffee intake and the risk of hypertension. *J Hypertens, 27*(8), 1594–1601.

Pendergrast, M. (1999). *Uncommon grounds: The history of coffee and how it transformed our world*. New York: Basic Books.

Perera, V., Gross, A. S., & McLachlan, A. J. (2012). Measurement of CYP1A2 activity: A focus on caffeine as a probe. *Curr Drug Metab, 13*(5), 667–678.

Popat, R. A., Van Den Eeden, S. K., Tanner, C. M., Kamel, F., Umbach, D. M., Marder, K., et al. (2011). Coffee, ADORA2A, and CYP1A2: The caffeine connection in Parkinson's disease. *Eur J Neurol, 18*(5), 156–765.

Reissig, C. J., Strain, E. C., & Griffiths, R. R. (2009). Caffeinated energy drinks—a growing problem. *Drug Alcohol Depend, 99*(1–3), 1–10.

Renda, G., Zimarino, M., Antonucci, I., Tatasciore, A., Ruggieri, B., Bucciarelli, T., et al. (2012). Genetic determinants of blood pressure responses to caffeine drinking. *Am J Clin Nutr, 95*(1), 241–248.

Retey, J. V., Adam, M., Khatami, R., Luhmann, U. F., Jung, H. H., Berger, W., et al. (2007). A genetic variation in the adenosine A2A receptor gene (ADORA2A) contributes to individual sensitivity to caffeine effects on sleep. *Clin Pharmacol Ther, 81*(5), 692–698.

Rogers, P. J., Heatherley, S. V., Mullings, E. L., & Smith, J. E. (2013). Faster but not smarter: Effect of caffeine and caffeine withdrawal on alertness and performance. *Psychopharmacol (Berl), 226*(2), 229–240.

Rogers, P. J., Hohoff, C., Heatherley, S. V., Mullings, E. L., Maxfield, P. J., Evershed, R. P., et al. (2010). Association of the anxiogenic and alerting effects of caffeine with ADORA2A and ADORA1 polymorphisms and habitual level of caffeine consumption. *Neuropsychopharmacol, 35*, 1973–1983.

Schuh, K. J., & Griffiths, R. R. (1997). Caffeine reinforcement: The role of withdrawal. *Psychopharmacol, 130*(4), 320–326.

Sigmon, S. C., Herning, R. I., Better, W., Cadet, J. L., & Griffiths, R. R. (2009). Caffeine withdrawal, acute effects, tolerance, and absence of net beneficial effects of chronic administration: Cerebral blood flow velocity, quantitative EEG, and subjective effects. *Psychopharmacology, 204*(4), 573–585.

Smith, A. P., Christopher, G., & Sutherland, D. (2013). Acute effects of caffeine on attention: A comparison of non-consumers and withdrawn consumers. *J Psychopharmacol, 27*(1), 77–83.

Solinas, M., Ferré, S., You, Z. B., Karcz-Kubicha, M., Popoli, P., & Goldberg, S. R. (2002). Caffeine induces dopamine and glutamate release in the shell of the nucleus accumbens. *J Neurosci, 22*(15), 6321–6324.

Somogyi, L. P. (2010). *Caffeine intake in the U. S. population*. Retrieved March 15, 2015, from *www.fda.gov/downloads/AboutFDA/CentersOffices/OfficeofFoods/CFSAN/CFSAN-FOIAElectronicReadingRoom/UCM333191.pdf.*

Strain, E. C., Mumford, G. K., Silverman, K., & Griffiths, R. R. (1994). Caffeine dependence syndrome: Evidence from case histories and experimental evaluations. *JAMA, 272*(13), 1043–1048.

Substance Abuse and Mental Health Services Administration Center for Behavioral Health Statistics and Quality. (2013). *The DAWN Report: Update on emergency department visits involving energy drinks: A continuing public health concern*. Rockville, MD: Author.

Sulem, P., Gudbjartsson, D. F., Geller, F., Prokopenko, I., Feenstra, B., Aben, K. K., et al. (2011). Sequence variants at CYP1A1–CYP1A2 and AHR associate with coffee consumption. *Hum Mol Genet, 20*(10), 2071–2077.

Svikis, D. S., Berger, N., Haug, N. A., & Griffiths, R. R. (2005). Caffeine dependence in combination with a family history of alcoholism as a predictor of continued use of caffeine during pregnancy. *Am J Psychiatry, 162*(12), 2344–2351.

Telch, J., Silverman, A., & Schmidt, N. B. (1996). Effects of anxiety sensitivity and perceived control on emotional responding to caffeine challenge. *J Anxiety Disord, 10*(1), 21–35.

Trabulo, D., Marques, S., & Pedroso, E. (2011). Caffeinated energy drink intoxication. *Emerg Med J, 28*, 712–714.

Uiterwaal, C. S., Verschuren, W. M., Bueno-de-Mesquita, H. B., Ocke, M., Geleijnse, J. M., Boshuizen, H. C., et al. (2007). Coffee intake and incidence of hypertension. *Am J Clin Nutr, 85*(3), 718–723.

U.S. Food and Drug Administration. (2013, May). FDA to investigate added caffeine. *FDA Consumer Health Information*, 1–2.

Weber, J. G., Ereth, M. H., & Danielson, D. R. (1993). Perioperative ingestion of caffeine and postoperative headache. *Mayo Clin Proc, 68*(9), 842–845.

Weng, X., Odouli, R., & Li, D. (2008). Maternal caffeine consumption during pregnancy and the risk of miscarriage: A prospective cohort study. *Am J Obstet Gynecol, 198*(3), 279e.1–279e.8.

Womack, C. J., Saunders, M. J., Bechtel, M. K., Bolton, D. J., Martin, M., Luden, N. D., et al. (2012). The influence of a CYP1A2 polymorphism on the ergogenic effects of caffeine use. *J Int Soc Sports Nutr, 9*(1), 7–12.

Wyatt, J. K., Cajochen, C., Ritz-De Cecco, A., Czeisler, C. A., & Dijk, D. (2004). Low-dose repeated caffeine administration for circadian-phase-dependent performance degradation during extended wakefulness. *Sleep, 27*(3), 374–381.

Yang, A. Palmer, A. A., & de Wit, H. (2010). Genetics of caffeine consumption and responses to caffeine. *Psychopharmacol, 211*(3), 245–257.

CHAPTER 11

Stimulants

RICHARD RAWSON
LARISSA J. MOONEY
WALTER LING

Stimulants in common use around the world range from caffeine to methamphetamine in terms of psychoactive potency. Stimulants activate the central and peripheral nervous systems and may be used to elevate mood, increase work productivity, and suppress fatigue and appetite. Virtually all the stimulants can be involved in substance use disorders (SUDs) as defined in DSM-5 (American Psychiatric Association, 2013). We discuss in this chapter the more widely used stimulants that are associated with the most serious consequences, excluding cocaine, which is covered in Chapter 12. We focus in this chapter on methamphetamine and other amphetamine-type stimulants (ATS) and include prescription stimulants such as methylphenidate. We also discuss in less detail emerging synthetic stimulant substances including the cathinones, such as mephedrone. Another substance with stimulant-type properties and ATS-like chemical structure is MDMA ("Ecstasy"), which is considered a hallucinogen and is therefore discussed in Chapter 9. Substances in the ATS group, such as amphetamine, dextroamphetamine, and methamphetamine, are characterized by their phenylethylamine structure. Structurally different substances, such as methylphenidate, fenethylline, and mephedrone, are also included in the ATS category and are discussed in this chapter because of their use profiles and their similarity in clinical manifestation. The plant-derived stimulants such as ephedra and khat also can produce stimulant-related disorders.

METHAMPHETAMINE AND OTHER ATS

Background

Plant-derived stimulants including coca, khat, tea, coffee, and a variety of other biologicals (e.g., ephedra) have been commonly used to stimulate the central nervous system (CNS) for thousands of years. In the past century, chemists and clandestine compounders have synthesized powerful stimulants, including the amphetamines. One of the most potent of this class of drugs is methamphetamine, first developed in 1893 and used in limited medical applications. No prescription was necessary to obtain amphetamine or methamphetamine until 1951 in the United States. Amphetamine-infused inhalers for relief of nasal congestion and cold symptoms were available over the counter into the mid-1960s.

Various ATS medications were commonly prescribed well into the late 1960s, especially Dexedrine (dextroamphetamine), which had long been used for alleviating symptoms of depression and for weight control and is still prescribed for the treatment of narcolepsy and attention-deficit/hyperactivity disorder (ADHD). The use of both licit and illicit methamphetamine escalated rapidly, with the street forms known as "speed" and "crank" becoming particularly popular in the 1950s and 1960s among many segments of society, from biker gangs to musicians to individuals trying to lose weight. The U.S. military provided dextroamphetamine to soldiers and pilots throughout the Vietnam War. Strict regulatory restrictions on the medical use of amphetamines were imposed during the early 1970s, and rates of use of pharmaceutical amphetamines decreased.

To supply the market for illicit ATS, motorcycle gangs became major producers of home laboratory-produced methamphetamine. Concurrent with the "crack" cocaine epidemic, the smoked form of methamphetamine called "ice" arrived in the United States from Asia in the mid-1980s but at first remained in a few urban areas in the western United States. During this same period, illicit production of powder methamphetamine expanded rapidly throughout the western United States. This form of methamphetamine was used via intranasal and injection routes of administration. During the late 1980s and into the 1990s, methamphetamine use trends included an eastward spread of methamphetamine production and use, and increasing numbers of methamphetamine smokers and high rates of use among specific groups, including individuals in rural areas and men who have sex with men.

The illicit manufacturing and marketing of ATS drugs focused on methamphetamine and involved small groups and individuals with a modicum of expertise, producing the drug in small quantities in "mom and pop" laboratories. During the late 1990s and into the early 21st century, Mexican drug cartels moved into the field of ATS distribution, expanding distribution to some southern and eastern U.S. regions. Beginning in 2003, some states imposed severe restrictions on access to pseudoephedrine, the primary precursor chemical for methamphetamine, followed by similar federal actions beginning in 2006. These regulatory measures reduced the production of methamphetamine in the United States and were associated with reductions in new users and use overall. Methamphetamine smuggled into the country from Mexico remains a consistent source of a high-grade and inexpensive product, however. In parts of the country without established drug trafficking networks, the availability and use of methamphetamine is substantially lower than during the mid-2000s.

Past-year ATS use in the United States was estimated at 1.3% of the population in 2013 (ages 15–64) (Substance Abuse and Mental Health Services Administration [SAMHSA], 2014a), and an estimated 469,000 individuals had stimulant dependence or abuse disorders. Most nationwide indicators have portrayed a stabilization or decline in numbers of methamphetamine users since the mid-2000s. For example, ATS treatment admissions increased from 5% to 9% of total admissions in 2005 but then decreased slightly to 7% in 2012 (SAMHSA, 2014b). Problems with ATS drugs continue to be more prevalent in some regions, particularly in the west. For example, 26.3% of addiction treatment admissions in California in 2011 were for ATS drugs (SAMHSA, 2013). Methamphetamine use also continues to be a major health concern for men who have sex with men.

The extent of ATS use and related problems is evident around the world, with an estimated 13.7 to 52.9 million ATS users in 2009 (United Nations Office on Drugs and Crime; UNODC, 2010). The demand for treatment related to ATS use is most common in Asia (UNODC, 2012), where ATS drugs are often used to improve work productivity and reduce appetite, distinct from the "recreational" use that is common in the United States; such use is referred to as "instrumental use" by the World Health Organization (National Addiction Research Centre, 1997; UNODC, 2013). Worldwide ATS abuse results in severe consequences, including ATS-related psychosis, which has been documented to be persistent and especially prevalent among young users and users by injection (Farrell, Marsden, Ali, & Ling, 2002). Stimulant use for intoxication beyond instrumental use is growing throughout the world, more so in some regions. For example, use of stimulants of all kinds (including the khat plant) is now rampant in the Middle East. Recent UNODC (2012) estimates indicate that 12 metric tons of amphetamine were seized in Saudi Arabia, out of a total of 24 tons seized around the world. Synthetic stimulants derived from nonamphetamine compounds have become popular in the Middle East, a region that suffers severe problems with stimulant abuse (UNODC, 2012). Notably, a long-outlawed drug called Captagon persists as a widely abused drug in most Arab countries. Originally composed of phenethylline (or fenethylline), Captagon was a stimulant prescribed for narcolepsy and ADHD; phenethylline metabolizes into amphetamine and theophylline. The virtually worldwide ban on manufacture of the drug in the 1980s did not stop its continued use and production, however, and it is extensively used in Middle Eastern countries. The "Captagon" widely used now is largely composed of ATS.

The picture of stimulant use in North America and around the world is one of constant change, with use patterns and drug preferences shifting as laws and regulations change, and even in response to chemical precursor availability. The rapid development of new stimulant preparations that have chemical variations sufficient to elude regulations is another sign of the difficulty in stemming the production of these easily manufactured compounds.

Mechanism of Action

ATS drugs facilitate the release of norepinephrine (NE) and dopamine from nerve terminals, resulting in a catecholamine surge that stimulates the sympathetic nervous system. ATS substances are ingested orally, intravenously, by smoking, or by "snorting." Similar to the use of cocaine, in the past decade smoking has been the most prevalent route of ATS administration, which is the most rapid means of delivering the drug to the brain. Because of its relatively low vaporization point, methamphetamine is readily smoked without complex preparation, as is required of cocaine, to produce a strong and virtually instant stimulant effect.

General actions of ATS drugs are similar to those of cocaine, but there are differences. Lacking action in the membrane ion channel, ATS substances do not have anesthetic activity, which reduces the risk of ATS drugs inducing some conditions (e.g., cardiac arrhythmias and seizures), but the peripheral sympathomimetic effects of ATS drugs may be more potent. The half-life of methamphetamine is 11–12 hours compared with 90 minutes for cocaine (Romanelli & Smith, 2006), and methamphetamine produces more severe and more durable physiological and subjective effects than cocaine (Newton, De La Garza, Kalechstein, & Nestor, 2005).

Physiological and Medical Effects

ATS administration in early phases of use produces acute dopaminergic stimulation of the brain's endogenous pleasure center, resulting in euphoria, increased sense of energy, alertness, and libido. Small to moderate doses result in vasoconstriction and elevated pulse and blood pressure. With increasingly frequent ATS use involving larger doses, the sympathomimetic effects are exaggerated and increased: dizziness, tremor, fever, dilated pupils, sweating, rapid breathing, rapid heartbeat, and high blood pressure. Continued chronic use of moderate dosages of ATS can result in movement disorders such as Parkinsonian features, including spontaneous muscle contractions and tremor. Longer term use is associated with depression, poor concentration, and fatigue.

The most salient and common medical conditions associated with ATS intoxication in emergency department settings include psychiatric symptoms, injury, skin infections, and dental pathology (Hendrickson, Cloutier, & McConnell, 2008). Acute ATS toxicity has been associated with fatalities resulting from drug-induced seizures, hypoxic stress, and cardiovascular complications (Davidson, Gow, Lee, & Ellinwood, 2001). Drug-induced hyperthermia (ensuing from methamphetamine's effects on the hypothalamus) can also result in death, which has been demonstrated in both preclinical and human research (Numachi et al., 2007). Cardiopulmonary consequences, including chest pain, hypertension, tachycardia, and breathing problems, are commonly associated with acute ATS toxicity in the emergency department (Richards et al., 1999). Acute coronary syndrome has been documented in 25% of methamphetamine users admitted to the emergency department for chest pain (Turnipseed, Richards, Kirk, Diercks, & Amsterdam, 2003) and may be associated with arrhythmias and cardiogenic shock (Wijetunga, Bhan, Lindsay, & Karch, 2004). Autopsy has revealed pulmonary edema and pulmonary hypertension in over 70% of ATS-related deaths (Karch, 2002).

Dermatological conditions such as cutaneous ulcers are common in ATS users and result from scratching or cutting in response to the sensation of bugs crawling below the skin (Bostwick & Lineberry, 2006). Injectors of ATS drugs may experience cellulitis and abscesses, and other users often experience burns and injuries that occur during manufacture of the drug, which involves highly caustic and explosive chemicals. Oral complications are also common in chronic ATS users, primarily among those who inject the drug. Common problems include caries, tooth fracture, gingivitis, and periodontitis (Shetty et al., 2010). In addition, ATS users often experience excessive tooth wear and temporomandibular joint syndrome related to bruxism, which may be a reaction to anxiety and restlessness, especially during early abstinence (Curtis, 2006).

Neurological complications of MA use include hyperkinetic and Parkinsonian movement disorders (Granado, Ares-Santos, & Moratalla, 2013), tonic-clonic seizures, and cerebrovasular accidents (Westover, Mcbride, & Haley, 2007). In addition, chronic methamphetamine use has been associated with reductions in striatal dopamine transporter (DAT) activity, which may correlate clinically with cognitive impairment (Volkow et al., 2001). Neurocognitive deficits associated with chronic methamphetamine use include episodic and working memory, executive functions, psychomotor task, and visuoconstruction problems (Scott et al., 2007). These deficits may worsen during early abstinence and persist for 9 months or longer, but recovery in DAT activity is observed with sustained abstinence (Volkow et al., 2001; Wang et al., 2004; Simon, Dacey, Glynn, Rawson, & Ling, 2004).

Psychiatric Effects

Following short-term use or episodic use of moderate dosages of ATS drugs, ATS use results in euphoria, diminished appetite, alertness, increased energy, and enhanced sexual drive. Long-term and/or high-dosage ATS use is associated with psychiatric symptoms, neurotoxicity, and medical conditions affecting multiple organ systems, as mentioned earlier (Albertson, Derlet, & Van Hoozen, 1999; Karch, 2002; Zweben et al., 2004). Behavioral manifestations may include agitation, grandiosity, hypervigilance, violence, impaired judgment, and impaired social or occupational functioning.

As troubling as the physical consequences of ATS use disorders are, the considerable impacts on psychological functioning and psychiatric health may be more severe and last longer. Several studies have indicated extensive psychiatric disorders among ATS abusers (Copeland & Sorenson, 2001; Glasner-Edwards, Mooney, et al., 2009; Shoptaw, Peck, Reback, & Rotheram-Fuller, 2003). Psychosis occurs in nearly 40% of methamphetamine-dependent individuals (Schuckit, 2006). Conditions induced by acute and long-term ATS use include anxiety, insomnia, irritability, paranoia, hallucinations, and delirium. The most common psychiatric disorders in ATS-dependent individuals include anxiety, mood, and psychotic disorders (Salo et al., 2011), and these conditions remain over extended periods. Three-year follow-up of methamphetamine-dependent adults after psychosocial treatment indicated that almost one-half of the sample had a current or recent psychiatric disorder (Glasner-Edwards, Mooney, et al., 2009). Depression symptoms among those at follow-up were correlated with increased likelihood of continued use of ATS (Glasner-Edwards, Marinelli-Casey, et al., 2009).

Common psychiatric symptoms reported among ATS users presenting to emergency departments include depression, anxiety, insomnia, and psychosis. Suicidal ideation and suicidal behaviors are also highly prevalent among individuals with ATS use disorders (McKetin, Lbman, Lee, Rosss, & Slade, 2011). Almost one-third of adults who had received psychosocial treatment for methamphetamine dependence reported at least one suicide attempt, which was more common among individuals with injection use, female gender, and severe depressive symptoms (Glasner-Edwards et al., 2008). Aggression and violence are prominent among ATS users (McKetin et al., 2014); 34.9% of ATS users in one study had committed a violent act while intoxicated on methamphetamine (Sommers, Baskin, & Baskin-Sommers, 2006). These and other effects of ATS use on society can be considerable; impacts include family disruption; child neglect and endangerment; and expenditure of resources for health care, social services, and law enforcement (Watanabe-Galloway et al., 2009).

Many severe-level users of ATS drugs develop psychosis that is directly related to the stimulant drugs and not definitively a manifestation of a preexisting underlying psychiatric disorder (McKetin, McLaren, Lubman, & Hides, 2006), although the latter may be one etiology. Psychosis related to ATS use, which may mimic schizophrenia, is more prevalent among individuals who either smoke or inject the drug intravenously and have a family history of psychiatric conditions. Symptoms of ATS psychosis include paranoia, delusions, and hallucinations (McKetin et al., 2006; Chen et al., 2005). One-third of individuals with psychotic symptoms related to ATS use have prolonged psychosis lasting more than 6 months (Ujike & Sato, 2004).

Variations in psychiatric symptoms are associated with differences in sensitivity to ATS, in amounts and/or frequency of use, and route of administration (Harris & Batki, 2000). The majority of ATS-related psychiatric symptoms may resolve within a week of ATS cessation, but prolonged psychiatric symptoms remain among other individuals, even among those with no history of mental illness (Chen et al., 2003). In a 3-year follow-up study of methamphetamine-dependent individuals after psychosocial treatment, the presence of a mental health diagnosis was associated with poorer functional outcomes and increased ATS use over time (Glasner-Edwards, Mooney, et al., 2009).

Treatment

In addition to exhibiting anxiety, depression, and psychosis, individuals presenting to emergency departments with acute ATS intoxication may be violent or suicidal (Richards et al., 1999; Albertson et al., 1999). Conservative care consists of placing nonthreatening individuals in a quiet, calm environment, while more agitated patients may require benzodiazepines or neuroleptics, and possibly gastric lavage and/or activated charcoal to promote clearance of the drug. While traditional antipsychotic medications (e.g., haloperidol) and benzodiazepines are effective in reducing symptoms of ATS psychosis and agitation, sometimes within an hour after administration, olanzapine and other medications appear to be more tolerable (Shoptaw, Kao, & Ling, 2009).

Craving and other postcessation symptoms ("withdrawal") are generally managed without extensive medication, although use of mild sedatives or sleep aids may be appropriate. Transient worsening of depression is common among ATS-involved individuals after binges and after cessation of the drug, and clinicians may determine a need for antidepressant therapy if symptoms persist. ATS cessation and supportive care (i.e., increased hydration, nutrition, rest) are largely adequate in most cases, depending on duration of use and level of intake, along with the presence of underlying psychiatric comorbidities that may complicate recovery.

Treatment for Consequences of Chronic Use and Dependence

Although the majority of ATS-related psychiatric symptoms resolve within a week of abstinence (Newton et al., 2005), prolonged psychiatric symptoms persist in some patients, even in the absence of a prior reported history of mental illness (Chen et al., 2003). Treatment of patients with recalcitrant psychiatric conditions related to extended periods of ATS use includes judicious use of antipsychotic or antidepressant medications to treat psychosis, depression, anxiety, or other psychiatric comorbidities.

Effective pharmacotherapy for treatment of ATS dependence has yet to be established or approved, although several medications have shown efficacy in early-phase studies. Naltrexone, an opioid antagonist, has shown promise in reducing drug use among people addicted to ATS (Jayaram-Lindstrom, Hammarberg, Beck, & Franck, 2008), although samples included amphetamine-dependent individuals, not specific users of the more potent methamphetamine form of ATS. Another medication that has shown partial efficacy in reducing use among methamphetamine-dependent individuals and helping to achieve abstinence is bupropion, an antidepressant used in smoking cessation therapy (Brensilver, Heinzerling, Swanson, & Shoptaw, 2012; Elkashef et al., 2008; Shoptaw et al., 2008; McCann & Li, 2012). Although effects on methamphetamine use outcomes have not been robust, post hoc analyses have suggested a possible effect in lower dose methamphetamine users (Shoptaw et al., 2008; Elkashef et al., 2008). Vigabatrin was found to have limited efficacy in reducing methamphetamine use in a small study in Mexico (Fechtner et al., 2006). Also of interest are modafinil, methylphenidate, and mirtazapine, although research trials have not consistently demonstrated clinical utility of these medications for treatment of ATS dependence.

More extensive research documentation and wider practical application have shown behavioral therapies to be effective for treatment of stimulant dependence, especially cognitive-behavioral therapy (CBT; Vocci & Montoya, 2009). Elements of CBT include individual or group counseling settings, family education, and motivational interviewing, much of it geared to prevention of relapse to drug use. Widely used versions of CBT have proven effective in reducing methamphetamine use during a 16-week trial in comparison to a "treatment as usual" condition (Rawson et al., 2004) and the therapy has been used as the behavioral treatment platform in many pharmacotherapy trials for ATS dependence (Elkashef et al., 2008).

Another behavioral approach, contingency management (CM), or motivational incentives, based on basic positive reinforcement principles, has been shown to produce significant reductions in methamphetamine use in multiple studies (Rawson et al., 2006; Roll et al., 2006). CM therapy involves providing specific tangible reinforcers or rewards that are contingent upon the performance of a desired behavior under a specified schedule of reinforcement. With methamphetamine users in treatment studies, the desired behavior measured has frequently been based on the provision of a drug-free urine sample. When methamphetamine users are rewarded for methamphetamine-negative urine specimens, their use of methamphetamine is reduced. CM can be combined with other psychotherapy or a medication (Shoptaw et al., 2006). At the present time, CM approaches have the strongest empirical support of all specific behavioral or pharmacological treatments for methamphetamine dependency.

PRESCRIPTION STIMULANTS

Background

Easily procured in the illegal "street" market, ATS drugs may also be purchased as legal medications prescribed for the treatment of ADHD and narcolepsy. Prescription stimulants have sometimes been diverted into the illegal market via large-scale thefts or, at an individual level, when prescribed medications are taken by individuals other than the patients for whom the drugs were intended. Anecdotal reports describe parents who have used ADHD medications (Adderall, Concerta) prescribed for their children.

Emerging literature has documented high prevalence rates of prescription stimulant misuse among younger populations: 5–9% of children in elementary through high school had used ATS drugs in the past year, and 5–35% of college-age individuals reported past-year use (Wilens et al., 2008). Up to 29% of respondents who were ATS users in high school and college also report selling or trading their medications for money or other drugs. Furthermore, nonmedical use of prescription ATS drugs is twice as likely among full-time college students as it is among individuals ages 18–22 who are not full-time students (SAMHSA, 2009).

Mechanism of Action

Many of the prescription stimulants are ATS drugs, which means they are quite similar to amphetamine and methamphetamine in their chemical structure and mechanism of action, as described earlier. Others, such as methylphenidate (Concerta), have somewhat different chemical and neurobiological aspects, while still acting sympathomimetically as CNS stimulants. Methylphenidate is similar in effects to ATS drugs, but its piperidine structure is distinct from ATS drugs. Like the ATS drugs, methylphenidate increases dopamine system activity but by different means. Methylphenidate binds the DAT and NE transporter, thus inhibiting reuptake of dopamine and NE (Sandoval et al., 2003; Volkow et al., 2002).

Physiological Effects

In addition to the negative physical and psychiatric consequences that may directly result from misuse of prescription stimulants, their use is often implicated in other substance misuse behaviors. For example, misuse of prescription stimulants frequently occurs with use of cocaine and Ecstasy (McCabe, Boyd, & Young, 2007), and with binge drinking and alcohol use disorders (McCabe, Cranford, & Boyd, 2006).

Treatment

Treatment approaches for acute intoxication, as well as use disorders involving the prescription ATS are the same as described earlier. The large number of young people who use prescription ATS indicates that particular attention should be paid to adolescents and young adults who present with medical conditions (e.g., anorexia, insomnia, pulmonary conditions, psychosis) that might be associated with undisclosed ATS use disorder. Understanding the possible drug-based etiology of such conditions requires a careful screening to elicit accurate information from the patient, who is likely to be reluctant to reveal drug use. In the case of psychosis, antipsychotics can be used, although no formal guidance is available on dosing or suitability for patient subtypes.

CATHINONES

Background

The cathinones consist of many chemical compounds created by legitimate and underground chemists in the process of manufacturing substances that are intended for recreational use as intoxicants, while avoiding legal sanctions until drug enforcement laws include such compounds. Most prevalent in the recent wave of cathinones include mephedrone, or 4-methylmethcathinone, and MDPV, or methylenedioxypyrovalerone. The group of substances has been commonly referred to as "bath salts" (or "plant food") because of the marketing of the substances in the form of packaged products with purported uses other than as intoxicants. Other common names include Meph, Drone, Meow-Meow, M-Cat, and Bubbles. In one retrospective study of cases presenting to poison control centers with exposure to cathinones, there were 37 street names identified in 236 patients (Spiller, Ryan, Weston, & Janson, 2011). That these substances are purveyed in "head shops" is indicative of their actual intended customer base and usage.

As with other clandestine drug preparations, the mephedrone substances and other drugs in the cathinone group require varying degrees of sophistication depending on the precursor chemicals that are available. Methcathinone requires oxidation of ephedrine (or pseudoephedrine), and N-methylephedrine, or N-methylpseudoephedrine, involves potassium permanganate dissolved in sulfuric acid. These distinctions are notable because a potential unintended outcome is that users of the latter are subject to manganese poisoning by the resulting product if it is not adequately purified. The prevalence of small-scale "mom-and-pop" manufacturing that was common in the case of methamphetamine and other ATS substance does not hold true for mephedrone and the other cathinones.

Use of mephedrone and similar compounds is extensive but understudied, especially in the United States. In Europe, the mephedrone drugs are fourth in popularity behind cannabis, cocaine, and Ecstasy (MDMA, 3,4-methylenedioxymethamphetamine) but their recent advent and rapid advance indicate a need for greater awareness of their increasing popularity. Estimates of prevalence rely on indirect indicators such as drug seizures and presentation of drugs for analysis at poison control centers; limited data show a rising trend in use in many parts of the United States and in most European nations. For example, data from the American Association of Poison Control Centers show an increase from zero calls for synthetic cathinones in 2009, to 304 in 2010, to 2,656 in 2012 (Mowry, Spyker, Cantilena, Bailey, & Ford, 2013).

Mechanism of Action

Like the ATS drugs, mephedrone and the other cathinone derivatives are CNS stimulants, but they are less potent due to their chemical structure inhibiting the molecular passage across the blood–brain barrier. No academic research has examined the pharmacokinetics or pharmacodynamics of the synthetic cathinones in humans (Hadlock et al., 2011). The cathinones appear to increase serotonin and dopamine in the nucleus accumbens in rat brains more so than do the ATS drugs (Kehr et al., 2011).

The drugs are ingested as tablets or snorted as powder, but some users also smoke the powder or dissolve it in water and spray the mixture onto mucous membranes (nose, mouth/throat, or even eyes). The dosage of mephedrone varies widely by report, ranging from 100 to 250 mg, but the half-life of the drug appears brief compared to the ATS drugs, requiring repeated dosing, as in the case of cocaine use. Typical use sessions may involve up to 1 gram of mephedrone, depending on purity and chemical variations. For example, other cathinone derivatives include more potent forms as p-methoxyphenethylamines (known as PMA and PMMA) and are highly potent at doses ~10 mg. Again, these are clinically derived observations from emergency departments and are not based on authoritative research.

Physiological Effects

Similar to the effects of ATS drugs, the cathinones produce sensations such as impaired perception, reduced motor control, disorientation, extreme paranoia, and violent episodes (Drug Enforcement Agency, 2007). Incidents with individuals who present at emergency departments for treatment of acute intoxication with the synthetic cathinones (e.g., mephedrone, MDPV) reveal symptoms that are similar to the sympathomimetic effects associated with ATS drugs, as described in previous sections. Given the lack of research in the area, information on psychiatric effects of synthetics such as mephedrone is derived from clinical reports of acute toxicity. Long-term physical and psychological consequences of use are unknown but potentially severe.

Treatment

Given the wide variation in chemical compounds that are included in the many "designer" ATS preparations obtained on the street, presentations involving "bath salts" and other forms of synthetic cathinones and similar substances should be addressed by reducing anxiety and ensuring the safety of the patient and others in the case of any violent or aggressive behaviors. Presentations for conditions (e.g., anxiety, violence, tachycardia, hallucinations) related to "bath salts" are increasing. As noted for treating acute toxicity involving ATS, use of benzodiazepines or neuroleptics is appropriate when indicated. In the case of persistent extreme agitation and other symptoms (e.g., tachycardia and hypertension), however, a consideration must include the possible presence of flephedrone or other fluorinated cathinones, which can affect metabolism of the preparation containing the other synthetic cathinones such as MDPV and mephedrone (Thornton, Gerona, & Tomaszewski, 2012). Making such a determination would require a toxicology assessment of the substance in question, if available. Gastric lavage or administration of charcoal may be useful in such cases.

OTHER STIMULANTS

Background

Naturally occurring stimulants provide rewarding effects and include substances such as coca, khat, tea, coffee, and a variety of other biologicals (e.g., ephedra). The occurrence of use disorders involving these other stimulants is negligible compared to prevalence of ATS use disorders, and associated consequences are not as severe or problematic. Caffeine is reviewed in detail in Chapter 10.

Khat, a plant native to the Middle East and Africa, historically was used as a mild intoxicant via oral ingestion and chewed or brewed in tea. Khat dependence is reported (Manghi et al., 2009), and use disorders involving khat are documented in the literature (Drug Enforcement Agency, 2011). Globally, it is estimated that approximately 10 million people are regular users of khat (WHO Expert Committee on Drug Dependence, 2006), but the prevalence of khat use in the United States is unknown. The U.S. Drug Enforcement Agency (2006) and other law enforcement agencies seized 47 tons of khat as unrefined plant matter in 2004. Use is more prevalent among some immigrant populations (from Arab and East African nations), and khat is not widely used in the general U.S. population.

Less common in recent years but still an ingredient in diet aids and energy pills (e.g., "Green Stinger," "Yellow Bullet") are extracts of the ephedra plant group, which contain ephedrine and pseudoephedrine as the active ingredient. These substances in the form of dietary supplements are banned from sale in the United States, but they are chemically synthesized for some medical uses (over-the-counter decongestant) and for illicit distribution; acquisition of these substances is possible via Internet-based purveyors domiciled in foreign countries. Because the U.S. Food and Drug Administration (FDA) ban dating back to 2004 did not ban all varieties of the entire plant (Nelson, 2004), forms of diet pills and energy pills containing *Ephedra viridis* extract from one variety of the plant are legal and widely available, whereas preparations including ephedra alkaloid or *Ephedra sinica* (also known by its traditional Chinese name, Ma Huang) are not legal.

Mechanisms of Action

Similar to ATS drugs, ephedra and ephedrine increase the activity of noradrenaline on adrenergic receptors. Khat's mechanism of action is the same as other cathinone-type substances, as noted earlier.

Physiological Effects

Basic CNS stimulant effects are produced by khat, with increased blood pressure and heart rate subsiding within a few hours for most people, but effects on sleep can persist in some individuals. Excessive consumption of khat causes thirst, hyperactivity, insomnia, loss of appetite, and psychosis (National Drug Enforcement Research Fund, 2011).

For khat users, mild depression is likely after extended periods of use. Khat may elicit manic behavior with delusions, paranoia, and hallucinations (Giannini & Castellini, 1982). Khat can cause damage to the nervous, respiratory, circulatory, and digestive systems (especially constipation) (Ali et al., 2010; Drug Enforcement Agency, 2011).

Use of ephedra has been associated with increased psychiatric disturbances, including psychosis, depression, agitation, and hallucinations, largely among individuals with preexisting conditions (Maglione et al., 2005).

Treatment

As noted earlier, the treatment for presentations involving acute intoxication and side effects caused by ingestion of plant-based stimulant preparations primarily relies on reducing anxiety and stabilizing CNS effects. Clearance of the substance may involve the usual methods, although resolution of symptoms occurs without intervention once the substance has been eliminated. Where the excessive use of khat has elicited more extreme psychiatric symptoms, however, the use of benzodiazepines may be appropriate.

SUMMARY

Among all the stimulants, methamphetamine is the ATS most broadly and consistently associated with the most damaging set of consequences and the most refractory use disorders. Historically, methamphetamine use has waxed and waned in subpopulations of user types, and prevalence has varied according to geographic region within the United States and around the world. Despite the severe problems and stark consequences of methamphetamine dependence and other ATS use disorders, drugs of this class have remained relatively available and unabated by interdiction and other law enforcement efforts. The ATS problem has never really "gone away"; the production methods, locations, and trafficking patterns change, but methamphetamine use remains a significant public health problem in some locations and some populations. Worldwide, the varieties of ATS and related substances appear to be expanding and diversifying. Thus, the development of effective harm reduction and treatment approaches is an ever-important effort to reduce the impacts of ATS use disorders in the legions of individuals who have become involved with the stimulant drugs.

In spite of almost two decades of effort, there are no efficacious pharmacotherapies for the treatment of ATS dependence. In 2015, we may be getting closer to effective, practical treatment approaches that would be broadly acceptable to clinicians, policymakers, and patients (Ling, Mooney, & Haglund, 2014). One such approach is a trial of combination pharmacotherapy that examines the depot naltrexone formulation plus bupropion, a medication proven to have partial efficacy for treatment of ATS use disorders. Bupropion, an antidepressant approved for smoking cessation treatment, has been shown to be effective in treatment of methamphetamine users with less severe addiction (McCann & Li, 2012).

A combination of medications deemed both suitable to address drug use disorders via a therapeutic effect on brain processes and useful in relieving symptoms of early abstinence (i.e., to reduce depression, craving) may prove to be a viable approach, especially as it reflects what is practiced by experienced, well-trained physicians who use such an "adaptive" regimen for their patients. If a rigorous and efficiently conducted clinical trial can establish research-proven efficacy and safety of combination pharmacotherapy, additional trials employing depot naltrexone plus other agents could extend the utility of this investigative platform, leading to more rapid and efficient examination of putative medications for treatment of ATS use disorders.

Clinical research and medication development efforts targeting ATS use disorders are making greater strides toward effectively addressing ATS problems, but this is only part of the effort. The primary burden falls on the shoulders of clinicians, especially those in primary care settings in which SUDs and related problems must be identified in the course of time-constrained contacts that inhibit elaborate screening for such problems. Recognition of underlying SUDs is necessary in order to intervene, if possible, before development of cognitive deficits and other physical and psychiatric conditions that ensue from long-term and high-severity ATS use. Most important is to consider the treatment of ATS use disorders in the same medical manner afforded to patients with other chronic, recurring diseases, emphasizing adequate duration of treatment. A harm reduction model may be more realistic in early-phase intervention for some patients than insistence on total abstinence, which may be unattainable.

Assessment techniques and practice tips are available, and clinicians should avail themselves of these useful tools. Examples of such resources follow:

- SAMHSA's *TIP 33: Treatment for Stimulant Use Disorders* (SAMHSA, 1999).
- *Matrix Intensive Outpatient Treatment for People with Stimulant Use Disorders* (SAMHSA, 2008). The Matrix Model of behavioral therapy was designed for treatment of substance use disorders: Evidence-based elements focus on relapse prevention, family and group therapies, drug education, and self-help participation. See extensive materials at *http://kap.samhsa.gov/products/manuals/matrix/index.htm.*
- *Best Practices in Addiction Treatment: A Workshop Facilitator's Guide.* This guide provides clinician-oriented information about evidence-based practices Download at *www.nattc.org/respubs/bpat/index.html.*
- *Methamphetamine Addiction, Treatment, and Outcomes: Implications for Child Welfare Workers* (Otero, Boles, Young, & Dennis, 2006).

REFERENCES

Albertson, T. E., Derlet, R. W., & Van Hoozen, B. E. (1999). Methamphetamine and the expanding complications of amphetamines. *West J Med, 170*, 214–219.
Ali, W. M., Zubaid, M., Al-Motarreb, A., Singh, R., Al-Shereiqi, S. Z., Shehab, A., et al. (2010).

Assocation of khat chewing with increased risk of stroke and death in patients presenting with acute coronary syndrome. *Mayo Clin Proc, 85,* 974–980.

American Psychiatric Association. (2000). *Diagnostic and statistical manual of mental disorders* (4th ed., text rev.). Washington, DC: Author.

American Psychiatric Association. (2013). *Diagnostic and statistical manual of mental disorders* (5th ed.). Arlington, VA: Author.

Bostwick, M. J., & Lineberry, T. W. (2006). The "meth" epidemic: Managing acute psychosis, agitation, and suicide risk. *Curr Psychiatry, 5*(11), 47–62.

Brensilver, M., Heinzerling, K. G., Swanson, A. N., & Shoptaw, S. J. (2012). A retrospective analysis of two randomized trials of bupropion for methamphetamine dependence: Suggested guidelines for treatment discontinuation/augmentation. *Drug Alcohol Depend, 125,* 169–172.

Chen, C. K., Lin, S. K., Sham, P. C., Ball, D., Loh, E. W., Hsiao, C. C., et al. (2003). Pre-morbid characteristics and co-morbidity of methamphetamine users with and without psychosis. *Psychol Med, 33*(8), 1407–1414.

Chen, C. K., Lin, S. K., Sham, P. C., Ball, D., Loh, E. W., & Murray, R. M. (2005). Morbid risk for psychiatric disorder among the relatives of methamphetamine users with and without psychosis. *Am J Med Genet B Neuropsychiatr Genet, 136*(1), 87–91.

Copeland, A. L., & Sorensen, J. L. (2001). Differences between methamphetamine users and cocaine users in treatment. *Drug Alcohol Depend, 62*(1), 91–95.

Curtis, E. K. (2006). Meth mouth: A review of methamphetamine abuse and its oral manifestations. *Gen Dent, 54*(2), 125–129.

Davidson, C., Gow, A. J., Lee, T. H., & Ellinwood, E. H. (2001). Methamphetamine neurotoxicity: Necrotic and apoptotic mechanisms and relevance to human abuse and treatment. *Brain Res Rev, 36*(1), 1–22.

Drug Enforcement Agency Fact Sheet. (2006). Khat. Retrieved from *www.dea.gov/pubs/pressrel/pr072606a.html.*

Drug Enforcement Agency Press Release. (2011). DEA Moves to emergency control synthetic stimulants: Agency will study whether to permanently control three substances. Retrieved April 2012, from *http://www.dea.gov/divisions/hq/2011/hq090711.shtml.*

Elkashef, A. M., Rawson, R. A., Anderson, A. L., Li, S. H., Holmes, T., Smith, E. V., et al. (2008). Bupropion for the treatment of methamphetamine dependence. *Neuropsychopharmacol, 33*(5), 1162–1170.

Farrell, M., Marsden, J., Ali, R., & Ling, W. (2002). Methamphetamine: Drug use and psychoses becomes a major public health issue in the Asia Pacific region. *Addiction, 97*(7), 771–772.

Fechtner, R. D., Khouri, A. S., Figueroa, E., Ramirez, M., Federico, M., Dewey, S. L., et al. (2006). Short-term treatment of cocaine and/or methamphetamine abuse with vigabatrin: Ocular safety pilot results. *Arch Ophthalmol, 124,* 1257–1262.

Giannini, A. J., & Castellani, S. (1982). A manic-like psychosis due to khat (Catha edulis Forsk.). *J Toxicol Clin Toxicol, 19*(5), 455–459.

Glasner-Edwards, S., Marinelli-Casey, P., Hillhouse, M., Ang, A., Mooney, L. J., Rawson, R., et al. (2009). Depression among methamphetamine users: Association with outcomes from the Methamphetamine Treatment Project at 3-year follow-up. *J Nervous Ment Dis, 197*(4), 225–231.

Glasner-Edwards, S., Marinelli-Casey, P., Hillhouse, M., Gonzales, R., Ang, A., et al. (2007). *Psychiatric illness as a predictor of post-treatment methamphetamine use.* Paper presented at the 69th annual meeting of the College on Problems of Drug Dependence, Quebec City, Canada.

Glasner-Edwards, S., Mooney, L. J., Marinelli-Casey, P., Hillhouse, M., Ang, A., Rawson, R., et al. (2008). Rick factors for suicide attempts in methamphetamine-dependent patients. *Am J Addict, 17,* 24–27.

Glasner-Edwards, S., Mooney, L. J., Marinelli-Casey, P., Hillhouse, M., Ang, A., Rawson, R. A., et al. (2009). Psychopathology in methamphetamine-dependent adults 3 years after treatment. *Drug Alcohol Rev, 29*(1), 12–20.

Granado, N., Ares-Santos, S., & Moratalla, R. (2013). Methamphetamine and Parkinson's disease. *Parkinsons Dis, 2013,* 308052.

Hadlock, G. C., Webb, K. M., McFadden, L. M., Chu, P. W., Ellis, J. D., Allen, S. C., et al. (2011). 4-Methylmethcathinone (mephedrone): Neuropharmacological effects of a designer stimulant of abuse. *J Pharmacol Exp Ther, 339*(2), 530–536.

Harris, D., & Batki, S. L. (2000). Stimulant psychosis: Symptom profile and acute clinical course. *Am J Addict, 9,* 28–37.

Hendrickson, R. G., Cloutier, R., & McConnell, K. J. (2008). Methamphetamine-related emergency department utilization and cost. *Acad Emerg Med, 15,* 23–31.

Jayaram-Lindström, N., Hammarberg, A., Beck, O., & Franck, J. (2008). Naltrexone for the treatment of amphetamine dependence: A randomized, placebo-controlled trial. *Am J Psychiatry, 165,* 1442–1448.

Karch, S. B. (2002). Synthetic stimulants. In S. B. Karch (Ed.), *Karch's pathology of drug abuse* (3rd ed., pp. 233–280). Boca Raton, FL: CRC Press.

Kehr, J., Ichinose, F., Yoshitake, S., Goiny, M., Sievertsson, T., Nyberg, F., et al. (2011). Mephedrone, compared to MDMA (Ecstasy) and amphetamine, rapidly increases both dopamine and serotonin levels in nucleus accumbens of awake rats. *Br J Pharmacol, 164*(8), 1949–1958.

Ling, W., Mooney, L., & Haglund, M. (2014). Treating methamphetamine abuse disorder. *Curr Psychiatry, 13*(9), 37–44.

Maglione, M., Miotto, K., Iguchi, M., Jungvig, L., Morton, S. C., & Shekelle, P. G. (2005). Psychiatric effects of ephedra use: An analysis of Food and Drug Administration reports of adverse events. *Am J Psychiatry, 162*(1), 189–191.

Manghi, R. A., Broers, B., Khan, R., Benguettat, D., Khazaal, Y., & Zullino, D. F. (2009). Khat use: Lifestyle or addiction? *J Psychoactive Drugs, 41*(1), 1–10.

McCabe, S. E., Boyd, C. J., & Young, A. (2007). Medical and nonmedical use of prescription drugs among secondary school students. *J Adolesc Health, 40,* 76–83.

McCabe, S. E., Cranford, J. A., & Boyd, C. J. (2006). The relationship between past-year drinking behaviors and nonmedical use of prescription drugs: Prevalence of co-occurrence in a national sample. *Drug Alcohol Depend, 84,* 281–288.

McCann, D. J., & Li, S. H. (2012). A novel, nonbinary evaluation of success and failure reveals bupropion efficacy versus methamphetamine dependence: Reanalysis of a multisite trial. *CNS Neurosci Ther, 18*(5), 414–418.

McKetin, R., Lubman, D. I., Lee, N. M., Ross, J. E., & Slade, T. N. (2011). Major depression among methamphetamine users entering drug treatment programs. *Med J Aust, 195*(3), S51–S55.

McKetin, R., Lubman, D. I., Najman, J. M., Dawe, S., Butterworth, P., & Baker, A. L. (2014). Does methamphetamine use increase violent behavior?: Evidence from a prospective longitudinal study. *Addiction, 109*(5), 798–806.

McKetin, R., McLaren, J., Lubman, D. I., & Hides, L. (2006). The prevalence of psychotic symptoms among methamphetamine users. *Addiction, 101*(10), 1473–1478.

Mooney, L. J., Glasner-Edwards, S., Marinelli-Casey, P., Hillhouse, M., Ang, A., Hunter, J., et al. (2009). Health conditions in methamphetamine-dependent adults 3 years after treatment. *J Addict Med, 3*(3), 155–163.

Mooney, L., Glasner-Edwards, S., Rawson, R. A., & Ling, W. (2009). Medical effects of methamphetamine use. In J. M. Roll, R. A. Rawson, & W. Ling (Eds.), *Methamphetamine addiction: From basic science to treatment.* New York: Guilford Press.

Mowry, J. B., Spyker, D. A., Cantilena, L. R., Bailey, J. E., & Ford, M. (2013). 2012 Annual report of the American Association of Poison Control Centers' National Poison Data System (NPDS): 30th annual report. *Clin Toxicol, 51,* 949–1229.

National Addiction Research Centre. (1997). Epidemiology and social context of amphetamine-type stimulant use. London: National Addiction Research Centre. Retrieved March 2015, from *http://libdoc.who.int/hq/1997/WHO_MSA_PSA_97.5_%28chp2%29.pdf.*

National Drug Enforcement Research Fund (NDERF). (2011). Law enforcement and khat: An analysis of current issues. Canberra, Australia: NDERF. Retrieved from *www.law.uq.edu. au/documents/khat/NDLERF40_khat.pdf*.

National Drug Intelligence Center. (2011). Synthetic cathinones (Bath Salts): An emerging domestic threat (U.S. Department of Justice *Situation Report*). Retrieved from *www.justice.gov/ archive/ndic/pubs44/44571/44571p.pdf*

Nelson, R. (2004). FDA issues alert on ephedra supplements in the USA. *Lancet, 363*(9403), 135.

Newton, T. F., De La Garza, R., II, Kalechstein, A. D., & Nestor, L. (2005). Cocaine and methamphetamine produce different patterns of subjective and cardiovascular effects. *Pharmacol Biochem Behav, 82*, 90–97.

Nordt, S. P., Vilke, G. M., Clark, R. F., Lee Cantrell, F., Chan, T. C., Galinato, M., et al. (2012). Energy drink use and adverse effects among emergency department patients. *J Community Health, 37*(5), 976–981.

Numachi, Y., Ohara, A., Yamashita, M., Fukushima, S., Kobayashi, H., Hata, H., et al. (2007). Methamphetamine-induced hyperthermia and lethal toxicity: Role of the dopamine and serotonin transporters. *Eur J Pharmacol, 572*(2–3), 120–128.

Otero, C., Boles, S., Young, N., & Dennis, K. (2006). *Methamphetamine addiction, treatment, and outcomes: Implications for child welfare workers.* Irvine, CA: National Center on Substance Abuse and Child Welfare.

Rawson, R. A., Marinelli-Casey, P., Anglin, M. D., Dickow, A., Frazier, Y., Gallagher, C., et al. (2004). A multi-site comparison of psychosocial approaches for the treatment of methamphetamine dependence. *Addiction, 99*, 708–717.

Rawson, R. A., McCann, M. J., Flammino, F., Shoptaw, S., Miotto, K., Reiber, C., & Ling, W. (2006). A comparison of contingency management and cognitive-behavioral approaches for stimulant-dependent individuals. *Addiction, 101*(2), 267–274.

Richards, J. R., Bretz, S. W., Johnson, E. B., Turnipseed, S. D., Brofeldt, B. T., & Derlet, R. W. (1999). Methamphetamine abuse and emergency department utilization. *West J Med, 170*(4), 198–202.

Roll, J. M., Petry, N. M., Stitzer, M. L., Brecht, M. L., Peirce, J. M., McCann, M. J., et al. (2006). Contingency management for the treatment of methamphetamine use disorders. *Am J Psychiatry, 163*, 1993–1999.

Romanelli, R., & Smith, K. M. (2006). Clinical effects and management of methamphetamine abuse. *Pharmacotherapy, 26*, 1148–1156.

Salo, R., Flower, K., Kielstein, A., Leamon, M. H., Nordahl, T. E., & Galloway, G. P. (2011). Psychiatric comorbidity in methamphetamine dependence. *Psychiatry Res, 186*(2), 356–361.

Sandoval, V., Riddle, E. L., Hanson, G. R., & Fleckenstein, A. E. (2003). Methylphenidate alters vesicular monoamine transport and prevents methamphetamine-induced dopaminergic deficits. *J Pharmacol Exp Ther, 304*, 1181–1187.

Schuckit, M. A. (2006). Comorbidity between substance use disorders and psychiatric conditions. *Addiction, 101*(Suppl. 1), 76–88.

Scott, J. C., Woods, S. P., Matt, G. E., Meyer, R. A., Heaton, R. K., Atkinson, J. H., et al. (2007). Neurocognitive effects of methamphetamine: A critical review and meta-analysis. *Neuropsychol Rev, 17*, 275–297.

Shetty, V., Mooney, L. J., Zigler, C. M., Belin, T. R., Murphy, D., & Rawson, R. (2010). The relationship between methamphetamine use and increased dental disease. *J Am Dent Assoc, 141*, 307–318.

Shoptaw, S., Heinzerling, K. G., Rotheram-Fuller, E., Steward, T., Wang, J., Swanson, A. N., et al. (2008). Randomized, placebo-controlled trial of bupropion for the treatment of methamphetamine dependence. *Drug Alcohol Depend, 96*, 222–232.

Shoptaw, S. J., Kao, U., & Ling, W. (2009, January 21). Treatment for amphetamine psychosis. *Cochrane Database Syst Rev, 1*, CD003026.

Shoptaw, S., Klausner, J. D., Reback, C. J., Tierney, S., Stansell, J., Hare, C. B., et al. (2006). A public health response to the methamphetamine epidemic: The implementation of contingency management to treat methamphetamine dependence. *BMC Public Health, 6*, 214.

Shoptaw, S., Peck, J., Reback, C. J., & Rotheram-Fuller, E. (2003). Psychiatric and substance dependence comorbidities, sexually transmitted diseases, and risk behaviors among methamphetamine-dependent gay and bisexual men seeking outpatient drug abuse treatment. *J Psychoactive Drugs, 35*(Suppl. 1), 161–168.

Simon, S. L., Dacey, J., Glynn, S., Rawson, R., & Ling, W. (2004). The effect of relapse on cognition in abstinent methamphetamine abusers. *J Subst Abuse Treat, 27*(1), 59–66.

Sommers, I., Baskin, D., & Baskin-Sommers, A. (2006). Methamphetamine use among young adults: Health and social consequences. *Addict Behav, 31*, 1469–1476.

Spiller, H., Ryan, M., Weston, R., & Janson, J. (2011). Clinical experience with and analytical confirmation of "bath salts" and "legal highs" (synthetic cathinones) in the United States. *Clin Toxicol (Phila), 49*(6), 499–505.

Substance Abuse and Mental Health Services Administration (SAMHSA). (1999). *Treatment for stimulant use disorders* (Treatment Improvement Protocol [TIP] Series, No. 33, Report No. [SMA] 09-4209). Rockville, MD: Author.

Substance Abuse and Mental Health Services Administration (SAMHSA). (2008). *Matrix intensive outpatient treatment for people with stimulant use disorders* (Pub. No. SMA13-4152). Rockville, MD: Author.

Substance Abuse and Mental Health Services Administration (SAMHSA). (2009). *Results from the 2008 National Survey on Drug Use and Health: National findings* (Office of Applied Studies, NSDUH Series H-36, HHS Publication No. SMA 09-4434). Retrieved from *http://archive.samhsa.gov/data/NSDUH/2k8nsduh/2k8Results.htm*.

Substance Abuse and Mental Health Services Administration (SAMHSA), Center for Behavioral Health Statistics and Quality. (2013). *Treatment Episode Data Set (TEDS): 2001–2011. State admissions to substance abuse treatment services.* BHSIS Series S-XX, HHS Publication No. (SMA) XX-XXXX. Rockville, MD: Author. Retrieved from *www.samhsa.gov/data/sites/default/files/TEDS2011St_Web/TEDS2011St_Web/TEDS2011St_Web.pdf*.

Substance Abuse and Mental Health Services Administration (SAMHSA). (2014a). *Results from the 2013 National Survey on Drug Use and Health: Summary of national findings* (NSDUH Series H-48, HHS Publication No. [SMA] 14-4863). Rockville, MD: Author. Retrieved from *www.samhsa.gov/data/sites/default/files/NSDUHresultsPDFWHTML2013/Web/NSDUHresults2013.pdf*.

Substance Abuse and Mental Health Services Administration (SAMHSA), Center for Behavioral Health Statistics and Quality. (2014b). *Treatment Episode Data Set (TEDS): 2002–2012. National admissions to substance abuse treatment services* (BHSIS Series S-71, HHS Publication No. [SMA] 14-4850). Rockville, MD: Author. Retrieved from *www.samhsa.gov/data/sites/default/files/TEDS2012N_Web.pdf*.

Thornton, S. L., Gerona, R. R., & Tomaszewski, C. A. (2012). Psychosis from a Bath Salt product containing flephedrone and MDPV with serum, urine, and product quantification. *J Med Toxicol, 8*(3), 310–313.

Turnipseed, S. D., Richards, J. R., Kirk, J. D., Diercks, D. B., & Amsterdam, E. A. (2003). Frequency of acute coronary syndrome in patients presenting to the emergency department with chest pain after methamphetamine use. *J Emerg Med, 24*, 369–373.

Ujike, H., & Sato, M. (2004). Clinical features of sensitization to methamphetamine observed in patients with methamphetamine dependence and psychosis. *Ann NY Acad Sci, 1025*, 279–287.

United Nations Office on Drugs and Crime (UNODC). (2010). Amphetamine-type stimulants—United Nations World Drug Report, 2009. Retrieved from *www.unodc.org/documents/wdr/WDR_2010/2.5_Amphetamine-type_stimulants.pdf*.

United Nations Office on Drugs and Crime (UNODC). (2012). United Nations World Drug Report, 2012. Retrieved from *www.unodc.org/unodc/data-and-analysis/WDR-2012.html*.

United Nations Office on Drugs and Crime (UNODC). (2013). *Patterns and trends of amphetamine-type stimulants and other drugs: Challenges for Asia and the Pacific*. Vienna: Author. Retrieved from *www.unodc.org/documents/scientific/2013_Regional_ATS_Report_web.pdf*.

U.S. Food and Drug Administration. (2010). FDA Press Release: FDA warning letters issued to four makers of caffeinated alcoholic beverages. Retrieved from *www.fda.gov/newsevents/newsroom/pressannouncements/2010/ucm234109.htm*.

Vocci, F., & Montoya, I. (2009). Psychological treatments for stimulant misuse, comparing and contrasting those for amphetamine dependence and those for cocaine dependence. *Curr Opin Psychiatry, 22*(3), 263–268.

Volkow, N. D., Chang, L., Wang, G. J., Fowler, J. S., Franceschi, D., Sedler, M., et al. (2001). Loss of dopamine transporters in methamphetamine abusers recovers with protracted abstinence. *J Neurosci, 21*, 9414–9418.

Volkow, N. D., Wang, G. J., Fowler, J. S., Logan, J., Franceschi, D., Maynard, L., et al. (2002). Relationship between blockade of dopamine transporters by oral methylphenidate and the increases in extracellular dopamine: Therapeutic implications. *Synapse, 43*, 181–187.

Wang, G. J., Volkow, N. D., Chang, L., Miller, E., Sedler, M., Hitzemann, R., et al. (2004). Partial recovery of brain metabolism in methamphetamine abusers after protracted abstinence. *Am J Psychiatry, 161*, 242–248.

Watanabe-Galloway, S., Ryan, S., Hansen, K., Hullsiek, B., Muli, V., et al. (2009). Effects of methamphetamine abuse beyond individual users. *J Psychoactive Drugs, 41*(3), 241–248.

Westover, A. N., Mcbride, S., & Haley, R. W. (2007). Stroke in young adults who abuse amphetamines or cocaine. *Arch Gen Psychiatry, 64*, 495–502.

Wijetunga, M., Bhan, R., Lindsay, J., & Karch, S. (2004). Acute coronary syndrome and crystal methamphetamine use: A case series. *Hawaii Med J, 63*, 8–13.

Wilens, T. E., Adler, L. A., Adams, J., Sgambati, S., Rotrosen, J., Sawtelle, R., et al. (2008). Misuse and diversion of stimulants prescribed for ADHD: A systematic review of the literature. *J Am Acad Child Adolesc Psychiatry, 47*(1), 21–31.

World Health Organization (WHO). (2006). *WHO Expert Committee on Drug Dependence 34th Report* (WHO Technical Report Series 942). Geneva: Author. Retrieved from *www.who.int/medicines/areas/quality_safety/WHO_TRS_942.pdf*.

Zweben, J. E., Cohen, J. B., Christian, D., Galloway, G. P., Salinardi, M., Parent, D., et al. (2004). Psychiatric symptoms in methamphetamine users. *Am J Addict, 13*, 181–190.

CHAPTER 12

Cocaine

EVARISTO AKERELE
NIRU NAHAR

Cocaine is the product obtained by processing the coca leaf. It is a stimulant that remains widely abused in the United States despite the tremendous resources applied to the eradication of the crop or interdiction of the drug. Cocaine remains a significant public health problem and the source of morbidity or mortality among its users, particularly those with a cocaine use disorder. In this chapter we review cocaine from a historical perspective before discussing the risks, the extent of use, pharmacology, effects, adverse outcomes, and treatment for cocaine use.

HISTORY AND ABORIGINAL USE

Coca leaves, the source of cocaine, have been chewed and ingested for thousands of years. The term "coca" may refer to any of the four cultivated plants that belong to the family Erythroxylaceae, which is native to western South America. Raw coca leaves, chewed or consumed as tea or "mate de coca," are rich in nutritional properties. Leaves of this plant have been chewed by Amerindian peoples for thousands of years, making coca one of the most venerable of "lifestyle drugs" (Flower, 2004), but aboriginal chewing or drinking of coca tea does not produce the euphoria experienced with cocaine. Pure cocaine was originally extracted from the leaf of the *Erythroxylum coca* bush. The alkaloid was first isolated and proposed as a local anesthetic in 1860. Karl Köller reported on the use of cocaine eye drops as a local anesthetic in 1884 (Markel, 2011). This was rapidly adopted, and the use of cocaine was soon extended to surgical practice. The physical and social harm caused by cocaine as a drug of abuse in the 20th and 21st centuries are the results of increased purity of illicit supplies of the drug (Ritter, 2010). This resulted from an extraction process based on manipulating its ionization, by altering the pH of aqueous "mulch" and extracting uncharged base into an organic solvent, which is then evaporated. Cocaine is now classified by the Drug Enforcement Agency as a Schedule II substance.

EPIDEMIOLOGY OF COCAINE USE AND COCAINE-RELATED DISORDERS

Overall the use of cocaine in the United States has dropped, and in some geographic or age-based groups, the rate of use is extremely lower than the peak rate in the 1980s. In the 12 or older age group, the trends are as follows: The prevalence of cocaine use dropped from 2.4 million in 2006 to 1.5 million in 2010. The incidence of cocaine use dropped from 1 million in 2002 to 637,000 in 2010. Similarly, the incidence of crack use declined from 337,000 to 83,000. The trend for the persons age 12 or older is downward for both initiates and current users (Substance Abuse and Mental Health Services Administration [SAMHSA], 2014).

Similarly, there has been a decline in cocaine use among high school students (Johnston, O'Malley, Bachman, & Schulenberg, 2010). The past-year usage levels reached their lowest point since the early 1990s. Significant declines in use were measured from 2008 to 2009 among 12th graders across all three survey categories: Lifetime use decreased from 7.2 to 6.0%; past-year use dropped from 4.4 to 3.4%; and past-month use dropped from 1.9 to 1.3%. Survey measures showed other positive findings among 12th graders as well; their perceived risk of harm associated with powder cocaine use increased significantly during the same period. Additionally, survey participants in the 10th grade reported significant changes, with past-month use falling from 1.2% in 2008 to 0.9% in 2009. The percentage of both adult and juvenile arrestees testing positive for cocaine in the Distrinct of Columbia peaked in 1988 in the midst of the cocaine epidemic, at 64 and 22%, respectively (CESAR Fax, 2012).

The trend for cocaine use among adults is similar, with one exception: Among young adults ages 18–25, the rate of current use of cocaine decreased from 2.0 to 1.5% over the years from 2002 to 2013 (SAMHSA, 2014). However, for adults ages 50–59, the rate of current illicit drug use increased from 2.7 to 5.8% between 2002 and 2010 (Figure 12.1).

The use of cocaine also varies with race and gender. The rate of current illicit drug use among Asians in 2010 was about 3.5%. The rate was 8.1% among Hispanics, 9.1% among whites, and 1.6% among blacks. In 2002 and 2003, Asians had the lowest rate of past-year cocaine use (0.7%) compared with other racial/ethnic groups. Asians also had the lowest rate of past-year crack cocaine use (0.1%) compared with other racial/ethnic groups. It would be interesting to explore some of the potential reasons for the difference in use across ethnic/racial groups (SAMHSA, 2014).

Data from Treatment Settings

There were 1.8 million admissions in 2008 (Treatment Episode Data Set [TEDS]; SAHMSA, 2008) for treatment of alcohol and drug abuse to publicly funded substance use disorders (SUDs) treatment programs that report to state administrative data systems. The treatment admissions were primarily for alcohol use disorder

222

III. SUBSTANCES OF ABUSE

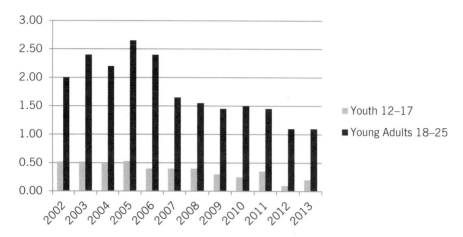

FIGURE 12.1. Percent of population using cocaine in the past month by year. Data from SAM-HSA (2014).

(41.4%). These were closely followed by visits for smoked cocaine (8.1%) and non-smoked cocaine (3.2%) (Figure 12.2). Most of the treatment seekers were white (60%), 21% were black, and 14% were Hispanic.

SAHMSA Data: 1995 versus 2005

The age of treatment seekers admitted for primary use of smoked cocaine increased between 1995 and 2005. Individuals admitted for treatment for smoked cocaine were primarily under age 35 (63%) in 1995; that percentage dropped to merely 32% of individuals under age 35 in 2005 (Figure 12.2).

Furthermore, the percentage of admissions who reported using cocaine for more than 10 years increased. The proportion of admissions who had smoked cocaine for more than 10 years increased from 32% in 1995 to 63% in 2005; the proportion of admissions who had inhaled cocaine for more than 10 years increased from 41% in 1995 to 49% in 2005.

In summary, the use of cocaine is dropping among individuals under age 35. However, for all forms of cocaine, there is an increase in the percentage of people who have used cocaine for more than 10 years. These data suggest that the popularity of cocaine among the young is dropping. However, for those who use cocaine, the duration of use is increasing.

Drug-Related Hospital Emergency Room Visits

Cocaine is plays a significant role in drug-related emergency room visits. The data from the 2008 Drug Abuse Warning Network (DAWN) report indicated that cocaine was involved in 482,188 of the nearly 2 million visits to emergency departments for drug misuse or abuse. This translates to almost one in four drug misuse or abuse emergency department visits (24%) that involved cocaine. In 2009, almost 1 million

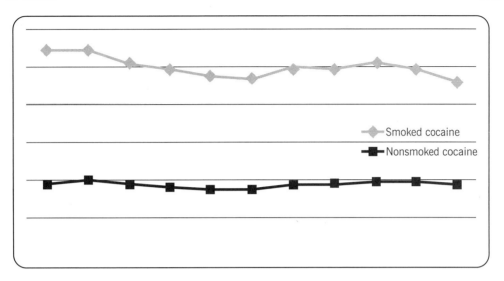

FIGURE 12.2. Percentage of primary cocaine admissions with route of administration. Data from SAMHSA (2007). Treatment Episode Data Set.

visits involved an illicit drug, either alone or in combination with other types of drugs. DAWN estimates that cocaine was involved in 422,896 emergency department visits. Rates for cocaine were highest in individuals ages 35–44; rates for heroin were highest among individuals ages 21–24; stimulant use was highest among those 25–29; and marijuana use was highest for those ages 18–20.

Cocaine has also become one of the primary drugs involved in drug-related emergency room deaths. According to the Centers for Disease Control and Prevention, among the deaths attributed to drug overdose, cocaine, heroin, and opioid painkillers are the most common substances involved. Cocaine overdoses caused over 6,000 deaths in 2006.

RISK FACTORS FOR SUBSTANCE USE DISORDER

Genetic epidemiological studies support a high degree of heritable vulnerability for cocaine use disorder. The data suggest that polymorphisms in the genes coding for dopamine receptors and transporter, and serotonin receptors and transporter, are apparently associated with the phenotypic expression of this vulnerability cocaine is used (Saxon, Oreskovich, & Brkanac, 2005).

Approximately one in five whites has a genetic variant that substantially increases the odds of being susceptible to cocaine use disorder. Among whites, one or both mutations were found in more than 40% of autopsied brain samples from people who had abused cocaine, compared to 19% of samples from people who lived drug-free. Overall, one in five samples from whites in the control group, and one in two to three whites in the cocaine overdose group, contained the genetic variant, compared to one in eight blacks (Moyer et al., 2011; Bilbao et al., 2008).

Bilbao et al. (2008) linked a version of the *CAMK4* gene with cocaine addiction after studying mice that had been genetically modified to alter the gene. One particular breed was affected more strongly by the drug and became addicted more quickly than others in the group. A series of genetic tests were run in humans to clarify the role of this gene; 670 individuals with cocaine use disorders were matched with more than 700 nonusers. Although 40% of nonusers carried the gene, it was found in 50% of individuals with cocaine use disorders. Individuals with cocaine use disorders are 25% more likely to carry the gene variant than nonusers of cocaine. The data suggest that genetic factors account for 70% of cocaine addiction.

PHARMACOLOGY

There are two chemical forms of cocaine that are abused: the water-soluble hydrochloride salt and the water-insoluble cocaine base, or freebase. Cocaine is generally sold on the street as a fine, white, crystalline powder; it is also known as "coke," "C," "snow," "flake," or "blow." Street dealers generally dilute it with inert substances such as cornstarch, talcum powder, or sugar, or with active drugs such as procaine (a chemically related local anesthetic) or amphetamine (NIDA, 2010). Some users combine cocaine with heroin in what is termed a "speedball."

When abused, the water-soluble hydrochloride salt, or powdered form of cocaine, can be injected or snorted. The water-insoluble cocaine base, or freebase form of cocaine, is processed with ammonia or sodium bicarbonate (baking soda) and water, then heated to remove the hydrochloride to produce a smokable substance. The freebase cocaine is referred to as "crack" in the streets due to the crackling sound heard when the mixture is smoked.

Powdered cocaine can be snorted or injected into the veins after it is dissolved in water. Cocaine base (crack) is smoked, either alone or with marijuana or tobacco. Cocaine is also abused in combination with opiates, such as heroin, a practice known as "speedballing." Although injecting into veins or muscles, snorting, and smoking are the common ways of using cocaine, all mucous membranes readily absorb cocaine. Cocaine users typically binge on the drug until they are exhausted or run out of cocaine.

The principal routes of cocaine administration are oral, intranasal, inhalation, and intravenous. Snorting is the process of inhaling cocaine powder through the nose, where it is absorbed into the bloodstream through the nasal tissues. The drug also can be rubbed onto mucous tissues. Smoking involves inhaling cocaine vapor or smoke into the lungs, where absorption into the bloodstream is as rapid as it is by injection. Injecting, which is the use of a needle to introduce the drug directly into the bloodstream, heightens the intensity of the drug's effects. The immediate euphoric effect is one of the reasons that crack became enormously popular in the mid-1980s.

The effects of cocaine use, such as increased energy, reduced fatigue, and mental alertness, depend on the route of drug administration. The faster cocaine is absorbed into the bloodstream and delivered to the brain, the more intense the high. Injecting or smoking cocaine produces a quicker, stronger high than snorting. On the other hand, faster absorption usually means shorter duration of action: The high from snorting cocaine may last 15–30 minutes, but the high from smoking it may last only 5–10 minutes.

Cocaethylene

A common pharmacokinetic-based issue is the increased risk when cocaine is taken combination with alcohol. Cocaine and alcohol are combined in the liver to produce cocaethylene (Harris, Everhart, Mendelson, & Jones, 2003). Cocaethylene, or ethyl-benzoylecgonine, is the ethyl ester of benzoylecgonine. Under normal circumstances, cocaine is metabolized to produce two biologically inactive metabolites, benzoylec-gonine and ecgonine methyl ester. When ethanol is present during the metabolism of cocaine, a portion of the cocaine undergoes transesterification with ethanol, instead of undergoing hydrolysis to water; this results in cocaethylene (Laizure, Mandrell, Gades, & Parker, 2003). Furthermore, ethanol slows the normal metabolism of cocaine. The resulting molecule acts like cocaine with slightly lesser potency but a longer half-life.

Cocaethylene then increases the level of serotonergic, noradrenergic, and dopaminergic neurotransmission by inhibiting the action of the serotonin transporter (SERT), norepinephrine transporter (NET), and dopamine transporter (DAT) which makes cocaethylene a serotonin–norepinephrine–dopamine reuptake inhibitor (SNDRI). Cocaethylene is more potent than cocaine at binding to the DAT; however, it is less potent at binding to the SERT and NET. It produces stimulant, euphoriant, anorectic, sympathomimetic, and local anesthetic effects. In most users, it produces more euphoria and possesses a longer duration of action than cocaine. Data suggest that it may be more cardiotoxic than cocaine and is associated with a greater risk of sudden death than cocaine alone (Bradberry et al., 1993; Jatlow et al., 1996).

Neurotransmitters and Behavioral Pharmacology

Cocaine acts by blocking the reuptake of certain neurotransmitters such as DAT, NET, and SERT (Cooper, Bloom, & Roth, 2003). By binding to the transporters that normally remove the excess of these neurotransmitters from the synaptic gap, cocaine prevents them from being reabsorbed by the neurons that released them and thus increases their concentration in the synapses. As a result, all the postsynaptic effects of dopamine, serotonin and norepinephrine are enhanced.

The effects of the enhanced postsynaptic dopamine, serotonin, and norepinephrine result from activation of the mesolimbic dopaminergic reward pathway via increased extraneuronal dopamine in the nucleus accumbens (Rang, Dale, Ritter, & Flower, 2007). The pathway is also activated by all drugs of dependence, including nicotine, ethanol, amphetamines, and opioids, as well as cocaine. Other forms of risk taking also activate this reward system. Cocaine penetrates mucous membranes following topical administration by spray, and its intense vasoconstrictor sympatho-mimetic action is an advantageous for anesthesia. In addition to its local anesthetic and central nervous system effects, cocaine enhances peripheral sympathetic neurotransmission by blocking uptake (Wood & Dargan, 2010). In the central nervous system, cocaine increases levels of dopamine, a brain neurotransmitter associated with pleasure and movement, in the brain's reward circuit (Koob & Volkow, 2010). The neural system most affected by cocaine is the ventral tegmental area (VTA) and the nucleus accumbens (in the midbrain). Nerve fibers originating in the VTA extend to the nucleus accumbens, one of the brain's key areas of reward. Rewards increase levels of the brain neurotransmitter dopamine, resulting in increased neural activity in the nucleus accumbens. Dopamine is usually then recycled back into the transmitting neuron from synapses by the DAT. When present, cocaine attaches to the DAT and blocks the usual recycling process. This results in a buildup of dopamine in the synapse, which contributes to the pleasurable effects of cocaine. Cocaine's yield of pleasurable feelings is primarily associated with one set of dopamine receptor, the D_3 receptor (Vorel et al., 2002).

Tolerance to cocaine may develop with repeated use (Small et al. 2009; NIDA, 2010a). In chronic cocaine consumers, the brain depends on exogenous drug to maintain the high degree of pleasure associated with the artificially elevated levels of some neurotransmitters in its reward circuits. The postsynaptic membrane may adapt to the high dopamine levels and manufacture new receptors. The resulting increased sensitivity produces depression and cravings if cocaine consumption ceases and dopamine levels return to normal (Canadian Institutes of Health Researches, Institute of Neurosciences, Mental Health and Addiction [INMHA], n.d.).

Chronic effects of cocaine abuse may change brain structure and function. These changes may account for the consolidation and structural reconfiguration of synaptic connections with exposure to cocaine (Mash et al., 2007) Adaptive hippocampal plasticity may be related to specific patterns of gene expression with chronic cocaine abuse. According to Mash et al., the data indicated that cocaine abusers had 151 gene transcripts up-regulated, while 91 gene transcripts were down-regulated. The primary cocaine-regulated transcript was RECK (reversion-inducing cysteine-rich protein with kazal motifs), in the human hippocampus. RECK is a membrane-anchored matrix metalloproteinase (MMP) inhibitor associated with regulation of extracellular matrix integrity and angiogenesis. Elevated RECK expression was associated with decreased active MMP9 protein levels in the hippocampus of individuals with cocaine use disorders. Extracellular matrix remodeling in the hippocampus may be a persisting effect of chronic abuse that contributes to the chronic relapsing nature of cocaine use disorder (Mash et al., 2007). Most brain regions may stop producing new neurons once the organ reaches full maturity. However, neurogenesis continues throughout life in the hippocampus (Pascual-Leone, Amedi, Fregni, & Merabet, 2005), a structure that is crucial to learning and memory. This process of neurogenesis can be affected by drug use.

Noonan, Choi, Self, and Eisch (2008; Mandyam et al., 2008), suggest that drugs of abuse may diminish production of new hippocampal neurons and thereby increase vulnerability to drug addiction. Noonan, Bulin, Fuller, and Eisch (2010) suggest that cocaine self-administration in adult rats is increased when production of hippocampal neurons is suppressed. Their results suggest that enhancing neurogenesis might be an effective strategy for treating drug abuse and preventing relapse. Cocaine self-administration in rats inhibits both cell proliferation and maturation in the hippocampus. When cocaine was no longer available and self-administration stopped, the rats that had previously self-administered the drug showed signs of enhanced maturity in new neurons, suggesting that abstinence may promote a compensatory response following drug-induced disruption of neurogenesis (Eisch et al., 2008).

Cocaine can also alter the production of several proteins (Hedges, Chakravarty, Nestler, & Meisel, 2009; Renthal et al., 2008; Wallace et al., 2008). These proteins include but are not limited to enzymes that influence DNA repair, cell death, stress resistance, metabolism, and aging. Probably the most interesting of these are two enzymes that belong to a group known as sirtuins, also known as "silent information regulators of transcription" (SIRTS). In experiments with mice, chemically boosting the activity of these enzymes intensified drug seeking (Renthal et al., 2009).

Another protein that may have a role in cocaine use disorder is delta-FosB, a transcription factor, one of a family of molecules that attach to a gene and accelerate or retard production of its protein. Chronic exposure to cocaine causes delta-FosB to accumulate in the striatum. This accumulation correlates with increased drug-seeking behaviors, probably by creating excesses or shortages of proteins in the nucleus accumbens and other areas of the striatum that support cognition and shape reward-related behaviors. Increased amounts of bound delta-FosB correlate with reduced proto-oncogene (c-Fos) production, as evidenced by lower levels of c-Fos messenger RNA (Alibhai, Green, Potashkin, & Nestler, 2007). The delta-FosB attracts an enzyme called histone deacetylase 1 (HDAC1) that causes DNA to be held more tightly against its protein scaffolding, resulting in less production of c-Fos.

CLINICAL FEATURES

Intoxication

Cocaine increases alertness, feelings of well-being and euphoria, energy and motor activity, and feelings of competence and sexuality. Its effects appear almost immediately after a single dose and disappear within a few minutes or an hour. Taken in small amounts, cocaine usually makes the user feel euphoric, energetic, talkative, and mentally alert, especially to the sensations of sight, sound, and touch. It can also temporarily decrease the need for food and sleep. Some users find that the drug helps them perform simple physical and intellectual tasks more quickly, although others experience the opposite effect.

The duration of cocaine's euphoric effects depends on the route of administration. The faster the drug is absorbed, the more intense the resulting high, but also the shorter the duration. The high from snorting is relatively slow to arrive, but it may last 15–30 minutes; in contrast, the effects from smoking are more immediate but may last only 5–10 minutes. The short-term physiological effects of cocaine use include constricted blood vessels and dilated pupils, and increased body temperature, heart rate, and blood pressure. Large amounts of cocaine may intensify the user's high but can also lead to bizarre, erratic, and violent behavior. Some cocaine users report feelings of restlessness, irritability, anxiety, panic, and paranoia. Users may also experience tremors, vertigo, and muscle twitches.

Overdose

The signs and symptoms of cocaine overdose are related to the psychological and stimulant effects of the drug. Use of cocaine causes tachyarrhythmia and a marked elevation of blood pressure, which can be life threatening. This can lead to death from respiratory failure, stroke, cerebral hemorrhage, or heart failure. Cocaine is also highly pyrogenic, because the stimulation and increased muscular activity cause greater heat production. Heat loss is inhibited by the intense vasoconstriction. Cocaine-induced hyperthermia may cause muscle cell destruction and myoglobinuria resulting in renal failure. The classic signs are hypertension, tachycardia, and tachypnea. This occurs with agitation, confusion, irritability, sweating, and hyperthermia. Sometimes seizures may occur.

Cocaine overdose can also present as a myocardial infarction with chest pain. This is thought to result from "spasm" of the coronary arteries that feed the heart muscle or from insufficient supply of blood flow to meet the needs of the stimulated heart muscle. Unfortunately, sudden death may also be the initial presentation to the emergency department; this is due to a lethal heart rhythm precipitated by cocaine consumption. It is important to avoid beta blockers.

Stroke, seizures, fever, infection, kidney failure, liver hepatitis, pneumonia, thrombophlebitis, and HIV are other potential complications of cocaine use and cocaine overdose. According to the Centers for Disease Control and Prevention, in 2005, 33,000 people died from cocaine overdose, which is a 60% increase since 1990. It is estimated that 70–80% of these were accidental deaths due to heart failure.

Acute cocaine-related toxicity is a common cause of presentation to accident and emergency departments. The clinical features of acute toxicity include tachycardia, dysrhythmias, agitation and aggressive behavior, hallucinations, dilated pupils, hypertonia, hyperreflexia, hyperpyrexia, acid–base disturbance, and arterial dissection. Extreme agitation associated with increased sympathetic outflow from the central nervous system coupled with blockade of peripheral noradrenaline transport by uptake (Wood & Dargan, 2010) may result in increased circulating noradrenaline concentrations. Acute hypertension and tachycardia can precipitate a catastrophic vascular event in patients with preexisting vascular disease. Some autopsy results indicate that fatal dysrhythmia is the likely cause of death from cocaine use.

The direct effects of cocaine on cardiac ion channels (voltage-gated sodium, potassium, and calcium channels) work in tandem with indirect sympathomimetic effects on the heart and the coronary vasculature to disrupt the co-coordinated electrical activity of the heart and produce potentially life-threatening dysrhythmias (O'Leary & Hancox, 2010). Hoffman (2010) suggested dysrhythmias in the setting of slow-on slow-off (Vaughan Williams Class IC) sodium channel blockade (with prolonged depolarization, characterized by prolongation of the QRS complex as the precursor to ventricular tachycardia, and on occasion a Brugada-like pattern on the electrocardiogram), potassium-channel blockade (QT prolongation, torsades de pointes) primarily of the inward potassium rectifier current, and catecholamine excess.

Chronic Use

Cocaine is a highly addictive drug. Cocaine addiction is considered a brain disease, because cocaine and drugs change the brain; they change its structure and how it works. These brain changes can be long-lasting and may lead to many harmful, often self-destructive, behaviors. In dependent individuals, the risk for relapse is high, even following long periods of abstinence, probably because of the brain changes. Studies (e.g., Gould, 2010) indicate that during periods of abstinence, the memory of the cocaine experience or exposure to cues associated with drug use can trigger tremendous craving and relapse to drug use. Brain images show decreased D_2 receptors in the brain of a person addicted to cocaine versus a nonuser (Volkow, Fowler, Wang, Baler, & Telang, 2009). The dopamine system is important for conditioning and motivation, and alterations such as this are likely responsible, in part, for the diminished sensitivity to natural rewards that develops with addiction. With repeated exposure to cocaine, the brain starts to adapt, and the reward pathway becomes less sensitive to natural reinforcers and to the drug itself. Tolerance may develop; at the same time, users may also become more sensitive to cocaine's anxiety-producing, convulsant, and other toxic effects.

Withdrawal

The symptoms are characterized by symptoms and signs that appear over a period of a few hours to several days after the cessation or reduction in heavy or prolonged use of cocaine. It consists of dysphoric mood and two or more of the following: fatigue, vivid and unpleasant dreams, insomnia or hypersomnia, increased appetite, and either psychomotor agitation or retardation. Cocaine craving and anhedonia are also present. Cocaine withdrawal peaks in 2–4 days with symptoms such as lowering of mood, fatigue, and general malaise lasting for several weeks.

COCAINE USE DISORDERS

DSM-5 (American Psychiatric Association, 2013) includes cocaine use disorder (a stimulant use disorder) among substance-related and addictive disorders. This diagnosis replaces the previous DSM diagnoses of cocaine abuse and cocaine dependence.

PSYCHIATRIC AND OTHER MEDICAL EFFECTS OF COCAINE

Psychiatric Comorbidity and Sequelae

Treatment of cocaine use disorder in comorbid populations is even more challenging. One potential solution might be to target such medication development toward specific subpopulations. Some data suggest that antipsychotics may be useful in the treatment of cocaine use disorder in individuals with schizophrenia (Akerele & Levin, 2007).

Cocaine use disorder may produce paranoia, and auditory and tactile hallucinations. Acute use can cause increased energy, mental alertness, tremors, reduced appetite, irritability, anxiety, panic, paranoia, violent behavior, psychosis, and feelings of exhilaration. Binge-patterned cocaine use may lead to irritability, restlessness, and anxiety.

Chronic use may cause many psychosocial problems such as changes in work-related habits and attitudes; lying, cheating, and stealing can become more rampant.

Medical Complications

Abusing cocaine has a variety of adverse effects on the body. Acute use increases heart rate, blood pressure, body temperature, metabolic energy, mental alertness, and causes tremors and reduced appetite.

Cocaine constricts blood vessels and dilates pupils. It can also cause headaches and gastrointestinal complications such as abdominal pain and nausea. Since cocaine tends to decrease appetite, chronic users can become malnourished as well. It can lead to weight loss, insomnia, cardiac or cardiovascular complications, stroke, seizures, addiction, and nasal septum perforation from snorting. Routes of administration of cocaine can produce different adverse effects. Regularly snorting cocaine, for example, can lead to loss of the sense of smell, nosebleeds, problems with swallowing, hoarseness, and an overall irritation of the nasal septum, which could result in a chronically inflamed, runny nose. Ingested cocaine can cause severe bowel gangrene due to reduced blood flow. This can result in death of cocaine traffickers called Mules. Mules ingest bags of cocaine to transport them across borders. The bags sometimes burst. The resulting intestinal gangrene may result in death. Persons who inject cocaine have puncture marks called "tracks," most commonly in their forearms, and may experience allergic reactions either to the drug or to some additive in street cocaine, which in severe cases can result in death.

Furthermore, drug intoxication and addiction can compromise judgment and decision making, and potentially lead to risky sexual encounters, needle sharing, and trading sex for drugs. Injecting cocaine can bring about severe allergic reactions and increased risk for contracting HIV/AIDS, the hepatitis C virus (HCV), and other blood-borne diseases. HCV has spread rapidly among injecting drug users (Hagan et al., 2007). Risk begins with the first injection, and within 2 years, nearly 40% of injecting drug users (IDUs) are exposed to HCV. By the time IDUs have been injecting for 5 years, their chances of being infected with HCV are between 50 and 80% (Academy for Educational Development, 2002). Cocaine-related deaths are often a result of cardiac arrest or seizure, followed by respiratory arrest.

Data (e.g., Lamy & Thibaut, 2010) indicate that babies born to mothers who abuse cocaine during pregnancy are more likely to be premature, have low birthweights, smaller head circumferences, and to be shorter than babies born to mothers who do not abuse cocaine. Multiple factors influence the effect of mothers' drug abuse on their babies. These factors include but are not limited to the amount and number of drugs abused, including nicotine; extent of prenatal care; possible neglect or abuse of the child; exposure to violence in the environment; socioeconomic conditions;

maternal nutrition; other health conditions; and exposure to sexually transmitted diseases. Exposure to cocaine during fetal development may also lead to later subtle, yet significant, deficits in some children, including deficits in some aspects of cognitive performance, information processing, and attention to tasks and abilities that are important for the realization of a children's full potential.

TREATMENT

Medical Treatments

Cocaine Intoxication/Overdose

Cocaine overdose is treated as a medical emergency due to the risk of cardiac toxicity. Physical cooling (ice, cold blankets, etc.) and acetaminophen may be used to treat hyperthermia, while specific treatments are then developed for any further complications. Sedation with agents such as diazepam (Valium) is recommended for the agitation, irritability, seizures, and hyperexcitable state. This also helps control the rapid heart rate and elevated blood pressure. If the body temperature is elevated, this is brought down with cold water, fans, cooling blankets, and acetaminophen. Specific therapies are geared to the specific complaint or system involved. For example, if the cocaine overdose has led to a true heart attack, clot-dissolving medications called "thrombolytic drugs" may be used. Further testing with cardiac catheterization may be done. If this test shows a blocked vessel, a balloon angioplasty may also be done. Treatment depends on the presenting complaint and organ system involved. There is no officially approved, specific antidote for cocaine overdose, and although some drugs (e.g., dexmedetomidine and rimcazole) have been found to be useful for treating cocaine overdose in animal studies, no formal human trials have been carried out. In addition, a history of high blood pressure or cardiac problems puts the patient at high risk of cardiac arrest or stroke, and requires immediate medical treatment.

Withdrawal from cocaine may not be as unstable as withdrawal from alcohol. However, withdrawal from any chronic substance abuse is very serious. There is a risk of suicide or overdose. Symptoms usually disappear over time. Individuals may benefit from anxiolytics, antidepressants, and so forth. Almost half of all people who are addicted to cocaine also have a mental disorder (Falck, Wang, Siegal, & Carlson, 2004). These conditions should be suspected and treated. When cocaine use disorder is diagnosed and treated, relapse rates are dramatically reduced.

Chronic Cocaine Use Disorder

Like any drug addiction, this is a complex disease that involves biological changes in the brain, as well as many social, familial, and other environmental problems. Therefore, treatment of cocaine addiction must be comprehensive, and strategies need to assess the neurobiological, social, and medical aspects of the patient's drug abuse. Moreover, patients who have a variety of addictions often have other, co-occurring mental disorders that require additional behavioral or pharmacological interventions.

Currently, there are no U.S. Food and Drug Administration (FDA)-approved medications for treating cocaine use disorder. Behavioral interventions—particularly, cognitive-behavioral therapy—have been shown to effectively decrease cocaine use and prevent relapse.

A significant number of medications have been evaluated for the treatment of cocaine use disorder. Randomized controlled trials (RCTs) focusing on the use of antidepressants (ADs), carbamazepine (CBZ), dopamine agonists (DAs), and other drugs used in the treatment of cocaine dependence showed mixed results (de Lima, de Oliveira, Soares, Reisser, & Farrell, 2002). Most studied drugs were ADs (20 studies), Das, and CBZ. Data were very heterogeneous, with dropout rates within the studies between 0 and 84%. A nonsignificant trend favoring CBZ was found in terms of dropouts, and results from one trial suggest that patients taking fluoxetine are less likely to drop out. The main efficacy outcome reported in the studies was the presence of cocaine metabolites in the urine. No significant results were found, regardless the type of drug or dose used for all relevant outcomes assessed. Currently, the data do not support the clinical use of CBZ, ADs, DAs, disulfiram, mazindol, phenytoin, nimodipine, lithium and NeuRecover-SA in the treatment of cocaine dependence.

Several medications marketed for other diseases (e.g., vigabatrin, modafinil, tiagabine, disulfiram, and topiramate) show promise and have been reported to reduce cocaine use in controlled clinical trials. Among these, disulfiram (used to treat alcoholism) has produced the most consistent reductions in cocaine abuse. On the other hand, new knowledge of how the brain is changed by cocaine is directing attention to novel targets for medications development. Compounds that are currently being tested for addiction treatment take advantage of underlying cocaine-induced adaptations in the brain that disturb the balance between excitatory (glutamate) and inhibitory (gamma-aminobutyric acid) neurotransmission (Schmidt & Pierce, 2010). Also, dopamine D_3 receptors (a subtype of dopamine receptor) constitute a novel molecular target of high interest. Medications that act at these receptors are now being tested for safety in humans. Finally, a cocaine vaccine that prevents entry of cocaine into the brain holds great promise for reducing the risk of relapse.

In addition to treatments for addiction, medical treatments are being developed to address the acute emergencies that result from cocaine overdose each year. Modafinil, a medication used to treat narcolepsy and related disorders, dramatically improves sleep among recently abstinent cocaine abusers. Cocaine abusers treated with modafinil for 16 days demonstrated improvements in several characteristics of sleep, including total sleep time (Morgan, Pace-Schott, Pittman, Stickgold, & Malison, 2010). Better sleep may boost patients' attention, memory, and mood—helping them benefit from behavioral therapy for addiction. The new results, the first to show modafinil's sleep-enhancing effects in abstinent drug abusers, extend the team's previous finding that during early abstinence, cocaine abusers demonstrate disrupted sleep without being aware of it. If the beneficial effects of modafinil are verified, clinicians may incorporate the medication into addiction treatment.

In deep brain stimulation, a stream of electrical pulses delivered to the brain's reward center curbs the power of a cocaine injection to spur rats to drug seeking (Vassoler et al., 2013). Findings suggest that deep brain stimulation of the nucleus accumbens shell holds promise as a therapy for severe cocaine addiction. Deep brain stimulation of a different brain region has benefited patients with Parkinson's disease, and the technique is also being tested as a potential therapy for severe depression that does not improve with medication. The disadvantage of this modality is that it involves an invasive technique.

The cocaine vaccine consists of a small amount of the drug chemically bonded to a protein, derived from cholera toxin, that stimulates the immune system to produce antibodies. Anti-cocaine antibodies latch onto cocaine molecules in the bloodstream, forming drug–antibody complexes that are too large to pass through the fine-grained tissue filter that enwraps and protects the brain (Orson, Kinsey, Singh, Wu, & Kosten, 2009). If the vaccinated person develops enough antibodies to capture and hold onto most of the cocaine molecules circulating in the blood, the drug will not produce the euphoria or other psychoactive effects that reinforce drug taking and addiction. For the first placebo-controlled test of the vaccine's ability to reduce cocaine use among people who are addicted to the drug, the researchers recruited 115 men and women who were seeking treatment at an outpatient clinic after having abused cocaine for about 15 years. The study participants were taking cocaine, on average, three times daily, 3 days per week. All of these individuals were also dependent on opioids and had initiated methadone maintenance therapy 2 weeks prior to their first dose of the cocaine vaccine or placebo. This population was chosen because the patients came to the clinic daily to receive their doses of methadone, thereby increasing the likelihood that they would be available for injections, as well as urine and blood tests, and would remain in the study for its full 24-week duration. Although their individual responses varied, vaccine recipients reduced their cocaine use more quickly than placebo recipients. A subgroup of vaccinated patients generated levels of antibodies that were sufficient to block cocaine's effects, and during the period of peak antibody production, they submitted more drug-free urine samples than participants in the placebo group or those who did not respond strongly to the vaccine (Martell et al., 2009). With further refinement to increase response, a vaccine might someday be available as a therapy for cocaine abuse.

Behavioral and Psychosocial Treatments

Behavioral treatments help patients engage in the treatment process, modify their attitudes and behaviors related to drug abuse, and increase healthy life skills. These treatments can also enhance the effectiveness of medications and help people stay in treatment longer. Treatment for drug abuse and addiction can be delivered in many different settings, using a variety of behavioral approaches. Many behavioral treatments for cocaine addiction have proven to be effective in both residential and outpatient settings. Behavioral therapies are often the only available and effective treatments for many drug problems, including stimulant addictions. However, the integration of behavioral and pharmacological treatments may ultimately prove to be the most effective approach.

There are a variety of psychotherapy programs available for outpatients. Most of the programs involve individual or group drug counseling. Some programs also offer other forms of behavioral treatment such as the following:

- Cognitive-behavioral therapy (CBT): Helps patients recognize, avoid, and cope with the situations in which they are most likely to abuse drugs.
- Motivational interviewing: A useful tool to assess the readiness of individuals to change their behavior and enter treatment.
- Contingency management/motivational incentives: Useful for positive reinforcement to encourage abstinence from drugs.
- Multidimensional family therapy: Developed for adolescents with drug abuse problems, as well as their families, addressing a range of influences on their drug abuse patterns and designed to improve overall family functioning.

CBT is an effective approach for preventing relapse. It focuses on helping cocaine-addicted individuals abstain and remain abstinent from cocaine and other substances. The underlying assumption is that learning processes play an important role in the development and continuation of cocaine abuse and addiction. These same learning processes can be harnessed to help individuals reduce drug use and successfully prevent relapse. This approach attempts to help patients recognize, avoid, and cope; that is, they recognize the situations in which they are most likely to use cocaine, avoid these situations when appropriate, and cope more effectively with a range of problems and behaviors associated with drug abuse. This therapy is also noteworthy because of its compatibility with a range of other treatments that patients may receive.

Contingency management/motivational incentives have shown positive results in cocaine-addicted populations. Motivational incentives may be particularly useful for helping patients achieve initial abstinence from cocaine and stay in treatment (Volkow, 2010). Programs use a voucher or prize-based system that rewards patients who abstain from cocaine and other drug use. On the basis of drug-free urine tests, the patients earn points, or chips, which can be exchanged for items that encourage healthy living, such as a gym membership, movie tickets, or dinner at a local restaurant. Furthermore, patients who abuse substances are better able to maintain desirable behaviors when they are rewarded daily or weekly, rather than when they are asked to focus solely on the ultimate goal of long-term recovery. In addition to abstinence, motivational incentives promote and reinforce multiple healthy behaviors, such as adherence to medication regimens, maintenance of regular exercise habit, job hunting, and other activities that support a drug-free lifestyle. Investigators are currently examining how to tailor incentive programs for adolescents and pregnant women (Alessi, Hanson, Wieners, & Petry, 2007).

The term "therapeutic community" describes a variety of short- and long-term residential, day treatment, and ambulatory programs. Residential treatment is particularly effective in antisocial individuals. The underlining principle in therapeutic communities is that drug abuse is a deviant behavior. This results from chronic deficits in social, educational, and economic skills. The individual either never learned these skills or somewhere along the line lost previously acquired skills. Thus, the goal of the therapeutic community is an overall reconstruction of personality and lifestyle, elimination of antisocial activity, and development of employability, including social and educational adaptation to civil society. Therapeutic communities are highly structured programs in which patients remain at a residence, typically for

6–24 months. Therapeutic communities differ from other treatment approaches principally in their use of the community treatment staff as a key agent of change to influence patient attitudes, perceptions, and behaviors associated with drug use. Patients in therapeutic communities may include those with relatively long histories of drug addiction, involvement in serious criminal activities, and seriously impaired social functioning. Therapeutic communties are now also being designed to accommodate the needs of women who are pregnant or have children. The focus of the therapeutic community is on the resocialization of the patient to a drug-free, crime-free lifestyle.

Community-based self-help recovery groups such as the 12-step program Cocaine Anonymous may also be helpful to people trying to sustain abstinence. Participants may benefit from supportive fellowship and from sharing with others who experience common problems and issues.

It is important that patients receive services that match all of their treatment needs. For example, if a patient is unemployed, it may be helpful to provide vocational rehabilitation or career counseling along with addiction treatment. If a patient has marital problems, it may be important to offer couple counseling.

CONCLUSION AND FUTURE DIRECTIONS

Cocaine use disorder is a significant public health issue. It costs the United States more than $600 billion annually in increased health care costs, crime, and lost productivity, not to mention the incalculable effects on individuals, families, and whole communities (NIDA, 2011). In spite of significant efforts by federal authorities, cocaine production has decreased only slightly. However, it is encouraging that the use of cocaine among the young is declining. Cocaine still accounts for 25% of emergency department presentations for drug-related visits. Pharmacological treatment remains elusive despite multiple promising agents. The primary modality of treatment is currently psychosocial. One modality for developing treatment is to target patients prior to the development of a cocaine use disorder. The primary goal of research should be identifying markers for individuals in the preuse disorder stage and developing modalities to prevent the progression to cocaine use disorder.

REFERENCES

Academy for Educational Development. (2002). Hepatitis C virus and HIV coinfection. Retrieved May 21, 2012, from *www.cdc.gov/idu/hepatitis/ hepc_and_hiv_co.pdf.*

Akerele, E. O., & Levin, F. R. (2007). Schizophrenia and cocaine and/or cannabis dependence: Double-blind treatment study comparing olanzapine to risperidone. *Am J Addict, 16,* 260–268.

Alessi, S. M., Hanson, T., Wieners, M., & Petry, N. M. (2007). Low-cost contingency management in community clinics: Delivering incentives partially in group therapy. *Exp Clin Psychopharmacol, 15*(3), 293–300.

Alibhai, I. N., Green, T. A., Potashkin, J. A., & Nestler, E. J. (2007). Regulation of fosB and ΔfosB mRNA expression: In vivo and in vitro studies. *Brain Res, 1143,* 22–33.

American Psychiatric Association. (2013). *Diagnostic and statistical manual of mental disorders* (5th ed.). Arlington, VA: Author.

Bilbao, A., Parkitna, J. R., Engblom, D., Perreau-Lenz, S., Sanchis-Segura, C., Schneider, M., et al. (2008). Loss of the Ca2+/calmodulin-dependent protein kinase type IV in dopaminoceptive neurons enhances behavioral effects of cocaine. *Proc Natl Acad Sci USA, 105*(45), 17549–17554.

Bradberry, C. W., Nobiletti, J. B., Elsworth, J. D., Murphy, B., Jatlow, P., & Roth, R. H. (1993). Cocaine and cocaethylene: Microdialysis comparison of brain drug levels and effects on dopamine and serotonin. *J Neurochem, 60*(4), 1429–1435.

Canadian Institutes of Health Researches, Institute of Neurosciences, Mental Health and Addiction (INMHA). (n.d.). The brain from top to bottom: How drugs affect neurotransmitters. Retrieved May 8, 2012, from *http://thebrain.mcgill.ca/flash/i/i_03/i_03_m/i_03_m_par/i_03_m_par_cocaine.html*.

CESAR Fax. (2012, March 12). Percentage of D.C. arrestees testing positive for cocaine reaches lowest level in more than 20 years; documents end of cocaine epidemic. *21*(10). Retrieved from *http://www.cesar.umd.edu/cesar/cesarfax/vol21/21–10.pdf*.

Cooper, J. R., Bloom, F. E., & Roth, R. H. (2003). *The biochemical basis of neuropharmacology* (8th ed.). New York: Oxford University Press.

de Lima, M. S., de Oliveira Soares, B. G., Reisser, A. A., & Farrell, M. (2002). Pharmacological treatment of cocaine dependence: A systematic review. *Addiction, 97*(8), 931–949.

Eisch, A. J., Cameron, H. A., Encinas, J. M., Meltzer, L. A., Ming, G. L., & Overstreet-Wadiche, L. S. (2008). Adult neurogenesis, mental health, and mental illness: Hope or hype? *J Neurosci, 28*(46), 11785–11791.

Falck, R. S., Wang, J., Siegal, H. A., & Carlson, R. G. (2004). The prevalence of psychiatric disorder among a community sample of crack cocaine users: An exploratory study with practical implications. *J Nerv Ment Dis, 192*(7), 503–507.

Flower, R. (2004). Lifestyle drugs: Pharmacology and the social agenda. *Trends Pharmacol Sci, 25*, 182–185.

Gould, T. J. (2010). Addiction and cognition. *Addict Sci Clin Pract, 5*(2), 4–14.

Hagan, H., Des Jarlais, D. C., Stern, R., Lelutiu-Weinberger, C., Scheinmann, R., Strauss, S., et al. (2007). HCV synthesis project: Preliminary analyses of HCV prevalence in relation to age and duration of injection. *Int J Drug Policy, 18*, 341–351.

Harris, D. S., Everhart, E. T., Mendelson, J., & Jones, R. T. (2003). The pharmacology of cocaethylene in humans following cocaine and ethanol administration. *Drug Alcohol Depend, 72*(2), 169–182.

Hedges, V. L., Chakravarty, S., Nestler, E: J., & Meisel, R. L. (2009). Delta FosB overexpression in the nucleus accumbens enhances sexual reward in female Syrian hamsters. *Genes Brain Behav, 8*(4), 442–449.

Hoffman, R. S. (2010). Treatment of patients with cocaine-induced arrhythmias: Bringing the bench to the bedside. *Br J Clin Pharmacol, 69*, 448–457.

Jatlow, P., McCance, E. F., Bradberry, C. W., Elsworth, J. D., Taylor, J. R., & Roth, R. H. (1996). Alcohol plus cocaine: The whole is more than the sum of its parts. *Ther Drug Monit, 18*(4), 460–464.

Johnston, L. D., O'Malley, P. M., Bachman, J. G., & Schulenberg, J. E. (2010). *Monitoring the Future national results on adolescent drug use: Overview of key findings, 2009* (DHHS Publication No. 10-7583). Bethesda, MD: NIDA.

Koob, G. F., & Volkow, N. D. (2010). Neurocircuitry of addiction. *Neuropsychopharmacol, 35*(1), 217–238.

Laizure, S. C., Mandrell, T., Gades, N. M., & Parker, R. B. (2003). Cocaethylene metabolism and interaction with cocaine and ethanol: Role of carboxylesterases. *Drug Metab Dispos, 31*(1), 16–20.

Lamy, S., & Thibaut, F. (2010). Psychoactive substance use during pregnancy: A review. *L'Encephale, 36*(1), 33–38.

Mandyam, C. D., Wee, S., Crawford, E. F., Eisch, A. J., Richardson, H. N., & Koob, G. F. (2008).

Varied access to intravenous methamphetamine self-administration differentially alters adult hippocampal neurogenesis. *Biol Psychiatry, 64*(11), 958–965.

Markel, H. (2011). Über coca: Sigmund Freud, Carl Koller, and cocaine. *JAMA, 305*(13), 1360–1361.

Martell, B. A., Orson, F. M., Poling, J., Mitchell, E., Rossen, R. D., Gardner, T., et al. (2009). Cocaine vaccine for the treatment of cocaine dependence in methadone-maintained patients: A randomized double-blind placebo-controlled efficacy trial. *Arch General Psychiatry, 66*(10), 1116–1123.

Mash, D. C., ffrench-Mullen, J., Adi, N., Qin, Y., Buck, A., & Pablo, J. (2007). The gene expression in human hippocampus from cocaine abusers identifies genes which regulate extracellular matrix remodeling. *PLoS ONE, 2*(11), e1187.

Morgan, P. T., Pace-Schott, E., Pittman, B., Stickgold, R., & Malison, R. T. (2010). Normalizing effects of modafinil on sleep in chronic cocaine users. *Am J Psychiatry, 167*(3), 331–340.

Moyer, R. A., Wang, D., Papp, A. C., Smith, R. M., Duque, L., Mash, D. C., et al. (2011). Intronic polymorphisms affecting alternative splicing of human dopamine D2 receptor are associated with cocaine abuse. *Neuropsychopharmacol, 36*, 753–762.

National Institute on Drug Abuse (NIDA). (2010a). Cocaine: Drug facts, revised. Retrieved from *www.drugabuse.gov/publications/drugfacts/cocaine.*

National Institute on Drug Abuse (NIDA), Medications Development. (2011, November). The burden of drug abuse and addiction. Retrieved May 10, 2012, from *http://m.drugabuse.gov/sites/default/files/medicationsdev.pdf.*

National Institute on Drug Abuse (NIDA), Research Report Series (2010b). Cocaine abuse and addiction. Retrieved March 5, 2012, from *www.drugabuse.gov/sites/default/files/rrcocaine.pdf.*

Noonan, M. A., Bulin, S. E., Fuller, D. C., & Eisch, A. J. (2010) Reduction of adult hippocampal neurogenesis confers vulnerability in an animal model of cocaine addiction. *J Neurosci, 30*(1), 304–315.

Noonan, M. A., Choi, K. H., Self, D. W., & Eisch, A. J. (2008). Withdrawal from cocaine self-administration normalizes deficits in proliferation and enhances maturity of adult-generated hippocampal neurons. *J Neurosci, 28*(10), 2516–2526.

O'Leary, M. E., & Hancox, J. C. (2010). Role of voltage-gated sodium, potassium and calcium channels in the development of cocaine-associated cardiac arrhythmias. *Br J Clin Pharmacol, 69*, 427–442.

Orson, F. M., Kinsey, B. M., Singh, R. A. K., Wu, Y., & Kosten, T. R. (2009). Vaccines for cocaine abuse. *Hum Vaccin, 5*(4), 194–199.

Pascual-Leone, A., Amedi, A., Fregni, F., & Merabet, L. B. (2005). The plastic human brain cortex. *Annl Rev Neurosci, 28*, 377–401.

Rang, H. P., Dale, M. M., Ritter, J. M., & Flower, R. J. (2007). *Rang and Dale's pharmacology* (6th ed.). London: Elsevier Churchill Livingstone.

Renthal, W., Carle, T. L., Maze, I., Covington, H. E., III, Truong, H. T., Alibhai, I., et al. (2008). Delta FosB mediates epigenetic desensitization of the c-fos gene after chronic amphetamine exposure. *J Neurosci, 28*(29), 7344–7349.

Renthal, W., Kumar, A., Xiao, G., Wilkinson, M., Covington, H. E., III, Maze, I., et al. (2009). Genome-wide analysis of chromatin regulation by cocaine reveals a novel role for sirtuins. *Neuron, 62*(3), 335–348.

Ritter, J. M. (2010). Dysrhythmias associated with cocaine overdose. *Br J Clin Pharmacol, 69*(5), 423–424.

Saxon, A. J., Oreskovich, M. R., & Brkanac, Z. (2005). Genetic determinants of addiction to opioids and cocaine. *Harvard Rev Psychiatry, 13*(4), 218–232.

Schmidt, H. D., & Pierce, R. C. (2010). Cocaine-induced neuroadaptations in glutamatetransmission: Potential therapeutic targets for craving and addiction. *Ann NY Acad Sci, 1187*, 35–75.

Small, A. C., Kampman, K. M., Plebani, J., De Jesus Quinn, M., Peoples, L., & Lynch, K. G. (2009). Tolerance and sensitization to the effects of cocaine use in humans: A retrospective study of long-term cocaine users in Philadelphia. *Subst Use Misuse, 44*(13), 1888–1898.

Substance Abuse and Mental Health Services Administration (SAMHSA). (2014). *Results from the 2013 National Survey on Drug Use and Health: Summary of national findings* (NSDUH Series H-48, HHS Publication No. [SMA] 14-4863). Rockville, MD: Author.

Substance Abuse and Mental Health Services Administration (SAMHSA) Office of Applied Studies, Drug and Alcohol Services Information System. (2007, September 13). The DASIS Report: Cocaine Route of Administration Trends: 1995–2005. Retrieved March 3, 2012, from *www.samhsa.gov/data/2k7/cracktx/cracktx.htm*.

United Nations Office on Drugs and Crime (UNODC). (2009). World Drug Report 2009. Retrieved March 7, 2012, from *www.unodc.org/documents/wdr/wdr_2009/wdr2009_eng_web.pdf*.

Vassoler, F. M., Schmidt, H. D., Gerard, M. E., Famous, K. R., Ciraulo, D. A., Kornetsky, C., et al. (2013). Deep brain stimulation of the nucleus accumbens shell attenuates cocaine priming-induced reinstatement of drug seeking in rats. *J Neurosci, 33*(36), 14446–14454.

Volkow, N. (2010, December). NIDA note. Retrieved May 8, 2012, from *https://www.drugabuse.gov/news-events/nida-notes/2010/12/incentives-promote-abstinence*.

Volkow, N. D., Fowler, J. S., Wang, G. J., Baler, R., & Telang, F. (2009). Imaging dopamine's role in drug abuse and addiction. *Neuropharmacol, 56*(Suppl. 1), 3–8.

Vorel, S. R., Ashby, C. R., Jr., Paul, M., Liu, X., Hayes, R., Hagan, J. J., et al. (2002). Dopamine D_3 receptor antagonism inhibits cocaine-seeking and cocaine-enhanced brain reward in rats. *J Neurosci, 22*(21), 9595–9603.

Wallace, D. L., Vialou, V., Rios, L., Carle-Florence, T. L., Chakravarty, S., Kumar, A., et al. (2008). The influence of DeltaFosB in the nucleus accumbens on natural reward-related behavior. *J Neurosci, 28*(41), 10272–10277.

Wood, D. M., & Dargan, P. I. (2010). Putting cocaine use and cocaine-associated cardiac arrhythmias into epidemiological and clinical perspective. *Br J Clin Pharmacol, 69*, 443–447.

CHAPTER 13

Sedatives/Hypnotics and Benzodiazepines

ROBERT L. DuPONT
WILLIAM M. GREENE
CAROLINE M. DuPONT

The sedatives and the hypnotics, especially the benzodiazepines, are widely used in medical practice in the treatment of anxiety, insomnia, and epilepsy, as well as for several other indications (Baldessarini, 2001). The combination of abuse by alcoholics and drug addicts and the withdrawal symptoms on discontinuation leads to the view that these are "addictive" drugs (DuPont, 2000; Juergens & Cowley, 2003). The pharmacology and the epidemiology of sedatives and hypnotics are reviewed in this chapter, in which we focus on the needs of the clinician.

A *sedative* lowers excitement and calms the awake patient, whereas a *hypnotic* produces drowsiness and promotes sleep. The nonbenzodiazepine sedatives generally depress central nervous system activity in a continuum, depending on the dose, beginning with calming and extending progressively to sleep, unconsciousness, coma, surgical anesthesia, and ultimately to fatal respiratory and cardiovascular depression. Sedatives share this spectrum of effects with many other compounds including general anesthetic agents, a variety of aliphatic alcohols, and ethyl alcohol. At lower doses, sedatives can cause impaired cognitive and motor functioning (including slurred speech and staggering). Sedation is a side effect of many other medicines, including antihistamines and neuroleptics.

The benzodiazepines were recognized in animal experiments in the 1950s for their ability to produce "taming" without apparent sedation. Chlordiazepoxide (Librium), the first benzodiazepine used in clinical practice, was introduced in 1961. Of the more than 3,000 additional benzodiazepines that have been synthesized, about 50 have been used clinically (Baldessarini, 2001). Several of the benzodiazepines, including alprazolam (Xanax), diazepam (Valium), lorazepam (Ativan), and clonazepam (Klonopin) are among not only the most widely prescribed medicines for anxiety but also the most frequently prescribed medicines worldwide. Xanax topped the list at over 46 million prescriptions for the drug in 2010 (see Table 13.1). All of the benzodiazepines are now off-patent, so none are promoted by pharmaceutical companies. Generic versions of these medicines are widely used and relatively inexpensive. After the intense controversies in medicine and in the media surrounding first the introduction of Valium in the 1960s and Xanax in the 1980s, there is far less media attention on the benzodiazepines today despite their continued widespread use in medical practice. For this reason, some of the references to the most controversial areas are from the period when the uses of these medicines were vigorously debated.

The benzodiazepines resemble the other sedatives except that they do not produce surgical anesthesia, coma, or death even at high doses except when co-administered with other agents that suppress respiration. The benzodiazepines can be antagonized by specific agents that do not block the effects of other sedatives. The benzodiazepine antagonists do not produce significant effects in the absence of the benzodiazepines. These properties distinguish the benzodiazepines from the other sedatives and produce a margin of safety that has led to the widespread use of benzodiazepines (Charney, Minic, & Harris, 2001).

EPIDEMIOLOGY

The National Comorbidity Survey Replication (NCS-R; 2007a, 2007b) found that 19.1% of the population had an anxiety disorder in the past 12 months and 31.2% had a lifetime history of an anxiety disorder. These studies established that anxiety disorders are the most prevalent class of mental disorders over a 12-month period of time. Using the standard human capital approach to estimate the social costs of illnesses in 1994, the anxiety disorders produced an estimated total social cost of $65 billion (DuPont, DuPont, & Rice, 2002). Of this total only $15 billion was the cost of all treatments, while $50 billion was due to lost productivity as a result of the often seriously disabling nature of the anxiety disorders. For comparison, in 2002 the economic cost of schizophrenia was an estimated $62.7 billion (Wu et al., 2005).

TABLE 13.1. Estimated Total Prescriptions (in Thousands) Dispensed for Selected Benzodiazepines, 2004 to 2010, and Change from 2004 to 2010

Generic name	Brand name	2004	2005	2006	2007	2008	2009	2010	Delta 2004–2010
alprazolam	Xanax	32,779	34,230	37,327	40,914	43,586	44,467	46,201	+40.9%
lorazepam	Ativan	18,436	19,002	19,789	21,022	22,043	22,436	23,429	+27.1%
clonazepam	Klonopin	15,564	16,763	18,152	20,078	21,846	23,090	23,085	+48.3%
diazepam	Valium	11,822	12,093	12,764	13,460	13,870	13,957	14,584	+23.4%
temazepam	Restoril	7,150	7,570	7,396	7,878	7,911	9,001	10,517	+47.1%
triazolam	Halcion	1,223	...	...	...	...	...	...	...

Note. . . . , No data available. Data from Top 200 Drugs, Resource Guide; available at *http://drugtopics.modernmedicine.com.*

The benzodiazepines were introduced in the 1960s as being comparatively problem free compared to the barbiturates, which they rapidly replaced. Their popularity reached unprecedented levels in the early 1970s. However, a powerful backlash, labeled the "social issues," that emerged did cause a drop in the use of the benzodiazepines during the 1980s even though there was a rise in the prevalence of the disorders for which they are used (DuPont, 1986, 1988).

As the benzodiazepines became more controversial, and as various regulatory approaches were employed to limit their use in medical practice, there was a danger that clinicians would revert to the older and generally more toxic sedatives and hypnotics, which, in the era of the benzodiazepines, had become unfamiliar (Juergens & Cowley, 2003). Thus, there is more than historical interest in looking at these earlier sedatives, because for some younger medical practitioners, they are new medicines. The use of sedatives and hypnotics for the treatment of anxiety and insomnia in patients with addiction to alcohol and other drugs entails additional risks, especially when the benzodiazepines are used (Handelsman, 2002).

For more than three decades the federal government has tracked the rates of self-reported nonmedical use of a variety of drugs within the United States, primarily via two ongoing surveys. Monitoring the Future (MTF), a survey of high school students, currently tracks illicit use of "tranquilizers" (primarily benzodiazepines) and "sedatives" (primarily barbiturates) (Johnston, O'Malley, Bachman, & Schulenberg, 2012). The National Survey on Drug Use and Health (NSDUH), formerly known as the National Household Survey on Drug Abuse (NHSDA), is a survey of Americans age 12 and up that also tracks the use of tranquilizers and sedatives (Substance Abuse and Mental Health Services Administration [SAMHSA], 2011b). Neither survey identifies "benzodiazepines" specifically. Since 1975, MTF data revealed a general trend of steadily declining tranquilizer and sedative use until about 1992, at which point these agents experienced a slight resurgence until the early to mid-2000s, at which point they resumed a decline in use (Johnston et al., 2012). Perceived availability has continued a slow steady decline since 1975 (Johnston et al., 2012). In 2010, the NSDUH estimated the percentage of Americans, 12 years of age and older, who had used a tranquilizer nonmedically during the prior 30 days as 0.9%, up from 0.8% in 2009, and 0.7% in 2008 (SAMHSA, 2011b). Past-month nonmedical use of sedatives in this group has remained steady from 2007 through 2010 at 0.1%. In 2010, the estimated total number of Americans age 12 and up with nonmedical use of tranquilizers and sedatives was 2.16 million and 374,000, respectively (SAMHSA, 2011b). A series of national surveys tracking the medical use of the benzodiazepines indicated that their use peaked in 1976, and by the late 1980s it fell about 25% from that peak rate (DuPont, 1988). A survey of medical use of the benzodiazepines, administered in 1979 (near the peak of benzodiazepine use in the United States), indicated that 89% of Americans age 18 years and older had not used a benzodiazepine within the previous 12 months. Of those who had used a benzodiazepine, most (9.5% of all adults) had used the benzodiazepine either less than every day or for less than 12 months, or both, whereas a minority (1.6% of the adult population) had used a benzodiazepine on a daily basis for 12 months or longer. This long-term user group was two-thirds female; 71% were ages 50 or older, and most had chronic medical problems as well as anxiety (DuPont, 1988).

Of the individuals with anxiety disorders in a large community sample, three-fourths were receiving no treatment at all, including not using a benzodiazepine (DuPont, 1988). The 1.6% of the population who were chronic benzodiazepine users can be compared to the then-estimated 19.1% of the population (NCS-R, 2007a) suffering from anxiety disorders at any 12-month period. This statistic led many observers to conclude that not only are benzodiazepines not overprescribed but they also may actually be underprescribed because of the reluctance of both physician and patients to use these medicines (Mellinger & Balter, 1981).

Recent national estimates of drug-related emergency department (ED) visits highlighted by the Drug Abuse Warning Network (DAWN) are concerning both for the high prevalence of adverse reactions related to benzodiazepine use and the steep upward trend. From 2004 to 2009, estimated ED visits involving nonmedical use of benzodiazepines increased from 143,546 to 312,931; estimated ED visits involving adverse reactions to benzodiazepines increased from 14,214 to 63,494; and estimated ED visits involving detox services for benzodiazepines increased from 14,717 to 48,769 (SAMHSA, 2011a). Alprazolam (Xanax) tops the list in all these categories. In 2009, of all ED visits involving nonmedical use of pharmaceuticals (1,079,683), 33.6% of these involved anxiolytics, sedatives, or hypnotics (SAMHSA, 2011a).

DISTINGUISHING MEDICAL AND NONMEDICAL USES OF BENZODIAZEPINES

Nonmedical benzodiazepine use is different from, and far less common than, medical use of the benzodiazepines. Nonmedical use of benzodiazepines is a small, but significant, part of the overall nonmedical drug problem in the nation. Nonmedical use of benzodiazepines is almost always part of a pattern of abuse of alcohol and other drugs. The benzodiazepines are seldom used nonmedically as the only substance of abuse. To understand the place of the benzodiazepines in contemporary medical practice, it is important to separate appropriate medical use from inappropriate nonmedical use. Five characteristics distinguish medical from nonmedical use of all controlled substances, including the benzodiazepines.

1. *Intent.* Is the substance used to treat a diagnosed medical problem, such as anxiety or insomnia, or is it used to get high (or to treat the complications of the nonmedical use of other drugs)? Typical medical use of a benzodiazepine or other controlled substance occurs without the use of multiple nonmedical drugs, whereas nonmedical use of benzodiazepines is usually polydrug abuse. Although alcoholics and drug addicts sometimes use the language of medicine to describe their reasons for using controlled substances nonmedically, "self-administration" or "self-medication" of an intoxicating substance outside the ordinary practice boundaries of medical care is a hallmark of drug abuse (DuPont, 1998).

2. *Effect.* What is the effect of the controlled substance use on the user's life? The only acceptable standard for medical use is that it helps the user live a better life. Typical nonmedical drug use is associated with deterioration in the user's life, even

though continued use and denial of the negative consequences of this use are nearly universal.

3. *Control.* Is the substance use controlled only by the user, or does a fully knowledgeable physician share the control of the drug use? Medical drug use is controlled by the physician, as well as the patient, whereas typical nonmedical use is solely controlled by the user.

4. *Legality.* Is the use legal or illegal? Medical use of a controlled substance is legal. Nonmedical drug use of controlled substances, including benzodiazepines, is illegal.

5. *Pattern.* What is the pattern of the controlled substance use? Typical medical use of controlled substances is similar to the use of the penicillin or aspirin in that it occurs in a medically reasonable pattern to treat an easily recognized health problem other than addiction. Typical use of nonmedical drugs (e.g., alcohol, marijuana, or cocaine), in contrast, takes place at parties or in other social settings. Medical substance use is stable and at a moderate dose level. Nonmedical use of a controlled substance is usually polydrug abuse at high and/or unstable doses (Juergens & Cowley, 2003).

The use of benzodiazepines to treat anxiety generates physician concerns that are similar to the concerns about the use of opiates to treat pain, because, like the opiates, the benzodiazepines are widely abused by drug addicts and alcoholics. In addition, there is concern, again as exists for the opiates, that any medical use of the benzodiazepines is "addicting." For this reason many physicians are reluctant to use benzodiazepines and, if they do use them, they are reluctant to use them over long periods of time. These concerns are reinforced by the difficulties physicians have identifying substance use disorders (SUDs) in their patients. In other words, because of concern over the risks of abuse and addiction, this category of medicines is often avoided entirely, and when these medicines are used, they are used in subtherapeutic doses and for unnecessarily brief periods of time.

In this chapter care is taken to distinguish between medical and nonmedical use of benzodiazepines. A variety of strategies are described to identify and manage the nonmedical use of benzodiazepines. We call attention to the common presentations of anxious patients, with the goal of assisting the prescribing physician in rapid and reliable identification of nonmedical use, or abuse, of the benzodiazepines.

Many anxious patients have a history of medical benzodiazepine use. Anxious patients without addiction generally report relatively low-dose use of benzodiazepines, as described later in this chapter, no dose escalation over time, and good results in reducing their anxiety. These non-addicted anxious patients report no or very limited alcohol use and no use of illegal drugs. In contrast, substance abusers who seek benzodiazepines report that in their earlier use of a benzodiazepine, they experienced dose escalation to high doses and only limited, but nonetheless valued, antianxiety benefits from their benzodiazepine use. These patients often report heavy alcohol and illegal drug use; however, they may minimize this use.

Less commonly seen is the anxious patient who has never taken a benzodiazepine. Almost without exception, first-time patients who are not alcoholics or drug addicts report that they are very sensitive to medicines. They report that most medicines they have used for anxiety and other conditions produced undesirable side effects and were discontinued after one or two doses. They ask their physicians for the lowest dose of whatever medicine is prescribed, including the benzodiazepine. They worry about the potential addiction and sedating effects of benzodiazepines. If they accept a prescription (and many do not), they commonly do not take any of it, or they cut the already low prescribed dose in half because of their concern over these potential side effects. It is often difficult to get anxious patients to take any medicine, including a benzodiazepine, because their excessive worry, the hallmark of an anxiety disorder, is applied to any medicine they are given, including a benzodiazepine.

In striking contrast to this picture, drug addicts and alcoholics who seek an initial prescription for a benzodiazepine for anxiety immediately want high doses. Then they are likely to raise the dose beyond the physician-recommended dose. They seldom report excessive sensitivity to any medicine, but they do say that many medicines have been ineffective. While this contrast in presentations is far from universal, it is common and provides the prescribing physician with valuable information about the risks of abuse of the benzodiazepine. Patients show their risk potential in their own behavior in dealing with the physician.

Another word of advice to prescribing physicians: The identification of an SUD is an important therapeutic opportunity, one that should not be missed. Helping the patient with an SUD recognize the disease and successfully manage this lifelong and potentially fatal disease is both intensely challenging and greatly rewarding.

MEDICAL USE AND ABUSE

The benzodiazepines are among the most widely prescribed psychotropic medicines in the world. The World Health Organization (WHO; 1988) labeled them "essential drugs" that should be available in all countries for medical purposes, and several benzodiazepines have remained on the list ever since (WHO, 2011). Of the widely used psychotropic drugs, they are among the least likely to cause any adverse effects, including serious medical complications and death.

Workplace drug testing is often limited to identification of marijuana, cocaine, morphine/codeine, amphetamine/methamphetamine, phencyclidine (PCP), and more recently, Ecstasy. However, benzodiazepines and barbiturates are sometimes added to the test panel. Laboratory positive test results from patients with legitimate prescriptions for benzodiazepines and barbiturates are reported to employers by medical review officers (MROs) as negative, as are other laboratory results that reflect appropriate medical treatment with other controlled substances (MacDonald, DuPont, & Ferguson, 2003).

Several important health concerns about benzodiazepine use that are unrelated to addiction have been expressed, especially about the long-term use of benzodiazepines, including the effects on the brain, the possibility of cerebral atrophy associated with prolonged benzodiazepine use, and other problems, such as memory loss and personality change (Golombok, Moodley, & Lader, 1988; American Psychiatric Association Task Force on Benzodiazepine Dependence, Toxicity, and Abuse, 1990).

Though the clinical implications remain unclear, a recent meta-analysis examining cognitive performance in long-term users of benzodiazepines suggests impairment across broad domains of cognitive function (Barker, Greenwood, Jackson, & Crowe, 2004a). Benzodiazepine-related cognitive dysfunction is generally thought to resolve after drug discontinuation, but evidence exists for measurable impairment even 6 months after discontinuation (Barker, Greenwood, Jackson, & Crowe, 2004b). For the majority of patients, this likely has minimal clinical significance.

SUDs VERSUS PHYSICAL DEPENDENCE

SUDs are mental disorders defined in the fifth edition of the *Diagnostic and Statistical Manual of Mental Disorders* (DSM-V; American Psychiatric Association, 2013). Categorization of these disorders is based on the number of symptoms that lead to clinically significant impairment or distress: mild (two to three criteria), moderate (four to five criteria) and severe (six or more criteria). Sample criteria include out-of-control drug use, use outside social and medical sanctions, continued use despite clear evidence of drug-caused problems, and a drug-centered lifestyle. Physical, or physiological, dependence is defined by the presence of either tolerance or withdrawal, and is merely an expected state of neuroadaptation. Physical dependence may, but often does not, accompany SUDs. The appropriate treatment for moderate or severe SUDs is commonly specialized additional treatment followed by prolonged participation in one of the 12-step programs and/or other ongoing support and care. The appropriate treatment for physical dependence, in clear contrast, is gradual dose reduction to permit biological adaptation to lower doses of the substance, leading to zero dosing.

A patient who seeks to continue using a medicine because it is helpful is no more demonstrating "drug-seeking behavior" than is a patient who finds eyeglasses helpful in the treatment of myopia demonstrating "glasses-seeking behavior" if deprived of a corrective lens. SUDs are characterized by use despite problems caused by that use (loss of control) and by denial (and dishonesty)—neither of which is seen in appropriate medical treatment (DuPont & Gold, 1995).

Precisely the same confusion of medically trivial physical dependence with a serious SUD occurs in regard to the use of opiates in the treatment of severe pain. Many patients and many physicians undertreat severe pain because they are unable to distinguish physical dependence, the benign pharmacological fact of neuroadaptation in medical patients, from the abuse of opiates by drug addicts, a malignant biobehavioral disorder (Savage, 2003).

PHARMACOLOGY

In this section, the sedatives and hypnotics are divided for convenience into three groups: the barbiturates, "other sedatives and hypnotics," and the benzodiazepines. Later in the chapter, we discuss the newer agents, which are alternatives to the benzodiazepines.

Barbiturates

Barbital was introduced into medical practice in 1903, phenobarbital, in 1912. Their rapid success led to the development of over 2,000 derivatives of barbituric acid, with dozens being used in medical practice. The only sedatives to precede the barbiturates were the bromides and chloral hydrate, both of which were in widespread use before the end of the 19th century.

The most commonly used barbiturates today are secobarbital (Seconal), pentobarbital (Nembutal), amobarbital (Amytal), butabarbital (Butisol), butalbital (Fioricet/Fiorinal), mephobarbital (Mebaral), and phenobarbital (Luminal). Secobarbital and pentobarbital are short-term in their duration of action. Amobarbital, butabarbital, and butalbital have intermediate durations, while mephobarbital and phenobarbital have long-term durations of action. Ultrashort-acting barbiturates are used as anesthetics, but not in outpatient medicine.

Barbiturates reversibly suppress the activity of all excitable tissue; the central nervous system (CNS) is particularly sensitive to these effects. Except for the antiepileptic effects of phenobarbital, there is a low therapeutic index for the sedative effects of the barbiturates, with general CNS depression being linked to the desired therapeutic effects. The amount of barbiturates that can cause a fatal overdose is well within the usual size of a single month's prescription. A common problem with the medical use of barbiturates for both sedation and hypnosis is the rapid development of tolerance, with a common tendency of medical patients to raise the dose on chronic administration. The barbiturates affect the gamma-aminobutyric acid (GABA) system, producing both a cross-tolerance to other sedating drugs, including alcohol and the benzodiazepines, and a heightened risk of fatal overdose reactions (Charney et al., 2001).

Other Sedatives and Hypnotics

Over the course of the 20th century several medicines with diverse structures were used as sedatives and hypnotics. In general, the pharmacological properties of these medicines resembled the barbiturates. They produced profound CNS depression with little or no analgesia. Their therapeutic index was low and their abuse potential was high, similar to the barbiturates. Chloral hydrate (Notec), ethchlorvynol (Placidyl), ethinamate (Valmid), glutethimide (Doriden), meprobamate (Miltown, Equanil), methyprylon (Noludar), and paraldehyde (Paral) belong in this class of seldom-used medicines that does not include medicines that have a useful place in contemporary medical practice.

Despite the continued widespread use of antihistamines to treat insomnia, the U.S. Food and Drug Administration (FDA), noting the prominent sedative side effects encountered in the administration of antihistamines (including doxylamine, diphenhydramine, and pyrilamine), concluded that the antihistamines are not consistently effective in the treatment of sleep disorders. Tolerance rapidly develvops to the sedating effects of these medicines, and the antihistamines can produce paradoxical stimulation. In addition, the antihistamine doses currently approved for the treatment of allergies are inadequate to induce sleep. Antihistamines used to treat sleep disorders can produce daytime sedation because of their relatively long half-lives (Charney et al., 2001).

The use of sedating antidepressants such as trazodone (Desyrel) and amitripty-line (Elavil) to treat insomnia at dose levels lower than are effective for the treatment of depression, like the use of sedating antihistamines for this indication, can be clini-cally problematic, since these agents may be both less effective and more likely to pro-duce undesirable side effects (especially in producing daytime sedation) than benzodi-azepines in this indication (Mendelson et al., 2001). However, trazodone can play an important role in the successful management of detoxification from other sedative/hypnotics (e.g., alprazolam), because insomnia is a hallmark symptom of withdrawal, and because medicines without abuse potential are strongly preferred in this group. Evidence suggests that patients undergoing sedative detoxification may be more likely to remain sedative-free when given trazodone (Rickels et al., 1999). Recently, a new formulation of very low-dose doxepin (Silenor) has been approved for use as a hyp-notic. A novel agent recently approved for insomnia, ralmeteon (Rozerem), acts as an agonist at melatonin receptors, and lacks the abuse potential and motor/cogni-tive impairment seen with many other hypnotics on the market (Johnson, Suess, & Griffiths, 2006).

Benzodiazepines

The identification of the benzodiazepine receptors in 1977 began the modern era of benzodiazepine research, establishing this class as the best understood of the psychi-atric medicines. GABA receptors are membrane-bound proteins divided into three subtypes, $GABA_A$, $GABA_B$, and $GABA_C$ receptors. The $GABA_A$ receptors, where benzodiazepines bind, comprise five subunits that together form the chloride chan-nel that primarily mediates neuronal excitability (seizures), rapid mood changes, and clinical anxiety, as well as sleep. The effects of benzodiazepines are reversed by benzodiazepine antagonists, one of which—flumazenil—is used clinically to rapidly reverse the effects of benzodiazepine overdoses (Charney et al., 2001). The benzo-diazepine receptors, part of the GABA system, are found in approximately 30% of CNS synapses and in all species above the level of the shark, demonstrating their fundamental biological importance.

Like other classes of psychotropics, there are pharmacological differences among the individual benzodiazepines that have clinical significance, such that they cannot be used interchangeably. These pharmacological differences among the benzodiaz-epines include the rapidity of onset (distributional half-life), persistence of active drug and/or metabolite in the body (elimination half-life), major metabolic breakdown pathways (conjugation vs. oxidation), and specific molecular structure (e.g., alpra-zolam has a unique triazolo ring that may account for some differences in its clinical effects) (Charney et al., 2001). Table 13.2 summarizes these differences for the most widely used benzodiazepines. Clinically important pharmacological characteristics are summarized as they relate to the use and abuse of the benzodiazepines (Chouin-ard, Lefko-Singh, & Teboul, 1999). Benzodiazepines may produce some clinically relevant effects by mechanisms that do not involve GABA-mediated chloride con-ductance (Burt & Kamatchi, 1991). The benzodiazepines have only a slight effect on rapid eye movement (REM) sleep, but they do suppress deeper, Stage 4 sleep. Although this effect is probably of no clinical significance in most settings, diazepam has been used successfully to prevent "night terrors" that arise in Stage 4 sleep.

TABLE 13.2. Pharmacological Characteristics of Benzodiazepines

Generic name	Trade name	Onset of action after oral administration	Rate of metabolism	Metabolized primarily by liver oxidation	Active metabolites	Elimination half-life (hr)	Maximum usual dose (mg/day)
Used primarily to treat anxiety							
alprazolam	Xanax	Intermediate	Intermediate	Yes	Yes	12–15	4
chlordiazepoxide hydrochloride	Librium	Intermediate	Long	Yes	Yes	5–30	100
clonazepam[a]	Klonopin	Fast	Long	Yes	No	26–30	2
clorazepatea dipotassium[a]	Tranxene	Fast	Long	Yes	Yes	36–200	60
diazepam[a,b]	Valium	Fast	Long	Yes	Yes	20–50	40
halazepam	Paxipam	Intermediate	Long	Yes	Yes	50–100	160
lorazepam	Ativan	Intermediate	Short	No	No	10–14	6
oxazepam	Serax	Slow	Short	No	No	5–10	60
prazepam	Centrax	Slow	Long	Yes	Yes	36–200	60
Used primarily to treat insomnia							
estazolam	ProSom	Fast	Short	Yes	No	10–24	2
flurazepam hydrochloride	Dalmane	Intermediate	Long	Yes	Yes	40–100	30
quazepam	Doral	Fast	Long	Yes	Yes	20–120	30
temazepam	Restoril	Intermediate	Short	No	Yes	8–12	30
triazolam	Halcion	Intermediate	Short	Yes	No	2–5	0.25

[a]Approved to treat epilepsy.
[b]Approved as a muscle relaxant.

Speed of Onset

The most important distinction among the benzodiazepines in the substance abuse context is the speed of onset, which is a significant factor in abuse potential (Griffiths & Weerts, 1997). Those benzodiazepines with a slow onset (either because they are slowly absorbed or they must be metabolized to produce an active substance) have a relatively lower abuse potential. Those that rapidly reach peak brain levels after oral administration are relatively more likely to produce euphoria and are therefore more likely to be abused by alcoholics and drug addicts. Alprazolam and diazepam have relatively rapid onset of action and are therefore among the most effective producers of euphoria. In contrast, the more slow-acting benzodiazepines, such as oxazepam (Serax) and prazepam (Centrax), appear to have lower abuse potentials.

Clorazepate and prazepam, with inactive parent compounds, are also less likely to be abused for their euphoric effects because of slower onset of action. Oxazepam and the other slower-onset benzodiazepines, like phenobarbital compared to other barbiturates and codeine compared to other opiates, appear to have relatively low abuse potential.

The relative rapid onset of diazepam does not mean that it is more likely than other benzodiazepines to lead to abuse by medical patients who have no addiction history. On the other hand, the pharmacology of the benzodiazepines suggests that, for patients with a history of addiction to alcohol and other drugs, diazepam and alprazolam may be more likely to be abused than oxazepam, clorazepate, or prazepam (Griffiths & Weerts, 1997).

Some serious students of the pharmacology of benzodiazepines believe that abuse is no more likely for diazepam than for oxazepam (Woods, Katz, & Winger, 1988). Addicts' greater liking for diazepam in some studies, in this view, is the result of the dose: Raise the dose of oxazepam in the double-blind studies, and the liking scores of oxazepam are indistinguishable from those of diazepam. In contrast, other well-respected researchers are convinced that diazepam, lorazepam, and alprazolam have greater abuse potential—not solely because of dosage factors—because of their more rapid absorption and penetration of the blood–brain barrier due to greater lipid solubility (Griffiths & Sannerud, 1987).

Metabolic Pathways

The metabolic pathways of the various benzodiazepines are important clinically, because those benzodiazepines that are metabolized by oxidation in the liver may alter the effects of other drugs. This is illustrated by the "boosting" effect of some benzodiazepines when used by methadone-maintained patients. Although the pharmacology of this effect is not well understood, it appears that simultaneous use of a benzodiazepine (e.g., most commonly diazepam or alprazolam) that competes with methadone for oxidative pathways in the liver produces higher peak levels of methadone in the blood (and brain) shortly after methadone administration. Thus, prior use of some benzodiazepines may enhance brain reward for an hour or so after oral methadone dosages.

Benzodiazepines primarily metabolized via conjugation are not as dependent on intact liver functioning, so they are less likely to raise methadone plasma levels or to build up plasma levels of the active benzodiazepine in patients with compromised liver function (e.g., cirrhosis, hepatitis). The benzodiazepines metabolized by conjugation include lorazepam, oxazepam, and temazepam. Thus, these are less "liked" by methadone-maintained patients and are the recommended agents to be used in patients with compromised hepatic function.

Oxazepam is both a slow-onset and a conjugated benzodiazepine, making it perhaps the best choice for methadone-maintained patients who are treated with a benzodiazepine. On the other hand, oxazepam has a short elimination half-life, which means it must be taken three or four times a day for continuous therapeutic effects. Oxazepam is no less likely to produce physical dependence (including difficulties on discontinuation) than any other benzodiazepine. Oxazepam is a widely used benzodiazepine in Europe (but not in the United States), where it is commonly abused by drug addicts and alcoholics. Thus, whatever benefit oxazepam may possess for alcoholics and drug addicts compared to other benzodiazepines is relative and not absolute (DuPont, 1988).

Persistence

Persistence of the benzodiazepine (or an active metabolite) in the body is important clinically, because it governs the rapidity of onset of withdrawal symptoms after the last dose in people who have used benzodiazepines for prolonged periods. The benzodiazepines with shorter elimination half-lives are more likely to produce early and pronounced withdrawal symptoms on abrupt discontinuation, whereas those with longer elimination half-lives generally produce more delayed and somewhat attenuated withdrawal symptoms. In general, alprazolam, lorazepam, and oxazepam are more rapidly eliminated than are clorazepate, diazepam, flurazepam, and prazepam. Thus, the benzodiazepines with shorter elimination half-lives are more likely to produce acute withdrawal on abrupt cessation after prolonged use. Clonazepam has a longer elimination half-life than alprazolam or lorazepam, so it is less likely to produce interdose withdrawal symptoms and it is more appealing as a withdrawal agent (for the same reason, methadone and phenobarbital are attractive as agents in opiate withdrawal and sedative/hypnotic withdrawal, respectively).

When discontinuing benzodiazepine treatment abruptly, the speed of onset and the severity of symptoms are greater for benzodiazepines with shorter elimination half-lives (e.g., alprazolam or lorazepam) than for those with a longer half-life (e.g., clonazepam). However, abrupt discontinuation is not an appropriate medical treatment for benzodiazepine discontinuation after prolonged, daily use, especially when higher benzodiazepine doses are used. When short-acting benzodiazepines are withdrawn gradually over several weeks or longer, they do not produce more symptoms of withdrawal than do longer-acting benzodiazepines (Sellers et al., 1993).

Although a long half-life may be beneficial in reducing the speed of onset and severity of benzodiazepine withdrawal on abrupt discontinuation, it can be more problematic in other situations. An increase in motor vehicle crash involvement was found in older adults using long half-life benzodiazepines, whereas those using shorter half-life benzodiazepines showed no increase in the probability of crashes compared to people of the same age who did not use a benzodiazepine (Hemmelgarn, Suissa, Huang, Boivin, & Pinard, 1997; Wang, Bohn, Glynn, Mogun, & Avorn, 2001).

Reinforcement

Three additional aspects of benzodiazepine pharmacology are relevant to the treatment of addicted patients: reinforcement, withdrawal, and tolerance. Reinforcement is the potential for these medicines to be abused or "liked" by alcoholics and drug addicts. In controlled studies, benzodiazepines are not reinforcing or "liked" by either normal or anxious subjects. For example, normal and anxious subjects, given a choice between placebos and benzodiazepines, more often choose the placebo in double-blind acute dose experiments, or they show no preference (Woods, Katz, & Winger, 2000; Roy-Byrne & Cowley, 1991). In contrast, subjects with a history of addiction in studies prefer benzodiazepines—especially at high doses—to placebo (Ashton, 1997). Studies have demonstrated that people with a history of addiction show a greater preference for intermediate-acting barbiturates and stimulants, as well as narcotics, than for benzodiazepines. Thus, the benzodiazepines are reinforcing for alcoholics and drug addicts (though not for anxious people or for those who do not have a history of addiction). The benzodiazepines are relatively weak reinforcers compared to opiates, stimulants, and barbiturates, among alcoholics and drug addicts.

This research confirms the common clinical observation that among addicted people, benzodiazepines are rarely drugs of choice for euphoric effects (DuPont, 1984, 1988). Although it remains unclear why alcoholics and drug addicts react differently to benzodiazepines than do normal or anxious subjects, this phenomenon exists with all abused drugs. It is not limited to the benzodiazepines. Normal subjects do not generally "like" drugs of abuse, including stimulants, narcotics, and even alcohol, in double-blind studies. Whether addicted people either learn to like the intoxicated feeling or have some innate (perhaps genetically determined) difference that explains this characteristic response to alcohol and controlled substances remains an unanswered question of importance to the prevention of addiction.

When it comes to the outpatient treatment of anxiety in patients with a history of addiction, the use of controlled substances, including benzodiazepines, is generally contraindicated. A number of alternative treatments for anxiety are available, including psychotherapy (especially cognitive-behavioral therapy), meditation/self-relaxation techniques, biofeedback, eye movement desensitization and reprocessing (EMDR), and the various pharmacological options that we discuss later in this chapter. As a general principle, the use of psychotropic medicines, whether controlled substances (e.g., benzodiazepines) or noncontrolled substances (e.g., antidepressants or antipsychotics), is unlikely to produce a therapeutic benefit for the actively using addicted patient. Stable abstinence is required for these antianxiety medicines to produce therapeutic results.

For patients who have been stable in recovery (including recovering alcoholics) and need treatment for anxiety, it is advisable not to use benzodiazepines as first-line therapy, and only when the severity of the condition warrants the risk. In such cases, benzodiazepine should not be used unless the physician can be sure that the patient uses the benzodiazepine only as prescribed and in the absence of any nonmedical drug use, including alcohol use. Many recovering people who have used benzodiazepines successfully in the treatment of their anxiety disorders have not had their sobriety threatened by the use of benzodiazepines. We have seen many more patients in recovery who do not want to use any controlled substance, and who have done well with their anxiety problems without using a benzodiazepine (Ciraulo et al., 1996; Sattar & Bhatia, 2003).

If a benzodiazepine is to be used by a recovering person, it may be prudent to use one of the slow-onset medicines (e.g., clonazepam, oxazepam, clorazepate, or prazepam), and to include a family member as well as the sponsor from a 12-step fellowship in the therapeutic alliance to help ensure that there is no abuse of the benzodiazepine or any other drug, including alcohol.

Withdrawal

All of the medicines that influence the GABA system show cross-tolerance and similar withdrawal patterns. Because of cross-tolerance within this class of sedatives and hypnotics, an alcoholic or barbiturate addict can be withdrawn under medical supervision using a benzodiazepine. For the same reason, phenobarbital can be used to manage benzodiazepine withdrawal (Wesson, Smith, & Ling, 2003).

The sedatives/hypnotics withdrawal syndrome, including the potential for withdrawal seizures on abrupt discontinuation, is also a phenomenon of this class of medicines. This syndrome commonly includes anxiety, insomnia, tremors, excessive perspiration, hypertension, tachycardia, nausea, vomiting, illusions, and hallucinations, and it may even progress to the point of seizure, delirium, or death. This phenomenon argues against abrupt discontinuation of any of these medicines after daily use for more than a few weeks, especially withdrawal from high doses of a benzodiazepine. A common pattern of benzodiazepine use for anxious patients is as-needed dosing, so on many days there is no benzodiazepine use or the benzodiazepine is used at very low doses (e.g., a total of 10 mg or less of diazepam or the equivalent of another benzodiazepine). Abrupt cessation from these intermittent and low doses is seldom problematic; on the one hand, there is seldom a need for abrupt discontinuation. On the other hand, abrupt cessation of the benzodiazepines, along with the other sedatives and hypnotics, at higher doses can cause withdrawal seizures, because they are potent antiepileptic drugs that raise the seizure threshold. Medicines that raise the seizure threshold when abruptly discontinued produce a rebound drop in the seizure threshold that may cause seizures, even in people who have not previously had an epileptic seizure.

Tolerance

Tolerance is rapid, and all but complete, to the sedative and to the euphoric effects of the benzodiazepines on repeated oral administration at a steady dose level for even a few days. This rapidly developing tolerance for both sedation and euphoria/reward is seen clinically when these medicines are used to treat anxiety. Patients often experience sedation or drowsiness when they take their first few benzodiazepine doses, but within a few days of steady dosing, the symptoms of sedation lessen and, for most patients, disappear. This early sedation can be significant in the context of driving an automobile or in other safety-related situations. It is desirable for physicians to warn patients of this possibility in initial dosing with a benzodiazepine and to urge caution in hazardous situations.

By contrast, tolerance to the antianxiety and antipanic effects of the benzodiazepines is virtually nonexistent. Non-alcoholic or non-drug-addicted medical patients who use a benzodiazepine to treat chronic anxiety obtain substantial beneficial effects at standard, low doses. They do not escalate their benzodiazepine doses beyond common therapeutic levels, even after they have taken benzodiazepines every day for many years.

This distinction between rapid tolerance to the sedating and the euphoric effects and the absence of tolerance to the antianxiety effects of benzodiazepines is important for the clinician. Patients who use benzodiazepines to get high typically add other substances and escalate their benzodiazepine dose over time. People who use benzodiazepines to get high not only use them at dramatically higher doses than anxious patients who are not substance abusers but also they often use the benzodiazepines by snorting (nasal insufflation) and intravenous injection rather than orally. This commonly observed pattern reflects the existence of tolerance to the euphoric effects of benzodiazepines among addicted people and the less rewarding effects of oral administration at lower doses, because it produces slower onset and lower brain levels of the drug. In contrast, typical medical patients using benzodiazepines for their antianxiety effects take them orally at low and stable doses, without the addition of other drugs, including alcohol.

Some patients who use benzodiazepines daily, even after a long time, do escalate their dose beyond the common level, add other drugs (especially alcohol), and/or have poor clinical responses to their benzodiazepine use (i.e., inadequate suppression of anxiety). These patients typically have a personal and/or a family history of addiction to alcohol and other drugs. These same patients sometimes have unusual difficulty in discontinuing their use of benzodiazepines. This group of problems with long-term high-dose benzodiazepine use is frequently seen in substance abuse treatment programs, reinforcing the view in the addiction field that benzodiazepines are ineffective, problem-generating medications, especially after long-term, high-dose use. This pattern of problems is, in our experience, uncommon in the typical medical or psychiatric practices dealing with anxious patients who do not have a history of addiction. In these settings, the typical anxious patients using benzodiazepines do so without dose escalation, even over decades, without problems resulting from their benzodiazepine use and with continuing excellent responses. Nevertheless, when problems do occur, the best clinical response is discontinuation of benzodiazepine use. For some patients, this requires medically supervised detoxification in an inpatient setting, often with simultaneous attention to commonly co-occurring SUDs.

IDENTIFICATION OF PROBLEMS
AMONG LONG-TERM BENZODIAZEPINE USERS

Physicians frequently encounter patients, or family members of patients, who are concerned about the possible adverse effects of long-term use of a benzodiazepine in the treatment of anxiety or insomnia. In helping to structure the decision making for such a patient, we use the Benzodiazepine Checklist (DuPont, 1986; see Table 13.3). There are four questions to be answered by patients and physicians together:

1. *Diagnosis.* Is there a current diagnosis that warrants the prolonged use of a prescription medicine? The benzodiazepines are serious medicines that should only be used for serious illnesses.

2. *Medical and nonmedical substance use.* Is the dose of the benzodiazepine the patient is taking reasonable? Is the clinical response to the benzodiazepine favorable? Is there any use of nonmedical drugs, such as cocaine or marijuana? Is there any excessive use of alcohol (e.g., everyday drinking or more than two drinks on any day)? Are there other medicines being used that can depress brain function?

3. *Toxic behavior.* Is the patient free of evidence of slurred speech, staggering, accidents, memory loss, or other mental deficits or other evidence of sedation?

4. *Family monitor.* Does the family confirm that there is a good clinical response and no adverse reactions to the patient's use of a benzodiazepine? Because people who abuse drugs deny drug-caused problems and often lie to their doctors, and because many family members are concerned about long-term benzodiazepine use, we generally ask that a family member come to the office at least once with the patient who is taking a benzodiazepine for a prolonged period. This gives us an opportunity to confirm with the family member, while the patient is present, that use of the benzodiazepine produces a therapeutic benefit without problems. If there is a problem of toxic behavior or abuse of other drugs, we are more likely to identify it when we speak with the patients' family members; if not, we have an opportunity to educate and reassure both the patients and their family members when they are seen together. Clinicians

---

TABLE 13.3. Benzodiazepine Checklist for Long-Term Use

1. *Diagnosis.* Is there a current diagnosis that warrants the prolonged use of a prescription medicine?

2. *Medical and nonmedical substance use.* Is the dose of the benzodiazepine the patient is taking reasonable? Is the clinical response to the benzodiazepine favorable? Is there any use of nonmedical drugs, such as cocaine or marijuana? Is there any excessive use of alcohol (e.g., a total of more than fourteen drinks a week, or more than two drinks a day)? Are there other medicines being used that can depress the functioning of the CNS?

3. *Toxic behavior.* Is the patient free of evidence of slurred speech, staggering, accidents, memory loss, or other mental deficits or evidence of sedation?

4. *Family monitor.* Does the family confirm that there is a good clinical response and no adverse reactions to the patient's use of a benzodiazepine?

Standard for continued benzodiazepine use: a "yes" to all four questions.

---

also should not hesitate to require random urine drugs screens in long-term benzodiazepine patients. This is not a violation of the doctor–patient relationship, but rather the standard of care to identify substance abuse.

Most patients using benzodiazepines without a history of addiction produce four "yes" answers to these four questions. Even a single "no" answer deserves careful review and may signal the need to discontinue the benzodiazepine. After completion of the Benzodiazepine Checklist, if there is clear evidence that the long-term benzodiazepine use is producing significant benefits and no problems, and if the patient wants to continue using the benzodiazepine (which, in our experience, are common circumstances for chronically anxious patients), then we have no hesitancy in continuing to prescribe a benzodiazepine, even for the patient's lifetime.

On the other hand, many anxious patients, even when they have good responses without problems, want to stop using benzodiazepines. Other patients do not want to stop using a benzodiazepine, but they do show signs of poor clinical response or trouble with benzodiazepine use. In either case, discontinuation is in order. Benzodiazepine withdrawal is an achievable goal for all patients.

Some critics of benzodiazepines, including Stefan Borg and Curtis Carlson of St. Goran's Hospital in Stockholm, Sweden (Allgulander, Borg, & Vikander, 1984), have expressed concerns about the possibility that benzodiazepine use may lead to alcohol problems in patients without a prior history of alcohol abuse, especially in women. The simple advice to a long-term medical user of a benzodiazepine is not to use alcohol or to use alcohol only occasionally, and never have more than one or two drinks in 24 hours. Most anxious patients who do not have a prior history of addiction either do not use alcohol at all or they use it only in small amounts. Because the Benzodiazepine Checklist helps the physician, the patient, and the patient's family identify any problems (including alcohol abuse) at early stages, it facilitates constructive interventions.

LONG-TERM DOSE AND ABUSE

One clinical observation helps the physician identify among benzodiazepine users the people with anxiety who have addiction problems. Most anxious medical users of benzodiazepines have used these medicines at low and stable doses over time, often for many years, with good clinical responses. Dose is a critical and distinguishing variable in long-term benzodiazepine use. People who are addicted to alcohol and other drugs commonly abuse benzodiazepines in high and unstable doses; anxious patients who are not addicted do not. People with active addiction seldom report a good clinical response to low and stable doses of benzodiazepines.

We use a simple assessment of dose level: If the patient's typical benzodiazepine dose level is stable at or below one-half the ordinary clinical maximum dose of the prescribed benzodiazepine, as recommended in the *Physicians' Desk Reference* (PDR Network, 2011) or in the package insert approved by the FDA for the prescribed benzodiazepine, we call this the "green light" benzodiazepine dose zone. Thus, patients whose daily benzodiazepine dose is stable at or less than 2 mg of alprazolam, 20 mg of diazepam, 5 mg of lorazepam, 4 mg of clonazepam, or 60 mg of oxazepam, are in the relatively safe or green-light zone.

The "red light" or danger zone is above the FDA-approved maximum daily dose (e.g., above 4 mg of alprazolam or 40 mg of diazepam). Except in the treatment of panic, when doses up to two or three times the FDA maximum for chronic anxiety are occasionally needed, it is unusual to see an anxious non-alcohol- or non-drug-abusing patient taking benzodiazepine doses that are this high. Most patients with panic disorder, after a few months of treatment, are able to do well (with good panic suppression) in the green-light zone, without the physician or the patient making any effort to limit or restrict the benzodiazepine dose level. If vigilance and control are required by the physician to limit the benzodiazepine dose to levels below the maximum recommended doses, this is a poor prognostic sign and a signal that addiction to alcohol and other drugs may be a confounding, comorbid disorder.

One common clinical challenge is to see a patient, a family member, or sometimes a physician or therapist who is concerned about "tolerance" and "addiction" because the patient feels compelled to raise the dose of the benzodiazepine over time. In our experience, such worries among patients who lack a personal history of addiction to alcohol or other nonmedical drugs are usually the result of benzodiazepine underdosing rather than evidence of addiction. Although some patients with such a presentation are more comfortable taking no medicine at all, most need education about the proper dose of the benzodiazepine. Once the benzodiazepine dose is raised to an ordinary therapeutic level (e.g., well within the green-light zone), the patient usually feels much better in terms of his or her symptoms of an anxiety disorder and has no inner pressure to raise the benzodiazepine dose further.

Within the addicted population, several patterns of benzodiazepine abuse have been identified. The most common pattern is the use of a benzodiazepine to reduce the adverse effects of the abuse of other, more preferred drugs. Typical is the suppression of a hangover and other withdrawal phenomena from alcohol use with a benzodiazepine. Patients waking up in the morning after an alcoholic binge may take 10–40 mg or more of diazepam, for example, "just to face the day."

Other common patterns of nonmedical use are to use the benzodiazepines (often alprazolam or lorazepam) concomitantly with stimulants (often cocaine or methamphetamine) to reduce the unpleasant experiences of the stimulant use, and/or to use benzodiazepines (often triazolam [Halcion]) to treat the insomnia that accompanies stimulant abuse. Use of benzodiazepines (e.g., alprazolam or diazepam) to "boost" the high of methadone used to treat opiate addiction is common.

Benzodiazepines are occasionally used as primary drugs of abuse, in which case they are typically taken orally at high doses, though they may be crushed and snorted via nasal insufflation as well. Addicted patients report using doses of 20–100 mg or more of diazepam or the equivalent doses of other benzodiazepines, for example, at one time. Such high-dose oral use is often repeated several times a day for long periods or on binges. Although, in our experience, such primary benzodiazepine abuse without simultaneous use of other drugs is unusual, it does occur.

Daily use of benzodiazepines, even when there is no dose escalation and no abuse of alcohol or other drugs nonmedically, has led to controversy. Clinical experience has shown that even over long periods of daily use, the benzodiazepines typically do not lose their efficacy or produce significant problems for most patients. An example of this experience was a study of 170 adult patients treated for a variety of sleep disorders continuously with a benzodiazepine for 6 months or longer over a 12-year period. The study found sustained efficacy, with low risk of dose escalation, adverse effects, or abuse (Schenck & Mahowald, 1996).

DISCONTINUATION OF BENZODIAZEPINE USE

Discontinuation of sedatives and hypnotics, including the benzodiazepines, can be divided into three categories: (1) long-term low-dose benzodiazepine use, (2) high-dose benzodiazepine abuse and multiple drug abuse, and (3) high-dose abuse of non-benzodiazepine sedatives and hypnotics (especially intermediate-acting barbiturates). The first group of patients can usually be discontinued on an outpatient basis. Some of the second and even the third group can be treated as outpatients, but many will require inpatient care. Inpatient discontinuation today with managed care is generally reserved for patients who fail at outpatient discontinuation and for those who demonstrate acutely life-threatening loss of control over their drug use. The pharmacological management of inpatient benzodiazepine withdrawal from nontherapeutically high doses of these medicines is covered in standard texts dealing with inpatient detoxification (Ries, Miller, Fiellin, & Saitz, 2009; Wesson et al., 2003). Refer to Table 13.4 for a list of common sedatives/hypnotics dose equivalents, which may prove useful in the context of detoxification or switching agents.

With respect to withdrawal from benzodiazepines in the context of addiction treatment, the most common problem of addiction treatment professionals is that some of their patients who take benzodiazepines also suffer from underlying anxiety disorders and panic attacks. When these patients stop taking a benzodiazepine, they experience a short-term rebound increase in these distressing symptoms. These rebound symptoms, including panic attacks, are difficult for the patients and their physicians to separate from withdrawal symptoms, because the symptoms and time course are similar and both types of symptoms occur at low benzodiazepine doses and peak during the first or second drug-free week.

Most patients who take benzodiazepines at prescribed dose levels can discontinue using them with quite moderate symptoms if the dose reduction is gradual (Busto, Simpkins, & Sellers, 1983; Rickels, Schweizer, Csanalosi, Case, & Chung, 1988). One study indicated that about half of long-term benzodiazepine users could stop with no withdrawal symptoms (Tyrer, Rutherford, & Huggett, 1981). However, some patients who stop benzodiazepine use, especially after use for many years, do have withdrawal symptoms that are either prolonged or severe (Noyes, Garvey, Cook, & Perry, 1988). About one-third of medical patients with long-term use of a benzodiazepine have clinically significant withdrawal symptoms, even after gradual tapering, and about one in eight patients stopping a benzodiazepine will have prolonged and/or severe symptoms (DuPont, 1988). In any case, discontinuation symptoms (except for abrupt cessation, which can produce seizures and is not indicated) from benzodiazepines are usually "distressing but not dangerous" (DuPont et al., 1992; Sellers et al., 1993).

TABLE 13.4. Common Sedative/Hypnotic Dose Equivalents

Class	Generic name	Trade name	Dose (mg)
Benzodiazepines	diazepam	Valium	10
	alprazolam	Xanax, Niravam	0.5–1
	lorazepam	Ativan	2
	clonazepam	Klonopin	1–2
	chlordiazepoxide	Librium	25
	clorazepate	Tranxene	7.5
	oxazepam	Serax	10–15
	temazepam	Restoril	15
	triazolam	Halcion	0.25
	flurazepam	Dalmane	15
Barbiturates	phenobarbital	n/a	30
	pentobarbital	Nembutal	100
	secobarbital	Seconal	100
	butalbital	Fiorinal, Fioricet	100
	amobarbital	Amytal	100
Related compounds	carisoprodol	Soma	700
	meprobamate	Miltown, Equanil	1,200
	chloral hydrate	Noctec	500
	methaqualone	Quaalude	300
	ethchlorvynol	Placidyl	500
	zolpidem	Ambien	20
	zaleplon	Sonata	20
	eszopiclone	Lunesta	3

Note. Adapted with permission from Greene and Gold (2014).

There are a number of useful publications on the diagnosis and treatment of chronic anxiety (DuPont, Spencer, & DuPont, 2004; Spencer, DuPont, & DuPont, 2004; Ross, 1994; Davidson, 2003). The benzodiazepines can be used to treat either acute or chronic anxiety, as well as the panic attacks that are commonly associated with anxiety disorders. The benzodiazepines can be used either as needed or every day, and they can be used either alone or with other medicines, most often with antidepressants (Davidson, 1997).

Because all of the benzodiazepines have been off-patent for years, there was an interest in the development of new, patentable delivery mechanisms for two of the most widely used benzodiazepines (Stahl, 2003). Alprazolam became available in an extended release formulation (Xanax XR). It had the advantage of slower onset of action, which reduces initial sedation in the hour or two after administration. Slower onset of action also lowers the abuse potential of Xanax XR, since it is the rapid onset of action that triggers the brain reward that addicts seek. This newer formulation of alprazolam permits once-a-day, or at most twice-a-day, dosing and reduces the risk of "clock watching," which can be seen with frequent dosing throughout the day.

Clonazepam was reformulated into an orally disintegrating tablet, Klonopin Wafers, for easier oral administration without having to swallow a pill. In the new formulations of these two benzodiazepines, the manufacturers moved in opposite directions to maximize two different therapeutic effects. Xanax XR has a slower onset and longer duration of action to smooth the brain level of alprazolam for 24-hour/day effectiveness. Sublingual clonazepam has been reformulated to overcome the problems some patients have swallowing pills and to have more rapid onset of action.

NEWER SEDATIVE AND HYPNOTIC AGENTS

Three novel nonbenzodiazepine hypnotic agents have been introduced, the so-called "Z drugs." Zolpidem (Ambien), zaleplon (Sonata), and eszopiclone (Lunesta) are rapid-onset, short-duration of action medicines that act on the benzodiazepine receptors of the GABA system. They have been shown to reduce insomnia and have gained widespread popularity, but exactly how effective they are remains unclear. In a large Phase 3 trial of eszopiclone, the active drug group reported falling asleep only 15 minutes faster than the placebo group (Schwartz & Woloshin, 2009). These agents have largely replaced the benzodiazepines as hypnotic medicines, although they lack the anxiolytic, anticonvulsant, and muscle-relaxant properties of the benzodiazepines (Scharf, Mayleben, Kaffeman, Krall, & Ochs, 1991). Zolpidem and zaleplon are reinforcing to alcoholics and drug addicts, underscoring the fact that the abuse potential of these drugs appears to be similar to that of the benzodiazepines. These medicines impair memory and performance of complex tasks in ways that are similar to the acute effects of benzodiazepines. They do not affect Stage 4 sleep, as do the benzodiazepines.

Both zaleplon and zolpidem are effective in relieving sleep-onset insomnia, and both have been approved by the FDA for use up to 7–10 days at a time. Both medicines clinically appear to have sustained hypnotic activity over longer periods of time. Zolpidem has a half-life of about 2 hours, which is consistent with therapeutic activity over a typical 8 hours of sleep. Zaleplon has a 1-hour half-life that offers the possibility of dosing in the middle of the night for broken sleep. For this reason, zaleplon is approved both for bedtime use and in midsleep periods of insomnia. Eszopiclone's serum levels peak between 1.0 and 1.3 hours, and it has an elimination half-life of about 6 hours (Halas, 2006). Unlike its peers, eszopiclone has no FDA-recommended limit for duration of use.

ALTERNATIVE AGENTS

As it became apparent that GABA-ergic, noradrenergic, and serotonergic systems all play roles in the pathophysiology of anxiety disorders, a variety of alternatives to the sedatives/hypnotics became available to treat both anxiety and insomnia. Propranolol, a beta-blocker known to inhibit norepinephrine, has long been used to treat performance-related anxiety and panic, and is being investigated for use in the treatment of posttraumatic stress disorder (PTSD; Brunet et al., 2008). Buspirone (Buspar), a serotonin partial agonist and dopamine–norepinephrine antagonist, has been shown to reduce anxiety in generalized anxiety disorder, but it does not suppress panic attacks and is not used as a primary treatment of obsessive–compulsive disorder (OCD). Buspirone is not abused by alcoholics and drug addicts, and it does not produce withdrawal symptoms on abrupt discontinuation. Like the antidepressants, buspirone requires several weeks of daily dosing to produce antianxiety effects, which are less dramatic from the patients' point of view than are the effects produced by the benzodiazepines (Sussman & Stein, 2002).

In recent years the antiepileptic medicines, including valproate (Depakote) and gabapentin (Neurontin), have been used as augmenting agents in the treatment of anxiety (Lydiard, 2002). Since 2007, pregabalin (Lyrica) has been approved for the treatment of generalized anxiety disorder in Europe.

The antidepressants as a class have been shown to possess antipanic and antianxiety effects, opening a new range of uses for these medicines in the treatment of anxiety disorders. The selective serotonin reuptake inhibitors (SSRIs) have emerged as the first-line treatment for many anxiety disorders (DuPont, 1997; Jefferson, 1997; Davidson, 2003). Options available today include sertraline (Zoloft), escitalopram (Lexapro), citalopram (Celexa), fluoxetine (Prozac), paroxetine (Paxil), and luvoxamine (Luvox). Serotonin–norepinephrine reuptake inhibitors (SNRIs), including venlafaxine (Effexor), duloxetine (Cymbalta), and desvenlafaxine (Pristiq), are also now being used with increased frequency in the successful management of anxiety disorders (Dell'Osso, Buoli, Baldwin, & Altamura, 2010). Although the earlier antianxiety and anti-insomnia medicines focused exclusively on the benzodiazepine receptors in the GABA system, recognition of the importance of serotonin and norepinephrine neurotransmitters in the management of anxiety and insomnia, and the success of buspirone have stimulated a search for a new generation of antianxiety medicines that are not controlled substances (e.g., they are not abused by alcoholics and drug addicts). Recognition of the withdrawal symptoms associated with abrupt discontinuation of some antidepressants (especially those with shorter half-lives and more anticholinergic properties) has shown that withdrawal is not limited to controlled substances (DuPont, 1997).

Atypical antipsychotic use for off-label indications, including anxiety and insomnia, has exploded over the past decade (Boodman, 2012). There is good evidence to support the use of atypicals in certain situations, such as using risperidone (Risperdal) as an adjunct in refractory OCD (Hollander, Baldini Rossi, Sood, & Pallanti, 2003; Pfanner et al., 2000). Despite the potential for serious side effects (metabolic syndrome, extrapyramidal symptoms, even cardiac problems and sudden death) these medicines have come into common use for a variety of unapproved conditions. A recent Cochrane review analyzed existing randomized controlled trials of quetiapine (Seroquel), risperidone (Risperdal), and olanzapine (Zyprexa), for use in common anxiety disorders (not including OCD), and found a positive effect only with quetiapine, no advantage over antidepressants, and high dropout rates due to side effects (Depping, Komossa, Kissling, & Leucht, 2010). The use of atypicals for the management of routine anxiety/insomnia remains controversial. At this time, cautious prudence warrants judicious use of these agents in select patients for whom other options have failed. The atypical antipsychotics offer an alternative to the benzodiazepines to suppress anxiety on an as-needed basis for patients with SUDs.

REFERENCES

Allgulander, C., Borg, S., & Vikander, B. (1984). A 4–6 year follow-up of 50 patients with primary dependence on sedative and hypnotic drugs. *Am J Psychiatry, 141,* 1580–1582.

American Psychiatric Association. (2013). *Diagnostic and statistical manual of mental disorders* (5th ed.). Arlington, VA: Author.

American Psychiatric Association Task Force. (1990). *Benzodiazepine dependence, toxicity, and abuse.* Washington, DC: American Psychiatric Association.

Ashton, C. H. (1997). Benzodiazepine dependency. In A. Baum, S. Newman, J. Weinman, R. West, & C. McManus (Eds.), *Cambridge handbook of psychology and medicine* (pp. 376–380). Cambridge, UK: Cambridge University Press.

Baldessarini, R. J. (2001). Depression and anxiety disorders. In J. G. Hardman & L. E. Limbird (Eds.), *Goodman and Gilman's the pharmacological basis of therapeutics* (10th ed., pp. 447–483). New York: McGraw-Hill.

Barker, M. J., Greenwood, K. M., Jackson, M., & Crowe, S. F. (2004a). Cognitive effects of long-term benzodiazepine use: A meta-analysis. *CNS Drugs, 18*(1), 37–48.

Barker, M. J., Greenwood, K. M., Jackson, M., & Crowe, S. F. (2004b). Persistence of cognitive effects after withdrawal from long-term benzodiazepine use: A meta-analysis. *Arch Clin Neuropsychol, 19*(3), 437–454.

Boodman, S. G. (2012, March 12). Antipsychotic drugs grow more popular for patients without mental illness. *The Washington Post.* Available at *www.washingtonpost.com/national/health-science/antipsychotic-drugs-grow-more-popular-for-patients-without-mental-illness/2012/02/02/gIQAH1yz7R_story.html.*

Brunet A., Orr, S. P., Tremblay, J., Robertson, K., Nader, K., & Pitman, R. K. (2008). Effect of post-retrieval propranolol on psychophysiologic responding during subsequent script-driven traumatic imagery in post-traumatic stress disorder. *J Psychiatric Res, 42*(6), 503–506.

Burt, D. R., & Kamatchi, G. L. (1991). GABA receptor subtypes: From pharmacology to molecular biology. *FASEB J, 5,* 2916–2923.

Busto, U., Simpkins, J., & Sellers, E. M. (1983). Objective determination of benzodiazepine use and abuse in alcoholics. *Br J Addict, 48,* 429–435.

Charney, D. S., Minic, S. J., & Harris, R. A. (2001). Hypnotics and sedatives. In J. G. Hardman & L. E. Limbird (Eds.), *Goodman and Gilman's the pharmacological basis of therapeutics* (10th ed., pp. 399–427). New York: McGraw-Hill.

Chouninard, G., Lefko-Singh, K., & Teboul, E. (1999). Metabolism of anxiolytics and hypnotics: Benzodiazepines, buspirone, zopliclone, and zolpidem. *Cell Mol Neurobiol, 19,* 533–552.

Ciraulo, D. A., Sarid-Segal, O., Knapp, C., Ciraulo, A. O., Greenblatt, D. J., & Shader, R. I. (1996). Liability to alprazolam abuse in daughters of alcoholics. *Am J Psychiatry, 153,* 956–958.

Davidson, J. (2003). *The anxiety book.* New York: Penguin/Putnam.

Davidson, J. R. T. (1997). Use of benzodiazepines in panic disorder. *J Clin Psychiatry, 58*(Suppl. 2), 26–31.

Dell'Osso, B., Buoli, M., Baldwin, D. S., & Altamura, A. C. (2010). Serotonin–norepinephrine reuptake inhibitors (SNRIs) in anxiety disorders: A comprehensive review of their clinical efficacy. *Hum Psychopharmacol, 25*(1), 17–29.

Depping, A. M., Komossa, K., Kissling, W., & Leucht, S. (2010). Second-generation antipsychotics for anxiety disorders. *Cochrane Database Syst Rev, 12,* CD008141.

DuPont, R. L. (1984). *Getting tough on gateway drugs: A guide for the family.* Washington, DC: American Psychiatric Press.

DuPont, R. L. (1986). *Benzodiazepines: The social issues.* Rockville, MD: Institute for Behavior and Health.

DuPont, R. L. (Ed.). (1988). Abuse of benzodiazepines: The problems and the solutions. *Am J Drug Alcohol Abuse, 14*(Suppl. 1), 1–69.

DuPont, R. L. (1997). The pharmacology and drug interactions of the newer antidepressants. *Essential Psychopharmacol, 2,* 7–31.

DuPont, R. L. (1998). Addiction: A new paradigm. *Bull Menninger Clin, 62,* 231–242.

DuPont, R. L. (2000). *The selfish brain: Learning from addiction* (rev. ed.). Center City, MN: Hazelden.

DuPont, R. L., DuPont, C. M., & Rice, D. P. (2002). Economic costs of anxiety disorders. In D. J. Stein & E. Hollander (Eds.), *Textbook of anxiety disorders* (pp. 475–483). Washington, DC: American Psychiatric Press.

DuPont, R. L., & Gold, M. S. (1995). Withdrawal and reward: Implications for detoxification and relapse prevention. *Psychiatr Ann, 25,* 663–668.

DuPont, R. L., Spencer, E. D., & DuPont, C. M. (2004). *The anxiety cure: An eight step program for getting well* (rev. ed.). New York: Wiley.

DuPont, R. L., Swinson, R. P., Ballenger, J. C., Burrows, G. D., Noyes, R., Rubin, R. T., et al. (1992). Discontinuation effects of alprazolam after long-term treatment of panic-related disorders. *J Clin Psychopharmacol, 12,* 352–354.

Golombok, S., Moodley, P., & Lader, M. (1988). Cognitive impairment in long-term benzodiazepine users. *Psychol Med, 18,* 365–374.

Greene, W. M., & Gold, M. S. (2014). Drug abuse. In E. T. Bope & R. Kellerman (Eds.), *Current therapy 2014* (pp. 1118–1122). Philadelphia: Elsevier.

Griffiths, R. R., & Sannerud, C. A. (1987). Abuse of and dependence on benzodiazepines and other anxiolytic/sedative drugs. In H. Meltzer, B. S. Bunney, & J. T. Coyle (Eds.), *Psychopharmacology: The third generation of progress* (pp. 1535–1541). New York: Raven Press.

Griffiths, R. R., & Weerts, E. M. (1997). Benzodiazepine self-administration in humans and laboratory animals—implications for problems of long-term use and abuse. *Psychopharmacol, 134*(1), 1–37.

Halas, C. J. (2006). Eszopiclone. *Am J Health Syst Pharm, 63*(1), 41–48.

Handelsman, L. (2002). Anxiety in the context of substance abuse. In D. J. Stein & E. Hollander (Eds.), *Textbook of anxiety disorders* (pp. 441–448). Washington, DC: American Psychiatric Publishing.

Hemmelgarn, B., Suissa, S., Huang, A., Boivin, J.-F., & Pinard, G. (1997). Benzodiazepine use and the risk of motor vehicle crash in the elderly. *JAMA, 278,* 27–31.

Hollander, E., Baldini Rossi, N., Sood, E., & Pallanti, S. (2003). Risperidone augmentation in treatment-resistant obsessive–compulsive disorder: A double-blind, placebo-controlled study. *Int J Neuropsychopharmacol, 6*(4), 397–401.

Jefferson, J. W. (1997). Antidepressants in panic disorder. *J Clin Psychiatry, 58*(Suppl. 2), 20–25.

Johnson, M. W., Suess, P. E., & Griffiths, R. R. (2006). Ramelteon: A novel hypnotic lacking abuse liability and sedative adverse effects. *Arch Gen Psychiatry, 63*(10), 1149–1157.

Johnston, L. D., O'Malley, P. M., Bachman, J. G., & Schulenberg, J. E. (2012). *Monitoring the Future national results on adolescent drug use: Overview of key findings, 2011.* Ann Arbor: Institute for Social Research, The University of Michigan.

Juergens, S. M., & Cowley, D. S. (2003). The pharmacology of benzodiazepines and other sedative–hypnotics. In A. W. Graham, T. K. Schultz, M. F. Mayo-Smith, & R. K. Ries (Eds.), *Principles of addiction medicine* (3rd ed., pp. 119–139). Chevy Chase, MD: American Society of Addiction Medicine.

Lydiard, R. B. (2002). Pharmacotherapy for panic disorder. In D. J. Stein & E. Hollander (Eds.), *Textbook of anxiety disorders* (pp. 257–272). Washington, DC: American Psychiatric Publishing.

MacDonald, D. L., DuPont, R. L., & Ferguson, J. L. (2003). The role of the medical review officer. In A. W. Graham, T. K. Schultz, M. F. Mayo-Smith, & R. K. Ries (Eds.), *Principles of addiction medicine* (3rd ed., pp. 1405–1419). Chevy Chase, MD: American Society of Addiction Medicine.

Mellinger, G. D., & Balter, M. B. (1981). Prevalence and patterns of use of psychotherapeutic drugs: Results from a 1979 national survey of American adults. In G. Tognoni, C. Bellan-tuono, & M. Lader (Eds.), *Epidemiological impact of psychotropic drugs* (pp. 117–135). Amsterdam: Elsevier.

Mendelson, W. B., Roth, T., Casella, J., Roehrs, T., Walsh, J., Woods, J. H., et al. (2001, May). *Report on a conference: The treatment of chronic insomnia: Drug indication, chronic use and abuse liability.* Presented at the NCDEU meeting, Phoenix, AZ.

National Comorbidity Survey Replication (NCS-R). (2007a). *NCS-R 12-month prevalence of DSM-IV/WMH-CIDI disorders by sex and cohort.* Boston: Harvard School of Medicine. Available at *www.hcp.med.harvard.edu/ncs/ftpdir/ncs-r_12-month_prevalence_estimates. pdf.*

National Comorbidity Survey Replication (NCS-R). (2007b). *NCS-R lifetime prevalence of DSM-IV/WMH-CIDI disorders by sex and cohort.* Boston: Harvard School of Medicine. Available at *www.hcp.med.harvard.edu/ncs/ftpdir/ncs-r_lifetime_prevalence_estimates.pdf.*

Noyes, R., Garvey, M. J., Cook, B. L., & Perry, P. J. (1988). Benzodiazepine withdrawal: A review of the evidence. *J Clin Psychiatry, 49,* 382–389.

PDR Network. (2011). *Physicians' desk reference.* Montvale, NJ: Author.

Pfanner, C., Marazziti, D., Dell'Osso, L., Presta, S., Gemignani, A., Milanfranchi, A., et al. (2000). Risperidone augmentation in refractory obsessive–compulsive disorder: An open-label study. *Int Clin Psychopharmacol, 15*(5), 297–301.

Rickels, K., Schweizer, E., Csanalosi, I., Case, G. W., & Chung, H. (1988). Long-term treatment of anxiety and risk of withdrawal. *Arch Gen Psychiatry, 45,* 444–450.

Rickels, K., Schweizer, E., Garcia-Espana, F., Case, G., DeMartinis, N., & Greenblatt, D. (1999). Trazodone and valproate in patients discontinuing long-term benzodiazepine therapy: Effects on withdrawal symptoms and taper outcome. *Psychopharmacology, 141*(1), 1–5.

Ries, R. K., Miller, S. C., Fiellin, D. A., & Saitz, R. (Eds.). (2009). *Principles of addiction medicine* (4th ed.). Chevy Chase, MD: American Society of Addiction Medicine.

Ross, J. (1994). *Triumph over fear: A book of help and hope for people with anxiety, panic attacks, and phobias.* New York: Bantam Books.

Roy-Byrne, P. P., & Cowley, D. S. (Eds.). (1991). *Benzodiazepines in clinical practice: Risks and benefits.* Washington, DC: American Psychiatric Press.

Sattar, S. P., & Bhatia, S. (2003). Benzodiazepines for substance abusers. *Curr Psychiatry, l2*(5), 25–34.

Savage, S. R. (2003). Principles of pain management in the addicted patient. In A. W. Graham, T. K. Schultz, M. F. Mayo-Smith, & R. K. Ries (Eds.), *Principles of addiction medicine* (3rd ed., pp. 1405–1419). Chevy Chase, MD: American Society of Addiction Medicine.

Scharf, M. B., Mayleben, D. W., Kaffeman, M., Krall, R., & Ochs, R. (1991). Dose–response effects of zolpidem in normal geriatric subjects. *J Clin Psychiatry, 52,* 77–83.

Schenck, C. H., & Mahowald, M. W. (1996). Long-term, nightly benzodiazepine treatment of injurious parasomnias and other disorders of disrupted nocturnal sleep in 170 adults. *Am J Med, 100,* 333–337.

Schwartz, L. M., & Woloshin, S. (2009). Lost in transmission—FDA drug information that never reaches clinicians. *N Engl J Med, 361*(18), 1717–1720.

Sellers, E. M., Ciraulo, D. A., DuPont, R. L., Griffiths, R. R., Kosten, T. R., Romach, M. K., et al. (1993). Alprazolam and benzodiazepine dependence. *J Clin Psychiatry, 54*(Suppl.), 64–74.

Spencer, E. D., DuPont, R. L., & DuPont, C. M. (2004). *The anxiety cure for kids: A guide for parents.* New York: Wiley.

Stahl, S. M. (2003). At long last, long-lasting psychiatric medications: An overview of controlled-released technologies. *J Clin Psychiatry, 64*(4), 355–356.

Substance Abuse and Mental Health Services Administration (SAMHSA). (2011a). Drug Abuse Warning Network, 2009: National estimates of drug-related emergency department visits (HHS Publication No. [SMA] 11-4659, DAWN Series D-35). Rockville, MD: Author.

Substance Abuse and Mental Health Services Administration (SAMHSA). (2011b). *Results from the 2010 National Survey on Drug Use and Health: Summary of national findings* (NSDUH Series H-41, HHS Publication No. [SMA] 11-4658). Rockville, MD: Author.

Sussman, N., & Stein, D. J. (2002). Pharmacotherapy for generalized anxiety disorder. In D. J. Stein & E. Hollander (Eds.), *Textbook of anxiety disorders* (pp. 135–141). Washington, DC: American Psychiatric Publishing.

Tyrer, P., Rutherford, D., & Huggett, D. (1981). Benzodiazepine withdrawal symptoms and propranolol. *Lancet, 1,* 520–522.

Wang, P. S., Bohn, R. L., Glynn, R. J., Mogun, H., & Avorn, J. (2001). Hazardous benzodiazepine regimens in the elderly: Effects of half-life, dosage, and duration on risk of hip fracture. *Am J Psychiatry, 158,* 892–898.

Wesson, D. R., Smith, D. E., & Ling, W. (2003). Pharmacologic interventions for benzodiazepine and other sedative–hypnotic addiction. In A. W. Graham, T. K. Schultz, M. F. Mayo-Smith, & R. K. Ries (Eds.), *Principles of addiction medicine* (3rd ed., pp. 721–735). Chevy Chase, MD: American Society of Addiction Medicine.

Woods, J. H., Katz, J. L., & Winger, G. (1988). Use and abuse of benzodiazepines: Issues relevant to prescribing. *JAMA, 260,* 3476–3480.

Woods, J. H., Katz, J. L., & Winger, G. (2000). Abuse and therapeutic use of benzodiazepines and benzodiazepine-like drugs. In F. E. Bloom & D. J. Kupfer (Eds.), *Psychopharmacology: The fourth generation of progress.* Brentwood, TN: American College of Neuropsychopharmacology.

World Health Organization. (1988). *The use of essential drugs: Third report of the World Health Organization expert committee* (WHO Technical Report Series No. 770). Geneva: Author.

World Health Organization. (2011, March). *WHO Model Lists of Essential Medicines.* Geneva: Author. Available at *http://whqlibdoc.who.int/hq/2011/a95053_eng.pdf.*

Wu, E. Q., Birnbaum, H. G., Shi, L., Kessler, R. C., Moulis, M., & Aggarwal, J. (2005). The economic burden of schizophrenia in the United State. *J Clin Psychiatry, 66*(9), 1122–1129.

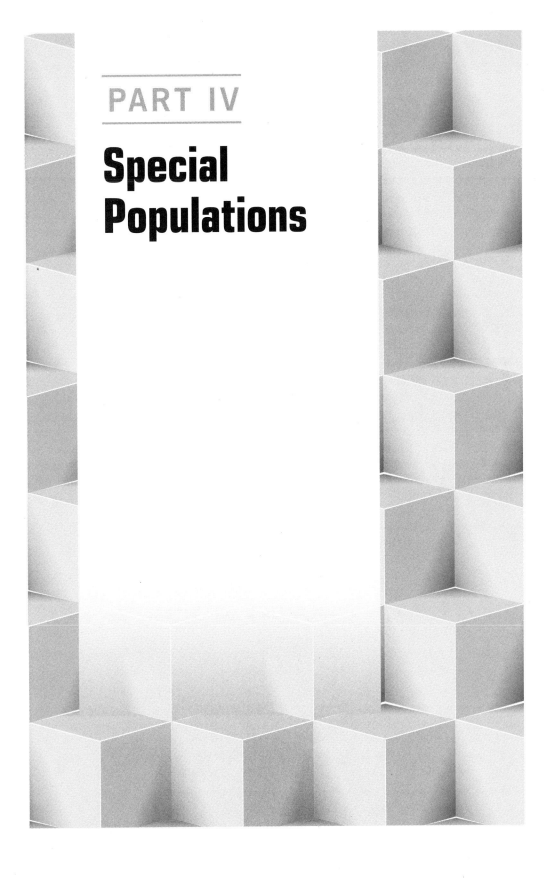

PART IV

Special Populations

CHAPTER 14

Polysubstance Use, Abuse, and Dependence

RICHARD N. ROSENTHAL
PETROS LEVOUNIS
ABIGAIL J. HERRON

DEFINING MULTIPLE SUBSTANCE USE

Diagnostic Approaches

Historical Definitions

The term "polysubstance dependence" originated in the DSM nomenclature only in 1987, with the introduction of DSM-III-R. Prior to this, DSM-III (American Psychiatric Association, 1980) had the diagnostic category "mixed substance abuse," in which there were criteria for diagnosing substance abuse, but either the substances could not be identified or the abuse involved "*so many* substances that the clinician *prefers*" to treat them as a combination rather than define a specific disorder for each substance (emphasis added). In addition, in DSM-III, there was an attempt to create clinically meaningful diagnostic categories with respect to dependence on multiple substances, hence the diagnoses "Dependence on a Combination of Opioid and other Non-alcoholic Substances," an early nod to the high prevalence of use of multiple substances among heroin users, and "Dependence on a Combination of Substances, excluding Opioids and Alcohol." In parallel with the DSM-III diagnosis for multiple substance abuse, each of these multiple dependence criteria applied only if the substances could not be identified, or the dependence involved *so many* substances that the clinician *preferred* to treat them as a combination rather than define a specific disorder for each substance. This concept is what underlies the typical, non-DSM use of the term "polysubstance dependence." In DSM-III-R (American Psychiatric Association, 1987), the concept of polysubstance dependence was formally introduced. The imprecise DSM-III concept of "so many" substances was dropped in favor of a threshold number of substances, and clinician "preference" was eliminated as an option to making such diagnoses. DSM-III-R polysubstance dependence stipulated that the person meet criteria due to repeated use of at least three substance categories as a group over half a year, excluding caffeine and nicotine, but not meet diagnostic criteria of dependence for any specific substance.

In DSM-IV, the concept of polysubstance dependence was more specific (American Psychiatric Association, 1994). However, the DSM-IV version allowed for two different ways to interpret the diagnosis. The first diagnostic concept of polysubstance dependence in DSM-IV was at least three groups of substances repeatedly used by the patient during 12 months that, as a group, comprised dependence criteria, but in which there is no specific drug that independently qualified for substance dependence. Any substance for which the patient satisfies criteria for dependence should be given that diagnosis independently of other substances used. A second, more exclusive DSM-IV concept of polysubstance dependence was three or more classes of drugs used by the patient without dependence on any one drug, but the sum of the criteria met for all drugs used was three or more.

The definition of polysubstance dependence was clarified somewhat in DSM-IV-TR (American Psychiatric Association, 2000). However, there were still two possible interpretations with DSM-IV-TR relative to polysubstance dependence. One schema focuses on episodes of indiscriminate use of a variety of substances that each met one criterion, but when added together met three or more dependence criteria; the other is that full dependence criteria were only met when the drug classes used were grouped together as a whole (First & Pincus, 2002). That stated, polysubstance dependence was a relatively rare disorder as defined by DSM-IV, and the formal diagnosis was used infrequently by clinicians and researchers (Schuckit, Smith, et al., 2001).

Although there was a diagnostic category of "mixed substance abuse" in DSM-III (American Psychiatric Association, 1980), there was no diagnosis of polysubstance abuse in DSM-IV-TR (American Psychiatric Association, 2000). There may not be many people who abuse multiple substances over time with clinically significant impact, for whom no single substance is sufficient to meet formal abuse criteria. This is because one needed to meet only one of the four DSM-IV criteria to pass the threshold for a substance abuse diagnosis related to that particular substance. However, it is conceivable that one could meet a criterion for substance abuse based on use of multiple substances, but not on one in particular. For example, a person could have two arrests for driving under the influence, one for alcohol and the other for cannabis, in the same year.

Changes in Diagnostic Criteria for DSM-5

Changes to DSM-5 involve a major shift in the classification of substance use disorders (SUDs). DSM-III and DSM-IV used a dichotomous concept in which dependence was considered a biological process distinct from consequences of use, leading to separate diagnoses of dependence and abuse (Edwards & Gross, 1976). A number of studies identified problems with this classification system. Several indicated that abuse was not a prodromal phase of dependence (Hasin, Grant, & Endicott, 1990; Hasin, Van Rossem, McCloud, & Endicott 1997; Grant, Stinson, & Harford, 2001; Schuckit et al., 2008; Schuckit, Danko, et al., 2001). The frequency with which alcohol abuse was diagnosed by meeting a single criterion for hazardous use (driving while intoxicated) was also highlighted as a weakness (Hasin, Paykin, Endicott, & Grant, 1999; Hasin & Paykin, 1999). Additionally, there was the problem of "diagnostic orphans," in which individuals were subthreshold for dependence, having met one or two criteria but none for abuse, and were therefore not diagnosed with any formal SUD (Hasin & Paykin, 1998, 1999; Pollock & Martin, 1999; Ray, Miranda, Chelminski, Young, & Zimmerman, 2008; Degenhardt, Lynskey, Coffey, & Patton, 2002; Lynskey & Agrawal, 2007; Martin, Chung, & Langenbucher, 2008).

This led to the development of the concept that abuse and dependence be combined into a single disorder of graded severity, with two criteria required to make a diagnosis. The work group also recommended the elimination of the legal problems criterion and addition of craving, for a total of 11 criteria, with severity specifiers of "mild" for two to three criteria, "moderate" for four to five, and "severe" for six or more.

For polysubstance use, one implication is that it will be more difficult to attribute symptoms to multiple substances over a 12-month period without making independent SUD diagnoses specific to each class of substances. For formal diagnosis, one simply has to record all the substances separately. Thus, the term "polysubstance dependence" has been eliminated as a formal disorder. But the clinical significance of polysubstance dependence is alive and well, and warrants significant attention from a practicing clinician.

Descriptive Approaches: Polydrug Use or Polysubstance Use?

Most broadly, the literature frequently describes "polydrug use" or "polysubstance use." This nondiagnostic designation generally describes the use of multiple substances rather than framing the use and its effects in clinical terms, which is the intent of diagnosis. As such, "polydrug use" describes, at minimum, the use of multiple substances, whether licit or illicit. In the treatment research literature, "polydrug use" is often used to describe the lifetime number of drugs regularly used to a threshold SUD, in addition to the index substance (Ball, Carroll, Babor, & Rounsaville, 1995; Feingold, Ball, Kranzler, & Rounsaville, 1996). However, in other than addiction or mental health treatment settings, the expression "polysubstance use" or "polysubstance abuse" is frequently meant to describe use by subjects of as few as two substances, such as cocaine and alcohol, alcohol and cannabis, or opiates and cocaine (Birnbach, Browne, Kim, Stein, & Thys, 2001; Ross, Kohler, Grimley, & Bellis, 2003).

In an effort to further distinguish patterns of use, Grant and Hartford (1990) framed polydrug use either as "simultaneous," which is the use of multiple drugs at the same occasion, or "concurrent," which is the use of different substances on different occasions. Use of different substances is common in patients with alcohol dependence or substance dependence (Caetano & Weisner, 1995), the majority of whom use substances simultaneously (Staines, Magura, Foote, Deluca, & Kosanke, 2001; Olthuis, Darredeau, & Barrett, 2013). Longitudinal studies in community samples are able to discriminate between simultaneous and concurrent polydrug use, but a differential impact upon subsequent health outcomes including psychological distress, physical symptoms, and services utilization has not been identified (Earley-wine & Newcomb, 1997).

Clinicians and researchers use the term "polysubstance dependence" more frequently as shorthand for patients for whom DSM-IV criteria suggest that the patient fulfill independent dependence criteria for several different substances. Conway, Kane, Ball, Poling, and Rounsaville (2003) call this construct "polysubstance involvement." According to DSM-IV (American Psychiatric Association, 1994, 2000), these patients should have a diagnosis of substance dependence for each substance for which the person meets criteria. Because there is room for misinterpretation between the formal DSM-IV concept of polysubstance dependence and the more frequently used broad concept of use of multiple substances that is also described as "polysubstance dependence," we use in this chapter the convention "multiple substance use disorders" to denote the latter, broad concept, reserving the former for cases in which a formal DSM-based diagnosis applies. "Multiple SUDs" here denotes that the identified subject or sample has two or more formal SUD diagnoses, at least meeting criteria for substance abuse, or meets it by reasonable proxy, such as seeking treatment. "Multiple substance dependence" means that the identified subject or sample meets formal or reasonable proxy criteria for two or more substance dependence disorders.

EPIDEMIOLOGY

Readers of the research and clinical addiction literature face a problem in understanding what is meant by terms used to describe multiple SUDs in a specific sample population. These terms are variously given as "polysubstance abuse," "polydrug abuse," "polyaddiction," and "multiple-drug dependence." As stated earlier, "polysubstance abuse," in a narrow DSM-IV perspective, is relatively unlikely to occur, especially in clinical settings, where patients are likely to meet criteria for several SUD diagnoses. On the other hand, the terms "polysubstance abuse" and "polydrug abuse" are frequently used by clinicians and researchers as descriptors of multiple drug use in populations of patients who have an index diagnosis of substance dependence, such as opioid dependence, and who meet at least DSM substance abuse criteria for the other substances.

The use of differing phraseology to describe use of multiple drugs is not limited to the domain of mental health and addiction clinicians and researchers. Cause of death statements from medical examiners and coroners often contain terms such as "polydrug toxicity," "polypharmacy," "multiple drug poisoning," and "polypharmaceutical overdose" to describe multiple-drug-induced deaths (Cone et al., 2004).

Population-Based Studies

When considered in community samples, the presence of an SUD diagnosis elevates lifetime risks of additional SUD diagnoses (Regier et al., 1990; Compton, Thomas, Stinson, & Grant, 2007). In the National Comorbidity Study (NCS), more than 40% of individuals with DSM-III-R alcohol dependence had, excluding nicotine dependence, co-occurring drug abuse or dependence (Kessler et al., 1997). Between 13 and 18% of those with alcohol abuse also have a co-occurring lifetime drug use disorder (Kessler et al., 1997). Lifetime drug use disorder was also present in 21.5% of subjects (odds ratio [OR] = 7.1) with an alcohol use disorder identified in the Epidemiologic Catchment Area Survey (ECA; Regier et al., 1990). In addition, among individuals with a nonalcohol SUD in the ECA study, 47.3% also had a lifetime alcohol use disorder. Excluding nicotine dependence, which was not surveyed in the ECA, individuals with cocaine abuse/dependence have the strongest risk (84.8%; OR = 36.3) of any group with an SUD for an additional alcohol use disorder (Regier et al., 1990). In the ECA, the associated use disorder for barbiturates, opiates, amphetamines, and hallucinogens demonstrates an OR for an additional lifetime alcohol use disorder of 10.0 or more (Regier et al., 1990).

However, if one tries to understand the temporal relationship between classes of substances used, lifetime diagnoses do not easily allow for the attribution that the use of multiple substances is temporally co-emergent. Using this threshold to determine multiple substance abuse may lower its specificity and therefore overestimate its prevalence. Past-year prevalence rates are more likely than lifetime rates to provide higher specificity for identifying persons with concurrent multiple substance use in a subpopulation identified as having two or more SUDs. There are only a few national surveys that have presented past-year data on substance use comorbidity. The National Epidemiologic Survey on Alcohol and Related Conditions (NESARC) demonstrated, as would be expected, dramatically increased 12-month risk of any drug use disorders among respondents with alcohol dependence compared to those with no alcohol dependence (OR = 9.8) (Hasin, Stinson, Ogburn, & Grant, 2007) and similar risk for any 12-month alcohol use disorders among those with drug dependence (OR = 15.0) (Compton et al., 2007). In addition, data from the annual National Survey on Drug Use and Health (NSDUH; Substance Abuse and Mental Health Services Administration [SAMHSA], 2011b) offer an important source of epidemiological data on substance dependence using criteria specified in DSM-IV.

Adolescents

Adolescent substance users are a subgroup identified as being at high risk for concurrent polysubstance use and, with that, progression to hazardous use, abuse, or dependence (Brook, Brook, Zhang, Cohen, & Whiteman, 2002). The NSDUH, formerly titled the National Household Survey on Drug Abuse (NHSDA), includes subjects from age 12 and offers community substance use data on adolescents who are not typically covered in other national surveys. Compared with older age groups, younger users in treatment settings are more likely to report polydrug use (SAMHSA, 2003). Although males overall are more likely than females to use or be dependent on alcohol, cannabis, or cocaine, Kandel, Chen, Warner, Kessler, and Grant (1997), using NHSDA data to determine abuse and dependence by proxy, demonstrated that these gender differences for rates of use and dependence rates among users are largely attenuated among adolescents. Adolescent girls who use alcohol or illicit drugs are at higher risk for dependence than adolescent boys, and among female users of alcohol, cannabis, or cocaine, the rates of dependence are the highest in adolescents as compared with older age groups. The 2010 NSDUH results show that among individuals ages 12–17, 6.9% of males and 7.7% of females had past-year substance dependence or abuse versus 12.2% of males and 5.8% of females among individuals age 18 or older (SAMHSA, 2011b).

Clinical Samples

In treatment samples, multiple SUDs are common but typically underdiagnosed (Ananth, Vandeater, Kamal, & Brodsky, 1989; Rosenthal, Hellerstein, & Miner, 1992). In a review of 69,891 admissions to publicly funded treatment programs in Tennessee between 1998 and 2004, Kedia, Sell, and Relvea (2007) found that poly-drug use was reported in 48.7% of admissions. In general, the risk for comorbid substance and other mental disorder diagnoses is increased when comparing clinical to community samples, and the highest rates of comorbid SUDs and other mental disorders are typically found in institutional populations, including psychiatric units, substance abuse programs, and jails and prisons (Regier et al., 1990; Kokkevi & Stefanis, 1995; Jordan, Schlenger, Fairbank, & Caddell, 1996; Hien, Zimberg, Weisman, First, & Ackerman, 1997). This is due in part to the selection bias that the people who are most likely admitted to treatment programs have impairment due to their drug use. Because of higher severity, they are at higher risk than other drug users for an additional substance use diagnosis (Rosenthal, Nunes, & Le Fauve, 2012).

Comorbidity of various SUDs and other mental disorders tends to cluster among certain subsets of the general population, such that more than half of the lifetime alcohol, drug, and mental disorders diagnoses can be found among about 14% of the population (Kessler et al., 1994). In any year, almost 59% of the community sample with an alcohol, drug, or other mental (ADM) disorder meet criteria for three or more lifetime ADM disorders (Kessler et al., 1994). Therefore, as compared to the community, treatment settings that aggregate those with an SUD are also most likely to cluster people at highest risk for multiple SUDs. This is borne out in large-scale family genetics studies. For example, in the Collaborative Study on the Genetics of Alcoholism (COGA), among 1,212 subjects recruited from addiction treatment centers with definite alcohol dependence, 62% had an additional diagnosis of cannabis and/or cocaine dependence (Bierut et al., 1998).

Treatment Episode Data Set (TEDS) data consistently reveal that about half of treatment admissions have reported multiple SUDs. Fifty-six percent of all 2006 TEDS admissions reported abuse of multiple substances, with alcohol, marijuana and cocaine the most common secondary substances. Alcohol was reported in 61% of all admissions (40% as the primary substance), marijuana was reported in 37% of admissions (16% as primary), and cocaine was reported in 32% of all admissions (14% as primary) (SAMHSA, 2008). This means that in addition to the index substance for which the patient was admitted to treatment, a substantial portion of patients are also abusing other substances. The SAMHSA-sponsored National Survey of Substance Abuse Treatment Services (N-SSATS) demonstrated that of the 1,172,841 people receiving treatment in 12,532 responding facilities in 2010, 42.5% (n = 498,671) were being treated for abuse or dependence on alcohol and at least one other substance (SAMHSA, 2011a). Thirty-one percent were in treatment for drug use disorders only, while the remaining 21% were in treatment for alcohol use disorders only.

Multiple SUDs

The increased risk of comorbidity among treatment-seeking populations over that of the general population has clinical implications for the outcome of treatment (Rosenthal & Westreich, 1999). Patients with multiple SUDs have greater difficulty achieving remission in intensive addiction treatment (Ritsher, Moos, & Finney, 2002). In addition, a history of multiple substance use predicts relapse to drugs in addiction treatment follow-up studies (Walton, Blow, & Booth, 2000). Among patients in treatment for SUDs in the 2-year follow-up study by Walton and colleagues, subjects (n = 241) self-reported their current primary substances of choice. Forty-one percent indicated alcohol as the sole drug of abuse. Among the 59.1% who were polysubstance users, the drug of choice was alcohol (79.1%), cocaine (72.7%), marijuana (48.2%), stimulants (8.6%), sedatives (13.7%), heroin (9.4%), opiates (16.5%), and hallucinogens (5.0%).

Nicotine and Multiple SUDs

Nicotine dependence has not been traditionally thought of in the context of treating drug-abuse problems, even among clinicians trained in addiction treatment. Consequently, when multiple SUDs are considered, the discussion usually does not include whether the person referred to is a habitual smoker. Nonetheless, over 90% of patients in methadone maintenance treatment are current tobacco smokers, a reasonable proxy for nicotine dependence (Clemmey, Brooner, Chutuape, Kidorf, & Stitzer, 1997). Similarly, 90% of patients in alcoholism inpatient treatment are current smokers (Beatty, Blanco, Hames, & Nixon, 1997). Thus, even among patients identified as having only one current SUD, these patients are, in fact, multiply drug dependent.

Multiple Substance Use among Alcoholics

The concurrent abuse of alcohol and drugs is a significant problem. Alcohol and drug use disorders frequently overlap, and there are high rates of nonalcohol SUDs among patients in treatment for alcohol use disorders (Beatty et al., 1997). The NESARC study found 12-month prevalence rates of 7.35% for alcohol use disorders only, 0.9% for drug use disorders only, and 1.1% for comorbid alcohol and drug use disorders. The 12-month prevalence of treatment seeking was significantly higher in those with comorbid alcohol and drug use disorders, 21.76%, compared with 6.06% for those with an alcohol use disorder only, and 15.63% for those with a drug use disorder only (Stinson et al., 2005). The NESARC study also found that individuals with both alcohol and drug use disorders had lower rates of remission than those with either alcohol or drug use disorders, but not both (Karno, Grella, Niv, Warda, & Moore, 2008). Results from the 2010 NSDUH indicated a similar prevalence when looking at past-year dependence or abuse. Twenty-two million persons age 12 or older met criteria for past substance dependence or abuse in the past year (8.7% of the population age 12 or older). Of these, 2.9 million had dependence or abuse of alcohol and illicit drugs (approximately 1.1%), 4.2 million had dependence or abuse of illicit drugs only, and 15 million had dependence or abuse of alcohol only (SAMHSA, 2011b).

Multiple Substance Use among Injecting Heroin Users

Injection drug use (IDU) is highly correlated with use of multiple substances. Heroin IDUs frequently use multiple drugs in addition to nicotine, such as alcohol, benzodiazepines, cannabis, and amphetamines, and there do not appear to be differences between treatment and nontreatment samples with regard to the number of either lifetime or current dependence diagnoses (Darke & Ross, 1997; Dinwiddie, Cottler, Compton, & Abdallah, 1996; Kidorf, Brooner, King, Chutuape, & Stitzer, 1996). Early polysubstance use also correlates with later IDU. Trenz et al. (2012) showed that individuals with early onset polysubstance use had higher rates of IDU than those who initiated use later. Darke and Ross (1997) recruited a nonrandom sample of 222 Australian heroin injectors, half of whom were in methadone treatment, and found that they had used a mean of 5.3 different classes of substances in the prior 6 months, and 40% had three or more current DSM-III-R dependence diagnoses. Injecting drugs increases the risk for comorbid substance dependence. Dinwiddie and colleagues (1996) found elevated lifetime rates of alcohol, amphetamine, sedative/hypnotic opiate, and hallucinogen dependence among IDUs compared to non-IDUs with a substantial drug use history.

Severity of psychopathology also appears to be highly associated with multiple substance use. Compared to users of cocaine alone, compulsive simultaneous users of cocaine and heroin ("speedball") have higher Minnesota Multiphasic Personality Inventory (MMPI) scores on Depression and Trait Anxiety with more severe psychopathology (Malow, West, Corrigan, Pena, & Lott, 1992). With frequent use of this combination, cocaine abusers who are using opiates to reduce the jitters and "crash" of intravenous cocaine use likely increase the risk of heroin dependence in this population (Levin, Foltin, & Fischman, 1996).

Darke and Ross (1997) demonstrated in a sample of Australian heroin IDUs that heroin use is correlated strongly with not only multiple substance use but also comorbid psychiatric disorders. Among IDUs, the extent and severity of non-substance-related psychopathology is a strong and linear predictor of the extent of multiple substance dependence. The prevalence of current mood and/or anxiety disorders was about 55%, with 25% having both a current mood and anxiety disorder—in each case clearly greater than the prevalence in the general population (Darke & Ross, 1997; Kessler et al., 1994). Darke and Ross (1997) also found a significant positive correlation between the number of lifetime drug dependence diagnoses and the number of lifetime comorbid psychiatric diagnoses in IDUs, and a similar positive correlation ($p < .001$) for current disorders. Although a causal attribution cannot be made, the onset of the mood or anxiety disorder preceded the onset of the heroin dependence in 60–80% of cases, suggesting that use of multiple drugs addresses untreated, underlying psychiatric disorders. However, the increased prevalence of multiple substance dependence in persons with more severe psychopathology might be due to shared genetic vulnerability; attempts to manage mood and anxiety thorough self-medication; or disturbances in motivation, judgment, and behavior directly due to psychopathology that increase vulnerability to addiction. In addition, it can be argued that multiple drug use can itself result in a broad range of psychiatric sequelae.

Gender Issues

In the general population, significantly more men than women across ethnic groups (white, black, Hispanic) either use or are dependent on alcohol, cannabis, or cocaine (Kandel, Chen, Warner, Kessler, & Grant, 1997). Women who use nicotine, however, are more likely to meet dependence criteria than men (Kandel et al., 1997). In general, women with SUDs have higher rates of other psychiatric comorbidity compared to men (Rosenthal et al., 2012). Yet in examining gender effects in opioid dependence, in a study of heroin users, there did not appear to be a gender-based difference in risk for dependence on multiple substances, which may be related to the equivalent risk of mental disorders in this subpopulation (Darke & Ross, 1997). In the general population, there were clear gender differences in the risk for anxiety and mood disorders, with the relative risk for females about double that for males (Kessler et al., 1994). In multiple-substance-dependent IDUs, who clearly had high disorder severity, there appeared to be no difference by gender in either the lifetime prevalence of mood and anxiety disorders or the prevalence of anxiety disorders. Only the rate of depressive disorders was significantly elevated for females over males (Darke & Ross, 1997).

PERSONALITY CORRELATES

In community samples, 28.6% of individuals with a current alcohol use disorder and 47.7% of those with a current drug use disorder have at least one personality disorder (PD; Grant et al., 2004). Furthermore, of individuals with at least one PD, 16.4% had a current alcohol use disorder and 6.5% had a current drug use disorder. PDs are associated with poorer treatment outcome for patients with alcohol dependence and drug dependence (Helzer & Pryzbeck, 1988; Rounsaville, Dolinsky, Babor, & Meyer, 1987). In various treatment settings, patients with SUDs screened with standard instruments met criteria for PDs, with 57–73% having at least one PD diagnosis and 35–50% having at least two PD diagnoses (Kleinman et al., 1990; Kranzler, Satel, & Apter, 1994; Marlowe et al., 1995; Rounsaville et al., 1998; Skinstad & Swain, 2001). PD diagnoses are associated with an increased risk of multiple substance use in IDUs (Darke, Williamson, Ross, Teeson, & Lynskey, 2004).

Categorical Personality Disorders

Individuals with the "Cluster B" PDs (antisocial, borderline, narcissistic, histrionic), as described in DSM-IV (American Psychiatric Association, 1994) demonstrate elevated rates of SUDs (Mors & Sorenson, 1994). Conversely, patients with SUDs have an elevated rate of Cluster B PDs, and patients dependent on multiple substances are more likely to be diagnosed with Cluster B PDs than non-multiple-substance-dependent subjects (Skinstad & Swain, 2001). For example, in 370 patients with heterogenous SUDs, Rounsaville and colleagues (1998) found that 57% had an DSM-III-R PD diagnosis, of which 45.7% were Cluster B, including 27% with antisocial personality disorder (ASPD) and 18.4% with borderline personality disorder (BPD).

Antisocial Personality Disorder

The risk of ASPD among drug-dependent individuals in community samples is 29 times that of the general population, and rates of ASPD among IDUs range between 35 and 71% (Regier et al., 1990; Dinwiddie et al., 1996; Darke et al., 2004; Agrawal, Lynskey, Madden, Bucholz, & Heath, 2007). ASPD appears to be a risk factor for multiple substance dependence. For example, patients who meet dependence criteria for both cocaine and alcohol have higher psychiatric severity and are more likely to have ASPD than patients with cocaine dependence only (Cunningham, Corrigan, Malow, & Smason, 1993). Among clinical populations, sociopathy among substance abusers is associated with high treatment dropout and poorer treatment outcome (Leal, Ziedonis, & Kosten, 1994; Woody, McLellan, Luborsky, & O'Brien, 1985). Tómasson and Vaglum (2000) followed 100 treatment-seeking alcoholics with ASPD for 28 months in a European study: 47% of the cohort had multiple SUDs, and they had more prior admissions and were more frequently involved in fights. The route of drug administration also is associated with elevated risk of ASPD. Compared to non-IDUs with a substantial drug use history, rates of ASPD are elevated in IDUs (Dinwiddie et al., 1996). Increased social deviance is a factor that likely increases risk of access to hard drugs. However, the specific contribution of ASPD to SUD risk is less clearly delineated. Family genetics studies suggest that familial aggregation of SUDs is largely independent of ASPD (Bierut et al., 1998; Merikangas et al., 1998).

Borderline Personality Disorder

Although ASPD has been the PD that is traditionally diagnosed in patients with SUDs, and is typically believed to be responsible for the higher risk of self- and other-harmful behaviors in this population, evidence suggests that some proportion of the risk for multiple substance use, as well as suicide attempts and psychiatric severity, is associated with BPD (Darke et al., 2004). Trull, Sher, Minks-Brown, Durbin, and Burr (2000) reviewed 26 studies of the comorbidity of BPD and SUDs and found rates of BPD that ranged from 5 to 65%. Much of the variability between studies was due to different instruments used and populations studied. However, the rate across studies was 57.4%; thus, it is clear that the prevalence of BPD was elevated among patients with SUDs (Trull et al., 2000). BPD is present in 18–34% percent of cocaine abusers in treatment settings and 46% of injection heroin users in and out of treatment (Kleinman et al., 1990; Kranzler et al., 1994; Marlowe et al., 1995; Darke et al., 2004). In a study of injection heroin users, 46% of the sample met criteria for BPD, including 38% who also met criteria for comorbid ASPD, yet there appeared to be little increased risk for harmful behaviors among IDUs with ASPD compared to those without ASPD (Darke et al., 2004).

Dimensional Approaches

In addition to the increased rates of SUD in persons with categorically defined PDs compared to controls, there are personality dimensions that may be predictive of increased risk for SUDs. Moreover, those with multiple SUDs tend to have more severe personality pathology, as measured on dimensional constructs, than do users of single substances, independent of drug of choice (Pedersen, Clausen, & Lavik, 1989; McCormick, Dowd, Quirt, & Zegarra, 1998). Multiple substance-dependent individuals tend to have high levels of two personality characteristics particularly related to behavioral disinhibition—impulsivity and sensation seeking (see review in Conway et al., 2003). Those with multiple substance dependence score lower in measures of behavioral inhibition (constraint) than those who prefer to use alcohol, cocaine, or cannabis singly (Conway, Swendson, Rounsaville, & Merikangas, 2002).

Impulsivity

Impulsivity/disinhibition appears to be a major factor in both SUD and BPD. Though impulsivity is associated with polysubstance use (O'Boyle & Barratt, 1993), and in addition to the risks for polysubstance abuse attributable to BPD as described earlier, impulsivity appears to be more elevated in comorbid BPD–SUD than in either disorder alone (Kreudelbach, McCormick, Schulz, & Grueneich, 1993; Morgenstern, Langenbucher, Labouvie, & Miller, 1997). As such, impulsivity may explain some of the increased risk in substance users with BPD for polydrug use and its sequelae. In an analysis of the association between personality and substance use in a nonclinical population screened for alcohol use or PDs, partialing out trait impulsivity significantly reduced the correlation between BPD or ASPD and the risk for an SUD, suggesting that at least part of the association between SUDs and personality may be due to underlying personality traits such as impulsivity (Casillas & Clark, 2002). On the balance, increased morbidity in polysubstance abusers might also be explained by a constitutional insensitivity to negative feedback from the environment. The poor performance of multiple subjects with SUDs on the Gambling Task suggests a heightened tendency to continue reinforced behavior in the context of increasing negative consequences (Grant, Contoreggi, & London, 2000).

Novelty Seeking

A related personality trait that consistently has been linked with vulnerability to development of an SUD is novelty or sensation seeking. Among children, those with higher sensation seeking are more likely to declare an intention to use alcohol and to have symptoms of substance abuse as adults (Cloninger, Sigvardsson, & Bohman, 1988; Webb, Baer, & McKelvey, 1995). Generally, persons with SUDs exhibit higher levels of this trait than do those without SUDs, whether they abuse alcohol or other substances (Conway et al., 2002). Moreover, users of multiple substances tend to have even higher levels of sensation seeking, such that the greater the involvement in multiple-substance dependence, the greater behavioral disinhibition (Pedersen et al.,

1989; Conway et al., 2003). Conversely, the high sensation seekers among cocaine-dependent individuals are more likely to have multiple SUDs (Ball, Carroll, & Rounsaville, 1994). Conway and colleagues (2003) demonstrated that the number of lifetime substance dependence diagnoses among 325 individuals in addiction treatment was positively and linearly associated with broad psychological measures of behavioral disinhibition. Compared to patients who were dependent upon one substance, those who were dependent upon two or more substances had higher scores on several different instruments used to rate behavioral undercontrol. All other things being equal (e.g., access, economic status), the more disinhibited the person with a vulnerability to substance dependence, the more likely it is that thresholds for contact with multiple drugs will be breached, and that vulnerability is linked to use of multiple drugs.

Other Characteristics

Multiple substance-dependent patients in treatment report lower mean levels of self-efficacy and higher mean levels of temptation regarding substance use in comparison to patients who are dependent only on alcohol (Edens & Willoughby, 1999). In addition to the increased impulsivity and sensation seeking of patients with multiple SUDs compared to patients without multiple SUDs, the former score higher on all measures of hostility and aggression (McCormick & Smith, 1995).

Typological Approaches

Another important development in elucidating the relationship between patterns of substance use and both categorical and dimensional approaches to measuring personality is the recognition of characteristic patterns, typically grouped into two broad categories among substance abusers, designated Types A and B (Ball, Kranzler, Tennen, Poling, & Rounsaville, 1998). Earlier classification systems in reference to alcoholism had a similar typology, variously referred to as Types 1 and 2 (Cloninger, 1987), developed out of measures in family genetic studies, or Types A and B (Babor et al., 1992), which developed through cluster analyses of a somewhat broader set of patient characteristics. Feingold and colleagues (1996), using a schema analogous to that of Babor et al. (1992) replicated the A/B classification in 521 subjects chosen from the community, inpatient and outpatient drug treatment programs, or outpatient psychiatric treatment programs. The subjects were grouped by presence of alcohol, cocaine, marijuana, or opiate abuse or dependence, and the authors found a consistent 60:40 ratio of Type A to Type B for each of the drug groups, suggesting clusters of personality characteristics that are independent of drug of choice. Similarly, in 370 patients in treatment for alcoholism, cocaine, or opiate dependence, Ball and colleagues (1998) replicated the A/B classification and also found a 60:40 Type A to Type B ratio. Type A substance abusers had less multiple drug use, as well as an older age of onset, fewer years of heavy use, less family history of substance abuse, less impulsivity, and less severe substance abuse. Type B substance abusers tended to have more severe characteristics than type A, scoring higher on the personality dimensions of neuroticism, novelty seeking, and harm avoidance. They also had a higher prevalence of multiple substance abuse, earlier age of onset, more childhood psychiatric symptoms, a higher incidence of all Cluster B PDs, and more family histories of substance abuse (Ball et al., 1998). The Type B profile is quite common in methadone patients, in whom there is a greater prevalence of ASPD than in the general population (Brooner, King, Kidorf, Schmidt, & Bigelow, 1997).

With respect to the issue at hand, compared to drug abusers who are categorized as Type A, Type B is predictive of multiple SUDs. This is an important refinement in the assessment of drug abusers: Since multiple SUDs do not occur in non-substance-abusing populations, this distinction gives some predictive power in the target subpopulation of those with SUDs. As described earlier, ASPD in persons with SUD is predictive of multiple SUDs, injection drug use, and higher severity; an earlier study indicated that ASPD is one of the best predictors of Type B membership among cocaine abusers (Ball et al., 1995). However, Ball et al. (1998) found that the basis for A/B distinctions in personality dimensions and disorders among the 370 patients in their study remained much the same when the cluster analysis was controlled for presence of ASPD. The typological distinction not only has heuristic value, but Type B patients also have more severe SUDs and relapse more quickly after addiction treatment than do Type A patients (Babor et al., 1992; Ball et al., 1995). In addition, the more frequent family history of SUD and early onset in the Type B patients is consistent with a stronger genetic component compared with late-onset Type A patients.

GENETIC AND FAMILY STUDIES

Vulnerability to substance abuse has general genetic, familial, and nonfamilial environmental factors, as well as factors that appear to be specific to a particular class of substances. A family history of substance abuse is one of the strongest risk factors for development of an SUD (Merikangas et al., 1998). Studies have demonstrated that there are genetic influences on the risk for substance abuse (Tsuang et al., 1996) and that, at least among men, abusing one category of drug is associated with a marked increase in the probability of abusing other classes of drugs (Tsuang et al., 1998). One of the strongest predictors for presence of an SUD is the presence of another SUD (Bierut et al., 1998).

Much of the evidence for the heritability of the general and specific vulnerability for an SUD is taken from studies of familial aggregation. Bierut and colleagues (1998) compared siblings of probands with alcohol dependence with those of a control group for the presence of lifetime SUDs. Not only were the siblings of alcoholic probands more likely to have a lifetime alcohol use disorder, but they also had an increased risk of cannabis, cocaine, and nicotine dependence. Fifty percent of the alcohol-dependent siblings of alcohol-dependent probands had an additional diagnosis of cannabis and/or cocaine dependence. It is compelling with respect to understanding the risk for multiple substance dependence that the siblings of cannabis-dependent probands had an increased risk of cannabis dependence, siblings of cocaine-dependent probands had an increased risk for cocaine dependence, and siblings of habitual smokers were at higher risk for nicotine dependence (Bierut et al., 1998). In another study, Tsuang et al. (1998) demonstrated that there is a general drug abuse vulnerability factor with genetic, family, and nonfamily environmental components that is shared across all drugs of abuse, in addition to genetic factors that appear to be unique for most classes of drug abuse. So, although there appear to be nongenetic general and specific factors for familial transmission of vulnerability to SUDs, multiple SUDs among probands render increased vulnerability to multiple SUDs in relatives at least through both drug-specific and common genetic factors.

NEUROPSYCHOLOGICAL IMPACT OF MULTIPLE SUDs

As compared with non-polysubstance-using drug abusers, those with multiple SUDs demonstrate the greatest degree of chronic neuropsychological impairment, and recover the least function with long-term abstinence (Beatty et al., 1997; Medina, Shear, Schafer, Armstrong, & Dyer, 2004). This may be due in part to the increased cumulative exposure of the brain to drugs and alcohol: Multiple substance users tend to use as much of a particular substance (e.g., alcohol or cocaine) as those who use only alcohol or cocaine (Selby & Azrin, 1998). Polysubstance users show high levels of impairment in executive functioning, particularly in working memory (Verdejo-García & Pérez-García, 2007; Fernández-Serrano, Pérez-García, Perales, & Verdejo-García, 2010). Selby and Azrin (1998) conducted a comprehensive neuropsychological battery with 355 prison inmates classified by DSM-IV criteria into four groups: those with alcohol use disorders, cocaine use disorders, multiple SUDs, and no history of an SUD. The multiple SUDs and the alcohol groups demonstrated more significant impairment on most measures than the cocaine or no-drug groups, but the multiple SUDs group performed worse than the cocaine-alone, alcohol-alone, or no SUD groups on measures of short-term memory, long-term memory, and visual motor ability. Beatty and colleagues (1997) found analogous results in their neuropsychological evaluation of spatial cognition in multiple SUD and non-multiple-SUD inpatient alcoholics who had at least 3 weeks of sobriety. Patients with multiple SUDs had more significant impairment of geographical knowledge requiring place localization, over and above the impairment of the alcoholics compared to controls on all other measures of visuospatial perception, construction, learning, and memory. After 3 weeks of sobriety, alcoholics with multiple SUDs, compared with alcoholics without multiple SUDs, also demonstrated greater memory deficits in tests of recall (Bondi, Drake, & Grant, 1998). The heavy cocaine users among the alcoholics had the worst deficits, suggestive of subcortical dysfunction due to small vessel infarcts. Subjects with multiple SUDs also demonstrated more impaired decision making through poor performance on the Gambling Task than non-drug-using controls (suggesting dysfunction of the ventromedial prefrontal cortex; Bechara, 1999; Grant et al., 2000).

Given the neuropsychological effects of multiple SUDs described earlier, it is important to recognize that baseline cognitive function also has a role in vulnerability to multiple SUDs. Premorbid intellectual functioning is a predictor of drug use: Compared to matched non-drug-using controls, multiple substance users were demonstrated to have lower fourth-grade Iowa Test composite and individual scores on Vocabulary, Reading, Language, Work–Study Skills, and Mathematics subtests (Block, Erwin, & Ghoneim, 2002).

SPECIAL POPULATIONS

Opioid Dependence and Opioid Maintenance Treatment

Polydrug use is the norm among heroin users. In a study of 329 primary heroin users by Darke and Hall (1995), the most prevalent drugs used during the preceding 6 months were tobacco (94%), cannabis (84%), alcohol (78%), benzodiazepines (64%), amphetamines (42%), cocaine (24%), and hallucinogens (22%); the mean number of drug classes used was 5.2. However, it appears that as they grow older, illicit drug users reduce their range of drugs: Age is inversely correlated in IDUs with the number of current dependence diagnoses, and young males who are not in treatment and who inject amphetamines are at higher risk for polysubstance use (Darke & Hall, 1995; Darke & Ross, 1997).

Cocaine Use

The use of cocaine by patients in methadone or buprenorphine maintenance treatment programs was reported to be as high as 73% in a sample of 1,038 newly admitted patients in 15 methadone clinics in New York City (Magura, Kang, Nwakeze, & Demsky, 1998). Contrary to popular belief, the simultaneous use of intravenous heroin and cocaine ("speedball") does not result in a novel set of experiences, nor does it reinforce the effects of either drug when used alone, especially when cocaine and heroin are used in high doses. Cocaine, however, has been shown to alleviate some symptoms of opioid withdrawal, and as such may be used in a self-medicating pattern, as mentioned earlier (Leri, Bruneau, & Stewart, 2003).

Cannabis Use

Cannabis use among patients in methadone treatment programs has been investigated to answer the practical question of whether cannabinoid-positive urine toxicology examinations predict poor treatment outcome. Both an Israeli study (Weizman, Gelkopf, Melamed, Adelson, & Bleich, 2004) and review of the three U.S. studies (Epstein & Preston, 2003) suggest that cannabis use is not a risk factor for treatment outcome of methadone-maintained outpatients. The authors concluded that cannabinoid-positive urines do not need to be a major focus of clinical attention.

Overdose

In examining both fatal and nonfatal heroin overdoses, the majority of cases involve simultaneous use of alcohol, benzodiazepines, and tricyclic antidepressants (TCAs), such that the toxicology of heroin overdose is probably best described as "polydrug toxicity" (Darke & Zador, 1996; Darke & Hall, 2003). In fatal heroin overdoses, alcohol has been used more than 50% of the time (Darke & Hall, 2003). The mechanism of action for the overdose appears to be the synergistic effect of the various depressants on the central nervous system, leading to respiratory collapse. This is further collaborated by autopsy findings of an inverse relationship between alcohol and morphine blood concentrations; in the presence of alcohol, lower levels of morphine are sufficient to result in death (Darke & Hall, 2003). In a study by Darke and Ross (2000) in Sydney, Australia, both fatal and nonfatal heroin overdoses were linked to concomitant use of TCAs but not selective serotonin reuptake inhibitors (SSRIs), despite the fact that heroin users in Australia predominantly use SSRIs instead of TCAs.

Adolescents and "Club Drugs"

Although club drugs, including MDMA (3,4-methylenedioxymethamphetamine), ketamine, and GHB (gamma-hydroxybutyrate), originally got their name from nightclubs and raves, they are now used in both club and nonclub settings (Rosenthal & Solhkhah, 2013). Overall, studies of typical MDMA users reveal high rates of multiple drug use (Parrott, Milani, Parmar, & Turner, 2001; Parrott, Sisk, & Turner, 2000; Rodgers, 2000; Schifano, Di Furia, Forza, Minicuci, & Bricolo, 1998). Among treatment seekers, heavy MDMA use is associated with increased psychopathology (Parrott et al., 2000; Schifano et al., 1998). In addition to use of alcohol and cannabis, the heavier the MDMA use, the more likely the co-use of stimulants and hallucinogens (Scholey et al., 2004). MDMA as a sole drug of abuse is an uncommon phenomenon; it is therefore a reasonable proxy for abuse of multiple substances (Rodgers, 2000).

Club Drugs and the Circuit Scene

Circuit parties are large-scale dance events, primarily for gay men, where use of multiple drugs is prevalent. Participants often travel from all over the country, and sometimes overseas, to attend these large gatherings that bring together several thousand gay men. MDMA, ketamine, GHB, cocaine, methamphetamine, and alcohol are the most frequently used substances. Studies indicate high rates of simultaneous drug use at circuit parties (Mansergh et al., 2001; Mattison, Ross, Wolfson, Franklin, & San Diego HIV Neurobehavioral Research Group, 2001; Lee, Galanter, Dermatis, & McDowell, 2003; Lee & Levounis, 2008). The average number of substances ingested by responders on the day of the circuit party studied by Lee et al. (2003) was 2.4, with a range of 0 to 7. Most people report that using drugs during a circuit party enhances the dancing experience, relieves inhibitions, and improves sex. Substance use and sex can become connected to the point that sex itself can trigger cravings (Levounis & Ruggiero, 2006). Others describe multiple substance use as self-medication for depressed mood, anxiety, social isolation, or stress associated with living with HIV disease or AIDS (Levounis, Drescher, & Barber, 2012). Some participants report a synergistic effect between drugs, as in the case of the MDMA and ketamine combination that according to some users results in a more intense "high," while others feel that ketamine prolongs the effect of MDMA.

Multiple Substance Use and HIV Risk

Multiple substance use has become a great concern in the gay community in the context of the crystal methamphetamine epidemic and the rising incidence of HIV transmission among gay men in large urban environments. In a study of 214 individuals utilizing a Massachusetts Department of Health van service targeting men who have sex with men (MSM), participants reporting polysubstance use were more likely to be infected with HIV (OR = 4.62; p = .03). They were also nine times more likely to report having unprotected sex in the 12 months prior to study enrollment (adjusted OR = 9.53; p = .007) compared to nonpolysubstance-using MSM (Mimiaga et al., 2008). It is reasonable to suspect that an important personality factor may be involved, such as behavioral dyscontrol in the form of impulsivity or sensation seeking. When disinhibiting drugs such as alcohol and GHB are taken together, a person who has high trait impulsivity is even more likely to engage in risky behavior. For example, Cook et al. (2001) identified gay men recently infected with syphilis in Liverpool, UK, and found that 61% had used GHB as an aphrodisiac in the context of unprotected sex.

The association of multiple substance use and HIV raises medical concerns in terms of both HIV transmission and treatment. Sexual disinhibition and increased risk of HIV transmission have been correlated with substance use, and particularly to stimulants, not only in the gay community but also in a variety of other settings (Levounis, Galanter, Dermatis, Hamowy, & DeLeon, 2002). These findings support the hypothesis that multiple substance use may directly result in increased rates of unsafe sex and HIV seroconversion. In terms of HIV treatment, club drugs such as MDMA and GHB interact with protease inhibitors, resulting in dangerously high levels of the club drugs (Harrington, Woodward, Hooton, & Horn, 1999). Furthermore, patients often fail to adhere to complicated HIV pharmacological regimens during intoxication with or withdrawal from a variety of different drugs of abuse (Lee et al., 2003).

TREATMENT CONSIDERATIONS

At its simplest, treating patients with chronic multiple SUDs requires a focus on each disorder separately, in addition to providing the patient with a coherent overall rationale and approach to addiction treatment. Although multiple SUDs have a net negative impact on treatment outcome, Abellanas and McLellan (1993) have shown that patients with multiple SUDs report generally similar motivation for change across drugs of abuse, which means that their desire to modify their substance use remains consistent across substances. Motivational interviewing is an essential element in both engaging the polysubstance-using patient in treatment and promoting treatment adherence (Miller & Rollnick, 1991; Levounis & Arnaout, 2010). An additional issue is the specific impact of other substance use on recovery for a particular SUD. Treatment is therefore best constructed with a bottom-up approach, using evidence-based approaches where available (Rosenthal, 2004) rather than assuming that optimal treatment should be largely psychotherapeutic or pharmacotherapeutic. For example, there is a clear evidence base for the use of methadone as an agonist therapy for stabilization of opioid dependence (Ciraulo, 2003). However, there is not good evidence that an adequate dose of methadone for treating opioid dependence will suffice in treating cocaine abuse or dependence. Since there is no approved pharmacotherapy for cocaine use disorders at present, the optimal therapy should come from the behavioral treatments, which also have an evidence base. As such, the approach to treating patients with opioid dependence and cocaine dependence should have both pharmacotherapeutic and psychotherapeutic components.

In the acute setting, multiple SUDs present the treatment team with significant challenges. Given a patient's complicated history of recent and chronic use of multiple substances, the clinician in the emergency room or the detoxification unit often struggles to make treatment priorities out of a constellation of signs and symptoms that may be the result of intoxication or withdrawal from a number of substances. Given the frequent occurrence of multiple substance use diagnoses (particularly between alcohol and other drugs), any attempt to attribute observed findings associated with comorbid substance use to a single substance or class of substances is often difficult, if not impossible. Intoxication from stimulants may result in psychotic symptoms, but so does withdrawal from sedatives. Lethargy is not only a classic sign of opioid intoxication but also a consequence of stimulant withdrawal. A patient who currently uses both benzodiazepines and crystal methamphetamine and presents with seizures may be either acutely intoxicated with methamphetamine or suffering from severe benzodiazepine withdrawal, or both. Furthermore, the serious psychosocial complications of multiple SUDs adds significantly to the difficulty in treating the already confusing biological manifestations of the illness. As in the case of relapse prevention, the successful management of acute multiple substance use relies primarily on identification and treatment of each intoxication and withdrawal syndrome separately. For example, patients with serious withdrawal from heroin and alcohol typically require both opioid agonists (e.g., methadone or buprenorphine) and benzodiazepines (e.g., chlordiazapoxide or lorazepam), with particular attention to potential synergistic effects between the two classes of medications.

REFERENCES

Abellanas, L., & McLellan, A. T. (1993). "Stage of change" by drug problem in concurrent opioid, cocaine, and cigarette users. *J Psychoactive Drugs, 25*, 307–313.

Agrawal, A., Lynskey, M. T., Madden, P. A., Bucholz, K. K., & Heath, A. C. (2007). A latent class analysis of illicit drug abuse/dependence: Results from the National Epidemiological Survey on Alcohol and Related Conditions. *Addiction, 102*(1), 94–104.

American Psychiatric Association. (1980). *Diagnostic and statistical manual of mental disorders* (3rd ed.). Washington, DC: Author.

American Psychiatric Association. (1987). *Diagnostic and statistical manual of mental disorders* (3rd ed., rev.). Washington, DC: Author.

American Psychiatric Association. (1994). *Diagnostic and statistical manual of mental disorders* (4th ed.). Washington, DC: Author.

American Psychiatric Association. (2000). *Diagnostic and statistical manual of mental disorders* (4th ed., text rev.). Washington, DC: Author.

Ananth, J., Vandeater, S., Kamal, M., & Brodsky, A. (1989). Missed diagnosis of substance abuse in psychiatric patients. *Hosp Community Psych, 40*, 297–299.

Babor, T. F., Hofmann, M., DelBoca, F. K., Hesselbrock, V., Meyer, R. E., Dolinsky, Z. S., et al. (1992). Types of alcoholics: I. Evidence for an empirically derived typology based on indicators of vulnerability and severity. *Arch Gen Psychiatry, 49*, 599–608.

Ball, S. A., Carroll, K. M., Babor, T. F., & Rounsaville, B. J. (1995). Subtypes of cocaine abusers: Support for a Type A–Type B distinction. *J Consult Clin Psychol, 63*, 115–124.

Ball, S. A., Carroll, K. M., & Rounsaville, B. J. (1994). Sensation seeking, substance abuse, and psychopathology in treatment-seeking and community cocaine abusers. *J Consult Clin Psychol, 62,* 1053–1057.

Ball, S. A., Kranzler, H. R., Tennen, H., Poling, J. C., & Rounsaville, B. J. (1998). Personality disorder and dimension differences between Type A and Type B substance abusers. *J Pers Disord, 12,* 1–12.

Beatty, W. W., Blanco, C. R., Hames, K. A., & Nixon, S. J. (1997). Spatial cognition in alcoholics: Influence of concurrent abuse of other drugs. *Drug Alcohol Depend, 44,* 167–174.

Bechara, A. (1999). Different contributions of the human amygdala and ventromedial prefrontal cortex to decision-making. *J Neurosci, 19,* 5473–5481.

Bierut, L. J., Dinwidie, S. H., Begleiter, H., Crowe, R. R., Hesselbrock, V., Nurnberger, J. I., et al. (1998). Familial transmission of substance dependence: Alcohol, marijuana, cocaine and habitual smoking. *Arch Gen Psychiatry, 55,* 982–988.

Birnbach, D. J., Browne, I. M., Kim, A., Stein, D. J., & Thys, D. M. (2001). Identification of polysubstance abuse in the parturient. *Br J Anaesth, 87*(3), 488–490.

Block, R. I., Erwin, W. J., & Ghoneim, M. M. (2002). Chronic drug use and cognitive impairments. *Pharmacol Biochem Behav, 73,* 491–504.

Bondi, M. W., Drake, A. I., & Grant, I. (1998). Verbal learning and memory in alcohol abusers and polysubstance abusers with concurrent alcohol abuse. *J Int Neuropsychol Soc, 4,* 319–328.

Brook, D. W., Brook, J. S., Zhang, C., Cohen, P., & Whiteman, M. (2002). Drug use and the risk of major depressive disorder, alcohol dependence, and substance use disorders. *Arch Gen Psychiatry, 59*(11), 1039–1044.

Brooner, R. K., King, V. L., Kidorf, M., Schmidt, C. W., & Bigelow, G. E. (1997). Psychiatric and substance use comorbidity among treatment seeking opioid abusers. *Arch Gen Psychiatry, 54,* 71–80.

Caetano, R., & Weisner, C. (1995). The association between DSM-III-R alcohol dependence, psychological distress and drug use. *Addiction, 90,* 351–359.

Casillas, A., & Clark, L. A. (2002). Dependency, impulsivity, and self-harm: Traits hypothesized to underlie the association between Cluster B personality and substance use disorders. *J Pers Disord, 16,* 424–436.

Ciraulo, D. A. (2003). Outcome predictors in substance use disorders. *Psychiatric Clin N Am, 26*(2), 381–409.

Clemmey, P., Brooner, R., Chutuape, M. A., Kidorf, M., & Stitzer, M. (1997). Smoking habits and attitudes in a methadone maintenance treatment population. *Drug Alcohol Depend, 44,* 123–132.

Cloninger, C. R. (1987). A systematic method for clinical description and classification of personality variants. *Arch Gen Psychiatry, 44,* 573–588.

Cloninger, C. R., Sigvardsson, S., & Bohman, M., (1988). Childhood personality predicts alcohol abuse in young adults. *Alcohol Clin Exp Res, 12,* 494–505.

Compton, W. M., Thomas, Y. F., Stinson, F. S., & Grant, B. F. (2007). Prevalence, correlates, disability, and comorbidity of DSM-IV drug abuse and dependence in the United States: Results from the National Epidemiologic Survey on Alcohol and Related Conditions. *Arch Gen Psychiatry, 64*(5), 566–576.

Cone, E. J., Fant, R. V., Rohay, J. M., Caplan, Y. H., Ballina, M., Reder, R. F., et al. (2004). Oxycodone involvement in drug abuse deaths: II. Evidence for toxic multiple drug–drug interactions. *J Anal Toxicol, 28*(7), 616–624.

Conway, K. P., Kane, R. J., Ball, S. A., Poling, J. C., & Rounsaville, B. J. (2003). Personality, substance of choice, and polysubstance involvement among substance dependent patients. *Drug Alcohol Depend, 71,* 65–75.

Conway, K. P., Swendson, J. D., Rounsaville, B. J., & Merikangas, K. R. (2002). Personality, drug of choice, and comorbid psychopathology among substance abusers. *Drug Alcohol Depend, 65,* 225–234.

Cook, P. A., Clark, P., Bellis, M. A., Ashton, J. R., Syed, Q., Hoskins, A., et al. (2001). Re-emerging syphilis in the UK: A behavioral analysis of infected individuals. *Commun Dis Public Health,* *4,* 253–258.

Cunningham, S. C., Corrigan, S. A., Malow, R. M., & Smason, I. H. (1993). Psychopathology in inpatients dependent on cocaine or alcohol and cocaine. *Psychol Addict Behav, 7,* 246–250.

Darke, S., & Hall, W. (1995). Levels and correlates of polydrug use among heroin users and regular amphetamine users. *Drug Alcohol Depend, 39,* 231–235.

Darke, S., & Hall, W. (2003). Heroin overdose: Research and evidence-based intervention. *J Urban Health, 80*(2), 189–200.

Darke, S., & Ross, J. (1997). Polydrug dependence and psychiatric comorbidity among heroin injectors. *Drug Alcohol Depend, 48,* 135–141.

Darke, S., & Ross, J. (2000). The use of antidepressants among injecting drug users in Sydney, Australia. *Addiction, 95,* 407–417.

Darke, S., Williamson, A., Ross, J., Teesson, M., & Lynskey, M. (2004). Borderline personality disorder, antisocial personality disorder and risk-taking among heroin users: Findings from the Australian Treatment Outcome Study (ATOS), *Drug Alcohol Depend, 74*(1), 77–83.

Darke, S., & Zador, D. (1996). Fatal heroin overdose: A review. *Addiction, 91,* 1765–1772.

Degenhardt, L., Lynskey, M., Coffey, C., & Patton, G. (2002). Diagnostic orphans' among young adult cannabis users: Persons who report dependence symptoms but do not meet diagnostic criteria. *Drug Alcohol Depend, 67,* 205–212.

Dinwiddie, S. H., Cottler, L., Compton, W., & Abdallah, A. B. (1996). Psychopathology and HIV risk among injection drug users in and out of treatment. *Drug Alcohol Depend, 43,* 1–11.

Earleywine, M., & Newcomb, M. D. (1997). Concurrent versus simultaneous polydrug use: Prevalence, correlates, discriminant validity and prospective effects on health outcomes. *Exp Clin Psychopharmacol, 5,* 353–364.

Edens, J. F., & Willoughby, F. W. (1999). Motivational profiles of polysubstance-dependent patients: Do they differ from alcohol-dependent patients? *Addict Behav, 24,* 195–206.

Edwards, G., & Gross, M. (1976). Alcohol dependence: Provisional description of a clinical syndrome. *BMJ, 1,* 1058–1061.

Epstein, D. H., & Preston, K. L. (2003). Does cannabis use predict poor outcome for heroin-dependent patients on maintenance treatment?: Past findings and more evidence against. *Addiction, 98,* 269–279.

Feingold, A., Ball, S. A., Kranzler, H. R., & Rounsaville, B. J. (1996). Generalizability of the Type A/Type B distinction across different psychoactive substances. *Am J Drug Alcohol Abuse, 22,* 449–462.

Fernández-Serrano, M. J., Pérez-García, M., Perales, J. C., & Verdejo-García, A. (2010). Prevalence of executive dysfunction in cocaine, heroin and alcohol users enrolled in therapeutic communities. *Eur J Pharmacol, 626*(1), 104–112.

First, M. B., & Pincus, H. A. (2002). The DSM-IV Text Revision: Rationale and potential impact on clinical practice. *Psychiatr Serv, 53,* 288–292.

Grant, B., & Hartford, T. (1990). Concurrent and simultaneous use of alcohol with sedatives and tranquilizers: Results of a national survey. *J Subst Abuse, 2,* 1–14.

Grant, B. F., Stinson, F. S., Dawson, D. A., Chou, S. P., Ruan, W. J., & Pickering, R. P. (2004). Co-occurrence of 12-month alcohol and drug use disorders and personality disorders in the United States: Results from the National Epidemiologic Survey on Alcohol and Related Conditions. *Arch Gen Psychiatry, 61,* 361–368.

Grant, B. F., Stinson, F. S., & Harford, T. C. (2001). Age at onset of alcohol use and DSM-IV alcohol abuse and dependence: A 12-year follow-up. *J Subst Abuse, 13,* 493–504.

Grant, S., Contoreggi, C., & London, E. D. (2000). Drug abusers show impaired performance in a laboratory test of decision making. *Neuropsychologia, 38,* 1180–1187.

Harrington, R. D., Woodward, J. A., Hooton, T. M., & Horn, J. R. (1999). Life-threatening interactions between HIV-1 protease inhibitors and the illicit drugs MDMA and gamma-hydroxybutyrate. *Arch Int Med, 159,* 2221–2224.

Hasin, D., & Paykin, A. (1998). Dependence symptoms but no diagnosis: Diagnostic "orphans" in a community sample. *Drug Alcohol Depend, 50*, 19–26.

Hasin, D., & Paykin, A. (1999). Dependence symptoms but no diagnosis: diagnostic "orphans" in a 1992 national sample. *Drug Alcohol Depend, 53*, 215–222.

Hasin, D., Paykin, A., Endicott, J., & Grant, B. (1999). The validity of DSM-IV alcohol abuse: Drunk drivers vs. all others. *J Stud Alcohol, 60*, 746–755.

Hasin, D., Van Rossem, R., McCloud, S., & Endicott, J. (1997). Alcohol dependence and abuse diagnoses: Validity in community sample heavy drinkers. *Alcohol Clin Exp Res, 21*, 213–219.

Hasin, D. S., Grant, B., & Endicott, J. (1990). The natural history of alcohol abuse: Implications for definitions of alcohol use disorders. *Am J Psychiatry, 147*, 1537–1541.

Hasin, D. S., Stinson, F. S., Ogburn, E., & Grant, B. F. (2007). Prevalence, correlates, disability and comorbidity of DSM-IV alcohol abuse and dependence in the United States: Results from the National Epidemiologic Survey on Alcohol and Related Conditions. *Archives of General Psychiatry, 64*, 830–842.

Helzer, J. E., & Pryzbeck, T. R. (1988). The co-occurrence of alcoholism with other psychiatric disorders in the general population and its impact on treatment. *J Stud Alcohol, 49*, 219–224.

Hien, D., Zimberg, S., Weisman, S., First, M., & Ackerman, S. (1997). Dual diagnosis subtypes in urban substance abuse and mental health clinics. *Psychiatr Serv, 48*, 1058–1063.

Jordan, B. K., Schlenger, W. E., Fairbank, J. A., & Caddell, J. M. (1996). Prevalence of psychiatric disorders among incarcerated women: II. Convicted felons entering prison. *Arch Gen Psychiatry, 53*, 513–519.

Kandel, D., Chen, K., Warner, L. A., Kessler, R. C., & Grant, B. (1997). Prevalence and demographic correlates of symptoms of last year dependence on alcohol, nicotine, marijuana and cocaine in the U.S. population. *Drug Alcohol Depend, 44*(1), 11–29.

Karno, M. P., Grella, C. E., Niv, N., Warda, U., & Moore, A. A. (2008). Do substance type and diagnosis make a difference?: A study of remission from alcohol- versus drug-use disorders using the National Epidemiologic Survey on Alcohol and Related Conditions. *J Stud Alcohol Drugs, 69*(4), 491–495.

Kedia, S., Sell, M. A., & Relvea, G. (2007). Mono- versus polydrug abuse patterns among publicly funded clients. *Subst Abuse Treat Prev Policy, 2*, 33.

Kessler, R. C., Crum, R. M., Warner, L. A., Nelson, C. B., Schulenberg, J., & Anthony, J. C. (1997). Lifetime co-occurrence of DSM-III-R alcohol abuse and dependence with other psychiatric disorders in the National Comorbidity Study. *Arch Gen Psychiatry, 54*, 313–321.

Kessler, R. C., McGonagle, K. A., Zhao, S., Nelson, C. B., Hughes, M., Eshelman, S., et al. (1994). Lifetime and 12-month prevalence of DSM-III-R psychiatric disorders in the United States: Results from the National Comorbidity Study. *Arch Gen Psychiatry, 51*, 8–19.

Kidorf, M., Brooner, R. K., King, V. L., Chutuape, M. A., & Stitzer, M. L. (1996). Concurrent validity of cocaine and sedative dependence diagnoses in opioid-dependent outpatients. *Drug Alcohol Depend, 42*, 117–123.

Kleinman, P. H., Miller, A. B., Millman, R. B., Woody, G. E., Todd, T., Kemp, J., et al. (1990). Psychopathology among cocaine abusers entering treatment. *J Nerv Ment Dis, 178*, 442–447.

Kokkevi, A., & Stefanis, C. (1995). Drug abuse and psychiatric comorbidity. *Compr Psychiatry, 36*, 329–333.

Kranzler, H. R., Satel, S., & Apter, A. (1994). Personality disorder and associated features in cocaine-dependent inpatients. *Compr Psychiatry, 35*, 335–340.

Kruedelbach, N., McCormick, R. A., Schulz, S. C., & Grueneich, R. (1993). Impulsivity, coping styles, and triggers for craving in substance abusers with borderline personality disorder. *J Pers Disord, 7*, 214–222.

Leal, J., Ziedonis, D., & Kosten, T. (1994). Antisocial personality disorder as a prognostic factor for pharmacotherapy of cocaine dependence. *Drug Alcohol Depend, 35*, 31–35.

Lee, S. J., Galanter, M., Dermatis, H., & McDowell, D. (2003). Circuit parties and patterns of drug use in a subset of gay men. *J Addict Dis, 22*(4), 47–60.

Lee, S. J., & Levounis, P. (2008). Gamma hydroxybutyrate: An ethnographic study of recreational use and abuse. *J Psychoactive Drugs, 40*(3), 245–253.

Leri, F., Bruneau, J., & Stewart, J. (2003). Understanding polydrug use: Review of heroin and cocaine co-use. *Addiction, 98,* 7–22.

Levin, F. R., Foltin, R. W., & Fischman, M. W. (1996). Pattern of cocaine use in methadone-maintained individuals applying for research studies. *J Addict Dis, 15,* 97–106.

Levounis, P., & Arnaout, B. (Eds.). (2010). *Handbook of motivation and change: A practical guide for clinicians.* Arlington, VA: American Psychiatric Publishing.

Levounis, P., Drescher, J., & Barber, M. E. (Eds.). (2012). *The LGBT casebook.* Arlington, VA: American Psychiatric Publishing.

Levounis, P., Galanter, M., Dermatis, H., Hamowy, A., & DeLeon, G. (2002). Correlates of HIV transmission risk factors and considerations for interventions in homeless, chemically addicted and mentally ill patients. *J Addict Dis, 21*(3), 61–72.

Levounis, P., & Ruggiero, J. S. (2006). Outpatient management of crystal methamphetamine dependence among gay and bisexual men: How can it be done? *Prim Psychiatry, 13,* 75–80.

Lynskey, M. T., & Agrawal, A. (2007). Psychometric properties of DSM assessment of illicit drug abuse and dependence: Results from the National Epidemiologic Survey on Alcohol and Related Conditions (NESARC). *Psychol Med, 37,* 1345–1355.

Magura, S., Kang, S. Y., Nwakeze, P. C., & Demsky, S. (1998). Temporal patterns of heroin and cocaine use among methadone patients. *Subst Use Misuse, 33,* 2441–2467.

Malow, R. M., West, J. A., Corrigan, S. A., Pena, J. M., & Lott, W. C. (1992). Cocaine and speedball users: Differences in psychopathology. *J Subst Abuse Treat, 9,* 287–292.

Mansergh, G., Colfax, G. N., Marks, G., Rader, M., Guzman, R., & Buchbinder, S. (2001). The circuit party men's health survey: Findings and implications for gay and bisexual men. *Am J Public Health, 91,* 953–958.

Marlowe, D. B., Husband, S. D., Lamb, R. J., Kirby, K. C., Iguchi, M. Y., & Platt, J. J. (1995). Psychiatric comorbidity in cocaine dependence: Diverging trends, Axis II spectrum and gender differentials. *Am J Addict, 4,* 70–81.

Martin, C. S., Chung, T., & Langenbucher, J. W. (2008). How should we revise diagnostic criteria for substance use disorders in DSM-V? *J Abnorm Psychol, 117*(3), 561–575.

Mattison, A. M., Ross, M. W., Wolfson, T., Franklin, D., & San Diego HIV Neurobehavioral Research Group. (2001). Circuit party attendance, club drug use, and unsafe sex in gay men. *J Subst Abuse, 31,* 119–126.

McCormick, R. A., Dowd, E. R., Quirt, S., & Zegarra, J. H. (1998). The relationship of NEO-PI performance to coping styles, patterns of use, and triggers for use among substance abusers. *Addict Behav, 23,* 497–507.

McCormick, R. A., & Smith, M. (1995). Aggression and hostility in substance abusers: The relationship to abuse patterns, coping style, and relapse triggers. *Addict Behav, 20,* 555–562.

Medina, K. L., Shear, P. K., Schafer, J., Armstrong, T. G., & Dyer, P. (2004). Cognitive functioning and length of abstinence in polysubstance dependent men. *Arch Clin Neuropsychol, 19*(2), 245–258.

Merikangas, K. R., Stolar, M., Stevens, D. E., Goulet, J., Preisig, M. A., Fenton, B., et al. (1998). Familial transmission of substance use disorders. *Arch Gen Psychiatry, 55,* 973–979.

Miller, W. R., & Rollnick, S. (1991) *Motivational interviewing: Preparing people to change addictive behavior.* New York: Guildford Press.

Mimiaga, M. J., Reisner, S. L., Vanderwarker, R., Gaucher, M. J., O'Connor, C. A., Medeiros, M. S., et al. (2008). Polysubstance use and HIV/STD risk behavior among Massachusetts men who have sex with men accessing Department of Public Health mobile van services: Implications for intervention development. *AIDS Patient Care STDS, 22*(9), 745–751.

Morgenstern, J., Langenbucher, J., Labouvie, E., & Miller, K. J. (1997). The comorbidity of alcoholism and personality disorders in a clinical population: Prevalence rates and relation to alcohol typology variables. *J Abnorm Psychol, 106,* 74–84.

Mors, O., & Sorensen, L. V. (1994). Incidence and comorbidity of personality disorders among first ever admitted psychiatric patients. *Eur Psychiatry, 9*, 175–184.

O'Boyle, M., & Barratt, E. S. (1993). Impulsivity and DSM-III-R personality disorders. *Pers Indiv Differ, 14*, 609–611.

Olthuis, J. V., Darredeau, C., & Barrett, S. P. (2013). Substance use initiation: The role of simultaneous polysubstance use. *Drug Alcohol Rev, 32*(1), 67–71.

Parrott, A. C., Milani, R., Parmar, R., & Turner, J. J. D. (2001). Ecstasy polydrug users and other recreational drug users in Britain and Italy: Psychiatric symptoms and psychobiological problems. *Psychopharmacol, 159*, 77–82.

Parrott, A. C., Sisk, E., & Turner, J. (2000). Psychobiological problems in heavy "ecstasy" (MDMA) polydrug users. *Drug Alcohol Depend, 60*, 105–110.

Pedersen, W., Clausen, S. E., & Lavik, N. J. (1989). Patterns of drug use and sensation seeking among adolescents in Norway. *Acta Psychiat Scand, 79*(4), 386–390.

Pollock, N. K., & Martin, C. S. (1999). Diagnostic orphans: Adolescents with alcohol symptoms who do not qualify for DSM-IV abuse or dependence diagnoses. *Am J Psychiatry, 156*(6), 897–901.

Ray, L. A., Miranda, R., Jr., Chelminski, I., Young, D., & Zimmerman, M. (2008). Diagnostic orphans for alcohol use disorders in a treatment-seeking psychiatric sample. *Drug Alcohol Depend, 96*, 187–191.

Regier, D. A., Farmer, M. E., Rae, D. S., Locke, B. Z., Keith, S. J., Judd, L. L., et al. (1990). Comorbidity of mental disorder with alcohol and other drug abuse: Results from the Epidemiologic Catchment Area (ECA) Study. *JAMA, 264*, 2511–2518.

Ritsher, J. B., Moos, R. H., & Finney, J. W. (2002). Relationship of treatment orientation and continuing care to remission among substance abuse patients. *Psychiatr Serv, 53*(5), 595–601.

Rodgers, J. (2000). Cognitive performance amongst recreational users of "ecstasy." *Psychopharmacol, 151*, 19–24.

Rosenthal, R. N. (2004). Concepts of evidence based practice. In A. R. Roberts & K. R. Yeager (Eds.), *Evidence-based practice manual: Research and outcome measures in health and human services* (pp. 20–29). New York: Oxford University Press.

Rosenthal, R. N., Hellerstein, D. J., & Miner, C. R. (1992). Integrated services for treatment of schizophrenic substance abusers: Demographics, symptoms, and substance abuse patterns. *Psychiatric Q, 63*, 3–26.

Rosenthal, R. N., Nunes, E. V., & Le Fauve, C. (2012). Implications of epidemiological data for identifying persons with substance use and other mental disorders. *Am Journal Addict, 21*, 97–103.

Rosenthal, R. N., & Solhkhah, R. (2013). Club drugs and synthetic cannabinoid agonists. In H. R. Kranzler, D. A. Ciraulo, & L. R. Zindel (Eds.), *Clinical manual of addiction psychopharmacology* (2nd ed.). Washington, DC: American Psychiatric Publishing.

Rosenthal, R. N., & Westreich, L. (1999). Treatment of persons with dual diagnoses of substance use disorder and other psychological problems. In B. S. McCrady & E. E. Epstein (Eds.), *Addictions: A comprehensive guidebook* (pp. 439–476). New York: Oxford University Press.

Ross, L., Kohler, C. L., Grimley, D. M., & Bellis, J. (2003). Intention to use condoms among three low-income, urban African American subgroups: Cocaine users, noncocaine drug users, and non-drug users. *J Urban Health, 80*(1), 147–160.

Rounsaville, B. J., Dolinsky, Z. S., Babor, T. F., & Meyer, R. E. (1987). Psychopathology as a predictor of treatment outcome in alcoholism. *Arch Gen Psychiatry, 44*, 505–513.

Rounsaville, B. J., Kranzler, H. R., Ball, S., Tennen, H., Poling, J., & Triffleman, E. (1998). Personality disorders in substance abusers: Relation to substance use. *J Nerv Ment Dis, 186*, 87–95.

Schifano, F., Di Furia, L., Forza, G., Minicuci, N., & Bricolo, R. (1998). MDMA ("ecstasy") consumption in the context of polydrug abuse: A report on 150 patients. *Drug Alcohol Depend, 52*, 85–90.

Scholey, A. B., Parrott, A. C., Buchanan, T., Heffernan, T. M., Ling, J., & Rodgers, J. (2004). Increased intensity of ecstasy and polydrug usage in the more experienced recreational ecstasy/MDMA users: A WWW study. *Addict Behav, 29,* 743–752.

Schuckit, M. A., Danko, G. P., Raimo, E. B., Smith, T. L., Eng, M. Y., Carpenter, K. K., et al. (2001). A preliminary evaluation of the potential usefulness of the diagnoses of polysubstance dependence. *J Stud Alcohol, 62,* 54–61.

Schuckit, M. A., Danko, G. P., Smith, T. L., Bierut, L. J., Bucholz, K. K., Edenberg, H. J., et al. (2008). The prognostic implications of DSM-IV abuse criteria in drinking adolescents. *Drug Alcohol Depend, 97,* 94–104.

Schuckit, M., Smith, T. L., Danko, G. P., Bucholz, K. K., Reich, T., & Bierut, L. (2001). Five-year clinical course associated with DSM-IV alcohol abuse or dependence in a large group of men and women. *Am J Psychiatry, 158,* 1084–1090.

Selby, M. J., & Azrin, R. L. (1998). Neuropsychological functioning in drug abusers. *Drug Alcohol Depend, 50,* 39–45.

Skinstad, A. H., & Swain, A. (2001). Comorbidity in a clinical sample of substance abusers. *Am J Drug Alcohol Abuse, 27*(1), 45–64.

Staines, G. L., Magura, S., Foote, J., Deluca, A., & Kosanke, N. (2001). Polysubstance use among alcoholics. *J Addict Dis, 20,* 53–69.

Stinson, F. S., Grant, B. F., Dawson, D. A., Ruan, W. J., Huang, B., & Saha, T. (2005). Comorbidity between DSM-IV alcohol and specific drug use disorders in the United States: Results from the National Epidemiologic Survey on Alcohol and Related Conditions. *Drug Alcohol Depend, 80,* 105–116.

Substance Abuse and Mental Health Services Administration (SAMHSA). (2011a). *National Survey of Substance Abuse Treatment Services (N-SSATS): 2010 data on substance abuse treatment facilities* (DASIS Series S-59, HHS Publication No. [SMA] 11-4665). Rockville, MD: Author.

Substance Abuse and Mental Health Services Administration (SAMHSA). (2011b). *Results from the 2010 National Survey on Drug Use and Health: Summary of national findings* (NSDUH Series H-41, HHS Publication No. [SMA] 11-4658). Rockville, MD: Author.

Substance Abuse and Mental Health Services Administration, Office of Applied Studies. (2003). *Treatment Episode Data Set (TEDS): 1992–2001* (National Admissions to Substance Abuse Treatment Services, DASIS Series: S-20, DHHS Publication No.[SMA] 03-3778). Rockville, MD: Author.

Substance Abuse and Mental Health Services Administration, Office of Applied Studies. (2008). *Treatment Episode Data Set (TEDS): 1996–2006* (National Admissions to Substance Abuse Treatment Services, DASIS Series: S-43, DHHS Publication No. [SMA] 08-4347). Rockville, MD: Author.

Tómasson, K., & Vaglum, P. (2000). Antisocial addicts: The importance of additional Axis I disorders for the 28-month outcome. *Eur Psychiatry, 15*(8), 443–449.

Trenz, R. C., Scherer, M., Harrell, P., Zur, J., Sinha, A., & Latimer, W. (2012). Early onset of drug and polysubstance use as predictors of injection drug use among adult drug users. *Addict Behav, 37*(4), 367–372.

Trull, T. J., Sher, K. J., Minks-Brown, C., Durbin, J., & Burr, R. (2000). Borderline personality disorder and substance use disorders: A review and integration. *Clin Psychol Rev, 20*(2), 235–253.

Tsuang, M. T., Lyons, M. J., Eisen, S. A., Goldberg, J., True, W., Lin, N., et al. (1996). Genetic influences on DSM-III-R drug abuse and dependence: A study of 3,372 twin pairs. *Am J Med Genet, 67,* 473–477.

Tsuang, M. T., Lyons, M. J., Meyer, J. M., Doyle, T., Eisen, S. A., Goldberg, J., et al. (1998). Co-occurrence of abuse of different drugs in men: The role of drug-specific and shared vulnerabilities. *Arch Gen Psychiatry, 55,* 967–972.

Verdejo-García, A., & Pérez-García, M. (2007) Profile of executive deficits in cocaine and heroin polysubstance users: Common and differential effects on separate executive components. *Psychopharmacol (Berl), 190*(4), 517–530.

Walton, M. A., Blow, F. C., & Booth, B. M. (2000). A comparison of substance abuse patients' and counselors' perceptions of relapse risk: Relationship to actual relapse. *J Subst Abuse Treat, 19*(2), 161–169.

Webb, J. A., Baer, P. E., & McKelvey, R. S. (1995). Development of a risk profile for intentions to use alcohol among fifth and sixth graders. *J Am Acad Child Adolesc Psychiatry, 34,* 772–778.

Weizman, T., Gelkopf, M., Melamed, Y., Adelson, M., & Bleich, A. (2004). Cannabis abuse is not a risk factor for treatment outcome in methadone maintenance treatment: A 1-year prospective study in an Israeli clinic. *Aust N Z J Psychiatry, 38,* 42–46.

Woody, G. E., McLellan, A. T., Luborsky, L., & O'Brien, C. P. (1985). Sociopathy and psychotherapy outcome. *Arch Gen Psychiatry, 42,* 1081–1086.

CHAPTER 15

Co-Occurring Substance Use Disorders and Other Psychiatric Disorders

BENJAMIN C. SILVERMAN
LISA M. NAJAVITS
ROGER D. WEISS

Determining better ways to identify and treat individuals with co-occurring substance use disorders (SUDs) and other psychiatric disorders has become increasingly important from clinical, research, and policy perspectives. Several observations have driven this imperative: (1) Co-occurring SUDs with other psychiatric disorders are prevalent (Conway, Compton, Stinson, & Grant, 2006; Kessler et al., 1996; Regier et al., 1990; Swendsen et al., 2010) and associated with worse clinical and functional outcomes than either SUDs or other psychiatric disorders alone (Hser et al., 2006; Mueller et al., 1994; Ritsher et al., 2002); (2) many people with these co-occurring disorders do not receive adequate treatment (Substance Abuse and Mental Health Services Administration [SAMHSA], 2002); and (3) compared to psychiatric patients without co-occurring SUDs, patients with co-occurring disorders tend to use more costly treatments such as emergency and hospital care (Dickey & Azeni, 1996; Mark, 2003). Together, these observations have led to the development of specific new treatments designed or adapted for this population.

Within SUD populations, multiple SUDs are common (Conway et al., 2006; Kessler et al., 1997; Regier et al., 1990; Swendsen et al., 2010). While these individuals also may be considered "dually diagnosed," this chapter focuses exclusively on patients who have an SUD plus a non-SUD co-occurring psychiatric disorder. We refer to non-SUD psychiatric disorders simply as "psychiatric disorders" to distinguish them from SUDs. Additionally, this chapter excludes co-occurring nicotine dependence and psychiatric disorders, a topic that is important and broad enough to require independent attention (Ziedonis et al., 2008; see Chapter 6, this volume).

In this chapter, we review psychosocial and psychopharmacological treatments for patients with co-occurring SUDs and other psychiatric disorders.

EPIDEMIOLOGY

Studies in SUD and psychiatric treatment-seeking populations (McLellan & Druley, 1977; Ross et al., 1988) have suggested high prevalence rates of co-occurring SUDs and psychiatric disorders. However, treatment-seeking samples may not be representative of community populations, since they tend to have higher rates of comorbidity and may have more severe manifestations of the disorder for which they are seeking treatment. Thus, epidemiological studies of prevalence rates in community populations are important in assessing the true comorbidity prevalence rate.

The National Epidemiologic Survey on Alcohol and Related Conditions (NESARC) is the largest and most recent study to date that examines the epidemiology of SUDs and co-occurring psychiatric disorders in a community sample. Conducted in 2001–2002, with a follow-up reinterview wave carried out in 2004–2005, NESARC specifically sought out data on co-occurring conditions, asking questions about alcohol, tobacco, and other substance use, along with inquiries on psychiatric/psychological disorders, family history and medical conditions, and gambling, among others. Data were collected from randomly selected individuals based on household data from the 2000 Census, with an 81% response rate. NESARC results demonstrate that SUDs and psychiatric disorders are commonly co-occurring in community populations (Compton et al., 2007; Hasin et al., 2007; Hasin & Kilcoyne, 2012). When adjusted for other sociodemographic factors, lifetime alcohol use disorder was significantly associated with mood disorders (odds ratio [OR] = 2.4), anxiety disorders (OR = 2.3), and personality disorders (OR = 2.8). Likewise, 12-month and lifetime drug use disorders were significantly associated with alcohol use disorders, nicotine dependence, and mood, anxiety, and personality disorders (ORs = 2.2–9.0).

The two previous major psychiatric epidemiological studies, the Epidemiologic Catchment Area (ECA) study (Regier et al., 1990) and the National Comorbidity Study (NCS), carried out from 1990 to 1992 (Kessler et al., 1996), similarly demonstrate that co-occurring SUDs and psychiatric disorders are prevalent in community populations. Methodological advancements of the NCS included an expanded scope of the community sample (e.g., the ECA sampled from within five U.S. communities; the NCS sampled nationally representative households) and an advanced version of the *Diagnostic and Statistical Manual of Mental Disorders* (i.e., DSM-III-R; American Psychiatric Association, 1987). Also, while both studies surveyed most of the more common psychiatric disorders, the ECA did not include posttraumatic stress disorder (PTSD), whereas the NCS did. Neither epidemiological survey included Axis II disorders other than antisocial personality disorder. Despite these limitations and differences between the two studies, their results were often qualitatively similar, although the magnitude of their estimates differed somewhat at times. Among persons with psychiatric disorders, the ECA estimated that 30% had a co-occurring SUD. The prevalence varied by diagnosis, however; co-occurring SUDs were most common in individuals with antisocial personality disorder, followed by those with bipolar I disorder. In SUD populations, the ECA and NCS estimated that over half would experience psychiatric disorders in their lifetime. These lifetime estimates do not merely reflect rare or historical periods in an individual's history; the 12-month comorbidity prevalence rate of these disorders was also quite high. For example, the NCS estimated that over 33% of those with bipolar disorder experienced an SUD within 12 months, followed by nearly 20% of those with major depression and 15% of those with an anxiety disorder. From 2001 to 2003, a substantial portion (87.6%) of the NCS study population was reinterviewed in the National Comorbidity Survey–2 (NCS-2; Swendsen et al., 2010), allowing for updated diagnostic assessments (i.e., based on DSM-IV-TR; American Psychiatric Association, 2000) and demonstrating significant prospective risks posed by baseline mental disorders for the onset of SUDs in the follow-up time frame.

In Australia, the 2007 National Survey of Mental Health and Wellbeing (NSMHWB) revealed similarly high rates of comorbidity compared to the U.S. surveys, with 25.4% of individuals with an anxiety, affective, or SUDs having at least one other class of disorder (Teesson, Slade, & Mills, 2009). In particular, the NSMHWB estimated that individuals with an alcohol use disorder were more than twice as likely to have an anxiety disorder and were 4.5 times more likely to have any mental disorder compared to the rest of the sample (Teesson et al., 2010).

THE RELATIONSHIP BETWEEN SUBSTANCE ABUSE AND PSYCHOPATHOLOGY

While determining which disorder is primary in patients with co-occurring SUDs and psychiatric disorders can be useful in clinical research, it may provide little benefit in the clinical management of these patients. Patients with two disorders typically require treatment for both. In patients with co-occurring cannabis dependence and psychosis, for example, it is interesting scientifically to consider whether cannabis use led to the development or earlier onset of psychotic illness or vice versa (Moore et al., 2007), but clinically, patients require both SUD and psychiatric treatment to be helped most effectively. On the other hand, the exception is patients who present with temporary psychiatric symptoms caused by the substance use or its withdrawal, which resolve with treatment; an example of this would be psychosis induced by methamphetamine use (Grelotti, Kanayama, & Pope, 2010).

Meyer (1986) offered a now-classic framework to consider six possible ways in which SUD and other psychopathology may be related:

1. *Psychopathology may be a risk factor for SUDs.* As described previously, studies of patient and community samples indicate that the risk of having a co-occurring SUD is elevated in persons with psychiatric disorders. For example, dopaminergic dysfunction in patients with schizophrenia has been hypothesized to increase their risk of SUDs—particularly cocaine use disorders (Green et al., 1999; Smelson et al., 2002b). Another theory, widely known as the "self-medication hypothesis" (Khantzian, 1989, 1997; Khantzian & Albanese, 2008), suggests that psychopathology leads patients to use substances in an attempt to decrease unwanted psychiatric symptoms.

For example, a patient with insomnia due to PTSD nightmares may use alcohol or marijuana to induce sleep. Although research has not found direct connections between particular psychopathological symptoms and specific substances (rather, patients tend to misuse a wide variety of substances to "treat" a range of symptoms), the general principle is an important one. It is discussed in more detail in the next item.

2. *Psychiatric disorders and co-occurring SUDs may serve to modify the course of each other in terms of symptomatology, rapidity of onset, and response to treatment.* Also, as we described more below, there is considerable evidence that comorbidity is associated with worse outcomes. For example, there is evidence that patients with schizophrenia and co-occurring SUDs do not respond as well to similar doses of first-generation antipsychotic medications as those without SUDs (Bowers et al., 1990).

3. *Psychiatric symptoms may result from chronic intoxication.* Drug and alcohol use can result in a variety of psychiatric symptoms, such as depression, anxiety, euphoria, psychosis, and dissociative states. Most such symptoms disappear, however, within hours (e.g., cocaine-induced paranoia; Satel et al., 1991) to weeks (e.g., alcohol-induced anxiety or depression; Brown et al., 1991; Brown & Schuckit, 1988).

4. *Long-term substance use can lead to psychiatric disorders that may not remit.* Alcohol-induced, long-term cognitive changes, such as those seen in alcohol-induced persisting dementia, exemplify one way in which chronic use of a substance can create enduring change.

5. *Substance abuse and psychopathological symptoms may be meaningfully linked.* Some individuals may use alcohol or drugs in ways that enhance their psychiatric symptoms. For example, patients with antisocial personality disorder who seek disinhibition and aggression may use alcohol or cocaine, and patients with bipolar disorder may use cocaine or other stimulants to augment a euphoric mood (Weiss et al., 1986, 1988).

6. *The SUD and psychiatric disorder may be unrelated.* The presence of two disorders within an individual does not imply a causal link. For example, both alcohol dependence and depressive disorders are common in the general population; many people with both disorders are not depressed because they drink, nor do they drink because they are depressed. As another example, Brunette et al. (1997) studied the relationship between severity of substance abuse and severity of schizophrenic symptoms in patients diagnosed with both disorders, and found weak relationships and no consistent patterns of relationships between the two sets of symptoms.

The "Self-Medication Hypothesis"

One potential explanation for the increased prevalence rate of co-occurring SUDs among patients with psychiatric disorders has been the "self-medication hypothesis" (Khantzian, 1985, 1997; Khantzian & Albanese, 2008), which postulates that certain drugs may be particularly reinforcing for particular patients because of their specific psychopathology.

Two fundamental assumptions underlie this hypothesis: first, that substances are abused to relieve psychological pain, not just to create euphoria; and second, that there is specificity between patients' "drug of choice" and the particular intolerable emotions or symptoms that they are attempting to alleviate. For example, patients with social anxiety may be drawn to alcohol to decrease their symptoms, while patients who are prone to violence and anger outbursts may prefer the calming effects of opioids to the potentially disinhibiting effects of alcohol. Another recently discussed example might be the high prevalence of nicotine use in patients with schizophrenia, who might be drawn to smoking cigarettes (due to biological predispositions based on alterations in nicotinic acetylcholine receptors) as a way to modulate antipsychotic medication side effects or to self-medicate negative symptoms and cognitive deficits (Dalack et al., 1998; Winterer, 2010).

A major criticism of the self-medication hypothesis has been its heavy reliance on anecdotal data from patients in psychotherapy and the relative paucity of empirical studies testing it (Aharonovich et al., 2001). Additionally, intoxicants may produce very different effects acutely compared to the effects of chronic administration. Studies of individuals with heroin (Meyer & Mirin, 1979), cocaine (Post et al., 1974), and alcohol (Mendelson & Mello, 1966) use disorders have indicated a dichotomy between the acute effects of these drugs in producing euphoria or tension relief and the chronic or high-dose effects in producing dysphoria. Several researchers have sought to test empirically the self-medication hypothesis in larger samples. The results have tended not to support the specificity of using a particular addictive substance to alleviate specific psychopathology or mood states (Aharonovich et al., 2001; Weiss, Griffin, et al., 1992). However, while not necessarily a validation of the theory that patients use addictive substances to alleviate certain mood states, there is evidence that treating a co-occurring psychiatric disorder (Cornelius et al., 1997; Greenfield et al., 1998) and remission of its symptoms (Hasin et al., 1996) can improve SUD outcomes.

Other Theories

Weiss (1992) suggests three additional mechanisms by which psychopathology can make an individual more vulnerable to SUDs.

1. *Psychopathology may interfere with an individual's judgment or ability to appreciate consequences.* Individuals with psychiatric disorders may be more vulnerable to SUDs, because the impaired judgment that is often present in many psychiatric syndromes can interfere with one's ability or willingness to understand or change one's behavior. For example, severely depressed patients may have insight regarding the destructive effect of their drinking but continue to drink due to the pessimism about the possibility and value of change that is part of their depressive disorder. Similarly, the recklessness, irritability, and grandiosity of patients with mania or hypomania may interfere with their capacity to appreciate the harmful nature of their substance use.

2. *Psychopathology may accelerate the process of substance dependence by leading to more dysphoria either during chronic use or early abstinence.* It is possible

that patients with underlying psychopathology may experience more dysphoria from chronic substance use or more severe withdrawal symptoms when discontinuing drugs or alcohol. Although this potential mechanism has received little study, there is some evidence that cocaine abusers with major depressive disorder may report more severe mood symptoms during abstinence compared to cocaine abusers without depression (Gawin & Kleber, 1986).

3. *Psychopathology may reinforce the social context of drug use.* Some patients with severe psychiatric illness may be drawn to a drug-using subculture because they feel it facilitates socialization or a new peer group. For example, some patients with schizophrenia have described using substances to socialize or be accepted by peers, even though substances increased the risk of psychosis (Drake et al., 1989; Spencer et al., 2002).

Thus, multiple possible motivations and causes contribute to the initiation and maintenance of problematic alcohol and drug use in patients with psychiatric disorders.

DIAGNOSING PSYCHIATRIC DISORDERS IN PATIENTS WITH SUDs

The task of determining whether a patient is suffering from a substance-induced disorder or an independent psychiatric disorder can be complicated and has not been well-studied (Morojele et al., 2012; Torrens et al., 2011). Substances of abuse can cause a wide range of psychiatric symptoms. Clinicians evaluating such patients need to determine whether the disturbance is independent of substance use or related to intoxication or withdrawal. For example, when examining a patient who has a long history of alcohol dependence and depressive symptoms, it can be difficult to determine whether the depressive symptoms result from the direct pharmacological effects of alcohol, the many losses experienced as a result of the alcohol use, feelings of discouragement about the inability to stop drinking, or an independent mood disorder. Other etiologies, such as metabolic disturbances, head trauma, and personality disorders, must also be considered in the differential diagnosis of depressive symptoms in alcohol-dependent patients (Jaffe & Ciraulo, 1986). In a recent study, Torrens et al. (2011) compared risk factors for substance-induced versus independent psychiatric disorders in a population with co-occurring SUDs and psychiatric disorders. They found that mood and anxiety disorders were more likely to be independent. Subjects recruited from nontreatment setting were more likely to have substance-induced disorders than were subjects recruited from a treatment setting (OR = 3.5).

Given these considerations, one could ideally establish diagnostic rules to assist in determining whether a psychiatric syndrome is due to substance use or represents a separate and independent disorder. For example, some clinicians may establish a rule that a patient must be abstinent from alcohol and drugs for at least 4 weeks before one can make a diagnosis. Unfortunately, one does not always have the luxury of observing such lengthy abstinent periods (either by historical report or in the present) in which to assess this. In such circumstances, guidelines, as opposed to strict rules, can be helpful. For example, several studies have observed that for alcohol-dependent patients with major depressive disorder, treating the depression can have a positive impact on drinking (Cornelius et al., 1997; Greenfield et al., 1998). Thus, while DSM-5 (American Psychiatric Association, 2013) criteria for substance-induced depressive disorder suggest at least 4 weeks of symptom persistence during abstinence before a clinician can diagnose an independent depressive disorder, it also notes that clinicians can diagnose an independent disorder if other convincing factors are in place (e.g., a history of recurrent non-substance/medication-related episodes or symptoms that preexisted before onset of substance use). Certain disorders, such as eating disorders and PTSD, can be diagnosed readily, even in the context of substance use or withdrawal, since their symptoms do not closely resemble substance-related syndromes. Indeed, for a diagnosis such as PTSD, which tends to be underdiagnosed in patients with SUDs, the greater danger is to delay diagnosis; waiting for a period of abstinence may prevent needed treatment for the co-occurring disorder (Najavits, 2004).

Finally, clinicians should consider whether the patient's symptoms are what would be expected upon discontinuation of the abused substance. If there is considerable overlap between the observed symptoms and what one would expect from the drug discontinuation syndrome, then the clinician should wait until (1) the symptoms resolve, or (2) no longer are consistent with what would be expected with drug cessation (i.e., the syndrome one would expect to see after 1 week versus 1 month of alcohol abstinence). Alternatively, if there is little overlap between the symptoms observed and the expected abstinence syndrome (e.g., bulimia nervosa in an opioid-dependent patient), then the diagnosis can be made without waiting for an extended abstinent period.

DIAGNOSING SUDs IN PATIENTS SEEKING TREATMENT FOR PSYCHIATRIC DISORDERS

Co-occurring SUDs are often overlooked in patients seeking treatment for psychiatric disorders. The first step in the accurate diagnosis of SUDs is systematically to ask the patient about the presence of substance use. Structured clinical assessments have been demonstrated to improve detection of SUDs compared to routine assessment in outpatient severe and persistently mentally ill (SPMI; Breakey et al., 1998) and inpatient (Albanese et al., 1994) populations; they have also outperformed urine toxicology testing (Albanese et al., 1994). Unfortunately, the increasing acuity of patients on inpatient units and the demanding time constraints of outpatient psychiatric practice (Woodward et al., 1991) may pose challenges to the systematic assessment of SUDs. In one outpatient study, combining multiple standardized clinical instruments improved rates of detection but raised similar concerns about time constraints of routine clinical work and resultant underdetection (Wusthoff et al., 2011). In another outpatient study, adding the four-item CAGE (Cut down, Annoyed, Guilty, Eye-opener) Questionnaire (Ewing, 1984) improved the sensitivity of detecting SUDs from 62 to 97% in an SPMI population (Breakey et al., 1998). However, self-report alone, without urine toxicology, can also lead to underdetection of substance use (Claassen et al., 1997).

Finally, contingencies play an important role in patients' willingness to self-report substance use. If patients are repeatedly encouraged to be honest in their self-reports, and if they are told (and more importantly, if they believe) that there will be no negative consequences of reporting use (e.g., being discharged from a treatment program or reported to a probation officer or employer), then they are more likely to be forthcoming in reporting their use. If, however, they are concerned that there will be negative consequences, then they are less likely to do so. Thus, self-reports of use in an emergency department, where a patient is unlikely to know the clinician and will probably not believe (whether it is true or not) that there will be no negative consequences for disclosing use, are likely to be suspect. However, in an outpatient treatment setting, in which a patient has an opportunity to build a relationship with a clinician or treatment team, and perhaps sees other patients self-disclosing and benefiting from that disclosure, self-reports are likely to be more valid (Weiss et al., 1998).

TREATMENT OF PATIENTS WITH CO-OCCURRING SUDs AND OTHER PSYCHIATRIC DISORDERS

Association between Co-Occurring Disorders and Treatment Outcome

In both SUD and psychiatric treatment-seeking populations, patients with co-occurring SUDs and psychiatric disorders typically experience worse outcomes than their "singly diagnosed" peers (Ritsher et al., 2002; Schaar & Oejehagen, 2001; Najavits et al., 2007). However, there are specific populations in which the evidence is mixed, such as populations with SPMI (Farris et al., 2003; Gonzalez & Rosenheck, 2002) and antisocial personality disorder (Cacciola et al., 1995; Kranzler et al., 1996). The effect of other psychiatric disorders on SUD outcomes may vary by SUD type. For example, whereas co-occurring major depression appears to predict worse alcohol outcomes (Brown et al., 1998; Greenfield et al., 1998), there is less evidence for its predicting worse cocaine outcomes (McKay et al., 2002; Rohsenow et al., 2002).

There is also evidence (albeit somewhat inconsistent) that gender may play a role in mediating the effect of co-occurring psychiatric disorders on SUD outcome. Major depression in men has been associated with worse SUD outcome (Compton et al., 2003; Rounsaville et al., 1987), although this is not a consistent finding (Kranzler et al., 1996; Powell et al., 1992). In contrast, some studies suggest that female gender has been associated with similar or better SUD outcomes among patients with co-occurring psychiatric disorders (Compton et al., 2003; Rounsaville et al., 1987), except for phobia, which was associated in one study with worse SUD outcome in women (Compton et al., 2003). Finally, whereas antisocial personality disorder in men has been associated with worse outcomes (Compton et al., 2003; Kranzler et al., 1996), the evidence in women has been mixed (Compton et al., 2003; Rounsaville et al., 1987).

A Heterogeneous Population

Since patients with co-occurring disorders comprise a heterogeneous population, it follows that their treatment should perhaps reflect that heterogeneity (Weiss, Mirin, et al., 1992); a "one size fits all" approach therefore will likely not be optimal. However, providing group treatments tailored to patients with some degree of diagnostic homogeneity (e.g., patients with bipolar disorder and SUDs) can be a difficult strategy to implement if one is unable to recruit a large enough clinical population for these groups. Similarly, even within diagnostically homogeneous groups, considerable heterogeneity in illness severity and functioning may still exist. Ries et al. (1997) have suggested a conceptual approach that divides patients with co-occurring SUDs and psychiatric disorders into four major subgroups, according to the severity (i.e., major or minor) of each disorder. Although this is a somewhat crude way to classify patients, it may be helpful in developing an outpatient group treatment program for patients with co-occurring disorders.

An additional consideration is that not all patients are similar in terms of insight regarding their SUD, nor are they similarly ready to address it. Thus, patients who cannot decide whether to address their substance use may do better in a group focused on resolving that issue, as opposed to a group in which all participants are actively engaged in treatment and making lifestyle changes to support sobriety. We know of no studies, however, that have tested this idea empirically. It is possible, for example, that having a mix of patient severity levels in one group gives patients the opportunity to learn from those further along in their recovery. This is a central principle of Alcoholics Anonymous, and it appears to have strong anecdotal support. Treatments that focus on particular co-occurring diagnoses (e.g., bipolar patients with SUDs) also have not been directly compared to more general thematic groups (e.g., co-occurring disorder groups that are more general, encompassing a wide variety of diagnoses). Thus, it remains an empirical question how the heterogeneity of patients with co-occurring SUDs and psychiatric disorders should best be addressed within the realistic constraints of specific clinical settings.

Sequential, Parallel, and Integrated Treatment Models

There are three major models in which patients with co-occurring SUDs and psychiatric disorders are treated: sequential, parallel, and integrated treatment. We discuss each below.

In *sequential treatment*, the more acute condition is treated first, followed by the less acute co-occurring disorder. Often, this sequential approach is attempted when one condition is perceived to be more acute than another. Sometimes, however, it may occur because of the perception that one condition is secondary to another, that staff may not be trained to treat it, or because the condition is perceived as iatrogenic and must be addressed at the start of treatment. Historically, PTSD was perceived in these ways until quite recently, for example (Najavits et al., 2008). When sequential treatment does occur, the same staff may treat both disorders or the second disorder may be treated after transfer to a different program or facility. For example, a patient with mania and a cocaine use disorder needs mood stabilization before initiating substance abuse treatment. Conversely, a patient with major depression and alcohol withdrawal delirium is not in a position to discuss treatment adherence to antidepressant medication. Instead, this issue is best addressed when the patient is more stable (i.e., when the delirium has been fully treated and has subsided). Although sequential treatment has the advantage of providing an increased level of attention to the more acute disorder, a typical disadvantage of this model is that patients are often transferred to different clinicians to address the less acute disorder, and the interrelationship between the two disorders may never be adequately addressed.

In *parallel treatment*, both disorders are treated simultaneously, but not by the same treatment team. For example, a patient may receive treatment for an SUD in an addiction treatment program and for a psychiatric disorder in a mental health clinic. Typically, staff members of each program are very well-versed in their own areas of expertise, but not in the other. However, major cross-training efforts relative to co-occurring disorders have improved this situation in the past decade. The different treatment programs may also have different treatment philosophies, which may be confusing to the patient (Mueser et al., 1992; Ridgely et al., 1990). For example, in SUD treatment programs, clinicians may attribute psychiatric symptoms (e.g., depression and anxiety) to substance use; when a patient attempts to obtain relief, the clinician may view this as "drug-seeking" behavior. Alternatively, staff members in psychiatric programs may tend to minimize the importance of substance use and not stress its potential negative consequences.

Unfortunately, patients treated in parallel or sequential programs often have different experiences based on the treatment settings they enter. The two different programs may provide patients with different feedback on the relationship between their substance use and psychological symptoms. Patients in these situations are then left to attempt to integrate these sometimes disparate approaches themselves. In these circumstances, patients may be accused of "manipulating" and "splitting staff" when they present information obtained in one program that is contradictory to another.

In *integrated treatment*, the management of both disorders occurs in one treatment setting, and the same clinician or team of clinicians manages both illnesses. Integrated treatment has become increasingly interesting to researchers and clinicians, fostered by the belief that it is more effective than the other treatment models described earlier.

Integrated Behavioral Therapies for Patients with Co-Occurring Disorders

Integrated psychosocial treatments have been developed for diverse patient populations with co-occurring SUDs and psychiatric disorders, including patients with severe and persistent mental illness (Drake et al., 2001; McHugo et al., 1999), depression (Brown et al., 2006; Lydecker et al., 2010; Cornelius et al., 2011); bipolar disorder (Weiss et al., 2000, 2007, 2009; Weiss & Connery, 2011), personality disorders (Ball, 1998; Linehan et al., 2002), and anxiety disorders such as PTSD (Brady et al., 2001; Najavits et al., 1998; Najavits, 2002; Mills et al., 2012), obsessive–compulsive disorder (Fals-Stewart & Schafer, 1992), social phobia (Randall et al., 2001), and suicidal patients (Esposito-Smythers et al., 2011). We describe here some examples of the many interventions developed, limiting our discussion to treatments with an evidence base of at least one randomized controlled clinical trial, in an effort to be illustrative rather than comprehensive.

Integrated Group Therapy

Integrated group therapy (IGT) for bipolar disorder and substance abuse, developed by Weiss and Connery (2011) and colleagues (Weiss et al., 2000, 2007, 2009), is a manual-based group psychotherapy based on cognitive-behavioral therapy (CBT) principles, intended for patients with co-occurring bipolar disorder and SUDs, and focused on the relationship between mood symptoms and substance use or abstinence. Arranged around a "central recovery rule" of maintaining abstinence and adherence to prescribed medications, IGT takes into account the essential link between these two behaviors in this traditionally difficult-to-treat population. IGT has had three positive trials, including two randomized controlled trials (RCTs) in which it outperformed standard group drug counseling (Weiss et al., 2000, 2007, 2009); in the most recent study, IGT led to decreased substance use, increased likelihood and rate of achieving abstinence, and increased rates of "good clinical outcome," a composite measure of substance use and mood simultaneously (Weiss et al., 2009).

Seeking Safety

Seeking Safety (SS; Najavits, 2002; Najavits et al., 1998) involves a phase-based framework for PTSD and SUD recovery in which *safety* is defined the first stage of treatment. In SS, safety is the overarching goal: helping clients attain safety in their relationships, thinking, behavior, and emotions. It is a present-focused, CBT approach focused on psychoeducation and coping skills, and designed for flexible use: group or individual format; both genders; all settings (e.g., outpatient, inpatient, residential); all types of trauma and substances; and any clinician. It offers up to 25 topics, each representing a safe coping skill, such as Asking for Help, Compassion, Setting Boundaries in Relationships, Taking Good Care of Yourself, Creating Meaning, Coping with Triggers, Healing from Anger, and Detaching from Emotional Pain (Grounding). The topics can be conducted in any order, using as few or as many as are possible within the available time frame. It strives to be emotionally engaging, with simple, humanistic language, a quotation to start each session, and interactive exercises (for additional details, see the website *www.seekingsafety.org*). SS has had positive outcomes in RCTs including male veterans (Boden et al., 2012) and adolescent girls (Najavits et al., 2006), and is the only model thus far to outperform a control on both PTSD and SUDs (see Najavits & Hien, 2013, for a review of the points covered here). Studies of full-dose SS have shown more positive outcomes than partial-dose SS. The largest study of SS to date was conducted as part of the National Institute on Drug Abuse Clinical Trials Network. That study, despite being a partial-dose of SS (less than half the model) found that at end of treatment SS outperformed the comparison of Women's Health Education (WHE) on therapeutic alliance, HIV risk, and eating disorder symptoms, as well as eight out of nine secondary analyses focused on subsamples of the study (including heavy stimulant users and alcohol misusers) (Ruglass et al., 2012). In main outcomes, PTSD in both SS and WHE patients improved; SUDs improved in neither SS nor WHE, but the study was underpowered to detect SUD outcomes (i.e., over 45% of the sample was abstinent from substances at baseline; Hien et al., 2009). More research is warranted, especially in light of recent consistent results showing that exposure-based PTSD treatment has not outperformed less-intensive controls at end of treatment in four recent RCTs for PTSD–SUD samples (Foa et al., 2013; Mills et al., 2012; Sannibale et al., 2013; van Dam, Ehring, Vedel, & Emmelkamp, 2013; for a summary see Najavits, 2013).

Integrated Dual Disorders Treatment

Integrated dual disorders treatment (IDDT; Drake et al., 2001) focuses on providing mental health and SUD treatment concurrently by a team of interdisciplinary, cross-trained clinicians within the same program. Additional features include assertive community outreach; stagewise interventions that are determined by the client's stage of recovery (engagement, persuasion, active treatment, and relapse prevention); provision of a wide range of ancillary services; time-unlimited services; and motivational interventions. The model has had various positive outcomes for patients with schizophrenia and SUD, when compared to treatment as usual (TAU), for example (Morrens et al., 2011).

Dialectical Behavior Therapy

Dialectical behavior therapy (DBT) is a CBT approach designed for patients with borderline personality disorder. It has four key modules: mindfulness, distress tolerance, emotion regulation, and interpersonal effectiveness. It uses a conceptual approach from applied behavior analysis, "chain analysis," to identify sequential events that form the behavior sequence. It relies on a combination of group therapy, individual therapy, and, for the clinician, peer supervision and support. DBT organizes treatment into stages and targets that are strongly adhered to so as to promote effective outcomes, first addressing behaviors that could lead to the patient's death (e.g., suicide), then behaviors that could lead to premature termination from therapy, then behaviors that destroy the quality of life, and then addressing the need for alternative skills. DBT for substance abusers (Dimeff & Linehan, 2008) is a modified version of DBT for patients with SUDs to promote abstinence and reduce relapse. There have been numerous research studies of DBT, including a meta-analysis that found moderately positive effects for the model; it has been studied in some SUD samples as well, with modest positive results (Linehan et al., 1999, 2002; Harned et al., 2008; Dimeff & Linehan, 2008; see also *www.behavioraltech.org*).

Motivational Interviewing/Motivational Enhancement

Motivational interviewing (MI), developed by Miller and Rollnick (1991, 2002), utilizes theory derived from several psychotherapeutic models: systems, client-centered, CBT, and social psychology. MI is also called "motivational enhancement therapy" (MET), because it is often a brief treatment, conducted in as few as two sessions, sometimes aimed at helping the patient accept other psychotherapy (e.g., CBT). Guide-lines for modifying MI in patients diagnosed with SUDs and psychotic disorders have been published (Carey et al., 2001; Martino et al., 2002). Recent randomized pilot trials of MI in diverse populations with co-occurring disorders suggest that MI may improve the likelihood of making the transition to outpatient treatment (Swanson et al., 1999), improve SUD outcomes (Graeber et al., 2003), and decrease psychiatric hospitalization (Daley & Zuckoff, 1998). A recent review on the application of MI to various mental health disorders co-occurring with SUDs, including anxiety, depres-sion, and eating disorders, suggest promise but also needs further study, with more rigorous scientific testing (Westra et al., 2011). In recent years, too, MET has often been combined with CBT to improve outcomes, including studies addressing comor-bidity (e.g., Easton et al., 2012; Cornelius et al., 2011).

Overall Issues in Comorbidity Behavioral Therapies

The past several decades have seen remarkable progress in attending to co-occurring disorders. Various novel and creative approaches have been developed and tested in outcome trials. However, conclusions at this point are mixed and further research is warranted.

First, more research is needed to compare integrated versus single, sequential, or parallel treatment approaches. In general, research on manualized behavioral therapies for SUDs consistently find that they do not outperform each other (Car-roll & Rounsaville, 2007; Imel et al., 2008; Sellman, 2010), and certain integrated approaches may not necessarily outperform single-diagnosis approaches (Torchalla et al., 2012; Donald et al., 2005). Yet integrated treatments may have other virtues beyond just outcomes: They may increase engagement, may be perceived as highly relevant, may be easier to implement or teach, or be of lower cost than single, sequen-tial, or parallel approaches.

Second, it is important to note that results have sometimes been surprising. Some studies indicate either no difference in SUD outcomes between co-occurring versus non-co-occurring treatment (e.g., Mills et al., 2012; Schadé et al., 2008; Ball, 2007) or worse outcomes (e.g., Randall et al., 2001). Many factors may play into the het-erogeneity of findings, including methodology issues (Horsfall et al., 2009), who conducts the study (e.g., the treatment developer or independent scientists), and the nature of the treatments themselves. More research with high-quality treatments and study designs are needed. Also, there are encouraging new treatment developments, including the burgeoning technology-based approaches, such as computer-delivered care (e.g., Kelly et al., 2012).

SELF-HELP GROUPS AND INDIVIDUALS WITH CO-OCCURRING SUDs AND PSYCHIATRIC DISORDERS

As in other substance-using populations (Miller et al., 1997; Ritsher et al., 2002), self-help group attendance has been associated with improved substance use outcomes in populations with co-occurring SUDs and psychiatric disorders (Brooks & Penn, 2003; Ritsher et al., 2002). Whether this is a reflection of self-help groups' improving outcomes directly or a self-selection bias (i.e., patients attending self-help groups may be more likely to remain abstinent because they are more motivated) is unclear.

Despite the fact that self-help groups are both free of charge and geographically accessible (Kurtz, 1997), many patients with co-occurring disorders do not attend these meetings (Noordsy et al., 1996). Some clinicians may be reluctant to recommend self-help groups to patients with co-occurring disorders because of concerns that self-help group members might express negative attitudes towards psychotropic medication (Humphreys, 1997). However, recent research indicates that while this sometimes occurs (Noordsy et al., 1996), it is not prevalent (Meissen et al., 1999). Moreover, official Alcoholics Anonymous (AA; 1984) literature states that psychiatric medication, when legitimately prescribed, is appropriate. When educating patients about the interaction between psychiatric symptoms, drug and alcohol use, and medications, clinicians should inform patients that while some self-help group members may criticize the use of medications, this contradicts official AA policy.

Clinicians may also be concerned that these groups only focus on SUDs (Humphreys, 1997) and may therefore not be as helpful to patients who are struggling with other psychiatric disorders. Recent research suggests that some patients and AA contacts (i.e., persons listed in the AA directories as experienced members) agree (Meissen et al., 1999; Noordsy et al., 1996). However, by encouraging patients to focus on obtaining what AA and similar groups offer, and not expecting AA to provide services outside of its stated mission, clinicians can help patients with co-occurring disorders to take advantage of these groups.

To address some of the concerns described earlier, several dual focus self-help groups have emerged for participants with co-occurring SUDs and psychiatric disorders (e.g., Double Trouble in Recovery, Dual Recovery Anonymous, and Dual Disorders Anonymous; Bogenschutz et al., 2006; Magura et al., 2003). Similar to the literature on self-help groups in the SUD population, positive associations have been found between attendance at dual focus self-help groups and abstinence (Magura et al., 2003), as well as psychiatric/quality of life (Magura et al., 2002) outcomes. Again, whether this is a result of self-selection bias regarding the characteristics of patients who attend these meetings is unclear.

General Treatment Themes for Patients with Co-Occurring SUDs and Psychiatric Disorders

Because of the limitations of the empirical literature described earlier regarding psychosocial treatments, it may be helpful to draw on general recommendations provided by various writers on this subject (Bellack & DiClemente, 1999; Carey, 1995; Drake et al., 2001; Drake & Mueser, 2000; Najavits et al., 1996; Rounsaville & Carroll, 1997; Ziedonis et al., 2000; Najavits, 2002; Najavits & Capezza, 2014). Although treatment modalities differ, some common themes can help guide clinicians who must decide how to intervene with their patients. The suggestions are as follows:

- Be empathic and provide support for the difficulty of living with two disorders, but also emphasize accountability (e.g., the presence of a psychiatric disorder is not an excuse to use substances).
- Assist patients in setting a goal to stop substance use. Explore patients' perceptions of the relationship between their substance use and their psychiatric disorders. As part of this process, also explore the longer-term relationship between the two (e.g., an individual may report drinking to reduce social anxiety and initially feel better, then feel worse the following day) and discuss the advantages of a substance-free life.
- Educate patients and their family members about the symptoms of both disorders, and the causal connections between them.
- Monitor symptoms of both disorders and how they interact over time (including the use of biological measures such as urine screens for substance use when indicated).
- Monitor adherence to medications, since nonadherence is a significant risk for relapse.
- To improve functioning and foster the rewards of abstinence, assist patients in developing social, relationship, or vocational skills.
- Attend to patient safety, including attention to the human immunodeficiency virus (HIV) and suicidality, both of which have been found to be increased in patients with co-occurring disorders (Mahler, 1995; Weiss & Hufford, 1999).
- Have available resources to refer patients to self-help groups for each disorder.
- Discuss with patients what to do and whom to call in case of emergency.
- Provide positive reinforcement for improvements, however small, in each disorder.
- For patients who have had significant periods of recovery, acknowledge these successes and, in a positive way, ask them how they accomplished it. Doing so reminds patients of prior successes and can mitigate the feelings of hopelessness and discouragement that often accompany relapse.
- Take a relapse history to help identify triggers to relapse (e.g., discontinuing medications or treatment, engaging in high-risk behaviors such as socializing where alcohol is present).
- Expect occasional breaks in treatment attendance, and engage in active outreach.
- Recognize that patients may be more motivated to work on one disorder than the other, and may need encouragement to attend to both.
- Understand that the clinician too may feel more connection or engagement with one disorder over the other. For example, depression may evoke more sympathy than an SUD.
- Be aware of subtypes and subpopulations even within a particular comorbidity. For example, treatment of depression–SUD comorbidity may differ based on whether psychotic symptoms are present; based on age (e.g., adolescent vs. geriatric), and so forth.
- Provide referral to additional treatments and conduct a thorough assessment of case management needs, including treatment of physical health problems.

PHARMACOTHERAPY FOR PATIENTS WITH CO-OCCURRING SUDs AND OTHER PSYCHIATRIC DISORDERS

The literature regarding when to prescribe pharmacotherapy for patients with co-occurring disorders has evolved considerably in the past 20 years. Previous consensus in the field reflected reluctance to prescribe psychotropic medications in this population, in part based on methodologically flawed studies. For example, older studies examining the use of antidepressants in alcoholics often did not use standardized methods to assess the depressed population, had inadequate dosing or duration of antidepressants, and sometimes measured mood or drinking outcomes, but not both (Ciraulo & Jaffe, 1981). More recently, integrated pharmacological and psychosocial treatments have been increasingly accepted and are now often provided to patients as standard care. However, few trials have integrated novel psychosocial treatments with novel pharmacotherapies, and most treatments instead either focus on new pharmacological or new psychosocial interventions. In spite of this, clinical practice and more recent research have emphasized the importance of integrating pharmacological and psychotherapeutic treatment options.

Major Depression

Multiple meta-analyses of antidepressant medication efficacy in patients with co-occurring depression and SUDs have examined both mood and SUD outcomes (Iovieno et al., 2011; Nunes & Levin, 2004; Torrens et al., 2005). Results have shown mixed efficacy of antidepressants in this population, with better outcomes on depressive measures (comparable to results seen in patients with depression alone) than substance use outcomes, and without clear evidence to suggest use of one particular agent. Studies that required at least 1 week of abstinence before treating the depression yielded larger effect sizes and lower placebo response, suggesting that requiring even 1 week of abstinence before initiating medication treatment can successfully screen out transient depressive symptoms. Studies that exhibited better depression outcomes as a result of antidepressants also showed decreased quantity of substance use, and best outcomes occurred in studies combining antidepressants with psychotherapy. One such study used fluoxetine and CBT in depressed alcoholics, with improved depression and drinking outcomes (Cornelius et al., 1997). In another study, combining sertraline and CBT led to less drinking and improved depression compared to placebo (Moak et al., 2003). One study showed efficacy for desipramine in improving depression scores and length of abstinence from alcohol in a 6-month, double-blind, placebo-controlled trial (Mason et al., 1996). In a single-site trial, Pettinati et al. (2010) found that a combination of sertraline and naltrexone led to improved drinking outcomes and reduced depression compared to either sertraline or naltrexone alone, indicating that this combination may have value for the depressed and actively drinking patient. Most studies examining use of antidepressants in patients with co-occurring depression and cocaine use disorders have shown some effectiveness in antidepressant outcomes but little impact on cocaine use (Torrens et al., 2005). Some evidence suggests that stimulating antidepressants (e.g., tricyclics and bupropion) are preferred for treating depression in the context of cocaine use disorders (Rounsaville,

2004). Although antidepressants have been studied in patients with co-occurring depression and opioid use disorders, mostly in patients receiving methadone maintenance treatment, most studies have shown no improvement in outcomes of either illness (Nunes & Levin, 2004). An exception might be the tricyclic antidepressants imipramine and doxepin, which in this population have shown some benefit in reducing substance use, likely indirectly via positive effects on depression (Nunes et al., 1998; Nunes & Levin, 2004; Titievsky et al., 1982).

Bipolar Disorder

Although face validity would suggest that stabilizing mania or hypomania in patients with bipolar disorder would improve impulse control and judgment, and would therefore lead to decreased substance use, the literature is thin regarding the efficacy of mood-stabilizing medications on bipolar and SUD outcomes. A number of open-label prospective trials using medications for patients with an SUD and a bipolar or bipolar spectrum disorder have been conducted (i.e., with lithium, anticonvulsants, and antipsychotics), with results generally showing improvements in mood symptoms but inconclusive or unclear results regarding SUD outcomes (Brady et al., 1995; Brown et al., 2002, 2003a, 2003b; Calabrese et al., 2001; Gawin & Kleber, 1984; Geller et al., 1998; Nunes et al., 1990). An open-label pilot trial by Gawin and Kleber (1984) indicated that lithium may be effective in reducing cocaine use in patients with cyclothymia and cocaine abuse. However, an open-label trial of lithium in patients with bipolar spectrum disorders and cocaine abuse (Nunes et al., 1990) demonstrated little efficacy in mood or cocaine outcome measures. An open-label trial with valproate in patients with bipolar disorder and an SUD (Brady et al., 1995) resulted in improvement in mood and substance use measures. An open trial of lithium plus valproate in patients with rapid-cycling bipolar I or II disorder and alcohol, cannabis, and/or cocaine dependence (Calabrese et al., 2001) showed improvement in mood symptoms and a 25% remission rate in SUDs after 6 months. Open-label trials of lamotrigine (Brown et al., 2003a) and quetiapine (Brown et al., 2002) in patients with bipolar disorder and cocaine dependence suggest that these medications may be associated with improved mood symptoms and cocaine craving, although not with significant reductions in cocaine use. An add-on RCT of citicoline (Brown et al., 2007) in this same population resulted in decreased cocaine use and no changes in mood. Several double-blind, placebo-controlled studies assessing the efficacy of mood stabilizers or antipsychotic medications in patients with bipolar disorder and SUDs have been conducted (Brady et al., 2002; Brown et al., 2008, 2012; Geller et al., 1998; Salloum et al., 2005). Geller et al. (1998) conducted a double-blind, placebo-controlled, 6-week trial of lithium in adolescents with bipolar disorder and substance dependence, and found lithium to be efficacious for outcomes in both disorders (Geller et al., 1998). Brady et al. (2002) compared carbamazepine in cocaine-dependent individuals with and without a co-occurring affective disorder (note that less than half of the sample with affective disorders had bipolar I disorder, bipolar II disorder, or cyclothymia) in a 12-week, double-blind, placebo-controlled trial. The affective disorder group treated with carbamazepine showed a nonstatistically significant trend toward less cocaine use, while treatment with carbamazepine did not have any impact on individuals without affective disorders. In a 24-week, double-blind, placebo-controlled trial, Salloum et al. (2005) randomized 59 patients with bipolar disorder and alcohol dependence receiving lithium carbonate and psychosocial interventions to also receive valproate or placebo. Mood symptoms improved in both groups, while patients in the lithium plus valproate group had significantly fewer heavy drinking days. In a 10-week, double-blind, placebo-controlled trial, Brown et al. (2012) compared lamotrigine to placebo in 120 outpatients with bipolar disorder, depressed or mixed mood state, and cocaine dependence. No difference in mood symptoms occurred between the groups, and lamotrigine was associated with a decrease in the amount of money spent on cocaine (though without a significant difference in urine drug screen results). Two double-blind, placebo-controlled trials administering quetiapine to patients with alcohol dependence and bipolar I disorder (treated with mood stabilizers) resulted in no improvement over placebo in measures of alcohol use (Brown et al., 2008; Stedman et al., 2010). Generally speaking, the results of all of these trials confirm the safety and effectiveness of mood stabilizers in improving psychiatric symptoms in patients with co-occurring disorders, but fewer data objectively demonstrate a decrease in substance use, and results of most trials can be seen as preliminary.

Schizophrenia

Most of the literature on the pharmacological treatment of patients with schizophrenia and SUDs is limited to retrospective or open-label prospective studies, often with small sample sizes and/or lacking comparison groups. For example, an open trial of desipramine added to antipsychotic treatment in an integrated dual diagnosis relapse prevention program showed promise in reducing cocaine use and improving psychiatric symptoms (Ziedonis et al., 1992). Two open-label trials have found the first-generation depot antipsychotic flupenthixol deconoate to decrease cocaine (Levin et al., 1998b) and alcohol (Soyka et al., 2003) use in patients diagnosed with schizophrenia and SUDs. Multiple preliminary reports suggest the potential benefit of second-generation antipsychotic medications such as clozapine, olanzapine (Littrell et al., 2001; Smelson et al., 2006), risperidone (Smelson et al., 2002a; Rubio et al., 2006), quetiapine (Brown et al., 2003b), and aripiprazole (Beresford et al., 2005) in improving substance use outcomes in populations with co-occurring schizophrenia, though no conclusive data support the efficacy of first- or second-generation antipsychotic agents over the other (Petrakis, Leslie, et al., 2006; San et al., 2007; Sayers et al., 2005). Generally speaking, the atypical antipsychotic clozapine has shown the most promise in the treatment of patients with schizophrenia and SUDs (Buckley et al., 1994; Drake et al., 2000; Green et al., 2003; San et al., 2007; Lybrand & Caroff, 2009; Zimmet et al., 2000). In one RCT (enrolling 31 patients with co-occurring schizophrenia and cannabis use disorder), clozapine treatment was associated with decreased cannabis use compared to other antipsychotic medications, though without differences in symptoms or functioning (Brunette et al., 2011). The unique pharmacological receptor activity of clozapine may correct underlying reward system deficits of patients with schizophrenia and SUDs (Green et al., 1999, 2008; LeDuc & Mittleman, 1995). Additionally, when administered in low doses (50 mg or less) to normal volunteers, clozapine has been shown to attenuate the subjective high and rush associated with cocaine, as well as its pressor effect (Farren et al., 2000). In one naturalistic study, Drake et al. (2000) prospectively followed 151 patients with schizophrenia or schizoaffective disorder and co-occurring SUDs for 3 years. At the conclusion of the study, of the 36 patients who received treatment with clozapine, 79% were in remission from alcohol use disorder, compared to only 33.7% of those not taking clozapine. Despite these encouraging findings, evidence from normal study volunteers suggests that low-dose clozapine may increase cocaine blood levels and cause near-syncope (Farren et al., 2000). To our knowledge, however, no case reports or studies have documented clinically significant syncopal episodes in patients with schizophrenia and stimulant use disorders who are prescribed clozapine. Thus, while the introduction of second-generation antipsychotics is encouraging with regard to potential to improve SUD outcomes in this population with co-occurring disorders, well-designed controlled trials are needed to establish safety, tolerability, and efficacy in this population.

Anxiety Disorders

The use of benzodiazepines in populations with SUDs and co-occurring psychiatric disorders is controversial. This issue has been explored almost exclusively in populations with anxiety and alcohol use disorders. The prevalence of benzodiazepine use in patients with alcohol use disorders is greater than in the general population but comparable to that in populations with psychiatric disorders (Ciraulo et al., 1988). Clinicians are often understandably concerned that prescribing benzodiazepines to these patients may lead to either a worsening of the alcohol use disorder, the development of a benzodiazepine use disorder, or potentiation of the benzodiazepine effect when combined with alcohol. Preliminary evidence from case reports (Adinoff, 1992) and a prospective naturalistic study (Mueller et al., 1996) suggests that there may be a carefully selected subpopulation of patients with co-occurring alcohol use and anxiety disorders for whom long-term prescription of benzodiazepine may not affect sobriety or result in benzodiazepine misuse. However, it may not improve outcomes either. For example, a retrospective naturalistic study of veterans with PTSD and SUDs found that physicians were less likely to prescribe benzodiazepines for those with SUDs (Kosten et al., 2000). While those with prescribed benzodiazepines did not have worse outcomes, chronic benzodiazepine treatment (independent of a co-occurring SUD) did not improve anxiety or social functioning in these patients either. Similarly, Brunette et al. (2003) followed SPMI patients with SUDs annually for 6 years and found that the rate of benzodiazepine prescribing was high (up to 43%), but it was not associated with differences in substance use remission, hospitalization, or, interestingly, reductions in anxiety or depression. Also, unsurprisingly, patients prescribed benzodiazepines were more likely to abuse them than those who were not prescribed them. While controlled trials are needed to explore these issues more fully, the findings from these reports add further to concerns that the long-term use of benzodiazepines in these populations perhaps offers the risk of abuse or dependence without great potential for clinical benefit.

Another pharmacological alternative in this population is buspirone, which does not have abuse potential. Thus far, there have been three double-blind, placebo-controlled studies of buspirone in patients with alcohol dependence and anxiety—either generalized anxiety disorder (GAD; Tollefson et al., 1992), GAD and "other nonpanic anxiety" (Malcolm et al., 1992), or "anxious alcoholism" (Kranzler et al., 1994). Two of the studies found that buspirone was associated with improvements in anxiety and alcohol use outcomes (Kranzler et al., 1994; Tollefson et al., 1992). Although there have been concerns that buspirone's antianxiety effect is more limited in patients with a prior history of benzodiazepine use (Schweizer et al., 1986), a pooled analysis of eight placebo-controlled, randomized trials of patients with GAD (DeMartinis et al., 2000) indicated that patients with either remote (defined as at least 1 month duration) or no prior benzodiazepine treatment experienced improved anxiolysis, fewer adverse events, and clinical improvement similar to that on benzodiazepines compared to patients with recent benzodiazepine treatment. Thus, patients who have not received benzodiazepines for at least 1 month may benefit from buspirone. An RCT of buspirone for patients with co-occurring opioid dependence (on methadone maintenance treatment) and anxiety found that buspirone did not significantly reduce anxiety symptoms, though was associated with trends toward decreased depressive symptoms and slowed relapse rates (McRae et al., 2004).

In patients with co-occurring PTSD and SUDs, one RCT indicated that certain subtypes of patients might benefit from selective serotonin reuptake inhibitor (SSRI) treatment (Brady et al., 2005). In 94 patients with current alcohol dependence and PTSD randomly assigned to receive sertraline or placebo for 12 weeks, those participants with less severe alcohol dependence and earlier-onset PTSD had significantly fewer drinks per drinking day. The SSRI paroxetine has similarly been found to be effective in one randomized, placebo-controlled trial in patients with co-occurring social anxiety disorder and alcohol dependence (Randall, Johnson, et al., 2001). Participants receiving paroxetine showed improvements in anxiety and alcohol dependence symptoms. A follow-up randomized, placebo-controlled trial in patients with co-occurring social anxiety disorder and alcohol dependence (Thomas et al., 2008) found paroxetine to be effective in decreasing social anxiety and self-reported use of alcohol for self-medication purposes (i.e., to cope in order to engage with others in social settings), though it did not correlate with decreases in overall alcohol use.

Attention-Deficit/Hyperactivity Disorder

Although stimulants have been the most extensively studied treatment for adult attention-deficit/hyperactivity disorder (ADHD; Levin et al., 1999), there are concerns that in populations with co-occurring SUDs and psychiatric disorders, they may worsen the course of the SUDs or be subject to abuse themselves (Gawin et al., 1985). At the same time, it has also been observed that a childhood history of ADHD worsens outcomes for cocaine dependence (Carroll & Rounsaville, 1993). Therefore, improving a patient's difficulties with inattention and hyperactivity may have beneficial effects on substance abuse as well (Levin et al., 1999). Consistent with this, prospective studies of children who received stimulant treatment for ADHD indicate that stimulants have a protective effect against future development of SUDs as an adult (Wilens, 2003; Mannuzza et al., 2003).

Although not as well-studied as stimulants, nonstimulant medications that lack abuse potential are possible alternatives in the treatment of ADHD. In adult populations, bupropion (Wilens et al., 2002) desipramine (Wilens et al., 1996), and atomoxetine (Michelson et al., 2003) have undergone double-blind, placebo-controlled studies and have demonstrated effectiveness in the treatment of hyperactivity and inattention. Little research on these medications, however, has included patients with active SUDs. In one RCT of atomoxetine, adults with ADHD and alcohol abuse or dependence (Wilens et al., 2008) showed clinically significant improvement in ADHD symptoms with atomoxetine compared to placebo, but no difference in time to relapse of heavy drinking. In a single-blind trial of bupropion for adults with ADHD and cocaine abuse (Levin et al., 2002) and an open-label study of venlafaxine, patients with ADHD and alcohol use disorder (Upadhyaya et al., 2001) showed improvements in hyperactivity and inattention, as well as substance use outcomes. In a single-blind trial of sustained-release bupropion, adults with ADHD and SUDs (of all types) showed clinically significant reductions in ADHD symptoms but not SUD markers (Wilens et al., 2010). These results need to be replicated in larger, more rigorous studies.

Clinical trials of methylphenidate in adults with ADHD and a history of cocaine use disorders have also shown promising results. Both open-label trials of long-acting methylphenidate (Castaneda et al., 2000; Levin et al., 1998) and a double-blind, placebo-controlled study of regular methylphenidate (Schubiner et al., 2002) in adults with ADHD and cocaine dependence have all been consistent in that ADHD symptoms improved and no escalation of the stimulant dose was observed. However, while the open trial by Levin et al. (1998a) observed reductions in cocaine craving and use, Schubiner et al. (2002) found no evidence of improved cocaine outcomes in their double-blind, placebo-controlled trial. In a follow-up double-blind, placebo-controlled trial of sustained-release methylphenidate in adults with ADHD and cocaine dependence (all of whom also received weekly individual CBT), Levin et al. (2007) found no difference between methylphenidate and placebo relative to ADHD symptoms (though the majority of both groups showed > 30% improvements in symptoms). Cocaine-positive urine samples, however, decreased significantly in the methylphenidate group, especially among those who also had improvements in ADHD symptoms. In another RCT, Levin et al. (2006) compared sustained-release methylphenidate or sustained-release bupropion to placebo in adults with ADHD and opioid dependence on methadone maintenance; they found no significant differences in ADHD symptoms (with improvement noted in all treatment groups), along with no increase in cocaine use among any groups. In one double-blind, placebo-controlled pilot study of sustained-release methylphenidate, 24 adults with ADHD and amphetamine dependence (abstinent at time of enrollment) showed improvement in self-rated ADHD symptoms in both groups (not statistically different), as well as no differences in drug use, craving for amphetamine, or retention in treatment (Konstenius et al., 2010). In a small crossover trial of sustained release methylphenidate (Szobot et al., 2008), adolescents with ADHD and co-occurring SUDs had more improvement in ADHD symptoms than patients receiving placebo. A multisite trial of adolescents with ADHD and SUDs, however, found no more reduction of ADHD or SUD symptoms in those receiving osmotic-release methylphenidate than in those receiving placebo (Riggs et al., 2011). There was no worsening in substance use, however. Despite limited evidence that stimulants may be safely used in this population to treat ADHD without worsening SUD outcomes (and perhaps improving them), their use in these patients remains controversial.

What to Do When the Pharmacological Treatment for the Co-Occurring Psychiatric Disorder Has Abuse Potential

As evidenced in numerous studies, treating a co-occurring psychiatric disorder can often result in positive outcomes in reducing substance use, as well as improvements in the specific psychiatric disorder for which it is prescribed. However, what if the pharmacological treatment has the potential to worsen or create a new SUD? This dilemma is often considered in treating patients with SUDs and co-occurring anxiety disorders or ADHD, when clinicians ask themselves, "Is it safe to prescribe stimulants/benzodiazepines for this patient?"

Pharmacotherapies that do not have abuse potential should be considered first-line treatments before prescribing stimulants or benzodiazepines in these populations (Ciraulo & Nace, 2000; Levin et al., 1999), and it is important that patients receive adequate trials (i.e., dose and duration) of these medications before they are abandoned. Psychosocial treatments with demonstrated efficacy should also be tried before prescribing an abusable medication. For example, CBT has demonstrated efficacy for anxiety disorders (Beck, Wright, Newman, & Liese, 1993) and should be explored before prescribing a benzodiazepine. If these first-line treatments fail to improve the anxiety or ADHD symptoms, then the following guidelines are suggested when prescribing stimulants or benzodiazepines in these patient populations (Ciraulo & Nace, 2000; Levin et al., 1999):

- *Select preparations that limit the potential for abuse.* Medications with longer half-lives or sustained-release preparations have lower abuse potential and are therefore preferable in these populations. Select as low a dose as possible. For benzodiazepines, avoid as-needed-basis prescribing in lieu of a fixed dosing schedule. Limit the number of pills given with each prescription, keep a log of the pills prescribed, and check state-based prescription monitoring programs to minimize potential for doctor shopping (i.e., obtaining prescriptions for controlled substances from multiple providers at the same time). Frequent patient contact can help the clinician assess whether the medication is helpful, as well as whether it is being overused.
- *Use objective measures to document improvements.* For example, using a standardized assessment such as the Adult Behavior Checklist (Murphy & Barkley, 1996) or the Beck Anxiety Inventory (Beck, Epstein, Brown, & Steer, 1988) can help document improvements (or the lack thereof).
- *Monitor substance use.* Patients should be asked about alcohol and drug use,

and other sources of information (urine screens, collateral information from family members) should be strongly considered.

- *Enlist family members' help in supporting and monitoring the patient.* Verify the efficacy and appropriate use of the medication with family members.
- *Patients should safeguard medications.* While the patient may not abuse the medication, family members, roommates, or friends may.
- *Monitor prescriptions.* Keep careful track of the number of pills prescribed, check prescription monitoring programs, and beware of warning signs of abuse such as premature requests for refills, "lost prescriptions," or prescriptions obtained from multiple providers in a short period of time. These usually indicate overuse of the medication.

Pharmacotherapy Targeting Substance Dependence in Populations with Co-Occurring SUDs and Other Psychiatric Disorders

Although pharmacotherapies aimed specifically at decreasing alcohol or drug use (e.g., naltrexone, disulfiram, acamprosate) have been proven and accepted to be efficacious in improving SUD outcomes in non-dually diagnosed populations, their application in populations with co-occurring disorders has lagged behind. Recent data on their safety and potential efficacy in co-occurring populations may be helpful in increasing their use (Petrakis et al., 2005). For example, concerns that disulfiram may cause or exacerbate psychosis (Mueser et al., 2003) has contributed to a reluctance to prescribe it in patients with SPMI (Kingsbury & Salzman, 1990). Published case reports (Brenner et al., 1994), case series (Kofoed et al., 1986; Mueser et al., 2003), and RCTs (Petrakis, Nich, et al., 2006), however, have described its tolerability and potential benefit for improving alcohol outcomes. Additionally, evidence suggests that naltrexone may similarly improve drinking outcomes in patients with alcohol dependence and schizophrenia (Batki et al., 2002; Petrakis et al., 2004), bipolar disorder (Sonne & Brady, 2000; Brown et al., 2009), and major depression (Salloum et al., 1998; Petrakis et al., 2007). In one randomized, placebo-controlled trial, Petrakis et al. (2004) successfully treated 31 patients with schizophrenia and comorbid alcohol abuse or dependence for 12 weeks in an outpatient setting using naltrexone or placebo, in addition to patients' neuroleptic medication. Patients receiving naltrexone had significantly fewer drinking days, less heavy drinking days, and decreased cravings, with no changes in schizophrenia symptoms or status. Additionally, among male military veterans with alcohol dependence and PTSD, naltrexone and disulfiram were found to be more effective than placebo in reducing alcohol consumption (Petrakis, Poling, et al., 2006). Both naltrexone and disulfiram alone were associated with reduced alcohol consumption, though the combination did not confer extra benefit and was associated with more side effects in the PTSD group. Additionally, disulfiram showed more benefit than naltrexone in reducing PTSD symptoms in this study. In a randomized, controlled, 8-week trial of acamprosate in patients with co-occurring alcohol dependence and bipolar disorder (types I and II), acamprosate was well tolerated, without any worsening in depressive or manic symptoms and with some benefit on alcohol outcomes among completers in the last 2 weeks of the trial (Tolliver, Desantis, Brown, Prisciandaro, & Brady, 2012).

FUTURE DIRECTIONS

In the approximately 30 years since researchers and clinicians in the mental health and addictions fields first noted the high prevalence rate of comorbidity and worse outcomes in populations with co-occurring SUDs and psychiatric disorders, important strides have been made in further understanding the epidemiology and sequelae of these disorders, as well as the critical need to develop specific treatments for these populations. Significant progress has been made in developing new treatments, testing them with increasing methodological rigor, and developing optimal treatment methods for these often poorly served patient populations. In the next decade, we are hopeful that this continued research effort will translate into improved treatment methods and outcomes in these patients. Some important future directions include the need for practice guidelines relevant to SUD comorbidity; how to address comorbidity based on different treatment settings (e.g., primary care vs. specialty care); and increased attention to diagnostic decision making when symptom profiles of particular comorbidities overlap (e.g., substance misuse is part of the borderline personality disorder diagnosis). We are hopeful that the next decade will see continued research efforts that will translate into improved clinical care of these patients.

ACKNOWLEDGMENTS

This work was supported by Grant Nos. K24 DA022288 (to Roger D. Weiss), U10 DA15831 (to Roger D. Weiss), and R43DA026649 (to Lisa M. Najavits) from the National Institute on Drug Abuse; Grant Nos. W81XWH-10-2-0173 and W81XWH-10-2-0174 from the Department of Defense (to Lisa M. Najavits); and Department of Veterans Affairs Merit Grant Nos. SPLA-06-S09 and NEUA-001-08S (to Lisa M. Najavits).

REFERENCES

Adinoff, B. (1992). Long-term therapy with benzodiazepines despite alcohol dependence disorder. *Am J Addict, 1*(4), 288–293.
Aharonovich, E., Nguyen, H. T., et al. (2001). Anger and depressive states among treatment-seeking drug abusers: Testing the psychopharmacological specificity hypothesis. *Am J Addict, 10*(4), 327–334.
Albanese, M. J., Bartel, R. L., et al. (1994). Comparison of measures used to determine substance abuse in an inpatient psychiatric population. *Am J Psychiatry, 151*(7), 1077–1078.
Alcoholics Anonymous. (1984). *The AA member: Medications and other drugs* (brochure). New York: Alcoholics Anonymous World Services.
American Psychiatric Association. (1987). *Diagnostic and statistical manual of mental disorders* (3rd ed., rev.). Washington, DC: Author.
American Psychiatric Association. (2000). *Diagnostic and statistical manual of mental disorders* (4th ed., text rev.). Washington, DC: Author.
American Psychiatric Association. (2013). *Diagnostic and statistical manual of mental disorders* (5th ed.). Arlington, VA: Author.
Ball, S. A. (1998). Manualized treatment for substance abusers with personality disorders: Dual focus schema therapy. *Addict Behav, 23*(6), 883–891.
Ball, S. A. (2007). Comparing individual therapies for personality disordered opioid dependent patients. *J Pers Disord, 21*(3), 305–321.

Batki, S. L., Dimmock, J., et al. (2002). *Directly observed naltrexone treatment of alcohol dependence in schizophrenia: Preliminary analysis.* San Francisco: Research Society on Alcoholism.

Beck, A. T. (1979). *Cognitive therapy of depression.* New York: Guilford Press.

Beck, A. T., Epstein, N., Brown, G., & Steer, R. A. (1988). An inventory for measuring clinical anxiety: Psychometric properties. *J Consult Clin Psychol, 56,* 893–898.

Beck, A. T., Wright, F. D., Newman, C. F., & Liese, B. S. (1993). *Cognitive therapy of substance abuse.* New York: Guilford Press.

Bellack, A. S., & DiClemente, C. (1999). Treating substance abuse among patients with schizophrenia. *Psychiatr Serv, 50*(1), 75–80.

Beresford, T., Clapp, L., et al. (2005). Aripiprazole in schizophrenia with cocaine dependence. A pilot study. *J Clin Psychopharmacol, 25,* 363–366.

Boden, M. T., Kimerling, R., et al. (2012). Seeking Safety treatment for male veterans with a substance use disorder and post-traumatic stress disorder symptomatology. *Addiction, 107*(3), 578–586.

Bogenschutz, M. P., Geppert, C. M., et al. (2006). The role of twelve-step approaches in dual diagnosis treatment and recovery. *Am J Addict, 15*(1), 50–60.

Bowers, M. B., Mazure, C. M., et al. (1990). Psychotogenic drug use and neuroleptic response. *Schizophr Bull, 16*(1), 81–85.

Brady, K. T., Dansky, B. S., et al. (2001). Exposure therapy in the treatment of PTSD among cocaine-dependent individuals: Preliminary findings. *J Subst Abuse Treat, 21*(1), 47–54.

Brady, K. T., Sonne, S. C., et al. (1995). Valproate in the treatment of acute bipolar affective episodes complicated by substance abuse: A pilot study. *J Clin Psychiatry, 56*(3), 118–121.

Brady, K. T., Sonne, S. C., et al. (2002). Carbamazepine in the treatment of cocaine dependence: Sub-typing by affective disorder. *Exp Clin Psychopharmacol, 10*(3), 276–285.

Brady, K. T., Sonne, S. C., et al. (2005). Sertraline in the treatment of co-occurring alcohol dependence and posttraumatic stress disorder. *Alcohol Clin Exp Res, 29*(3), 395–401.

Breakey, W. R., Calabrese, L., et al. (1998). Detecting alcohol use disorders in the severely mentally ill. *Commun Ment Health J, 34*(2), 165–174.

Brenner, L. M., Karper, L. P., et al. (1994). Short-term use of disulfiram with clozapine. *J Clin Psychopharmacol, 14*(3), 213–215.

Brooks, A. J., & Penn, P. E. (2003) Comparing treatments for dual diagnosis: Twelve-step and self-management and recovery training. *Am J Drug Alcohol Abuse, 29*(2), 359–383.

Brown, E. S., Carmody, T. J., et al. (2009). A randomized, double-blind, placebo-controlled pilot study of naltrexone in outpatients with bipolar disorder and alcohol dependence. *Alcohol Clin Exp Res, 33*(11), 1863–1869.

Brown, E. S., Garza, M., et al. (2008). A randomized, double-blind, placebo-controlled add-on trial of quetiapine in outpatients with bipolar disorder and alcohol use disorders. *J Clin Psychiatry, 69*(5), 701–705.

Brown, E. S., Gorman, A. R., et al. (2007). A randomized, placebo-controlled trial of citicoline add-on therapy in outpatients with bipolar disorder and cocaine dependence. *J Clin Psychopharmacol, 27*(5), 498–502.

Brown, E., Jejtek, V. A., et al. (2002). Quetiapine in bipolar disorder and cocaine dependence. *Bipolar Disord, 4*(6), 406–411.

Brown, E., Jejtek, V. A., et al. (2003a). Lamotrigine in patients with bipolar disorder and cocaine dependence. *J Clin Psychiatry, 64*(2), 197–201.

Brown, E., Jejtek, V. A., et al. (2003b). Cocaine and amphetamine use in patients with psychiatric illness: A randomized trial of typical antipsychotic continuation or discontinuation. *J Clin Psychopharmacol, 23,* 384–388.

Brown, E. S., Sunderajan, P., et al. (2012). A randomized, double-blind, placebo-controlled, trial of lamotrigine therapy in bipolar disorder, depressed or mixed phase and cocaine dependence. *Neuropsychopharmacol, 37*(11), 2347–2354.

Brown, R. A., Monti, P. M., et al. (1998). Depression among cocaine abusers in treatment: Relation to cocaine and alcohol use and treatment outcome. *Am J Psychiatry, 155*(2), 220–225.

Brown, S. A., Glasner-Edwards, S. V., et al. (2006). Integrated cognitive behavioral therapy versus twelve-step facilitation therapy for substance-dependent adults with depressive disorders. *J Psychoactive Drugs, 38*(4), 449–460.

Brown, S. A., Irwin, M., et al. (1991). Changes in anxiety among abstinent male alcoholics. *J Stud Alcohol, 52*(1), 55–61.

Brown, S. A., & Schuckit, M. A. (1988). Changes in depression among abstinent alcoholics. *J Stud Alcohol, 49*(5), 412–417.

Brunette, M. F., Dawson, R., et al. (2011). A randomized trial of clozapine versus other antipsychotics for cannabis use disorder in patients with schizophrenia. *J Dual Diagn, 7*(1–2), 50–63.

Brunette, M. F., Mueser, K. T., et al. (1997). Relationships between symptoms of schizophrenia and substance abuse. *J Nerv Ment Dis, 185*(1), 13–20.

Brunette, M. F., Noordsy, D. L., et al. (2003). Benzodiazepine use and abuse among patients with severe mental illness and co-occurring substance use disorders. *Psychiatr Serv, 54*(1), 1395–1401.

Buckley, P., Thompson, P., et al. (1994). Substance abuse among patients with treatment-resistant schizophrenia: Characteristics and implications for clozapine therapy. *Am J Psychiatry, 151*(3), 385–389.

Cacciola, J. S., Alterman, A. I., et al. (1995). Treatment response of antisocial substance abusers. *J Nerv Ment Dis, 183*, 166–171.

Calabrese, J. R., Shelton, M. D., et al. (2001). Bipolar rapid cycling: Focus on depression as its hallmark. *J Clin Psychiatry, 62*(Suppl. 14), 34–41.

Carey, K. B. (1995) Treatment of substance use disorders and schizophrenia. In A. F. Lehman & L. B. Dixon (Eds.), *Double jeopardy: Chronic mental illness and substance use disorders* (pp. 85–108). Chur, Switzerland: Harwood.

Carey, K. B., Purnine, D. M., et al. (2001). Enhancing readiness-to-change substance abuse in persons with schizophrenia: A four-session motivation-based intervention. *Behav Modif, 25*(3), 331–384.

Carroll, K. M., & Rounsaville, B. J. (1993). History and significance of childhood attention deficit disorder in treatment-seeking cocaine abusers. *Compr Psychiatry, 34*, 75–86.

Carroll, K. M., & Rounsaville, B. J. (2007). A vision of the next generation of behavioral therapies research in the addictions. *Addiction, 102*(6), 850–862.

Castaneda, R., Levy, R., et al. (2000). Long-acting stimulants for the treatment of attention-deficit disorder in cocaine-dependent adults. *Psychiatr Serv, 51*(2), 169–171.

Ciraulo, D. A., & Jaffe, J. H. (1981). Tricyclic antidepressants in the treatment of depression associated with alcoholism. *J Clin Pharmacol, 1*, 146–150.

Ciraulo, D. A., & Nace, E. P. (2000). Benzodiazepine treatment of anxiety or insomnia in substance abuse patients. *Am J Addict, 9*(4), 276–284.

Ciraulo, D. A., Sands, B. F., et al. (1988). Critical review of the liability of benzodiazepine abuse among alcoholics. *Am J Psychiatry, 145*(12), 1501–1506.

Claassen, C. A., Gilfillan, S., et al. (1997). Substance use among patients with a psychotic disorder in a psychiatric emergency room. *Psychiatr Serv, 48*(3), 353–358.

Compton, W. M., Cottler, L. B., et al. (2003). The role of psychiatric disorders in predicting drug dependence treatment outcomes. *Am J Psychiatry, 160*(5), 890–895.

Compton, W. M., Thomas, Y. F., et al. (2007). Prevalence, correlates, disability, and comorbidity of DSM-IV drug abuse and dependence in the United States: Results from the National Epidemiologic Survey on Alcohol and Related Conditions. *Arch Gen Psychiatry, 64*, 566–576.

Conway, K. P., Compton, W., Stinson, F. S., & Grant, B. F. (2006). Lifetime comorbidity of DSM-IV mood and anxiety disorders and specific drug use disorders: Results from the National Epidemiologic Survey on Alcohol and Related Conditions. *J Clin Psychiatry, 67*(2), 247–257.

Cornelius, J. R., Douaihy, A., et al. (2011). Evaluation of cognitive behavioral therapy/motivational enhancement therapy (CBT/MET) in a treatment trial of comorbid MDD/AUD adolescents. *Addict Behav, 36*(8), 843–848.

Cornelius, J. R., Salloum, I. M., et al. (1997). Fluoxetine in depressed alcoholics: A double-blind, placebo-controlled trial. *Arch Gen Psychiatry, 54*(8), 700–705.

Dalack, G. W., Healy, D. J., et al. (1998). Nicotine dependence in schizophrenia: Clinical phenomena and laboratory findings. *Am J Psychiatry, 155*(11), 1490–1501.

Daley, D. C., & Zuckoff, A. (1998). Improving compliance with the initial outpatient session among discharged inpatient dual diagnosis clients. *Soc Work, 43*, 470–473.

DeMartinis, N., Rynn, M., et al. (2000). Prior benzodiazepine use and buspirone response in the treatment of generalized anxiety disorder. *J Clin Psychiatry, 61*(2), 91–94.

Dickey, B., & Azeni, H. (1996). Persons with dual diagnoses of substance abuse and major mental illness: Their excess costs of psychiatric care. *Am J Public Health, 86*(7), 973–977.

Dimeff, L. A., & Linehan, M. M. (2008). Dialectical behavior therapy for substance abusers. *Addict Sci Clin Pract, 4*(2), 39–47.

Donald, M., Dower, J., et al. (2005). Integrated versus non-integrated management and care for clients with co-occurring mental health and substance use disorders: A qualitative systematic review of randomised controlled trials. *Soc Sci Med, 60*(6), 1371–1383.

Drake, R. E., Essock, S. M., et al. (2001). Implementing dual diagnosis services for clients with severe mental illness. *Psychiatr Serv, 52*(4), 469–476.

Drake, R. E., & Mueser, K. T. (2000). Psychosocial approaches to dual diagnosis. *Schizophr Bul, 26*(1), 105–118.

Drake, R. E., Osher, F. C., et al. (1989). Alcohol use and abuse in schizophrenia: A prospective community study. *J Nerv Ment Dis, 177*, 408–414.

Drake, R. E., Xie, H., et al. (2000). The effects of clozapine on alcohol and drug use disorders among patients with schizophrenia. *Schizophr Bull, 26*(2), 441–449.

Easton, C. J., Oberleitner, L. M., et al. (2012). Differences in treatment outcome among marijuana-dependent young adults with and without antisocial personality disorder. *Am J Drug Alcohol Abuse, 38*(4), 305–313.

Esposito-Smythers, C., Spirito, A., et al. (2011). Treatment of co-occurring substance abuse and suicidality among adolescents: A randomized trial. *J Consult Clin Psychol, 79*(6), 728–739.

Ewing, J. A. (1984). Detecting alcoholism: The CAGE questionnaire. *JAMA, 252*, 1905–1907.

Fals-Stewart, W., & Schafer, J. (1992). The treatment of substance abusers diagnosed with obsessive–compulsive disorder: An outcome study. *J Subst Abuse Treat, 9*(4), 365–370.

Farren, C. K., Hameedi, F. A., et al. (2000). Significant interaction between clozapine and cocaine in cocaine addicts. *Drug Alcohol Depend, 59*(2), 153–163.

Farris, C., Brems, C., et al. (2003). A comparison of schizophrenic patients with or without coexisting substance use disorder. *Psychiatr Q, 74*(3), 205–222.

Foa, E. B., Yusko, D. A., et al. (2013). Concurrent naltrexone and prolonged exposure therapy for patients with comorbid alcohol dependence and PTSD: A randomized clinical trial. *JAMA, 310*(5), 488–495.

Gawin, F. H., & Kleber, H. D. (1984). Cocaine abuse treatment: Open pilot trial with desipramine and lithium carbonate. *Arch Gen Psychiatry, 41*, 903–909.

Gawin, F., & Kleber, H. D. (1986). Abstinence symptomatology and psychiatric diagnoses in cocaine abusers: Clinical observations. *Arch Gen Psychiatry, 43*, 107–113.

Gawin, F., Riordan, C., et al. (1985). Methylphenidate treatment of cocaine abusers without attention deficit disorder: A negative report. *Am J Drug Alcohol Abuse, 11*(3–4), 193–197.

Geller, B., Cooper, T. B., et al. (1998). Double-blind and placebo-controlled study of lithium for adolescent bipolar disorders with secondary substance dependency. *J Am Acad Child Adolesc Psychiatry, 37*(2), 171–178.

Gonzalez, G., & Rosenheck, R. A. (2002). Outcomes and service use among homeless persons with serious mental illness and substance abuse. *Psychiatr Serv, 53*(4), 437–446.

Graeber, D. A., Moyers, T. B., et al. (2003). A pilot study comparing motivational interviewing and an educational intervention in patients with schizophrenia and alcohol use disorders. *Commun Ment Health J, 39*(3), 189–202.

Green, A. I., Burgess, E. S., et al. (2003). Alcohol and cannabis use in schizophrenia: Effects of clozapine vs. risperidone. *Schizophr Res, 60*(1), 81–85.

Green, A. I., Noordsy, D. L., et al. (2008). Substance abuse and schizophrenia: Pharmacotherapeutic intervention. *J Subst Abuse Treat, 34*(1), 61–71.

Green, A. I., Zimmet, S. V., et al. (1999). Clozapine for comorbid substance use disorder and schizophrenia: Do patients with schizophrenia have a reward-deficiency syndrome that can be ameliorated by clozapine? *Harv Rev Psychiatry, 6*(6), 287–296.

Greenfield, S. F., Weiss, R. D., et al. (1998). The effect of depression on return to drinking: A prospective study. *Arch Gen Psychiatry, 55*(3), 259–265.

Grelotti, D. J., Kanayama, G., & Pope, H. G. (2010). Remission of persistent methamphetamine-induced psychosis after electroconvulsive therapy: Presentation of a case and review of the literature. *Am J Psychiatry, 167*(1), 17–23.

Harned, M. S., Chapman, A. L., et al. (2008). Treating co-occurring Axis I disorders in recurrently suicidal women with borderline personality disorder: A 2-year randomized trial of dialectical behavior therapy versus community treatment by experts. *J Consult Clin Psychol, 76*(6),1068–1075.

Hasin, D. S., & Kilcoyne, B. (2012). Comorbidity of psychiatric and substance use disorders in the United States: Current issues and findings from the NESARC. *Curr Opin Psychiatry, 25,* 165–171.

Hasin, D. S., Stinson, F. S., et al. (2007). Prevalence, correlates, disability, and comorbidity of DSM-IV alcohol abuse and dependence in the United States: Results from the National Epidemiologic Survey on Alcohol and Related Conditions. *Arch Gen Psychiatry, 64,* 830–842.

Hasin, D. S., Tsai, W.-Y., et al. (1996). The effects of major depression on alcoholism: Five-year course. *Am J Addict, 5*(2), 144–155.

Hien, D. A., Wells, E. A., et al. (2009). Multisite randomized trial of behavioral interventions for women with co-occurring PTSD and substance use disorders. *J Consult Clin Psychol, 77*(4), 607–619.

Horsfall, J., Cleary, M., et al. (2009). Psychosocial treatments for people with co-occurring severe mental illnesses and substance use disorders (dual diagnosis): A review of empirical evidence. *Harv Rev Psychiatry, 17*(1), 24–34.

Hser, Y. I., Grella, C., et al. (2006). Utilization and outcomes of mental health services among patients in drug treatment. *J Addict Dis, 25*(1), 73–85.

Humphreys, K. (1997). Clinicians' referral and matching of substance abuse patients to self-help groups after treatment. *Psychiatr Serv, 48*(11), 1445–1449.

Imel, Z., Wampold, B., et al. (2008). Distinctions without a difference: Direct comparisons of psychotherapies for alcohol use disorders. *Psychol Addict Behav, 22,* 533–543.

Iovieno, N., Tedeschini, E., et al. (2011). Antidepressants for major depressive disorder and dysthymic disorder in patients with comorbid alcohol use disorders: A meta-analysis of placebo-controlled randomized trials. *J Clin Psychiatry, 72*(8), 1144–1151.

Jaffe, J. H., & Ciraulo, D. A. (1986). Alcoholism and depression. In R. E. Meyer (Ed.), *Psychopathology and addictive disorders* (pp. 293–320). New York: Guilford Press.

Jeffery, D. P., Ley, A., et al. (2000). Psychosocial treatment programmes for people with both severe mental illness and substance misuse. *Cochrane Database Syst Rev, 2,* CD001088.

Kelly, P. J., Kay-Lambkin, F. J., et al. (2012). Study protocol: A randomized controlled trial of a computer-based depression and substance abuse intervention for people attending residential substance abuse treatment. *BMC Public Health, 12,* 113.

Kessler, R. C., Crum, R. M., et al. (1997). Lifetime co-occurrence of DSM-III-R alcohol abuse and dependence with other psychiatric disorders in the National Comorbidity Survey. *Arch Gen Psychiatry, 54*(4), 313–321.

Kessler, R. C., Nelson, C. B., et al. (1996). The epidemiology of co-occurring addictive and mental disorders: Implications for prevention and service utilization. *Am J Orthopsychiatry, 66*(1), 17–31.

Khantzian, E. J. (1985). The self-medication hypothesis of addictive disorders: Focus on heroin and cocaine dependence. *Am J Psychiatry, 142*(11), 1259–1264.

Khantzian, E. J. (1989). Addiction: Self-destruction or self-repair? *J Subst Abuse Treat, 6*(2), 75.

Khantzian, E. J. (1997). The self-medication hypothesis of substance use disorders: A reconsideration and recent applications. *Harv Rev Psychiatry, 4*(5), 231–244.

Khantzian, E. J., & Albanese, M. J. (2008). *Understanding addiction as self medication: Finding hope behind the pain.* Lanham, MD: Rowman & Littlefield.

Kingsbury, S. J., & Salzman, C. (1990). Disulfiram in the treatment of alcoholic patients with schizophrenia. *Hosp Community Psychiatry, 41*(2), 133–134.

Kofoed, L., Kania, J., et al. (1986). Outpatient treatment of patients with substance abuse and coexisting psychiatric disorders. *Am J Psychiatry, 143*(7), 867–872.

Konstenius, M., Jayaram-Lindström, N., et al. (2010) Sustained release methylphenidate for the treatment of ADHD in amphetamine abusers: A pilot study. *Drug Alcohol Depend, 108*(1–2), 130–133.

Kosten, T. R., Fontana, A., et al. (2000). Benzodiazepine use in posttraumatic stress disorder among veterans with substance abuse. *J Nerv Ment Dis, 188*(7), 454–459.

Kranzler, H. R., Burleson, J. A., et al. (1994). Buspirone treatment of anxious alcoholics: A placebo-controlled trial. *Arch Gen Psychiatry, 51*(9), 720–731.

Kranzler, H. R., Del Boca, F. K., et al. (1996). Comorbid psychiatric diagnosis predicts three-year outcomes in alcoholics: A posttreatment natural history study. *J Stud Alcohol, 57*(6), 619–626.

Kurtz, L. F. (1997). *Self-help and support groups: A handbook for practitioners.* Thousand Oaks, CA: Sage.

LeDuc, P., & Mittleman, G. (1995). Schizophrenia and psychostimulant abuse: A review and re-analysis of clinical evidence. *Psychopharmacology, 121*(4), 407–427.

Levin, F. R., Evans, S. M., et al. (1998a). Methylphenidate treatment for cocaine abusers with adult attention-deficit/hyperactivity disorder: A pilot study. *J Clin Psychiatry, 59*(6), 300–305.

Levin, F. R., Evans, S. M., et al. (1998b). Flupenthixol treatment for cocaine abusers with schizophrenia: A pilot study. *Am J Drug Alcohol Abuse, 24*(3), 343–360.

Levin, F. R., Evans, S. M., et al. (1999). Practical guidelines for the treatment of substance abusers with adult attention-deficit hyperactivity disorder. *Psychiatr Serv, 50*(8), 1001–1003.

Levin, F. R., Evans, S. M., et al. (2002). Bupropion treatment for cocaine abuse and adult attention-deficit/hyperactivity disorder. *J Addict Dis, 21*(2), 1–16.

Levin, F. R., Evans, S. M., et al. (2006). Treatment of methadone-maintained patients with adult ADHD: Double-blind comparison of methylphenidate, bupropion and placebo. *Drug Alcohol Depend, 81*(2), 137–148.

Levin, F. R., Evans, S. M., et al. (2007). Treatment of cocaine dependent treatment seekers with adult ADHD: Double-blind comparison of methylphenidate and placebo. *Drug Alcohol Depend, 87*(1), 20–29.

Linehan, M. M., Dimeff, L. A., et al. (2002). Dialectical behavior therapy versus comprehensive validation therapy plus 12-step for the treatment of opioid dependent women meeting criteria for borderline personality disorder. *Drug Alcohol Depend, 67*(1), 13–26.

Linehan, M. M., Schmidt, H., et al. (1999). Dialectical behavior therapy for patients with borderline personality disorder and drug-dependence. *Am J Addict, 8*, 279–292.

Littrell, K. H., Petty, R. G., et al. (2001). Olanzapine treatment for patients with schizophrenia and substance abuse. *J Subst Abuse Treat, 21*(4), 217–221.

Lybrand, J., & Caroff, S. (2009). Management of schizophrenia with substance use disorders. *Psychiatr Clin N Am, 32*, 821–833.

Lydecker, K. P., Tate, S. R., et al. (2010). Clinical outcomes of an integrated treatment for depression and substance use disorders. *Psychol Addict Behav, 24*(3), 453–465.

Magura, S., Laudet, A. B., et al. (2002). Adherence to medication regimens and participation in dual-focus self-help groups. *Psychiatr Serv, 53*(3), 310–316.

Magura, S., Laudet, A. B., et al. (2003). Role of self-help processes in achieving abstinence among dually diagnosed persons. *Addict Behav, 28*(3), 399–413.

Mahler, J. (1995). HIV, substance use, and chronic mental illness. In A. F. Lehman & L. B. Dixon (Eds.), *Double jeopardy: Chronic mental illness and substance use disorders* (pp. 159–175). Chur, Switzerland: Harwood.

Malcolm, R., Anton, R. F., et al. (1992). A placebo-controlled trial of buspirone in anxious inpatient alcoholics. *Alcohol Clin Exp Res, 16*(6), 1007–1013.

Mannuzza S., Klein, R. G., et al. (2003). Does stimulant treatment place children at risk for adult substance abuse?: A controlled, prospective follow-up study. *J Child Adolesc Psychopharmacol, 13*(3), 273–282.

Mark, T. L. (2003). The costs of treating persons with depression and alcoholism compared with depression alone. *Psychiatr Serv, 54*(8), 1095–1097.

Martino, S., Carroll, K., et al. (2002). Dual diagnosis motivational interviewing: A modification of motivational interviewing for substance-abusing patients with psychotic disorders. *J Subst Abuse Treat, 23*(4), 297–308.

Mason, B. J., Kocsis, J. H., et al. (1996). A double-blind, placebo-controlled trial of desipramine for primary alcohol dependence stratified on the presence or absence of major depression. *JAMA, 275,* 761–767.

McHugo, G. J., Drake, R. E., et al. (1999). Fidelity to assertive community treatment and client outcomes in New Hampshire dual disorders study. *Psychiatr Servs, 50*(6), 818–824.

McKay, J. R., Pettinati, H. M., et al. (2002). Relation of depression diagnoses to 2-year outcomes in cocaine-dependent patients in a randomized continuing care study. *Psychol Addict Behav, 16*(3), 225–235.

McLellan, A. T., & Druley, K. A. (1977). Non-random relation between drugs of abuse and psychiatric diagnosis. *J Psychiatr Res, 13*(3), 179–184.

McRae, A. L., Sonne, S. C., et al. (2004). A randomized, placebo-controlled trial of buspirone for the treatment of anxiety in opioid-dependent individuals. *Am J Addict, 13*(1), 53–63.

Meissen, G., Powell, T. J., et al. (1999). Attitudes of AA contact persons toward group participation by persons with a mental illness. *Psychiatr Serv, 50*(8), 1079–1081.

Mendelson, J. H., & Mello, N. K. (1966). Experimental analysis of drinking behavior of chronic alcoholics. *Ann NY Acad Sci, 133,* 828–845.

Meyer, R. E. (1986). How to understand the relationship between psychopathology and addictive disorders: Another example of the chicken and the egg. In R. E. Meyer (Ed.), *Psychopathology and addictive disorders.* New York: Guilford Press.

Meyer, R. E., & Mirin, S. M. (1979). *The heroin stimulus: Implications for a theory of addiction.* New York: Plenum.

Michelson, D., Adler, L., et al. (2003). Atomoxetine in adults with ADHD: Two randomized, placebo-controlled studies. *Biol Psychiatry, 53*(2), 112–120.

Miller, N. S., Ninonuevo, F. G., et al. (1997). Integration of treatment and posttreatment variables in predicting results of abstinence-based outpatient treatment after one year. *J Psychoactive Drugs, 29*(3), 239–248.

Miller, W. R., & Rollnick, S. (1991). *Motivational interviewing: Preparing people to change addictive behavior.* New York: Guilford Press.

Miller, W. R., & Rollnick, S. (2002). *Motivational interviewing: Preparing for change* (2nd ed.). New York: Guilford Press.

Mills, K. L., Teesson, M., et al. (2012). Integrated exposure-based therapy for co-occurring posttraumatic stress disorder and substance dependence: A randomized controlled trial. *JAMA, 308*(7), 690–699.

Moak, D. H., Anton, R. F., et al. (2003). Sertraline and cognitive behavioral therapy for depressed alcoholics: Results of a placebo-controlled trial. *J Clin Psychopharmacol, 23*(6), 553–562.

Moore, T. H., Zammit, S., et al. (2007). Cannabis use and risk of psychotic or affective mental health outcomes: A systematic review. *Lancet, 370*(9584), 319–328.

Morojele, N. K., Saban, A., et al. (2012). Clinical presentations and diagnostic issues in dual diagnosis disorders. *Curr Opin Psychiatry, 25*, 181–186.

Morrens, M., Dewilde, B., et al. (2011). Treatment outcomes of an integrated residential programme for patients with schizophrenia and substance use disorder. *Eur Addict Res, 17*(3), 154–163.

Mueller, T. I., Goldenberg, I. M., et al. (1996). Benzodiazepine use in anxiety disordered patients with and without a history of alcoholism. *J Clin Psychiatry, 57*(2), 83–89.

Mueller, T. I., Lavori, P. W., et al. (1994). Prognostic effect of the variable course of alcoholism on the 10-year course of depression. *Am J Psychiatry, 151*(5), 701–706.

Mueser, K. T., Bellack, A. S., et al. (1992). Comorbidity of schizophrenia and substance abuse: Implications for treatment. *J Consult Clin Psychol, 60*(6), 845–856.

Mueser, K. T., & Fox, L. (2002). A family intervention program for dual disorders. *Community Ment Health J, 38*(3), 253–270.

Mueser, K. T., Noordsy, D. L., et al. (2003). Disulfiram treatment for alcoholism in severe mental illness. *Am J Addict, 12*(3), 242–252.

Murphy, K. R., & Barkley, R. A. (1996). Prevalence of DSM-IV symptoms of ADHD in adult licensed drivers. *J Atten Disord, 1*, 147–161.

Najavits, L. M. (2002). *Seeking Safety: A treatment manual for PTSD and substance abuse.* New York: Guilford Press.

Najavits, L. M. (2004). Assessment of trauma, PTSD, and substance use disorder: A practical guide. In J. P. Wilson & T. Keane (Eds.), *Assessing psychological trauma and PTSD.* New York: Guilford Press.

Najavits, L. M. (2013). Therapy for posttraumatic stress and alcohol dependence. *JAMA, 310*(22), 2457–2458.

Najavits, L. M., Capezza, N. M. (2014). Depression and PTSD comorbidity. In S. Richards & M. O'Hara (Eds.), *The Oxford handbook of depression and comorbidity.* New York: Oxford University Press.

Najavits, L. M., Gallop, R. J., et al. (2006). Seeking Safety therapy for adolescent girls with PTSD and substance use disorder: A randomized controlled trial. *J Behav Health Serv Res, 33*(4), 453–463.

Najavits, L. M., Harned, M. S., et al. (2007). Six-month treatment outcomes of cocaine-dependent patients with and without PTSD in a multisite national trial. *J Stud Alcohol, 68*, 353–361.

Najavits, L. M., & Hien, D. (2013). Helping vulnerable populations: A comprehensive review of the treatment outcome literature on substance use disorder and PTSD. *J Clin Psychol, 69*(5), 433–479.

Najavits, L. M., Ryngala, D., et al. (2008). Treatment for PTSD and comorbid disorders: A review of the literature. In E. B. Foa, T. M. Keane, M. J. Friedman, & J. Cohen (Eds.), *Effective treatments for PTSD: Practice guidelines from the International Society for Traumatic Stress Studies.* New York: Guilford Press.

Najavits, L. M., Weiss, R. D., et al. (1996). Group cognitive-behavioral therapy for women with PTSD and substance use disorder. *J Subst Abuse Treat, 13*(1), 13–22.

Najavits, L. M., Weiss, R. D., et al. (1998). "Seeking Safety": Outcome of a new cognitive-behavioral psychotherapy for women with posttraumatic stress disorder and substance dependence. *J Trauma Stress, 11*(3), 437–456.

Noordsy, D. L., Schwab, B., et al. (1996). The role of self-help programs in the rehabilitation of persons with severe mental illness and substance use disorders. *Community Ment Health J, 32*(1), 71–81.

Nunes, E. V., & Levin, F. R. (2004). Treatment of depression in patients with alcohol or other drug dependence: A meta-analysis. *JAMA, 291*(15), 1887–1896.

Nunes, E. V., McGrath, P. J., et al. (1990). Lithium treatment for cocaine abusers with bipolar spectrum disorders. *Am J Psychiatry, 147*(5), 655–657.

Nunes, E. V., Quitkin, F. M., et al. (1998). Imipramine treatment of opiate-dependent patients with depressive disorders: A placebo-controlled trial. *Arch Gen Psychiatry, 55*(2), 153–160.

Petrakis, I., Leslie, D., et al. (2006). Atypical antipsychotic medication and substance use-related outcomes in the treatment of schizophrenia. *Am J Addict, 15*, 44–49.

Petrakis, I., Nich, C., et al. (2006). Psychotic spectrum disorders and alcohol abuse: A review of pharmacotherapeutic strategies and a report on the effectiveness of naltrexone and disulfiram. *Schizophr Bull, 32*(4), 644–654.

Petrakis, I., O'Malley, S., et al. (2004). Naltrexone augmentation of neuroleptic treatment in alcohol abusing patients with schizophrenia. *Psychopharmacol, 172*(3), 291–297.

Petrakis, I., Poling, J., et al. (2005). Naltrexone and disulfiram in patients with alcohol dependence and comorbid psychiatric disorders. *Biol Psychiatry, 57*(10), 1128–1137.

Petrakis, I., Poling, J., et al. (2006). Naltrexone and disulfiram in patients with alcohol dependence and comorbid post-traumatic stress disorder. *Biol Psychiatry, 60*(7), 777–783.

Petrakis, I., Ralevski, E., et al. (2007). Naltrexone and disulfiram in patients with alcohol dependence and current depression. *J Clin Psychopharmacol, 27*(2), 160–165.

Pettinati, H. M., Oslin, D. W., et al. (2010). A double-blind, placebo-controlled trial combining sertraline and naltrexone for treating co-occurring depression and alcohol dependence. *Am J Psychiatry, 167*, 668–675.

Post, R. M., Kotin, J., et al. (1974). The effects of cocaine on depressed patients. *Am J Psychiatry, 131*, 511–517.

Powell, B. J., Penick, E. C., et al. (1992). Outcomes of co-morbid alcoholic men: A 1-year follow-up. *Alcohol Clin Exp Res, 16*(1), 131–138.

Randall, C. L., Johnson, M. R., et al. (2001). Paroxetine for social anxiety and alcohol use in dual-diagnosed patients. *Depress Anxiety, 14*(4), 255–262.

Randall, C. L., Thomas, S., et al. (2001). Concurrent alcoholism and social anxiety disorder: A first step toward developing effective treatments. *Alcohol Clin Exp Res, 25*(2), 210–220.

Regier, D. A., Farmer, M. E., et al. (1990). Comorbidity of mental disorders with alcohol and other drug abuse. Results from the Epidemiologic Catchment Area (ECA) Study. *JAMA, 264*(19), 2511–2518.

Ridgely, S., Goldman, H. H., et al. (1990). Barriers to the care of persons with dual diagnoses: Organizational and financing issues. *Schizophr Bull, 16*(1), 123–132.

Ries, R. K., Sloan, K., et al. (1997). Dual diagnosis: concept, diagnosis, and treatment. In D. Dunner (Ed.), *Current psychiatric therapy* (pp. 173–180). Philadelphia: Saunders.

Riggs, P. D., Winhusen, T., et al. (2011). Randomized controlled trial of osmotic-release methylphenidate with cognitive-behavioral therapy in adolescents with attention-deficit/hyperactivity disorder and substance use disorders. *J Am Acad Child Adolesc Psychiatry, 50*(9), 903–914.

Ritsher, J. B., McKellar, J. D., et al. (2002). Psychiatric comorbidity, continuing care and mutual help as predictors of five-year remission from substance use disorders. *J Stud Alcohol, 63*(6), 709–715.

Rohsenow, D. J., Monti, P. M., et al. (2002). Brief coping skills treatment for cocaine abuse: 12-month substance use outcomes. *J Consult Clin Psychol, 68*(3), 515–520.

Ross, H. E., Glaser, F. B., et al. (1988). The prevalence of psychiatric disorders in patients with alcohol and other drug problems. *Arch Gen Psychiatry, 45*(11), 1023–1031.

Rounsaville, B. J. (2004). Treatment of cocaine dependence and depression. *Biol Psychiatry, 56*, 803–809.

Rounsaville, B. J., & Carroll, K. M. (1997). Individual psychotherapy for drug abusers. In J. H.

Lowinson, P. Ruiz, R. B. Millman, & J. G. Langrod (Eds.), *Substance abuse: A comprehensive textbook* (pp. 430–439). Baltimore, MD: Williams & Wilkins.

Rounsaville, B. J., Dolinsky, Z. S., et al. (1987). Psychopathology as a predictor of treatment outcome in alcoholics. *Arch Gen Psychiatry, 44*(6), 505–513.

Rubio, G., Martinez, I., et al. (2006). Long-acting injectable risperidone compared with zuclopenthixol in the treatment of schizophrenia with substance abuse comorbidity. *Can J Psychiatry, 51*(8), 531–539.

Ruglass, L. M., Miele, G. M., et al. (2012). Helping alliance, retention, and treatment outcomes: A secondary analysis from the NIDA Clinical Trials Network Women and Trauma Study. *Subst Use Misuse, 47*(6), 695–707.

Salloum, I. M., Cornelius, J. R., et al. (1998). Naltrexone utility in depressed alcoholics. *Psychopharmacol Bull, 34*(1), 111–115.

Salloum, I. M., Cornelius, J. R., et al. (2005). Efficacy of valproate maintenance in patients with bipolar disorder and alcoholism: A double-blind placebo-controlled study. *Arch Gen Psychiatry, 62*(1), 37–45.

San, L., Arranz, B., et al. (2007). Antipsychotic drug treatment of schizophrenic patients with substance abuse disorders. *Eur Addict Res, 13*, 230–243.

Sannibale, C., Teesson, M., et al. (2013). Randomized controlled trial of cognitive behaviour therapy for comorbid post-traumatic stress disorder and alcohol use disorders. *Addiction, 108*, 1397–1410.

Satel, S., Southwick, S., et al. (1991). Clinical features of cocaine-induced paranoia. *Am J Psychiatry, 148*, 495–499.

Sayers, S., Campbell, E., et al. (2005). Cocaine abuse in schizophrenic patients treated with olanzapine versus haloperidol. *J Nerv Ment Dis, 193*, 379–386.

Schaar, I., & Oejehagen, A. (2001). Severely mentally ill substance abusers: An 18-month follow-up study. *Soc Psychiatry Psychiatr Epidemiol, 36*(2), 70–78.

Schadé, A., Marquenie, L. A., et al. (2008). The effectiveness of anxiety treatment on alcohol-dependent patients with a comorbidphobic disorder: A randomised controlled trial. *Tijdschr Psychiatr, 50*(3),137–148.

Schubiner, H., Downey, K. K., et al. (2002). Double-blind placebo-controlled trial of methylphenidate in the treatment of adult ADHD patients with comorbid cocaine dependence. *Exp Clin Psychopharmacol, 10*(3), 286–294.

Schweizer, E., Rickels, K., et al. (1986). Resistance to the anti-anxiety effect of buspirone in patients with a history of benzodiazepine use. *N Engl J Med, 314*(11), 719–720.

Sellman, D. (2010). The 10 most important things known about addiction. *Addiction, 105*(1), 6–13.

Smelson, D. A., Losonczy, M. F., et al. (2002a). Risperdone decreases craving and relapses in individuals with schizophrenia and cocaine dependence. *Can J Psychiatry, 47*(7), 671–675.

Smelson, D. A., Losonczy, M. F., et al. (2002b). An analysis of cue reactivity among persons with and without schizophrenia who are addicted to cocaine. *Psychiatr Serv, 53*(12), 1612–1616.

Smelson, D. A., Ziedonis, D., et al. (2006). The efficacy of olanzapine for decreasing cue-elicited craving in individuals with schizophrenia and cocaine dependence: A preliminary report. *J Clin Psychopharmacol, 26*, 9–12.

Sonne, S. C., & Brady, K. T. (2000). Naltrexone for individuals with comorbid bipolar disorder and alcohol dependence. *J Clin Psychopharmacol, 20*(1), 114–115.

Soyka, M., Aichmüller, C., et al. (2003). Flupenthixol in relapse prevention in schizophrenics with comorbid alcoholism: Results from an open clinical study. *Eur Addict Res, 9*(2), 65–72.

Spencer, C., Castle, D., et al. (2002). Motivations that maintain substance use among individuals with psychotic disorders. *Schizophr Bull, 28*(2), 233–247.

Stedman, M., Pettinati, H. M., et al. (2010). A double-blind, placebo-controlled study with quetiapine as adjunct therapy with lithium or divalproex in bipolar I patients with coexisting alcohol dependence. *Alcohol Clin Exp Res, 34*(10), 1822–1831.

Substance Abuse and Mental Health Services Administration (SAMHSA). (2002). *Report to*

Congress on the prevention and treatment of co-occurring substance abuse disorders and mental disorders. Washington, DC: U.S. Department of Health and Human Services.

Swanson, A. J., Pantalon, M. V., et al. (1999). Motivational interviewing and treatment adherence among psychiatric and dually diagnosed patients. *J Nerv Ment Dis, 187*(10), 630–635.

Swendsen, J., Conway, K. P., et al. (2010). Mental disorders as risk factors for substance use, abuse and dependence: results from the 10-year follow-up of the National Comorbidity Survey. *Addiction, 105*(6), 1117–1128.

Szobot, C. M., Rohde, L. A., et al. (2008). A randomized crossover clinical study showing that methylphenidate-SODAS improves attention-deficit/hyperactivity disorder symptoms in adolescents with substance use disorder. *Braz J Med Biol Res, 41*(3), 250–257.

Teesson, M., Hall, W., et al. (2010). Prevalence and correlates of DSM-IV alcohol abuse and dependence in Australia: Findings of the 2007 National Survey of Mental Health and Wellbeing. *Addiction, 105*(12), 2085–2094.

Teesson, M., Slade, T., & Mills, K. (2009). Comorbidity in Australia: Findings of the 2007 National Survey of Mental Health and Wellbeing. *Aust N Z J Psychiatry, 43*(7), 606–614.

Thomas, S. E., Randall, P. K., et al. (2008). A complex relationship between co-occurring social anxiety and alcohol use disorders: What effect does treating social anxiety have on drinking? *Alcohol Clin Exp Res, 32*(1), 77–84.

Titievsky, J., Seco, G., et al. (1982). Doxepin as adjunctive therapy for depressed methadone maintenance patients: A double-blind study. *J Clin Psychiatry, 43*(11), 454–456.

Tollefson, G. D., Montague-Clouse, J., et al. (1992). Treatment of comorbid generalized anxiety in a recently detoxified alcoholic population with a selective serotonergic drug (buspirone). *J Clin Pharmacol, 12*(1), 19–26.

Tolliver, B. K., Desantis, S. M., et al. (2012). A randomized, double-blind, placebo-controlled clinical trial of acamprosate in alcohol-dependent individuals with bipolar disorder: A preliminary report. *Bipolar Disord, 14*(1), 54–63.

Torchalla, I., Nosen, L., et al. (2012). Integrated treatment programs for individuals with concurrent substance use disorders and trauma experiences: A systematic review and meta-analysis. *J Subst Abuse Treat, 42*(1), 65–77.

Torrens, M., Fonseca, F., et al. (2005). Efficacy of antidepressants in substance use disorders with and without comorbid depression: A systematic review and meta-analysis. *Drug Alcohol Depend, 78*(1), 1–22.

Torrens, M., Gilchrist, G., et al. (2011). Psychiatric comorbidity in illicit drug users: Substance-induced versus independent disorders. *Drug Alcohol Depend, 113*(2–3), 147–156.

Upadhyaya, H. P., Brady, K. T., et al. (2001). Venlafaxine treatment of patients with comorbid alcohol/cocaine abuse and attention-deficit/hyperactivity disorder: A pilot study. *J Clin Psychopharmacol, 21*(1), 116–117.

van Dam, D., Ehring, T., et al. (2013). Trauma-focused treatment for posttraumatic stress disorder combined with CBT for severe substance use disorder: A randomized controlled trial. *BMC Psychiatry, 13*(1), 172.

Weiss, R. D. (1992). The role of psychopathology in the transition from drug use to abuse and dependence. In M. Glantz & R. Pickens (Eds.), *Vulnerability to drug abuse* (pp. 137–148). Washington, DC: American Psychological Association.

Weiss, R. D., & Connery H. S. (2011). *Integrated group therapy for bipolar disorder and substance abuse.* New York: Guilford Press.

Weiss, R. D., Griffin, M. L., et al. (1992). Drug abuse as self-medication for depression: An empirical study. *Am J Drug Alcohol Abuse, 18*(2), 121–129.

Weiss, R. D., Griffin, M. L., et al. (2000). Group therapy for patients with bipolar disorder and substance dependence: Results of a pilot study. *J Clin Psychiatry, 61*(5), 361–367.

Weiss, R. D., Griffin, M. L., et al. (2007). A randomized trial of integrated group therapy versus group drug counseling for patients with bipolar disorder and substance dependence. *Am J Psychiatry, 164*(1), 100–107.

Weiss, R. D., Griffin, M. L., et al. (2009). A "community-friendly" version of integrated group therapy for patients with bipolar disorder and substance dependence: A randomized controlled trial. *Drug Alcohol Depend, 104*(3), 212–219.

Weiss, R. D., & Hufford, M. R. (1999). Substance abuse and suicide. In D. Jacobs (Ed.), *Harvard Medical School guide to assessment and intervention in suicide* (pp. 300–310). New York: Simon & Schuster.

Weiss, R. D., Mirin, S. M., et al. (1986). Psychopathology in chronic cocaine abusers. *Am J Drug Alcohol Abuse, 12*(1–2), 17–29.

Weiss, R. D., Mirin, S. M., et al. (1988). Psychopathology in cocaine abusers: Changing trends. *J Nerv Ment Dis, 176*(12), 719–725.

Weiss, R. D., Mirin, S. M., et al. (1992). The myth of the typical dual diagnosis patient. *Hosp Community Psychiatry, 43*(2), 107–108.

Weiss, R. D., Najavits, L. M., et al. (1998). Validity of substance use self-reports in dually diagnosed outpatients. *Am Journal Psychiatry, 155*(1), 127–128.

Westra, H. A., Aviram, A., et al. (2011). Extending motivational interviewing to the treatment of major mental health problems: Current directions and evidence. *Can J Psychiatry, 56*(11), 643–650.

Wilens, T. E. (2003). Does the medicating of ADHD increase or decrease the risk for later substance abuse? *Rev Bras Psiquatr, 25*(3), 127–128.

Wilens, T. E., Adler, L. A., et al. (2008). Atomoxetine treatment of adults with ADHD and comorbid alcohol use disorders. *Drug Alcohol Depend, 96*(1–2), 145–154.

Wilens, T. E., Biederman, J., et al. (1996). Six-week, double-blind, placebo-controlled study of desipramine for adult attention deficit hyperactivity disorder. *Am J Psychiatry, 153*(9), 1147–1153.

Wilens, T. E., Prince, J. B., et al. (2010). An open trial of sustained release bupropion for attention-deficit/hyperactivity disorder in adults with ADHD plus substance use disorders. *J ADHD Related Disord, 1*(3), 25–35.

Wilens, T. E., Spencer, T. J., et al. (2002). A controlled clinical trial of bupropion for attention deficit hyperactivity disorder in adults. *Am J Psychiatry, 158*(2), 282–288.

Winterer, G. (2010). Why do patients with schizophrenia smoke? *Curr Opin Psychiatry, 23*(2), 112–119.

Woodward, B., Fortgang, J., et al. (1991). Underdiagnosis of alcohol dependence in psychiatric inpatients. *Am J Drug Alcohol Abuse, 17*(4), 373–388.

Wusthoff, L. E., Waal, H., et al. (2011). Identifying co-occurring substance use disorders in community mental health centres: Tailored approaches are needed. *Nord J Psychiatry, 65*, 58–64.

Ziedonis, D., Hitsman, B., et al. (2008). Tobacco use and cessation in psychiatric disorders: National Institute of Mental Health report. *Nicotine Tob Res, 10*(12), 1691–1715.

Ziedonis, D., Richardson, T., et al. (1992). Adjunctive desipramine in the treatment of cocaine abusing schizophrenics. *Psychopharmacol Bull, 28*(3), 309–314.

Ziedonis, D., Williams, J., et al. (2000). Management of substance abuse in schizophrenia. *Psychiatr Ann, 30*(1), 67–75.

Zimmet, S. V., Strous, R. D., et al. (2000). Effect of clozapine on substance use in patients with schizophrenia and schizoaffective disorder: A retrospective study. *J Clin Psychopharmacol, 20*(1), 94–98.

CHAPTER 16

Gambling Disorder and Other "Behavioral" Addictions

LIANA R. N. SCHREIBER
MARC N. POTENZA
JON E. GRANT

Several behavioral problems have been hypothesized as having similarities to substance addictions and are referred to as "behavioral addictions." These behaviors involve short-term rewards that may engender persistent behaviors despite knowledge of adverse consequences (i.e., diminished control over the behavior). Diminished control is a core defining concept of psychoactive substance dependence or addiction (Potenza, 2006). The concept of behavioral addictions has some scientific and clinical heuristic value but remains controversial (Grant, Brewer, & Potenza, 2006).

Although which behaviors to include as behavioral addictions is still open for debate (Holden, 2010), the behaviors that have received the most research attention include gambling disorder, kleptomania, compulsive buying, compulsive sexual behavior, and Internet addiction. In the hope of contributing to this debate, we review in this chapter the evidence for similarities between behavioral addictions and substance use disorders (SUDs) and identify areas of uncertainty that warrant future research. It seems increasingly important that individuals involved in the prevention and treatment of SUDs have a current understanding of these behavioral addictions, and the potential for future research findings to guide prevention and treatment efforts for addictions in general.

CORE FEATURES OF BEHAVIORAL AND DRUG ADDICTIONS

Behavioral and drug addictions share common core qualities: (1) repetitive or compulsive engagement in a behavior despite adverse consequences; (2) diminished control

over the problematic behavior; (3) an appetitive urge or craving state prior to engagement in the problematic behavior; and (4) a hedonic quality during the performance
of the problematic behavior. These features have led to a description of behavioral
addictions as "addictions without the drug."

Clinical similarities between behavioral addictions and SUDs are best reflected
in the diagnostic criteria for gambling disorder. Criteria for gambling disorder (GD)
share common features with those for substance dependence (American Psychiatric
Association, 2013), including aspects of tolerance, withdrawal, repeated unsuccessful attempts to cut back or stop, and impairment in major areas of life functioning
(Blanco, Moreyra, Nunes, Saiz-Ruiz, & Ibanez, 2001). Epidemiological data also
support a relationship between GD and SUDs, with high rates of co-occurrence in
each direction (Potenza, Fiellin, Heninger, Rounsaville, & Mazure, 2002). Phenomenological data further support a relationship between behavioral and drug addictions; for example, high rates of GD and SUDs have been reported during adolescence
and young adulthood (Chambers & Potenza, 2003), and the telescoping phenomenon
(reflecting the more rapid progression from initial to problematic behavioral engagement in women as compared with men) initially described for alcoholism has been
applied to GD (Potenza, Steinberg, et al., 2001; Hernandez-Avila, Rounsaville, &
Kranzler, 2004). Emerging biological data, such as those identifying common genetic
contributions to alcohol use and gambling disorders (Slutske et al., 2000; Grant,
Kushner, & Kim, 2002), and common brain activity changes underlying gambling
urges and drug cravings (Hodgins, Stea, & Grant, 2011; Leeman & Potenza, 2012),
provide further support for a shared relationship between GD and SUDs.

EPIDEMIOLOGY

Arguably the best data on the prevalence of behavioral addictions exist for GD.
Approximately 0.4 to 1.6% of individuals in the United States meet criteria for GD
(National Opinion Research Center, 1999; Petry, Stinson, & Grant, 2005). Rates of
problem gambling, a less severe form of disordered gambling than GD (not presently
included among psychiatric classifications), have been estimated at an additional
3–5% of the general adult population (Hodgins et al., 2011). As with SUDs, higher
rates of problem gambling and GD have been reported in males, particularly during
adolescence and young adulthood.

Although no large-scale epidemiological studies have assessed the prevalence
of many other behavioral addictions in the general population, smaller community
studies indicate that these behaviors are present to varying degrees. A survey of college students (N = 791) indicated that three individuals (0.38%) met DSM-IV criteria
for kleptomania, and 3.44% reported symptoms consistent with the proposed criteria
for compulsive sexual behavior (Odlaug & Grant, 2010). The estimated prevalence
of compulsive buying based on a random digit dialing telephone survey in the United
States was 5.8% (Koran, Faber, Aboujaoude, Large, & Serpe, 2006). Worldwide,
Internet addiction has been estimated to have a prevalence rate of 1–14% (Block,
2008; Park, Kim, & Cho, 2008; Tsitsika et al., 2009; Bakken, Wenzel, Götestam,

Johansson, & Øren, 2009), although lower rates of 0.3–0.7% have been reported in the United States (Shaw & Black, 2008).

GAMBLING DISORDER

Clinical Characteristics

GD shares many features with SUDs. Gambling behavior usually begins in childhood or adolescence, with males tending to start at an earlier age (Auger, Lo, & O'Loughlin, 2012; Rahman et al., 2012; Chambers & Potenza, 2003; Grant & Kim, 2001a). Higher rates of GD are observed in men, with a telescoping phenomenon observed in females (Nelson, LaPlante, LaBrie, & Shaffer, 2006; Tavares et al., 2003). GD has been described as a chronic, relapsing condition (Potenza, Kosten, & Rounsaville, 2001). High rates of GD in adolescents and young adults suggest a natural history similar to that observed with SUDs (Chambers & Potenza, 2003).

Other gender-related differences in GD have been described. Female, compared with male gamblers, tend to have problems with nonstrategic forms of gambling, such as slot machines and bingo, whereas men are more likely than women to have problems with strategic forms, such as sports and card gambling (Potenza, Steinberg, et al., 2001; Blanco, Hasin, Petry, Stinson, & Grant, 2006; Odlaug, Marsh, Kim, & Grant, 2011). As is the case for SUDs and specific substances, further investigation is needed to determine how problems from specific forms of gambling might relate to prevention and treatment efforts. Both female and male gamblers report that advertisements are a common trigger of their urges to gamble, although females are more likely to report that feeling bored or lonely may also trigger their urges to gamble (Grant & Kim, 2001a; Ladd & Petry, 2002).

As with SUDs, financial and marital problems are common (Dowling, Smith, & Thomas, 2009; Grant, Schreiber, Odlaug, & Kim, 2010) and often include illegal behaviors, such as stealing, embezzlement, and writing bad checks (Grant & Potenza, 2007; Ledgerwood, Weinstock, Morasco, & Petry, 2007). Findings of similar cognitive features in GD and SUDs have also been reported (Brewer & Potenza, 2008); for example, both groups have been found to display rapid temporal discounting of rewards and to perform disadvantageously on decision-making tasks (Bechara, 2003; Hodgins et al., 2011). Furthermore, Goudriaan, Oosterlaan, de Beurs, and van den Brink (2006) found that similar cognitive deficits (i.e., poor inhibition, time estimation, cognitive flexibility, and planning) were found in both individuals with GD and those with alcohol dependence, although Lawrence, Luty, Bogdan, Sahakian, and Clark (2009a, 2009b) found more severe deficits in individuals with alcohol use problems than in those with gambling problems.

Co-Occurring Disorders

Patients with GD have high rates of lifetime mood (50–76%) and anxiety (16–41%) disorders (Erbas & Buchner, 2012; Petry et al., 2005; Black & Moyer, 1998; Crockford & el-Guebaly, 1998). Elevated rates of compulsive buying, compulsive sexual behavior, and intermittent explosive disorder have also been found (Black & Moyer, 1998; Grant & Kim, 2001a).

High rates of co-occurrence have been reported for SUDs (including nicotine dependence) and GD, with the highest odds ratios generally observed between gambling and alcohol use disorders (Cunningham-Williams, et al., 1998; Welte, et al., 2001; Petry, Stinson, & Grant, 2005). A Canadian epidemiological survey estimated that the relative risk for an alcohol use disorder is increased 3.8 fold when disordered gambling is present (Grant, Kushner, & Kim, 2002), and odds ratio ranging from 3.3 to 23.1 have been reported between GD and alcohol abuse/dependence in U.S. population-based studies (Cunningham-Williams, Cottler, Compton, & Spitznagel, 1998; Welte, Barnes, Wieczorek, Tidwell, & Parker, 2001).

Treatment

Although no medication has received regulatory approval in any jurisdiction as a treatment for gambling disorders, there have been 18 double-blind, placebo-controlled trials of various pharmacological agents (opioid antagonists, glutamatergic agents, antidepressants, mood stabilizers) for the treatment of GD (Hodgins et al., 2011). Given the high rates of placebo response often observed in treatment trials of GD, we focus in this section on findings from double-blind, placebo-controlled trials.

A meta-analysis of 16 pharmacological treatment trials, published between 2000 and 2006, found that compared to placebo, pharmacological trials were significantly more effective at reducing gambling symptomatology (Pallesen et al., 2007). However these results need careful interpretation due to studies reporting high subject attrition rates and placebo response, as well as treatment trials published since 2006.

Opioid Antagonists

Given their ability to modulate dopaminergic transmission in the mesolimbic pathway, opioid receptor antagonists (naltrexone, nalmefene) have been investigated in the treatment of GD. Two double-blind, placebo-controlled studies of naltrexone (Kim, Grant, Adson, & Shin, 2001; Grant, Kim, & Hartman, 2008) and two multicenter double-blind, placebo-controlled trials of nalmefene (Grant, Potenza, et al., 2006; Grant, Odlaug, Potenza, Hollander, & Kim, 2010) suggest the efficacy of opioid antagonists in reducing the intensity of urges to gamble, and gambling thoughts and behaviors. Pooled analyses of those who responded to opioid antagonists demonstrated significant reduction in gambling urges, particularly among participants with a positive family history of alcohol dependence (Grant, Kim, Hollander, & Potenza, 2008).

Antidepressants

Most studies of antidepressants in GD have focused on selective serotonin reuptake inhibitors (SSRIs). Fluvoxamine demonstrated mixed results in two placebo-controlled, double-blind studies—one 16-week crossover study supporting its efficacy at an average dose of 207 mg/d (Hollander et al., 2000), and a different 6-month, parallel-arm study with high dropout rates that found no significant difference in response to active or placebo drug (Blanco, Petkova, Ibanez, & Saiz-Ruiz, 2002). Similarly, paroxetine at doses between 20 and 60 mg/d (average end-of-study dose = 52 mg/d) demonstrated efficacy in one placebo-controlled, double-blind study (Kim, Grant, Adson, Shin, & Zaninelli, 2002), but a 16-week, multicenter study of paroxetine did not find a statistically significant difference between active drug and placebo (48% of individuals showing a positive response to placebo, 59% to active drug; Grant et al., 2003).

Currently, the only non-SSRI antidepressant examined for GD is bupropion, which has not been found superior to placebo (35.7 and 47.1% of those on active medication and placebo, respectively, reported "much" or "very much" improvement on the Clinical Global Improvement Impression Scale); however, these results are complicated by a high noncompletion rate of 43.6% and a small sample size (Black et al., 2007).

Mood Stabilizers

A double-blind study found sustained-release lithium carbonate superior to placebo in 29 bipolar-spectrum pathological gamblers over 10 weeks (Hollander, Pallanti, Allen, Sood, & Rossi, 2005). Bipolar spectrum disorders were defined as including DSM-IV diagnoses of bipolar II disorder, bipolar disorder not otherwise specified, and cyclothymia, and mood swings that occurred at times unrelated to gambling urges/behavior. Topiramate, however, was not found to reduce gambling behavior or urges significantly in a sample of 42 subjects with GD enrolled in a 14-week double-blind, randomized study (Berlin et al., 2013).

Antipsychotics

Olanzapine, an atypical antipsychotic drug, was not significantly different from placebo in the treatment of nonpsychotic pathological gamblers (Fong, Kalechstein, Bernhard, Rosenthal, & Rugle, 2008; McElroy, Nelson, Weldge, Kaehler, & Keck, 2008). Typical antipsychotic drugs have not been examined in the treatment of GD, although they have been associated with increasing gambling-related motivations in individuals with GD (Zack & Poulos, 2007). As individuals with psychotic disorders frequently experience GD (Desai & Potenza, 2009), trials investigating the efficacy and tolerability of medications in targeting PG-related thoughts and behaviors in this population are needed.

Other Agents

Because improving glutamatergic tone in the nucleus accumbens has been implicated in reducing reward-seeking behaviors in addictions (Li, Xi, & Markou, 2013; Kalivas, Lalumiere, Knackstedt, & Shen, 2009; Kalivas, Volkow, & Seamans, 2005), N-acetyl cysteine, an amino acid and glutamate-modulating agent, has been studied in the treatment of GD and has demonstrated positive effects on urges and gambling behavior (Grant, Kim, & Odlaug, 2007). Based on existing data on subgroups of individuals with GD, a pharmacotherapy treatment algorithm has been proposed (Bullock & Potenza, 2012).

Psychotherapy

Multiple behavioral treatments have been investigated (Hodgins et al., 2011). A meta-analysis using 22 randomized psychological treatment trials (mainly behavioral, cognitive, and cognitive-behavioral formats) published between 1968 and 2004, revealed that psychological treatments were more effective than not receiving treatment, event after a follow-up period averaging 17 months (Pallesen, Mitsem, Kvale, Johnsen, & Molde, 2005). Cognitive therapy focuses on changing the patient's beliefs regarding perceived control over randomly determined events. Case reports have demonstrated success with cognitive therapy (Ladouceur, Sylvain, Legate, Giroux, & Jacques, 1998), and further support is derived from three randomized trials. In the first, individual cognitive therapy resulted in reduced gambling frequency and increased perceived self-control over gambling when compared with a wait-list control group (Sylvain, Ladouceur, & Boisvert, 1997). A second trial that included relapse prevention also produced improvement in gambling symptoms compared to a wait-list group (Ladouceur et al., 2001). A third trial that evaluated the efficacy of cognitive intervention in a group format found that group cognitive treatment significantly reduced GD severity compared to a control condition (Ladouceur et al., 2003).

Cognitive-behavioral therapy (CBT) has also been used to treat GD. In one randomized trial, Echeburua, Baez, and Fernandez-Montalvo (1996) compared four groups: (1) individual stimulus control and *in vivo* exposure with response prevention, (2) group cognitive restructuring, (3) a combination of 1 and 2, and (4) a wait-list control. At 12 months, rates of abstinence or minimal gambling were higher in the individual treatment (69%) compared with group cognitive restructuring (38%) and the combined treatment (38%). More recent studies indicate that CBT is more efficacious than a referral to Gamblers Anonymous (Petry et al., 2006); internet-delivered CBT reduces GD severity significantly more than no treatment (Carlbring & Smit, 2008); and individualized CBT may be more effective than group CBT for treating GD (Dowling, Smith, & Thomas, 2007).

Brief interventions in the form of workbooks have also been studied. One study assigned gamblers to a workbook alone (the workbook included cognitive-behavioral and motivational enhancement techniques) or to the workbook in addition to one clinician interview (Dickerson, Hinchy, & England, 1990). Both groups reported significant reductions in gambling at a 6-month follow-up. Similarly, a separate study assigned gamblers to a workbook, a workbook plus a telephone motivational enhancement intervention, or a wait list. Compared to the workbook alone, those gamblers assigned to the motivational intervention and workbook reduced gambling throughout a 2-year follow-up period (Hodgins, Currie, & el-Guebaly, 2001; Hodgins, Currie, el-Guebaly, & Peden, 2004).

Two studies have investigated brief motivational interviewing. Hodgins, Currie, Currie, and Fick (2009) compared a wait-list control group to two brief motivational-interviewing groups (with and without six booster phone calls) and found that both treatment groups were effective in reducing gambling frequency and money lost.

Petry, Weinstock, Ledgerwood, and Morasco (2008) found that one session of motivational enhancement therapy plus three sessions of CBT significantly reduced gambling compared to a wait-list control group in a sample of 180 problem and pathological gamblers (60% of subjects were pathological gamblers).

In addition, three studies have tested aversion therapy and imaginal desensitization in randomized designs. In the first study, both treatments resulted in improvement in a small sample of patients (McConaghy, Armstrong, Blaszczynski, & Allcock, 1983). In the second study, 120 pathological gamblers were randomly assigned to aversion therapy, imaginal desensitization, *in vivo* desensitization, or imaginal relaxation. Participants receiving imaginal desensitization reported better outcomes at 1 month and up to 9 years later (McConaghy, Blaszczynski, & Frankova, 1991). Imaginal desensitization with motivational interviewing has also been found to be significantly more efficacious in reducing GD-related urges and behaviors than Gamblers Anonymous referrals. This treatment effect was largely maintained after 6 months of treatment cessation (Grant, Donahue, et al., 2009; Grant, Donahue, Odlaug, & Kim, 2011).

KLEPTOMANIA

Kleptomania was formally designated a psychiatric disorder in DSM-III, and the core features include (1) recurrent failure to resist an impulse to steal unneeded objects; (2) an increasing sense of tension before committing the theft; (3) an experience of pleasure, gratification or release at the time of committing the theft; and (4) stealing that is not performed out of anger, vengeance, or due to psychosis (DSM-5; American Psychiatric Association, 2013).

Clinical Characteristics

Kleptomania usually appears first during late adolescence or early adulthood (Grant & Kim, 2002a). The course is generally chronic, with waxing and waning of symptoms. Women are twice as likely as men to suffer from kleptomania (Grant & Kim, 2002a), to have a later age of onset, hoard stolen items, and to have a co-occurring eating disorder or other psychiatric illness (Grant & Potenza, 2008).

Like individuals with SUDs, most with kleptomania try unsuccessfully to stop. In one study, all participants reported increased urges to steal when trying to stop (Grant & Kim, 2002a). Most (77.3%) report a diminished ability to stop that often leads to feelings of shame and guilt (Grant & Kim, 2002a). Of married subjects, less than half had disclosed their behavior to their spouses due to shame and guilt (Grant & Kim, 2002a).

Although people with kleptomania often steal various items from multiple places, the majority steals from stores. In one study, 68.2% of patients reported that the value of stolen items had increased over time (Grant & Potenza, 2008), a finding that is suggestive of tolerance. Patients may keep, hoard, discard, gift, or return stolen items (McElroy, Pope, Hudson, Keck, & White, 1991). Many (64–87%) have been apprehended at some time due to their behavior (McElroy et al., 1991), and

15–23% report having been jailed (Grant, Odlaug, Davis, & Kim, 2009). Although the majority of the patients who were apprehended reported that their urges to steal were diminished after the apprehension, their symptom remission generally lasted only a few days or weeks (McElroy et al., 1991). Together, these findings demonstrate a continued engagement in the problematic behavior despite adverse consequences, a core feature of addiction.

Co-Occurring Disorders and Family History

High rates of other psychiatric disorders have been found in patients with kleptomania. Rates of lifetime comorbid affective disorders range from 38.9% (Grant & Kim, 2002a; Grant & Potenza, 2008) to 100% (McElroy et al., 1991). The rate of comorbid bipolar disorder has been reported as ranging from 9% (Grant & Kim, 2002a) to 60% (McElroy et al., 1991). Studies also indicate high lifetime rates of comorbid anxiety disorders (21.1–80.0%; Grant & Potenza, 2008; McElroy et al., 1991; McElroy, Hudson, Pope, Keck, & Aizley, 1992), impulse control disorders (20.0–47.4%; Grant & Potenza, 2008; Grant, 2003), SUDs (15.8–50.0%; Grant & Kim, 2002a; Grant & Potenza, 2008; McElroy et al., 1991), and eating disorders (13.7–60.0%; Grant & Potenza, 2008; McElroy et al., 1991).

Individuals with kleptomania are more likely than non-affected controls to have a first-degree relative with a psychiatric disorder (Grant, 2003). In addition, high rates of mood disorders (20–35%) and SUDs (15–20%) have been observed in first-degree relatives of patients with kleptomania (McElroy et al., 1991).

Treatment

Pharmacotherapy

Case reports, two small case series, and two open-label studies of pharmacotherapy have been performed for kleptomania. Given the high placebo responses rates observed in the treatment of impulse control disorders, findings from these studies should be interpreted cautiously. Various medications have been studied in case reports or case series, and several have been found effective: tolcapone, fluoxetine, nortriptyline, trazodone, clonazepam, valproate, lithium, fluvoxamine, paroxetine, and topiramate (Grant, 2011; Grant & Kim, 2002b).

Two open-label studies of kleptomania have been published. A trial of naltrexone for kleptomania involved 10 subjects in a 12-week, open-label study. Using a mean dose of 150 mg/d, medication resulted in a significant decline in the intensity of urges to steal, stealing thoughts, and stealing behavior (Grant & Kim, 2002b). Koran, Aboujaoud, and Gamel (2007) examined open-label escitalopram and found a high response rate (79%); however, in the double-blind discontinuation period, rates of relapse did not differ between escitalopram (43%) and placebo (50%).

Only one double-blind study that has been published assesses pharmacological treatment for kleptomania. In a sample of 25 subjects with kleptomania, naltrexone (mean dose of 117 mg/d) was significantly more effective in reducing stealing urges and behaviors in an 8-week randomized trial (Grant, Kim, & Odlaug, 2009).

Psychotherapy

Although multiple types of psychotherapies have been described in the treatment of kleptomania, no controlled trials exist in the literature. Forms of psychotherapy described in case reports as demonstrating success include psychoanalytic, insight-oriented, and behavioral (Goldman, 1991; McElroy et al., 1991). As no controlled trials of therapy for kleptomania have been published, the efficacies of these interventions are difficult to evaluate.

COMPULSIVE BUYING

Originally termed "oniomania" by Kraepelin and Bleuler, compulsive buying has been described for over a century (Christenson et al., 1994). Although not specifically recognized in DSM-5, the following diagnostic criteria have been proposed: (1) maladaptive preoccupation with or engagement in buying (evidenced by frequent preoccupation with or irresistible impulses to buy; or frequent buying of items that are not needed or not affordable; or shopping for longer periods of time than intended); (2) preoccupations, or the buying lead to significant distress or impairment; and (3) the buying does not occur exclusively during hypomanic or manic episodes (McElroy, Keck, Pope, Smith, & Strakowski, 1994).

Clinical Characteristics

As with other behavioral addictions and SUDs, the onset of compulsive buying appears to occur during late adolescence or early adulthood, although the full disorder may take several years to develop (Christenson et al., 1994; Black, 2007). Koran et al. (2006) estimated that about 5.8% of the U.S. population has lifetime prevalence compulsive buying. Unlike most substance abuse disorders, compulsive buying shows a female preponderance ranging from 80 to 95% in clinical samples (Black, 2007; Christenson et al., 1994; McElroy et al., 1994; Schlosser, Black, Repertinger, & Freet, 1994).

Compulsive buying is characterized by repetitive urges to shop that are most often unprovoked but may be triggered by being in stores. These urges may worsen during times of stress, emotional difficulties, or boredom. Urges are generally intrusive, and most patients attempt to resist them, although usually unsuccessfully. Even though purchased items are usually not exceptionally expensive, individuals with compulsive buying typically purchase items in large quantities (Black, 2007), which often results in large debts, marital or family disruption, and legal consequences (Christenson et al., 1994). Although the behavior is pleasurable and momentarily relieves the urges to shop, guilt, shame, and embarrassment generally follow buying episodes. Individuals with compulsive buying also report experiencing significantly increased negative affect and decreased positive affect before a buying episode, as well as a significant decrease in negative affect postbuying (Müller et al., 2012). Furthermore, these individuals report low quality of psychological well-being compared to those do not buy compulsively (Williams, 2012).

A positive interaction with salespeople is often described as a motivating factor in compulsive buying. The items bought vary considerably, and may include clothing, jewelry, books, and auto parts. Most items are not used or removed from the packaging, and many are given away, returned, or hoarded (Christenson et al., 1994).

Co-Occurring Disorders and Family History

Rates of co-occurring mood disorders range from 28 to 95% (Christenson et al., 1994; McElroy et al., 1994; Schlosser et al., 1994; Müller et al., 2012), with the mood disorder often preceding the compulsive buying by at least one year (Christenson et al., 1994). Lifetime histories of anxiety (41–80%), substance use (21–46%), eating (17–35%), and impulse control (21–40%) disorders are fairly common (Christenson et al., 1994; McElroy et al., 1994; Müller et al., 2012; Schlosser et al., 1994). High rates of personality disorders (60%) have also been found in individuals with compulsive buying. Most commonly observed are avoidant disorder (15%), obsessive-compulsive disorder (22%), and borderline personality disorder (15%) (Schlosser et al., 1994). In addition, individuals with compulsive buying frequently report having first-degree relatives with SUDs (25%), mood disorders (20%), or compulsive buying (10%), and they are significantly more likely than healthy controls to have a first-degree family member with one or more psychiatric disorders (Black, Repertinger, Gaffney, & Gabel, 1998).

Treatment

Pharmacotherapy

The effectiveness of pharmacotherapies in treating compulsive buying is beginning to be systematically investigated. Case reports and open-label studies have suggested that the following agents may be beneficial: nortriptyline, fluoxetine, bupropion, lithium, clomipramine, naltrexone, fluvoxamine, citalopram, and valproate (Black, Monahan, & Gabel, 1997; Koran, Bullock, Hartson, Elliott, & D'Andrea, 2002; McElroy et al., 1994).

In the first of two double-blind fluvoxamine studies, 37 subjects were treated for 13 weeks. Only nine out of 20 patients assigned to medication were responders (mean dose of 215 mg/d), and this rate did not differ significantly from that in the placebo group (eight out of 17 were responders) (Ninan et al., 2000). In the second double-blind study, Black, Gabel, Hansen, and Schlosser (2000) treated 23 patients for 9 weeks following a 1-week placebo lead-in phase. Using a mean dose of 200 mg/d, no differences in response rates were observed between the groups treated with active and placebo drug.

A double-blind study using citalopram, however, suggested the possible efficacy of SSRIs in treating compulsive buying. Open-label treatment for 7 weeks was followed by randomization of responders to medication or placebo for another 9 weeks. Patients taking active citalopram demonstrated statistically significant decreases in terms of the frequency of shopping, as well as the intensity of thoughts and urges concerning shopping (Koran, Chuong, Bullock, & Smith, 2003). However, in a more recent study with an identical research design, escitalopram was no more effective than placebo (Koran, Aboujaoude, Solvason, Gamel, & Smith, 2007).

There has been only one trial using a medication other than an antidepressant. Memantine, an N-methyl-D-aspartate receptor antagonist, was examined in a 10-week, open-label trial of nine individuals with compulsive buying. Eight of the nine subjects reported significantly reduced symptoms, such as time and money spent shopping per week (Grant, Odlaug, Mooney, O'Brien, & Kim, 2012).

Psychotherapy

Several case reports suggest that possible effective psychotherapeutic interventions might include exposure and response prevention, and supportive or insight-oriented psychotherapy (McElroy et al., 1994). Three randomized controlled studies indicated that CBT, using either an individual or group format, is more significantly effective than wait-list or telephone-guided self-help in reducing the frequency and duration of buying episodes, as well as overall compulsive buying severity (Mitchell, Burgard, Faber, Crosby, & de Zwaan, 2006; Müller et al., 2012, 2013).

INTERNET ADDICTION

Internet addiction is not currently recognized by DSM-5 (American Psychiatric Association, 2013) as a psychiatric disorder (Internet gaming disorder is included in the section "Conditions for Further Study") and valid, reliable diagnostic instruments have not been developed for an Internet addiction diagnosis (Weinstein & Lejoyeux, 2010). Tao and colleagues (2010), however, have recommended the following criteria for Internet addiction, which mirror those used for GD or SUDs: preoccupation with the Internet; withdrawal; increased tolerance for Internet use; inability to control Internet use; continuation of Internet use despite negative consequences; loss of interest in other activities; and using the Internet to relieve dysphoric mood states. Furthermore, Block (2008) has suggested that three subcategories exist for Internet addiction: excessive gaming, sexual preoccupations, and excessive e-mail/text messaging. Young, Pistner, O'Mara, and Buchann (2000) have suggested five subtypes of Internet addiction: cybersexual addiction, cyberrelational addiction, net compulsions, information overload, and computer addiction. However, some argue that Internet addiction does not require a new diagnostic categorization, that it is rather an addiction to the behaviors associated with Internet usage, such as sex or gaming (Yellowlees & Marks, 2007).

Clinical Characteristics

Researchers estimate that Internet addiction has a prevalence rate of 0.3–0.7% in the United States (Shaw & Black, 2008). Internet addiction has an age of onset between the late 20s and early 30s, and typically there is about a 10-year span between first use and problematic Internet use (Shaw & Black, 2008). Internet addiction also appears to be more prevalent in males (Shaw & Black, 2008; Ko et al., 2012).

Even though time spent online is not a discerning marker of Internet addiction, research has suggested that individuals with Internet problems typically spend 38–80 hours per week online (Young, 1995, 1996), and that they spend more time on the Internet for nonessential use (i.e., pleasure or personal use) compared to essential use (i.e., required for school or job functions) (Young, 1995; Shapira, Goldsmith, Keck, Khosla, & McElroy, 2000).

Personality variables, such as a high degree of novelty seeking and harm avoidance, have been associated with excessive use of the Internet (Ha et al., 2007; Ko et al., 2006; June, Sohn, So, Yi, & Park, 2007). Additionally, Young (1998) found that some may be drawn to the Internet due to the mental stimulation provided by the substantial amount of information available online, as well as the ability to be social without having face-to-face interactions with others and while remaining by oneself.

Problems associated with problematic Internet use include, but are not limited to, decreased academic performance, social/relational and occupational impairment, financial problems, and legal problems (Shapira et al., 2000). Research also indicates that individuals with Internet addiction may face health concerns, such as sleep deprivation, carpal tunnel syndrome, dry eyes, and headaches (Choi et al., 2009; Coniglio, Muni, Giammanco, & Pignato, 2007). Furthermore, in South Korea there were a series of 10 cardiopulmonary-related deaths in Internet cafés (Choi, 2007, as referenced in Block, 2008) and a game-related murder (Koh, 2007, as referenced in Block, 2008).

Co-Occurring Disorders and Family History

Like other addictions, Internet addiction frequently co-occurs with other psychiatric disorders, such as affective, anxiety, substance use, and impulse control disorders (Bai, Lin, & Chen, 2001; Shapira et al., 2000; Treur, Fábián, & Füredi, 2001; te Wildt, Putzig, Zedler, & Ohlmeier, 2007; Kratzer & Hegerl, 2008; Shaw & Black, 2008; Black, Belsare, & Schlosser, 1999). For example, a study of 20 individuals with problematic Internet use indicated that all subjects met DSM-IV criteria for an impulse control disorder not otherwise specified, as well as an additional lifetime DSM-IV Axis I diagnosis (Shapira et al., 2000). Additionally, high rates of personality disorders have been found in those with Internet addiction, most commonly borderline (24%), narcissistic (19%), and antisocial (19%; Black et al., 1999).

Shapira et al. (2000) reported that the majority (95%) of individuals with an Internet addiction reported a psychiatric family history, most commonly an affective disorder or an SUD.

Treatment

Currently, there is limited evidence regarding effective treatments for Internet addiction; however, both psychotherapy and psychopharmacology have been used to treat the behavior (Weinstein & Lejoyeux, 2010).

Pharmacotherapy

A small sample of 19 individuals with "compulsive–impulsive computer usage" was treated with 10 weeks of open-label escitalopram followed by a week of double-blind discontinuation. No significant differences were found between those receiving escitalopram and those receiving placebo (Hadley, Baker, & Hollander, 2006).

Another open-label study (Han et al., 2009) examined extended-release methylphenidate in 62 Korean children with Internet video game addiction and attention-deficit/hyperactivity disorder (ADHD). They found that after 8 weeks of treatment, daily duration of Internet use was significantly reduced, and this finding correlated with an increase in attention.

Shapira and colleagues (2000) reported that while only 35.7% of individuals using an antidepressant reported moderate or marked reduction in problematic Internet use, 58.3% of individuals with problematic Internet use reported a favorable response when taking a mood stabilizer.

Psychotherapy

No randomized clinical trials have assessed the efficacy of psychotherapy in Internet addiction. However, treatments that have utilized aspects of CBT, as well as marital and family therapy, and online self-help books and tapes, have been found to be helpful (Young, 2007; Shaw & Black, 2008).

COMPULSIVE SEXUAL BEHAVIOR

Compulsive sexual behavior (CSB), also termed "sexual addiction" and "hypersexual behavior," is characterized by an excessive, uncontrollable, culturally normative sexual behaviors, urges, and/or thoughts resulting in functional impairment and distress (Black, Kehrberg, Flumerfelt, & Schlosser, 1997; Coleman, 1992; Gerevich, Treuer, Danics, & Herr, 2005). In 1775, de Bienville published *Nymphomania or Dissertation concerning Furor Uterinus*, arguing that excessive sexual desire may be a product of the overstimulation of women's nerves through impure thoughts, consuming too much chocolate or rich food, or reading novels. About a century later, Krafft-Ebbing (1886/1927) in his book *Psychopathia Sexualis*, described the negative impact of excessive sexual behavior on life.

Similar to some of the other behavioral addictions, CSB is not currently recognized by DSM-5. The following diagnostic criteria have been proposed by Martin Kafka (2010): (1) intense, recurrent sexual fantasies, urges, or behaviors that are associated with at least three of following: (a) interference with life; (b) relief of dysphoric mood or stressful life events; (c) inability to control fantasies, urges, or behaviors; (d) disregard to negative consequences of sexual fantasies, urges, and behaviors to self or others; (2) frequent and intense sexual fantasies, urges, and behaviors associated with clinically significant distress or impairment in social, occupational, or other important life areas; and (3) sexual fantasies, urges, or behaviors not caused by an exogenous substance's (e.g., a drug of abuse or prescribed medication) direct physiological effect.

Clinical Characteristics

The estimated prevalence rate for CSB in the United States has ranged from 3 to 6% (Black, 2000; Carnes, 1991; Coleman, 1992; Kuzma & Black, 2008). A study revealed that 3.44% of college students reported symptoms consistent with the proposed criteria for CSB (Odlaug & Grant, 2010). Higher rates of CSB have been reported in sexual offenders and individuals with HIV (Marshall & Marshall, 2006), as well as in those who identify as homosexuals (Qualand, 1985; Parsons, 2005). The majority of individuals with CSB report being preoccupied with sexual fantasies, behaviors, or urges for over 60 minutes a day (Raymond, Coleman, & Miner, 2003).

Typically, and similar to the other behavioral addictions and SUDs, individuals develop CSB during late adolescence (Black, Kehrberg, et al., 1997; Kafka, 1997), and most who present for treatment are males (Black, Kehrberg, et al., 1997; Carnes, 1991; Raymond et al., 2003). Interestingly, females with CSB are more likely to have multiple sexual partners and lower relationship satisfaction than females who do not meet CSB criteria. Males with or without CSB, however, do not differ in terms of number of sexual partners or relationship satisfaction (Skegg, Nada-Raja, Dickson, & Paul, 2010).

Mood states, such as depression, happiness, or loneliness, may trigger CSB (Black, Kehrberg, et al., 1997; Kafka & Prentky, 1997). While engaging in CSB-related behaviors, some individuals report feelings of dissociation, while other report feeling important, powerful, excited, and gratified (Black, Kehrberg, et al., 1997; Kafka & Prentky, 1997). After engaging in activities, however, the majority feels a negative mood, such as shame and guilt (Black, Kehrberg, et al., 1997; Raymond et al., 2003; Reid, Stein, & Carpenter, 2011). Reid, Carpenter, and Lloyd (2009) found elevated rates of interpersonal sensitivity, depression, obsessiveness, and isolation in a sample of hypersexual individuals compared to controls. Additionally, many individuals report significant marital, occupational, and financial problems associated with sexual behavior (Coleman, Raymond, & McBean, 2003).

Co-Occurring Disorders and Family History

Co-occurring medical and psychiatric disorders are common in individuals with CSB. Medical sequelae from CSB may include pregnancy, sexually transmitted infections, HIV/AIDS, and physical injury due to repetitive sexual activities (e.g., anal and vaginal trauma, burns from overuse of a vibrator; Carnes, 1991; Coleman, 1992; Coleman et al., 2003). High rates of lifetime and current psychiatric comorbidity have also been documented in individuals with CSB, most commonly anxiety (50–96%, especially social phobia [21–42%]), and SUDs (64–71%; especially alcohol [63%], and cannabis [38%]), and mood disorders (39–71%; especially major depression [58%]; Raymond et al., 2003; Black, Kehrberg, et al., 1997). Personality disorders are also common, with studies revealing rates of 44–46% within the CSB population (Black, Kehrberg, et al., 1997; Raymond et al., 2003).

A family history of substance abuse and mental illness is also common. One study indicated that recovering sexual addicts report having at least one parent with a chemical dependency (46%), sexual addiction (36%), eating disorder (30%), or gambling problem (7%; Schneider & Schneider, 1996). Most individuals with CSB (87%) also have a family history of addiction (Carnes,1998).

Treatment

Pharmacotherapy

There is a dearth of research examining pharmacotherapies for CSB. Many pharmacological agents used to treat paraphilias have been used to treat CSB, due to their similar sexual-related characteristics (Krueger & Kaplan, 2002). These data, however, are largely case reports: naltrexone (Bostwick & Bucci, 2008; Grant & Kim, 2001b), naltrexone and SSRIs (Raymond, Grant, Kim, & Coleman, 2002), citalopram (Malladi & Singh, 2005), leuprolide acetate (Saleh, 2005), nefaxodone (Coleman, Gratzer, Nesvacil, & Raymond, 2000), clomipramine, and valproic acid (Gulsun, Vulcat, & Aydin, 2007), psychostimulants or bupropion (Kafka, 2000), and psychostimulant augmentation of SSRIs (Kafka & Hennen, 2000).

The only double-blind study that has been published for nonparaphilic CSB examined citalopram in 28 gay and bisexual men, and found significant treatment effects in regards to sexual desire and drive, masturbation frequency, and pornography use. However, groups did not differ in their reduction in risky sexual behavior (Wainberg et al., 2006).

Psychotherapy

Research suggests that cognitive-behavioral strategies (Penix Sbraga & O'Donohue, 2003; McConaghy, Armstrong, & Blaszczynksi, 1985) and psychodynamic psychotherapy (Cooper, Putnam, Planchon, & Boies, 1999; Goodman, 1998) may be helpful with this population. Couple therapy may also be helpful due to the negative impact CSB may have on the trust and intimacy in relationships (Brown, 1999).

In the only randomized study of psychotherapy for CSB, 20 subjects were randomized to either imaginal desensitization or covert sensitization. McConaghy and colleagues (1985) found that both interventions were effective in reducing CSB at 1-month and 1-year follow-up visits.

CONCLUSIONS

Behavioral addictions have historically received relatively little attention from clinicians and researchers. As such, our understanding of the basic features of these disorders is relatively primitive. Future research investigating behavioral addictions and their relationship to SUDs holds significant promise in advancing prevention and treatment strategies for addiction in general.

REFERENCES

American Psychiatric Association. (2000). *Diagnostic and statistical manual of mental disorders* (4th ed., text rev.). Washington, DC.

American Psychiatric Association. (2013). *Diagnostic and statistical manual of mental disorders* (5th ed.). Arlington, VA: Author.

Auger, N., Lo, E., & O'Loughlin, J. (2012). Risk of gambling onset in youth who are younger than same-grade peers. *Ann Epidemiol, 22*(5), 372–375.

Bai, Y. M., Lin, C. C., & Chen, J. Y. (2001). Internet addiction disorder among clients of a virtual clinic. *Psychiatr Serv, 52*(10), 1397.

Bakken, I., Wenzel, H., Götestam, K., Johansson, A., & Øren, A. (2009). Internet addiction among Norwegian adults: A stratified probability sample study. *Scand J Psychol, 50*(2), 121–127.

Bechara, A. (2003). Risky business: Emotion, decision-making, and addiction. *J Gambl Stud, 19*, 23–51.

Berlin, H. A., Braun, A., Simeon, D., Koran, L. M., Potenza, M. N., McElroy, S. L., et al. (2013). A double-blind, placebo-controlled trial of topiramate for pathological gambling. *World J Biol Psychiatry, 14*(2), 121–128.

Black, D. W. (2000). The epidemiology and phenomenology of compulsive sexual behavior. *CNS Spectrums, 5*(1), 26–72.

Black, D. W. (2007). A review of compulsive buying disorder. *World Psychiatry, 6*(1), 14–18.

Black, D. W., Arndt, S., Coryell, W. H., Argo, T., Forbush, K. T., Shaw, M. C., et al. (2007). Bupropion in the treatment of pathological gambling: A randomized, double-blind, placebo-controlled, flexible-dose study. *J Clin Psychopharmacol, 27*, 143–150.

Black, D. W., Belsare, G., & Schlosser, S. (1999). Clinical features, psychiatric comorbidity, and health-related quality of life in persons reporting compulsive computer use behavior. *J Clin Psychiatry, 60*, 839–843.

Black, D. W., Gabel, J., Hansen, J., & Schlosser, S. (2000). A double-blind comparison of fluvoxamine versus placebo in the treatment of compulsive buying disorder. *Ann Clin Psychiatry, 12*, 205–211.

Black, D. W., Kehrberg, L. L. D., Flumerfelt, D. L., & Schlosser, S. S. (1997). Characteristics of 36 subjects reporting compulsive sexual behavior. *Am J Psychiarty, 154*, 243–249.

Black, D. W., Monahan, P., & Gabel, J. (1997). Fluvoxamine in the treatment of compulsive buying. *J Clin Psychiatry, 58*, 159–163.

Black, D. W., & Moyer, T. M. (1998). Clinical features and psychiatric comorbidity of subjects with pathological gambling behavior. *Psychiatr Serv, 49*, 1434–1439.

Black, D. W., Repertinger, S., Gaffney, G. R., & Gabel, J. (1998). Family history and psychiatric comorbidity in persons with compulsive buying: Preliminary findings. *Am J Psychiatry, 155*, 960–963.

Blanco, C., Hasin, D. S., Petry, N., Stinson, F. S., & Grant, B. F. (2006). Sex differences in subclinical and DSM-IV pathological gambling: Results from the National Epidemiologic Survey on Alcohol and Related Conditions. *Psychol Med, 36*, 943–953.

Blanco, C., Moreyra, P., Nunes, E. V., Saiz-Ruiz, J., & Ibanez, A. (2001). Pathological gambling: Addiction or compulsion? *Seminars Clin Neuropsychiatry, 6*, 167–176.

Blanco, C., Petkova, E., Ibanez, A., & Saiz-Ruiz, J. (2002). A pilot placebo-controlled study of fluvoxamine for pathological gambling. *Ann Clin Psychiatry, 14*, 9–15.

Block, J. J. (2008). Issues for DSM-V: Internet addiction. *Am J Psychiatry, 165*, 306–307.

Bostwick, J. M., & Bucci, J. A. (2008). Internet sex addiction treated with naltrexone. *Mayo Clin Proc, 83*, 226–230.

Brewer, J. A., & Potenza, M. N. (2008). The neurobiology and genetics of impulse control disorders: Relationships to drug addictions. *Biochem Pharmacol, 75*(1), 63–75.

Brown, E. M. (1999). *Affairs: A guide to working through the repercussions of infidelity.* San Francisco: Jossey-Bass.

Bullock, S. A., & Potenza, M. N. (2012). Pathological gambling: Neuropsychopharmacology and treatment. *Curr Psychopharmacol, 1*(1), 67–85.

Carlbring, P., & Smit, F. (2008). Randomized trial of internet-delivered self-help with telephone support for pathological gamblers. *J Consult Clin Psychol, 76*(6), 1090–1094.

Carnes, P. (1991). *Don't call it love. Recovery from sexual addiction.* New York: Bantam.

Carnes, P. J. (1998). The obsessive shadow: Profiles in sexual addiction. *Prof Couns, 13*(1), 15–17, 40–41.

Chambers, R. A., & Potenza, M. N. (2003). Neurodevelopment, impulsivity, and adolescent gambling. *J Gambl Stud, 19,* 53–84.

Choi, K., Son, H., Park, M., Han, J., Kim, K., Lee, B., et al. (2009). Internet overuse and excessive daytime sleepiness in adolescents. *Psychiatry Clin Neurosci, 63*(4), 455–462.

Christenson, G. A., Faber, R. J., de Zwaan, M., Raymond, N. C., Specker, S. M., Ekern, M. D., et al. (1994). Compulsive buying: Descriptive characteristics and psychiatric comorbidity. *J Clin Psychiatry, 55,* 5–11.

Coleman, E. (1992). Is your patient suffering from compulsive sexual behavior? *Psychiatr Ann, 22,* 320–325.

Coleman, E., Gratzer, T., Nesvacil, L., & Raymond, N. C. (2000). Nefazodoneand the treatment of nonparaphilic compulsive sexual behavior: A retrospective study. *J Clin Psychiatry, 61,* 282–284.

Coleman, E., Raymond, N., & McBean, A. (2003). Assessment of compulsive sexual behavior. *Minn Med, 88*(7), 42–47.

Coniglio, M. A., Muni, V., Giammanco, G., & Pignato, S. (2007). Excessive internet use and internet addiction: Emerging public health issues. *Ig Sanita Pubbl, 63*(2), 127–136.

Cooper, A., Putnam, D. E., Planchon, L. A., & Boies, S. C. (1999). Online sexual compulsivity: getting tangled in the net. *Sex Addict Compulsivity, 6,* 79–104.

Crockford, D. N., & el-Guebaly, N. (1998). Psychiatric comorbidity in pathological gambling: A critical review. *Can J Psychiatry, 43,* 43–50.

Cunningham-Williams, R. M., Cottler, L. B., Compton, W. M., III, & Spitznagel, E. L. (1998). Taking chances: Problem gamblers and mental health disorders—results from the St. Louis Epidemiologic Catchment Area study. *Am J Public Health, 88,* 1093–1096.

de Bienville, D. T. (1775). *Nymphomania, or a dissertation concerning the furor uterinus: Clearly and methodically explaining the beginning, progress, and different causes of that horrible distemper* (E. S. Wilmot, Trans.). London: J. Bew.

Desai, R. A., & Potenza, M. N. (2009). A cross-sectional study of problem and pathological gambling in patients with schizophrenia/schizoaffective disorder. *J Clin Psychiatry, 70*(9), 1250–1257.

Dickerson, M., Hinchy, J., & England, L. S. (1990). Minimal treatments and problem gamblers: A preliminary investigation. *J Gambl Stud, 6,* 87–102.

Dowling, N., Smith, D., & Thomas, T. (2007). A comparison of individual and group cognitive-behavioral treatment for female pathological gambling. *Behav Res Ther, 45,* 2192–2202.

Dowling, N., Smith, D., & Thomas, T. (2009). The family functioning of female pathological gamblers. *Int J Ment Health Addict, 7,* 29–44.

Echeburua, E., Baez, C., & Fernandez-Montalvo, J. (1996). Comparative effectiveness of three therapeutic modalities in psychological treatment of pathological gambling: Long-term outcome. *Behav Cogn Psychother, 24,* 51–72.

Erbas, B., & Buchner, U. G. (2012). Pathological gambling: Prevalence, diagnosis, comorbidity, and intervention in Germany. *Dtsch Arztebl Int, 109*(10), 173–179.

Fong, T., Kalechstein, A., Bernhard, B., Rosenthal, R., & Rugle, L. (2008). A double-blind, placebo-controlled trial of olanzapine for the treatment of video poker pathological gamblers. *Pharmacol Biochem Behav, 89*(3), 298–303.

Gerevich, J., Treuer, T., Danics, Z., & Herr, J. (2005). Diagnostic and psychodynamic aspects of sexual addiction appearing as a non-paraphiliac form of compulsive sexual behavior. *J Subst Use, 10*(4), 253–259.

Goldman, M. J. (1991). Kleptomania: Making sense of the nonsensical. *Am J Psychiatry, 148,* 986–996.

Goodman, A. (1998). *Sexual addiction. An integrated approach.* Madison, CT: International Universities Press.

Goudriaan, A. E., Oosterlaan, J., de Beurs, E., & van den Brink, W. (2006). Neurocognitive functions in pathological gambling: A comparison with alcohol dependence, Tourette syndrome, and normal controls. *Addiction, 101,* 534–547.

Grant, J. E. (2003). Family history and psychiatry comorbidity in persons with kleptomania. *Compr Psych, 44*(6), 437–441.

Grant, J. E. (2011). Kleptomania treatment with tolcapone, a catechol-*O*-methyl-transferase (COMT) inhibitor. *Prog Neuropsychopharmacol Biol Psychiatry, 35*(1), 295–296.

Grant, J. E., Brewer, J. A., & Potenza, M. N. (2006). The neurobiology of substance and behavioral addictions. *CNS Spectrums, 11*(12), 924–930.

Grant, J. E., Donahue, C. B., Odlaug, B. L., & Kim, S. W. (2011). A 6-month follow-up of imaginal desensitization plus motivational interviewing in the treatment of pathological gambling. *Ann Clin Psychiatry, 23*(1), 3–10.

Grant, J. E., Donahue, C. B., Odlaug, B. L., Kim, S. W., Miller, M. J., & Petry, N. M. (2009). Imaginal desensitisation plus motivational interviewing for pathological gambling: Randomised controlled trial. *Br J Psychiatry, 195*(3), 266–267.

Grant, J. E., & Kim, S. W. (2001a). Demographic and clinical features of 131 adult pathological gamblers. *J Clin Psychiatry, 62,* 957–962.

Grant, J. E., & Kim, S. W. (2001b). A case of kleptomania and compulsive sexual behavior treated with naltrexone. *Ann Clin Psychiatry, 13,* 229–231.

Grant, J. E., & Kim, S. W. (2002a). Clinical characteristics and associated psychopathology of 22 patients with kleptomania. *Compr Psychiatry, 43,* 378–384.

Grant, J. E., & Kim, S. W. (2002b). Kleptomania: Emerging therapies target mood, impulsive behavior. *Curr Psychiatry, 1,* 45–49.

Grant, J. E., Kim, S. W., & Hartman, B. (2008). A double-blind, placebo-controlled study of the opiate antagonist naltrexone in the treatment of pathological gambling urges. *J Clin Psychiatry, 69,* 783–739.

Grant, J. E., Kim, S. W., Hollander, E., & Potenza, M. N. (2008). Predicting response to opiate antagonists and placebo in the treatment of pathological gambling. *Psychopharmacol (Berl), 200*(4), 521–527.

Grant, J. E., Kim, S. W., & Odlaug, B. L. (2007). N-acetyl cysteine, a glutamate-modulating agent, in the treatment of pathological gambling: A pilot study. *Biol Psychiatry, 62*(2), 652–657.

Grant, J. E., Kim, S. W., & Odlaug, B. L. (2009). A double-blind, placebo-controlled study of the opiate antagonist, naltrexone, in the treatment of kleptomania. *Biol Psychiatry, 65*(7), 600–606.

Grant, J. E., Kim, S. W., Potenza, M. N., Blanco, C., Ibanez, A., Stevens, L. C., et al. (2003). Paroxetine treatment of pathological gambling: A multi-center randomized controlled trial. *Int Clin Psychopharmacol, 18,* 243–249.

Grant, J. E., Kushner, M. G., & Kim, S. W. (2002). Pathological gambling and alcohol use disorder. *Alcohol Res Health, 26,* 143–150.

Grant, J. E., Odlaug, B. L., Davis, A. A., & Kim, S. W. (2009). Legal consequences of kleptomania. *Psychiatr Q, 80,* 251–259.

Grant, J. E., Odlaug, B. L., Mooney, M., O'Brien, R., & Kim, S. W. (2012). Open-label pilot study of memantine in the treatment of compulsive buying. *Ann Clin Psychiatry, 24*(2), 118–226.

Grant, J. E., Odlaug, B. L., Potenza, M. N., Hollander, E., & Kim, S. W. (2010). A multi-center, double-blind, placebo-controlled study of the opioid antagonist nalmefene in the treatment of pathological gambling. *Br J Psychiatry, 197*(4), 330–331.

Grant, J. E., & Potenza, M. N. (2007). Commentary: Illegal behavior and pathological gambling. *J Am Acad Psychiatry Law, 35*(3), 302–305.

Grant, J. E., & Potenza, M. N. (2008). Gender-related differences in individuals seeking treatment for kleptomania. *CNS Spectrums, 13*(3), 235–245.

Grant, J. E., Potenza, M. N., Hollander, E., Cunningham-Williams, R., Nurminen, T., Smits, G., et al. (2006). Multicenter investigation of the opioid antagonist nalmefene in the treatment of pathological gambling. *Am J Psychiatry, 163,* 303–312.

Grant, J. E., Schreiber, L., Odlaug, B. L., & Kim, S. W. (2010). Pathological gambling and bankruptcy. *Compr Psychiatry, 51*(2), 115–120.

Gulsun, M., Gulcat, Z., & Aydin, H. (2007). Treatment of compulsive sexual behaviour with clomipramine and valproic acid. *Clin Drug Investig, 27,* 219–223.

Ha, J. H., Kim, S. Y., Bae, S. C., Bae, S., Kim, H., Sim, M., et al. (2007). Depression and internet addiction in adolescents. *Psychopathology, 40*(6), 424–430.

Hadley, S. J., Baker, B. R., & Hollander, E. (2006). Efficacy of escitalopram in treatment of compulsive–impulsive computer use disorder (poster abstract). *Biol Psychiatry, 59,* 261S, No. 854.

Han, D., Lee, Y., Na, C., Ahn, J., Chung, U., Daniels, M., et al. (2009). The effect of methylphenidate on Internet video game play in children with attention-deficit/hyperactivity disorder. *Compr Psychiatry, 50*(3), 251–256.

Hernandez-Avila, C. A., Rounsaville, B. J., & Kranzler, H. R. (2004). Opioid-, cannabis- and alcohol-dependent women show more rapid progression to substance abuse treatment. *Drug Alcohol Depend, 74,* 265–272.

Hodgins, D. C., Currie, S. R., Currie, G., & Fick, G. H. (2009). Randomized trial of brief motivational treatments for pathological gamblers: More is not necessarily better. *J Consult Clin Psychol, 77*(5), 950–960.

Hodgins, D. C., Currie, S. R., & el-Guebaly, N. (2001). Motivational enhancement and self-help treatments for problem gambling. *J Consult Clin Psychol, 69, 50–57.

Hodgins, D. C., Currie, S. R., el-Guebaly, N., & Peden, N. (2004). Brief motivational treatment for problem gambling: A 24-month follow-up. *Psychol Addict Behav, 18,* 293–296.

Hodgins, D. C., Stea, J. N., & Grant, J. E. (2011). Gambling disorders. *Lancet, 378*(9806), 1874–1884.

Holden, C. (2010). Psychiatry: Behavioral addictions debut in proposed DSM-V. *Science, 327*(5968), 935.

Hollander, E., DeCaria, C. M., Finkell, J. N., Begaz, T., Wong, C. M., & Cartwright, C. (2000). A randomized double-blind fluvoxamine/placebo crossover trial in pathological gambling. *Biol Psychiatry, 47,* 813–817.

Hollander, E., Pallanti, S., Allen, A., Sood, E., & Rossi, N. (2005). Does sustained-release lithium reduce impulsive gambling and affective instability versus placebo in pathological gamblers with bipolar spectrum disorders? *Am J Psychiatry, 162,* 137–145.

June, K. J., Sohn, S. Y., So, A. Y., Yi, G. M., & Park, S. H. (2007). A study of factors that influence Internet addiction, smoking, and drinking in high school students. *Taehan Kanho Hakhoe Chi, 37*(6), 872–882. (in Korean)

Kafka, M. P. (1997). Hypersexual desire in males: An operational definition and clinical implications for males with paraphilias and paraphilia-related disorders. *Arch Sex Behav, 26*(5), 505–252.

Kafka, M. P. (2000). Psychopharmacologic treatments for nonparaphilic compulsive sexual behaviors. *CNS Spectrums, 5*(1), 49–59.

Kafka, M. P. (2010). Hypersexual disorder: A proposed diagnosis for DSM-V. *Arch Sex Behav, 39*(2), 377–400.

Kafka, M. P., & Hennen, J. (2000). Psychostimulant augmentation during treatment with selective serotonin reuptake inhibitors in men with paraphilias and paraphilia-related disorders: A case-series. *J Clin Psychiatry, 61,* 664–670.

Kafka, M. P., & Prentky, R. A. (1997). Compulsive sexual behavior characteristics. *Am J Psychiatry, 154*(11), 1632.

Kalivas, P. W., Lalumiere, R. T., Knackstedt, L., & Shen, H. (2009). Glutamate transmission in addiction. *Neuropharmacology, 56*(Suppl. 1), 169–173.

Kalivas, P. W., Volkow, N., & Seamans, J. (2005). Unmanageable motivation in addiction: A pathology in prefrontal–accumbens glutamate transmission. *Neuron, 45,* 647–650.

Kim, S. W., Grant, J. E., Adson, D. E., & Shin, Y. C. (2001). Double-blind naltrexone and placebo comparison study in the treatment of pathological gambling. *Biol Psychiatry, 49,* 914–921.

Kim, S. W., Grant, J. E., Adson, D. E., Shin, Y. C., & Zaninelli, R. M. (2002). A double-blind placebo-controlled study of the efficacy and safety of paroxetine in the treatment of pathological gambling. *J Clin Psychiatry, 63,* 501–507.

Ko, C.-H., Hsiao, S., Liu, C. G., Yen, J. U., Yang, M. J., & Yen, C. F. (2012). The characteristics of decision making, potential to take risks, and personality of college students with Internet addictions. *Psychiatry Res, 175*(1–2), 121–125.

Ko, C.-H., Yen, J. Y., Chen, C. C., Chen, S. H., Wu, K., & Yen, C. F. (2006). Tridimensional personality of adolescents with Internet addiction and substance use experience. *Can J Psychiatry, 51*(14), 887–894.

Koran, L. M., Aboujaoude, E. N., & Gamel, N. N. (2007). Escitalopram treatment of kleptomania: An open-label trial followed by double-blind discontinuation. *J Clin Psychiatry, 68,* 422–427.

Koran, L. M., Aboujaoude, E. N., Solvason, B., Gamel, N. N., & Smith, E. H. (2007). Escitalopram for compulsive buying disorder: A double-blind discontinuation study. *J Clin Psychopharmacol, 27*(2), 225–227.

Koran, L. M., Bullock, K. D., Hartston, H. J., Elliott, M. A., & D'Andrea, V. (2002). Citalopram treatment of compulsive shopping: An open-label study. *J Clin Psychiatry, 63,* 704–708.

Koran, L. M., Chuong, H. W., Bullock, K. D., & Smith, S. C. (2003). Citalopram for compulsive shopping disorder: An open-label study followed by double-blind discontinuation. *J Clin Psychiatry, 64,* 793–798.

Koran, L. M., Faber, R. J., Aboujaoude, E., Large, M. D., & Serpe, R. T. (2006). Estimated prevalence of compulsive buying in the United States. *Am J Psychiatry, 163,* 1806–1812.

Krafft-Ebbing, R. (1927). *Psychopathia sexualis* (F. J. Rebman, Trans.). New York: Rebman. (Original work published 1886)

Kratzer, S., & Hegerl, U. (2008). Is "Internet Addiction" a disorder of its own?: A study on subjects with excessive Internet use. *Psychiatr Prax, 35*(2), 80–83.

Krueger, R. B., & Kaplan, M. S. (2002). Behavioral and psychopharmacological treatment of the paraphilic and hypersexual disorders. *J Psychiatr Pract, 8,* 21–32.

Kuzma, J. M., & Black, D. W. (2008). Epidemiology, prevalence, and natural history of compulsive sexual behavior. *Psychiatr Clin N Am, 31,* 603–611.

Ladd, G. T., & Petry, N. M. (2002). Gender differences among pathological gamblers seeking treatment. *Exp Clin Psychopharmacol, 10,* 302–309.

Ladouceur, R., Sylvain, C., Boutin, C., Lachance, S., Doucette, C., & Leblond, J. (2003). Group therapy for pathological gamblers: A cognitive approach. *Behav Res Ther, 41*(5), 587–596.

Ladouceur, R., Sylvain, C., Boutin, C., Lachance, S., Doucette, C., Leblond, J., et al. (2001). Cognitive treatment of pathological gambling. *J Nerv Ment Dis, 189,* 774–780.

Ladouceur, R., Sylvain, C., Legate, H., Giroux, I., & Jacques, C. (1998). Cognitive treatment of pathological gamblers. *Behav Res Ther, 36,* 1111–1120.

Lawrence, A. J., Luty, J., Bogdan, N. A., Sahakian, B. J., & Clark, L. (2009a). Impulsivity and response inhibition in alcohol dependence and problem gambling. *Psychopharmacol, 207*(1), 163–172.

Lawrence, A. J., Luty, J., Bogdan, N. A., Sahakian, B. J., & Clark, L. (2009b). Problem gamblers share deficits in impulsive decision-making with alcohol-dependent individuals. *Addiction, 104*(6), 1006–1015.

Ledgerwood, D. M., Weinstock, J., Morasco, B. J., & Petry, N. M. (2007). Clinical features and treatment prognosis of pathological gamblers with and without recent gambling-related illegal behavior. *J Am Acad Psychiatr Law, 35,* 294–301.

Leeman, R. F., & Potenza, M. N. (2012). Similarities and differences between pathological gambling and substance use disorders: A focus on impulsivity and compulsivity. *Psychopharmacology, 219*(2), 469–490.

Li, X., Xi, Z. X., & Markou, A. (2013). Metabotropic glutamate 7 (mGlu7) receptor: A target for medication development for the treatment of cocaine dependence. *Neuropharmacol, 66,* 12–23.

Malladi, S. S., & Singh, A. N. (2005). Hypersexuality and its response to citalopram in a patient with hypothalamic hamartoma and precocious puberty. *Int J Neuropsychopharmacol, 8,* 1–2.

Marshall, L. E., & Marshall, W. L. (2006). Sexual addiction in incarcerated sexual offenders. *Sex Addict Compulsivity, 13,* 377–390.

McConaghy, N., Armstrong, M. S., & Blaszczynski, A. (1985). Expectancy, covert sensitization and imaginal desensitization in compulsive sexuality. *Acta Psychiatr Scand, 72,* 176–187.

McConaghy, N., Armstrong, M. S., Blaszczynski, A., & Allcock, C. (1983). Controlled comparison of aversive therapy and imaginal desensitization in compulsive gambling. *Br J Psychiatry, 142,* 366–372.

McConaghy, N., Blaszczynski, A., & Frankova, A. (1991). Comparison of imaginal desensitization with other behavioral treatments of pathological gambling: A two to nine year follow-up. *Br J Psychiatry, 159,* 390–393.

McElroy, S. L., Hudson, J. I., Pope, H. G., Keck, P. E., & Aizley, H. G. (1992). The DSM-III-R impulse control disorders not elsewhere classified: Clinical characteristics and relationship to other psychiatric disorders. *Am J Psychiatry, 149,* 318–327.

McElroy, S. L., Keck, P. E., Pope, H. G., Smith, J. M. R., & Strakowski, S. M. (1994). Compulsive buying: A report of 20 cases. *J Clin Psychiatry, 55,* 242–248.

McElroy, S. L., Nelson, E. B., Weldge, J. A., Kaehler, L., & Keck, P. E., Jr. (2008). Olanzapine in the treatment of pathological gambling: A negative randomized placebo-controlled trial. *J Clin Psychiatry, 69*(3), 433–440.

McElroy, S. L., Pope, H. G., Hudson, J. I., Keck, P. E., & White, K. L. (1991). Kleptomania: A report of 20 cases. *Am J Psychiatry, 148,* 652–657.

Mitchell, J. E., Burgard, M. B., Faber, R., Crosby, R. D., & de Zwaan, M. (2006). Cognitive behavioral therapy for compulsive buying disorder. *Behav Res Ther, 44*(12), 1859–1865.

Müller, A., Arikian, A., Swaan, M., & Mitchell, J. E. (2013). Cognitive-behavioural group therapy versus guided self-help for compulsive buying disorder: A preliminary study. *Clin Psychol Psychother, 20*(1), 28–35.

Müller, A., Mitchell, J. E., Crosby, R. D., Cao, L., Johnson, J., Claes, L., et al. (2012). Mood states preceding and following compulsive buying episodes: An ecological momentary assessment study. *Psychiatry Res, 200*(2–3), 575–580.

National Opinion Research Center. (1999). *Overview of the national survey and community database research on gambling behavior: Report to the National Gambling Impact Study Commission.* Chicago: Author.

Nelson, S. E., LaPlante, D. A., LaBrie, R. A., & Shaffer, H. J. (2006). The proxy effect: Gender and gambling problem trajectories of Iowa gambling treatment program participants. *J Gambl Stud, 22,* 221–240.

Ninan, P. T., McElroy, S. L., Kane, C. P., Knight, B. T., Castor, L. S., Rose, S. E., et al. (2000). Placebo-controlled study of fluvoxamine in the treatment of patients with compulsive buying. *J Clin Psychopharmacol, 20,* 362–366.

Odlaug, B. L., & Grant, J. E. (2010). Impulse-control disorders in a college sample: Results from the self-administered Minnesota Impulse Disorders Interview (MIDI). *Prim Care Companion J Clin Psychiatry, 12*(2), e1–e5.

Odlaug, B. L., Marsh, P. J., Kim, S. W., & Grant, J. E. (2011). Strategic vs nonstrategic gambling: Characteristics of pathological gamblers based on gambling preference. *Ann Clin Psychiatry, 23*(2), 105–112.

Pallesen, S., Mitsem, M., Kvale, G., Johnsen, B. H., & Molde, H. (2005). Outcome of psychological treatments of pathological gambling: A review and meta-analysis. *Addiction, 100*(10), 1412–1422.

Pallesen, S., Molde, H., Arnestad, H. M., Laberg, J. C., Skutle, A., Iversen, E., et al. (2007). Outcome of pharmacological treatments of pathological gambling: A review and meta-analysis. *J Clin Psychopharmacol, 27*(4), 357–364.

Park, S. K., Kim J. Y., & Cho, C. B. (2008). Prevalence of Internet addiction and correlations with family factors among South Korean adolescents. *Adolescence, 43,* 895–909.

Parsons, J. T. (2005). HIV-positive gay and bisexual men. In S. C. Kalichman (Ed.), *Positive prevention: Reducing HIV transmission among people living with HIV/AIDS* (pp. 99–133). New York: Kluwer.

Penix Sbraga, T., & O'Donohue, W. T. (2003). *The sex addiction workbook: Proven strategies to help you regain control of your life.* Oakland, CA: New Harbinger.

Petry, N. M., Ammerman, Y., Bohl, J., Boersch, A., Gay, H., Kadden, R., et al. (2006). Cognitive-behavioral therapy for pathological gamblers. *J Consul Clin Psychol, 74*(3), 555–567.

Petry, N. M., Stinson, F. S., & Grant, B. F. (2005). Comorbidity of DSM-IV pathological gambling and other psychiatric disorders: Results from the National Epidemiologic Survey on Alcohol and Related Conditions. *J Clin Psychiatry, 66,* 564–574.

Petry, N. M., Weinstock, J., Ledergwood, D. M., & Morasco, B. (2008). A randomized trial of brief interventions for problem and pathological gamblers. *J Consult Clin Psychol, 76,* 318–328.

Potenza, M. N. (2006). Should addictive disorders include non-substance-related conditions? *Addiction, 101*(Suppl. 1), 142–151.

Potenza, M. N., Fiellin, D. A., Heninger, G. A., Rounsaville, B. J., & Mazure, C. M. (2002). Gambling: An addictive behavior with health and primary care implications. *J Gen Intern Med, 17,* 721–732.

Potenza, M. N., Kosten, T. R., & Rounsaville, B. J. (2001). Pathological gambling. *JAMA, 286,* 141–144.

Potenza, M. N., Steinberg, M. A., McLaughlin, S. D., Wu, R., Rounsaville, B. J., O'Malley, S. S. (2001). Gender-related differences in the characteristics of problem gamblers using a gambling helpline. *Am J Psychiatry, 158*(9), 1500–1505.

Quadland, M. C. (1985). Compulsive sexual behavior: Definition of a problem and an approach to treatment. *J Sex Marital Ther, 11*(2), 121–132.

Rahman, A. S., Pilver, C. E., Desai, R. A., Steinberg, M. A., Rugle, L., Krishnan, S., et al. (2012). The relationship between age of gambling onset and adolescent problematic gambling severity. *J Psychiatr Res, 46*(5), 675–683.

Raymond, N. C., Coleman, E., & Miner, M. H. (2003). Psychiatric comorbidity and compulsive/impulsive traits in compulsive sexual behavior. *Compr Psychiatry, 44*(5), 370–380.

Raymond, N. C., Grant, J. E., Kim, S. W., & Coleman, E. (2002). Treatment of compulsive sexual behaviour with naltrexone and serotonin reuptake inhibitors: Two case studies. *Int Clin Psychopharmacol, 17,* 201–205.

Reid, R. C., Carpenter, B. N., & Lloyd, T. Q. (2009). Assessing psychological symptom patterns of patients seeking help for hypersexual behavior. *Sex Relation Ther, 24*(1), 47–63.

Reid, R. C., Stein, J. A., & Carpenter, B. N. (2011). Understanding the roles of shame and neuroticism in a patient sample of hypersexual men. *J Nerv Ment Dis, 199,* 263–267.

Saleh, F. (2005). A hypersexual paraphilic patient treated with leuprolide acetate: A single case report. *J Sex Marital Ther, 31,* 433–444.

Schlosser, S., Black, D. W., Repertinger, S., & Freet, D. (1994). Compulsive buying: Demography, phenomenology, and comorbidity in 46 subjects. *Gen Hosp Psychiatry, 16,* 205–212.

Schneider, J. P., & Schneider, B. H. (1996). Couple recovery from sexual addiction/co addiction: Results of a survey of 88 marriages. *Sex Addict Compulsivity, 3*(2), 111–126.

Shapira, N. A., Goldsmith, T. D., Keck, P. E., Jr., Khosla, U. M., & McElroy, S. L. (2000). Psychiatric features of individuals with problematic internet use. *J Affect Disord, 57,* 267–272.

Shaw, M., & Black, D. S. (2008). Internet addiction: Definition, assessment, epidemiology, and clinical management. *CNS Drugs, 22*(5), 353–365.

Skegg, K., Nada-Raja, S., Dickson, N., & Paul, C. (2010). Perceived "out of control" sexual behavior in a cohort of young adults from the Dunedin Multidisciplinary Health and Development Study. *Arch Sex Behav, 39*, 968–978.

Slutske, W. S., Eisen, S., True, W. R., Lyons, M. J., Goldberg, J., & Tsuang, M. (2000). Common genetic vulnerability for pathological gambling and alcohol dependence in men. *Arch Gen Psychiatry, 57*, 666–673.

Sylvain, C., Ladouceur, R., & Boisvert, J. M. (1997). Cognitive and behavioral treatment of pathological gambling: A controlled study. *J Consult Clin Psychol, 65*, 727–732.

Tao, R., Huang, X., Wang, J., Zhang, H., Zhang, Y., & Li, M. (2010). Proposed diagnostic criteria for Internet addiction. *Addiction, 105*(3), 556–564.

Tavares, H., Martin, S. S., Lobo, D. S., Silveira, C. M., Gentil, V., & Hodgins, D. C. (2003). Factors at play in faster progression for females pathological gamblers: An exploratory analysis. *J Clin Psychiatry, 64*(4), 433–438.

te Wildt, B. T., Putzig, I., Zedler, M., & Ohlmeier, M. D. (2007). Internet dependency as a symptom of depressive mood disorders. *Psychiatr Prax, 34*(Suppl. 3), S318–S322. (in German)

Treur, T., Fábián, Z., & Füredi, J. (2001). Internet addiction associated with features of impulse control disorder: Is it a real psychiatric disorder? *J Affect Disord, 66*(2–3), 283.

Tsitsika, A., Critselis, E., Kormas, G., Filippopoulou, A., Tounissidou, D., Freskou, A., et al. (2009). Internet use and misuse: A multivariate regression analysis of the predictive factors of Internet use among Greek adolescents. *Eur J Pharmacol, 168*, 655–665.

Wainberg, M. L., Muench, F., Morgenstern, J., Hollander, E., Irwin, T. W., Parsons, J. T., et al. (2006). A double-blind study of citalopram versus placebo in the treatment of compulsive sexual behaviors in gay and bisexual men. *J Clin Psychiatry, 67*, 1968–1973.

Weinstein, A., Lejoyeux, M. (2010). Internet addiction or excessive Internet use. *Am J Drug Alcohol Abuse, 36*, 277–283.

Welte, J., Barnes, G., Wieczorek, W., Tidwell, M. C., & Parker, J. (2001). Alcohol and gambling pathology among U.S. adults: Prevalence, demographic patterns and comorbidity. *J Stud Alcohol, 62*, 706–712.

Williams, A. D. (2012). Quality of life and psychiatric work impairment in compulsive buying: Increased symptom severity as a function of acquisition behaviors. *Compr Psychiatry, 53*(6), 822–828.

Yellowlees, P., & Marks, S. (2007). Problematic internet use or internet addiction? *Comput Hum Behav, 23*(3), 1447–1453.

Young, K. S. (1995). Internet addiction: Symptoms, evaluation, and treatment. Retrieved May 18, 2012, from *www.netaddiction.com/articles/symptoms.html*.

Young, K. S. (1996). Internet addiction: The emergence of a new clinical disorder. Retrieved May 18, 2012, from *www.netaddiction.com/articles/newdisorder.html*.

Young, K. S. (1998). *Caught in the net.* New York: Wiley.

Young, K. S. (2007). Cognitive behavioral therapy with Internet addicts: Treatment outcomes and implications. *Cyberpscyhol Behav, 10*(5), 671–679.

Young, K., Pistner, M., O'Mara, J., & Buchann, J. (2000). Cyber-disorders: The mental health concern for the new millennium. *Cyberpsychol Behav, 3*, 475–479.

Zack, M., & Poulos, C. X. (2007). A D_2 antagonist enhances the rewarding and priming effects of a gambling episode in pathological gamblers. *Neuropsychopharmacol, 32*, 1678–1686.

CHAPTER 17

Substance Abuse in Minority Populations

JOHN FRANKLIN

This chapter highlights psychosocial and clinical issues in the treatment of addictive disorders in African Americans, Hispanic Americans, Asian Americans, and Native Americans. Cultural competency of caregivers in treatment programs is vital but often lacking (Westermeyer, 2008). Substantial knowledge gaps still exist in minority substance abuse, and continued research in this area is needed. The growing ethnic diversity of the United States makes the significance of these issues even greater. According to the 2010 census, Hispanics make up 16.3% of the population; African Americans, 12.6%; Asian Americans/ Pacific Inlanders, 4.8%; Native Americans and Alaska Natives, 0.9%; and European Americans, 72.4% (U.S. Bureau of the Census, 2011). The fastest growing ethnic groups are Hispanics and Asian Americans. The Hispanic group increased 43% between the 2000 and 2010 census, also increased was the Asian American group. It is estimated that by 2060, the non-Hispanic white population in the United States will be a minority. This chapter reviews selected data on addictive disorders in minority populations. One important caveat is that today many people report being of mixed race, and the importance of this factor should be clearly acknowledged, but it is not discussed in any detail in this chapter.

Data for substance abuse in minorities come from numerous sources: the National Household Survey on Drug Abuse, the National Longitudinal Survey of Youth, Monitoring the Future, American Indian/Alaskan Native Statistics, and the Dawn Abuse Warning Network, to name a few. According to the 2010 National Survey on Drug Use and Health, among persons age 12 and older, 10.7% of African Americans, 9.1% of whites, 8.1 % of Hispanics, and 3.5% of Asians had past-month illicit drug use. Whites reported 56.7% current alcohol use, blacks reported 42.8%, Hispanics reported 41.8%, Asians reported 38.4%, and American Indian/Alaska Natives reported 36.6%. Binge drinking was reported in 24% of whites, 19.8% of blacks, 25.1% of Hispanics, 24.7% of American Indian/Alaska Natives, and 12.4%

of Asians. The rate of heavy use was highest for whites, followed by American Indians/Alaska Natives, Hispanics, blacks, and Asians. Twelve-month substance dependence disorder was 8.9% for whites, 8.2% for blacks, 9.7% for Hispanics, and 16% for American Indians/Alaska Natives (National Survey on Drug Use and Health, 2011). Heavy alcohol use peaked in the 20s then declined among white men.

Divisions along ethnic lines can be complicated by variations in country of origin, tribal affiliation, religious and spiritual orientation, and political and economic conditions. These differences may influence the clinical presentation and therapeutic needs of the patient. Other variables include socioeconomic status, educational level, occupational stability, dwelling situation, marital status, family of origin, and age.

Thus, a middle-class African American woman with a college degree and stable employment, dwelling in a reasonably safe neighborhood, may share a daily world outlook toward the future that is more similar to that of a European American woman with a similar background than to that of a single, unemployed African American mother dwelling in an inner city. A first-generation Mexican immigrant may have different risk factors for substance abuse than someone who is a U.S. native. Experiences within different Asian cultural groups can be vastly different. There are scant but increasing data regarding differences in biological vulnerability for substance abuse between ethnic groups (Nielson et al., 2010; Ittiwut et al., 2012; Du & Wan, 2009; Ehlers, Gilder, & Phillips 2008; Ehlers, Phillips, Gizer, Gilder, & Wilhelmsen, 2010, Ehlers, Phillips, Gizer, Gilder, & Yehuda, 2013; Gizer, Edenberg, Gilder, Wilhelmsen, & Ehlers, 2011; Ray, Bujarski, Chin, & Miotto, 2012; Duranceaux et al., 2008; Luczak et al. 2006; Cook et al., 2005; Hendershot, MacPherson, Myers, Carr, & Wall, 2005; Chan, McBride, Thomasson, Ykenney, & Crabb, 1994; Goldman et al., 1993; Berrettini & Persico, 1996).

SUBSTANCE USE AMONG MINORITY ADOLESCENTS

Ethnic differences in the prevalence, age of onset, gender, lifetime trajectory, service utilization, and medical and psychosocial consequences of substance use disorders (SUDs) have been reported. Adolescents have a 15% prevalence of having an SUD (Swendsen et al., 2012). Several recent studies have reported racial/ethnic differences in adolescent substance use and their consequences. Native American adolescents have been reported to have the highest prevalence of illegal substance use (47.5%). In analysis of the 2008 National Survey on Drug Use, adolescents in Native American, multiple race/ethnicity, and whites groups had elevated rates of substance-related disorders compared to African Americans and Asians (Wu, Woody, Yang, Pan, & Blazer, 2011). Hispanic youth may have the earliest initial use, and white adolescents have the highest rate of decreased use over time. Whites are generally younger than blacks at onset of drinking, and they progress to alcohol dependence faster (Alvanzo et al., 2011). Low parental education may be more of a risk factor for white kids than it is for African American or Hispanic children (Bachman et al., 2011). Asian American college students who are heavy drinkers may have higher developmental risk for later dependence (Iwamoto, Takamatsu, & Castellanos, 2012) There may be different cofactors among ethnic groups that make them vulnerable to the misuse of prescription drugs (Harrell & Broman, 2009; Green, Zebrak, Robertson, Fothergill, & Ensminger, 2012). Black youth, in contrast to whites, may initiate the use of cannabis before the use of cigarettes (Vaughn, Wallace, Perron, Copeland, & Howard, 2008). A recent longitudinal study of a cohort of inner-city, black children in Chicago reported less church attendance and extraversion, increasing risk of later cocaine and cannabis use (Fothergill, Ensminger, Green, Robertson, & Juon, 2009). Similarly, an increased number of conduct problems may lower the onset of drinking in black youth. Black youth are more likely than white youth to be arrested for drug offenses despite being less likely to use drugs. This disparity in the legal system can have long-lasting negative effects on black youth (Kakade et al., 2012). Black adolescents may be less prone to use inhalants (Nonnemaker, Crankshaw, Shive, Hussin, & Farrelly, 2011). However, by age 30, most racial/ethnic differences in substance use rates disappear (Chen & Jacobson, 2011).

Despite comparable prevalence of alcohol use and alcohol use disorders, and higher severity, blacks and Hispanics report increased social consequences of heavy drinking compared to whites and have lower levels of private insurance service utilization (Chartier & Caetano, 2011; Mulia, Zemore, & Greenfield, 2008; Marsh, Cao, Guerrero, & Shin, 2009). Treatment utilization among ethnic groups is equivalent, however. This may be the consequence of different rates of incarceration and more publically funded treatment among blacks and Latinos. Black substance users, however, compared to whites, receive less treatment for psychiatric comorbidities (Keyes et al., 2008). Blacks and Hispanics are exposed to greater social disadvantages of poverty, discrimination, and stigma, and these factors are associated with problem drinking (Smith, Dawson, Goldstein, & Grant, 2010; Mulia et al., 2008).

Asians with lower incomes suffer from effects of discrimination and this is a risk factor for substance use in that group, as may be low education in Hispanics (Lo & Cheng, 2012).

In black adolescents, effects of perceived racism on anger and self-control may correlate with increased substance use (Gibbons et al., 2012). School dropout rates have been associated with injection drug use in blacks; dropout rates should be targeted for intervention (Obot, Hubbard, & Anthony, 1999; Obot & Anthony, 2000).

SUBSTANCE ABUSE AMONG MINORITY WOMEN

African American families produce more alcohol abstainers than do European and Hispanic American families. African American women may express more conservative drinking norms (Herd, 1989). African American women may have eventual rates of heavy drinking comparable to that of European Americans; however, they report fewer social and personal problems. African American, Asian American, and Latin American women may be more insulated from alcohol-related social problems by their families, communities, and churches. A larger proportion of African American women, however, experience alcohol-related health problems than do European-American cohorts (Herd, 1989). One study of African American and Native American pregnant women indicated that African American women exhibit higher rates of fetal alcohol syndrome. These findings may be attributed to issues such as nutrition and access to health care. Concurrent illicit drug use may also be a contributing factor. A substantially higher percentage of American Indian/Alaska Native women drink compared to European American, African Americans, or Hispanics. There are higher rates of cocaine use in African American and Hispanic women compared to Asian or European American women. Among heroin and cocaine abusers, African American women woman have higher rates of sexually transmitted diseases (STDs) and different risk factors for use (Cavanaugh et al., 2011). Younger Hispanic women are more likely than European American women to abstain, though there is a one-sided convergence with increasing acculturation. For example, in one study, 75% of Mexican immigrant women abstained from alcohol, whereas 38% of third-generation Mexican American women were abstainers (Gilbert, 1991). American-born Hispanic women are more likely to report moderate to heavy drinking than their immigrant cohorts. Mexican American women who use substances suffer significantly higher lifetime rates of physical and sexual assault (Lown & Vega, 2001).

African American women in treatment often have myriad needs: employment, child care, treatment for victimization, and psychiatric symptoms. Personal losses such as death of loved ones, separation, and loss of child custody have a profound impact on drug use in African American women. Women in substance abuse treatment are oversampled in terms of sexual abuse. In a study of 1,272 randomly selected women in a jail with predominantly women of color, 8% had a comorbidity of severe mental disorder and substance abuse (Abram, Teplin, & McClelland, 2003). Life stress has been found to be a strong correlate of crack cocaine use in African-American women (Boyd, Guthrie, Pohl, Whitmarsh, & Henderson, 1994), as is gang affiliation in women. Child care has traditionally been a major obstacle to substance abuse treatment but especially for minorities, although this is not unique to ethnic minorities. Financial restriction is a fundamental barrier to treatment for women, with added hardship for women belonging to ethnic minority groups.

Supportive networks are important to substance abuse recovery irrespective of child care needs. A strong focus on the development of supports is indicated in the treatment of addicted women. Isolation among addicted women occurs for multiple reasons and include feelings of shame and guilt, and depression. Minority women may experience double stigma. Social networks should be a strong focus of recovery for addicted minority women. It may be necessary to utilize extended family, as well as supports outside the family. Respect for family systems is especially important in treating Hispanic women (Langrod, Alksne, Lowinson, & Ruiz, 1981).

SUBSTANCE ABUSE AMONG AFRICAN AMERICANS

As with all general ethnic/racial categories, African Americans are not a monolithic group. Important differences may be evidence between rural and urban folks and county of origin (Broman, Neighbors, Delva, Torres, & Jackson, 2008; Gibbons et al., 2007). Using 1-month prevalence data, compared to white teens of similar age, African American teens ages 12–17 drink heavily less often, 0.7 versus 3.4%. However, by age 26, heavy use of alcohol is similar, 7.8% in blacks versus 7.1% in whites. Heavy use among black men is relatively low in the early years, but it peaks in the middle age before declining (Herd, 1990). One hypothesis is that issues of racism and limited opportunities become more evident as blacks mature into adulthood. Strong pro-black racial identity maybe an important protective factor against adolescent substance use (Stock, Gibbons, Walsh, & Gerrard, 2011). Higher levels of posttraumatic stress disorder (PTSD) maybe an added risk factor for alcohol use in blacks (Williams, Jayawickreme, Sposato, & Foa, 2011). The factors involved in the later onset of heavy alcohol use in blacks and the subsequent rise in alcohol use need further research.

Diagnostic screening instruments for substance abuse in African-Americans have been shown to be valid (Duncan, Duncan, & Strycker, 2002). In a large inpatient sample, African-Americans were found to have later onset of use but earlier onset of alcohol-related problems (Hesselbrack, Hesselbrock, Segal, Schuckit, & Bucholz, 2003). African Americans appear to have worse health outcomes with moderate alcohol use and achieve lower occupational attainment (Sloan & Grossman 2011). In addition, the prevalence of alcohol-related problems in black men indicates significant differences in psychosocial distress compared to that of white men (Herd, 1994). The greatest differences between the groups are found in scores for loss of control, symptomatic drinking, binge drinking, health problems, and problems with friends and relatives. Blacks and whites had similar drinking patterns, as measured by frequency and maximum amounts consumed. Black men were significantly less permissive in attitudes toward alcohol use in particular situations, such as driving a car or spending time with small children in a parental role. Further analyses showed that the higher rates of alcohol-related problems were not fully accounted for by social and demographic differences between black and white men.

An earlier study by Herd (1990), reporting on data from a 1984 national survey, showed similar findings of greater alcohol-related problems among black men than white men in the past year. The exception was drunk driving, in which white men scored higher. Black men scored higher on symptoms of physical dependence and health problems. Here the rates of frequent heavy drinking were lower, not higher, for black men. Limited financial resources and access to health care likely contributed to the higher prevalence of alcohol-related health problems in black men. Blacks may be at higher risk for hepatic damage and cirrhosis from drinking (Singh & Hoyert, 2000). Herd (1994) suggests that this finding may represent a longer duration of heavy use, as opposed to more discrete phases of heavy alcohol use seen in white men. The body, it is hypothesized, is less resilient to alcohol toxicity at older ages. Binge alcohol use is associated with increased risky sexual behavior and increased STDs in black men (Raj et al., 2009).

Several studies have indicated that lower socioeconomic status seems to have a more profound influence on alcohol-related problems for black men compared to white men (Barr, Farrell, Barnes, & Welte, 1993; Herd, 1994; Jones, 1989; Jones-Webb, Hsiao, & Hannan,1995). Black men of lower socioeconomic status may experience more overt forms of discrimination and may be more likely to reside in communities in which there is more police surveillance. Group norms may be predictive of problematic alcohol use in African-Americans (Jones-Webb et al., 1995). Greater ethnic identity may be protective against problematic drinking (Herd & Grube,

1996). In addition, lower neighborhood cohesion has been associated with adolescent drug and alcohol problems.

Polymorphism of the ADH2*3 alcohol dehydrogenase metabolic enzyme may play role in alcohol expectations in African Americans (Ehlers, Carr, Betancourt, & Montane-Jaime, 2003). Lower P3 amplitudes during event-related potentials have also been reported in alcoholic African Americans (Ehlers et al., 2008). The association of alcohol use and hypertension may be particularly problematic in African American men. The association between hypertension and illicit drug use has also been reported (Kim, Dennison, Hill, Bone, & Levine, 2000). Ziedonis, Rayford, Bryant, and Rounsaville (1994) have reported on differential rates of lifetime psychiatric comorbidity in African American and European American cocaine addicts: European Americans have significantly higher rates of lifetime depression, alcohol dependence, attention deficits, and conduct disorders; African Americans often exhibit significant general coping skills but fewer treatment resources than European Americans (Walton, Blow, & Booth, 2001). There is some evidence that substance abuse in European Americans may be associated with greater underlying psychopathology, whereas African Americans may have greater social and environmental factors. Early initiation of sexual activity may be predictive of later substance abuse in African Americans (Stanton et al., 2001).

Illicit Drug Use

Historically, a greater proportion of blacks abstain from illicit drug use than do whites. This difference is especially pronounced in 12- to 25-year-olds. However, public databases such as the Client Data Acquisition Process and Drug Abuse Warning Network (DAWN; 2012) suggest that blacks and Hispanics are overrepresented in categories of heroin and cocaine use. Since the 1980s, we have seen up-and-down patterns of perceived harm among high school students. However, data still show a higher overall prevalence of illicit drug use in blacks (10.5%) versus whites (9.5%) (NSDUH: Substance Abuse and Mental Health Services Administration, 2014). Higher rates of marijuana and cocaine use account for the difference. In the 1998 NHSDA survey, blacks had higher prevalence of marijuana (5 percent v. 6.6 percent) and cocaine (0.7 vs. 1.3%) (NHSDA, 2000). The gap between whites' and blacks' adolescent marijuana use has disappeared. Blacks have higher rates of marijuana use by age 20 (Reardon & Buka, 2002). Also, emerging from epidemiological studies is a somewhat higher concentration of heroin use among blacks compared to whites. The NSDUH: Substance Abuse and Mental Health Services Administration (2014) indicated that past-month use of any illicit drug is higher for whites between ages 12 and 25, and higher for blacks from age 26 and up.

As with alcohol, illicit drug use appears to take a greater toll on African Americans' health, as measured by emergency department data. African Americans are overrepresented, as a percentage of the population, in emergency department visits. European Americans represent 50% of emergency department visits for illicit drugs compared to 30% for African Americans and 11% for Hispanics (DAWN, 2010). However, DAWN data are derived from large cities, where African American populations are proportionally high and may represent an overrepresentation of emergency department visits. African Americans are more likely than European Americans to be treated and released rather than hospitalized. The 2010 NHSDA survey indicated that cocaine is the primary drug leading to the emergency department visits for African Americans. African Americans are also overrepresented in the medical examiners' morbidity data. They account for 30% of drug-related deaths, while making up 23% of the population of the cities surveyed in DAWN. Cocaine is the most frequent cause of death (48.5%), followed by heroin and morphine. Much of the data about hard core drug use comes from similar information derived from public facilities. These data may seriously underestimate the persons who obtain alternative treatment for medical and psychosocial problems.

Literature reviewed by Brown, Alterman, Rutherford, Cacciola, and Zaballero (1993) suggests that correlates of heroin abuse may be educational impairment, poor employment history, history of legal problems (including incarceration), and possibly psychiatric problems. African Americans appear to be more closely scrutinized in primary care settings in terms of treating pain (Becker et al., 2011). Differences exist between African Americans requesting buprenorphine vs. methadone and presenting for public sector treatment. Women and people who are less likely to inject, prefer buprenorphine (Mitchell et al., 2011). A national sample (Kandel & Davies, 1991) indicated that early sexual intercourse was associated with elevated lifetime cocaine use among all ethnic groups; and that cocaine use correlates with daily marijuana use (defined by use at least 20 times in the last 30 days).

Low condom use among cocaine, marijuana, and alcohol abusers may be a risk factor for HIV among African Americans (Timpson, Williams, Bowen, & Keel, 2003). Cocaine use contributes to intracerebral bleeds, renal failure, chest pain, and myocardial infarctions. In addition, the severity of asthma exacerbation, with drug use, seems to be worse in African Americans (Rome, Lippmann, Dalsey, Taggart, & Pomerantz, 2000). Several groups are also studying strategies to decrease cigarette smoking in African Americans (Okuyemi, Ahluwalia, Richter, Mayo, & Resnicow, 2001; Ahluwalia, Harris, Catley, Okuyemi, & Mayo, 2002).

A coarse reading of this literature might imply that there is some intrinsic nature to the ethnic groups that accounts for differences in patterns of drug use. Lillie-Blanton, Anthony, and Schuster (1993) regrouped participants according to neighborhood rather than race or ethnicity, holding constant social and environmental risk factors that likely influenced the racial comparisons and applied this design to the apparent differences in crack cocaine use among European Americans, Hispanics, and African Americans. This interesting analysis revealed that the odds ratios did not vary significantly among the ethnic groups. Being African American did not place individuals at higher risk for crack use. Though this analysis does not refute the epidemiological findings of the study, it does suggest that the apparent differences may be more a product of social conditions, including availability of drugs, than issues intrinsic to ethnicity. Drug trafficking, often concentrated in minority neighborhoods, is a risk factor for use.

Among African American and European Americans, there may be differences in mu receptor polymorphisms (Crowley et al., 2003). However, strong evidence has yet to established that these gene findings are associated with actual drug use (Kranzler

Gelernter, O'Malley, Hernandez-Avila, & Kaufman, 1998). One report indicated no association between particular dopamine receptor alleles and cocaine dependence in African Americans (Gelernter, Kranzler, & Satel, 1999. Negative findings have also been reported for the association between serotonin transporter polymorphisms and aggression in African Americans with cocaine dependence (Patkar et al. 2002). One study indicated no increased genetic risk for addiction in persons with African heritage (Ducci et al., 2009).

The "war on drugs" and other pressures have resulted in overrepresentation in jails and prisons of African Americans arrested for drug-related charges (Wood, Werb, Marshall, Montaner, & Kerr, 2009). Inequalities in criminal sentencing may indicate subtle racism. For example, the differential sentencing for crack cocaine use, which is more prevalent in African American communities than powder cocaine, has been a matter of national debate. Recent laws have been enacted to mitigate some of these disparities in sentencing.

Prevention and Treatment Issues

Access to treatment is a problem for African Americans (Zule et al., 2008). There is low retention of African-American youth in clinical research trials (Magruder, Ouyang, Miller, & Tilley, 2009). Some argue that prevention and treatment of substance abuse and HIV in African American communities must recognize and address institutional racism, sociopolitical exploitation, patterns of drug distribution, limited employment opportunities, and African Americans' coping strategies (Agar & Reisinger, 2002). Gainful employment is a particularly powerful intervention. Neighborhood poverty in African Americans, compared to that in European Americans, may have a greater impact on sense of general well-being (Ludwig et al., 2012). Neighborhood perception of lack of safety and negative peer effects can increase risk for depression and drug use (Zule et al., 2008; Reitzel et al., 2012; Fite, Wynn, Lochman, & Wells, 2009). Many in the African American community stress the issues of self-help and community empowerment to combat divisive elements leading to drug and alcohol use. As a result, network therapy may have a particular role in more distressed communities. In a large Veterans Administration (VA) residential study, African Americans had similar rates of program participation but tended to do better in aftercare programs with greater African American staff presence (Rosenheck & Seibyl, 1998). Friedman and Glassman (2000), using data from the National Collaborative Study, found that social and peer relationship problems predicted 18.8% of the variance for future substance use in an urban adolescent population.

Standard treatment approaches are certainly effective for African Americans. In a National Institute on Drug Abuse (NIDA) Clinical Trials Network randomized controlled trial (RCT) of motivational enhancement therapy, African American women fared better than African American men (Montgomery, Burlew, Kosinski, & Forcehimes, 2011). Several RCTs have shown that cognitive-behavioral treatment and other smoking cessation techniques are effective with African Americans (Webb, 2008; Webb, de Ybarra, Baker, Reis, & Carey, 2010). One study, however, indicated that the combination of bupropion, nicotine patch, and counseling was less effective in African Americans (Covey et al., 2008), and another indicated negative effects for the use of varenicline in African American smokers (Nollen et al., 2011). In both clinical and laboratory studies, the use of naltrexone to decrease alcohol consumption may be less efficacious in African Americans (Ray & Oslin 2009; Plebani, Oslin, & Lynch, 2011). African American adolescents maybe disproportionately referred to restrictive environments for treatment in comparison to European American adolescents (Feaster et al., 2010).

Pro-black attitudes and awareness of racial oppression have been associated with negative substance use attitudes (Gary & Berry, 1985). Strong ethnic identity may protect against substance abuse and should be incorporated into treatment programs, especially for adolescents (Longshore, Grills, & Annon, 1999). However, James, Kim, and Armijo (2000) reported a positive association between high levels of cultural identity and heavy drug use. Culturally sensitive interventions have been shown to enhance getting people into treatment and improving outcomes (Dushay, Singer, Weeks, Rohena, & Gruber, 2010; Longshore et al., 1999). There is no question that the standard treatment approaches highlighted in the rest of this book can readily be applied to all ethnic groups. Standard cognitive-behavioral treatments have been shown to be as effective for African Americans as for European Americans (Milligan, Nich, & Carroll, 2004). Computer-based prevention strategies have also been found to be effective for African American girls (Schinke, Fang, Cole, & Cohen-Cutler, 2011).

Misdiagnosis of psychiatric comorbidities in African Americans can limit treatment effectiveness (Baker & Bell, 1999). There is an association between substance abuse and suicide in African Americans, but it may be less robust than in European American men (Garlow, 2002). The core features of loss of control and compulsivity that characterize a drug abuser or alcoholic are not dissimilar between ethnic groups. However, as we continue to tailor treatment to individuals, racial and cultural factors have to be addressed.

Should programs in primarily African American communities be especially designed to promote cultural sensitivity? In some sense this goes on naturally; the feel, look, and language of an Alcohol Anonymous (AA) meeting in an African American community is different from that in a European American self-help group. AA had its beginnings in the Oxford movement and was initially for middle-class European Americans. However, the church and spiritual dimensions of African American life are integral aspect of black culture, and it is not surprising that AA has been successfully transplanted to the black community. There have been attempts to develop and describe culturally sensitive mental health facilities (Deitch & Solit, 1993; Rowe & Grills, 1993). These attempts often are trapped in a quagmire of definitions of culture, race, and what is crucial to a culturally relevant program. Culturally relevant programs might promote positive racial and cultural identity, enhance self-esteem, increase self-determination, and appreciate traditional African American values. Afrocentric values stress relationships, verbal fluidity, emotional expressiveness, and spirituality. A study of substance abuse programs, using the National Drug Abuse Treatment System Survey, suggests that culturally competent treatment is holistic, emphasizing employment, spiritual strength, and physical health (Howard, 2003). Programs that hire staff members who mirror the patients' ethnic background may minimize racial bias. In addition, knowledge of African American history and culture is a component of a culturally competent program (Howard, 2003; Reizel et al., 2012).

Research questions related to primary hypotheses that especially address ethnic concerns are needed. There may be dimensions to an all-black treatment program that go beyond variables currently thought to be important. Blacks' ethnic biological differences, if any exist, need further work. Differences in health outcome and possibly medication responses need further consideration. The issue of matching or nonmatching of therapist or patients along racial and ethnic dimensions has been a subject of considerable discussion in mental health and has a role in the substance abuse field. Matching of racial and cultural attributes between therapist and client may enhance empathy or in some cases result in an overidentification with the client on the part of the therapist. Empathy and respect of others' cultural norms are essential components of any discussion of cultural sensitivity.

SUBSTANCE ABUSE AMONG HISPANIC AMERICANS

Hispanics comprise a heterogeneous group, including Mexican Americans, Puerto Ricans, Cuban Americans, and others. As with other ethnic groups, a greater number of Hispanic men drink alcohol and use drugs than do Hispanic women. Mexican American men were more likely to abstain than other Hispanic men. However, they drank more heavily and reported more alcohol-related problems. The "prevention paradox" is that binge drinkers who drink more moderate amounts, on whole, cause more public health problems than the smaller percentage of Hispanics who drink more heavily (Caetano & Mills, 2011). This observation may have important public health consequences. The Mexican Americans living near the Mexico–U.S. border may have higher rates of drinking compared other U.S. –Mexican residents (Maldonado-Molina and Delcher 2012, Caetano, Mills, & Vaeth,. 2012). All Hispanic groups, with the exception of Cubans, have twice the rate of liver cirrhosis compared to European Americans (Stinton, 2001; Yoon, Yi, & Thomson, 2011). Puerto Rican men have the highest prevalence of illicit drug use (10%) versus Mexican Americans (5%) (NSDUH: Substance Abuse and Mental Health Services Administration, 2011). Self-reported rates of drinking and driving are highest in Hispanics and European Americans (Caetano & Clark, 2000). Also, Latinos and African Americans have higher rate of overdose deaths. Cuban men had fewer abstainers, a smaller proportion of heavy drinkers, and fewer alcohol-related problems. Drinking increases with education and income for both sexes (Caetano, 1989). Although Hispanic men have higher rates of injection drug use (IDU), in Hispanic men IDU is in decline (Pouget, Friedman, Cleland, Tempalski, & Cooper, 2012). In New York City, cocaine and opiate positive urine results in victims of firearms deaths are highest in Latino men (Galea, Ahern, Tardiff, Leon, Vlahov, 2002).

Illicit Drug Use and Alcohol Use Disorder

According to the 2010 NHSDA for all age groups except 12–17, Hispanics had the fewest members in the "ever used any illicit drug" category as compared to European

Americans and African Americans. Hispanics were more likely to binge-drink and use more heavily. Caetano and Medina-Mora (1990) compared the drinking patterns of Mexican Americans and Mexicans living in Mexico. A more permissive attitude about alcohol use is associated with acculturation (Myers et al., 2011). Alcohol use increased with acculturation in Mexican men and woman. However, Mexican Americans reported fewer alcohol-related problems than did Mexican men living in Mexico. Data derived from the 2005 National Alcohol Survey, which represented predominately Mexican Americans, indicated that high acculturation is associated with drinking only in men with higher incomes (Karriker-Jaffe & Zemore, 2009). Acculturation effects families, which has impact on adolescent mental health and substance abuse (Buchanan & Smokowski, 2011). First-generation Hispanic youth have been reported to have lower rates of driving under the influence (DUI) compared to second- and third-generation Hispanic youth (Maldonado-Molina, Reingle, Jennings, & Prado, 2011). Perceived discrimination toward Mexican-born adolescents in the United States is associated with increased substance abuse and permissive attitudes (Kulis, Marsiglia, & Nieri, 2009). Positive parent–child attachment, peer influence, and strong ethnic identification may be mitigating factors (Kopak, Chen, Haas, & Gillmore, 2012; Prado et al., 2009; Ndiaye, Hecht, Wagstaff, & Elek, 2009). For Mexican women born in the United States, abstention rates steadily decreased and rates of infrequent drinking steadily increased with acculturation. This pattern is not seen in Mexican-born women living in the United States (Caetano & Medina-Mora, 1990). Hispanic women in women-only treatment centers report greater mental health and criminal justice problems on admission (Hser, Hunt, Evans, Chang, & Messina, 2012). Similarly, in south Florida, U.S.-born Hispanic young adults have increased rates of substance abuse and mental health problems compared to Hispanic immigrants. In the National Latino and Asian American Study, U.S.-born Mexicans had higher rates of mental health disorder compared to Cubans and other immigrants (Alegria et al., 2008). Substance abuse comorbidity in Latinos with schizophrenia is related to U.S. immigration status, depression, and unemployment (Jiménez-Castro et al., 2010), although Latinos' overall rates of dual diagnosis are one-fourth lower than that of the general U.S. population (Vega, Canino, Cao, & Alegria, 2009). Inhalant use is reported to be high among Hispanic youth in southwestern border states. Polymorphism of the alcohol dehydrogenase 2 gene and P450 2E1 has been reported to contribute to development of alcoholism in Mexican American men (Konishi et al., 2003).

Treatment Issues

Among people of need, Hispanics and African Americans, compared to European Americans, have greater unmet need for alcohol and drug abuse treatment. Hispanics receive active treatment 22.4% of the time and African Americans, 25%, versus European Americans, 37%. One study using data from the 2005 U.S. National Alcohol Survey reported that Latino women have particular problems with treatment underutilization that may be related to greater sense of stigma (Zemore, Mulia, Yu, Borges, & Greenfield, 2009). In the state of Massachusetts, Latinos are one-third less likely to enter residential treatment (Lundgren, Amodeo, Ferguson, & Davis, 2001).

Hispanics, despite higher intravenous drug use compared to European Americans, enroll less often in methadone maintenance, and this may be partly related to greater shame associated to methadone use in Hispanic men (Zaller, Bazazi, Velazquez, & Rich, 2009). In Los Angeles County, Guerrero, Cepeda, Duan, and Kim (2012) found that Cubans and Puerto Ricans used more opiates and cocaine compared to other Latinos, and despite being more educated, were less likely to complete substance abuse treatment. Language can be the most concrete barrier to adequate treatment for Hispanics in communities without adequate Spanish-speaking facilities. However, cultural sensitivity is not guaranteed by just speaking the language. Tools have been developed to assess the overall cultural competency of treatment centers for Hispanic clients (Shorkey, Windsor, & Spence, 2009). In a secondary analysis of data from the Clinical Network's Motivational Enhancement Therapy trial, Suarez-Morales et al. (2010) found that client–therapist matching of birthplace and acculturation did not make a difference in outcome. Language matching had a modest effect for alcohol abusers only (Carroll et al., 2009). Spanish-speaking male staff must also be able to treat female clients with respect and sensitivity to sexual, family, and childrearing issues. A number of authors (e.g., Szapocznik & Fein, 1995) identify family issues as being perhaps the most important component of addiction treatment of Hispanic clients.

Gfroerer and De La Rosa (1993) found that parents' attitudes and use of drugs, licit or illicit, played an important role in the drug use behavior of 12- to 17-year-old Hispanic youth. Parents need to be informed clearly and honestly about their influence. Also, the role of family should be well understood by treatment staff. Each family member has a function within the family. If properly educated, the family members can each provide support using their already established role. Some of the traditional roles according to Langrod et al. (1981) are to esteem older adults for their wisdom, the father for his authority, the mother for her devotion, and children for their future promise. Denial of alcoholism may be extensive in Hispanic fathers who drink only on the weekend and fulfill work obligations. Szapocznik and Fein (1995) include the cultural tradition of interdependence with extended family made up of uncles, aunts, cousins, and lifelong friends. Basically, the functional family does include any person who has day-to-day contact with and a role in the family. The family is an important resource and must be integrated into the treatment.

SUBSTANCE ABUSE AMONG ASIAN AMERICANS

People of Asian heritage make up nearly 4.8 % of the U.S. population according to U.S. Bureau of the Census (2011). The largest group is Chinese Americans (22.8%), followed by Asian Indians (19.4%), Filipinos (17.4%), Koreans (9.7%), and Vietnamese (10.6%); Japanese as a group constitute 5.2%, although counted as mixed with other races, the Japanese are 13.9%. Countries of Asian immigration include Mongolia, Pakistan, Nepal, Bangladesh, Burma, Thailand, Cambodia, Malaysia, and Singapore, and others. Many languages, cultures, and political systems are represented. Most of the world's major religions are represented, including Buddhism, Hinduism, Judaism, Christianity, and Islam. These religions have varying views regarding alcohol use. Alcohol use is prohibited in the Moslem teachings. Hinduism and Buddhism suggest avoidance of alcohol and other mind-altering substances. The Judeo-Christian perspective is more lenient and incorporates alcohol use into some religious ceremonies. These views affect the way the society, the family, and the problem drinker deal with the concept and acceptance of alcoholism. The acceptance and availability of treatment for individuals also have an impact.

The well-described "flushing " reaction in some Asian people has been linked to variations of aldehyde dehydrogenase isoenzymes. The reaction occurs because of a limited ability to degrade acetaldehyde to acetic acid. The toxic acetaldehyde is responsible for the flushing, headache, nausea, and other symptoms with alcohol use that are estimated to occur in 47–85% of Asians (U.S. Department of Health and Human Services, 1993). This was thought to explain the lower rates of alcohol abuse among Asians. The ALDH2*2 allele has been found to be protective against experiencing alcohol-related blackouts in Asian American college students (Luczak et al., 2006). However, studies have shown that sociocultural factors also play a substantial role in alcohol use within this population (Johnson & Nagoski, 1990; Newlin, 1989).

Some databases on alcoholism in ethnic/minority populations do not include information on Asian Americans. The Epidemiologic Catchment Area (ECA) study placed Asian Americans in the "other" category. Two national studies that do survey Asians as a specific category are DAWN and NHSDA (National Institute on Drug Abuse, 1990). The percentage of past-month use among Asian/Pacific Islanders is 2.8%, the lowest among the major ethnic groups. The 1-month prevalence in Native Hawaiians and other Pacific Islanders is 6.2% versus Asians at 2.7%. However, the Korean subgroup of Asians has a 6.9% prevalence rate, similar to African Americans. Groups of the same ethnic origin that live in different regions of the country can manifest different risk factors for abuse (Kim, Kim, & Nochajski, 2010). The available research literature is mostly described as community based or it pertains to specific subgroups within the Asian American community, such as students. Given these limitations, a number of studies indicate that there is significant variation in drinking patterns among the different Asian groups. There is some evidence that rates of heavy drinking is higher for Filipino Americans and Japanese Americans, followed by Korean Americans and Chinese Americans: 29.0, 28.9, 25.8, and 14.2%, respectively (Kitano & Chi, 1989). The breakdown by sex found heavy drinking in 11.7% of Japanese women, 3.5% of Filipino women, and 0.8% of Korean women, whereas Chinese women registered near zero. Filipinos who self-report unfair treatment in the United States report more illegal prescription drug and alcohol abuse (Gee, Delva, & Takeuchi, 2007). Asian American alcohol abuse has been associated with reported unfair treatment and low ethnic identification (Chae et al., 2008) A more recent study of 1,575 Asian American college undergraduates indicated that Japanese students had the highest rate of alcohol binging, followed by Filipino, Korean, and Chinese students (Iwamoto et al., 2012). Asian American drug users, once identified, may have more persistent drug use disorders compared to non-Hispanic whites (Xu et al., 2011). Interestingly, there is a Japanese AA-like organization called the All Nippon Sobriety Association.

Potential treatment problems in the Asian American community begin with the lack of acceptance of alcoholism and drug addictions as treatable illnesses. Ja and Aoki (1993) wrote about the typical chain of events in the life of an intact Asian family when substance abuse begins to appear. Often substance abuse problems are ignored or denied with the hope that they will disappear. Also, the family will make efforts to conceal it from the community to avoid embarrassment and shame. Prevention or early treatment is unlikely in this family and community dynamic. When denial is overwhelming, the family breaks down and may resort to shaming and other attempts at punishment. The family may also turn to extended family members and elders, basically moving gradually outward from the nuclear family to the external community. There is a deep sense of failure on the part of the family by the time members resort to outside professional help. It is not uncommon at this point to have the family members completely turn over the alcoholic or addict and resist participation themselves. The client is often still in denial and resistant to treatment until an alliance with staff is facilitated. As with other ethnic groups, when culturally competent care is available, service utilization improves (Yu, Clark, Chandra, Dias, & Lai, 2009).

Asian Americans represent 1.3% of patients in publicly funded treatment entering treatment for the first time; stimulants are the major drug of abuse (Wong & Barnett, 2010). New treatment approaches have been shown to be adaptable to Asian Americans. A family Web-based, mother–daughter substance abuse prevention program has been reported to be efficacious (Fang, Schinke, & Cole, 2010). There are many alternative medicine treatment approaches, such as traditional herbs and acupuncture. Some alternative treatments have shown scientific promises; others have not (Lu et al., 2009).

Treatment barriers begin with ignorance about the actual extent of drug and alcohol problems in the Asian American community. Asians are thought of by many as model immigrants. The 1960s brought in a large wave of educated and skilled Asian professionals. Migration since the 1970s has resulted in people with less education and fewer language and work skills immigrating to the United States (Varma & Siris, 1996). Many of them entered as refugees from war-ravaged countries. Poverty, overcrowded domiciles, discrimination, and other social problems are present in the lives of Asian Americans; however, documentation of these problems is sparse. This notion of "model" immigrant may be hurting the Asian American community from outside and within. It also lends itself to the denial within the community and amplifies the elements of shame and embarrassment felt by the family.

Better documentation of the extent of drug and alcohol abuse in the Asian American population, ideally, would enhance the funding for culturally sensitive education and treatment. Education at the community level is needed to foster awareness and acceptance, and assist in prevention (Wooksoo, Isok, & Nochajski, 2010). Treatment programs that target Asian Americans might consider the insular and private style of the Asian American family. Also essential is recognition of the dominance of the family and community over the psychological and social needs of the individual. An acceptance of these differences would decrease conflict between the family and treatment personnel. This show of respect for their values may facilitate the family's participation in the treatment. A treatment goal for all individuals should be reintegration back into the family and community, if at all possible.

SUBSTANCE ABUSE AMONG NATIVE AMERICANS

American Indians often more appropriately self-identify as Native Americans and First Nations. There are more than 200 Native American tribes that have a differential use of illicit substances. Studies show that American Indian/Alaska Native youth have twice the prevalence of cigarette, alcohol, marijuana, and cocaine use than Hispanics, blacks or whites. Alcohol abuse is recognized as a significant problem among Native Americans. The CAGE questionnaire (Cut down, Annoyed, Guilty, Eye-opener), however, has not been particularly useful in Native American samples (Saremi et al., 2001). Conduct disorder has been found to be a significant risk factor for alcohol dependence in Navajo Indians (Kunitz, 2008). In a Michigan Monitoring the Future study, Native American adolescents had the highest levels of tobacco, alcohol, and illicit drug use (Wallace et al., 2002). The fluctuating pattern of drug use among American Indians mirrors the larger adolescent culture (Beauvais, Jumper-Thurman, & Burnside, 2008). Age of first onset maybe a particular risk factor for alcohol and drug dependence in Native Americans (Kunitz, 2008). A recent study indicates that greater income supplements from casinos may lower substance abuse risk in Native Americans adolescents (Costello, Erklani, Copeland, & Angold, 2010). However, the recent increase in Indian-owned casinos has offered not only monetary opportunities but also the possibilities of increased gambling and substance abuse. In a large inpatient sample, Alaska Native men and women had earlier onsets of alcohol dependence (Hesselbrack, Hesselbrock, Segal, Schuckit, & Bucholz, 2003). American Indian/Alaska Native youth may also participate in more risky behaviors (Frank & Lester, 2002) in references. The *Morbidity and Mortality Weekly* report (Centers for Disease Control and Prevention, 2009) found that the highest rate of suicides during alcohol intoxication were among American Indians/Alaska Natives (37%). Age-adjusted alcohol-related deaths and years of potential life lost are significantly higher than those in the general population (Centers for Disease Control and Prevention, 2008). Although the alcohol mortality rate for Native Americans was three- to fourfold the national average, recent evidence indicates that there has been a decrease in mortality since 1969 (Burns, 1995). This drop seems to be in concert with the doubling of alcohol treatment services by the Indian Health Service in the 1980s.

Illicit drug use among Native Americans is less clear because of poor data available. The use of hallucinogens has an important role in some Native American religious rituals. Peyote and mescaline has been use by Native American in spiritual exercises for years but can have toxic effects, as reported by poison control centers (Carstairs & Cantrell, 2010). Increases in the P3 component of the event-related potential have been reported in Native American cannabis-dependent users (Ehlers et al., 2008). The heterogeneity of Native American cultures is plainly evident and further discourages simplistic discussions of Indian culture. The "firewater" myth states that alcohol introduced to Native Americans by white settlers produced exaggerated biological effects in such persons. Garcia-Andrade, Wall, and Ehlers (1997) found less subjective intoxication among nonalcoholic mission Indian men with greater Native American heritage. The same researchers implicate alcohol expectancy and metabolism rates as possible differential effects among tribes (Wall, Garcia-Anrade, Thomasson, Cole, & Ehlers, 1996; Garcia-Andrade et al., 1997).

Native Americans share a belief in the unity and sacredness of all nature. An individual or ethnic group may be more or less familiar with its own culture. Confrontation approaches, successful to many Anglo programs, may cause Native Americans to shy away. Risk factors for alcohol and drug use in Native Americans parallel many of the same issues of other disenfranchised groups. Attempts at assimilation of Native Americans, in the context of isolation from mainstream opportunities, has contributed to further cultural stress. Six-month remissions rates from alcohol dependence have increased significantly in Native American communities, reported to be a high as 59% (Gilder, Lau, Corey, & Ehlers, 2008). Being a woman, and being older and married are associated with better outcomes. Traditional healing methods are treatment tools in this population and may be used alongside other best practices (Coyhis and Simonelli, 2008). More local intervention and attention to culturally relevant treatment is needed (Dickerson & Johnson, 2011; Gone & Calf Looking, 2011; Gone, 2011). Interventions that use traditional healing and spirituality combined with more standard cognitive-behavioral therapy and contingency management models may bridge the best of both worlds, although challenges remain (Novins et al., 2011; Novins et al., 2012). Resistance to, and mistrust of evidenced based medicine and research still exists in these communities (Larios, Wright, Jernstrom, Lebron, & Sorensen, 2011). Traditional sweat lodge treatments are increasingly being used again for treatment. Heart disease and alcohol use beforehand are contraindicated for sweat lodge treatment (Livingston 2010). In an RCT, naltrexone alone and with sertraline has been used effectively in rural Alaska Natives (O'Malley et al., 2008). The breakdown of Native American culture, a factor that allowed alcohol to take a foothold, has been reversing in recent years. Self-determination and a return to traditional spiritual and healing beliefs have helped springboard alternative indigenous models of alcohol and drug recovery.

REFERENCES

Abram, K. M., Teplin, L. A., & McClelland, G. M. (2003). Comorbidity of severe psychiatric disorders and substance use disorders among women in jail. *Am J Psychiatry, 160*(5), 1007–1010.

Agar, M., & Reisinger, H. S. (2002). A heroin epidemic at the intersection of histories: The 1960s epidemic among African Americans in Baltimore. *Med Anthropol, 21*(2), 115–156.

Ahluwalia, J., Harris, K. J., Catley, D., Okuyemi, K. S., & Mayo, M. S. (2002). Sustained-release bupropion for smoking cessation in African americans: A randomized controlled trail. *JAMA, 288*(4), 468–474.

Alegria, M., Canino, G., Shrout, P. E., Woo, M., Duan, N., Vila, D., et al. (2008). Prevalence of mental illness in immigrant and non-immigrant U.S. Latino groups. *Am J Psychiatry, 165,* 359–369.

Alvanzo, A. H., Storr, C. L., La Flair, L., Green, K. M., Wagner, F. A., & Crum, R. M. (2011).

Race/ethnicity and sex differences in progression from drinking initiation to the development of alcohol dependence. *Drug Alcohol Depend, 118*(2–3), 375–382.

Bachman, J. G., O'Malley, P. M., Johnston, L. D., Schulenberg, J. E., & Wallace, J. R. (2011). Racial/ethnic differences in the relationship between parental education and substance use among U.S. 8th-, 10th-, and 12th-grade students: Findings from the Monitoring the Future project. *J Stud Alcohol Drugs, 72*(2), 179–185.

Baker, F. M., & Bell, C. C. (1999). Issues in the psychiatric treatment of African Americans. *Psychiatr Serv, 50*(3), 362–368.

Barr, K. E. M., Farrell, M. P., Barnes, G. M., & Welte, J. W. (1993). Race, class and gender differences in substance abuse: Evidence of a middle-class/under-class polarization among black males. *Soc Probl, 403*, 314–327.

Beauvais, F., Jumper-Thurman, P., & Burnside, M. (2008). The changing patterns of drug use among American Indian students over the past thirty years. *Am Indian Alsk Native Ment Health Res, 15*(2), 15–24.

Becker, W. C., Starrels, J. L., Moonseong, H., Xuan, L., Weiner, M. G., & Turner, B. J. (2011). Racial differences in primary care opioid risk reduction strategies. *Ann Fam Med, 9*(3), 219–225.

Berrettini, W. H., & Persico, A. M. (1996). Dopamine D_2 receptor gene polymorphisms and vulnerability to substance abuse in African Americans. *Biol Psychiatry, 40*, 144–147.

Boyd, C., Guthrie, B., Pohl, J., Whitmarsh, J., & Henderson, D. (1994). African American women who smoke crack cocaine: Sexual trauma and the mother–daughter relationship. *J Psychoactive Drugs, 26*(3), 243–247.

Broman, C. L., Neighbors, H. W., Delva, J., Torres, M., & Jackson, J. S. (2008). Prevalence of substance use disorders among African Americans and Caribbean Blacks in the National Survey of American Life. *Am J Public Health, 98*(6), 1107–1114.

Brown, L. S., Jr., Alterman, A. I., Rutherford, M. J., Cacciola, J. W., & Zaballero, A. R. (1993). Addiction Severity Index Scores of four racial/ethnic and gender groups of methadone maintenance patients. *J Subst Abuse, 5*(3), 269–279.

Buchanan, R. L., & Smokowski, P. (2011). Pathways from acculturation stress to substance use among Latino adolescents. *Subst Use Misuse, 44*(5), 740–762.

Burns, T. R. (1995). How does IHS relate administratively to the high alcoholism mortality rate? *Am Indian Alsk Native Ment Health Res, 6*(3), 31–45.

Caetano, R. (1989). Drinking patterns and alcohol problems in a national sample of U.S. Hispanics. In D. L. Spiegler, D. A. Tate, S. S. Aitken, & C. M. Christian (Eds.), *Alcohol use among U.S. ethnic minorities: Proceedings of a conference on the epidemiology of alcohol use and abuse among ethnic minority groups* (NIAAA Research Monograph No. 18, DHHS Publication No. ADM 89-1435, pp. 147–162). Washington, DC: U.S. Government Printing Office.

Caetano, R., & Clark, C. L. (2000). Hispanics, Blacks, and Whites driving under the influence of alcohol: Results from the 1995 National Alcohol Survey. *Accid Anal Prev, 32*(1), 57–64.

Caetano, R., & Medina-Mora, M. E. (1990). Reasons and attitudes toward drinking and abstaining: A comparison of Mexicans and Mexican-Americans. In *Epidemiologic trends in drug use: Community epidemiology work group proceedings, June, 1990* (pp. 173–191). Rockville, MD: National Institute of Drug Abuse.

Caetano, R., & Mills, B. (2011). The Hispanic Americans Baseline Alcohol Survey (HABLAS): Is the prevention paradox applicable to alcohol problems across Hispanic national groups? *Alcohol Clin Exp Res, 35*(7), 1256–1264.

Caetano, R., Mills, B., & Vaeth, P. C. (2012). Alcohol consumption and binge drinking among U.S.–Mexico border and non-border Mexican Americans. *Alcohol Clin Exp Res, 36*(4), 677–685.

Carroll, K. M., Martino, S., Ball, S. A., Nich, C., Frankforter, T., Anez, L. M., et al. (2009). A multisite randomized effectiveness trial of motivational enhancement therapy for Spanish-speaking substance users. *J Consult Clin Psychol, 77*(5), 993–999.

Carstairs, S. D., & Cantrell, F. L. (2010). Peyote and mescaline exposures: A 12-year review of a statewide poison center database. *Clin Toxicol, 4*, 350–353.

Cavanaugh, C. E., Floyd, L. J., Penniman, T. V., Hulbert, A., Gaydos, C., & Latimer, W. W. (2011). Examining racial/ethnic disparities in sexually transmitted diseases among recent heroin-using and cocaine-using women. *J Womens Health (Larchmt), 20*(2), 197–205.

Centers for Disease Control and Prevention. (2008). Alcohol-attributable deaths and years of potential life lost among American Indians and Alaska Natives—United States, 2001–2005. *Morb Mortal Wkly Rep, 57*(34), 938–941.

Centers for Disease Control and Prevention. (2009). Alcohol and suicide among racial/ethnic populations: 17 states, 2005–2006. *Morb Mortal Wkly Rep, 58*(23), 637–641.

Chae, D., Takeuchi, D., Barbeau, E., Bennett, G., Lindsey, J., Stoddard, A., et al. (2008). Alcohol disorders among Asian Americans: Associations with unfair treatment, racial/ethnic discrimination, and ethnic identification (the National Latino and Asian Americans study, 2002–2003). *J Epidemiol Commun Health, 62*(11), 973–979.

Chan, R. J., McBride, A. W., Thomasson, H. R., Ykenney, A., & Crabb, D. W. (1994). Allele frequencies of the preproenkephalin A (PENK) gene CA repeat in Asians, African-Americans, and Caucasians: Lack of evidence for different allele frequencies in alcoholics. *Alcohol Clin Exp Res, 18*(3), 533–535.

Chartier, K. G., & Caetano, R. (2011). Trends in alcohol services utilization from 1991–1992 to 2001–2002: Ethnic group differences in the U.S. population. *Alcohol Clin Exp Res, 35*(8), 1485–1497.

Chen, P., & Jacobson, K. C. (2011). Developmental trajectories of substance use from early adolescence to young adulthood: Gender and racial/ethnic differences. *J Adolesc Health, 50*(2), 154–163.

Cook, T., Luczak, S., Shea, S., Ehlers, C., Carr, L., & Wall, T. (2005). Associations of ALDH2 and ADH1B genotypes with response to alcohol in Asian Americans (English). *J Stud Alcohol, 66*(2), 196–204.

Costello, E., Erkanli, A., Copeland, W., & Angold, A. (2010). Association of family income supplements in adolescence with development of psychiatric and substance use disorders in adulthood among an American Indian population. *JAMA, 303*(19), 1954–1960.

Covey, L. S., Botello-Harbaum, M., Glassman, A. H., Masmela, J., Loduca, C., Salzman, V., et al. (2008). Smokers' response to combination bupropion, nicotine patch, and counseling treatment by race/ethnicity. *Ethn Dis, 18*(1), 59–64.

Coyhis, D., & Simonelli, R. (2008). The Native American healing experience. *Subst Use Misuse, 43*(12–13), 1927–1949.

Crowley, J. J., Oslin, D. W., Patkar, A. A., Gottheil, E., DeMaria, P. A. Jr., O'Brien C. P., et al. (2003). A genetic association study of the mu opiod receptor and severe opioid dependence. *Psychiatr Genet, 13*(3), 169–173.

Data Acquisition Process and Drug Abuse Warning Network (DAWN) Substance Abuse and Mental Health Services Administration. (2012). *Drug Abuse Warning Network, 2010: National estimates of drug-related emergency department visits* (HHS Publication No. [SMA] 12-4733, DAWN Series D-38). Rockville, MD: Author.

Deitch, D., & Solit, R. (1993). International training for drug abuse treatment and the issue of cultural relevance. *J Psychoactive Drugs, 25*(1), 87–95.

Dickerson, D. L., & Johnson, C. L. (2011). Design of a behavioral health program for urban American Indian/Alaska Native youths: A community informed approach. *J Psychoactive Drugs, 43*(4), 337–342.

Du, Y., & Wan, Y. J. (2009). The interaction of reward genes with environmental factors in contribution to alcoholism in Mexican Americans. *Alcohol Clin Exp Res, 33*(12), 2103–2112.

Ducci, F., Roy, A., Shen, P. H., Yuan, Q., Yuan, N. P., Hodgkinson, C. A., et al. (2009). Association of substance use disorders with childhood trauma but not African genetic heritage in an African American cohort. *Am J Psychiatry, 166*, 1031–1040.

Duncan, S. C., Duncan, T. E., & Strycker, L. A. (2002). A multilevel analysis of neighborhood context and youth alcohol and drug problems. *Prev Sci, 3*(2), 87–95.

Duranceaux, N., Schuckit, M., Luczak, S., Eng, M., Carr, L., & Wall, T. (2008). Ethnic differences in level of response to alcohol between Chinese Americans and Korean Americans. *J Stud Alcohol Drugs, 69*(2), 227–234.

Dushay, R. A., Singer, M., Weeks, M. R., Rohena, L., & Gruber, R. (2010). Lowering HIV risk among ethnic minority drug users: Comparing culturally targeted intervention to a standard intervention. *Am J Drug Alcohol Abuse, 27*(3), 501–524.

Ehlers, C. L., Carr, L., Betancourt, M., & Montane-Jaime, K. (2003). Association of the ADH2*3 allele with greater alcohol expectancies in African-American young adults. *J Stud Alcohol, 64*(2), 176–181.

Ehlers, C. L., Gilder, D. A., & Phillips, E. (2008). P3 components of the event-related potential and marijuana dependence in Southwest California Indians. *Addict Biol, 13*, 130–142.

Ehlers, C., Phillips, E., Gizer, I., Gilder, D., & Wilhelmsen, K. (2010). EEG spectral phenotypes: Heritability and association with marijuana and alcohol dependence in an American Indian community study. *Drug Alcohol Depend, 106*(2–3), 101–110.

Ehlers, C., Phillips, E., Gizer, I., Gilder, D., & Yehuda, R. (2013). Lifetime history of traumatic events in an American Indian community sample: Heritability and relation to substance dependence, affective disorder, conduct disorder and PTSD. *J Psychiatr Res, 47*(2), 155–161.

Fang, L., Schinke, S. P., & Cole, K. C. A. (2010). Preventing substance use among early Asian-American adolescent girls: Initial evaluation of a web-based, mother– daughter program. *J Adolesc Health, 47*, 529–532.

Feaster, D., Robbins, M., Henderson, C., Horigian, V., Puccinelli, M., Burlew, A., et al. (2010). Equivalence of family functioning and externalizing behaviors in adolescent substance users of different race/ethnicity. *J Subst Abuse Treat, 38*(Suppl. 1), S113–S124.

Fite, P. J., Wynn, P., Lochman, J. E., & Wells, K. C. (2009). The influence of neighborhood disadvantage and perceived disapproval on early substance use initiation. *Addict Behav, 34*, 769–771.

Fothergill, K., Ensminger, M., Green, K., Robertson, J., & Juon, H. S. (2011). Pathways to adult marijuana and cocaine use: A prospective study of African Americans from age 6 to 42. *J Health Soc Behav, 50*(1), 65–81.

Frank, M. L., & Lester, D. (2002). Self-destructive behaviors in American Indian and Alaska Native high school youth. *Am Indian Alsk Native Ment Health Res, 10*(3), 24–32.

Friedman, A. S., & Glassman, K. (2002). Family risk factors versus peer risk factors for drug abuse: A longitudinal study of an African-American urban community sample. *J Subst Abuse Treat, 18*(3) 267.

Friese, B., Grube, J. W., Seninger, S., Paschall, M. J., & Moore, R. S. (2009). Drinking behavior and sources of alcohol: Differences between Native American and White youths. *J Stud Alcohol Drugs, 72*(1), 53–60.

Galea, S., Ahern, J., Tardiff, K., Leon, A. C., & Vlahov, D. (2002). Drugs and firearm deaths in New York City, 1990–1998. *J Urban Healt, 79*(1), 70–86.

Garcia-Andrade, C., Wall, T. L., & Ehlers, C. L. (1997). The firewater myth and response to alcohol in mission Indians. *Am J Psychiatry, 154*(7), 983–988.

Garlow, S. J. (2002). Age, gender and ethnicity differences in patterns of cocatin and ethanol use preceding suicide. *Am J Psychiatry, 159*(4), 615–619.

Gary, L., & Berry, G. (1985). Predicting attitudes toward substance use in a black community. *Community Ment Health J, 21*, 45–51.

Gee, G. C., Delva, J., & Takeuchi, D. T. (2007). Relationships between self-reported unfair treatment and prescription medication use, illicit drug use, and alcohol dependence among Filipino Americans. *Am J Public Health, 97*(5), 933–940.

Gelernter, J., Kranzler, H., & Satel, S. L. (1999). No association between D$_2$ dopamine receptor

(DRD2) alleles or haplotypes and cocain dependence or severity of cocaine dependence in European- and African-Americans. *Biol Psychiatry, 45*(3), 340–345.

Gfroerer, J., & De La Rosa, M. (1993). Protective and risk factors associated with drug use among Hispanic youth. *J Addict Dis, 12*(2), 87–107.

Gibbons, F. X., O'Hara, R. E., Stock, M. L., Gerrard, M., Weng, C., & Wills, T. A. (2012). The erosive effects of racism: Reduced self-control mediates the relation between perceived racial discrimination and substance use in African American adolescents. *J Pers Soc Psychol, 102*(5), 1089–1104.

Gibbons, F. X., Reimer, R. A., Gerrard, M., et al. (2007). Rural-urban differences in substance use among African-American adolescents. *J Rural Health, 23*(Suppl. 22-8).

Gilbert, M. J. (1991). Acculturation and changes in drinking patterns among Mexican-American women. *Alcohol Health Res World, 15*(3), 234–238.

Gilder, D., Lau, P., Corey, L., & Ehlers, C. (2008). Factors associated with remission from alcohol dependence in an American Indian community group. *Am J Psychiatry, 165*(9), 1172–1178.

Gizer, I., Edenberg, H., Gilder, D., Wilhelmsen, K., & Ehlers, C. (2011). Association of alcohol dehydrogenase genes with alcohol-related phenotypes in a Native American community sample. *Alcohol Clin Exp Res, 35*(11), 2008–2018.

Goldman, D., Brown, G. L., Albaugh, B., Robin, R., Goodson, S. Trunzo, M., et al. (1993). DRD2 dopamine receptor genotype, linkage disequilibrium, and alcoholism in American Indians and other populations. *Alcohol Clin Exp Res, 17*(2), 199–204.

Gone, J. P. (2011). The red road to wellness: Cultural reclamation in a Native First Nations community treatment center. *Am J Community Psychol, 47*(1–2), 187–202.

Gone, J. P., & Calf Looking, P. E. (2011). American Indian culture as substance abuse treatment: Pursuing evidence for a local intervention. *J Psychoactive Drugs, 43*(4), 291–296.

Green, K., Zebrak, K., Robertson, J., Fothergill, K., & Ensminger, M. (2012). Interrelationship of substance use and psychological distress over the life course among a cohort of urban African Americans. *Drug Alcohol Depend, 123*(1–3), 239–248.

Guerrero, E. G., Cepeda, A., Duan, L., & Kim, T. (2012). Disparities in completion of substance abuse treatment among Latino subgroups in Los Angeles County, CA. *Addict Behav, 37*(10), 1162–1166.

Harrell, Z., & Broman, C. (2009). Racial/ethnic differences in correlates of prescription drug misuse among young adults. *Drug Alcohol Depend, 104*(3), 268–271.

Hendershot, C., MacPherson, L., Myers, M., Carr, L., & Wall, T. (2005). Psychosocial, cultural and genetic influences on alcohol use in Asian American youth. *J Stud Alcohol, 66*(2), 185–195.

Herd, D. (1989). The epidemiology of drinking patterns and alcohol-related problems among U.S. blacks. In D. Spiegler, D. Tate, D. S. Aitkens, & C. Christian (Eds.), *Alcohol use among U. S. ethnic minorities* (NIAAA Research Monograph No. 18, DHHS Publication No. ADM 89-1435, pp. 3–50). Washington, DC: U.S. Government Printing Office.

Herd, D. (1990). Subgroup differences in drinking patterns among black and white men: Results from a national survey. *J Stud Alcohol, 51*(3), 221–232.

Herd, D. (1994). Predicting drinking problems among black and white men: Results from a national survey. *J Stud Alcohol, 55*, 61–71.

Herd, D., & Grube, J. (1996). Black identity and drinking in the U.S.: A national study. *Addiction, 91*(6), 845–857.

Hesselbrock, M. N., Hesselbrock, V. M., Segal, B., Schuckit, M. A., & Bucholz, K. (2003). Ethnicity and psychiatric comorbidity among alcohol-dependent persons who receive inpatient treatment: African Americans, Alaska Natives, Caucasians and Hispanics. *Alcohol Clin Exp Res, 27*(8), 1368–1373.

Howard, D. L. (2003). Culturally competent treatment of African-American clients among a national sample of outpatient substance abuse treatment units. *J Subst Abuse Treat, 24*(2), 103–113.

Hser, Y., Hunt, S., Evans, E., Chang, Y., & Messina, N. (2012). Hispanic parenting women in women-only versus mixed-gender drug treatment: A 10-year prospective study. *Addict Behav, 37*(6), 729–735.

Ittiwut, C., Yang, B., Kranzler, H., et al. (2012). GABRG1 and GABRA2 variation associated with alcohol dependence in African Americans. *Alcohol Clin Exp Res, 36*(4), 588–593.

Iwamoto, D., Takamatsu, S., & Castellanos, J. (2012). Binge drinking and alcohol-related problems among U.S.-born Asian Americans. *Cultur Divers Ethnic Minor Psychol, 18*(3), 219–227.

Ja, D., & Aoki, B. (1993). Substance abuse treatment: Cultural barriers in the Asian-American community. *J Psychoactive Drugs, 25*(1), 61–71.

James, W. H., Kim, G. K., & Armijo, E. (2000). The influence of ethnic identity on drug use among ethnic minority adolescents. *J Drug Educ, 30*(3), 265–280.

Jiménez-Castro, L., Hare, E., Medina, R., Raventos, H., Nicolini, H., Mendoza, R., et al. (2010). Substance use disorder comorbidity with schizophrenia in families of Mexican and Central American ancestry. *Schizophr Res, 120*(1–3), 87–94.

Johnson, R. C., & Nagoski, C. T. (1990). Asians, Asian-Americans, and alcohol. *J Psychoactive Drugs, 22*(1), 45–52.

Jones, R. J. (1989). *The socio-economic context of alcohol use and depression: Results from a national survey of black and white adults.* Presented at the 15th annual Ketil Bruun Alcohol Epidemiology Symposium, Maastricht, The Netherlands.

Jones-Webb, R., Hsiao, C., & Hannan, P. (1995). Relationships between socioeconomic status and drinking problems among black and white men. *Alcohol Clin Exp Res, 19*(3), 623–627.

Kakade, M., Duarte, C. S., Liu, X., Fuller, C. J., Drucker, E., Hoven, C. W., et al. (2012). Adolescent substance use and other illegal behaviors and racial disparities in criminal justice system involvement: Findings from a US national survey. *Am J Public Health, 102*(7), 1307–1310.

Kandel, D. B., & Davies, M. (1991). Cocaine use in a national sample of U.S. youth (NLSY): Epidemiology, predictors, and ethnic patterns. In C. Schade & S. Schober (Eds.), *The epidemiology of cocaine use and abuse* (NIDA Research Monograph No. 110, pp. 151–188). Washington, DC: U.S. Government Printing Office.

Karriker-Jaffe, K., & Zemore, S. (2009). Associations between acculturation and alcohol consumption of Latino men in the United States. *J Stud Alcohol Drugs, 70*(1), 27–31.

Keyes, K., Hatzenbuehler, M., Alberti, P., Narrow, W., Grant, B., & Hasin, D. (2008). Service utilization differences for Axis I psychiatric and substance use disorders between white and black adults. *Psychiatr Serv, 59*(8), 893–901.

Kim, M. T., Dennison, C. R., Hill, M. N., Bone, L. R., & Levine, D. M. (2000). Relationship of alcohol and illicit drug use with high blood pressure care and control among urban hypertensive black men. *Ethn Dis, 10*(2), 175–183.

Kim, W., Kim, I., & Nochajski, T. H. (2010). Risk and protective factors of alcohol use disorders among Filipino Americans: Location of residence matters. *Am J Drug Alcohol Abuse, 36*(4), 214–219.

Kitano, H. H. L., & Chi, I. (1989). Asian Americans and alcohol: The Chinese, Japanese, Koreans, and Filipinos in Los Angeles. In D. Spiegler, D. Tate, S. Aitkens, & C. Christian (Eds.), *Alcohol use among U.S. ethnic minorities* (NIAAA Research Monograph No. 18, DHHS Publication No. ADM 89-1435, pp. 373–382). Washington, DC: U.S. Government Printing Office.

Konishi, T., Calvillo, M., Leng, A. S., Feng, J., Lee, T., Lee, H., et al. (2003). The ADH3*2 and CYP2E1 c2 alleles increase the risk of alcoholism in Mexican-American me. *Exp Mol Pathol, 74*(2), 183–189.

Kopak, A., Chen, A., Haas, S., & Gillmore, M. (2012). The importance of family factors to protect against substance use related problems among Mexican heritage and White youth. *Drug Alcohol Depend, 124*(1–2), 34–41.

Kranzler, H. R., Gelernter, J., O'Malley, S., Hernandez-Avila, C. A., & Kaufman, D. (1998). Association of alcohol or other drug dependence with alleles of the mu opioid receptor gene (OPRM1). *Alcohol Clin Exp Res, 22*(6), 1356–1359.

Kulis, S., Marsiglia, F., & Nieri, T. (2011). Perceived ethnic discrimination versus acculturation stress: Influences on substance use among Latino Youth in the Southwest. *J Health Soc Behav, 50*(4), 443–459.

Kunitz, S. J. (2008). Risk factors for polydrug use in a Native American population. *Subst Use Misuse, 43*(3–4), 331–339.

Langrod, J., Alksne, L., Lowinson, J., & Ruiz, P. (1981). Rehabilitation of the Puerto Rican addict: A cultural perspective. *Int J Addict, 16*(5), 841–847.

Larios, S. E., Wright, S., Jernstrom, A., Lebron, D., & Sorensen, J. L. (2011). Evidence-based practices, attitudes, and beliefs in substance abuse treatment programs serving American Indians and Alaska Natives: A qualitative study. *J Psychoactive Drugs, 43*(4), 355–359.

Lillie-Blanton, M., Anthony, J., & Schuster, C. R. (1993). Probing the meaning of racial/ethnic group comparisons in crack cocaine smoking. *JAMA, 296*(8), 993–997.

Livingston, R. (2010). Medical risks and benefits of the sweat lodge. *J Altern Complement Med, 6*, 617–619.

Lo, C. C., & Cheng, T. C. (2012). Discrimination's role in minority groups' rates of substance-use disorder. *Am J Addict, 21*(2), 150–156.

Longshore, D., Grills, C., & Annon, K. (1999). Effects of a culturally congruent intervention on cognitive factors related to drug-use recovery. *Subst Use Misuse, 34*(9), 1223–1241.

Lown, A. E., & Vega, W. A. (2001). Alcohol abuse and dependence among Mexican-American women who report violence. *Alcohol Clin Exp Res, 25*(10), 1479–1486.

Lu, L., Liu, Y., Zhu, W., Shi, J., Liu, Y., Ling, W., et al. (2009). Traditional medicine in the treatment of drug addiction. *Am J Drug Alcohol Abuse, 35*(1), 1–11.

Luczak, S., Shea, S., Hsueh, A., Chang, J., Carr, L., & Wall, T. (2006). ALDH2*2 is associated with a decreased likelihood of alcohol-induced blackouts in asian american college students (English). *J Stud Alcohol, 67*(3), 349–353.

Ludwig, J., Duncan, G., Gennetian, L., Katz, L., Kessler, R., Kling, J., et al. (2012). Neighborhood effects on the long-term well-being of low-income adults. *Science, 337*(6101), 1505–1510.

Lundgren, L., Amodeo, M., Ferguson, F., Davis, K. & Schilling, R. (2001). Racial and ethnic differences in drug treatment entry of injection drug users in Massachusetts: Detoxification only, residential treatment, and methadone. *J Subst Abuse Treat, 21*, 145–153.

Magruder, K. M., Ouyang, B., Miller, S., & Tilley, B. C. (2009). Retention in under-represented minorities in substance abuse treatment. *Clin Trials, 6*, 252–260.

Maldonado-Molina, M. M., & Delcher, C. (2012). Commentary on Caetano, Mills, and Vaeth (2012): The role of context on alcohol consumption among Mexican Americans. *Alcohol Clin Exp Res, 36*(4), 566–567.

Maldonado-Molina, M. M., Reingle, J. M., Jennings, W. G., & Prado, G. (2011). Drinking and driving among immigrant and US-born Hispanic young adults: Results from a longitudinal and nationally representative study. *Addict Behav, 36*(4), 381–388.

Marsh, J. C., Cao, D. D., Guerrero, E. E., & Shin, H. C. (2009). Need-service matching in substance abuse treatment: racial/ethnic differences. *Eval Program Plann, 32*(1), 43–51.

Milligan, C. O., Nich, C., & Carroll, K. M. (2004). Ethnic differences in substance abuse treatment retention, compliance, and outcome from two clinical trials. *Psychiatr Serv, 55*(2), 167–173.

Mitchell, S. G., Kelly, S., Gryczynski, J., Myers, C., Jaffe, J., O'Grady, K., et al. (2011). African American patients seeking treatment in the public sector: Characteristics of buprenorphine vs. methadone patients. *Drug Alcohol Depend, 122*(1–2), 55–60.

Montgomery, L., Burlew, A., Kosinski, A. S., & Forcehimes, A. A. (2011). Motivational enhancement therapy for African American substance users: A randomized clinical trial. *Cultur Divers Ethnic Minor Psychol, 17*(4), 357–365.

Mulia, N., Ye, Y., Zemore, S., & Greenfield, T. (2008). Social disadvantage, stress, and alcohol use among black, Hispanic, and white Americans: Findings from the 2005 U.S. National Alcohol Survey. *J Stud Alcohol Drugs, 69*(6), 824–833.

Myers, R., Chou, C., Sussman, S., Baezconde-Garbanati, L., Pachon, H., & Valente, T. (2011). Acculturation and substance use: Social influence as a mediator among Hispanic alternative high school youth. *J Health Soc Behav, 50*(2), 164–179.

National Institute on Drug Abuse. (1990). *National Household Survey on Drug Abuse.* Rockville, MD: Author.

Ndiaye, K., Hecht, M. L., Wagstaff, D. A., & Elek, E. (2009). Mexican-heritage preadolescents' ethnic identification and perceptions of substance use. *Subst Use Misuse, 44*(8), 1160–1182.

Newlin, D. B. (1989). The skin-flushing response: Autonomic, self-report and conditioned responses to repeated administrations of alcohol in Asian men. *J Abnorm Psychol, 98,* 421–425.

Nielson, D., Harmon, S., Yuferov, V., et al. (2010). Ethnic diversity of DNA methylation in the OPRM1 promoter region in lymphocytes of heroin addicts. *Hum Genet, 127,* 639–649.

Nollen, N. L., Cox, L., Nazir, N., Ellerbeck, E. F., Owen, A., Pankey, S., et al. (2011). A pilot clinical trial of varenicline for smoking cessation in black smokers. *Nicot Tobacco Res, 13*(9), 868–873.

Nonnemaker, J. M., Crankshaw, E. C., Shive, D. R., Hussin, A. H., & Farrelly, M. C. (2011). Inhalant use initiation among U.S. adolescents: Evidence from the National Survey of Parents and Youth using discrete-time survival analysis. *Addict Behav, 36*(8), 878–881.

Novins, D. K., Aarons, G. A., Conti, S. G., Dahlke, D., Daw, R., Fickenscher, A., et al. (2011). Use of the evidence base in substance abuse treatment programs for American Indians and Alaska Natives: Pursuing quality in the crucible of practice and policy. *Implement Sci, 6*(1), 63–74.

Novins, D., Boyd, M., Brotherton, D., Fickenscher, A., Moore, L., & Spicer, P. (2012). Walking on: Celebrating the journeys of Native American adolescents with substance use problems on the winding road to healing. *J Psychoactive Drugs, 44*(2), 153–159.

Obot, I. S., & Anthony J. C. (2000). School dropout and injecting drug use in a national sample of white non-Hispanic American adults. *J Drug Edu, 30*(2), 145–155.

Obot, I. S., Hubbard, S., & Anthony, J. C. (1999). Level of education and injecting drug use among African Americans. *Drug Alcohol Depen, 55*(1–2), 177–182.

Okuyemi, K. S., Ahluwalia, J. S., Richter, K. P., Mayo, M. S., & Resnicow, K. (2001). Differences among African-American light, moderate and heavy smokers. *Nicotine Tob Res, 3*(1), 45–50.

O'Malley, S. S., Robin, R. W., Levenson, A. L., GreyWolf, I., Chance, L. E., Hodgkinson, C. A., et al. (2008). Naltrexone alone and with sertraline for the treatment of alcohol dependence in Alaska Natives and non-natives residing in rural settings: A randomized controlled trial. *Alcohol Clin Exp Res, 32*(7), 1271–1283.

Patkar, A. A., Berrettini, W. H., Hoehe, M., Hill, K. P., Gottheil, E., Thornton, C. C., et al. (2002). No association between polymorphisms in the serotonin transporter gene and susceptibility to cocaine dependence among African-American individuals. *Psychiatr Genet, 12*(3), 161–164,

Plebani, J. G., Oslin, D. W., & Lynch, K. G. (2011). Examining naltrexone and alcohol effects in a minority population: Results from an initial human laboratory study. *Am J Addict, 20*(4), 330–336.

Pouget, E. R., Friedman, S. R., Cleland, C. M., Tempalski, B. B., & Cooper, H. F. (2012). Estimates of the population prevalence of injection drug users among hispanic residents of large US metropolitan areas. *J Urban Health Bull NY Acad Med, 89*(3), 527–564.

Prado, G., Huang, S., Schwartz, S. J., Maldonado-Molina, M., Bandiera, F., de la Rosa, M., et al. (2009). What accounts for differences in substance use among U.S.-born and immigrant

Hispanic adolescents?: Results from a longitudinal prospective cohort study. *J Adolesc Health, 45*(2), 118–125.

Raj, A., Reed, E., Santana, C., Walley, A. Y., Welles, S. L., Horsburgh, C. R., et al. (2009). The associations of binge alcohol use with HIV/STI risk and diagnosis among heterosexual African American men. *Drug Alcohol Depend, 101*(1–2), 101–106.

Ray, L., Bujarski, S., Chin, P., & Miotto, K. (2012). Pharmacogenetics of naltrexone in Asian Americans: A randomized placebo-controlled laboratory study. *Neuropsychopharmacol, 37*(2), 445–455.

Ray, L., & Oslin, D. (2009). Naltrexone for the treatment of alcohol dependence among African Americans: Results from the COMBINE Study. *Drug Alcohol Depend, 105*(3), 256–258.

Reardon, S. F., & Buka, S. L. (2002). Differences in onset and persistence of substance abuse and dependence among Whites, Blacks, and Hispanics. *Public Health Reports 117*(Suppl. 1), S51–S59.

Reitzel, L. R., Vidrine, J. I., Businelle, M. S., Kendzor, D. E., Cao, Y., Mazas, C. A., et al. (2012). Neighborhood perceptions are associated with tobacco dependence among African American smokers. *Nicot Tobacco Res, 14*(7), 786–793.

Rome, L. A., Lippmann, M. L., Dalsey, W. C., Taggart, P., & Pomerantz, S. (2000). Prevalence of cocaine use and its impact on asthma exacerbation in an urban population. *Chest, 117*(5), 1324–1329.

Rosenheck, R., & Seibyl, C. L. (1998). Participation and outcome in a residential treatment and work therapy program for addictive disorders: The effects of race. *Am J Psychaiarty, 155*(8), 1029–1034.

Rowe, D., & Grills, C. (1993). African-centered drug treatment: An alternative conceptual paradigm for drug counseling with African-American clients. *J Psychoactive Drugs, 25*(1), 21–33.

Saremi, A., Hanson, R. L., Williams, D. E., Roumain, J., Robin, R. W., Long, J. C., et al. (2001). Validity of the CAGE questionnaire in an American Indian population. *J Stud Alcohol, 62*(3), 294–300.

Schinke, S. P., & Fang, L., Cole, K. C., & Cohen-Cutler, S. (2011). Preventing substance use among Black and Hispanic adolescent girls: Results from a computer-delivered, mother–daughter intervention approach. *Subst Use Misuse, 46*(1), 35–45.

Shorkey, C., Windsor, L., & Spence, R. (2009). Assessing culturally competent chemical dependence treatment services for Mexican Americans. *J Behav Health Serv Res, 36*(1), 61–74.

Singh, G. K., & Hoyert, D. L. (2000). Social epidemiology of chronic liver disease and cirrhosis mortality in the United States, 1935–1997: Trends and differentials by ethnicity, socioeconomic status and alcohol consumption. *Hum Biol, 72*(5), 801–820.

Sloan, F., & Grossman, D. (2011). Alcohol consumption in early adulthood and schooling completed and labor market outcomes at midwife by race and gender. *Am J Public Health, 101*(11), 2093–2101.

Smith, S., Dawson, D., Goldstein, R., & Grant, B. (2010). Examining perceived alcoholism stigma effect on racial-ethnic disparities in treatment and quality of life among alcoholics. *J Stud Alcohol Drugs, 71*(2), 231–236.

Stanton, B., Li, X., Pack, R., Cottrell, L., Harris, C., & Burns, J. M. (2002). Longitudinal influence of perceptions of peer and parental factors on African-American adolescent risk involvement. *J Urban Health, 79*(4), 536–548.

Stock, M. L., Gibbons, F. X., Walsh, L. A., & Gerrard, M. (2011). Racial identification, racial discrimination, and substance use vulnerability among African American young adults. *Pers Soc Psychol Bull, 37*(10), 1349–1361.

Suarez-Morales, L., Martino, S., Bedregal, L., McCabe, B. E., Cuzmar, I. Y., Paris, M., et al. (2010). Do therapist cultural characteristics influence the outcome of substance abuse treatment for Spanish-speaking adults? *Cultur Divers Ethnic Minor Psychol, 16*(2), 199–205.

Substance Abuse and Mental Health Services Administration. (2011). *Results from the 2010*

National Survey on Drug Use and Health: Summary of national findings (NSDUH Series H-41, HHS Publication No. [SMA] 11-4658). Rockville, MD: Author.

Substance Abuse and Mental Health Services Administration. (2014). *Results from the 2013 National Survey on Drug Use and Health: Summary of national findings* (NSDUH Series H-48, HHS Publication No. [SMA] 14-4863). Rockville, MD: Author.

Swendsen, J., Burstein, M., Case, B., Conway, K., Dierker, L., & He, J. (2012). Use and abuse of alcohol and illicit drugs in US adolescents: Results of the National Comorbidity Survey–Adolescent Supplement. *Arch Gen Psychiatry, 69*(4), 390–398.

Szapocznik, J., & Fein, S. (1995). *Issues in preventing alcohol and other drug abuse among Hispanic/Latino families* (CSAP Cultural Competence Series 2, DHHS Publication No. [SMA] 95-3034). Washington, DC: U.S. Government Printing Office.

Timpson, S. C., Williams, M. L., Bowen, A. M., & Keel, K. B. (2003). Condom use behaviors in HIV-infected African American crack cocaine users. *Subst Abuse 24*(4), 211–220.

U.S. Bureau of the Census. (2011). *Current Population Reports.* Washington, DC: U.S. Government Printing Office.

U.S. Department of Health and Human Services. (1993, September). *Alcohol and health.* Alexandria, VA: Editorial Experts.

Varma, S., & Siris, S. (1996). Alcohol abuse in Asian Americans. *Am J Addict, 5*(2), 136–143.

Vaughn, M., Wallace, J., Perron, B., Copeland, V., & Howard, M. (2008). Does marijuana use serve as a gateway to cigarette use for high-risk African-American youth? *Am J Drug Alcohol Abuse, 34*(6), 782–791.

Vega, W. A., Canino, G., Cao, Z., & Alegria, M. (2009). Prevalence and correlates of dual diagnoses in U.S. Latinos. *Drug Alcohol Depend, 100*(1–2), 32–38.

Wall, T. L., Garcia-Andrade, C., Thomasson, H. R., Cole, M., & Ehlers, C. L. (1996). Alcohol elimination in Native American mission Indians: An investigation of interindividual variation. *Alcohol Clin Exp Res, 20*(7), 1159–1164.

Wallace, J. M., Jr., Bachman, J. G., O'Malley, P. M., Johnston, L. D., Schulenberg, J. E., & Cooper, S. M. (2002). Tobacco, alcohol, and illicit drug use: Racial and ethnic differences among U.S. high school seniors, 1976–2000. *Public Health Rep, 117*(Suppl. 1), S67–S75.

Walton, M. A., Blow, F. C., & Booth, B. M. (2001). Diversity in relapse prevention needs: Gender and race comparisons among substance abuse treatment patients. *Am J Drug Alcohol Abuse, 27*(2), 225–240.

Webb, M. S. (2008). Treating tobacco dependence among African Americans: A meta-analytic review. *Health Psychol, 27*(Suppl. 3), S271–S282.

Webb, M. S., de Ybarra, D., Baker, E. A., Reis, I. M., & Carey, M. P. (2010). Cognitive-behavioral therapy to promote smoking cessation among African American smokers: A randomized clinical trial. *J Consult Clin Psychol, 78*(1), 24–33.

Westermeyer, J. (2008). A sea change in the treatment of alcoholism. *Am J Psychiatry, 165*(9), 1093–1095.

Williams, M., Jayawickreme, N., Sposato, R., & Foa, E. B. (2012). Race-specific associations between trauma cognitions and symptoms of alcohol dependence in individuals with comorbid PTSD and alcohol dependence. *Addict Behav, 37*(1), 47–52.

Wong, W., & Barnett, P. G. (2010). Characteristics of Asian and Pacific Islanders admitted to U.S. drug treatment programs in 2005. *Public Health Rep, 125*(2), 250–257.

Wood, E., Werb, D., Marshall, B., Montaner, J., & Kerr, T. (2009). The war on drugs: A devastating public-policy disaster. *Lancet, 373*(9668), 989–990.

Wooksoo, K., Isok, K., & Nochajski, T. H. (2010). Risk and protective factors of alcohol use disorders among Filipino Americans: Location of residence matters. *Am J Drug Alcohol Abuse, 36*(4), 214–219.

Wu, L., Woody, G., Yang, C., Pan, J., & Blazer, D. (2011). Racial/ethnic variations in substance-related disorders among adolescents in the United States. *Arch Gen Psychiatry, 68*(11), 1176–1185.

Xu, Y., Okuda, M., Hser, Y., Hasin, D., Liu, S., & Grant, C. B. (2011). Twelve-month prevalence of psychiatric disorders and treatment-seeking among Asian Americans/Pacific Islanders in the United States: Results from the National Epidemiological Survey on Alcohol and Related Conditions (English). *J Psychiatr Res, 45*(7), 910–918.

Yoon, Y., Yi, H., & Thomson, P. (2011). Alcohol-related and viral hepatitis C-related cirrhosis mortality among hispanic subgroups in the united states, 2000–2004. *Alcohol Clin Exp Res, 35*(2), 240–249.

Yu, J., Clark, L., Chandra, L. P., Dias, A., & Lai, T. F. (2009). Reducing cultural barriers to substance abuse treatment among Asian Americans: A case study in New York City. *J Subst Abuse Treat, 37*(4), 398–406.

Zaller, N. D., Bazazi, A. R., Velazquez, L. L., & Rich, J. D. (2009). Attitudes toward methadone among out-of-treatment minority injection drug users: Implications for health disparities. *Int J Environ Res Public Health, 6*(2), 787–797.

Zemore, S. E., Mulia, N., Yu, Y., Borges, G., & Greenfield, T. K. (2009). Gender, acculturation, and other barriers to alcohol treatment utilization among Latinos in three national alcohol surveys. *J Subst Abuse Treat, 36*(4), 446–456.

Ziedonis, D., Rayford, B., Bryant, K. J., & Rounsaville, B. (1994). Psychiatric comorbidity in white and African-American cocaine addicts seeking substance abuse treatment. *Hosp Community Psychiatry, 45*(1), 43–49.

Zule, W. A., Morgan-Lopez, A. A., Lam, W. K. K., Wechsberg, W. M., Luseno, W. K., & Young, S. K. (2008). Perceived neighborhood safety and depressive symptoms among African American crack users. *Subst Use Misuse, 43*(3–4), 445–468.

CHAPTER 18

Addiction in the Workplace

LAURENCE WESTREICH

This chapter provides a broad overview of the management of addiction in the workplace for occupational psychiatrists, as well as clinicians who treat employed patients. When evaluating and treating addiction, practitioners of occupational psychiatry occupy a middle ground between their obligation to assist the employee and to represent the best interests of the employee's (and their own) employer. This "dual agency" (Robertson & Walter, 2008) describes the inevitable tension between roles for the occupational psychiatrist, which must be managed very carefully to respect the expectations, rights, and obligations of all involved.

Treating clinicians are usually responsible only for treating their patients, but may have some legal and ethical obligations if their patients endanger others or themselves. And in those circumstances in which a patient has directed the treating clinician to contact an employer, a basic understanding of the relevant labor issues and laws is helpful.

Mere substance use, even outside the physical workplace, may affect some sensitive professional or "zero-tolerance" positions, as is the case with pilots, professional athletes, or individuals covered by U.S. Department of Transportation guidelines. For other workplaces, only substance use or effects during work hours are relevant. This chapter reviews the full range of addiction issues that may arise in the workplace, but the nosological distinctions between substance use disorders, misuse, and dependence are addressed elsewhere (American Psychiatric Association, 2013; Galanter & Kleber, 2008). Occupational interactions with compulsive behaviors such as Internet addiction, gambling, and sex addiction are also addressed.

Often the interests of the employee and employer are exactly aligned: Both value quick treatment and a return to work. However, sometimes these interests diverge or are only partially aligned. For instance, when an employee wishes to continue working but is not fit for duty, the occupational psychiatrist must make uncomfortable decisions that may directly affect the employee's livelihood. A similar tension exists for occupational psychiatrists who monitor impaired professionals: The duty to treat the patient may conflict with a duty to protect the public from an impaired physician, for instance. Although some employee assistance programs (EAPs) manage this tension by taking on an "arms-length" relationship with the employer and keeping all clinical information private, in other scenarios, there is no possibility of such a separation. However they are managed, these dilemmas are common when occupational psychiatrists work with addiction, and best practices dictate that these conundrums be addressed thoughtfully, honestly, and in full view of all involved.

This chapter reviews available data on addiction in the workplace, the broad legal implications of evaluating employees with apparent drug or alcohol use, and the role of EAPs in the workplace management of addiction. The legal, practical, and laboratory basics of workplace drug testing are described. A description of the special issues facing substance-using professionals and athletes is followed by concluding recommendations for managing addiction in the workplace. Although this chapter's focus is on the practical issues in workplace addiction, workplace intervention will be shown to be powerful—if somewhat circumscribed by law—forces for bringing the addicted person to recovery.

DATA ON ADDICTION IN THE WORKPLACE

Data on workplace addiction reveal a surprisingly high prevalence of workplace drug and alcohol problems, and behavioral addictions in the workplace. The National Survey on Drug Use and Health, an annual survey of the civilian noninstitutionalized U.S. population (Larson, Eyerman, Foster, & Gfoerer, 2007), reveals that for all full-time workers, the prevalence of past-month illicit drug use was 8.2%. Nineteen percent of full-time workers in the age 18–25 group acknowledged using illicit drugs in the past month, and this percentage dropped in older age groups: 10.3% of 26- to 34-year-old, 7.0% of 35- to 49-year-old, and 2.6% of 50- to 64-year-old full-time workers acknowledged past-month illicit drug use. Of all full-time workers, 8.8% acknowledged heavy drinking in the past month, defined as "drinking five or more drinks on the same occasion on 5 or more days in the past 30 days."

Drug and alcohol use by employees profoundly affects productivity: Shand and Fawcett (2003) demonstrated that drug and alcohol users are two to three times more likely to be absent from work than nonusers. Drug users were found to claim illness benefits at a rate three times that of nonusers, and to file five times as many worker's compensation claims. Between 20 and 25% of accidents documented in this study involved intoxicated persons injuring themselves or others. Contrary to stereotypes about "laziness" among heavy drug and alcohol users, many are employed either part-time or full-time. In fact, the workplace may function as a respite from other stressors, or from the chaos of a life filled with addiction and its consequences. Epstein and Preston (2011) found that when they questioned a cohort of 79 employed methadone-maintained individuals who misused heroin and cocaine, being at work was associated with lower stress, greater happiness, and lower drug craving. Although beyond the scope of this chapter, the dual diagnosis of mental illness and addiction is as common in the workplace as it is elsewhere (Brown & Bennett, 2004), and it raises difficulties in diagnosis, management, and treatment.

Despite the ubiquity of Internet usage in the workplace, and the widespread understanding that the Internet can provoke compulsive behaviors, few reliable data on the subject exist. As early as 1996, one survey of 1.000 U.S. companies demonstrated that more than half of the executives surveyed believed that Internet usage was slowing rather than speeding up their employees' productivity. (Robert Half International, 1996).

WORKPLACE ADDICTION AND THE LAW

Changing societal views about addiction correlate with changes in the relevant labor law: In some circumstances, changing cultural mores produce new law, and in others, new law affects perception of addiction. In both cases, employers and employees must comply with the relevant statues, and addicted people should be aware of their changing set of rights and obligations.

One groundbreaking regulation was the Drug Free Workplace Act of 1988 (U.S. House of Representatives, 1988). Although technically only mandatory for businesses that receive federal grants or contracts of more than $100,000, the Act has promoted workplace rules, programs, and attitudes that are useful for many businesses that technically are not covered. For instance, responses to the Drug-Free Workplace Act (Substance Abuse and Mental Health Services Administration, 1989) have included the evolution of five main components for a successful drug-free workplace program. First, a written policy disseminated to all employees can set the boundaries and structure of a successful program. Second, employee education about addiction, drugs, and how to manage potential problems can generate a sense of group cohesiveness in addressing the issues. Third, supervisor education focused on clarifying the agreed-upon policy, adhering to the relevant laws, referring affected workers, and helping workers in recovery return to the workplace lends a sense of focus to the program. Fourth, an effective EAP can help employees with a broad range of social and psychological problems in addition to addiction, thereby improving the collaborative atmosphere in the workplace. Finally, a drug testing program lends a sense of seriousness and consequence to the drug-free workplace program. By doing drug testing and attaching consequences to positive tests, employers underline their commitment to safety in the workplace and the health of their employees and customers. (EAPS and drug testing are reviewed in more depth below.)

Without regular modification, however, no workplace drug program can remain effective. (DuPont & Martin, 2012). The advent of new drugs of abuse, such as bath salts, or emerging trends in drug use, such as the last decade's sharp uptick in prescription drug abuse, demonstrates that any drug program, in the workplace or elsewhere, must be dynamic and engaged with changes in the presentation of addiction. Other challenges include the controversy over medical marijuana and the differences between state and federal laws. Similarly, the quite pointed efforts of illicit chemists to develop drugs that are unfindable in standard workplace tests pose difficulties for testers and untold dangers for those who ingest these substances.

While the Drug-Free Workplace Act and private programs based on it were designed to provide a safe and drug-free workplace, the 1990 Americans with Disabilities Act (ADA) was passed to protect the employment rights of disabled persons, including, in some circumstances, those who use or are addicted to drugs and alcohol (Westreich, 2002). The ADA protects the rights of job applicants or employees from discrimination based on any known disability, or the perception of that disability, and provides reasonable accommodations for a disabled or impaired employee to fulfill the necessary job functions. The ADA underscores the importance of employment tests that measure the important requirements of the job rather than an applicant or prospective employee's disability. Importantly, applicants or employees who are unqualified for the position with or without accommodations are *not* protected by the ADA.

Regarding addiction, this lack of ADA protection for inability to perform the essential work functions plays out most obviously for the employee who comes to work intoxicated, in withdrawal, or otherwise impaired by a substance of abuse. That employee benefits from no ADA protection, because the problem is the inability to perform the job function rather than the actual condition itself, addiction. If there is not workplace intoxication, the alcohol-dependent person who notifies his or her employer of the problem and fulfills the other requirements of the ADA would be protected against job discrimination. By contrast, the courts have ruled that illicit drug use is protected only if the drug use is not "current"; however, the definition of "current" is very much disputed. One judge opined that "current" drug use "does not require that a drug user have a heroin syringe in his arm or a marijuana bong in his mouth at the exact moment contemplated. Instead, in this context, the plain meaning of 'currently' is broader" (*Shaffer v. Preston Memorial Hosp. Corp.*, 1996). Needless to say, the judge in this case did not extend ADA protection to the complainant. The courts have consistently narrowed ADA protection for addicted and drug/alcohol-using persons over the years: A labor lawyer would be a necessary consultant for any person concerned with ADA protection for addiction.

The specific needs of a particular position are often relevant to ADA protection. For instance, official guidance from the U.S. Department of Justice (1997) on the hiring of police officers notes that applicants may be denied a position if they acknowledge the casual use of drugs or current use of drugs, but they may not be denied a position if they acknowledge a history of drug addiction. (That would be a covered disability.) Also, preemployment drug and alcohol testing is allowed under the ADA. Given the demands on police officers, this sort of guidance is quite helpful, and it is the sort of advice that potential employers need to receive from knowledgeable attorneys and/or human resources personnel.

EMPLOYEE ASSISTANCE PROGRAMS

EAPs in the workplace can have enormous positive effects for those who are addicted to drugs or alcohol, and even for employees who simply misuse drugs or alcohol. Although initially developed for the assessment of addiction issues, most EAPs now provide treatment or referrals for a wide variety of psychiatric conditions and family problems. Clinicians who work in EAPs—EAP professionals—may come from a variety of disciplines, including psychology, social work, and professional counseling. One professional organization, the Employee Assistance Professionals Association, offers a widely accepted credential for EAP professionals. (Certified Employee Assistance Professional [CEAP] Program, 2011).

In addition to ensuring a standardized level of knowledge and skill for CEAPs, professional certification provides for ongoing education on psychiatric conditions and treatment techniques. The CEAP program includes requirements for work experience, continuing education, and mentoring.

In regard to addiction and drug and alcohol use, the successful EAP should be well integrated into the workplace, supported by management, and have clear boundaries for confidentiality. As with other workplace responses to addiction, the confidentiality that the employee may expect needs to be clearly defined to all involved. These confidentiality parameters are necessarily different in different situations and work environments. For some "zero-tolerance" occupations such as pilot or physician, an EAP professional might be obliged to report any addiction or substance misuse, an unfortunate but sometimes inevitable parameter. Other workplaces or occupations might allow for a full assurance of confidentiality in any employee–EAP discussion.

One study of EAP usage by 852 hourly and salaried employees (Delaney, Grube, & Ames, 1998) showed a clear link between supervisor support for the EAP and the likelihood that the employee would avail him or herself of the EAP's services. In addition, union membership, social support for the EAP, and employee belief in it, correlated with higher levels of EAP utilization. Unfortunately, however, those employees who reported drinking during work hours were relatively unlikely to report willingness to seek assistance from the EAP. Although this reluctance is understandable if one considers the level of denial likely present in employees who drink on the job, the finding reflects a disconnect between the EAP in this study and the employees who need it most.

Providing evidence-based and effective psychological assessment and treatment to those employees who need it is a primary function of most EAPs; nowhere is this more obvious than for the addictive disorders. Enlightened employers who support their EAPs can render an enormous service to their employees, as well as protect the workplace from the legal, physical, and emotional damage that addiction can wreak. Preemptively educating and screening employees for substance use problems is one compassionate and inarguable approach to promoting employee health. One innovative model involves telephone screening of employees and, if necessary, referral for treatment.(McPherson, Goplerud, Derr, Mickenberg, & Courtemanche, 2010) Using a method well established in the clinical sphere, screening, brief intervention and referral to treatment (SBIRT), the researchers screened 295 workers from a large financial firm who presented to the EAP for a variety of issues. In this (admittedly self-selected) group, the most common self-reported problems were stress–anxiety–panic (38%) and depression (19%), followed by an alcohol use problem (6%) and a substance use problem (1%). In contrast to the self-report, the clinician's use of the Alcohol Use Disorders Identification Test (AUDIT) revealed that fully 40% of the subjects prescreened positive for hazardous alcohol use, and all of these subjects received a brief intervention at the level deemed appropriate by the EAP clinician.

Even given the high cost of workplace alcohol and drug problems, employers must evaluate the cost-effectiveness of EAP responses to the problem. One preliminary study (Cowell, Bray, & Hinde, 2012) found that alcohol screening by EAP professionals, when delivered during a regular counseling session, cost $0.64, and the delivery of any needed brief intervention was $2.52, with both costs consisting mostly of the EAP professional's time. The authors found that "the low costs for the current study suggest that only modest gains in outcomes would likely be needed to justify delivering SBI in an EAP setting" (p. 55). Although EAP clinicians assess a wide variety of psychological problems, the available evidence suggests that a well-run and management-supported EAP can deliver tremendous benefits in the evaluation and treatment of drug- and alcohol-using employees.

DRUG AND ALCOHOL TESTING IN THE WORKPLACE

Drug and alcohol testing in the workplace is an increasingly accepted method of deterring drug and alcohol use, or at least deflecting it from the particular workplace and hours when the testing is being done. Preliminary data show that testing programs do in fact discourage drug use and are probably cost-effective in doing so (French, Roebuck, & Alexandre, 2004). Given the legal framework for workplace drug and alcohol testing, and the presumptive good effects of that testing, the devil remains in the details. Unless a workplace testing program is carefully designed and well managed, the results are prone to be confusing, unintended consequences result, and may be challenged legally. Also, given the potential consequences of a positive workplace drug test, there is a substantial illicit market in methods for delivering false-positive results. One intrepid—and illegal—website offers synthetic urine, fake penises for deceiving test observers, and heat packs for keeping the fake urine at body temperature (Whizzinator Website, n.d.).

The well-designed workplace testing program results from a collaboration of medical, scientific, and legal professionals who can construct a program that addresses particular issues for the workplace in question. For instance, the workplace testing program should have a distinct goal or set of goals. Is the goal of the program to prevent workplace accidents? Assist employees with addiction problems? Satisfy federally mandated guidelines? Generate good publicity for management or a union? Or prevent employees from taking unfair advantage of banned performance-enhancing drugs? Although all of these goals might seem similar, they actually necessitate different sorts of programs with different protocols.

Home testing by an untrained person—which can be done by any concerned parent who picks up a testing kit at the local pharmacy—is prone to error and misinterpretation, and has no place in the occupational sphere. Home testing by a trained professional using calibrated instruments can be productive but is expensive and complicated to administer. However, this sort of testing away from the workplace can mitigate the substantial embarrassment and inconvenience associated with testing, especially if the test is a saliva test for alcohol, for instance. Any testing that is designed for a legal or employment setting must be forensic-quality testing, with a clear chain of custody between testee, collector, laboratory, and reporter. That is, all who are involved with the testing must be prepared to defend under cross-examination the provenance of the particular sample being tested, its transportation and storage, and the testing methods.

In addition to the testing itself, there must be a clear protocol in place for choosing when to test, whom to test, and what body fluids to test. Any discrimination against a particular person or class of people discredits the entire process and would call into question the validity of a particular test result. For instance, preemployment testing, while not considered a medical test and therefore allowed under the ADA, should be applied fairly and with a clear protocol for which potential employees are tested. All job applicants might be tested, or persons who are chosen randomly, or those who are applying for safety-sensitive positions.

Other sorts of workplace drug testing include "reasonable cause" testing, random testing, postaccident testing, periodic testing, and rehabilitation testing. One person's reasonable cause might not suffice for another person, especially if one person involved is a representative for the employee! Some workplaces define "reasonable cause" as simply a supervisor's suspicion, while others require actual legal involvement or mention in the news media. Random testing must be truly random to avoid both the taint of discrimination and making the testing time predictable and easy for a drug user to beat. Although postaccident testing seems obvious, a sensible testing protocol defines the seriousness of an accident that would necessitate a test, the time frame within which a test must be done, and the procedure for confirming that the test is completed properly and within the agreed-upon time frame. Testing employees on a scheduled basis has little value in the employment sphere, because all but the most disorganized drug and alcohol users will easily evade the test. Rehabilitation testing, for the purpose of measuring the effectiveness of addiction treatment, can generate significant rewards in the occupational setting, with the dual purpose of promoting abstinence for the employee and protecting the workplace from drug and alcohol use.

The medical review officer (MRO) is a physician who is specifically trained and licensed by the Department of Health and Human Services to oversee workplace drug testing (Medical Review Officer Certification Council, Swotinsky, & Smith, 2010). Originally developed in the U.S. military for assessment of soldiers' drug tests, the set of skills possessed by MROs includes test selection, review of the chain of custody, laboratory knowledge of specific tests and, perhaps most importantly, a sophisticated knowledge of the ever-changing set of new intoxicants and methods for skirting drug tests. Although the U.S. Department of Transportation and most laboratories require that forensic testing only be released to a licensed MRO, many nonmandated employers choose to retain an MRO to ensure that their testing is well-conceived and managed.

BEHAVIORAL ADDICTIONS

The behavioral addictions, also known as "process addictions" (Shaffer, 1996), are broadly defined as compulsive participation in a behavior that harms the patient physically, emotionally, or otherwise. These sorts of compulsive behaviors are insidious in the occupational environment, since the behaviors themselves are often innocuous, natural, or simply irrelevant to an employee's work. While employers can absolutely prohibit drug or alcohol use during work hours or for some period of time beforehand, it is impractical or impossible to forbid the ingestion of food, use of the Internet, gambling, shopping, or sexual behaviors.

Internet usage is necessary in many, if not most, modern-day workplaces, but the Internet can be problematic for some users. Even without mentioning behaviors such as gambling or viewing pornography, which employers can ban, excessive use of the Internet for non-work-related activities is problematic and can become compulsive. (Murali & George, 2007; Young, 1999). Typical complaints include physical ailments such as carpal tunnel syndrome and back pain, as well as depression and simple loneliness. Although many employers monitor Internet use by their employees, it is simply impossible to monitor all use, all the time, and to decide which e-mail is relevant to work, and how relevant that e-mail is. The boundary between devotion to work and actual addiction to the Internet is murky, and it takes a savvy supervisor to confront an employee and refer that individual for help, whether for professional supervision on appropriate workplace behavior, or psychological assistance. The most commonly used paradigms for compulsive Internet usage include cognitive-behavioral techniques and support groups.

Compulsive Internet usage in the workplace can manifest as habitual shopping or gambling, but sexual compulsivity in the workplace is most likely to be explosive and detrimental to the employee and employer, whether the employee acts out uncontrollable sexual behaviors physically or they are only Internet-based. Internet sex addiction can mean different things to different people, but it has been defined as consisting of excessively (1) seeking out online material for masturbatory use, (2) arranging meetings with others for sexual contact, or (3) buying sexually related goods that can be used offline (Dunn, Seaburne-May, & Gatter, 2012). Although none of these behaviors is itself illegal, the behaviors breach the boundaries of most workplaces and would result in a reprimand, if not sanctions, for the employee. Given the ease, ubiquity, and supporting case law (*United States of America v. Jeffrey Brian Ziegler*, 2007) for employer monitoring of employee Internet use, the employee who engages in any of these behaviors is by definition taking an unreasonable risk in pursuit of sexual gratification.

Experts in sexual compulsivity have noted that the "workaholic" may find sexual addiction an exhilarating addition to the compulsive work behavior (Carnes, 1992). As with sexual compulsivity in other venues, the behavior decreases any chances for actual intimacy and endangers the person's emotional and physical health. But in the occupational setting, sexual acting out can result in termination from the position or, in some situations, legal sanctions. Although employee manuals may provide an outline of behavior considered inappropriate in the workplace, for the behavioral addictions, supervisory personnel must exercise individual judgment in confronting employees with these sorts of compulsive behaviors.

ZERO-TOLERANCE EMPLOYEES: PROGRAMS FOR IMPAIRED PROFESSIONALS

Some employees receive "zero-tolerance" for substance use or addiction, based on the theory that the extensive harm individuals such as commercial pilots, truck drivers, or physicians might cause justifies a strict and inflexible standard. However, despite the apparent commonsense nature of this standard, fairness and practicality dictate that workplace drug and alcohol programs generate thoughtful responses to such employees who use, or are accused of using, banned or regulated substances.

There is ample evidence that substance use by these sorts of employees causes serious problems. In one study (Li et al., 2011) of aviation employees between 1995 and 2005, 4,977 employees were tested under a postaccident protocol, while 1,129,922 employees were tested randomly over the same time period. Although the prevalence of postaccident drug tests positive for marijuana, amphetamines, opiates, or phencyclidine was very low (1.82%), that percentage was three times the positive rate on random tests (64%). Also, this study did not measure alcohol use, an arguably more common phenomenon among aviation employees.

According to the Federal Aviation Administation (FAA; 2012), pilot errors increase dramatically at the 0.04% blood alcohol concentration (BAC). When the FAA studied 338 aviation fatalities in 1993, 12.7% involved a BAC of 0.02% or more, while 8.9% had a BAC greater than 0.4%. For this reason, Federal Aviation Regulation CFR 91.17 (2006) has put into place the 8-hour "bottle to throttle rule."

> No person may act or attempt to act as a crewmember of a civil aircraft (1) Within 8 hours after the consumption of any alcoholic beverage; (2) While under the influence of alcohol; (3) While using any drug that affects the person's faculties in any way contrary to safety; or (4) While having an alcohol concentration of 0.04 or greater in a blood or breath specimen. Alcohol concentration means grams of alcohol per deciliter of blood or grams of alcohol per 210 liters of breath.

Although the harm they cause is perhaps not as dramatic as the damage potential of intoxicated pilots, physicians are similarly given a public trust that entails a high degree of vigilance with regard to impairment. Most states have programs for managing impaired physicians, most commonly for drug- and alcohol-related reasons, and protecting patients; similarly, programs run by the state or physician groups help foster good treatment of these impaired physicians and promote a monitored return to practice.

In 2011, the Federation of State Medical Boards (FSMB) published a document that codified best practices in the management of physicians impaired by drugs or alcohol, or other causes. The policy differentiates between physician health programs (PHPs) run by physicians themselves, and state medical boards, with the recommendation that these two types of entities collaborate on their mutual goals of assisting impaired physicians and protecting patients. The document also promotes the use of standard diagnoses and an assessment of relapse that focuses on the potential to affect public safety, and advocates a voluntary track for physicians who request assistance, as well as a mandated track for physicians who are required by a state medical board to have treatment.

The recovery rate for physicians with addiction problems is higher than that of the general public, probably because of the important value physicians attach to their work, and the near-certainty that they will lose their medical license if they relapse while under the supervision of a PHP or state medical board. In a study of 904 physicians admitted to PHPs in 16 states, DuPont et al. (2009) found that 78% of the addicted physicians had no positive drug or alcohol tests during the 5-year period of the study. The authors believe that the excellent outpatient and inpatient care offered to the participants, along with mandated participation in peer-led support groups such as Alcoholics Anonymous and Narcotics Anonymous led to these excellent outcomes.

ADDICTION AMONG ATHLETES

Competitive athletics can be considered a workplace with its own idiosyncratic norms and obligations, whether the athletes are professionals or amateurs. Although professional athletes may have additional protections if they are represented by a union or protected by U.S. Federal Labor Law in the form of the National Labor Relations Board (NLRB), almost all athletes have duties that other employees do not. These obligations may consist of a ban on the use of substances or medications that are perfectly legal and uncontrolled for others, or the acceptance of a drug testing program that would seem draconian or overly intrusive in another setting.

After many years of denial and protesting his innocence, the competitive cyclist Lance Armstrong was recently relieved by the International Cycling Union of his seven Tour-de-France Gold Medals for doping violations (Macur, 2012). The intense media and public pressure in this case reveal the symbolic importance of "clean" competition, and well as the powerful forces that may pressure the athlete into cheating. Armstrong's case, and many others, demonstrates that both elite athletes and those on the cusp of success are vulnerable to the temptations of using illicit performance-enhancing drugs (PEDs) and techniques.

Substance use in the sports workplace can be divided into drug use that is clearly for the enhancement of athletic performance (e.g., anabolic androgenic steroids), substance use that is certainly addictive (cocaine), and a middle category that may be both (amphetamine). Although all legitimate sports organizations, professional and amateur, have banned the use of PEDs, many of these substances are widely available to athletes, as is the advice of amateur pharmacologists on how to use the substances effectively. While the hazards of these PEDs should be an overriding reason to eschew their use, many athletes are willing to take substantial risks in order to achieve success, even to the point or risking dangerous physical and emotional side effects, and disgrace if they are caught. Also, many young users of PEDs are taking them simply for enlarged muscle size rather than improved function: Bodybuilders and adolescent boys trying to impress others are in this category. For the physician who treats athletes, the control of PED use presents at least one important dilemma, in that the physician's patient-athlete may be at risk of punishment if the physician reveals the PED use (Green, 2006). For prescribing physicians outside the world of sports, the prescription of a PED may seem like a simple off-label prescription of a medication, as commonly practiced in modern medicine. Some sports physicians argue that given the common use of PEDs, they should be simply allowed and managed rather than prohibited (Millar, 1994). However, organized sports organizations are becoming increasingly unforgiving of athletes who are prescribed banned substances, even by a legitimately trained and licensed physician: The final responsibility is the athlete's.

Use of addictive drugs by athletes—most commonly marijuana and cocaine—is usually treated differently in the sports workplace, at least initially. Users of these substances are assumed to need help rather than being viewed simply as cheating—a view that is usually correct. Despite the contention that marijuana may actually benefit performance in some situations, most commonly the marijuana-using athlete is using the drug for consciousness-changing or frank addiction. Similarly, the addictive aspects of cocaine are far more prominent than any performance-enhancing attributes. So athletes found to be using either of these substances are generally referred for treatment by sports organizations rather than sanctioned. (Sanctions might be imposed for a failure to attend treatment or continuing positive drug tests.) Athletes do become addicted to other substances of abuse, such as opioids, benzodiazepines, and hallucinogens other than marijuana, and these individuals would also be referred to treatment rather than immediately sanctioned.

Some addictive and banned substances also have legitimate therapeutic purposes, most commonly stimulant medications, such as the various methylphenidate and amphetamine preparations available for treating attention-deficit/hyperactivity disorder. In order to allow legitimately diagnosed athletes to use their needed medications, most sport organizations grant therapeutic use exemptions (TUEs) for use of the particular medication in questions. TUE policies across sport usually have four main criteria that must be fulfilled in order for the athlete to receive an exemption. (Westreich, 2011) First, the athlete must experience some significant impairment to his or her health without the medication. Second, the medication must confer no additional advantage to the athlete above and beyond his or her ability to perform before the relevant medical condition emerged, a sensible but totally unverifiable requirement. Third, there must be no reasonable alternative to the medication. Finally, use of the medication cannot be the result of previous use of a banned substance. This situation would arise most commonly in the case of the athlete who, because of his use of anabolic–androgenic steroids, requests an exemption for the therapeutic use of testosterone.

As the preceding paragraph should suggest, the ethical dilemmas regarding doping in the sport workplace are abundant, not the least of which is the question of what exactly is wrong with attempting to enhance performance with substances in the first place. As pointed out by ethicist T. H. Murray (2008), this is a legitimate question with some important answers. Athletes in a sport in which PED use occurs face an essential choice: They must either compete without the use of illicit PEDs in the expectation that they will lose to a competitor who chooses to cheat, they could discontinue competing at a competitive level, or they may join the cheaters and hope for the best. The ultimate task of anti-PED drug programs in sports is to provide a fourth alternative, thus allowing athletes to compete with the—necessarily incomplete— assurance that they are competing on a level playing field.

CONCLUSIONS

Addiction in the workplace provokes many quandaries at the interface between psychiatry and the law. However, the skillful practitioner can design effective and transparent responses to addiction in the occupational environment that lead to the best possible outcomes for all involved. Sometimes these outcomes involve the protection of employees and clients by forestalling drug or alcohol use in the workplace, and sometimes they result in a successful therapeutic intervention with the addicted person. While the goal of the occupational psychiatrist is not simply to treat addiction, often the added incentive of job loss or jeopardy results in the employee receiving the necessary treatment.

Although the inevitable dilemma of dual agency confronts the occupational psychiatrist working with addiction in the workplace, this challenge can be managed ethically, within the bounds of the law, and with respect for the addicted person. Clinicians involved with EAPs can design effective prevention, identification, and treatment programs for addiction that are a credit to the employer and the employee. Drug and alcohol testing programs can be similarly designed to promote workplace safety, while allowing the addicted or drug- or alcohol-using employee to obtain the necessary treatment, with a return to work as an expected outcome. The special circumstances of "zero-tolerance" employees, and athletes, can also be addressed in the most productive and fair manner possible. By working together, addiction treatment professionals and those familiar with labor laws can fashion these sorts of complicated but enormously important protocols.

REFERENCES

American Psychiatric Association. (2013). *Diagnostic and statistical manual of mental disorders* (5th ed.). Arlington, VA: Author

Brown, S. A., & Bennett, M. E. (2004). Dual diagnosis. In J. C. Thomas & M. Hersen (Eds.), *Psychopathology in the workplace* (pp. 59–74). New York: Brunner/Routledge.

Carnes, P. (1992). *Out of the shadows, understanding sexual addiction.* Center City, MN: Hazelden Press.

CEAP Candidate Information. (2011). Retrieved October 4, 2012, from *www.eapassn.org/i4a/pages/index.cfm?pageid=3456#intro.*

Cowell, A. J., Bray, J. W., & Hinde, B. A. (2012). The cost of screening and brief intervention in employee assistance programs. *J Behav Health Serv Res, 39*(1), 55–67.

Delaney, W., Grube, J. W., & Ames, G. M. (1998). Predicting likelihood of seeking help through the employee assistance program among salaried and union hourly employees. *Addiction, 93*(3), 399–410.

Dunn, N., Seaburne-May, M., & Gatter, P. (2012). Internet sex addiction: A license to lust? *Adv Psychiatr Treat, 18,* 270–277.

DuPont, R. L., & Martin, D. M. (2012). A new challenge for drug-free workplace programs. *Occup Health Saf, 81*(2), 32, 34.

DuPont, R. L., McClellan, A. T., White, W. L., et. al. (2009). Setting the standard for recovery: Physicians' health programs. *J Subst Abuse Treat, 36,* 1159–1171.

Epstein, D. H., & Preston, K. L. (2011). TGI monday?: Drug-dependent outpatients report lower stress and more happiness at work than elsewhere. *Am J Addict, 21,* 189–192.

Federal Aviation Administration (FAA). (2012). Alcohol and flying: A deadly combination. Retrieved October, 30, 2012, from *www.faa.gov/pilots/safety/pilotsafetybrochures.*

Federal Aviation Regulation CFR 91.17. (June 15, 2006). Final Rule, Docket No. 2004-19835.

Federation of State Medical Boards (FSMB). (2011). Policy on Physician Impairment. Retrieved October 27, 2012, from *www.csam-asam.org/sites/default/files/pdf/misc/fsmb2011.pdf.*

French, M. T., Roebuck, M. C., & Alexandre, P. K. (2004). To test or not to test: Do workplace drug testing programs discourage employee drug use? *Soc Sci Res, 33,* 45–63.

Galanter, M., & Kleber, H. (Eds.). (2008). *Substance abuse treatment.* Washington, DC: American Psychiatric Press.

Green, G. A. (2006). Doping control for the team physician: A review of drug testing procedures in sport. *Am J Sports Med, 34*(10), 1690–1698.

Larson, S. L., Eyerman, J., Foster, M., & Gfoerer, J. (2007) *Worker substance use and workplace policies and problems.* Rockville, MD: SAMHSA, Office of Applied Studies.

Li, G., Baker, S. P., Zhao, Q., et al. (2011). Drug violations and aviation accidents: Findings from the US mandatory drug testing programs. *Addiction, 106,* 1287–1292.

Macur, J. (2014, March 2). End of the ride for Lance Armstrong. *New York Times,* p. SP1.

McPherson, T. L., Goplerud, E., Derr, D., Mickenberg, J., & Courtemanche, S. (2010). Telephonic screening and brief intervention for alcohol misuse among workers contacting the employee assistance program: A feasibility study. *Drug Alcohol Rev, 29,* 641–646.

Medical Review Officer Certification Council, Swotinsky, R. B., & Smith, D. R. (Eds.). (2010). *The medical review officer's manual* (4th ed.). Beverly Farms, MA: OEM Press.

Murali, V., & George, V. (2007). Lost online: An overview of internet addiction. *Adv Psychiatr Treat, 13,* 24–30.

Murray, T. H. (2008). Doping in sport: Challenges of medicine, science, and ethics. *J Int Med, 264,* 95–98.

Millar, A. P. (1994). Licit steroid use—hope for the future. *Br J Sp Med, 28*(2), 79–83.

Robert Half International. (1996, October 10). Surf's up!: Is productivity down? [Press release].

Robertson, M. D., & Walter, G. (2008). Many faces of the dual-role dilemma in psychiatric ethics. *Aust N Z J Psychiatry, 42*(3), 228–235.

Shaffer, H. J. (1996). Understanding the means and objects of addiction: Technology, the Internet, and gambling. *J Gamb Stud, 12* (4), 461–469.

Shaffer v. Preston Memorial Hosp. Corp., 107 F. 3d. 274 (4th Cir., 1996).

Shand, F., & Fawcett, J. (2003). *Guidelines for the treatment of alcohol problems.* Canberra, Australia: Commonwealth Department of Health and Aging.

Substance Abuse and Mental Health Services Administration (SAMHSA). (1989). Components of a drug-free workplace. Retrieved October 8, 2012, from *http://workplace.samhsa.gov/fedpgms/pages/modelplan508.pdf.*

United States of America v. Jeffrey Brian Ziegler, 474 F.3d 1184 (9th Cir., January 30, 2007).

U.S. Department of Justice, Civil Rights Division, Disability Rights Section. (1997). Questions and answers: The Americans with Disabilities Act and hiring police officers. Retrieved October 7, 2012, from *www.ada.gov/copsq7a.pdf.*

U.S. House of Representatives. (1988). Drug-Free Workplace Act of 1988, U.S.C. 701-707.

U.S. House of Representatives. (1998). Drug-Free Workplace Act of 1998, U.S.C. 105-584.

Westreich, L. (2002). Addiction and the Americans with Disabilities Act. *J Am Acad Psychiatry Law, 30*(3), 355–363.

Westreich, L. (2011). Anabolic androgenic steroids. In J. Lowinson, P. Ruiz, & J. Langrod (Eds.), *Substance abuse: A comprehensive textbook* (3rd ed.). New York: Williams & Wilkins.

Whizzinator Website. (n.d.). Retrieved October 23, 2012, from *www.thewhizzinator.com/lifestyle-products.*

Young, K. S. (1999). Internet addiction: Symptoms, evaluation, and treatment. In L. VandeCreek & T. L. Jackson (Eds.), *Innovations in clinical practice* (Vol. 17, pp.19–31). Sarasota, FL: Professional Resource Press.

CHAPTER 19

Forensic Approaches to Substances of Abuse

AVRAM H. MACK

Behavioral health clinicians today are facing an increasing role in the legal system in a variety of contexts. There are many reasons for this, including increases in litigation, prison populations, substance abuse, and professional interest in forensic psychiatry. People who misuse substances often must contend with lawsuits, prosecution, psychiatric commitment, interpersonal conflicts, and violence—all of which may require their clinicians to become involved with the legal system to some degree. Increasingly clinicians need to view any documentation through the critical lens that is a part of forensic work (e.g., signing disability applications). Because of the growth of systems for mandated treatment as "diversion" from judicial interventions, many more addiction psychiatrists may find themselves formally engaged in forensic psychiatry. As a result, these clinicians must develop a working familiarity with the legal system as it relates to the issues they will face with their patients.

Clinicians who deal with substance use disorders (SUDs) need to understand forensic issues in order to practice with skill and to communicate effectively in legal settings. The purpose of this chapter is to guide the general or addiction psychiatrist with respect to the legal context of practice regarding substances of abuse. The aim here is to provide a basic framework for forensic approaches to substances of abuse. The chapter highlights a variety of legal settings in which a clinician might be asked to provide an opinion, and I discuss important considerations to help guide the clinician in each. For a discussion of legal issues that arise in clinical care (e.g., confidentiality, Tarasoff duties, or liability reduction), rather than in judicial settings, the reader is directed to Lifson and Simon (1998) or Gutheil and Appelbaum (2007).

LEGAL AND ETHICAL ISSUES REGARDING SUBSTANCE USE IN CLINICAL CARE

The topics presented in this section include situations that arise in clinical care or when addiction experts are asked for consultation.

Preventing Misuse of Controlled Substances

Misuse of controlled substances has become increasingly common and in most instances occurs when the substances have been provided by friends or family members. Controlled substance misuse is less common when individuals acquire the drugs from a doctor, the Internet, or through stealing. One likely reason for this distinction is that getting controlled substances from a friend or relative may lead to accidental overdoses. Several institutions and governments have begun to try to combat misuse. Many colleges and universities are creating "contracts" with students who are taking stimulant medications, with requirements to be compliant with treatment recommendations and with the risk of disciplinary action due to noncompliance. Some clinicians, especially those who frequently treat pain, have developed a "uniform" approach to any recipient of a controlled substance prescription (Gourlay, Heit, & Almahrezi, 2005). And most states have now developed electronically based monitoring programs—in New York State, physicians prescribing controlled substances are required to check this system before each prescription.

Few methods are more effective than a real clinical relationship with the patient, however. And in that sense, it is the new patient who might deserve added scrutiny; emergency supplies can be limited to one day's worth. Psychiatrists should also be mindful of other principles as a guide: (1) When prescribing a controlled substance, the patient should be reminded of his or her responsibilities in controlling the medication and safety disposing of unused portions; (2) treatment should not be "open-ended," and reassessment should be ongoing; (3) the actual process of prescribing should include informed consent and proper documentation of all required information on the prescription, which may vary across states; and (4) clinicians should always remain cognizant that there are situations in which they should stop prescribing. This should be done where stopping the medications is in a patient's best interests and referrals are made where appropriate.

Confidentiality

The stringent laws governing the release of information about patients and substance use were developed to reduce stigma and to ensure that individuals do not avoid treatment if they are concerned about revelations. Federal law 42 CFR Part 2 contains regulations that should be reviewed, and one should integrate these requirements into universal approaches for releasing information. Electronic medical record systems, including those to be involved in Health Information Exchange systems used by individual practitioners and by organizations, need to address these issues as well. Consent requirements under 42 CFR Part 2 require patient consent in some situations where the Health Insurance Portability and Accountability Act of 1996 (HIPAA) does not (Brooks, 1997). Clinicians need to know whether or not their practice is governed by 42 CFR or the HIPAA "Privacy Rule," or neither (see *www.samhsa.gov/healthprivacy/docs/samhsapart2-hipaacomparison2004.pdf*).

Impaired Professionals

Interactions with impaired professionals in any profession need to be handled carefully. Many local medical organizations have built peer structures around impaired professionals. The individual physician may have a duty to report an impaired peer, but that depends on state law in some cases. Addiction experts may be called on to provide opinions about the fitness of professionals in law enforcement and public safety (the rate of alcohol use disorders among urban police officers in one city was higher than that in the general population [Ballenger et al., 2010]), attorneys, transportation workers, and others).

Reporting Abuse or Neglect

Clinicians have requirements to report abuse or neglect, and this applies to persons misusing substances of abuse. All states have requirements regarding maltreatment of children; many have such laws regarding maltreatment of older adults. Such reports are exceptions to the HIPAA Privacy Rule and to CFR 42 confidentiality and privacy rules. This is important when considering the possibility that children who spend time near parents who are misusing substances are at greater risks than other children for neglect or abuse. Or, from another vantage point, child abuse and domestic violence are both more common in substance users than in the general population (see the section on "Violence and Aggression"), which means that such reporting is not uncommon. It is notable that the HIPAA Privacy Rule allows an exception to confidentiality only for initial reporting rather than responses to follow-up questions.

Mandated Treatment in Criminal and Civil Settings

Between functioning as a clinician and as a forensic expert, the physician plays a part in a growing number of settings in which treatment is mandated by a body of authority (usually a court). Depending on the jurisdiction and the authoritative body, the names of the governing laws and standards may have different names and verbiage despite sharing common objectives and similar procedures.

Court-ordered treatment has two major trajectories, and they represent different goals, although the end result may be the same. The first involves systems designed to move disordered criminal offenders out of the justice system and into treatment. The other major category of court-ordered treatment consists of the laws that provide for the involuntary commitment (inpatient or outpatient) of patients whose disorders endanger themselves or others (Monahan et al., 2005). Many of these systems are exclusive for either substance use or psychiatric treatment, and many jurisdictions have systems for only one of these two realms of treatment. A central dilemma for all of these programs is whether treatment of addictions is possible when forced on the individual (given the success of these programs, however, this dilemma should spur important academic thought about the value of coercion in addiction treatment generally). Psychiatrists with knowledge of addictions can play a major role in these proceedings, and judges are often receptive to the psychiatrists' insights.

Criminal Diversion

"Diversion" refers to institutions, practices, and laws that divert criminal offenders who have a mental disorder or an SUD out of the standard criminal justice system and into alternative programs. Diversion may occur at many different points in the criminal process, including prearrest, prearraignment, pretrial, in lieu of punishment, or after some punishment. A comprehensive review of the rationales for, and the many types of, diversion programs can be found in a volume by the Council of State Governments (2002). The core feature of diversion is that an authority releases the offender from further blame or from punishment in exchange for the offender's engagement in treatment. Typically, the offender must express to the authority (police, prosecutor, or judge) a voluntary willingness to engage in treatment. Because of the conditional aspect of diversion, there is often a question as to whether such expressed willingness reflects a genuine wish for treatment or instead is used simply to avoid criminal proceedings.

Drug courts are one type of diversion found in a limited number of jurisdictions. Drug courts mandate treatment and seem to have low recidivism rates and lead to education, cost savings, and drug-free infants (Carey et al., 2006). These programs are generally for nonviolent offenders with less serious charges (e.g., misdemeanors). These institutions may protect the patient or the public from violence or accidents, and they may reduce expenditures on incarceration or hospitalization, but some states require that a mental disorder other than an SUD be present. However, drug courts' limited focus can obscure the presence of a psychiatric disorder, and those involved should advocate for awareness and diagnosis in such cases (Hagedorn & Willenbring, 2003). Some have called for the growth of co-occurring courts that deal with persons who have both major mental disorders and SUDs.

Involuntary Treatment

Mandated treatment exists in some jurisdictions for those with serious and pervasive SUDs who have been or will likely become dangerous to themselves or others. Various states, counties, and the federal government have been developing ways in which to intervene (Gerbasi et al., 2000). Thomsen and Appelbaum (2002) have commented on the valid legal basis for this approach. In 1962, the U.S. Supreme Court ruled in *Robinson v. California* that "a state might establish a program of compulsory treatment for those addicted to narcotics. Such a program might require periods of involuntary confinement, and penal sanctions might be imposed for failure to comply with established treatment procedures."

As of 1997, 31 states and the District of Columbia had statutes specifically allowing involuntary treatment or commitment for substance-dependent individuals. This treatment can be inpatient, outpatient, or partial hospitalization. The criteria and process for commitment vary by state but usually require a judicial hearing in which the individual's or the community's safety is believed to be endangered by the refusal of the patient to receive treatment. Even in states in which these statutes exists, many clinicians and families (and even judges or attorneys) are unaware of them and, as a result, fail to avail themselves of the legal avenues in place to facilitate patients' entry into or compliance with essential treatment and care.

Treatment in Correctional Settings

A significant segment of the U.S. population is currently under criminal justice supervision, and most of these individuals have active SUDs or dual diagnoses (Karberg & Mumola, 2006). Throughout the world, an SUD preceding incarceration occurs at rates much higher than in the community (Fazel et al., 2008). "Correctional" is a broad term that refers to the settings in which individuals in the criminal justice system are supervised through the judicial process. This can mean not only institutions of incarceration (jails or prisons) but also supervision either before a trial (pretrial release), as a part of punishment (probation), or as a condition of early release from incarceration (parole or supervised release). Because of the variety of correctional contexts, psychiatrists must be prepared to advise on screening and treatment, make recommendations for release conditions, and become a part of the treatment for those reentering the community. Both the American Psychiatric Association (2000) and the National Commission on Correctional Health Care (2003) have developed guidelines for correctional facilities, and the Office of Juvenile Justice and Delinquency Prevention (2005) has created guidelines for clinicians who come into contact with incarcerated minors.

Incarceration is a setting in which the individual is removed from the community, and the attention that needs to be given by addiction specialists at the various stages of incarceration varies according to the setting and its purpose. Broadly speaking, individuals occupy three very different incarceration ecologies: (1) lockup (on arrest); (2) jail (following arraignment, during trial, prior to sentencing, or in sentences of up to 1 year); and (3) prison (postsentencing for more than 1 year). Substance-related disorders may appear at any point in the incarceration process, and ongoing, focused surveillance should be a part of every correctional system. For example, appropriate short-term clinical attention may be needed to treat the aggression of intoxication, reducing the potential for morbidity and mortality associated with intoxication (e.g., cocaine) or withdrawal (e.g., alcohol).

Proper recognition of SUDs can lead to long-term benefits for the institution and for society. Research has established that focused, rehabilitation-oriented treatment for addiction leads to favorable outcomes following incarceration, including decreased drug use and criminal activity and improved overall functionality (Gendreau, 1996; Mateyoke-Scrivner et al., 2004). The outcomes improve even more significantly when appropriate aftercare is provided (Griffith et al., 1999). A recent study in England reported a substantial decline in criminal activity in individuals with SUDs following voluntary participation in either residential or outpatient treatment programs (Gossop et al., 2005). Unfortunately, in reality, the typical levels of available psychiatric and medical services differ greatly among these settings (Weinstein et al., 2005). Psychiatrists should be advocates for ensuring that appropriate services are available at these various stages.

Screening

Many individuals who are arrested have been using a drug of abuse just prior to their arrest, and may be carrying such substances at the time. Accordingly, it is imperative that the intake process include a careful examination of the individual for intoxication, overdose, or active withdrawal from any substance—particularly alcohol, benzodiazepines, or other sedatives. Ironically, for long-term users who are not actively intoxicated or in withdrawal, the opportunity to be referred to rehabilitation programs can be missed at screening. The clinician should use all available data, including testing and medical history, to guide more detailed screening.

An SUD necessitates further, specialized medical assessment for associated pathology, such as infectious disease, cardiac injury, or thromboembolic events or the potential for these conditions (Baillargeon et al., 2003). Screening for SUDs also must be geared to detect comorbid psychiatric conditions, which are common in the addicted incarcerated population. The burden of drug or alcohol use disorders among women is at least as great, if not greater, in incarcerated women. (Binswanger et al., 2010).

Treatment and Rehabilitation

The correctional setting provides the opportunity for abstinence, treatment, and possibly rehabilitation. Several studies have shown that residential treatment (or "therapeutic community") during incarceration followed by continued care in the community led to reduction in criminal recidivism and substance relapse (Mitchell, Wilson, & MacKenzie, 2007). However, because of the lack of standardized and validated clinical assessment tools in correctional facilities, little information is available about the treatment needs of inmates. SUDs in this population are often accompanied by a variety of other concerns, including mental health issues, associated medical conditions, unemployment, and lack of education, which make successful treatment and recovery more difficult; these issues typically are not addressed by currently available resources (Belenko & Peugh, 2005).

The available resources for long-term treatment of addictions vary greatly among the incarcerated. Unfortunately, most prison systems do not address addiction in long-term inmates, and when available, long-term residential programs fail to address treatment issues of inmates with shorter terms of incarceration (Belenko & Peugh, 2005). In some systems, addiction is addressed only in the last months of incarceration, most commonly through psychoeducation (Chandler, Fletcher, & Volkow, 2009). Some groups also offer ongoing Alcoholics Anonymous meetings, education, and group and individual psychotherapies. Many jails do not provide adequate detoxification, and few provide adequate treatment services.

The lack of access to adequate treatment for addicted and mentally ill people in the general population contributes to the large number of arrested individuals. Some individuals who are imprisoned still find access to substances of abuse, and in these cases, short-term detoxification may be the appropriate first step. Several institutions have had success in using opioid agonists for incarcerated populations. However, there has been some concern over the misuse of prescribed substances, leading one system to remove quetiapine from its formulary (Tamburello, Lieberman, Baum, & Reeves, 2012).

Contingency management (CM), which is a form of psychotherapy, has support as a method for treating abuse of many different substances. It utilizes incentives, even somewhat directly countering the interest to use, and is divided into three basic principles: (1) frequently monitoring for change in the behavior desired, (2) reinforcement of the desired behavior, and (3) withholding positive reinforcers when it does not occur. Recent data indicate CM's effectiveness in the treatment of stimulant dependence (McDonnell et al., 2013) in a randomized controlled trial of contingency management for stimulant use in community mental health patients with serious mental illness. And CM has been studied in cocaine abusers with and without legal problems, and its success in both groups indicates that it is a promising avenue for those in the correctional setting (Petry, Rash, & Easton, 2011).

Nonincarceration Correctional Settings

The risks of ongoing substance use are significant both for persons referred directly to probation and those released after some period of incarceration. This time period is a critical opportunity for individuals to maintain abstinence while in the community. For those who are being released from incarceration, the risk of continued use exists regardless of whether the release is sudden, planned, or after a short time or a long time. Local justice systems are largely ill-equipped to create a solid plan for care and monitoring. Upon discharge, both those with SUDs only and those with SUDs and comorbid psychiatric conditions are at high risk for relapse, which may affect criminality as well. One Scottish study found that of the increased deaths after release, many had injection drug use, especially with HIV (Bird & Hutchinson, 2003). Data indicate that psychosocial aspects of reentry are the most important factors in reducing relapse and recidivism (Rounds-Bryant, Motivans, & Pelissier, 2004).

Addiction psychiatrists may work with parole boards, probation officers, or pretrial service agencies to mandate treatment following release. Depending on the prevailing law, parole, probation, or pretrial agencies may mandate treatment by referring the case to the court or by referring parolees to mandated treatment. When asked by a court to suggest a treatment plan for the parolee, the addiction psychiatrist should offer multiple modes of multidisciplinary treatment and surveillance. One should consider residential, group, or day treatment; medication management; and other treatment possibilities. The period of treatment should be for a minimum of 1 year. Random screens are best done twice weekly. Attendance at activities should be required. The clinician should reevaluate at regular intervals.

Forensic Psychiatric Expertise on Substances of Abuse

Behavioral Toxicology: Substances and the Risk of Violence, Injury, or Altered Mental State

The possibility of undesired or inappropriate behavior in the context of intoxication on, or withdrawal from, an abused substance is important in many cases. However, this varies according to the substance. Courts can be greatly assisted by physicians and other specialists who can distill the differences among the substances: one can term this "forensic psychiatric toxicology," in which a trained expert may be knowledgeable about assessment of the individual and the substances intoxicating him or her at the levels of external behavior, as well as pharmacology. One must be able to protect one's opinions in the face of defeating oversimplification and generalizations by other parties.

VIOLENCE AND AGGRESSION

"Aggression" is defined as overt behavior with the intent to inflict noxious stimulation or to behave destructively toward another organism. "Violence" is aggression among humans. "Hostility" is defined as unfriendly human attitudes, including tantrums, irritability, refusal to cooperate, and suspicion. All of these behaviors can be problematic, and substances of abuse may promote these behaviors in a variety of ways.

Substances of abuse may promote aggression, hostility, or violence by heightening physiological or psychological states, including anxiety, paranoia, confusion, agitation, irritability, grandiosity, sensation, motor reactivity, or vigilance. The effects of substances on such behaviors are independent of major mental disorder (Steadman et al., 1998). Substances may effect aggression, hostility, or violence during intoxication or withdrawal, during a substance-induced psychiatric or neurological state, or as a result of the comorbidity that comes with use. These effects vary according to the particular substance: Intoxication may be associated with irritability, grandiosity, poor judgment, confusion, or psychosis, all of which may lead to aggression. Withdrawal also might include agitation, delirium (which often includes violence, albeit disorganized), or anxiety. Substance-induced psychiatric states (mental disorders caused by ongoing use of a substance) might create conditions with some increased risk of violence, including reversible or irreversible cognitive deficits, mood disorders, psychosis, or seizures. Finally, comorbid conditions add to risk of violence (Steadman et al., 1998; Swanson, 1994), especially when the patient fails to adhere to treatment or has a personality disorder as a comorbid condition.

Crime is distinct from violence in that it is a social construct. Crime is also linked to substance use, but the two do not share as close a causal relationship as violence and substance abuse. Of the people arrested for violent offenses, 70% test positive for substances of abuse (Sinha & Easton, 1999). Evidence suggests that alcohol use commonly precedes or accompanies violence between sexes, especially among male perpetrators (Leonard & Quigley, 1999), and that the risk of child abuse and child neglect increases when substances are used (Schuck & Widom, 2003). In the United States, 34% of the risk for community violence is attributable to substance use (Swanson, 1994). Forty percent of the risk for homicide by Finnish men was found to be attributable to alcohol use (Eronen, Hakola, & Tiihonen, 1996).

COMORBID SUBSTANCE USE AND PSYCHIATRIC DISORDERS

There is a significant difference in the dangerousness associated with severe mental disorders when substance abuse enters the picture. Investigation, particularly the MacArthur Violence Risk Assessment Study, indicates that persons with co-occurring substance use and psychiatric disorders are more frequently violent than those who have only one diagnosis or the other (Steadman et al., 1998; Swartz et al., 1998). The most important findings over the past decade indicate that violence is not usually associated with major mental disorders that occur in isolation: Perhaps only 4% of reported violence is the result of mental disorders (Swanson, 1994). However, when these mentally ill patients use substances, the risks of violence increase dramatically (Steadman et al., 1998). One explanation of this finding is that treatment noncompliance increases the risk of violence (Torrey 1994), and substance use increases treatment noncompliance (Swartz et al., 1998). This line of research has shown that substances are often involved in instances of violence among those with major mental disorders. The presence of conduct disorder confers an increased risk for initiation of use of all substances from ages 15–18, with less risk for alcohol abuse at age 18, but at age 21, risk for initiation remained elevated for the "club drugs" and cocaine, inhalants, and amphetamines (Hopfer et al., 2013).

SUBSTANCE-INDUCED PSYCHIATRIC DISORDERS

The possibility of substance-induced disorders, particularly sleep disorders or cognitive disorders, significantly adds to the potential ramifications of exposure to substances. For example, chronic caffeine-induced intoxication may lead to chronic deprivation of sleep and a greater potential for abnormal behavior than that due to the caffeine itself. Zolpidem is another substance that may induce abnormal sleep and therefore abnormal behavior (Daley, McNiel, & Binder, 2011).

ALCOHOL

The documented relationship between alcohol and aggression is based on epidemiological evidence (Murdoch, Pihl, & Ross, 1990) and "laboratory" evidence in which intoxication is effected in controlled environments (Bushman & Cooper, 1990), followed by situations engendering anger toward others. Note that individuals with antisocial personality disorder are 21 times more likely to develop alcohol use disorder (Moeller & Dougherty, 2001). Alcohol use can lead to physiological states that have risks of aggression. The finding of a gene that tends to be present in individuals with antisocial personality disorder, especially when substance dependence is present, is of interest (Li et al., 2012).

Alcohol intoxication causes behavioral disturbance and an adrenergic reaction. Withdrawal includes agitation, restlessness, or delirium in severe states. Neurological injuries or disease may be caused directly or indirectly by alcohol. Cognitive impairment may be a result of chronic use.

Given these and other scenarios, it is important to consider history and future risk of violence in those with heavy alcohol use. Continued evidence linking completed suicide with alcohol use highlights the need to assess patients carefully (Kolves et al., 2006). Some studies demonstrate that the intoxication phase tends to be more predictive of violence than the presence of a dependence diagnosis (Mulvey et al., 2006).

CANNABIS

Literature concerning cannabis, violence, and crime makes it increasingly clear that cannabis is not as benign as previously thought. Cannabis, which remains the most widely used illicit substance worldwide (United Nations, 1997), may increase the tendency to be violent or disruptive in heavy users who are experiencing withdrawal. A cannabis withdrawal syndrome with increased cortisol-releasing factor (Tanda, Pontieri, & Di Chiara, 1997) and aggression, restlessness, and irritability has been defined and recognized by some investigators (e.g., Budney et al., 2004). In addition, both youth and adult cannabis users frequently have comorbid psychiatric disorders.

Cannabis use is common among those who commit crimes. It is significantly associated with crimes involving weapons, as well as with reckless endangerment and attempted homicide (Friedman, Glassman, & Terras, 2001). Of all those convicted of homicide in New York State in 1984, marijuana was the most commonly used illicit drug (Spunt et al., 1994). Cannabis dependence is associated with increased violent crime (Arseneault et al., 2000). Finally, one study that compared the effect of drugs on the likelihood of violence between groups of youth of "high" and "low" delinquency found the only significant effect to be mediated by cannabis (Friedman, Terras, & Glassman, 2003). The possibility of relaxed prohibitions on cannabis use or possession has the risk of expanding all of these violent or problematic behaviors. Leading experts have stated that physicians who play a part in helping patients obtain "medical marijuana" are indirectly contributing to this on a societal level (Kleber & DuPont, 2012).

SEDATIVES/HYPNOTICS

Intoxication with sedatives/hypnotics, which are discussed by DuPont, Greene, and DuPont (Chapter 13, this volume), is not usually associated with violence, although periods of withdrawal may predispose individuals to agitation, anxiety, or irritability. They are, however, associated with the risk of injury due to their effects relative to arousal, falls, and motor coordination. There has been a growing recognition of the effects of the "Z" drugs, the soporifics that only partially activate the benzodiazepine receptor. The U.S. Food and Drug Administration (FDA) has warned clinicians to reduce the starting dose of this medication (Kuehn, 2013). Various episodes of harm and injury have been described as having been committed by individuals experiencing some effect (sometimes seen as somnambulism) of zolpidem, for example. And while some individuals have asserted that their conduct occurred through involuntary intoxication, others have fought against that by asserting that the condition was foreseeable and the defendant should have protected against the abnormal behavior (Daley et al., 2011).

COCAINE AND COCAETHYLENE

Cocaine is a substance that frequently is a consideration in courts for a number of reasons, including the risk of violence to others during the irritability or psychosis of intoxication, and of agitation during withdrawal. The effects of cocaine are greater when it has been converted to cocaethylene when alcohol impacts cocaine metabolism. With cocaethylene, alcohol creates prolonged and enhanced effects of cocaine. It is not just an extended amount of cocaine, it is also a biotransformation channel to a transesterification. It is actually less potent. But the mental state of someone on cocaethylene may be further impaired by longer periods of agitation, poor sleep, and the results of that. And human interactions have a greater time period in which to lead to problems. It also provides for a longer period of the stimulant effects of alcohol. The paranoia of cocaine lasts longer when combined with alcohol.

DISSOCIATIVE ANESTHETICS: N-METHYL-D-ASPARTATE RECEPTOR ANTAGONIST HALLUCINOGENS

Phencyclidine is a substance that comes up frequently in some cities, and experts understand the importance of its pharmacology. Data reflect increased risk of violence when other substances are used, including opioids (especially during withdrawal) and phencyclidine (PCP), in which the risk occurs during the agitation and confusion of intoxication. First, metabolism of PCP increases with chronic use, which is the opposite of the effect of cocaethylene. But that change has to do with pharmacokinetics, not behavior. Consulting an expert on substances of abuse ensure that the fact finder is not the victim of oversimplification. Additionally, PCP's intoxication may range in time, but that is a separate consideration from the severity of the intoxication. Furthermore, PCP's capacity to fluctuate in serum levels in a nonlinear fashion (due to lipophilicity and gastric reuptake) belies any assumptions. Knowledge of substances as pharmacological agents is key and will differentiate experts.

OTHER SUBSTANCES

Greater consumption of soft drinks, although they are not illicit substances, had a significant and strong association with both violence and weapon carrying among Boston high school students (Solnick & Hemenway, 2012). Classical (serotonergic) hallucinogens have been cited by defense attorneys as the basis of abnormal behavior as well, albeit without significantly beneficial legal outcomes in criminal matters.

Substance Use and SUDs in the Criminal Process

The criminal process begins with the prohibited action (the *actus reus*) and continues to prosecution of and assignment of blame (conviction) for the action. Along the way, various events in law enforcement or judicial settings call for decisions on how to proceed: whether to report an incident, whether to prosecute, under what crime to prosecute, whether the defendant may stand trial, whether he or she can be held responsible, whether he or she had—or could have had—the requisite "evil mind" (*mens rea*) or intent for that crime, what the punishment should be, and so forth. The opinion of the addiction expert may be helpful with any of these decisions. The criminal defendant's addictive disorder is particularly important in terms of the mitigation of responsibility when substance use treatment is mandated as an alternative to incarceration, or when the long-term medical or psychiatric effects of substances interfere with the defendant's ability to proceed in the criminal process. However, intoxication or addiction alone is almost never accepted as a complete defense in determining responsibility for a criminal act. Each state has laws that may relate to the potential for intoxication or addiction to be a mitigating factor for culpability in certain crimes. Potential experts should understand the nuances of these positions. In each state, laws define specific criteria that must be met as a part of any expert's opinion, and the expert must have a grasp of those legal requirements before engaging in any consultation.

CRIMINAL SETTING

In a few special situations, responsibility cannot be assigned to a criminal offender. These situations include "insanity," involuntary intoxication, and being otherwise incompetent (e.g., being a minor). Over time, case law and statutes have almost completely eliminated voluntary intoxication as a defense against responsibility for any crime. Involuntary intoxication, however, may be "exculpatory." This term reflects situations in which intoxication occurs via trickery, under duress, or as a result of a previously unknown vulnerability to an atypical reaction to a substance or side effect of medication (Myers & Vondruska, 1998). Some jurisdictions have specific guidelines and limitations for an acceptable involuntary intoxication defense (Downs & Billick, 2000).

Another possibly exculpatory condition is "settled insanity," a situation in which long-term use has led to a chronic brain injury that is different from acute intoxication or toxic psychosis (Slovenko, 1995). Some authors have debated which psychiatric diagnoses may be used when describing an individual with "settled insanity" (Leong, Leisenring, & Dean, 2007). Regardless of theory or apparent logic, when considering an opinion that an individual had settled insanity at the time of an offense, it is best to adhere to a neurological diagnosis or at least to recognized forms of permanent substance-induced conditions, and recall that some psychiatric conditions are known to be induced only by a limited set of substances. Furthermore, in such cases, it is essential to consider malingering. As an example one psychiatrist claimed that a previously healthy antisocial male professional fighter who killed while intoxicated on psilocybin suffered from DSM-IV hallucinogen-induced schizophrenia with onset at intoxication, with index intoxication at the time he killed. The diagnosis was theoretically possible, but the perpetrator's obvious lack of schizophrenia 2 years later diminished the credibility of his expert's opinion.

Although voluntary intoxication is not an excuse for criminal acts, it may alter the law under which the individual is prosecuted (Slovenko, 1995). When "specific intent" is required in order to be convicted of a particular charge (e.g., murder rather than manslaughter for a homicide), voluntary intoxication has been successfully used as a defense against intent (that the perpetrator could not have had the specific intent required for a murder conviction). In some states, when accidents occur while a person is intoxicated, the forensic psychiatrist is asked to investigate the presence or absence of *mens rea* when the substance was first ingested (Wagenaar & Toomey,

2002). The psychiatric expert must check with the attorney as to which charge is a specific intent crime and which rules apply in the relevant jurisdiction for that case.

The concept that an intoxicated offender or victim or witness may not be able to recall or comment on an act because he or she was in a state of "blackout" is very controversial in the legal context. This has been advanced as a defense for culpability and for *mens rea*. This condition is supported by little evidence-based medical information, but most addiction psychiatrists and laypeople are familiar with the clinical phenomenon. Forensic psychiatrists, especially those without much experience in addiction psychiatry, may misuse, inappropriately downplay or identify, or otherwise misapply the term "blackout." Concerns about malingering have fed doubt in the courtroom about whether and how the occurrence of a blackout can be clearly determined. One study revealed that blackouts can occur during criminally relevant behavior, but they rarely occurred at blood alcohol concentrations of less than 250 mg/100 ml. A good approach is to seek objective data such as blood alcohol concentrations and to analyze the nature of the offense, because blood alcohol concentrations high enough to produce blackouts also would likely impair fine motor control and make it difficult to perform acts such as firing at a target from a far distance (van Oorsouw et al., 2004). It is important to distinguish this effect of intoxication from amnesia: A blackout is a period for which memory is not ever recorded, whereas in amnesia, previously known information is forgotten.

Other substances may affect the memory of witnesses or perpetrators, such as hallucinogens, alcohol, and a variety of sedatives/hypnotics. When the individual asserts that he or she was intoxicated, retrospective laboratory samples can be of assistance, particularly hair. Hair sampling can also be used to distinguish between single- and long-term use of various sedatives/hypnotics (Kintz, Villain, & Cirimele, 2006).

In some situations, intoxication alone may directly establish a defendant as guilty. Crimes such as driving while intoxicated or driving under the influence are called "strict liability crimes." For such charges, *mens rea* is not required for a conviction; the *actus reus* is simply the driving while intoxicated. All that is required is evidence that the legal standard for intoxication was met. Some states have mandated maximum sentences in cases in which death results from a driver who was driving while intoxicated or driving under the influence. These sentences are applied even if the influence by the substance is shown to have played a minimal role in the events leading to the death.

Substances of abuse also affect victims and witnesses of crimes, particularly in terms of memory, as well as threatening behaviors. Among victims of sexual assault, for example, insufficient memory of a sexual assault may be the result of a self-induced substance-based state, as in the case of blackouts or basic sedation or confusion due to the substance. The "date rape" drug gamma-hydroxybutyric acid (GHB), which is also a treatment for narcolepsy, is one such sedating substance that is found in "drug-facilitated sexual assault." One study of emergency department patients indicated that around 20% of all such assaults occur with some such facilitation (Mont et al., 2009). In terms of witnesses (and victims are witnesses, too), the possibility of intoxication or other impairment at the time of the witnessing may be argued in court, and experts can be asked to give information as appropriate.

SENTENCING RECOMMENDATIONS

Following a criminal conviction, a defendant enters the sentencing phase of the legal process. In various jurisdictions, psychiatric opinions may play an important role in the sentencing phase. The psychiatrist can wield great influence in identifying SUDs and in making clear recommendations for treatment both during a sentence and after the sentence is completed. A recent case in the federal system, *United States v. Booker* (2005), provided leeway for U.S. district court judges to diverge from sentencing guidelines if the presence of psychiatric disorders (including SUDs) substantially affected some part of the criminal behavior. This case has been challenged, but it remains in effect.

Civil Matters and Family Law

Civil law is the part of the judicial system that addresses conduct and conflict in a wide range of noncriminal human interactions—from family issues, such as divorce and custody to personal injury, negligence, wills, and estates. Individuals involved in such matters may be encumbered by addictions. As in criminal proceedings, the psychiatrist may be asked to play a role in civil cases as either a fact supplier or an expert witness. The psychiatrist may be asked to place substance use in the context of past behavior or to make predictions about future behavior. I review several frequently visited topics in this section. For issues relating to the workplace, see Mack, Kahn, and Frances (2005).

FAMILY AND MATRIMONIAL LAW

In disputes over divorce, custody, guardianship, adoption, or child safety, the substance use of any involved party commonly arises as a significant issue. The fiercely adversarial nature of these proceedings often impedes the formation of a valid picture. In such situations, the evaluating psychiatrist functions best when appointed by the court rather than being retained by either opposing side. It is crucial to evaluate all involved parties. Appropriate consent must be obtained before the examination of a minor. The psychiatrist is often asked to comment on the substance use of parents and its effects on the child. Although the presence of an SUD does not necessarily mean lack of parental fitness, it certainly is a factor that should be considered. Recommendations for custody and visitation may be made with substance abuse treatment as a condition.

PERSONAL INJURY

Substance abuse issues often arise when one party that alleges injuries sues another party for damages. Either side may allege that the other was intoxicated at the time of the injury and seek the help of a psychiatrist to establish or to negate such claims. The effect of long-term addiction also may be raised. Injured parties may blame the party that provided the substance of abuse. Many cases have exposed the liability of bars, bartenders, and parents of minors (Mack et al., 2005). For example, parents who allow a minor to serve alcohol or to use alcohol on their premises may be breaking the law and are exposing themselves to civil liability. Sexual harassment cases may be brought to either criminal or civil settings, and addictions may also be raised as an issue in such cases. Product liability assertions have been brought against makers of medications (e.g., zolpidem) for damages effected while a person was intoxicated on the medication.

DISABILITY

People who claim a disability based on an addiction may raise their claims with either a private insurance company or the federal government. In these cases, addiction psychiatrists are routinely called on to serve as experts. They may be retained by the individual claiming disability or by the insurance company for an "independent medical examination." If the case goes to court, expert testimony will be included. Any physician who completes paperwork certifying disability should consider the possibility that he or she may be called to testify about his or her findings in court. Management of addictions in patients with chronic pain complaints is clinically complex; this complexity translates into the expert question of whether returning to work is possible. The treating psychiatrist should consider referring a patient for consultation with an addiction psychiatrist or pain expert when faced with such a question.

OTHER AREAS

An addiction psychiatrist may have special expertise in other areas of civil law. In medical malpractice cases, a patient may allege that a physician caused him or her to become addicted to substances, or a patient may claim that his or her physician was impaired by substances. Of the impaired physicians in state health and recovery programs, 50–70% are there because of SUDs. Because workplace actions frequently lead to legal consequences, the addiction psychiatrist is frequently involved in consultation regarding the workplace (Wagenaar, 2001). The presence of substance use is frequently a part of retrospective challenges to testamentary capacity (Shulman, Cohen, & Hull, 2005; Spar & Garb, 1992).

Substance Use and Administrative Law

The term "administrative law" refers to the expectations, due process procedures, and practices of various regulatory bodies with oversight over the status of individuals involved in professions, athletics, the military, and other areas of social activity. For example, when a state medical board investigates a physician, it adheres to its own regulations and requirements, and this process falls within the category of administrative law. In some cases, military or other administrative law proceedings require psychiatric input concerning addiction. These include noncivil and noncriminal institutions such as athletic, security, licensing, or ethics bodies. The English Civil Aviation Authority or the U.S. Federal Aviation Administration may hold hearings on pilots' licenses, and entry into sensitive government employment may be barred by a history of substance use alone. Driver's license questions are usually handled in general criminal courts, but decisions on noncriminal aspects of driving may be decided by administrative bodies in some states.

Each institution or organization has different interests when considering substance use. Administrative bodies may seek evidence about a licensee's degree of substance use and its effect on ability to perform, or other bodies may be attempting to determine whether the individual should be offered employment. The critical tool for the expert is the language of the regulations or statutes under which the individual is being scrutinized. This ranges from the person being "alcoholic" to having been intoxicated with a blood alcohol level greater than 0.04% (above which airplane flying is impaired; Dave, 2004). In some cases, the forensic expert is asked by an employer to perform a "fitness for duty" evaluation; in other cases, an individual who is in the process of losing his or her status has the right to bring forth evidence (in the form of an expert's opinion) that he or she does not have problems with substances. When their opinions are in opposition to the interests of the individual, forensic experts often weather a great deal of scrutiny and criticism because the livelihood or other special aspects of the individual's life are at stake.

Substance Use in Litigation

When clinicians are asked to respond to specific questions of an authority, they must pay special attention to the process by which they answer such questions. The particular process underlying a clinician's responses should ensure that the response is consistent with the ideals of the American Academy of Psychiatry and the Law (2005): honesty and objectivity. Considerations of this process are discussed below.

COMMUNICATING PSYCHIATRIC INFORMATION TO LEGAL BODIES

What does "forensic" actually mean? Its definition highlights the work of the forensic psychiatrist: "Forensic (adj.). Used in or suitable to courts of law or public debate" (Garner, 2003). The distinctions between forensic work and clinical care help to clarify the role of the forensic psychiatrist working as an expert in a legal setting.

Forensic and clinical psychiatry have some fundamental differences that are important to understand. Although both fields are based on solid knowledge of current medical information and, where appropriate, careful assessment of the individual and his or her mental state, they differ in their objectives. Forensic psychiatry consists of specific statements concerning psychiatric conditions in response to specific questions. The forensic psychiatrist's obligation to "strive for objectivity" diverges from the clinician's interest in altruistic clinical intervention. Engaging in forensic practice requires an understanding of how to create, communicate, and protect one's findings and opinions in manners suitable to courts or other such institutions.

Basic Legal Settings. In order to communicate effectively in a legal setting and with legal authorities, the clinician must be familiar with basic rules and features of U.S. law, as well as the particular rules applied by the local jurisdiction (Group for the Advancement of Psychiatry, 1991; Gutheil, 1998; Rosner, 2003). When a psychiatrist becomes involved as an expert in a legal case, his or her duty is to provide objective, truthful information and protect it from misuse or distortion by any other parties or witnesses. Typically, cases in which a psychiatrist is retained as an expert are adversarial, and the forensic expert must understand his or her limited but thoughtful role in the case: to render an opinion that is as unbiased and unassailable as possible.

Fact versus Expert Witness. Professionals who testify in a deposition, hearing, or trial may do so as witnesses of facts or as experts. It is important to maintain the distinction between these roles, and clinicians must think ahead about which role they are being asked to perform. A clinician who is asked to describe his or her patient or to produce a patient's medical records is serving as a fact witness. This is very different from the expert, who, in cases of crime or litigation, has been asked to give an independent opinion related to the legal questions at hand. In judicial settings, any duly trained clinician can qualify as an expert witness by virtue of his or her education, training, and experience. Clinicians should be wary of serving as experts in cases involving their own patients, because doing so almost always affects both the patient's treatment and the clinician's ability to render truly objective opinions. Occasionally, individuals seeking a shortcut to a physician's testimony pose as bona fide patients and later attempt to use the medical record (which is a legal document) to their benefit. One common context that arises is when a parent in a custody battle requests that the clinician testify on his or her behalf. To do so, however, would violate the guidelines of the American Psychiatric Association and the American Association of Psychiatry and Law, as it would inject transference and countertransference into the therapeutic relationship with both the patient and his or her parents. The reader is referred to Gutheil (1998) for further details on this question of "wearing two hats."

Distinctions between Medical Diagnoses and Legal Definitions. What purpose does a forensic opinion serve for the legal system? It provides an objective explanation of an area of expertise to attorneys, judges, and juries. When communicating in a legal setting, the forensic psychiatrist must ensure that his or her language can be understood by a lay audience, while upholding its clinical validity. Some terms are easily misused in adversarial settings or even in laws and regulations. For example, unlike the medical use of "narcotic" to refer to an opioid, one standard law dictionary defines narcotic as "an addictive drug. A drug that is controlled or prohibited by law" (Garner, 2003). The clinician communicating with nonmedical bodies must work to ensure that relevant, yet correct, language is used and that the proper definitions are established.

The potential for misuse of language is particularly heightened in diagnosis. In forensic situations, it is essential to use diagnostic terms that are accepted by all parties. "Addiction" has been a word that carries biological, behavioral, and social connotations. It should not be misused in a legal context. Among physicians, "addiction" has been interchangeable with a diagnosis of substance dependence. Some experts also use "addiction" to distinguish dependence on illicit substances from chemically induced dependence by medications. However, the medical community also has come to consider the possibility of food, gambling, and sexual intercourse as activities of "addiction." Attorneys, clients, and some doctors may apply the suffix "-ism" to any behavior they wish to portray as compulsive or uncontrollable. Caution is necessary when "addiction" is used to discuss behaviors beyond substances of abuse, because there has been a backlash to the expanding application of this word.

In most jurisdictions, the standard is the current classification of mental disorders, DSM-5 (American Psychiatric Association, 2013). Courts and attorneys frequently misunderstand DSM SUD diagnoses and need the expert to provide clarification. The new terminology of addictive disorders and the unification of "dependence" and "abuse" may lead to improvements or distractions in describing disturbances in the use of substances of abuse.

DSM-5 has an imperfect fit with the needs of courts: For example, the court often asks the expert for predictions on the future, or degree of dangerousness, neither of which has a DSM-5 category. This awkward fit reflects a problem for the psychiatrist in the courtroom, who must refrain from making predictions that cannot be quantified or validated. Courts also should be reminded that an abnormal finding on a test or an instrument does not imply a diagnosis.

"Chemical dependency" is a term that frequently arises in in probate or mental health courts that may commit individuals to emergency or long-term care. The law defines "chemical dependency" in terms of deleterious effects of alcohol or drug use, but it is typically not specifically tied to DSM-5 criteria. Physicians asked to comment on alleged chemical dependency must know the legal rather than simply the clinical criteria for this status. Addiction professionals need to be ready to interpret correctly the meaning of laboratory values related to substances of abuse. One also needs to be able to address which matrices are the most reliable, such as hair, saliva, sweat, urine or serum. Medical review officers (MROs) are specially trained addiction professionals who are knowledgeable about the handling of specimens and how to evaluate positive or negative test results. See Baron and Baron (Chapter 4, this volume) on drug testing or other resources for the newest advances in what is and what is not usable laboratory information.

CLINICAL ASSESSMENTS FOR LEGAL BODIES

Although courts or attorneys may ask for it, there is no such thing as a "complete psychiatric assessment." The expert psychiatrist must help the attorney or the court pose a specific question to be answered by his or her report and testimony. Every forensic psychiatric assessment must be done with a particular focus and a specific question in mind. The forensic assessment of a subject who abuses substances must include a thorough review of all history, including medical, psychiatric, and social function. Collateral sources of historical information are essential. Sinha and Easton (1999) have provided a useful guide for the forensic substance abuse evaluation.

In addition, standardized instruments and laboratory tests may be presented as past medical records, or they may be obtained by the expert. Use of standardized instruments, such as the Michigan Alcoholism Screening Test, is acceptable because this may provide normalized data with which to make comparisons. Laboratory studies may be important, depending on the time frame and setting, but it is essential to know what tests are being ordered and their significance. For example, a urine drug screen for alcohol gives different information than does a serum carbohydrate-deficient transferrin (CDT) test. In addition, sensitivity, specificity, and the potential for false-positive or false-negative results vary in each case; some addiction clinicians and many forensic psychiatrists are unaware of the qualities of each laboratory study and of the potential for false-positive results on a test such as the CDT (Fleming, Anton, & Spies, 2004). Even the presence of an abnormal CDT, liver enzyme, or macrocytic anemia level, and any other pathophysiological effects of exposure to alcohol, does not necessarily imply addiction or dependence, and such claims seem necessarily incomplete (Baron, Baron, & Baron, 2005). To ignore such possibilities is a disservice to the individual and to justice. There are significant concerns about miscommunication of positive ethyl glucuronide tests, and they are now seen as only one component of a testing program.

LIABILITY FOR THE FORENSIC EXPERT

Forensic expert work is just as susceptible to liability as any other area of practice. Although the specific risks may be different, any professional who performs high-stakes evaluations and must communicate them under great scrutiny (including legal requirements for honesty) faces many potential liabilities. It is hard enough to speak in a courtroom or even in front of a stenographer, but it is even more difficult to do so under oath, in a cross-examination, under criticism, with media attention, under the threat of complaints to professional or ethical boards, or even with accusations of perjury (which is a criminal offense) (Binder, 2002; Gold & Davidson, 2007). The forensic expert is always well served to be in the position of "friend to the Court," as is the case in drug courts, in which case he or she is asked to be a neutral expert rather than appearing to be beholden to one of the parties, but even that position is not a complete shield from criticism or accusations of bias.

Gutheil and Simon (2005) provide a review of the narcissistic vulnerabilities of the forensic expert that may impede his or her work in this field. The threat of complaints or lawsuits may increase in forensic settings in which the practitioner appears to have a conflict of interest. A good example includes "fitness for duty" examinations, in which it is clear that the examiner, who may hold the "key" to the evaluee's livelihood, has been hired by the organization or institution. Avoiding real or apparent conflicts of interest is one important step in protecting one's opinion or finding from attack.

CONCLUSION

Clinicians may be confronted with legal situations in which substance use plays an important role, and they must maintain a clear understanding of their responsibilities and obligations to their patient, retaining attorney, profession, and their own ethics and the law. One should never hesitate to clarify these issues through consultation with a peer, a local medical society, or an attorney. Involvement with the legal issues as they relate to addictive disorders is a complex yet potentially rewarding role one can play as a clinician. In this manner, mental health knowledge can be suitably and effectively conveyed to social institutions that need it.

REFERENCES

American Academy of Psychiatry and the Law. (2005). Ethics guidelines for the practice of forensic psychiatry. Retrieved April 13, 2007, from *www.aapl.org/pdf/ethicsgdlns.pdf.*

American Psychiatric Association. (2000). *Psychiatric services in jails and prisons* (2nd ed.). Washington, DC: Author.

American Psychiatric Association. (2013). *Diagnostic and statistical manual of mental disorders* (5th ed.). Arlington, VA: Author.

Arseneault, L., Moffitt, T., Caspi, A., et al. (2000). Mental disorders and violence in a total birth cohort: Results from the Dunedin study. *Arch Gen Psychiatry, 57,* 979–986.

Baillargeon, J., Wu, H., Kelley, M. J., et al. (2003). Hepatitis C seroprevalence among newly incarcerated inmates in the Texas correctional system. *Public Health, 117,* 43–48.

Ballenger, J. F,. Best, S. R., Metzler, T. J., et al. (2010). Patterns and predictors of alcohol use in male and female urban police officers. *Am J Addict. 20,* 21–29.

Baron, D., Baron, D. A., & Baron, R. (2005). Testing for substances. In R. Frances, S. I. Miller, & A. H. Mack (Eds.), *Clinical textbook of addictive disorders* (3rd ed., pp. 63–71). New York: Guilford Press.

Belenko, S., & Peugh, J. (2005). Estimating drug treatment needs among state prison inmates. *Drug Alcohol Depend, 77,* 269–281.

Binder, R. L. (2002). Liability for the psychiatrist expert witness. *Am J Psychiatry, 159,* 1819–1825.

Binswanger, I. A., Merrill, J. O., Krueger, P. M., et al. (2010). Gender differences in chronic medical, psychiatric, and substance-dependent disorders among jail inmates. *Am J Public Health, 100,* 476–482.

Bird, S. M., & Hutchinson, S. J. (2003). Male drugs-related deaths in the fortnight after release from prison: Scotland, 1996–99. *Addiction, 98,* 185–190.

Brooks, M. K. (1997). *Federal confidentiality regulations in substance abuse treatment and domestic violence* (TIPS 25). Washington, DC: SAMHSA.

Budney, A. J., Hughes, J. R., Moore, B. A., et al. (2004). Review of the validity and significance of cannabis withdrawal syndrome. *Am J Psychiatry, 161,* 1967–1977.

Bushman, B. J., & Cooper, H. M. (1990). Effects of alcohol on human aggression: An integrative research review. *Psychol Bull, 107,* 341–354.

Carey, S. M., Finigan, M., Crumpton, D., et al. (2006). California drug courts: Outcomes, costs, and promising practices—an overview of Phase II in a statewide study. *J Psychoactive Drugs, 3*(Suppl.), 345–356.

Chandler, R. K., Fletcher, B. W., & Volkow, N. (2009). Treating drug abuse and addiction in the criminal justice system: Improving public health and safety. *JAMA, 301,* 183–190.

Council of State Governments. (2002). *Criminal Justice/Mental Health Consensus Project.* New York: Author.

Daley, C., McNiel, D. E., & Binder, R. L. (2011). "I did *What?*": Zolpidem and the Courts. *J Am Acad Psychiatry Law, 39,* 535–542.

Dave, B. P. (2004). Flying under the influence of alcohol. *J Clin Forensic Med, 11,* 12–14.

Downs, L., & Billick, S. B. (2000). Involuntary intoxication. *J Am Acad Psychiatry Law, 28,* 368–369.

Eronen, M., Hakola, P., & Tiihonen, J. (1996). Mental disorders and homicidal behavior in Finland. *Arch Gen Psychiatry, 53,* 497–501.

Fazel, S., Bains, P., & Doll, H. (2008). Substance abuse and dependence among prisoners: A systematic review. *Addiction, 101,* 181–191.

Fleming, M. F., Anton, R. F., & Spies, C. D. (2004). A review of genetic, biological, pharmacological, and clinical factors that affect carbohydrate-deficient transferrin levels. *Alcohol Clin Exp Res, 28,* 1347–1355.

Friedman, A. S., Glassman, K., & Terras, B. A. (2001). Violent behavior as related to use of marijuana and other drugs. *J Addict Dis, 20*, 49–72.

Friedman, A. S., Terras, A., & Glassman, K. (2003). The differential disinhibition effect of marijuana use on violent behavior: A comparison of this effect on a conventional, non-delinquent group versus a delinquent or deviant group. *J Addict Dis, 22*, 63–78.

Garner, B. (2003). *Black's law dictionary* (8th ed.). St Paul, MN: Thomson, West.

Gendreau, P. (1996). Offender rehabilitation: What we know and what needs to be done. *Crim Justice Behav, 23*, 144–161.

Gerbasi, J., Bonnie, R., & Binder, R. (2000). Resource document on mandatory outpatient treatment. *J Am Acad Psychiatry Law, 28*, 127–144.

Gold, L. H., & Davidson, J. E. (2007). Do you understand your risk?: Liability and third-party evaluations in civil litigation. *J Am Acad Psychiatry Law, 35*(2), 200–210.

Gossop, M., Trakada, K., Stewart, D., et al. (2005). Reductions in criminal convictions after addiction treatment: 5-year follow-up. *Drug Alcohol Depend, 79*, 295–302.

Gourlay, D. L., Heit, H. A., & Almahrezi, A. (2005). Universal precautions in pain medicine: A rational approach to the treatment of chronic pain. *Pain Med, 6*(2), 107–112.

Griffith, J. D., Hiller, M. L., Knight, K., et al. (1999). A cost-effectiveness analysis of in-prison therapeutic community treatment and risk classification. *Prison J, 79*, 352–368.

Group for the Advancement of Psychiatry. (1991). Committee on Psychiatry and Law: The mental health professional and the legal system. *Rep Group Adv Psychiatry, 131*, 1–192.

Gutheil, T. G. (1998). *The psychiatrist in court: A survival guide.* Washington, DC: American Psychiatric Press.

Gutheil, T. G., & Appelbaum, P. S. (2007). *Clinical handbook of psychiatry and the law* (4th ed.). Philadelphia: Lippincott, Williams & Wilkins.

Gutheil, T. G., & Simon, R. I. (2005). Narcissistic dimensions of expert witness practice. *J Am Acad Psychiatry Law, 33*, 55–58.

Hagedorn, H., & Willenbring, M. (2003). Psychiatric illness among drug court probationers. *Am J Drug Alcohol Abuse, 29*, 775–788.

Hopfer, C., Salomonsen-Sautel, S., Mikulikch-Gilbertson, S., et al. (2013). Conduct disorder and initiation of substance use: A prospective longitudinal study. *J Am Acad Child Adolesc Psychiatry, 52*, 511–518.

Karberg, J. C., & Mumola, C. J. (2006). *Drug use and dependence, state and federal prisoners, 2004* (NCJ 209588). Washington, DC: U.S. Department of Justice, Bureau of Justice Statistics.

Kintz, P., Villain, M., & Cirimele, V. (2006). Hair analysis for drug detection. *Ther Drug Monit, 28*(3), 442–446.

Kleber, H. D., & DuPont, R. L. (2012). Physicians and medical marijuana. *Am J Psychiatry, 169*, 564–568.

Kolves, K., Varnik, A., Tooding, L. M., et al. (2006). The role of alcohol in suicide: A case–control psychological autopsy study. *Psychol Med, 36*, 923–930.

Kuehn, B. M. (2013). FDA warning: Driving may be impaired the morning following sleeping pill use. *JAMA, 309*, 645–646.

Leonard, K., & Quigley, B. (1999). Drinking and marital aggression in newlyweds: An event-based analysis of drinking and the occurrence of husband marital aggression. *J Stud Alcohol, 60*, 537–545.

Leong, G. B., Leisenring, S. E., & Dean, M. D. (2007). Commentary: Intoxication and settled insanity—unsettled matters. *J Am Acad Psychiatry Law, 35*, 183–187.

Li, D., Zhao, H., Kranzler, H. R., et al. (2012). Association of COL25A1 with comorbid antispcial personality disorder and substance dependence. *Biol Psychiatry, 71*, 733–740.

Lifson, L. E., & Simon, R. I. (1998). *The mental health practitioner and the law: A comprehensive handbook.* Cambridge, MA: Harvard University Press.

Mack, A. H., Kahn, J. P., & Frances, R. J. (2005). Addiction in the workplace. In R. J. Frances, S. I. Miller, & A. H. Mack (Eds.), *Clinical textbook of addictive disorders* (3rd ed., pp. 340–353). New York: Guilford Press.

Mateyoke-Scrivner, A., Webster, J. M., Staton, M., et al. (2004). Treatment retention predictors of drug court participants in a rural state. *Am J Drug Alcohol Abuse, 30,* 605–625.

McDonnell, M. G., Srebnik, D., Angelo, F., et al. (2013). Randomized controlled trial of contingency management for stimulant use in community mental health patients with serious mental illness. *Am J Psychiatry, 170,* 94–101.

Mitchell, O., Wilson, D. B., & MacKenzie, D. L. (2007). Does incarceration-based drug treatment reduce recidivism?: A meta-analytic synthesis of the research. *J Exp Criminol, 3,* 353–375.

Moeller, F. G., & Dougherty, D. M. (2001). Antisocial personality disorder, alcohol, and aggression. *Alcohol Res Health, 25,* 5–11.

Monahan, J., Redlich, A. D., Swanson, J., et al. (2005). Use of leverage to improve adherence to psychiatric treatment in the community. *Psychiatr Serv, 56,* 37–44.

Mont, J. D., MacDonald, S., Rotbard, N., et al. (2009). Factors associated with suspected drug-facilitated sexual assault. *Can Med Assoc J, 180,* 513–519.

Mulvey, E. P., Odgers, C., Skeem, J., et al. (2006). Substance use and community violence: A test of the relation at the daily level. *J Consult Clin Psychol, 74,* 743–754.

Murdoch, D., Pihl, R. O., & Ross, D. (1990). Alcohol and crimes of violence: Present issues. *Int J Addict, 25,* 1065–1081.

Myers, W. C., & Vondruska, M. A. (1998). Murder, minors, selective serotonin reuptake inhibitors, and the involuntary intoxication defense. *J Am Acad Psychiatry Law, 26,* 487–496.

National Commission on Correctional Health Care. (2003). *Standards for health services in prisons.* Chicago: Author.

Office of Juvenile Justice and Delinquency Prevention. (2005). Screening and assessing mental health and substance use disorders among youth in the juvenile justice system: A resource guide for practitioners. Retrieved March 6, 2005, from *www.ncjrs.org/pdffiles1/ojjdp/204956.pdf.*

Petry, N. M., Rash, C. J., & Easton, C. J. (2011). Contingency management treatment in substance abusers with and without legal problems. *J Am Acad Psychiatry Law, 39,* 370–378.

Robinson v. California, 370 U.S. 660 (1962).

Rosner, R. (2003). *Textbook of forensic psychiatry* (2nd ed.). New York: Oxford University Press.

Rounds-Bryant, J. L., Motivans, M. A., & Pelissier, B. M. (2004). Correlates of drug treatment outcomes for African American and white male federal prisoners: Results from the TRIAD Study. *Am J Drug Alcohol Abuse, 30,* 495–514.

Schuck, A. M., & Widom, C. S. (2003). Childhood victimization and alcohol symptoms in women: An examination of protective factors. *J Stud Alcohol, 64,* 247–256.

Shulman, K. I., Cohen, C. A., & Hull, I. (2005). Psychiatric issues in retrospective challenges of testamentary capacity. *Int J Geriatr Psychiatry, 20,* 63–69.

Sinha, R., & Easton, C. (1999). Substance abuse and criminality. *J Am Acad Psychiatry Law, 27,* 513–526.

Slovenko, R. (1995). *Psychiatry and criminal culpability.* New York: Wiley.

Solnick, S. J., & Hemenway, D. (2012). The "Twinkie" defense: The relationship between carbonated, non-diet soft drinks and violence perpetration among Boston high school students. *Inj Prev, 18,* 259–262.

Spar, J. E., & Garb, A. S. (1992). Assessing competency to make a will. *Am J Psychiatry, 149,* 169–174.

Spunt, B., Goldstein, P., Brownstein, H., et al. (1994). The role of marijuana in homicide. *Int J Addict, 29,* 195–213.

Steadman, H. J., Mulvey, E. P., Monahan, J., et al. (1998). Violence by people discharged from acute psychiatric inpatient facilities and by others in the same neighborhoods. *Arch Gen Psychiatry, 55,* 393–401.

Substance Abuse and Mental Health Services Administration (SAMHSA), Office of Applied Studies. (2006). *DAWN: Opiate-related drug misuse deaths in six states.* Rockville, MD: Author.

Swanson, J. W. (1994). Mental disorder, substance abuse, and community violence: An epidemiological approach. In J. Monahan & H. J. Steadman (Eds.), *Violence and mental disorder: Developments in risk assessment* (pp. 101–136). Chicago: University of Chicago Press.

Swartz, M. S., Swanson, J. W., Hiday, V. A., et al. (1998). Violence and severe mental illness: The effects of substance abuse and nonadherence to medication. *Am J Psychiatry, 155,* 226–231.

Tamburello, A. C., Lieberman, J. A., Baum, R. M., & Reeves, R. (2012). Successful removal of quetiapine from a correctional formulary. *J Am Acad Psychiatry Law, 40,* 502–508.

Tanda, G., Pontieri, F. E., & Di Chiara, G. (1997). Cannabinoid and heroin activation of mesolimbic dopamine transmission by a common μ1 opioid receptor mechanism. *Science, 276,* 2050–2054.

Thomsen Hall, K., & Appelbaum, P. (2002). The origins of commitment for substance abuse in the U.S. *J Am Acad Psychiatry Law, 30,* 33–45.

Torrey, E. F. (1994). Violent behavior by individuals with serious mental illness. *Hosp Community Psychiatry, 45,* 653–662.

United Nations. (1997). World Drug Report. Retrieved January 12, 2007, from *www.un.org/ga/20special/wdr/e_hilite.htm.*

United States v. Booker, 543 US 220 (2005).

van Oorsouw, K., Merckelbach, H., Ravelli, D., et al. (2004). Alcoholic blackout for criminally relevant behavior. *J Am Acad Psychiatry Law, 32,* 364–370.

Wagenaar, A. C. (2001). Liability of commercial and social hosts for alcohol-related injuries: A national survey of accountability norms and judgments. *Public Opin Q, 65,* 344–368.

Wagenaar, A. C., & Toomey, T. L. (2002). Effects of minimum drinking age laws: Review and analyses of the literature from 1960 to 2000. *J Stud Alcohol, 14*(Suppl.), 206–225.

Weinstein, H., Kim, D., Mack, A., et al. (2005). Prevalence and assessment of mental disorders in correctional settings. In C. Scott (Ed.), *Handbook of correctional mental health* (pp. 43–68). Washington, DC: American Psychiatric Publishing.

CHAPTER 20

Patients with Chronic Pain and Opioid Misuse

DEBORAH L. HALLER
SIDNEY H. SCHNOLL

NONMEDICAL USE OF OPIOID ANALGESICS

Opioid analgesics have been used for thousands of years to treat numerous ailments. Along with the known benefits of their use, it has long been known that products derived from opium and synthetic alternatives are subject to abuse. It has been a continuous challenge to find the correct balance between making the medications available to patients in need and reducing to the extent possible the nonmedical use and abuse. Over the past 20 years, the pendulum has swung from liberalization of use, because of the concerns regarding untreated and undertreated pain, to increased concern about abuse and the need for increased restrictions on use.

Data from the National Survey on Drug Use and Health (NSDUH) annual survey, reported from the Substance Abuse and Mental Health Services Administration (SAMHSA), show the prevalence rates of nonmedical use of prescription medications, with opioid analgesics being the primary contributor to that abuse. It should be noted, however, that the levels of nonmedical use have remained flat over the eight years between 2002 and 2010. This includes lifetime, past-year, and past-month nonmedical use, with past-year and past-month figures being similar.

In 2010, 2.7% of people age 12 and older reported "nonmedical" use of pharmaceuticals (opioid analgesics, tranquilizers, sedatives, and/or stimulants) within the prior 30 days; as noted earlier, this rate is identical to that obtained in 2002. Opioid analgesics accounted for the bulk of this overall rate, with population-based rates varying between 1.8 and 2.1% between the years 2002 and 2010, compared to those for all pharmaceuticals combined (2.5–2.9%), cocaine (0.6–1.0%), cannabis

(5.8–6.9%), and all illicit drugs (7.9–8.9%). More than half (55%) of nonmedical users of opioid analgesics obtained them from friends or relatives at no cost, although the original source for these drugs was a physician in 79.4% of cases. Another 17.3% of opioid analgesics were obtained directly from a doctor, 4.4% from a drug dealer, and 0.4% through Internet purchase. To summarize, within the general population, the prevalence of past-month nonmedical use of opioid analgesics has remained stable for a number of years, hovering around 2%. At the same time, opioid analgesics have become a prominent aspect of the nation's overall drug problem, with rates surpassing those for cocaine and heroin, while remaining lower than those for cannabis.

Several factors distinguish prescription from other drug abuse. One is the legality of the drugs (if obtained by prescription). The other is "diversion," in which drugs that are meant for distribution through the legal supply chain are instead transferred to the illegal supply chain and used illicitly. Most diversion of pharmaceutical medications occurs from the "medicine cabinet" at home, but there also is diversion at wholesale and retail levels, with prescription medications being redirected for distribution by drug dealers who also sell cocaine and heroin. Diversion also occurs within the confines of the health care delivery system, with occasional inappropriate actions ranging from manufacturers all the way to roommates of patients.

A number of proprietary surveillance systems have been developed to measure the diversion and nonmedical use of pharmaceuticals. These systems are product specific (brand name) and can measure rates of nonmedical use based on product availability and geographic location of the nonmedical use (Butler et al., 2008; Cicero et al., 2007). For example, by 2012, 49 states had enacted legislation, and over 40 states implemented prescription drug monitoring programs (PDMPs) designed to enhance the capacity of regulatory, law enforcement, and public health officials to collect and analyze controlled substance prescription data through centralized databases administered by state agencies. In this climate, it is not surprising that physicians have become more vigilant. This chapter reviews aspects of clinical care of individuals, but several epidemiological reviews have been published elsewhere on chronic pain patients with opioid addiction (Chabel, Erjavec, Jacobson, Mariano, & Chaney, 2007; Fleming, Balousek, Klessig, Mundt, & Brown, 2007; Haller & Acosta, 2010) and drug treatment patients with pain (Rosenblum et al., 2003; Jamison, Kauffman, & Katz, 2000). The literature indicates that individuals with pain and opioid dependence are prevalent in both medical clinics and drug treatment programs. Alcohol, other drug, and psychiatric comorbidity are common in this population, further complicating the clinical picture. Undertreatment of pain in substance abusers often leads to increased drug-seeking behavior and illicit drug use (Schnoll & Weaver, 2003).

PAIN INFORMATION FOR SUBSTANCE ABUSE CLINICIANS

Definition of Pain

The International Association for the Study of Pain (IASP) defines pain as "an unpleasant sensory and emotional experience associated with actual or potential tissue damage, or described in terms of such damage" (Merskey & Bogduk, 1994). This definition may confuse clinicians who are not pain experts, because it is not very specific and it encompasses more than the physical sensation that most people think of as pain. In reality, pain is a complex phenomenon that is subjective and therefore difficult to measure. Objective (laboratory) findings may or may not be present. Furthermore, the absence of physiological evidence of tissue damage cannot be construed to mean that the pain is not "real." According to the Taxonomy Committee of the International Association for Study of Pain (Merskey & Bogduk, 1994), when pain is reported in the absence of identifiable bodily damage, it may be psychologically driven; however, it still is pain.

It is critical for providers to understand pain, because it is the most common complaint for which people seek medical attention (Haddox et al., 1997). Although most pain is relatively short-lived, approximately 20% of Americans suffer from "chronic" pain of 3 months' duration or longer (Turk, 1996). Pain rates are even higher among those with addiction problems (Jamison et al., 2000; Rosenblum et al., 2003); some find their way into methadone clinics, where they are treated for opioid dependence, with the medication also providing some degree of pain relief, despite its being prescribed in a way that is not consistent with standards for pain management (i.e., daily dose as opposed to every 6–8 hours). Therefore, this segment of the pain population remains "hidden" to a large extent. Other substance abusers with pain are never properly diagnosed or treated. This is problematic since untreated or undertreated pain may provoke "drug-seeking" behavior as patients attempt to self-medicate their physical (as well as emotional) discomfort. Many individuals with chronic pain also experience some degree of functional interference that is evidenced across multiple domains to include problems with mobility or capacity to work, impaired sleep, mood disturbance and/or decreased interest in social interactions. Thus, the overarching concept of "quality of life," in addition to pain severity, always must be considered.

Pain Components

Pain has four components (somatic, emotional, cognitive, and behavioral) that influence its experience and expression. However, the relative contribution of these four components varies from person to person. The physical sensation of pain is "filtered" through prior experiences with injury and tissue damage and also is influenced by cultural beliefs and psychological makeup. Both emotions (e.g., depression, anxiety) and cognitions (e.g., "I can't control it, and it will never go away") mediate the physical sensation of pain, making it more or less tolerable and manageable. This multidimensional model explains why two people with similar injuries may respond in disparate ways; one may become disabled, while the other may remains functional. The model also explains why someone with a relatively minor injury may have a poor outcome compared to someone with a more severe injury. Unfortunately, many health care providers focus solely on the somatic component of pain, while underestimating the importance of feelings, beliefs, and behaviors. Failure to understand and appreciate how the other components of pain interact with the physical sensation of pain to produce the "experience" of pain often results in inadequate or inappropriate treatment of pain. In addition to having poor pain knowledge, many providers become impatient with patients who appear distressed, express feelings of helplessness and hopelessness, and/or display pain behaviors such as wincing, grimacing, and crying. Such patients are more likely to be dismissed by providers as psychiatric cases who are attention-seeking, demanding, and/or seeking secondary gain (e.g., disability benefits or access to opioid medications). Table 20.1 provides a listing of pharmacological and nonpharmacological interventions to address the four components of pain.

Physical Component

There are two types of physical pain, nociceptive and neuropathic. "Nociceptive pain" is the result of damage to the body caused by injury or disease. The damage can be located and often successfully treated, resulting in a diminution of pain. Injuries that cause nociceptive pain include broken bones, burns, and tumors. Neuropathic pain is more complicated, as it may not be associated with a specific injury. In the absence of a specific "pain generator," it also is more difficult to treat. Diabetic neuropathy and complex regional pain syndrome (also known as "reflex sympathetic dystrophy") and causalgia are examples of neuropathic pain. Another way of categorizing pain is typical vs. atypical. Typical pain is similar to nociceptive pain. Typical pain can be acute or prolonged. With onset of typical pain, there is a normal protective action, such as withdrawing one's hand from a hot stove or placing the body in a protective position to prevent or reduce pain ("guarding"). Chronic typical pain occurs with diseases such as back pain or arthritis. Atypical pain is similar to neuropathic pain. It is not protective and is usually prolonged or chronic. The origin of the pain can be from peripheral nerves; it likewise may be central, for example, following a stroke or other brain injury. This type of pain is difficult to diagnose and treat. Doctors often doubt the validity of atypical pain because they cannot identify a pain generator (source of pain). These patients often are assumed to have psychiatric problems, including somatoform disorders.

TABLE 20.1. Interventions for Chronic Pain

Intervention	Symptoms targeted	Treatment provider
Physical therapy, massage therapy, aquatherapy	Muscular pain, joint pain	Physical therapist, massage therapist, chiropractor
Surgery (including placement of hardware, stimulators, and pumps to deliver medications)	Orthopedic pain, nerve pain	Surgeon (orthopedist, neurosurgeon, anesthesiologist)
Nerve blocks, trigger point injections, acupuncture	Localized pain syndromes	Anesthesiologist or other pain specialist
Opioids and other medications	Pain, co-occurring psychiatric disorders	Physician, physician's assistant, nurse practitioner
Counseling, cognitive-behavioral therapy, biofeedback, hypnosis, support groups	Psychiatric disorders, emotional distress, cognitive distortions, functional interference, pain behavior, substance abuse	Psychologist, psychiatrist, social worker, peers (self-help)

PAIN PERCEPTION

It is important to recognize that pain has an adaptive function in that it alerts the organism to the fact that an injury has occurred and that care should be taken not to exacerbate the situation. There are four basic processes involved in pain perception. The first of these is "transduction," which is the process whereby a mechanical signal (the injury) is transformed first to a chemical, then to an electrical signal. The second process is "transmission"; after the sensation is transformed to an electrical signal, it is sent along the peripheral nerves to the spinal cord and ultimately to the brain, where "perception" occurs. More specifically, once the impulse reaches the brain, the type and nature of the pain is identified (e.g., the pain may be perceived as burning, sharp, or dull). Finally, "modulation" occurs when the brain sends information back down the spinal cord that may alter perception of the pain. Thus, a person's emotional state at the time of the painful impulse plays a role in perception.

ASPECTS OF PAIN

To characterize pain fully, a number of aspects must be considered. First is the "pain generator" (i.e., the cause of physical pain). Pain generators include both injuries and diseases. Examples of pain generators include broken bones, a cancerous tumor, rheumatoid arthritis, or an abscess. Patients whose pain complaints are vague or who have diagnoses that lack objective physical pathology (e.g., fibromyalgia) are more likely to be viewed as having "psychogenic" pain (Turk, 1996). Conversely, those with cancer-related (malignant) pain tend to be taken more seriously. In our society, there is less shame associated with having cancer than with having back pain, headaches, or other problems whose origin may be unclear. This is true even when the pain intensity and functional interference are comparable. As a result of this bias, patients with cancer find it easier to access opioid analgesics than do patients with pain due to other causes. They also are more likely to receive higher doses of medication, although some patients with cancer still remain undertreated.

Another consideration is duration of pain. The transition from acute to chronic pain occurs after 3 months and is more likely to occur when acute pain is poorly treated. Recovery from chronic pain is more difficult than recovery from acute pain, because patients are required to make major life adjustments. A related dimension is intermittent versus persistent pain. Both pain types (acute and chronic) may be either intermittent or persistent. While intermittent pain comes and goes, persistent pain is always there. The worst case scenario occurs when pain is both chronic and persistent, because these patients never experience any relief. In this situation, there often is significant emotional, cognitive, and behavioral involvement resulting in functional impairment. Patients with chronic, persistent pain often feel that they have little or no control over their situation. As demoralization sets in, pain behavior increases, with patients evidencing greater disability. In contrast, patients with short-term, intermittent pain tolerate their situation much better, because they know it will end, and because they have periods of respite. Not surprisingly, patients with diverse pain characteristics are treated differently. For instance, those with chronic, persistent pain are more likely to be maintained on longer-acting opioids on a "round-the-clock" schedule; in contrast, those with intermittent pain (even if chronic) generally are treated with shorter-acting opioids that they use only when the pain is bothersome. Patients with sporadic, intense pain (e.g., the pain of sickle cell disease or kidney colic) are particularly difficult to manage, because they require strong, round-the-clock medications, but for a more limited period of time.

The most commonly considered pain characteristic is severity. Pain varies in intensity, which means that it is worse at some times than at others. Pain often is worse in the morning, when medication has worn off, or in the evening, following a day's activities. It is rare for pain to be of constant intensity. An absence of variability in pain ratings also may signal a stronger psychological/emotional component. Because pain is a subjective experience, it is difficult to measure. The most frequent approach to measuring pain intensity is through use of visual analogue scales (VASs) that ask patients to rate their pain on a scale of 1 to 10, with 1 reflecting No pain and 10 the Worst pain imaginable. (Note: when measuring pain in young children, a 5-point "faces" scale is typically used; Hockenberry, Wilson, & Winkelstein, 2005.) The same scale is used to rate each of the following types of pain: (1) worst; (2) least; (3) typical; and (4) tolerable; tolerable pain is an important concept because it often is the goal of treatment. By repeatedly assessing pain during the course of treatment, the practitioner can gauge the effectiveness of whatever treatment is being delivered, including treatment with opioid analgesics. For instance, if adequate doses of opioid analgesics are given but the pain remains the same or worsens, this suggests that opioids may not be an appropriate treatment for that patient and their use should be reconsidered. In addition to pain intensity, pain quality is important. Patients describe their pain in different ways. Mostly they use adjectives that provide a flavor to what they are experiencing. For instance, it is common for patients to characterize their pain as sharp, dull, aching, stabbing, burning, cramping, nagging, and so forth. Some of these descriptors are helpful in making a diagnosis. For example, burning or shooting pain is most often related to neuropathic pain. Measures such as the McGill Pain Questionnaire (Melzack, 2005; Table 20.2) can help providers to assess pain quality.

It also is useful to consider which things make pain worse (triggers) and which ones abate it. This assessment may provide clues regarding functional limitations and what interventions may hold promise. For instance, patients who experience severe "flare-ups" of their pain after mowing the lawn or driving long distances in the car may need to limit such activities. "Pacing" is important, because some individuals who tend to overexert themselves then experience worsening pain as a consequence. Conversely, it is critical that patients with pain not avoid activities that have the potential to induce pain, because this may, inadvertently, result in increased dysfunction and disability. To assist clinicians in assessing these aspects of pain, commonly used measures of pain and functional interference are found in Table 20.2.

Emotional Component

In addition to the physical (somatic) component of pain, both emotional distress and psychopathology influence how people process, experience, and react to the physical sensation of pain. Patients who have a strong emotional response to pain (sadness,

TABLE 20.2. Measures of Pain Severity, Functional Interference, and Pain Behavior

Measure	Target behavior	No. of items	Administration	Source
National Institutes of Health pain intensity measures (visual analogue scales [VAS])	Pain severity (worst, best, right now, tolerable)	4	Evaluator-administered	Public domain (McCaffery & Beebe, 1993)
Numeric and VAS pain scales	Pain; interference	Numeric: 1 (rated 3–10); VAS: 1 (10 cm)	Self- or evaluator-administered	Public domain
Wong–Baker FACES Pain Rating Scale	Pain (for children and elderly)	1 (0–5)	Evaluator-administered	Hockenberry, Wilson, & Winkelstein (2005)
Brief Pain Inventory—Short Form (SF-MPQ-2)	Pain severity; location; interference	15 (descriptors: 0–3); present pain; VAS	Self-administered	Copyright M. D. Anderson Cancer Center (Dworkin et al., 2009)
West Haven–Yale Multidimensional Pain Inventory (WHYMPI)	Pain, interference, perceived life control, affective distress, perceived support from others, responses of others to patient's pain, coping style	61	Self- or computer-administered	Kerns, Turk, & Rudy (1985)
McGill Pain Questionnaire (MPQ)	Pain components: sensory, affective, evaluative (i.e., subjective experience of pain) and miscellaneous; pain location; pain intensity	20 (pain components); 1 (location); 1 (intensity); 3 (experience)	Self-report	Copyright 2009
Millon Behavioral Medicine Diagnostic (MBMD)	Behavioral health; pain; functioning; coping; psychiatric problems; recently added pain norms	165 (severity)	Paper and pencil; computer-administered; interpretive reports available	Pearson
Minnesota Multiphasic Personality Inventory (MMPI-II and RF)	Psychopathology; norms for patients with pain and disability available	478 (severity)	Paper and pencil; computer-administered; interpretive reports available	Pearson
University of Alabama Pain Scale (UAB Pain Behavior Scale)	Pain behavior	10	Observational	Richards, Nepomuceno, Riles, & Suer (1982)
Pain Behavior Checklist (PBC)	Pain behavior	16	Observational	Dirks, Wunder, Kinsman, McElhinny, & Jones (1993)

anxiety, fear, irritability) often are labeled as "psychiatric cases" whose pain is manufactured or exaggerated. They may receive inferior care, because their physical complaints are trivialized or misattributed to psychiatric problems. The situation is further exacerbated when the patient has an addiction problem. Substance abusers often are undertreated by providers who are concerned about prescribing medication for legitimate pain complaints. Fights revolving around access to pain medication may result in a therapeutic breach, with patients feeling they have to "beg for pain medicine" and doctors believing they are being manipulated. These situations are frustrating to both parties and have the potential to threaten the therapeutic alliance. Whether clinicians' attitudes have a negative effect on patients' subsequent behavior is unknown, but this should be investigated in future research.

Patients with pain often experience emotional distress. Depression, anxiety, fear, and irritability are especially common, as are feelings of low self-esteem, guilt, and shame. Patients often become socially isolated and lonely, withdrawing from meaningful aspects of life. Because of shifting responsibilities/roles within the family that often occur when someone becomes disabled, familial and marital conflicts can arise. Patients may feel diminished, dependent, and experience a fear of abandonment and/or lack of social support that further contribute to feelings of emotional distress. Comprehensive pain management programs frequently work with psychologists who conduct evaluations to determine how patients are coping with pain from a psychological standpoint. A number of standardized instruments may be used to assess psychological functioning, distress, and related concerns among patients with pain; several of these are detailed in Table 20.2. Any psychiatric or psychological factor may complicate pain and should be identified and addressed thoroughly.

Psychiatric disorders that have physical symptoms as part of their presentation are especially relevant to patients with pain.

Cognitive Component

The cognitive component of pain, including beliefs and perceptions about pain, frequently is overlooked by treating clinicians. Examples include the belief that the pain is never going to get any better and that there is no way to control or overcome it. Negative beliefs also may generalize to life in general, with patients adopting the belief that their lives are virtually over. Patients who doubt their ability to be instrumental in altering their situations and believe it is unlikely they ever will improve are less likely to put effort into rehabilitation and more likely to give up compared to those who believe that their situation can and will improve. In the absence of efforts to recover, their chances for recovery are reduced, creating a self-fulfilling prophesy. Furthermore, negative beliefs about pain and recovery can result in clinical depression characterized by feelings of hopelessness and helplessness. Finally, some patients with chronic pain develop somatic preoccupations (i.e., excessive attention to bodily discomforts and sensations). This can lead to a heightened sensitivity and attention to small, often insignificant bodily cues. For instance, patients with strong disease convictions (e.g., "I must have cancer") often continue to hold on to these beliefs, even when their status has improved. One way to approach the cognitive component of pain is through cognitive restructuring, such as in cognitive-behavioral therapy (CBT).

Behavioral Component

"Pain behavior" consists of signals that alert the observer to the fact that the individual is experiencing pain. These include vocal and nonvocal (shifting positions, moaning/groaning, wincing, limping, etc.) complaints of pain, restlessness, bracing, rubbing, and use of supportive devices such as canes and braces. Patients with pain often resist functional improvements because they believe that movement will exacerbate their pain. Unfortunately, absence of activity delays recovery and leads to increased disability. To complicate matters, some patients engage in pain behaviors for the purpose of secondary gain, whether on a fully conscious or less than fully conscious level. For example, when someone is disabled, family members often assume their responsibilities or treat them in a more caring way. Disability benefits (Social Security Disability Insurance [SSDI], Workers' Compensation) can be powerful incentives that inadvertently act to maintain dysfunctional behavior; patients receiving disability benefits for long periods of time are less likely ever to return to work. Pain behavior typically is evaluated through direct observation, and often is assessed both at rest and during movement.

In a study of the relationship between current and past-30-day pain severity ratings and pain behavior (measured by a 16-item checklist), Dirks, Wunder, Kinsman, McElhinny, and Jones (1993) found that gender, race, age, pain site, type of injury, duration of pain, legal representation, and evaluating clinician were not associated with "good agreement" between pain severity and pain behavior; however, patients who consciously exaggerating their pain (32% of sample) reported higher pain ratings and evidenced more discrepancies between their pain ratings and pain behavior than those without exaggerated pain. Severity of current pain was unrelated to pain behavior for conscious exaggerators; however, a moderately strong relationship was found between pain severity and pain behavior for those whose pain was not exaggerated. These findings confirm independence of pain intensity and pain behavior.

It is a good practice to observe the patient when he or she is unaware that you are doing so to determine to what extent pain behavior is maintained in the absence of an observer. Another method of evaluating the extent of pain behavior is by directing the patient to maintain a pain diary. In pain diaries, patients keep track of their daily activities and rate the severity of their pain while engaging in various tasks. Pain diaries should require the patient to record their use of pain medication, so that patterns of medication use may be determined. Self-monitoring is an excellent way of helping patients to become more aware of their behavioral patterns and it can be a useful strategy, even in the absence of a more formal behavioral treatment program. For some patients, becoming more aware of medication-taking behavior can influence medication taking, much in the way that monitoring calories can influence eating behavior.

Summary

Pain is a complex phenomenon with multiple components (somatic, emotional, cognitive, and behavioral). The relative contribution of these four components determines how people experience pain and also how they respond to it. The various aspects of pain (type, persistence, duration, severity, and quality) determine the relative salience of each of these components. For instance, a patient who has severe, persistent pain but a stoic nature, and believes strongly that he or she will recover, may be more functional than someone who has less severe, intermittent pain but is emotionally overwhelmed and feels hopeless about the chances for recovery. While the experience of pain is a private event, the expression of pain is public and has an impact on family, friends, and health care providers. When the patient with pain also is a substance abuser, the clinical picture is likely to be exaggerated. Patients are more likely to engage in aberrant medication-taking behaviors (AMTBs) in an effort to obtain more or stronger medication. Such behaviors can strain the doctor–patient relationship, making collaborative treatment more difficult. From the providers' perspective, drug-abusing patients can be time-consuming, demanding, manipulative, and difficult to manage. To avoid becoming involved in what could become a complicated treatment, providers may "overcorrect" in an effort to contain opioid misuse. Unfortunately, undertreatment of pain among substance abusers has the potential to stimulate drug-seeking behavior and other AMTBs, and to compromise the therapeutic relationship. For these reasons, it is essential that patients with comorbid pain and opioid

TABLE 20.3. Top 10 AMTBs Endorsed by Providers and Patients in Project Pain

Item	Provider	Rank	Patient	Rank
Has increased dose of pain medicine without first obtaining permission from doctor	57.1%	#1	71.4%	#1
Frequently requests more and stronger pain medicine	42.9%	#2	42.9%	#5
Is overly concerned about access to pain medicine	42.9%	#2		
Has expressed concern over own use of pain medicine	38.2%	#4	57.1%	#4
Has more than one doctor who prescribes pain medicine	37.1%	#5		
Admits that use of pain medicine is "out of control"	37.1%	#5		
Argues with providers regarding use of pain medicine	35.3%	#7	39.3%	#8
Manipulates doctors to get pain medicine	34.3%	#8		
Goes to emergency department to obtain pain medicine	34.3%	#8		
Uses recreational drugs	32.4%	#8		
Continues to take pain medicine, even though relief is minimal			67.9%	#2
Feels that he or she has been treated like an "addict" by medical providers			60.7%	#3
Borrows pain medicine from someone else			42.9%	#5
Family members/friends have complained about his or her use of pain medicine			42.9%	#5
Uses pain medicine to treat problems other than pain, such as sleeplessness or depression			39.3%	#9
Continues to take pain medicine despite side effects			39.3%	#9

dependence be carefully evaluated, and their treatment be designed on an individual basis to address those domains that are most affected. Table 20.3 on the preceding page provides a summary of the most commonly endorsed AMTBs for 36 patients with chronic noncancer pain who participated in a NIDA-funded study (Project Pain) focusing on opioid misuse during pain treatment. The study employed the "Problems with Pain Meds" checklist, which consists of 48 AMTBs in four categories (opioid misuse, behavioral problems, legal problems, and family concerns) that are endorsed by patients and providers separately (and then compared).

TREATMENT CONSIDERATIONS FOR COMORBID PAIN AND OPIOID USE DISORDERS

The handful of treatment studies that have been conducted in patients with comorbid pain and opioid dependence have yielded a few key findings that could inform future research. A 12-week intervention employing methadone and adherence counseling resulted in statistically significant and clinically important changes in pain, functional interference, and opioid use. However, outcomes were poorer for polydrug abusers. This is understandable given that the intervention was not designed to deal with drug problems other than opioid dependence. Patients with complex addiction problems likely require a longer, more intensive, and more addiction-focused approach. Given that methadone is a first-line treatment for opioid dependence and is widely used to treat chronic pain, its efficacy for concurrent treatment of these two disorders is not surprising. Still, use of methadone for this purpose requires considerable training. Because the effective dose range is broad, some patients require high doses. Unfortunately, higher than average doses and mixing of methadone with other drugs is associated with an increased risk for adverse events due to the difference between the pharmacokinetics and the pharmacodynamics of the drug. Accordingly, providers who lack experience with methadone may not wish to use it.

Although buprenorphine/naloxone (bup/nx) is preferable to methadone from a safety standpoint, its efficacy for treating pain and opioid dependence concurrently remains unclear. Inductions can be difficult, especially for patients previously maintained on longer-acting agonists. Patients do not do well when subjected to tapering regimens, although outcomes are no worse than those for patients without pain. The reported analgesic effects for bup/nx are not especially robust; in some instances, reductions in pain are statistically significant but lack clinical importance. Rigorous standards that are comparable to those employed in pain clinical trials should be employed to determine the efficacy of bup/nx for pain. While the buprenorphine transdermal patch (which is approved for pain but not for opioid dependence) might produce better outcomes, it has not been studied in this population. More research is needed to clarify for which patients these two medications may be appropriate and under what conditions. Unfortunately, current regulations (e.g., no provision for divided doses or for breakthrough medication) make it unlikely that methadone clients with pain-related problems could be adequately treated for both conditions in their opioid treatment programs (OTPs). As a consequence, these patients frequently obtain additional prescriptions (including for methadone) from outside providers, thus presenting an increased risk for overdose.

Many OTP clients have mild-to-moderate chronic pain coupled with severe addiction problems, typically involving heroin and other illicit drugs as well as opioid analgesics. In contrast, pain management patients tend to have moderate-to-severe pain but lower rates of illicit drug use disorders. Patients thus appear to select treatment settings based on their perceived "primary" problem. Because modern pain management strategies would be very difficult to implement in OTPs, due to rigid dispensing and other regulations, we focus in this section on the management of chronic pain in office-based treatment settings.

Treating chronic pain in the context of opioid abuse or dependence is a difficult proposition. The patients are complex, presenting with a unique mix of the four pain components (somatic, emotional, cognitive, and behavioral) and opioid dependence, as well as other substance abuse and psychiatric disorders. Because comorbidities make the clinical presentation worse and have a negative impact on outcomes, the more problems a patient has, the more difficult he or she will be to treat. To be successful, providers should be prepared to invest more time with these cases, seeing patients frequently and on a very regular schedule. Following a specific protocol is highly recommended, and enhanced monitoring strategies are indicated. In addition, providers need to become both educators and armchair therapists. Not all providers are equipped to provide this range of services themselves; therefore, many will need to coordinate care with other providers, including addictions clinicians and psychotherapists.

Even with safeguards in place, some patients probably should not be treated in the office setting. This decision should be made on a case-by-case basis, taking both patient and provider characteristics into consideration. Based on what currently is known, patients with the following comorbidities are poor candidates for office-based treatment, unless the provider is an addiction expert who has ready access to drug and psychiatric treatment facilities: (1) drug abuse problems that are sufficiently severe to require specialized treatment (e.g., alcohol, cocaine, methamphetamine, or benzodiazepines); (2) severe, unstable mental illnesses, such as major depression, bipolar disorder, or posttraumatic stress disorder (PTSD); (3) somatization disorders other than pain disorder (which is common in this population); (4) significant antisocial characteristics and/or a legal history that increases the risk for diversion. Neither should patients who refuse to (1) participate in adjunctive treatments, including drug counseling or psychotherapy; (2) be monitored for illicit drug via drug screens; or (3) sign an opioid contract (stating what will be expected of them and what the provider will do in return) be considered for office-based treatment. While opioid contracts do not alter behavior (Hariharan, Lamb, & Neuner, 2007) they provide a "framework" for collaborative work and prevent patients from later arguing that they were not informed about various policies and procedures (e.g., no early refills). Contracts also provide an "exit strategy" for patients who are nonadherent. To summarize, treatment should not be initiated without (1) a treatment protocol; (2) an opioid contract; (3) a monitoring system; and (4) and exit strategy.

Myths and Misconceptions about Opioid Abuse and Dependence

Many providers harbor misconceptions about substance abuse that influence their prescribing practices. The first is that *overuse of pain medication equals addiction,* which may or may not be true. Overuse is the most common AMTB, patients take more medication than has been prescribed at one time and/or take it more frequently than prescribed. Common reasons for overuse include wanting to achieve a desired effect (to get high), to treat problems other than pain (e.g., insomnia or anxiety), or to mitigate undertreatment. The primary consequence of overuse is that patients run out of medication early. Because prescriptions for Schedule II controlled substances cannot be refilled early, individuals who overuse their pain medication are "uncovered" for periods of time between prescriptions. Abrupt cessation of opioids during these uncovered periods results in increased pain, withdrawal symptoms in those who are physically dependent, and characteristic drug-seeking behaviors that include (1) increased requests for medication; (2) doctor shopping; (3) attempts to get the pharmacist to refill prescriptions early; (4) visits to the emergency department to obtain opioids; (5) borrowing pain medication from others; (6) buying prescription opioids on the street; and (7) heroin use. Although drug-seeking behavior frequently is interpreted as a sign of addiction, patients without addiction problems react similarly when undertreated—a phenomenon known as "pseudoaddiction." Although pseudoaddiction may be distinguished from true addiction by providing adequate doses of opioid medication, many providers are reticent to increase the dose in someone who is displaying AMTBs and may be an addict. In fact, they often do just the opposite: withholding medication, tapering the patient off opioids (for "noncompliance"), or terminating treatment altogether. These provider behaviors are likely to cause a therapeutic rupture, with patients feeling betrayed, misunderstood, and treated like addicts. To summarize, undertreatment is a provider problem whose primary cause is poor knowledge of pain management strategies coupled with concerns about addiction that include tolerance, hyperalgesia, dependence, addiction, diversion, relapse, and overdose (American Society of Anesthesiologists, 1997). It occurs in those with and without addiction problems and therefore should not be considered indicative of a substance use disorder (SUD) in the absence of other signs and symptoms.

Another common misconception is that *tolerance will lead to continual dose increases*. During the early phase of opioid therapy for pain, dose adjustments should be made based on feedback from the patient regarding how well the medication is working. Often, the starting dose more than doubles before the patient experiences relief. Unfortunately, many providers focus more on the magnitude of the dose than on the effectiveness of that dose. Once the patient has been stabilized, there is little need to raise the dose. Thus, tolerance does not continue to grow, although it does vary considerably from person to person. The exception to this is if the underlying disease (e.g., cancer) progresses or if medications are added to the regimen that decrease the effectiveness of the pain medication (e.g., some antiretrovirals); in these instances, the dose will need to be revisited. It is important to understand that the dose of opioid medication needed to treat pain is likely to be substantially higher than the dose needed to address addiction. Furthermore, when treating pain and opioid dependence concurrently, the dose is likely to be higher than when treating either disorder separately. To summarize, when treating moderate-to-severe chronic pain, the "effective" dose can vary greatly; high doses reflect tolerance but are not an indication of severity of addiction. The effective dose is far more important than the absolute dose.

The idea that *tolerance equals addiction* also is incorrect. "Tolerance" is a physiological phenomenon that occurs as the cells adapt to the presence of the drug. When a person is tolerant, it takes more medication to obtain the same degree of pain relief than previously was achieved at a lower dose. Tolerance is common among individuals who are maintained on opioids for pain. Furthermore, as tolerance develops, the dose of opioid medication that is needed to relieve pain increases. However, tolerance is not the same thing as "addiction," which is a behavioral disorder characterized by loss of control over drug use, craving, and other criteria. Tolerance is not necessary for a diagnosis of addiction, although most opioid abusers are tolerant. The vast majority of pain patients who are maintained on opioids are tolerant but not addicted. When patients have comorbid pain and opioid dependence (addiction), they display characteristics of both groups.

Another fallacy is the belief that *physical dependence equals addiction.* Like tolerance, physical dependence occurs as cells adapt to the presence of a drug; when the drug is abruptly withdrawn, a characteristic drug-class specific withdrawal syndrome occurs. For opioids, this is a flu-like syndrome that is uncomfortable (but not fatal). The withdrawal syndrome is the same for opioid analgesics as it is for heroin. Although physical dependence is one of the criteria considered when diagnosing addiction, this criterion alone is insufficient to make this diagnosis. In fact, patients may be both tolerant and dependent but not addicted.

Provider Characteristics That Influence Prescribing Practices

Provider attitudes, values, and beliefs also impact treatment decisions and associated outcomes. Those who are overly concerned about being manipulated by drug-seeking patients or who fear being monitored by state regulatory boards may undertreat as a safety precaution, even though this is likely to backfire, resulting in increased pain, functional interference and drug-seeking behaviors. Providers who believe that opioids are inherently bad, that addiction lies in the drug and not the person, or that opioid use is a sign of personal weakness, may be reticent to prescribe, even when this is clearly indicated. Some providers are simply fearful and therefore are reticent about prescribing opioids to patients with chronic pain, let alone to those at risk for abusing them. They may be concerned about new-onset (i.e., iatrogenic) addiction, although this is relatively rare in those without a history of substance abuse (Portenoy & Foley, 1986). A greater concern is posed by patients with past or current substance abuse problems, especially opioid abuse or dependence. These individuals, while at increased risk for abusing prescribed opioid analgesics, still may require them to treat severe chronic pain. In such instances, providers must realistically assess their capacity to provide the level of care that will be required for the patient to be adequately assessed and treated.

That said, providers who lack training in addiction medicine should not endeavor to treat individuals with remitted, partially remitted, or active opioid use disorders. Providers who wish to treat substance abusers with pain will need to modify their office and prescribing procedures to include additional safeguards, such as more frequent office visits, urine drug screens, and opioid contracts (Weaver & Schnoll, 2002). Another prerequisite is a formal relationship with an established drug treatment program to which patients can be referred should significant problems develop that cannot be managed in the office setting.

Providers should evaluate their personal situation when deciding whether to treat patients with comorbid pain and opioid dependence. Factors to be considered include (1) extent of training in pain management, opioid pharmacology, and substance abuse; (2) attitudes and beliefs about pain patients and addicts; (3) willingness to implement a treatment protocol to modify one's prescribing and office practices; and (4) relationships with both pain and addiction specialists who agree to serve as consultants or referral sources for complex patients who require more intensive treatment.

Although pain specialists typically are knowledgeable about pain and opioid pharmacology, they often lack training in the field of addictions. This deficit may result in failure to screen patients prior to initiating opioid therapy or to implement an appropriate structure for containing them (protocol, drug screen, and contract). When they get into trouble, they also have difficulty managing them. Although the appropriate structure for treating them may not be in place (protocol, drug screens, contract, etc.), they often respond to substance abuse by threatening the patient and/ or terminating the treatment. Although referrals to drug treatment may be made, this strategy often fails because pain patients typically do not see themselves as addicts. Should referral to ancillary drug treatment fail, the provider is then left in a very difficult situation, because such patients cannot be abandoned, yet are nearly impossible to refer. Conversely, if the provider elects to maintain the patient on opioids for pain, without the proper modifications to treatment (e.g., drug screens, counseling, pharmacotherapy for psychiatric disorders, opioid contracts), the treatment is likely to fail.

Complicating Factors

Nonopioid Substance Use

Another issue is use, misuse, and addiction with substances other than opioids. As previously noted, substance abuse comorbidity is common among those with pain and opioid dependence, and includes alcohol, pharmaceuticals, and street drugs such as cocaine. While drug–drug interactions can cause adverse reactions in patients who are maintained on opioid analgesics for pain, some of these substances have therapeutic value that rarely is recognized or appreciated. For example, some patients report that cannabis has analgesic properties when used in combination with opioids; the animal literature supports this claim (Welch & Stevens, 1992), but minimal research has been conducted in humans, and the findings have been equivocal (Campbell et al., 2001). More research is needed to determine whether cannabis should be considered as an adjunct to opioid therapy for pain. Although cocaine (and other stimulants) tend to exacerbate pain, they may increase analgesia and decrease sedation when used along with opioids (Forrest et al., 1977). Other drugs also may act in a synergistic fashion when taken with opioids, increasing their intoxicating and/or analgesic effects. While polypharmacy is a potential problem for this population, "supplementation" of prescribed opioids with opioids obtained from other sources is a particular threat. If mixed agonist–antagonist drugs or partial agonists such as buprenorphine are mixed with full agonist drugs like morphine or methadone, this may precipitate withdrawal. To ensure that supplementation is not occurring, providers are encouraged to conduct random urine toxicology screens. Unfortunately, standard drug screens have significant limitations. Most screens assess for morphine-based drugs such as codeine but do a poor job of detecting the most commonly abused opioid analgesics (hydrocodone and oxycodone). Furthermore, synthetic opioids such as fentanyl cannot be identified without costly laboratory tests. Patients who may supplement their prescribed opioid medication with nonmorphine-based drugs may require a "tailored" panel that employs more advanced detection methodology such as gas chromatography/mass spectrometry (GC/MS).

Diversion

Some providers may be concerned about diversion. While established drug abusers may attempt to infiltrate pain programs and doctors' offices to obtain access to drugs, this behavior is unlikely to go undetected for long, particularly if a "bogus" patient lacks a legitimate pain complaint. On the other hand, prescription pads may be stolen and/or prescriptions stolen. Another concern is that prescribed drugs will somehow end up on the street. While patients with legitimate pain are unlikely to share their pain medication with others, diversion from the family medicine chest is a distinct possibility if patients are careless. For this reason, patients must be educated about diversion and be encouraged to secure their medications in locked cabinets so that others will not appropriate them for illegal purposes. Should the clinician feel confident in his or her ability to overcome these potential barriers, certain guidelines that may prove helpful (highlighted below).

Problematic Prescribing Practices

Several common prescribing practices run counter to good management of chronic persistent pain. In most instances, providers are attempting to prescribe "responsibly" to avoid having their patients develop addiction problems, and to prevent being monitored by medical state boards for overprescribing. This generally translates into prescribing practices that are designed to limit access to opioids. Unfortunately, among patients with significant pain (including those with and without addiction problems), limiting access has the undesirable side effect of stimulating drug-seeking and other AMTBs, such as borrowing medications from family and friends. However, in the context of undertreatment, these behaviors cannot be viewed as addictive in nature.

Use of short-acting (as opposed to long-acting) opioids is a common practice. Because short-acting opioids have a more rapid onset and offset than long-acting opioids, they are more likely to produce euphoria that is reinforcing and may result in increased self-administration to get high. Use of short-acting agents also produces "mini-withdrawals" that encourage patients to take the medication at shorter intervals than prescribed. For example, short-acting opioids typically are prescribed every 4–6 hours, but wear off in 2–3 hours; thus, patients who redose early end up taking more throughout the day. For this reason, long-acting opioids such as MS Contin (morphine), OxyContin (oxycodone), Duragesic Patch (fentanyl), and methadone that last 8 or more hours are preferable when treating patients with chronic, persistent pain. The primary concern about prescribing long-acting opioids to patients with opioid use disorders is that higher doses of drug may be extracted from the delivery matrix and consumed at one time. This occurs when patients crush and snort long-acting medications or inject medications from transdermal patches. Altering the route of administration of a prescribed opioid is a sign of addiction that requires careful monitoring. Methadone does not have this problem, however. Recently, manufacturers of extended-release opioids have started to market their products in tamper-deterrent formulations. These can consist of matrices that are harder to crush or gel when placed in liquid, making them harder to insufflate (snort) or inject. Another approach is to add an opioid antagonist to the formulation that is sequestered unless the product is crushed, resulting in a blocking of the opioid effect following tampering.

Use of p.r.n. (as-Needed) Medication

The idea behind this dosing strategy is that patients will use less medication if they take it only when their pain is severe. Unfortunately, patients on p.r.n. dosing schedules often take more medication, because the pain is harder to treat once it becomes severe. A better strategy is to maintain patients on scheduled medications that are taken "round the clock" (regardless of pain level) to keep the pain at a more tolerable level. At the same time, good pain management often involves the use of "breakthrough" (p.r.n.) medication in situations when the pain is worse than usual or cannot be controlled by the usual dose. The amount of breakthrough medication provided should be limited, and patients should be required to document how often and under what circumstances they are using breakthrough medication in order to determine whether it is being utilized appropriately. If breakthrough medication is being regularly used for legitimate purposes, this likely indicates the need for a higher standard dose. Once the standard dose is stabilized, use of breakthrough medication should be minimal unless the patient has a progressive disease (e.g., cancer) with gradually increasing pain levels.

Giving the Lowest Possible Dose or Extending the Dosing Interval

Providers often attempt to maintain patients on the lowest possible dose as a means of preventing addiction; ironically, this practice may encourage AMTBs. When the dose is too low to "cover" the pain, patients experience increased pain and may engage in drug-seeking behavior to address this problem; in this situation, drug seeking is seen among both nonabusers and abusers. To avoid having patients go to the emergency department, "doctor shop," or borrow medications from friends, they should be provided adequate doses of medication that are prescribed at appropriate intervals to control pain.

Extending the Dosing Interval

The rationale for this practice basically is the same as that for providing the lowest dose possible (i.e., to keep the total daily dose [TDD] low and prevent addictive behaviors from emerging). Once again, good intentions can result in negative consequences for patients.

Dosing Issues for Patients with Comorbid Pain and Opioid Dependence

Patients with opioid use disorders are more likely to be undertreated than other patients with pain. There are several reasons for this. First, their level of opioid tolerance may not be taken into consideration when the dosage of pain medication is established. It is possible, for instance, for the provider to give too low a dose for pain to someone who has been maintained on a relatively high dose of methadone to treat addiction, because the provider does not appreciate that he or she is now treating two disorders simultaneously. While undertreating is less of a problem when patients receive separate treatment for pain and opioid dependence, this situation may result in overdose, especially if the two treatments are not coordinated.

Second, the provider may falsely assume that the patient's medication for addiction will also cover the pain. Third, the provider may be reticent about providing drugs with abuse liability to a known drug abuser, citing concerns about possible overdose, diversion, or other illegal activity. Undertreatment of pain in opioid-dependent individuals is particularly problematic, because it may lead to increased drug-seeking behavior in order to control pain, resulting in relapse (Savage et al., 2003).

TREATING PATIENTS WITH CHRONIC PAIN AND OPIOID USE DISORDERS

We designed previous sections of this chapter to educate readers about pain and opioid dependence, and to offer a rationale for office-based treatment for some, but not all, individuals with this particular comorbidity. In this section, we provide practical information about concurrent treatment of pain and addiction, which includes (1) selection criteria; (2) evaluation strategies; (3) components of treatment (protocols); (4) efficacy; and (5) management of complex cases (e.g., those with other addiction and/or psychiatric disorders).

Selection Criteria

Ideally, providers who wish to treat patients with chronic pain and opioid abuse or addiction (remitted, partially remitted, or active) should have training in both disorders, although this is rare. Many pain specialists have good knowledge of opioid pharmacology, yet lack the skills to deal with the behavioral disorder of addiction, making office-based treatment a challenge. Conversely, substance abuse specialists understand addiction but fail to appreciate the significance of pain and, in many cases, the need to treat patients with opioids and other medications. To treat these disorders concurrently, providers need to blend knowledge and borrow treatment strategies from both disciplines. For this reason, clinicians who hold rigid beliefs, are unwilling to learn and adopt new treatment approaches, and/or are inflexible about modifying their office practices and prescribing procedures, are not a good fit for co-treatment of pain and addiction.

Although chronic pain is common in participants in methadone maintenance treatment programs, many are not candidates for office-based treatment. Their addiction problems often are too severe to be managed in this setting (e.g., poly-drug abuse, intravenous [IV] drug use). Conversely, their pain problems typically are of mild-to-moderate intensity, raising the question of whether opioid therapy (for pain) is even necessary. The strict regulatory constraints under which opioid treatment programs (OTPs) operate make it virtually impossible to employ modern pain management strategies. Therefore, OTP patients who wish to receive office-based treatment for both their addiction and pain will need to be converted from methadone to buprenorphine or receive "split" treatment. Intentionally promoting "split" treatment (in which an OTP patient is sent to an outside provider for supplemental opioids for pain) is not recommended for reasons already described. More appropriate populations for office-based treatment are (1) patients with moderate-to-severe chronic pain who abuse opioid analgesics and are being treated in medical settings, and (2) opioid abusers with moderate-to-severe chronic pain who are seeking office-based treatment for addiction.

Within these two subgroups of patients with chronic pain and opioid dependence, additional criteria should be considered when deciding whether a particular individual is a candidate for opioid maintenance therapy for pain. First, individuals with nonopioid SUDs that are severe enough to warrant medical supervision, for instance, those with current alcohol, benzodiazepine, and/or cocaine dependence, are inappropriate. Exclusion of those with dependence syndromes is recommended, because the office setting provides inadequate structure for managing patients with severe addictive disorders; neither do the protocols address comanagement of other drug use disorders. Providers who wish to treat pain but find themselves needing to conduct sedative/hypnotic tapers are likely to have a difficult time. In contrast, many individuals with substance use disorders should be considered especially because they comprise a large segment of the population.

Another potentially problematic subgroup of patients is those with severe, unstable mental illnesses such as bipolar disorder or schizophrenia, although, if well-treated, they may become suitable candidates. Again, patients with less severe problems, especially depression and anxiety, which are prevalent in this population, should be considered, although ancillary interventions (e.g., antidepressants, psychotherapy) often are needed to optimize outcomes. While patients with somatic symptom disorder (with predominant pain) are appropriate for office-based treatment, however, those with other disorders that feature somatic concerns (e.g., psychological factors affecting other medical conditions) may be difficult to manage because their pain problems are part of a much larger picture of complaints and concerns, many of which lack objective evidence, making the need for opioid maintenance therapy less clear. Patients with certain personality disorders also may pose management problems; for instance, those with significant antisocial characteristics and/or a legal history are at increased risk for diversion. Those with borderline personality disorder may be prone to overdose and strained doctor–patient relations, although, at least theoretically, opioids may have a positive impact on emotional dysregulation (Bandelow, Schmahl, Falkai, & Wedekind, 2010). Patients with severe personality disorders often do poorly in settings that are relatively low intensity and lack a firm "holding environment" to address their behavioral disturbances. For this reason, the office setting likely is inadequate to contain those with Cluster B disorder and traits. Finally, patients who refuse to comply (or attempt to modify) the treatment frame should be excluded. This includes those who refuse to participate in adjunctive interventions (e.g., drug or psychiatric treatment), to be monitored for unauthorized drug use, and/ or to sign an opioid agreement.

Initial Evaluation

Prior to accepting a patient for opioid maintenance therapy, a comprehensive assessment should be completed. The "Screening and Assessment Algorithm" (National Institute on Drug Abuse [NIDA], 2012) provides a framework for collecting the information needed to make this decision: (1) pain severity/characteristics; (2) pain treatment history; (3) clinical interview; (4) history and physical; (5) laboratory findings; (6) urine toxicology; (7) risk factors for opioid abuse (substance abuse and mental health); and (8) results obtained from state prescription drug monitoring programs. Patients who are applying for this type of treatment must be advised that they will need to complete an evaluation to be considered. Those who are unable or unwilling to cooperate with the evaluation process should not be considered for treatment. While the evaluation should be completed in a timely way, the process often takes a few weeks to complete. It is important that clinicians not feel pressured to implement opioid therapy prior to completing the evaluation, because, once started, it can be very difficult to discontinue therapy should the evaluation results indicate problems. As part of the initial evaluation, the provider should consider employing any of a number of brief, valid, self-administered questionnaires designed to answer specific questions, for example, the risk for opioid analgesic abuse during pain therapy. Recommended measures are listed in Table 20.4.

Treatment Protocol

Before initiating opioid treatment for pain, one needs to decide on office policies and procedures. For instance, it is important to establish rules regarding when patients will be seen, how after hour's and emergency calls will be handled, refill policies, and so forth. At a minimum, the protocol should cover the following topics: (1) prescribing practices (selection of drug, dose titration, use of breakthrough medications etc.); (2) monitoring procedures (e.g., questionnaires, urine toxicology, pill counts, pain/medication diary); (3) consequences of unauthorized/ illicit substance use (e.g., how many positive tests or missed visits before treatment options are reconsidered); and (4) tapering and referral procedures should they become necessary. The protocol should be sufficiently detailed to allow another clinician to treat the patient if the primary provider is unable to do so.

TABLE 20.4. Measures of Opioid Anaglesic Abuse/Dependence and Risk for Addiction

Measure	Target behavior	No. of items	Administration	Source
Screener and Opioid Assessment for Patients with Pain (SOAPP V1); Screener and Opioid Assessment for Patients with Pain—Revised (SOAPP-R)	Risk for opiate analgesic abuse	5, 14, or 24	Self-administered	Available to registered users at *www.painedu.org*; copyright *painedu@inflexxion.com*
Current Opioid Misuse Measure (COMM)	Adherence to opioid therapy for pain	17	Self-administered	Available to registered users at *www.painedu.org*; copyright *painedu@inflexxion.com*
Problems with Pain Meds (PPM)	Aberrant medication-taking behaviors	41; five subscales	Self-administered (both patient and provider)	Available from the author (Haller)
Pain Medicine Questionnaire (PMQ)	Likelihood of prescription opioid abuse	26	Self-administered	Public domain (Adams et al., 2004)
Prescription Drug Use Questionnaire (PDUQ) and PDUQ-P	Designed to detect prescription pain medication addiction in chronic pain patients	Interviewer version: 42 items (39 scored); patient version: 31 items	Interviewer-administered; self-administered	Available in Compton, Darakjian, & Miotto (1998)

An important component of the treatment protocol is the opioid contract, which is a mutual agreement between the provider and patient that specifies what is expected of the patient (e.g., regular attendance, abstinence from unauthorized drugs) and what the provider will do for the patient in return. The agreement also stipulates the conditions of the treatment, for instance, that lost or stolen prescriptions may not be refilled, that dose adjustments will only be entertained during regularly scheduled office visits, or that patients will be required to enroll in drug treatment after three positive toxicology tests. Opioid agreements also constitute informed consent; once executed, patients should receive a copy to take home. Finally, contracts should specify what may happen if the patient is nonadherent or the treatment is ineffective. For example, the contract may stipulate that a taper may be initiated after three missed visits or three positive toxicology screens for illicit drugs. The contract also should specify the conditions under which a patient may be required to attend drug treatment. Attempts to link patients to ancillary drug treatment are more likely to be successful if continued access to opioids (for pain) is made contingent on program attendance. In contrast, attempts to transfer patients who have been unable/unwilling to comply with or benefit from office-based treatment may fail because patients identify as pain patients (not addicts) and see the goals of drug treatment programs as different from those of pain treatment. The agreement should not include imperatives, since these may limit discretion on the part of the provider, and if the provider does not carry out an imperative stated in the agreement, he or she might be cited for breach of contract.

Treatment Efficacy

Repeated assessments are needed to evaluate progress and determine whether the therapy is working, needs to be adjusted, or should be terminated. If pain and interference ratings are taken during regularly scheduled treatment visits, providers may use them to help guide treatment and adjust the dose in "real time" (i.e., during that visit, if indicated). Once the dose has stabilized, minimal adjustments will be needed. In addition, repeated measures' testing provides evidence of efficacy. By comparing the magnitude of change against recommended "benchmarks," it is possible to determine whether improvement is minimal, moderate, or substantial. Furthermore, one population may be compared with another, for example, pain outcomes for patients with and without opioid dependence may be compared. Studies conducted with nonaddicted patients with chronic pain have found that decreases of 1.7–2.0 points on a 10-point intensity scale are consistent with patient reports of "much improved" on quality-of-life measures (Farrar, Young, LaMoreaux, Werth, & Poole, 2001; Hanley, et al., 2006; Salaffi, Stancati, Silvestri, Ciapetti, & Grassi, 2004) In addition, the Initiative on Methods, Measurement, and Pain Assessment in Clinical Trials (IMMPACT) consensus panel has recommended measures and benchmarks for interpreting the magnitude of change in pain intensity for participants in clinical trials (Dworkin et al., 2008). Furthermore, patients view clinically important reductions in pain as follows: (1) minimal (1 VAS point or 10–20% reduction); (2) moderate (2 VAS points or 30–36% reduction); and (3) substantial ($\geq$ 4 VAS points or > 50% reduction). A reduction in pain of 50% often is equated with treatment success.

Managing Co-Occurring SUDs

As previously noted, substance abuse comorbidity is common in this population. While polydrug abuse complicates treatment, some (illicit) substances may have therapeutic value that rarely is recognized or appreciated. For example, patients often report that pain relief is enhanced when cannabis is used in combination with opioids. Although the animal literature supports this claim (Welch & Stevens,1992), minimal research has been conducted in humans and available findings have been equivocal (Campbell et al., 2001). Although more research is needed to determine whether cannabis should be considered as an adjunct to opioid therapy for pain, the availability of medical marijuana complicates the situation, because patients already have access to legal cannabis for treatment of pain in many states. Furthermore, as states legalize cannabis for recreational purposes, this likely will lead more patients to experiment on their own. Therefore, providers who practice in these states need to decide whether they will prescribed cannabis, ignore its use (if obtained from another provider), or restrict its use as part of the treatment agreement without the benefit of convincing effectiveness research. Another interesting interaction involves stimulants. Although cocaine and other stimulants tend to exacerbate pain, they may increase analgesia and decrease sedation when used along with opioids (Forrest et al., 1977). Other drugs also may act in a synergistic fashion when taken with opioids, increasing their intoxicating and/or analgesic effects.

"Supplementation" of prescribed opioids with those obtained from other sources, both licit and illicit, is another significant problem for this population. To ensure that this is not occurring, providers are encouraged to conduct random toxicology screens (although these will be of no help if the patient is abusing the prescribed drug). In addition, standard drug screens have significant limitations. Most assess for morphine-based drugs, such as codeine, but do a poor job of detecting commonly used opioid analgesics such as hydrocodone and oxycodone. Because synthetic opioids such as fentanyl cannot be identified without using costly laboratory tests, patients who are likely to supplement their prescribed opioid medication with non-morphine-based drugs may require a "tailored" panel that is confirmed by GC/MS or other, more specific laboratory tests.

Co-Occurring Psychiatric Disorders

Most patients with comorbid pain and opioid dependence have one or more psychiatric disorders. Depression and anxiety disorders are especially common, but some patients have serious mental illnesses, such as bipolar disorder or schizophrenia. Such patients are not appropriate candidates for opioid maintenance for pain unless they under the care of a psychiatrist and well-stabilized. Parenthetically, if the patient is nonadherent with psychiatric treatment, he or she also may be nonadherent with pain treatment. Many drugs that are used to treat psychiatric problems also are used to treat chronic pain, for example, anticonvulsants/mood stabilizers and certain antidepressants. Since therapeutic doses vary widely by indication, it is important to specify for which condition the medication is being prescribed. For example, small doses of amitriptyline frequently are used to facilitate sleep and increase analgesia at night, although doses of 25–100 mg are unlikely to address depression.

Guidelines for Prescribing Opioids for Pain to Substance Abusers

In general, medications and doses that are highly effective in treating pain are more likely to be associated with increased rates of diversion, morbidity, and mortality. Conversely, fewer adverse events are associated with less potent medications and lower doses, although pain relief is less. Providers must therefore weigh the "risk–benefit ratio" when deciding which medication is best suited for which patient. The other critical variable is the dose of medication to be used. This must be sufficient to provide pain relief, while also suppressing drug-seeking or supplementation. We hope that the following guidelines facilitate the decision-making process, so that treatment of a particular patient may be "optimized" while keeping the risk for AMTBs at a minimum.

Use of Long-Acting Opioids

Use of short-acting/immediate-release (IR) opioids to treat pain is a common practice. Unfortunately, because they have a more rapid onset and offset than long-acting opioids, they are more likely to produce euphoria, which encourages self-administration. Use of IR opioids also produces "mini-withdrawals" that lead patients to take medication more frequently than prescribed. For this reason, long-acting/extended-release (ER) opioids such as MS Contin (morphine), OxyContin (oxycodone), Duragesic Patch (fentanyl), and methadone that last for 8 or more hours are preferable when treating patients with persistent chronic pain. The primary concern with these medications is diversion, with higher doses of the drug being extracted from the delivery matrix and consumed at one time. This occurs when patients crush and snort long-acting medications or inject medications from transdermal patches. Altering the route of administration of a prescribed opioid is a clear sign of addiction that requires careful monitoring. Methadone does not have this problem, however. Recently developed and marketed tamper-deterrent formulations of ER medications that limit the ability to extract the active ingredient from the formulation or release an opioid antagonist to reduce the patient's ability to inject or insufflate (snort) the medication. These include: OxyContin (oxycodone), Hysingla (hydrocodone), Opana (oxymorphone), Nucynta (tapentadol), and Embeda (morphine/naltrexone). OxyContin, Hysingla, and Embeda have received Category 1, 2, and 3 labeling from the Food and Drug Administration (FDA) indicating that they are "expected to result in a meaningful reduction in abuse." Oxaydo (formerly Oxecta), an immediate release oxycodone formulation has also been granted category labeling from the FDA. In the future, the FDA may decide to not approve any new opioid product that is not in some form of abuse deterrent formulation or has such characteristics inherent in the molecule. The FDA may remove category labeling if the product does not result in reduction of nonmedical use.

Avoid p.r.n. Dosing

The idea behind "as needed" dosing is that patients will use less medication if they take it only when their pain is severe. Ironically, patients on p.r.n. dosing schedules often take more (not less) medication, because pain is harder to treat once it becomes severe, requiring higher doses. A better strategy is to maintain patients on scheduled medications that are taken "round the clock" to keep the pain at a more tolerable level. As noted earlier, use of ER medications for persistent pain is preferable.

Use Breakthrough Medication

Rescue medication should be available for use in situations in which pain is worse than usual or cannot be controlled by the usual dose. When used in this way, the medication is being used to treat "breakthrough" pain. IR opioids are appropriate to treat breakthrough pain because they provide more rapid relief (have a rapid onset). For instance, a reasonable regimen might include MS Contin (ER morphine) "round the clock" and MSIR (IR morphine) for rescue purposes. If the same medication is available in both long- and short-acting formulations, this can make monitoring easier, although this is not always possible. Patients who are taking breakthrough medication should be instructed to document how often and under what circumstances they are using it. In this way, the provider may evaluate whether use of breakthrough medication is appropriate or not. For instance, use of rescue medication after driving for many hours is appropriate, whereas use to combat emotional distress is not. When pain medication is taken for reasons other than intended (e.g., to deal with emotional distress), this constitutes nonmedical use or abuse. If breakthrough medication is being routinely (though appropriately) used, this suggests that a higher round-the-clock dose is needed. Once the round-the-clock dose has been established, the need for breakthrough medication should be minimal unless the patient has a progressive disease with gradually increasing pain levels.

Provide Adequate Doses at Appropriate Dosing Intervals

For several reasons, patients with comorbid pain and opioid dependence are more likely to be undertreated. Providers often fail to take tolerance into consideration when establishing the initial dose of pain medication; this is problematic, because tolerant patients require higher starting doses. Another contributing factor is providers' failure to appreciate that they are treating two disorders concurrently. As a general rule, patients with dual disorders require more medication than those with only one disorder. Undertreatment can occur despite good intentions. Providers try to keep the dose as low as possible to prevent addiction, although undertreatment results in unnecessary suffering and also can provoke drug-seeking behavior (Schnoll & Weaver, 2003). To avoid emergency department visits, "doctor shopping," and/or borrowing of drugs from friends or relatives, patients with comorbid pain and opioid dependence should be given adequate doses of medication at appropriate intervals both to manage pain and control AMTBs.

Avoid Multiple Providers

The risk for overdose, death, and drug–drug interactions increases when patients are receiving opioid analgesics from multiple sources. Most problems are the result of patients failing to tell one provider about the other out of fear that one or both prescriptions will be discontinued. However, even when clinicians are aware of one another's existence, they rarely work in concert. One provider may alter the medication regimen without the other's knowledge, resulting in too high or too low a dose. Incompatible medications (e.g., methadone and bup/nx) may be prescribed, leading to adverse consequences. When patients drop out of or are terminated from one or another treatment and this information is not communicated to the other provider, this may precipitate a withdrawal syndrome, despite patients' continued access to opioids. Patients and providers are understandably confused by the varyious regulations that govern the prescribing of methadone for addiction versus pain. When the same drug is being used for both indications, it is difficult to comprehend why the patient needs to stand on line in the methadone clinic to receive his or her daily dose of liquid methadone, while having access to a 30-day supply of tablet form methadone for self-administration purposes. This is yet another reason why "split" treatment is discouraged, although it may work in the rare situation in which the methadone provider is willing to take the patient on (privately) for pain management.

Select Appropriate Medications

Because there is considerable interpatient variability in opioid receptor response and because the pharmacokinetic and pharmacodynamic actions of opioids vary from person to person, providers need to be comfortable with more than one opioid medication. Several drugs may need to be tried before a good response is achieved. Also, after a patients is maintained on a drug for an extended period of time, it may lose effectiveness. When this occurs, pain providers often "switch" to another opioid medication. This strategy, known as "opioid rotation," requires a dose recalculation for the new opioid; conversion tables and equianalgesic doses are available to assist providers in achieving this objective. It is important, however, to start the patient on a low dose of the new medication to avoid an inadvertent toxic reaction. Most opioid conversion tables were developed under acute use conditions, not chronic use conditions. To optimize treatment, many patients require both regular and breakthrough medications. Although some medications (e.g., morphine and oxycodone) are available in both IR and ER forms, others are not. For this reason, providers may need to prescribe two medications, one for round-the-clock dosing and the other for breakthrough purposes. A listing of available ER and IR medications may be found in Table 20.5.

When treating patients with comorbid pain and opioid dependence, two medications immediately come to mind—methadone and buprenorphine. Both are approved for for opioid dependence, though in different formulations. Although providers often believe it is illegal to prescribe methadone to addicts outside the confines of an OTP, this is not true. Methadone may be prescribed for pain by clinicians with appropriate Drug Enforcement Agency (DEA) registration. When used for pain, methadone is dispensed at pharmacies the same as other drugs, usually a month's supply at a time. However, prescribing methadone to opioid-dependent individuals for pain should not be undertaken unless the provider is very experienced and has close ties to an OTP to which the patient may be referred for addiction treatment if necessary.

Bup/nx is a viable alternative to methadone for treating opioid addiction; however, its efficacy for treating pain in opioid-dependent individuals is less clear. While the sublingual formulation of bupenorphine is not approved for pain, "off-label" use of bup/nx for concurrent treatment of pain and opioid dependence is fairly common. (Heit & Gourlay, 2008) Although the transdermal formulation is approved for pain (7-day patch) and may be used in conjunction with bup/nx for breakthrough pain, there is no literature regarding this dosing strategy for pain patients with opioid use disorders. One potential issue with bup/nx is a potential ceiling effect. Because bup/nx is a partial agonist, its antagonist effects at higher doses limit its utility in those who require more medication than a dose equivalent to 80 mg of methadone (Ripamonti, 2012). However, for those who do not require high opioid doses for pain, bup/nx is an excellent analgesic. It is relatively long acting, but divided doses still are recommended due to its shorter analgesic half-life (Ripamonti, 2012). As with methadone,

TABLE 20.5. Drugs Used in the Treatment of Pain

Drug class	Examples	Symptoms targeted
Nonsteroidal anti-inflammatory drugs (NSAIDs)	ibuprofen (Motrin), naproxen sodium (Aleve), celecoxib (Celebrex), ketorolac tromethamine (Torradlo), diclofenac sodium (Voltaren), rofecoxib (Vioxx), ketoprofen (Orudis), indomethacin (Indocin), naproxen sodium (Anaprox), sulindac (Clinoril), piroxicam (Feldene), etodolac (Lodine), aspirin	Pain, inflammation
Anticonvulsants	gabapentin (Neurontin), carbamazepine (Tegretol), phenytoin (Dilantin), valproic acid (Depakote), topiramate (Topimax)	Nerve pain
Antidepressants	Tricyclic antidepressants (TCAs) such as amitriptyline (Elavil) and imipramine (Tofranil); selective serotonin reuptake inhibitors (SSRIs) such as fluoxetine (Prozac), sertraline (Zoloft); other antidepressants such as venlafaxine (Effexor), bupropion (Wellbutrin)	Pain, sleep disturbances, depression
Sedatives/ hypnotics	diazepam (Valium), chlordiazepoxide (Librium), alprazolam (Xanax), zolpidem tartrate (Ambien), clonazepam (Klonopin), lorazepam (Ativan)	Anxiety, sleep disturbance
Muscle relaxants	methocarbamol (Robaxin), diazepam (Valium), cyclobenzaprine (Flexeril), metaxalone (Skelaxin), carisoprodol (Soma)	Spasms
Opioids	propoxyphene (Darvon), acetaminophen plus codeine (Tylenol #3), oxycodone with acetaminophen (Percocet), meperidine (Demerol), hydromorphone hydrochloride (Dilaudid), hydrocodone bitartrate and acetaminophen (Vicodin), hydrocodone bitartrate plus acetaminophen (Lorcet), morphine immediate release (MS IR), morphine (MS Contin), oxycodone (OxyContin); methadone, fentanyl transdermal (Duragesic Patch), buprenorphine (Buprenex)	Pain
Local anesthetics	lidocaine, novacaine	Localized pain
Capsaicin	capsaicin (Zacin Cream)	Localized pain

no special license (including an X waiver) other than DEA registration is needed to prescribe buprenorphine for pain.

ANCILLARY BEHAVIORAL INTERVENTIONS

Even when providers implement recommended office and prescribing procedures, these may prove insufficient to control substance abuse. Before initiating a taper or transferring the patient to drug treatment for failure to adhere to the treatment contract, providers may wish to consider enhancing the treatment by adding one or more behavioral interventions. A number of evidence-based therapies for substance abuse are available, including cognitive-behavioral relapse prevention therapy (CBT/RP; Larimer, Palmer & Marlatt, 1999), motivational interviewing (MI; Miller & Rollnick, 2002; Substance Abuse and Mental Health Services Administration, 1999), and supportive expressive therapy (SE; Woody et al., 1983). Abstinence-based interventions such as individual drug counseling (IDC; Mercer & Woody, 1999) and 12-step facilitation therapy (TSF; Humphries, 1999), as well as attendance at 12-step self-help groups, may be useful in addressing nonopioid substance use. However, when patients who are being treated with opioids for pain simultaneously are enrolled in abstinence-based drug treatments, this can present a significant conflict, because the goals of treatment for pain and addiction are inconsistent. One addiction-focused behavioral intervention that can (and should) be delivered by prescribing clinicians is opioid adherence counseling, the elements of which include (1) execution of an opioid agreement; (2) psychoeducation about chronic pain and opioid analgesics; (3) self-monitoring through use of a diary tracking pain and medication use; and (4) frequent drug screens, along with personalized feedback regarding results. Motivation enhancement therapy (MET) interventions also can be helpful by addressing patients' ambivalence about changing their drug use behavior.

To achieve optimal outcomes, co-occurring psychiatric problems such as depression, anxiety, and personality disorders also require treatment. These problems are prevalent in patients with chronic pain, with and without addiction problems. If the prescribing physician has received psychiatric training and is capable of delivering behavioral interventions, he or she may be in a position to deliver behavioral as well as pharmacological treatments. Otherwise, patients need to be referred for psychiatric treatment based on the presenting problem. Many of the behavioral interventions that are used to treat addictive disorders also are used to treat pain and associated sequellae. CBT is used to combat distorted pain perceptions (e.g., that pain is uncontrollable) and target symptoms of depression. Additional strategies such as guided imagery, progressive muscle relaxation, biofeedback, mindfulness, and hypnosis can help to decrease pain, reduce stress, and provide patients with a sense of self-control. In addition to individual counseling, group therapy is used to treat both substance abuse and pain. Secondary to pain and functional interference, many patients decrease their involvement in social activities and become relatively isolated. Participation in group therapy can help them to reconnect with others, receive support, and work toward common goal of pain reduction and abstinence from other drugs. Although mutual self-help groups such as Alcoholics Anonymous (AA) or Narcotics Anonymous (NA) may be helpful, many patients resist this approach because they do not identify as substance abusers and are fearful of being criticized for using opioids to treat pain. While some 12-step groups may not welcome such individuals, other may appreciate the need for legitimate medical care and accept the patient's wish to achieve abstinence with regard to alcohol or other drugs. Finally, the Internet can serve as an additional source of support for substance abusers with chronic pain. There are numerous sites for pain patients to visit to learn about their pain disorders and connect with others who are suffering from the same painful conditions. For patients who are struggling to maintain adherence to the treatment protocol, group therapy can be an excellent, relatively low-cost option.

SUMMARY

Patients with chronic pain and opioid dependence can be successfully treated in office-based settings by trained clinicians who are willing to implement a treatment protocol that is designed to provide adequate treatment for pain, while actively managing co-occurring SUDs. Providers need to consider carefully patients who may be candidates for this type of treatment. Treatment should be aggressive. When patients experience difficulties, the protocol should guide decision making to include enhancing treatment to achieve the best result possible. Despite these efforts, some patients are unable to achieve preestablished treatment goals and objectives. These patients must be referred to higher intensity pain and addictions treatments to include agonist therapy and whatever pain treatments may be recommended by specialists. Although office-based treatment of pain and opioid dependence is an uncertain proposition, patients who respond to this approach will benefit from being treated by a provider who understands the importance of integrated care.

REFERENCES

Adams, L. L., Gatchel, R. J., Robinson, R. C., Polatin, P., Gajraj, N., Deschner, M., et al. (2004). Development of a self-report screening instrument for assessing potential opioid medication misuse in chronic pain patients. *J Pain Symptom Manage, 27,* 440–459.

American Society of Anesthesiologists Task Force on Pain Management. (1997). Practice guidelines for chronic pain management. *Anesthesiology, 86,* 995–1004.

Bandelow, B., Schmahl, C., Falkai, P., & Wedekind, D. (2010). Borderline personality disorder: A dysregulation of the endogenous opioid system? *Psychol Rev, 117,* 623–636.

Butler, S. F., Budman, S. H., Licari, A., Cassidy, T. A., Lioy, K., Dickinson, J., et al. (2008). National addictions vigilance intervention and prevention program (NAVIPPRO): A real-time, product-specific, public health surveillance system for monitoring prescription drug abuse. *Pharmacoepidemiol Drug Saf, 17*(12), 1142–1154.

Campbell, F. A., Tramer, M. R., Carroll, D., Reynolds, D. J. M., Moore, R. A., & McQuay, H. J. (2001). Are cannabinoids an effective and safe treatment option in the management of pain?: A qualitative, systematic review. *BMJ, 323,* 13–16.

Chabal, C., Erjavec, M. K., Jacobson, L., Mariano, A., & Chaney, E. (2007). Prescription opiate abuse in chronic pain patients: Clinical criteria, incidence, and predictors. *Clin J Pain, 13,* 150–155.

Cicero, T. J., Dart, R. C., Inciardi, J. A., Woody, G. E., Schnoll, S. H., & Muñoz, A. (2007). The development of a comprehensive risk-management program for prescription opioid analgesics: Researched, abuse, diversion and addiction-related surveillance (RADARS), *Pain Med, 8,*157–170.

Compton, P., Darakjian, J., & Miotto, K. (1998). Screening for addiction in patients with chronic pain and "problematic" substance use: Evaluation of a pilot assessment tool. *J Pain Symptom Manage, 16,* 355–363.

Dirks, J. F., Wunder, J., Kinsman, R., McElhinny, J., & Jones, N. F. (1993). A Pain Rating Scale and a Pain Behavior Checklist for clinical use: Development, norms, and the consistency score. *Psychother Psychosom, 59,* 41–49.

Dworkin, R. H., Turk, D. C., Revicki, D. A., Harding, G., Coyne, K. S., Peirce-Sandner, S., et al. (2009). Development and initial validation of an expanded and revised version of the Short-Form McGill Pain Questionnaire (SF-MPQ-2). *Pain, 144,* 35–42.

Dworkin, R. H., Turk, D. C., Wryrich, K. W., Beaton, D., Cleeland, C. S., Farrar, J. T., et al. (2008). Interpreting the clinical importance of treatment outcomes in clinical trials: IMMPACT recommendations. *J Pain, 9*, 105–121.

Farrar, J. T., Young, J. P., LaMoreaux, L., Werth, J. L., & Poole, R. M. (2001). Clincial importance of changes in chronic pain intensity measured on an 11-point numerical pain rating scale. *Pain, 94*, 149–158.

Fleming, M. F., Balousek, S. L., Klessig, C. L., Mundt, M. P., & Brown, D. D. (2007). Substance use disorders in a primary care sample receiving daily opioid therapy. *J Pain, 8*, 573–582.

Forrest, W. H., Jr., Brown, B. W., Jr., Brown, C. R., Defalque, R., Gold, M., Gordon, H. E., et al. (1977). Dextroamphetamine with morphine for the treatment of post-operative pain. *N Engl J Med, 296*, 712–715.

Haddox, J. D., Joranson, D., Angarola, R. T., Brady, A., Carr, D. B., Blonsky, R., et al. (1997). The use of opioids for the treatment of chronic pain: A consensus statement from the American Academy of Pain Medicine and the American Pain Society. *Clin J Pain, 13*, 6–8.

Haller, D. L., & Acosta, M. C. (2010). Characteristics of pain patients with opioid-use disorders. *Psychosomatics, 51*, 257–266.

Hanley, M. A., Jensen, M. P., Ehde, D. M., Robinson, L. R., Cardenas, D. D., Turner, J. A., et al. (2006). Clinically significant changes in pain intensity ratings in persons with spinal cord injury or amputation. *Clin J Pain, 22*, 25–31.

Hariharan, J., Lamb, G. C., & Neuner, J. M. (2007). Long-term opioid contract use for chronic pain management in primary care practice: A five year experience. *J Gen Int Med, 22*, 485–490.

Heit, H. A., & Gourlay, D. L. (2008). Buprenorphine: New tricks with an old molecule for pain management. *Clin J Pain, 24*, 93–97.

Hockenberry, M. J., Wilson, D., & Winkelstein, M. L. (2005). *Wong's essentials of pediatric nursing* (7th ed.). St. Louis, MO: Mosby.

Humphries, K. (1999). Professional interventions that facilitate 12-step self-help group involvement. *Alcohol Res Health, 23*, 93–98.

Jamison, R. N., Kauffman, J., & Katz, N. P. (2000). Characteristics of methadone maintenance patients with chronic pain. *J Pain Symptom Manage, 19*, 53–62.

Kerns, R. D., Turk, D. C., & Rudy, T. E. (1985). The West Haven–Yale Multidimensional Pain Inventory (WHYMPI). *Pain, 4*, 345–356.

Larimer, M. E., Palmer, R. S., & Marlatt, G. A. (1999). Relapse prevention: An overview of Marlatt's cognitive-behavioral model. *Alcohol Res Health, 23*, 151–160.

Manchikanti, L., Fellows, B., Damron, K. S., Pampati, V., & McManus, C. D. (2005). Prevalence of illicit drug among individuals with chronic pain in the Commonwealth of Kentucky: An evaluation of patterns and trends. *J KY Med Assoc, 10*(3), 55–62.

McCaffery, M., & Beebe, A. (1993). *Pain: Clinical manual for nursing practice*. Baltimore, MD: Mosby.

Melzack, R. (2005). McGill Pain Questionnaire: From description to measurement. *Anesthesiol, 103*, 199–202.

Mercer, D. E., & Woody, G. E. (1999, September). *An individual drug counseling approach to treat cocaine addiction: The Collaborative Cocaine Treatment Study Model* (Therapy Manuals for Drug Abuse Treatment [Manual 3], NIH Publication Number 99-4380). Washington, DC: National Institutes of Health.

Merskey, H., & Bogduk, N. (Eds.). (1994). *Classification of chronic pain descriptions of chronic pain syndromes and definitions of pain terms*. Seattle, WA: IASP Press.

Miller, W. R., & Rollnick, S. R. (2002). *Motivational interviewing: Preparing people for change* (2nd ed). New York: Guilford Press.

National Institute on Drug Abuse (NIDA). (2012). Screening and assessment algorithm: Algorithm for assessing patients with chronic pain for substance abuse/risk and for possible chronic opioid therapy. Retrieved October 31, 2012, from *www.opioidrisk.com/node/1829*.

Portenoy, R. K., & Foley, K. M. (1986). Chronic use of opioid analgesics in non-malignant pain: Report of 38 cases. *Pain, 25,* 171–186.

Richards, J. S., Nepomuceno, C., Riles, M., & Suer, Z. (1982). Assessing pain behavior: The UAB Pain Behavior Scale. *Pain, 14,* 393–398.

Ripamonti, C. L. (2012). Pain management. *Annals of Oncology, 23*(Suppl. 10), x294–x301.

Rosenblum, A., Joseph, H., Fong, C., Kipnis, S., Cleland, C., & Portenoy, R. K. (2003). Prevalence and characteristics of chronic pain among chemically dependent patients in methadone maintenance and residential treatment facilities. *JAMA, 289,* 2370–2378.

Salaffi, F., Stancati, A., Silvestri, C. A., Ciapetti, A., & Grassi, W. (2004). Minimal clinically important changes in chronic musculoskeletal pain intensity measured on a numerical rating scale. *Eur J Pain, 8,* 283–291.

Savage, S. R., Joranson, D. R., Covington, E. C., Schnoll, S. H., Heit, H. A., & Gilson, A. M. (2003). Definitions related to the medical use of opioids: Evolution towards universal agreement. *J Pain Symptom Manage, 26,* 655–667.

Schnoll, S. H., & Weaver, M. S. (2003). Addiction and pain. *Am J Addict, 12*(Suppl. 2), S27–S35.

Substance Abuse and Mental Health Services Administration (SAMHSA), Center for Substance Abuse Treatment. (1999). Enhancing motivation for change in substance abuse treatment. Retrieved from *www.motivationalinterview.org.*

Turk, D. C. (1996). Clinicians' attitudes about prolonged use of opioids and the issue of patient heterogeneity. *J Pain Symptom Manage, 11,* 218–230.

Weaver, M. F., & Schnoll, S. H. (2002). Opioid treatment of chronic pain in patients with addiction. *J Pain Palliative Care Pharmacother, 16,* 5–26.

Welch, S. P., & Stevens, D. L. (1992). Antinociceptive activity of intrathecally administered cannabinoids alone, and in combination with morphine, in mice. *J Pharmacol Exp Ther, 262,* 10–18.

Woody, G. E., Luborsky, L., McLellan, A. T., O'Brien, C. P., Beck, A. T., Blaine, J., et al. (1983). Psychotherapy for opiate addicts: Does it help? *Arch Gen Psychiatry, 40,* 639–645.

World Health Organization. (2011). *Ensuring balance in national policies on controlled substances: Guidance for availability and accessibility of controlled medicines.* Geneva, Switzerland: Author.

CHAPTER 21

Substance Use among Older Adults

STEVE KOH
ROBERT GORNEY
NICOLAS BADRE
DILIP V. JESTE

It is widely recognized that the fastest growing population in the United States is those above the age of 65. According to 2010 U.S. Census data, currently those age 65 years and older account for 13% of the total population (U.S. Census Bureau, 2012). It is estimated that by 2030, those above the age of 65 will account for more than 72 million individuals and make up 18% of the total population.

While there are few estimates of drug use in the current older adult population, as the younger cohorts age, it is expected that the prevalence of substance use will increase. One study looking at those age 50 years and older indicated that 60% use of alcohol, 2.6% use marijuana, and 0.41% use cocaine (Blazer & Wu, 2009). Importantly, whereas those above age 65 had 0.7% of marijuana use, those between ages 50 and 64 had 4% of use. Gfroerer, Penne, Pemberton, and Folsom (2003) used the National Household Survey on Drug Abuse to estimate the need for substance abuse treatment in older adults. They found that by 2020, the need will increase to 4.4 million individuals, which represents a 38% increase. Simoni-Wastila and Yang (2006) found a growing problem of prescription medication abuse. They estimated that there will be 2.7 million prescription drug abusers by 2020. What seems to be clear from these studies is that as younger population cohorts age, the prevalence of substance abuse and dependence will increase in the older population.

Despite the rising prevalence of alcohol and substance abuse in older adults, few are willing to seek treatment, and historically there has been a lack of emphasis on special needs of older adults in existing treatment programs (Barrick & Conners, 2002). Even among clinicians, there exists a form of ageism in which exploration of possible alcohol and substance misuse is not routinely done. This may be due to the lack of knowledge about the true prevalence of such abuse in older adults and/or the attitude that older adults are not impacted by alcohol and substance abuse. Even among our primary care colleagues, it is common for potential abuse history to be neglected in the older adult population. The low index of suspicion can lead to poor recognition and treatment of disorders. Some of the common barriers to identification of substance misuse in older people can be summarized in Table 21.1. Previous editions of the DSM have not acknowledged the special considerations pertaining to the older adult when delineating alcohol and substance misuse. These special considerations are summarized in Table 21.2.

Keeping in mind the rising prevalence of alcohol and substance abuse in the increasing age population, we review in this chapter the abuse of alcohol, benzodiazepines, opiates, and, briefly, other substances (e.g., tobacco, marijuana, and stimulants). The majority of this chapter deals with alcohol, which has the highest prevalence rate and the most research data. The sections review basic epidemiology, screening, substance effects, and treatment modalities, where appropriate.

ALCOHOL ABUSE IN OLDER ADULTS

Alcohol is one of the most widely used and misused substances in the older adult population. Currently it is recommend by the National Institute on Alcohol Abuse and Alcoholism (NIAAA; n.d.) that adults over age 65 drink no more than one standard drink per day (NIAAA Alcohol Alert No. 40). In this vein, it is recommended that older adults not consume more than two alcoholic drinks in any one sitting. Alcohol misuse can be defined here as meeting one of two definitions: at-risk drinkers

TABLE 21.1. Barriers in Identifying Substance Abuse in Older Adults

Clinicians' barriers

- Older-age-related assumptions (e.g., substance use is believed to be less prevalent in older age)
- Failure to recognize symptoms or to attribute symptoms to substance abuse (some symptoms of substance abuse maybe masked by other physical ailments)
- Problems in effectively screening for substance abuse in older adults
- Discomfort with addressing substance abuse with older adults
- Absence of collateral information from family members and caretakers

Older adults' barriers

- Symptoms attributed to getting old or to another illness
- Poor insight into their substance abuse and not voluntarily seeking help
- Stigma of seeking psychiatric help and of "addiction" and "substance abuse"
- Knowledge gap about how psychiatrists can help with substance abuse
- Reluctance of patients to report due to shame, denial, desire to continue using, pessimism about treatment and recovery
- Cognitive problems, including substance-induced amnesia, underlying dementia
- Family members and/or caretakers may not adequately report concerns of substance abuse

Note. Adapted with permission from Crome, Dar, Janikiewicz, Rao, and Tarbuck (2011).

TABLE 21.2. Some Barriers to Applying DSM Substance Abuse Criteria to Older Patients

Criteria	Special considerations for older adults
Tolerance	Older adults may have higher sensitivity even with lower intake (possibly due to changes in body fat distribution, changes to liver and kidney functions, etc.)
Withdrawal	Older adults who developed abuse late in life may not immediately show signs of physiological dependence
Taking larger amounts or over a longer period than intended	Increased cognitive impairment can interfere with self-monitoring; substance use itself can exacerbate cognitive impairment and self-monitoring
Unsuccessful efforts to cut down or control use	Older adults may no longer try to cut down or control use due to lifelong addiction or simply because they lack understanding of the negative impact of substance use
Spending much time to obtain and use substances and to recover from effects	Availability may be increased as some substances are readily available as prescriptions
Giving up activities due to use	Older adults may have fewer activities, making detection of problems more difficult
Continuing use despite physical or psychological problem caused by use	May not know or understand that problems are related to use, even after medical advice

Note. Adapted from Blow (1998).

(drinkers whose intake is eight or more drinks per week, but who do not meet abuse or dependence criteria), and those who meet alcohol use disorder criteria according to DSM-5 (American Psychiatric Association, 2013). In spite of the significant increases in public awareness and services for those individuals who misuse alcohol, little of that interest has translated into education or treatment programs specifically for older adults.

Older adults are likely to experience differences in blood alcohol concentration (BAC) in comparison with younger adults. Both the pharmacokinetics and pharmacodynamics of alcohol change as we age, resulting in higher BACs for similar ingested amounts of alcohol, effects that are often more pronounced in women. Additionally, as older adults tend to have more medical problems and more substantial medication burden, alcohol–medication interactions can yield serious and potentially life-threatening consequences in older adults (Moore, Blow, et al., 2011).

Epidemiology

The general consensus is that as people enter old age, their drinking tends to decline. However, there have been studies suggesting that the baby-boomer generation has higher rates of alcohol problems than previous generations (U.S. Department of Health and Human Services, 2000). An undetermined percentage of older adult alcoholics are first diagnosed in older age and may not have begun heavy drinking until older age. It has been suggested that the stresses of old age, including health problems, loss of independence, and loneliness, may be contributing factors in the use of alcohol as a coping mechanism, although these explanations for the development of late-onset-pattern heavy drinking may be an oversimplification (Gomberg, 2003).

A study by Breslow and Smothers (2004) indicated that between 10 and 15% of men and 5 and 7% of women age 65 years and older drink more than one alcoholic drink per day on average, and that the amount of alcohol during a drinking day decreases with increasing age but remains significant. A study that examined primary care patients age 65 and older indicated that 8–9% admitted to drinking more than one drink daily, with roughly half drinking more than two drinks daily or binge drinking, which is associated with depression, anxiety, and poor social support (Kirchner et al., 2007).

Historically, there have been gender-related changes in alcohol consumption into old age, such that women tend to curb their drinking as they age more than do men. It is unclear whether this pattern will continue as women from the baby-boomer generation enter older age. Older women are more likely to experience the adverse effects of heavier drinking, whether these are medical morbidity, social, psychological or physical effects, as their age-similar male counterparts, and are also more apt to have comorbid medical conditions, depression, anxiety, and abuse of psychoactive medications.

More research is warranted to better educate, screen, and treat the population in an age-specific manner. Researchers need to examine potential gender differences in these domains given that most of the alcohol use research in the older population has historically been done on men. Cultural and socioeconomic differences may play a role as well. There likely are inherent differences between the older adults who have misused alcohol in their earlier adult lives and those who develop problems with alcohol later in life, and these differences need to be further elucidated.

Screening

Screening for alcohol use disorders in older adults usually begins with an index of suspicion on the part of the health care provider. As with younger adults, this involves a thorough medical, psychiatric, social and family history; in addition, asking about alcohol and other substance use in terms of onset, current and past amounts consumed, frequency, binge habits, tolerance, and withdrawal symptoms is paramount in the initially stages of screening for alcohol problems. As people generally tend to minimize or underestimate their alcohol use, and as cognition is often affected both by aging and chronic alcohol use, older adults who drink heavily may not be able to give an accurate representation of their drinking patterns. Gathering collateral information from significant others and family is often helpful not only in determining the amount of alcohol use but also the potential psychosocial ramifications of that use. Laboratory findings such as elevated mean corpuscular volume (MCV) and gamma-glutamyl transferase (GGT) levels or laboratory values consistent with hepatic inflammation, such as elevated aspartate aminotransferase (AST) levels or cirrhosis, may be useful in the screening process and may be more sensitive in older adults. Elevated carbohydrate-deficient transferase, serum glucose, serum uric acid, and decreased albumin levels are also associated with chronic alcohol abuse in older people. For those older adults who drink heavily, it is useful to ask about withdrawal symptoms, a history of withdrawal seizures, or delirium, because this information may help to guide the therapeutic approach. As there is some overlap between commonly experienced medical and psychiatric symptoms in older adults and alcohol withdrawal, including insomnia, tremor, gastrointestinal (GI) upset, and anxiety, and because alcohol withdrawal can potentially be fatal, it is important to screen these patients carefully and recognize a temporal relationship between cessation and a marked decrease of alcohol use and symptoms.

Several tools for screening for alcohol use disorders have been developed with variable sensitivities and specificities in different populations (Adams, Barry, & Fleming, 1996; Clay, 1997; Moore, Blow, et al., 2011). Most studies that examine the validity of these screening tools in the older adult population have involved men and veteran populations. The CAGE Questionnaire contains four items (Cut down, Annoyed, Guilty, Eye-opener) and remains the most widely used tool for screening for alcohol use disorders in clinical practice (Moore, Seeman, Morgenstern, Beck, & Reuben, 2002), but it has variable sensitivity and specificity and has mainly been validated on a relatively narrow population. Using only the CAGE Questionnaire to screen for alcohol use disorders in the older adult population may be inadequate (Adams et al., 1996). The Short Michigan Alcohol Screening Test—Geriatric Version (SMAST-G) is a 10-item screening measure that likely picks up a subset of alcohol mis-users that the CAGE Questionnaire does not (Moore et al., 2002). A 10-item screening tool, the Alcohol Use Disorders Identification Test (AUDIT) is commonly used and has been validated in older adults. When considering screening tools for alcohol use disorders in the older adult population, one must keep in mind that these tools seem to vary in terms of ease of clinical use and sensitivity, specificity, and applicability to differing subsets of the population. It may be useful to employ more than one tool as a method to improve screening for alcohol use disorders (Moore et al., 2002).

Alcohol-Related Illness

Alcohol misuse is related to adverse effects in several physical health and psychiatric domains. Isolated acute alcohol intoxication can lead to increased risk of falls and potentially motor vehicle accidents that result in significant trauma, especially in conjunction with medication interactions or other substance misuse. Chronically, alcohol abuse and dependence are associated with multiple disease outcomes in several organ systems. The neurological and psychiatric, cardiovascular, pulmonary, gastrointestinal (e.g., liver and pancreas), endocrine, skeletal, hematopoietic, and immune systems may all be affected. In addition, chronic alcohol use is associated with some malignancies. Chronicity, amount of alcohol use, genetic predisposition, and psychosocial variables should also be considered when relating alcohol use to disease outcomes in older adults.

More than 90% of older adult subjects with a diagnosis of either alcohol abuse or dependence have a history of depression (Caputo et al., 2012) and, conversely, depressed older adults are three to four times more likely than nondepressed older adults to have an alcohol use disorder, with a prevalence of 15–30% in patients with late-life major depression (Devenand, 2002). Like depression, late-life anxiety disorders can both be a consequence of problematic alcohol use and a primary psychiatric illness. Generalized anxiety disorder is the most common type of anxiety disorder in the older adult population, and those with the disorder are more than twice as likely as those without an anxiety disorder to have a substance use disorder (SUD) (Mackenzie, Reynolds, Chou, Pagura, & Sareen, 2011).

The suicide rate is disproportionately high in the older adult population. SUDs, particularly alcohol abuse and dependence, are the second most common category of psychiatric disorders associated with completed suicide in the older population, following only depression (Blow, Brockmann, & Barry, 2004). Drinking among older adults elevates suicide risk through interactions with many factors that are more prevalent in this age group than in younger adults; factors include depressive symptoms, medical illness, negatively perceived health status, and low socioeconomic support. Together, alcohol misuse and comorbid psychiatric illness are a potentially lethal combination, accounting for a large number of suicides in late life, although the relationship between alcohol use and late-life suicide is a complex one that remains poorly defined and requires more research to understand the relationship so that we can better incorporate detection and prevention strategies for those at high risk.

It has long been established that alcohol alone causes changes in sleep patterns in adults, including decreased sleep latency, decreased Stage 4 restful sleep, and precipitation or worsening of sleep apnea (Wagman, Allen, & Upright, 1977). This compounds the natural sleep changes (decreased Stage 3, Stage 4, and rapid-eye-movement [REM] sleep) that occur in old age. Sleep disturbances are a common problem both in persons who misuse alcohol and those in early recovery from an alcohol use disorder. These problems are often more severe in older adults than in the younger population (Brower & Hall, 2001). Sleep apnea, common in both older adults and adults with problematic drinking, can be both potentiated and exacerbated by the use of alcohol. Treatment of insomnia in older alcoholic patients who are either still drinking or in early recovery (outside of the window of acute withdrawal) with benzodiazepines and benzodiazepine receptor agonists should be avoided if possible (benzodiazepine use for the treatment of sleep disorders in older adults is discussed below).

The relationship between alcohol use and cognition in older adults is still under investigation. Chronic alcohol use can lead to multiple types of cognitive dysfunction, characterized grossly as alcohol-associated dementia (AAD) and Wernicke–Korsakoff syndrome (WKS). Older alcoholics tend to have deficits related to both the frontal and prefrontal cortex areas (Oscar-Berman & Schendan, 2000). Although it is commonly thought that chronic alcohol misuse contributes to cognitive deficits in late life, AAD as a distinct illness has been difficult to study, because differentiating and relating it to other dementing illnesses common in older age have been challenging. AAD is thought to be a result of the direct neurotoxicity of alcohol on the brain.

WKS, in this context, stems from a thiamine deficiency often seen in chronic alcoholics, which leads to excessive glutamate release and subsequent neuronal damage. The clinical picture of WKS can be divided into the classic Wernicke's encephalopathy: ophthalmoplegia, gait ataxia, and confusion, and Korsakoff's psychosis, which clinically presents as hallucinations, amnesia, and confabulation. Deficits from

chronic alcohol use can be seen in many cognitive domains, including the perceptual–motor skills, visual–spatial functions, learning/memory, and abstraction and
problem solving (Parsons & Nixon, 1993).

Cardiovascular illnesses are commonly present in the older adult population and
are associated with alcohol use. The relationship between alcohol use in older adults
and cardiovascular disease is complex; research is being done on the topic to determine if light-to-moderate alcohol use confers some benefit. Heavy alcohol consumption has been associated with hypertension, cardiomyopathy, and arrhythmias.

Falls are a common problem in older adults for various reasons, including having risk factors such as cerebellar or vestibular dysfunction, poor vision and hearing,
muscle weakness, and orthostasis. Heavy alcohol use, either alone or in conjunction
with these potential risk factors, puts older adults at high risk of falls and significant
subsequent morbidity and mortality. Heavy drinking is associated with peripheral
neuropathies, putting those adults who consume heavy amounts of alcohol at risk for
orthostasis and sensorimotor neuropathies. Older adults who drink more than two
drinks per day have been shown to have higher risk of falls than older adults who
consume less (Mukamal et al., 2004). Hip fractures are a significant cause of morbidity and mortality in older adults, and are related to both risk of falls and low bone
mineral density. Both risk of falls and decreased bone mineral density are related to
heavy alcohol consumption in older adults.

Treatment

Prevention Strategies

Abuse prevention strategies should be considered in high-risk older adults and have
been found to be successful at curbing drinking patterns (Oslin et al., 2006). While
brief alcohol counseling strategies have been well studied in adults, there have been
fewer studies assessing brief alcohol interventions in older patients, and the results
have been mixed in terms of short- and long-term efficacy (Fleming, Manwell, Barry,
Adams, & Stauffacher, 1999; Gordon et al., 2003; Lin et al., 2010; Moore, Blow, et
al., 2011). Still, in 2004, the U.S. Preventive Services Task Force recommended that
routine alcohol screening be followed by brief alcohol counseling for all adults.

Formal Treatment

Nonpharmacological treatment for alcohol use disorders in older adults has been
found to be useful, notably when done in an age-targeted manner. There have been
several small studies with positive results examining the outcome of age-specific
treatment programs (Blow, Walton, Chermack, Mudd, & Brower, 2000). Twelve-step
programs, such as Alcoholics Anonymous (AA), have long been a successful mainstay
of treatment in the community. It remains unclear how effective 12-step groups are
in the older adult population, because it is difficult to study such highly variable settings; however, clearly, there are individuals who benefit from the programs.

For those older adults who meet criteria for an alcohol use disorder and wish to
abstain or reduce their drinking, medications should be considered to curb cravings.

There are potentially several populations of alcohol-dependent patients that are distinguishable based on craving (Oslin, Cary, Slaymaker, Colleran, & Blow, 2009), and it is possible that in the future we may have the ability to discern which patients may respond more favorably to medications targeting cravings.

Naltrexone is an opioid-receptor antagonist used in the treatment of alcohol dependence to reduce cravings and the reinforcing and/or positive emotional response to alcohol use. Although it has been studied primarily in younger patients, and its most robust effect seems to be on decreasing excessive or heavy drinking (Pettinati et al., 2006), smaller studies have indicated tolerability (Oslin, Liberto, O'Brien, Krois, & Norbeck, 1997) and some benefit (Oslin, Liberto, O'Brien, & Krois, 1997) in older adults in terms of preventing relapse. Because naltrexone is an opioid-receptor antagonist, it may limit the efficacy of prescribed opiate medications, which are commonly used in the older population. A long-acting, injectable form of the medication is available, but it is expensive compared with the oral form.

Acamprosate has been approved for the treatment of alcohol dependence and is thought to reduce cravings in part by affecting the reward pathway, but no studies have been done specifically with older adults. Disulfiram, which inhibits aldehyde dehydrogenase and prevents the metabolism of alcohol's primary metabolite, acetaldehyde, leading to unwelcome effects, is seldom used in older adults due to concerns about serious adverse side effects, including the disulfiram reaction, which may complicate general medical conditions such as heart disease.

Goals of research should include detailing appropriate pharmacological and nonpharmacological treatment strategies such that outcomes can be researched and measured.

Assessment and Management of Alcohol Withdrawal

The first steps in the prevention and management of alcohol withdrawal in older adults is to take a history and perform a physical examination, and to consider the patient's medications and medical comorbidities. The goal of the clinician treating a patient potentially in withdrawal from alcohol is patient safety, and preventing potentially serious complications such as seizure, delirium, and death. Supportive therapy should be initiated, because older adults are especially sensitive to disturbances associated with chronic alcohol use. This includes careful replacement of volume with normal saline; correction of electrolyte disturbances; prophylactic treatment of potential vitamin deficiencies with thiamine, folate, and a multivitamin; and considering the utilization of aspiration, fall and seizure precautions (Wan, Kyomen, Catic, & Tan, 2012). Strong consideration should be made for treatment of older adults in alcohol withdrawal in a highly monitored setting.

The Clinical Institute Withdrawal Assessment of Alcohol Scale, Revised (CIWA-Ar) is a guideline for administering pharmacological agents for the treatment of alcohol withdrawal based on a review of symptoms and physical examination findings (Sullivan, Sykora, Schneiderman, Naranjo, & Sellers, 1989). Because this guideline was validated on a younger population, it should not be relied upon as the sole clinical indicator for use of pharmacological interventions in the management of alcohol withdrawal in older adults, especially those with cognitive impairment. Rather, it may be useful to rely on objective measures such as vital sign instability to tailor treatment (Wan et al., 2012), although it is important to consider that dehydration, anxiety, and medications such as beta-blockers (Zechnich, 1982) can all potentially alter vital signs and obscure the diagnosis of delirium tremens. It is important to consider the entire clinical picture when treating alcohol withdrawal in older adults.

Many medications have been considered potentially helpful for treating alcohol withdrawal but the current "gold standard" of treatment is use of benzodiazepines. One should be judicious with the use of medication to treat alcohol withdrawal such that enough is used to treat signs and symptoms of withdrawal, with careful monitoring of the patient's condition through frequent measurement of vital signs, physical examinations, and review of symptoms, but not enough to overly sedate the patient and increase the risk of associated morbidity. Because older adults tend to be on a number of medications, medication interactions should be considered prior to initiating treatment.

Three commonly used benzodiazepines used to treat alcohol withdrawal are diazepam (half-life 20–100+ hours), chlordiazepoxide (half-life 5–30 hours), and lorazepam (half-life 9–16 hours). Traditionally, diazepam and chlordiazepoxide have been used because they require less frequent dosing and lead to fewer interdose symptoms. However the pharmacokinetics of these medications is altered not only as people age but also by hepatic dysfunction.

As it is relatively short acting and is metabolized via glucuronidation in the liver, lorazepam is the benzodiazepine of choice for treatment of alcohol withdrawal in older adults. It may be necessary to utilize longer acting benzodiazepines to prevent potential lapses in prophylactic coverage in those older adults who have a history of delirium tremens or withdrawal seizure (Wan et al., 2012).

Barbiturates can be used in a monitored setting if benzodiazepines have failed, but the risk is higher for respiratory depression and sedation, and because barbiturates are fat-soluble, they tend to be processed more slowly by older adults, who tend to have larger fat reservoirs. There are some promising data to suggest that anticonvulsants may be beneficial in treating alcohol withdrawal, either as a stand-alone option or as an adjunct to a benzodiazepine; however, there are limited prospective data on older adults at this time.

BENZODIAZEPINE ABUSE IN OLDER ADULTS

Epidemiology

Benzodiazepines comprise up to 23% of all prescriptions for older adults, which is the age group most prescribed benzodiazepines (Center for Substance Abuse Treatment, 1998). They are commonly prescribed in dosages exceeding recommended amounts for older adults. In nursing homes, these trends are amplified as the majority of residents receive benzodiazepines. Despite these tendencies, clinicians and academicians have lamented the fact that there is not enough research on benzodiazepines use in older adults, despite significant research on alcohol use.

It has long been known that older adults have increased sensitivity to benzodiaz-epines and slower metabolism of longer-acting agents. In general, all benzodiazepines increase risk of cognitive impairment, delirium, falls, fractures, and motor vehicle accidents in older adults. The Beers criteria, in particular, recommend the avoidance of benzodiazepines of any type for insomnia, agitation, or delirium in older patients; this leaves only seizure disorders, REM sleep disorders, benzodiazepine withdrawal, alcohol withdrawal, severe generalized anxiety disorder, periprocedural anesthesia, and end-of-life care as recommended uses of benzodiazepines in older adults (American Geriatrics Society, 2012).

Sleep disturbances are the most common indications for benzodiazepine pre-scriptions in older adults, comprising up to 59% of prescriptions (Bourgeois et al., 2012). Half of older adults report sleep problems. Risk factors for sleep disorders in older adults include female gender, single status, widowed or divorced, pluripathol-ogy, poor health, Alzheimer's disease, and psychotropic consumption. Pathophysiol-ogy of the increase in sleep disorders in older adults is hypothesized to be related to the decreased activity of the suprachiasmatic nucleus, contributing to the disruption of circadian rhythms in older adults, including the nocturnal secretion of endogenous melatonin. Another hypothesis attributes a significant role to the prescriptions given to older adults, in particular stimulants, antihypertensives, respiratory medications, chemotherapy, and decongestants, which all have been noted to cause insomnia (Nei-krug & Ancoli-Israel, 2010).

Anxiety is the second most common indication for benzodiazepine prescriptions in the older adults, with up to 17% of prescriptions for benzodiazepines having this indication (Bourgeois et al., 2012). More surprising is the finding that almost 50% of older adults are prescribed chronic benzodiazepines for anxiety disorder in the absence of concomitant antidepressant prescriptions, despite clear indications that benzodiazepines are not the preferred long-term treatment (Uchida et al., 2009). Risk factors for anxiety disorder in older adults include female gender, low socioeconomic status, family history, external locus of control, current level of perceived stress, poor primary support, and poor social support.

Problematic use of prescription drugs by older adults is usually unintentional, which makes statistical studies on the prevalence of abuse difficult. But the large number of hospitalizations as a result of the misuse of those medications is troubling. At the same time, increased and chronic use of benzodiazepines is associated with increased risk of hip fractures, and chronic use has been related to poor long-term health outcomes. Older adults with dementia, hypoalbuminemia, or chronic renal failure have been shown to be more prone to these adverse effects of benzodiazepines (Bogunovic & Greenfield, 2004).

Screening

Clinicians and patients may not recognize somnolence and fatigue as adverse effects but rather as a common process in aging. Cognitive impairment caused by benzodi-azepines may as well be dismissed as being secondary to age. Diagnostically, with-drawal from benzodiazepines can be misinterpreted by family members as an indica-tion of more severe dementia, requiring more benzodiazepines for agitation.

Prevention of misdiagnoses that lead to the prescription of benzodiazepines is essential. In particular, sleep disorders in older adults may easily be misdiagnosed. Sleep-disordered breathing and periodic limb movement syndromes are two common disorders of older adults for which nonbenzodiazepine evidence-based treatments exist. When symptoms suggest sleep-disordered breathing—high snoring severity, unintentional napping, and/or excessive daytime sleepiness—an overnight recording of the apnea–hypopnea index should be obtained. When the assessment suggests periodic limb movement disorder, an overnight polysomnogram with a calculated period limb movement index may be obtained (Neikrug & Ancoli-Israel, 2010).

Treatment, Including Alternatives in the Management of Sleep and Anxiety

There is little research on the appropriate methods to treat withdrawal, or to taper benzodiazepines, which are specific to older adults. However multisubstance studies indicate that older adults generally have better functional outcomes than do younger patients treated for substance abuse. Interestingly, some communities have enacted wide substance abuse programs targeting, in part, benzodiazepines abuse with individual and family counseling, recommendations about medication changes, and involvement in a peer support/education group. The results of these programs include reductions in depression, drug use, and hospital days, as well as hospital stays (Brennan, Nichol, & Moos, 2003).

In the management of insomnia in older adults, a variety of medications have been used, including antihistamines, antidepressants, anticonvulsants, and antipsychotics. More recently nonbenzodiazepine sedatives such as zolpidem have been shown to be safe and effective in older adults. However, despite their significant benefit in reducing abuse and treating sleep, they may lead to as many fractures, falls, and delirium (Finkle et al., 2011). Trazodone may also be considered an advantageous alternative, because it has a less anticholinergic effect but is sedating through antihistamine and alpha$_1$ blockade.

In 2005, the National Institutes of Health (NIH) declared that the risk of medicating primary insomnia in older adults outweighed the benefits; hence, numerous nonpharmaceutical tools have been studied that have significant impact on the sleep of older adults. For most older adults with primary insomnia, improvement of sleep hygiene is crucial. For older adults in nursing homes, several tools (e.g., limiting naps, adjusting medications, avoiding stimulants such as coffee, environmental improvements, examining sleep problems, and initiating specific treatment) have been shown to improve sleep. However, the high level of nighttime noise and ambient light in nursing homes may make the implementation of those tools more difficult. Finally, considering treatment for other common causes of insomnia in older adults is essential, including bright light therapy for circadian rhythm shifts, continuous positive airway pressure for sleep-disordered breathing, and dopamine agonist for restless legs syndrome or periodic limb movement disorder.

For the treatment of anxiety, several studies have questioned the lack of use of selective serotonin reuptake inhibitors (SSRIs) and serotonin–norepinephrine reuptake inhibitors (SNRIs) in older adults who are instead prescribed benzodiazepines, despite documented evidence of adverse effects of chronic benzodiazepine use. Nonetheless, the Beers criteria do point to risk associated with falls and SSRIs, and other studies point to their propensity to cause hyponatremia in older adults. More recently, a small randomized clinical trial demonstrated that both sertraline and buspirone appear effective and well tolerated in the treatment of anxiety in older adults (Mokhber, Azarpazhooh, Khajehdaluee, Velayati, & Hopwood, 2010). Pregabalin has also been shown to be a safe and effective alternative to benzodiazepines in the management of anxiety in older adults (Montgomery, Chatamra, Pauer, Whalen, & Baldinetti, 2008). Concerning nonpharmacological methods, conflicting data exists on the importance of cognitive-behavioral therapy, physical therapy, and other behavior approaches.

OPIATE ABUSE IN OLDER ADULTS

Epidemiology

As noted by the U.S. Department of Health, a large share of prescriptions for older adults are for psychoactive, mood-changing drugs that carry the potential for misuse, abuse, or dependency, including opiates. Opiates are also at risk of being prescribed by the multiple providers of older adults. Of older adults in the United States, 11.6% use opiates. In terms of abuse, opiates are second only to alcohol in older adults, accounting for up to 22% of inpatients admissions for substance abuse in older adults (Current Comment, 2003). Furthermore, older adults make up a large portion of patients receiving treatment for opiate abuse, and as much as one-third in some centers (Addiction Treatment Forum, 2003).

Chronic pain, which often leads to prescription of opiates, is widespread in older adults, with some studies indicating that the majority of older adults suffer from chronic pain, and up to 80% among those institutionalized (Lunde, Nordhus, & Pallesen, 2009). Despite these figures and the concern for opiate dependence, pain continues to be undertreated in older adults. At this time, there is no evidence for the long-term effectiveness of opiates for persistent, noncancerous pain conditions in older patients.

Opiates are found to be the psychoactive prescription most likely to lead to hospitalization for an adverse drug event in older adults. This is worrisome, because older adults comprise the age group most likely to die from opiate use and misuse due to poorer tolerance of its adverse effects. Commonly, respiratory depression is found to be the culprit of poor outcome and death.

Screening

In the assessment of pain, research indicates that cognitive impairment does not weaken validity of self-reported pain (Parmelee, Smith, & Katz, 1993). Nonetheless, tools have been developed to address pain appropriately, including that of older adults, such as the Screener and Opioid Assessment for Patients with Pain—Revised (SOAPP-R), which includes assessment of abuse potential. SOAPP-R has been recommended for use by the American Geriatrics Society (Butler, Fernandez, Benoit, Budman, & Jamison, 2008).

Treatment, Including Alternatives in the Management of Pain

Some communities have enacted wide substance abuse programs that in part target opiate-abusing individuals and families, recommend medication changes, and advocate involvement in a peer support/education group. The results of these programs include reduction of depression, drug use, and hospital days, as well as hospital stays (Brymer & Rusnell, 2000). In addition, others have examined the use of methadone as is commonly used in younger adults, and found that older adults were no different than their younger counterparts in terms of medical and psychiatric problems or employment, but did significantly better in treatment (Firoz & Carlson, 2004). These results are expected to translate in studies on naltrexone and buprenorphine. Despite these better outcomes, older methadone clients experience stigma associated with drug addiction, old age, psychotropic medication use, depression, poverty, race, and HIV status. These stigmas are believed to act as barriers to treatment, along with the pace of treatment interventions.

For the treatment of acute opiate withdrawal, few practitioners have enacted a specific regimen for older adults. Nonetheless, specialists tend to adjust utilization of medications considering risks associated with other general medical conditions, as well as greater blood pressure liability. In particular, clonidine is used in moderation and close attention is given to vital parameters and older adults' tolerability.

The treatment of pain in older adults is a complex problem due to medical comorbidities, the barriers to diagnosis, and the lack of obvious solutions. Alternatives to opiates can have significant adverse effects, in particular nonsteroidal anti-inflammatory drugs (NSAIDs), whose gastropathy often cause poor outcomes. Thus, the American Geriatric Society cautions about judicious use of NSAIDs, and instead recommends the prescription acetaminophen as the first line of treatment for pain in older adults (American Geriatrics Society Panel on Pharmacological Management of Persistent Pain in Older Persons, 2009). Despite some evidence for their effectiveness in the treatment of pain, tricyclics are considered to have significant adverse effects in the older population. SNRIs, as well as gabapentin and pregabalin, are considered more appropriate and may constitute a second-line agent or additional tool in combination with acetaminophen.

ABUSE OF OTHER SUBSTANCES IN OLDER ADULTS

Studies have confirmed that even in old age, use of alcohol increases rate of other substance use, and up to 15% of drug users had two or more drugs in the past year (Blazer & Wu, 2009). Stimulants and other substances, such as hallucinogens, are not well studied in older adults, but some researchers have attempted assess their prevalence rates. Blazer and Wu found that in their study population of persons age 50 and older, 0.41% were cocaine users. The other substances had very low prevalence:

0.11% used inhalants, 0.10% used hallucinogens, 0.11% used methamphetamine, and 0.05% used heroin. The data suggest that while use of non-alcohol illicit substances has low prevalence rates, over time, use will increase and require special attention by the clinician.

Older adults are less likely to quit smoking, and rates of use have not declined over time (Kleykamp & Heishman, 2011). It is also reported that older adults with nicotine dependence have comorbid anxiety and substance abuse, and even those without nicotine dependence have high rates of dependency symptoms (Sachs-Ericsson, Collins, Schmidt, & Zvolensky, 2011). Despite this, older smokers often receive suboptimal care and low rates of intervention. There are misconceptions about the smoking in older adults that need to be addressed by clinicians at all levels. Beliefs such as quitting smoking in older age has no benefit, smoking can help with chronic pain, or tobacco may help with mood or cognition problems should be avoided (Shi, Hooten, & Warner, 2011). Common pharmacological treatments for smoking cessation are nicotine replacement, bupropion, and varenicline. Although there have not been specific studies of their use in older populations, their effectiveness and dangers have been well documented. The most widely publicized adverse effect, suicidal behavior, needs to be kept in mind. Currently, it is believed that varenicline produces the highest risk of depression and suicidal behavior, followed by lower risk for bupropion and the lowest risk for nicotine (T. J. Moore, Furberg, Glenmullen, Maltsberger, & Singh, 2011). As the older adult population ages, it will be important to maintain keen vigilance over continuing tobacco use and provide optimal screening, prevention, and treatment modalities.

The use of marijuana is predicted to increase as the younger cohort ages. Blazer and Wu (2009) reported that while only 0.7% of persons age 65 and up use marijuana, this rate goes up to 4.0% in those between ages 50 and 64. DiNitto and Choi (2011) found that up to 23% of the younger older adult cohort (ages 50–64) had usage rate of at least half the days of the year and significantly higher psychological distress scores. These data indicate that as the younger older adult cohort population becomes older, the prevalence of marijuana use will increase. While there are studies showing adverse effects of marijuana use in adolescents and adulthood, the available data are insufficient to determine how its use impacts the older population. Even so, some studies specifically seem to implicate worse health outcome in the older adult population with use of marijuana. Aryana and Williams (2007) found marijuana use can potentially increase risk of myocardial infarction in older adults. Discovery of an endogenous cannabinoid system and evidence of it regulating neurodegenerative processes have led some to study whether marijuana can help to interrupt the pathological process in Alzheimer's disease. A Cochrane review on this issue indicates that no current evidence supports the effectiveness of cannabinoids in dementia treatment (Krishnan, Cairns, & Howard, 2009). While the number of studies on effective treatment of marijuana dependence is low, it is reported that behavioral treatments such as motivational enhancement therapy, cognitive-behavioral therapy, and contingency management are somewhat effective (Budney, Roffman, Stephens, & Walker, 2007). In summary, there is no evidence to suggest benefit of marijuana use in older adults' health, and negative impact of its use has been reported. Clinicians should routinely assess for marijuana use in the older adult population.

CONCLUSIONS

The population is aging, and as the younger cohort moves into older age, the prevalence of substance abuse and dependence will increase. Younger individuals have higher acceptance and use rates of substances, and the long-term effects of their use will become evident in the next decade. As the population ages, it is important to note the barriers to effective and efficient prevention, screening, and treatment of substance use in the older population. These barriers exist in forms of clinical and public ageism, poor understanding of the impact of substances, inadequate resources for tailored treatment access, and insufficient research information and data on older adult substance users. There is a need for increased clinical outreach and research on this increasingly emerging issue.

REFERENCES

Adams, W. L., Barry, K. L., & Fleming, M. F. (1996). Screening for problem drinking in older primary care patients. *JAMA, 276,* 1964–1967.

American Geriatrics Society. (2012). Beers Criteria Update Expert Panel: American Geriatrics Society updated Beers Criteria for potentially inappropriate medication use in older adults. *J Am Geriatr Soc, 60,* 616–631.

American Geriatrics Society Panel on Pharmacological Management of Persistent Pain in Older Persons. (2009). Pharmacological management of persistent pain in older persons. *J Am Geriatr Soc, 57,* 1331–1346.

American Psychiatric Association. (2013). *Diagnostic and statistical manual of mental disorders* (5th ed.). Arlington, VA: Author.

Aryana, A., & Williams, M. A. (2007). Marijuana as a trigger of cardiovascular events: Speculation or scientific certainty? *Int J Cardiol, 118,* 141–144.

Barrick, C., & Connors, G. J. (2002). Relapse prevention and maintaining abstinence in older adults with alcohol-use disorders. *Drugs Aging, 19*(8), 583–594.

Blazer, D. G., & Wu, L.-T. (2009). The epidemiology of substance use and disorders among middle aged and elderly community adults: National Survey on Drug Use and Health (NSDUH). *Am J Geriatr Psychiatry, 17*(3), 237–245.

Blow, F. C., Brockmann, L. M., & Barry, K. L. (2004). Role of alcohol in late-life suicide. *Alcohol Clin Exp Res, 28,* 48S–56S.

Blow, F. C., Walton, M. A., Chermack, S. T., Mudd, S. A., & Brower, K. J. (2000). Older adult treatment outcome following elder-specific inpatient alcoholism treatment. *J Subst Abuse Treat, 19,* 67–75.

Bogunovic, O. J., & Greenfield, S. F. (2004). Practical geriatrics: Use of benzodiazepines among elderly patients. *Psychiatr Serv, 55,* 233–235.

Bourgeois, J., Elseviers, M. M., Azermai, M., Van Bortel, L., Petrovic, M., & Vander Stichele, R. R. (2012). Benzodiazepine use in Belgian nursing homes: A closer look into indications and dosages. *Eur J Clin Pharmacol, 68,* 833–844.

Brennan, P. L., Nichol, A. C., & Moos, R. H. (2003). Older and younger patients with substance use disorders: Outpatient mental health service use and functioning over a 12-month interval. *Psychol Addict Behav, 17,* 42–48.

Breslow, R. A., & Smothers, B. (2004). Drinking patterns of older Americans: National Health Interview Surveys 1997–2001. *J Stud Alcohol, 65*(2), 232–240.

Brower, K. J., & Hall, J. M. (2001). Effects of age and alcoholism on sleep: A controlled study. *J Stud Alcohol, 62,* 335–343.

Brymer, C., & Rusnell, I. (2000). Reducing substance dependence in elderly people: The side effects program. *Can J Clin Pharmacol, 7,* 161–166.

Budney, A. J., Roffman, R., Stephens, R. S., & Walker, D. (2007). Marijuana dependence and its treatment. *Addict Sci Clin Pract, 4,* 4–16.

Butler, S. F., Fernandez, K., Benoit, C., Budman, S. H., & Jamison, R. N. (2008). Validation of the revised Screener and Opioid Assessment for Patients with Pain (SOAPP-R). *J Pain, 9,* 360–372.

Caputo, F., Vignoli, T., Leggio, L., Addolorato, G., Zoli, G., & Bernardi, M. (2012). Alcohol use disorders in the elderly: A brief overview from epidemiology to treatment options. *Exp Gerontol, 47*(6), 411–416.

Center for Substance Abuse Treatment. (1998). Substance abuse among older adults (TIP Series, No. 26). Rockville, MD: Substance Abuse and Mental Health Services Administration.

Clay, S. W. (1997), Comparison of the AUDIT and CAGE questionnaires in screening for alcohol use disorders in elderly primary care outpatients. *J Am Osteopath Assoc, 10,* 588–592.

Crome, I., Dar, K. Janikiewicz, S., Rao, T., & Tarbuck, A. (Eds.). (2011, June). *Our invisible addicts: First report of the Older Persons' Substance Misuse Working Group of the Royal College of Psychiatrists* (College Report CR 165). London: Royal College of Psychiatry.

Current comments—the further "graying of methadone." (2003). *Addiction Treatment Forum, 12,* 4–5.

Devanand, D. P. (2002). Comorbid psychiatric disorders in late life depression. *Biol Psychiatry, 52,* 236–242.

DiNitto, D. M., & Choi, N. G. (2011). Marijuana use among older adults in the USA: User characteristics, patterns of use, and implications for intervention. *Int Psychogeriatr, 23*(5), 732–741.

Finkle, W. D., Der, J. S., Greenland, S., Adams, J. L., Ridgeway, G., Blaschke, T., et al. (2011). Risk of fractures requiring hospitalization after an initial prescription for zolpidem, alprazolam, lorazepam, or diazepam in older adults. *J Am Geriatr Soc, 59,* 1883–1890.

Firoz, S., & Carlson, G. (2004). Characteristics and treatment outcome of older methadone-maintenance patients. *Am J Geriatr Psychiatry, 12,* 539–541.

Fleming, M. F., Manwell, L. B., Barry, K. L., Adams, W., & Stauffacher, E. A. (1999). Brief physician advice for alcohol problems in older adults: A randomized community-based trial. *J Fam Pract, 48,* 378–384.

Gfroerer, J., Penne, M., Pemberton, M., & Folsom, R. (2003). Substance abuse treatment need among older adults in 2020: The impact of the aging baby-boom cohort. *Drug Alcohol Depend, 69,* 127–135.

Gomberg, E. S. (2003). Treatment for alcohol-related problems: Special populations: Research opportunities. *Recent Dev Alcohol, 16,* 313–333.

Gordon, A. J., Conigliaro, J., Maisto, A. A., McNeil, M., Kraemer, K. L., & Kelley, M. E. (2003). Comparisons of consumption effects of brief interventions for hazardous drinking elderly. *Subst Use Misuse, 38,* 1017–1035.

Kirchner, J. E., Zubritsky, C., Cody, M., Coakley, E., Chen, H., Ware, J. H., et al. (2007). Consumption among older adults in primary care. *J Gen Intern Med, 22,* 92–97.

Kleykamp & Heishman. (2011). The older smoker. *JAMA, 306*(8), 876–877.

Krishnan, S., Cairns, R., & Howard, R. (2009). Cannabinoids for the treatment of dementia (Review). *Cochrane Database Syst Rev, 2,* CD007204.

Lin, J. C., Karno, M. P., Tang, L., Barry, K. L., Blow, F. C., Davis, J. W., et al. (2010). Do health educator telephone calls reduce at-risk drinking among older adults in primary care? *J Gen Intern Med, 25,* 334–339.

Lunde, L. H., Nordhus, I. H., & Pallesen, S. (2009). The effectiveness of cognitive and behavioural treatment of chronic pain in the elderly: A quantitative review. *J Clin Psychol Med Settings, 16,* 254–262.

Mackenzie, C. S., Reynolds, K., Chou, K. L., Pagura, J., & Sareen, J. (2011). Prevalence and correlates of generalized anxiety disorder in a national sample of older adults. *Am J Geriatr Psychiatry, 19,* 305–315.

Mokhber, N., Azarpazhooh, M. R., Khajehdaluee, M., Velayati, A., & Hopwood, M. (2010). Randomized, single-blind, trial of sertraline and buspirone for treatment of elderly patients with generalized anxiety disorder. *Psychiatry Clin Neurosci, 64,* 128–133.

Montgomery, S., Chatamra, K., Pauer, L., Whalen, E., & Baldinetti, F. (2008). Efficacy and safety of pregabalin in elderly people with generalised anxiety disorder. *Br J Psychiatry, 193,* 389–394.

Moore, A. A., Beck, J. C., Babor, T. F., Hays, R. D., & Reuben, D. B. (2002). Beyond alcoholism: identifying older, at-risk drinkers in primary care. *J Stud Alcohol, 63,* 316–324.

Moore, A. A., Blow, F. C., Hoffing, M., Welgreen, S., Davis, J. W., Lin, J. C., et al. (2011). Primary care-based intervention to reduce at-risk drinking in older adults: A randomized controlled trial. *Addiction, 106,* 111–120.

Moore, A. A., Seeman, T., Morgenstern, H., Beck, J. C., & Reuben, D. B. (2002). Are there differences between older persons who screen positive on the CAGE questionnaire and the Short Michigan Alcoholism Screening Test—Geriatric Version? *J Am Geriatr Soc, 50,* 858–862.

Moore, T. J., Furberg, C. D., Glenmullen, J., Maltsberger, J. T., & Singh, S. (2011). Suicidal behavior and depression in smoking cessation. *PLoS ONE, 6*(11), e27016.

Mukamal, K. J., Mittleman, M. A., Longstreth, W. T., Jr., Newman, A. B., Fried, L. P., & Siscovick, D. S. (2004). Self-reported alcohol consumption and falls in older adults: Cross-sectional and longitudinal analyses of the cardiovascular health study. *J Am Geriatr Soc, 52,* 1174–1179.

National Institute on Alcohol Abuse and Alcoholism. (n.d.). Alcohol and aging (Alcohol Alert No. 40). Retrieved from *http://pubs.niaaa.nih.gov/publications/aa40.htm.*

National Institutes of Health. (2005). National Institutes of Health State of the Science Conference statement on Manifestations and Management of Chronic Insomnia in Adults, June 13–15, 2005. *Sleep, 28,* 1049–1057.

Neikrug, A. B., & Ancoli-Israel, S. (2010). Sleep disorders in the older adult—a mini-review. *Gerontology, 56,* 181–189.

Oscar-Berman, M., & Schendan, H. E. (2000). Asymmetries of brain function in alcoholism: Relationship to aging. In L. Obler & L. T. Connor (Eds.), *Neurobehavior of language and cognition: Studies of normal aging and brain damage* (pp. 213–240). New York: Kluwer Academic.

Oslin, D. W., Cary, M., Slaymaker, V., Colleran, C., & Blow, F. C. (2009). Daily ratings measures of alcohol craving during an inpatient stay define subtypes of alcohol addiction that predict subsequent risk for resumption of drinking. *Drug Alcohol Depend, 103,* 131–136.

Oslin, D. W., Grantham, S., Coakley, E., Maxwell, J., Miles, K., Ware, J., et al. (2006). PRISM-E: Comparison of integrated care and enhanced specialty referral in managing at-risk alcohol use. *Psychiatric Serv, 57,* 954–958.

Oslin, D., Liberto, J. G., O'Brien, J., & Krois, S. (1997). Tolerability of naltrexone in treating older, alcohol-dependent patients. *Am J Addict, 6,* 266–270.

Oslin, D., Liberto, J. G., O'Brien, J., Krois, S., & Norbeck, J. (1997). Naltrexone as an adjunctive treatment for older patients with alcohol dependence. *Am J Geriatr Psychiatry, 5,* 324–332.

Parmelee, P. A., Smith, B., & Katz, I. R. (1993). Pain complaints and cognitive status among elderly institution residents. *J Am Geriatr Soc, 41,* 517–522.

Parsons, O. A., & Nixon, S. J. (1993). Neurobehavioral sequelae of alcoholism. *Neurol Clin, 11,* 205–218.

Pettinati, H. M., O'Brien, C. P., Rabinowitz, A. R., Wortman, S. P., Oslin, D. W., Kampman, K. M., et al. (2006). The status of naltrexone in the treatment of alcohol dependence: Specific effects on heavy drinking. *J Clin Psychopharmacol, 26,* 610–625.

Sachs-Ericsson, N., Collins, N., Schmidt, B., & Zvolensky, M. (2011). Older adults and smoking:

Characteristics, nicotine dependence and prevalence of DSM-IV 12-month disorders. *Aging Ment Health, 15*(1), 132–141.

Shi, Y., Hooten, M., & Warner, D. O. (2011). Effects of smoking cessation on pain in older adults. *Nicotine Tobacco Res, 13*(10), 919–925.

Simoni-Wastila, L., & Yang, H. K. (2006). Psychoactive drug abuse in older adults. *Am J Geriatr Pharmacother, 4*, 380–394.

Sullivan, J. T., Sykora, K., Schneiderman, J., Naranjo, C. A., & Sellers, E. M. (1989). Assessment of alcohol withdrawal: the revised clinical institute withdrawal assessment for alcohol scale (CIWA-Ar). *Br J Addict, 84*, 1353–1357.

Uchida, H., Suzuki, T., Mamo, D. C., Mulsant, B. H., Kikuchi, T., Takeuchi, H., et al. (2009). Benzodiazepine and antidepressant use in elderly patients with anxiety disorders: A survey of 796 outpatients in Japan. *J Anxiety Disord, 23*, 477–481.

U.S. Census Bureau. (2012). *The 2010 Statistical Abstract of the United States.* Washington, DC: Author.

U.S. Department of Health and Human Services. (2000). *Special Report to the U.S Congress on Alcohol and Health: Highlights from current research* (NIH Publication No. 00-1583). Washington, DC: National Institutes of Health, National Institute on Alcohol Abuse and Alcoholism.

U.S. Preventive Services Task Force. (2004). Screening and behavioral counseling interventions in primary care to reduce alcohol misuse: Recommendation statement. *Ann Intern Med, 140*, 554–556.

Wagman, A. M., Allen, R. P., & Upright, D. (1977). Effects of alcohol consumption upon parameters of ultradian sleep rhythms in alcoholics. *Adv Exp Med Biol, 85A*, 601–616.

Wan, S.-H., Kyomen, H. H., Catic, A. G., & Tan, Z. S. (2012). Identification and management of alcohol abuse and withdrawal in elders. *Clin Geriatr, 20*, 28–34.

Zechnich, R. J. (1982). Beta blockers can obsure diagnosis of delirium tremens. *Lancet, 8*, 1071–1072.

CHAPTER 22

HIV/AIDS and Substance Use Disorders

CHERYL ANN KENNEDY
STEVEN J. SCHLEIFER

Since human immunodeficiency virus/acquired immune deficiency syndrome (HIV/AIDS) erupted in a pandemic in 1981, it has been the focus of attention and remains a serious global public health threat. By 2013, an estimated 35 million persons were living with HIV/AIDS (PLWHA) worldwide, up 17% from 2001, representing new HIV infections and the effect of significant expansion of antiretroviral therapy (ART). Of people ages 15–24 years, HIV prevalence declined in most of the 24 countries with national prevalence of 1% or higher. An estimated 12.9 million people receive HIV treatment. Decreasing AIDS-related deaths and more PLWHA living longer and productive lives is a consequence of expanded treatment. Over 2.5 million AIDS-related deaths have been avoided since 1995 due to ART according to calculations by the United Nations Programme on HIV/AIDS (UNAIDS, 2014). Global trends hide important regional and cultural variations. Impressive as the overall gains are, only a handful of countries have achieved levels of HIV service coverage needed eventually to halt the epidemic (UNAIDS, 2014). Since 2000, the annual number of new AIDS diagnoses has remained fairly constant. The Centers for Disease Control and Prevention (CDC; 2012a) estimated that by the end of 2011, there were 1.3 million PLWHA in the United States, an increase from 2006. Of the new U.S. HIV infections in 2009, 9% were injection drug users (IDUs; CDC, 2012b), reflecting a significant reduction. About 75% of adults and adolescents living with AIDS are men, and researchers warn that sex partnerships with IDUs continue to be an understudied network-level risk factor for heterosexual HIV infection. Heterosexuals with no injection history who partner with IDUs are more than twice as likely to be HIV-infected; sex partnerships with IDUs play an important role in heterosexual HIV transmission in areas with large IDU populations (Jenness, Neaigus, Hagan, Murrill, & Wendell, 2012).

HIV/AIDS continues to affect minorities in the United States disproportionately, primarily African Americans and Latinos, who constitute 58% of the AIDS cases reported since 1981. IDU is a major factor in the spread of HIV in minority communities. Other factors include men who have sex with men (MSM) and heterosexual transmission. AIDS is the leading cause of death among African American men ages 25–44 (National Institute of Allergy and Infectious Diseases [NIAID], 2012). Links are clear between substance use and high-risk behaviors in non-injection drug user (NIDU) men and women, especially for stimulant users (Young & Shoptaw, 2013). Use of methamphetamine and other stimulants contribute to sexually risky behaviors, no matter the user's sexual orientation. A strong link exists between sexual risk and methamphetamine use in MSM, and among some heterosexual adults and youth. In 2010, the number of new infections in MSM showed a significant 12% increase from 2008. More troubling is that MSM represent about 4% of U.S. males, and in 2010 they accounted for 78% of new HIV infections in men and 63% of all new infections. The greatest increase in transmission rates in MSM occurred in the group ages 13–24 years (CDC, 2012a).

NIDUs of mind-altering substances (alcohol, other sedatives, stimulants, club and designer drugs) play an increasing, albeit less direct, role in HIV risk and disease progression. Impaired states influence sexual behavior and lead to risky practices that increase risk of HIV exposure. Once HIV is introduced into a community of IDUs, spread is ordinarily rapid. Drug-using populations fuel the epidemic around the world, and there is evidence that these individuals are at higher risk for accelerated and more severe neurocognitive dysfunction compared to non drug-using HIV-infected populations (Nath et al., 2002).

SUBSTANCE USE, PSYCHOSOCIAL STRESSORS, AND IMMUNE EFFECTS

Psychoactive substances can have immunosuppressive effects that increase infection risk or further compromise those with HIV (Palepu et al., 2003). Extensive psychosocial assessments have found associations between specific stressors, depression, and the course of HIV disease. Psychological distress was independently associated with shorter time to AIDS among HIV-infected IDUs, especially those with the lowest CD4 counts (Golub et al., 2003). The strongest predictor of poor adherence and lack of viral suppression in an ART adherence study of current and former drug users was active cocaine use. Depressive symptoms and use of alcohol or drugs to cope were predictive of nonadherence (Arsten et al., 2002). A longitudinal study of HIV-positive drug and alcohol users found strong temporal association of ART adherence and viral suppression when users switched to nonuse (Lucas, Gebo, Chaisson, & Moore 2002). Interventions to treat affective disorders in substance users may have both medical and psychosocial benefits.

NEUROCOGNITIVE AND NEUROPSYCHIATRIC COMPLICATIONS

Neurocognitive and neuropsychiatric disorders can develop in those with HIV at almost any point, whether they are symptomatic or not. Confounding signs and symptoms can arise from primary HIV infection; treatment side effects; comorbid conditions, including psychiatric disorders, substance use disorders (SUDs), or coinfection with hepatitis C virus (HCV); or other infections. As an aging demographic, HIV-infected people are confronting the chronic illnesses of older adults, including cardiovascular disease, diabetes, arthritis, dementia, and neoplasms. During 2005 in the United States, 15% of new infections and 24% of the HIV-positive population over 33 states were age 50 years or older (Althoff et al., 2010). Neuropsychiatric complications with cognitive, affective, and behavioral symptoms can be manifestations of HIV in the central nervous system (CNS): decline in motor function, executive skills, and information processing speed. These neurocognitive signs are the first sign of AIDS in 7–20% and impairment increases as the disease progresses (Reger, Welsh, Razani, Martin, & Boone, 2002). The neuropsychiatric impact can range from subtle signs to severe global impairment.

It is estimated that over 1 million persons in the United States have HIV-associated neurocognitive dysfunction (HAND; Ances, 2008). Neurologists group HAND in a hierarchy of severity of patterns of CNS involvement from asymptomatic neurocognitive impairment to minor neurocognitive disorder, to the more severe HIV-associated dementia (HAD). HAD is the same as AIDS dementia complex and HIV encephalopathy. The incidence of HAND is decreasing since ART, but prevalence continues to be high, and despite adequate immune suppression and virologic control, in some, neurocognitive disorders may persist (McArthur, Steiner, Sacktor, & Nath, 2010; Simioni et al., 2010). Dementia may be increasing in PLWHA, and HAND may now be the most common form of "young-age" dementia globally (Wright et al., 2008; Koutsilieri, Scheller, Sopper, ter Meulen & Riederer, 2002).

Although the Mini-Mental State Exam (Folstein, Folstein, & McHugh,1975) screens for cortical dementia, it should not be used alone, but with other simple tests that screen for the subcortical signs associated with HIV, such as poor performance on tests of movement, coordination, attention, concentration, mental flexibility, and reaction time. The HIV Dementia Scale (HDS; Power, Selnes, Grim, & McArthur, 1995) and the International Dementia Scale (Sacktor et al., 2005) are effective for rapid screening of the deficits associated with HIV. Deficits are best localized by neuropsychological testing and results can be used for design of remediation strategies (Antinori et al., 2007). Cognitive complaints may be a sign of depression (Vance, Ross, & Downs, 2008).

Differentiating the CNS effects of chronic drug and alcohol use is confounded by overlap of signs and symptoms with HIV neurocognitive deficits. Abnormal findings in attention, concentration, dexterity, language, verbal and nonverbal memory, sensory processing, abstraction, and problem solving have been demonstrated with chronic alcohol, cocaine, opiate, and polysubstance abuse (Ling, Compton, Rawson, & Wesson, 1996; DeRonchi et al., 2002). Persistent users of cannabis show neurocognitive decline over the lifespan from childhood to midlife (Meier et al., 2012).

Neuropathological studies comparing HIV-positive substance users to nonusers indicate marked severity of HIV encephalitis in users (Bell, Brettle, Chiswick, & Simmonds, 1998; Anthony, Arango, Stephens, Simmonds, & Bell, 2008), with significant loss of dopaminergic neurons in the substantia nigra (Reyes, Faraldi, Senseng, Flowers, & Fariello, 1991). Most drugs of abuse activate dopamine, and that destabilization yields a synergistic neurotoxicity when combined with HIV (Nath et al., 2002). Alcohol dependence has an additive effect on the cognitive deficits associated with HIV and, alcohol, like HIV, induces inflammatory processes in the brain leading to neurodegeneration that is likely driven by oxidative stress, overproduction of pro-inflammatory factors, and impairment of the blood–brain barrier and glutamate-associated neurotoxicity (Persidsky et al., 2011). HIV-associated neurotoxicity is comparable to that mediated by alcohol.

Evidence shows residual changes in serotonin and dopamine transmission in Ecstasy (3,4-methylenedioxymethamphetamine [MDMA]) users, with persistent functional deficits after periods of abstinence. Most consistent findings link MDMA with subtle cognitive impairments in memory and in motor and cognitive performance (Gouzoulis-Mayfrank & Daumann, 2009). Accurate diagnosis of co-occurring disorders is paramount in managing CNS dysfunction. Those with CNS compromise are sensitive to pharmacological effects, and psychotropic medication should be used for specific symptom management or for a known psychiatric disorder at the lowest effective doses with careful monitoring. Supportive, insight-oriented psychotherapy, neuropsychoeducation, and specific interventions designed to overcome deficits and assist with adherence (phone reminder alarms for dosing, multimedication prefill boxes, calendars, etc.) may help patients, caregivers, and others with coping and adaptation.

PSYCHIATRIC DISORDERS AND SUBSTANCE USE

Depression and anxiety disproportionately affect persons with HIV infection. Study methodology, populations studied, and psychiatric diagnostic methods vary, but on point-prevalence screening, 48–54% of HIV-positive individuals are depressed or anxious (Galvan, Burnam, & Bing, 2003) and 25–40% have anxiety or depressive disorders with drug use (Bing et al., 2001; Asch et al., 2003); when diagnostic instruments are used, 5–20% have anxiety or depression (Evans & Charney, 2003; Cruess et al., 2003). We found that HIV-positive persons with psychological distress are more likely to use drugs and alcohol, and less likely to practice safer sex (Kennedy et al., 1993).

HIV–HCV CO-INFECTION, RISK-TAKING BEHAVIOR, ALCOHOLISM, AND DEPRESSION

Around 3 million people live with chronic HCV according to the CDC (2012b), and an estimated 250,000 to 300,000 people are coinfected with HCV and HIV (from using drugs) representing about 25% of all PLWHA; about 10% are coinfected with hepatitis B virus (HBV); 80% of IDUs have HCV. Chronic HCV infection is the leading cause of death, after AIDS-related complications, among HIV-infected individuals in areas where ART is available (Weber et al., 2006). HIV co-infection exacerbates HCV disease, increasing the likelihood of cirrhosis and HCV-related mortality (CDC, 2013; de Lédinghen et al., 2008; Holmberg, Ly, & Xing, & 2012). HIV-positive individuals who are co-infected with HCV can be safely treated with

Many depression screening tools have been shown to be valid and reliable, but two questions can be an effective quick screen for detecting unrecognized depression (Chichinov, Wilson, & Enns, 1994):

1. "During the past month, have you often been bothered by feeling down, depressed, or hopeless?"
2. "During the past month, have you often been bothered by little interest or pleasure in doing things?"

Symptoms associated with depression include:

- Hopelessness, helplessness
- Depressed, negative feelings, "wanting to end it all"
- Guilt, no joy in anything
- Sleep disturbance
- Appetite, weight changes
- Restlessness, slowing
- Irritability
- Attention and concentration problems.

Some patients present with poor frustration tolerance, a change in treatment adherence or functioning, interpersonal problems, and unexplained medical complaints, including cognitive complaints (investigate for impairment). Acute intoxication, overdose, or withdrawal must be ruled out. Psychiatric conditions and SUDs commonly co-occur, and clinical opportunity dictates addressing both.

interferon (INF-alpha), but need monthly depression screening while on INF. Those with a depression or psychosis history can continue regular medications with careful monitoring (CDC, 2009; Douaihy, Hilsabeck, Assam, Jain, & Daley, 2008; Cooper, Giordano, Mackie, & Mills, 2010). All coinfected individuals should receive ART as well (CDC 2012c). New direct acting antiviral drugs for HCV are showing efficacy and low toxicity with interferon free regimens (Feeney & Chung, 2014).

Increasingly, incident HCV in HIV-infected MSM is associated with sexually risky behavior (Danta & Rodger, 2011; Matthews et al., 2011). Serosorting (HIV-positive individuals having sex with others with HIV) is associated with increased sexually transmitted infections (STIs) that increase susceptibility to HCV infection. Mucosal sexual trauma is frequently associated with bleeding, impacting HCV transmission (Schmidt et.al., 2011). In subpopulations of HIV-positive MSM, certain drugs (stimulants) may be nasally or rectally administered. These drugs enhance risk-taking behavior due to disinhibition and increase in pain threshold. Stimulants and novel "designer" drugs may be more likely to be used by groups of individuals who are apt to engage in traumatic sexual practices (Darrow et al., 2005; Colfax et al., 2004).

Acute alcohol exposure has demonstrable immune effects, and chronic users may only show modest effects due to adaptation unless they have developed liver disease or other medical comorbidity (Cook, 1998; Schleifer, Keller, Shiflet, Benton, & Eckholdt, 1999). The high comorbidity of alcoholism and depressive disorders, and the documented association between depressive disorders and altered immunity (Blume,

Douglas, & Evans, 2011), suggests that the immune effects of these disorders may interact additively or synergistically. Decreased natural killer (NK) cell activity in patients with alcoholism is worse in those with comorbid major depression (Irwin et al., 1990), and our group found that comorbid depression may account for many of the immune changes in alcoholics (Schleifer, Keller, & Czaja, 2003). Alcohol consumption is associated with reduced medication adherence and less effective antiviral activity (Hendershot, Stoner, Pantalone, & Simoni, 2009).

SUBSTANCE USE AND RISK OF HIV INFECTION

Many exposure and host factors influence seroconversion and disease progression in substance users, including altered baseline host immune capacity and viral load in the HIV-positive person. The presence of host-concurrent infections, most notably viral (herpes simplex, cytomegalovirus, the hepatitides), and bacterial infections in the bloodstream (endocarditis and others) may contribute to altered immunity. Mucosal breaches (STIs, traumatic sex) afford easy entry of microorganisms. Infections have increased prevalence in substance-using populations, and in those who use multiple drugs, risk effects may be synergistic. Alcohol use is associated with CNS inflammation that may exacerbate HAND syndromes, while stimulation of a cannabinoid receptor (CB_2) may have mitigating anti-inflammatory effects (Persidsky et al., 2011). Other factors impacting behavioral risk or compromised immune processes include malnutrition, general life stress, the stress of living with HIV (Evans et al., 1995), poor coping mechanisms, and depressive disorders. One study found that psychological distress was independently associated with shorter time to AIDS among HIV-infected IDUs, especially those with the lowest CD4 counts (Golub et al., 2003).

Widespread substance use presents a special threat to adolescent health and is associated with motor vehicle accidents, homicides, and suicides, as well as medical, psychological, and social morbidity (Singh, Kochaneck, & MacDorman, 1996). Substance use significantly increases adolescent risk behaviors for HIV transmission (Chan, Passetti, Garner, Lloyd, & Dennis, 2011). Cases of AIDS and rates of HIV infection are rapidly rising among adolescents, particularly in those from marginalized higher risk groups who do not easily access traditional services (CDC, 2012a; Kennedy & Eckholdt, 1997; Mofenson, & Flynn, 2000; Kennedy, Botwinik, Johnson, Ruranga, & Johnson, 2006).

Opioids

In addition to the high risk of HIV transmission in IDUs who share needles, compromised immune function from opioid exposure may add to risk of infection and disease progression. There is reduced lymphocyte stimulation in response to various mitogens in heroin addicts (Govitaprong, Suttitum, Kotchabhakdi, & Uneklabh, 1998). Opioids have a variety of effects that are primarily immunosuppressive (McCarthy, Wetzela, Slikera, Eisenstein, & Rogers, 2001). Chronic exposure to morphine may reduce HIV replication, while withdrawal, mediated by stress effects, can lead to acute immune suppression and disease exacerbation (Donahue & Vladhov, 1998).

Opioid addicts who enter methadone maintenance treatment are significantly less likely to become infected with HIV in the first place. (Metzger et al.,1993). For the infected, consistent participation in methadone maintenance is associated with more consistent use of ART (Sambamoorthi, Warner, Crystal, & Walkup, 2000). Office-based buprenorphine opioid substitution therapy or medication-assisted treatment (MAT) for detoxification and maintenance is comparable to methadone treatment, and there are few absolute contraindications (Kraus et al., 2011).

Opioids can serve as a "cofactor" for HIV infection of lymphocytes both as a function of opioid binding to T cell receptors (Wang & Ho, 2011) and through generalized suppressive effects on the immune system, increasing susceptibility to HIV and other infections (Goforth, Lupash, Brown, Tan, & Fernandez, 2004). Such considerations raise concerns about the ultimate benefits of MAT. Immunosuppressive effects may be mediated both by opiate-induced stimulation of the hypothalamic–pituitary–adrenal axis and by direct immunosuppressive effects with activation of opioid receptors on immune cells. In contrast, naltrexone and other opioid antagonists may have beneficial effects and may enhance the effects of antiviral agents (Gekker, Lokensgard, & Peterson, 2001; Wang et. al., 2006). It is less clear whether buprenorphine has immunosuppressive effects (Gomez-Flores & Weber, 2000).

Alcohol

Alcohol use is associated with HIV incidence (O'Leary & Harzenbuehler, 2009); the association appears to be related to both behavioral and immune factors. Stress, maladaptive behaviors and coping, and depression are highly prevalent in alcoholics and exacerbate HIV/AIDS risk behavior (Fisher, Bang, & Kapiga, 2007). Effects are nonspecific, but alcohol use is associated with a range of negative immunomodulatory effects involving cytokines (Cook, 1998; Schleifer, Keller, Shiflet, Benton, & Eckholdt, 1999; Hebert & Pruett, 2002). Alcoholism and medical morbidities often co-occur, and increased HIV risk may be related to alcohol-induced immune alterations associated with lack of viral suppression even when on ART (Chander, Lau, & Moore 2006), which can exacerbate secondary effects of HIV infection such as hepatotoxicity (Szabo & Zakhari, 2011).

Marijuana

The role of cannabis use in human disease remains unclear and is a subject of considerable debate. Smoked cannabis is associated with adverse pulmonary effects and susceptibility to infection (Friedman, Newton, & Klein, 2003). The findings are mixed regarding the contribution of marijuana to HIV progression (Sidney, Beck, Tekawa, Quesenberry, & Friedman, 1997, Abrams et al., 2003) and effects on immunity in HIV infected persons (Bredt et al., 2002). Massi, Vaccani, and Parolaro (2006) found enough evidence to suggest that the cannabinoid system significantly impacts almost every component of immune response and affects the cytokine network. Cannabinoids may play a beneficial role in offsetting CNS inflammatory effects in HIV-infected persons (Persidsky et. al., 2011). The use of cannabinoids as potentially useful adjuncts in the management of AIDS-related symptoms and syndromes, such as the AIDS wasting syndrome, nausea, vomiting, anorexia, and glaucoma, and for some state-based medical marijuana programs remains controversial.

Stimulants, Club Drugs, and Designer Drugs

Stimulant use, smoking crack cocaine, or injecting drugs incurs considerable risk for HIV through behavioral and immune-related mechanisms. Cocaine, especially crack, and methamphetamine are associated with increased progression of HIV disease partly as a function of decreased medication adherence (Baum et al., 2009; Moore, Keruly, & Chaisson, 2004; Booth, Kwiatkowski, & Chitwood, 2000). Cocaine and methamphetamine increase HIV replication and alter cytokine activity in HIV-infected cells (Gekker et al., 2006; Roth et al., 2002; Ellis et al., 2003; Yu et al., 2002). Methamphetamine is implicated in increased CNS inflammation in HIV-infected persons (Everall et al., 2005).

MDMA is long been associated with impulsive aggression (Gerra et al., 2000), including high-risk behaviors with numerous "one-night stands" (casual sexual relations), frequent visits to clubs that pose a high risk for multiple partners, and acquiring STIs including HIV (Klitzman, Greenberg, Pollack, & Dolezal, 2002). The combination of novelty seeking and impulsivity seen in some clubs with a high prevalence of substance use can lead to high-risk sexual behaviors, leading to HIV (Hayaki, Anderson, & Stein, 2006; Kjome et al., 2010). Cocaine is the drug of choice in club culture, along with ketamine, MDMA, cocaine, gamma-hydroxybutyric acid (GHB), methamphetamine, and lysergic acid diethylamide (LSD) (Parsons, Grov, & Kelly, 2009). More recent use of synthetic cannabinoids, mephedrones ("bath salts"), cathinones, and other novel "designer drugs" have complicated the medical issues since they have been little studied and are not captured by routine urine toxicology. Kalokhe et al. (2012) demonstrated that intimate partner violence (IPV) occurs frequently among HIV-infected crack users and is associated with outcomes known to facilitate HIV transmission and disease progression, including reduced utilization of outpatient HIV care, ART nonadherence, and new STI diagnoses.

Nicotine

Nicotine is not well studied relative to HIV risk and immune effects. Reports about the contribution of smoking (increased prevalence in PLWHA) to HIV infection and progression are conflicting (Furber, Maheswaran, Newell, & Carroll, 2007). The immunomodulatory effects of nicotine show that tobacco smoke can increase production of proinflammatory cytokines and decrease the levels of anti-inflammatory cytokines. It can lead to elevated IgE concentrations and activates macrophage and dendritic cell activity (Arnson, Shoenfeld, & Amital, 2010; Sopori, Kozak, Savage, Geng, & Kluger, 1998). Nicotine and HIV may compete for the same receptor, but the significance of this is unclear. Results of several studies have suggested an exacerbating and a protective role for nicotine or tobacco smoke in HIV disease, perhaps most importantly in the CNS (Giunta et al., 2004; Rock et al., 2008; Zhao et al., 2010). Other adverse health effects of nicotine will likely be of major importance in the aging PLWAH population.

DRUG ADDICTION TREATMENT FOR PLWHA

Treatment of alcohol and drug use in those with or at risk for HIV requires vigorous behavioral change strategies. AIDS education, prevention, and behavioral training are ongoing components of drug treatment. Use of diagnostic and general treatment principles such as those in DSM-5 (American Psychiatric Association [APA], 2013) and the *APA Practice Guideline for the Treatment of Patients with Substance Use Disorders* (2006), and widely used placement criteria of the American Society of Addiction Medicine (ASAM; 2013) should guide decisions. Drug addiction is chronic and may require continuous or repeated treatments. Substance use is associated with lack of adherence to ambulatory psychiatric care (Kennedy, Skurnick, & Lintott, 1994). In one 12-year study, 29% of persistent drug injectors had the highest mortality rates (Galai, Safaeian, Vlahov, Bolotin, & Celentano, 2003). Overall care of the HIV-infected person is improved by case management integration, and medical and substance use treatment (Knowlton et al., 2001). Cultural competency presents a primary hurdle for interventions aimed at altering risky behaviors. Community-based outreach programs have proved to be most effective (Kwiatowski, Booth, & Lloyd, 2000). For the users who cannot or will not enter treatment, specific counseling methods (motivational interviewing and contingency management) can be used to communicate effective harm reduction techniques. Emphasis must be placed on use of a new, sterile needle for each injection to prevent infections. Alcoholics, females, transgender persons, stimulant users, and adolescents need targeted counseling on sexual practices, especially when intoxicated (Kennedy, Johnson, Botwinick, & Johnson, 2002). Commercial sex work, often found to be linked with drug use to support habits (Edlin et al., 1994), or bartering sex to obtain drugs, further adds to risk by introducing multiple partners (Catania et al., 1995). Individuals with comorbid diagnoses are at the highest risk and often require wraparound services with many levels of support to change behaviors.

Drug-using populations fuel the HIV epidemic around the world. These individuals are at higher risk for accelerated, more severe neurocognitive dysfunction compared to non-drug-using HIV-infected populations (Nath et al., 2002). Alcohol and other drug users with HIV need regular screening (including urine) for psychiatric disorders and SUDs, and vice versa. Those who screen positive for mental illness or SUDs need referral to a qualified interprofessional team with a psychiatrist. Symptoms deserve a comprehensive, discipline-specific evaluation for accurate diagnosis and recommendations. Co-located MAT modalities (methadone, buprenorphine, naltrexone, etc.) and other, easily accessed specialty services can facilitate adherence (Korthuis et al., 2011).

HIV Testing

The CDC (2009) recommends screening for the presence of HIV in persons in substance use treatment programs and use of opt-out HIV screening in all health care settings, so that unidentified HIV-positive individuals can be linked with clinical and prevention services to further reduce HIV transmission. "Opt-out screening" is doing an HIV test after telling the individual that the test will be done; the person may elect to decline or defer. "Opt-in screening" requires the person to actively give permission. The opt-out method's efficacy was demonstrated when the number of infants born with HIV infection went from a high of 1,650 in 1991, to an estimated 144–236 infants in 2002 through opt-out testing policies in pregnancy treatment (CDC, 2009). Patients prefer routine testing rather than being perceived to be "at risk."

In 2012, the U.S. Food and Drug Administration (FDA) approved the first over-the-counter home-use rapid HIV test kit to detect the presence of antibodies to HIV-1 and HIV-2. The home collection of oral fluid gives test results within 20–40 minutes. Positive results need confirmation, and a negative result does not rule out HIV, especially with recent exposure. The test has the potential to identify previously undiagnosed HIV infections, particularly if used by those unlikely to use standard screening methods. The manufacturer of the approved in-home HIV test has a 24-hour/7 days a week telephone consumer support center for user education, information, and next steps (FDA, 2012).

Clinical Considerations

The use of antiretroviral regimens is recommended for all HIV-positive persons regardless of CD4 cell count, with modifications in the timing and choice of ART left to the provider (CDC, 2012b, CDC, 2014; Thompson et al., 2012). Evidence shows the harmful impact of ongoing HIV replication on AIDS and non-AIDS disease progression. The 2012 recommendations reflect data showing the benefit of ART in preventing secondary HIV transmission to others (CDC, 2012b). The many physical and emotional effects of HIV complicate the contemporaneous treatment of chemical dependency. Issues of death and dying can be prominent, and some individuals may be hopelessness and question the value or practicality of abstinence.

HIV-positive IDUs do not necessarily have more rapidly progressive HIV than NIDUs, but there is a disparity in treatment outcomes with delayed access to ART, other comorbid diseases, psychosocial barriers, and less long-term adherence. Active drug use should not be an absolute contraindication to ART. Comprehensive coordinated care from an interprofessional team can improve the patient–provider relationship by overcoming stigma and stereotypes and give adherence support to IDUs starting ART (Kennedy, Holland, Sarwin, Mundy, & Jones, 2000; Spire, Lucas, & Carrieri, 2007). Individuals who could be instrumental in motivating drug-addicted individuals may be burned out or, in the face of HIV, be reluctant to confront the SUD. Those with long-term addictions, multiple disabilities, or severe social needs may be marginalized and long-estranged from support mechanisms. Inconsistent compliance and subsequent crisis utilization alienates health care providers. Dismissal of the addiction problem may convey a dehumanizing message that life problems are no longer relevant for a patient because he or she is "terminal" and "hopeless."

HIV-related psychological needs are multifaceted. Anxiety and depression, often complicated by cravings, guilt feelings, denial, or cognitive impairment, frequently accompany HIV/AIDS. Suicidal ideation is common. Patients overwhelmed by illness, grief, and a sense of loss require a supportive, insight-oriented, and psychodynamically sound approach. Consultation–liaison (psychosomatic) and addiction psychiatrists can be particularly valuable in the care of patients with HIV, regardless of setting. Psychiatrists are in a unique position to help persons living with or dying of HIV/AIDS to receive the type and level of care desired (Kennedy & Hill, 1997). Significant others may benefit from referral to support groups; women have special issues and suffer more psychological distress than men (Kennedy, Skurnick, Jaffee, Foley, & Louria, 1994; Kennedy, Skurnick, Foley, & Louria, 1995).

Patients do best at centers with integrated care management, specialized services, and a positive track record with HIV. Pitfalls for mental health professionals, addictions counselors, and other staff include countertransference issues linked to fear of contagion; addictophobia; racism; fear of lesbian, gay, bisexual, or transgender (LGBT) persons; denial of helplessness; and the need for professional omnipotence. Therapists must monitor how overwhelming emotional issues impact, strain, or push traditional boundaries observed in psychotherapy.

Legal Issues

Confidentiality issues arise when treating individuals with drug addiction and HIV infection. Pascal (1987) points out that federal law protects the confidentiality of patient records for those persons under treatment for drug use. The Health Insurance Portability Assurance Act (HIPAA; 2003) provides for the electronic transmission of health information and medical record privacy and is the U.S. standards for the protection and privacy of personal health information. In acute health care delivery, disclosure outside the clinical setting is only permitted with the patient's written consent. Reporting of HIV status to public health authorities may be required in some states and may be disclosed without patient consent to the extent required by law.

Single parents of minor children, particularly pregnant women, have special needs around custody and care of children if they should become disabled or die prematurely. Future planning is best when timely and appropriate, and patients themselves prefer that physicians broach these subjects, and earlier rather than later in the disease process (Kennedy & Hill, 1997).

PREVENTION AND PUBLIC HEALTH

Prevention is the strongest defense against spread of this blood infection and STI. Behavioral change studies indicate that IDUs can reduce risk (Des Jarlais & Friedman, 1987). IDUs use whatever is available, sterile or otherwise. A large national survey of regulations of syringes and needles found that deregulation of syringe sale and possession would reduce the morbidity and mortality associated with bloodborne infections, including HIV, among IDUs, their sexual partners, and their children (Gostin, Lazzarini, Jones, & Flaherty, 1997). Regulations vary but despite a U.S. General Accounting Office (1993) report, other task force recommendations, and scientific studies that indicate a new infections plateau in IDUs where needle exchanges have been tried, the U.S. Congress reinstated a ban on federal funding of needle exchange programs that was overturned in 2009 (Federal Funding Ban, 2012).

Research has found that needle exchange programs are quickly adopted by IDUs and shows no increase in new users or increase in frequency of use (Watters, Estilo,

Prevention strategies to prevent HIV acquisition in IDUs include:

- Cessation of injection drug use, detoxification
- Cessation of needle sharing
- Needle exchange programs
- Harm reduction methods
- MAT: methadone, buprenorphine
- Drug-free treatment programs
- PrEP with ART
- Counseling to help disclose injection history
- Risk reduction training for those with IDU partners

Clark, & Lorvick, 1994). Lurie and Drucker (1997) estimated that from 4,000 to 10,000 HIV infections in the United States that cost between $250,000 and $500,000, and untold amounts of human misery, might have been prevented by needle exchange programs. Increasing condom use with this group should be a priority goal for HIV prevention programs. Multiple strategies are needed to prevent HIV acquisition and transmission in high-risk groups, and the CDC (2014) guideline for Pre-Exposure Prophylaxis, PrEP includes those at risk through injection of illicit drugs.

Male IDUs are important for the spread of HIV into the general population. Male IDUs reported a greater percentage of non-IDU heterosexual contacts than did female IDUs (Des Jarlais et al., 1987). Our group found that high-risk women in sero-discordant heterosexual relationships were more likely to insist on condom use if they were employed, and those couples who practiced safe sex at a study entry were less likely to relapse into unsafe behaviors in 6 months if the female was employed. Unsafe sexual practices, most notably anal sex, were implicated in HIV sexual transmission within heterosexual couples (Kennedy et al., 1993; Skurnick, Abrams, Kennedy, Valentin, & Cordell, 1998; Skurnick, Kennedy, et al., 1998).

CONCLUSION

IDUs and other drug users are primary sources of HIV transmission to other adults, adolescents, and children in the United States. Health care providers have a major responsibility to educate, promote prevention, and provide treatment to this group. HIV counseling, testing, and referral to drug treatment, mental health, and other health services must be accessible. Those drug users who are unable to abstain from injecting may benefit from harm reduction strategies. Public health measures may have to be addressed through policy change. Therapists and counselors involved in the treatment of drug-addicted individuals must be prepared to discuss explicitly issues of sexual orientation and safer sex, stressing use of barrier methods (condoms, dental dams), and LGBT issues, as well as openly discuss the effects of drug use and intoxication on sexual behavior and HIV risk. Integrated case management is required for quality care of addicted individuals. Professionals should be aware of the wide range of presenting signs and symptoms of HIV infection and other confounding infections or states (intoxication/withdrawal), as well as treatment choice options and difficult end-of-life decisions regarding care, treatments, and legal issues.

The extraordinary rates of HIV infection among substance users suggest that these individuals will use an increasing proportion of health care resources, particularly since HIV and addictions are chronic, ongoing conditions. Numerous behavioral epidemiological studies have shown that both injection-related risk factors (years of injecting drugs, type of drug injected, direct and indirect sharing of injection paraphernalia) and sex-related risk factors (lack of condom use, multiple sex partners, survival sex) lead to the spread of HIV, HBV, and HCV. Interrupting the spread of HIV requires increased capacity of outreach workers for IDUs, and increased and expanded access to health and social services for those who are using drugs or infected with HIV (Estrada, 2002). Treatment slots for those with HIV infection or AIDS will increase in demand. As HIV flourishes in drug users, the potential for spread into other segments of the population increases. For a successful battle against one part of the AIDS epidemic, additional resources for drug education, prevention, treatment, rehabilitation, and research are urgently needed.

REFERENCES

Abrams, D. I., Hilton, J. F., Leiser, R. J., Shade, S. B., Elbeik, T. A., Aweeka, F. T., et al. (2003). Short-term effects of cannabinoids in patients with HIV-1 infection: A randomized, placebo-controlled clinical trial. *Ann Intern Med, 139*(4), 258–266.

Althoff, K. N., Gebo, K. A., Gange, S. J., Klein, M. B., Brooks, J. T., Hogg, R. S., et al. (2010). CD4 count at presentation for HIV care in the United States and Canada: Are those over 50 years more likely to have a delayed presentation? *AIDS Res Ther, 15*(7), 45.

American Psychiatric Association. (2006). *American Psychiatric practice guideline for the treatment of patients with substance use disorders* (2nd ed.). Retrieved September 2, 2012, from *www.psychiatryonline.org*.

American Psychiatric Association. (2013). *Diagnostic and statistical manual of mental disorders* (5th ed.). Arlington, VA: Author.

American Society for Addiction Medicine. (2013). *ASAM criteria: Treatment criteria for addictive, substance-related and co-occurring conditions* (3rd ed.). Chevy Chase, MD: Author.

Ances, B. (2008). HIV-associated neurocognitive disorders in the era of highly active antiviral therapies. *Neurol Neurosurg.* Retrieved September 4, 2012, from *www.medscape.com*.

Anthony, I. C., Arango, J. C., Stephens, B., Simmonds, P., & Bell, J. E. (2008). The effects of illicit drugs on the HIV infected brain. *Front Biosci, 1*(13), 1294–1307.

Antinori, A., Arendt, G., Becker, J. T., Brew, B. J., Byrd, D. A., Cherner, M., et al. (2007). Updated research nosology for HIV-associated neurocognitive disorders. *Neurol, 69*(18), 1789–1799.

Arnson, Y., Shoenfeld, Y., & Amital, H. (2010). Effects of tobacco smoke on immunity, inflammation and autoimmunity. *J of Autoimmunity, 34*(3), J258–J265.

Arsten. J. H., Demas, P. A., Grant, R. W., Gourevitch, M. N., Farzadegan, H., Howard, A. A., et al. (2002). Impact of active drug use on antiretroviral therapy adherence and viral suppression in HIV-infected drug users. *J Gen Intern Med, 17*, 377–381.

Asch, S. M., Kilbourne, A. M., Gifford, A. L., Burnam, A., Turner, B., Shapiro, M. F., et al. (2003). Under diagnosis of depression in HIV: Who are we missing? *J Gen Intern Med, 18*, 450–460.

Baum, M. K., Rafie, C., Lai, S., Sales, S., Page, B., & Campa, A. (2009). Crack-cocaine use accelerates HIV disease progression in a cohort of HIV-positive drug users. *J Acquir Immune Defic Syndr, 50*(1), 93–99.

Bell, J. E., Brettle, R. P., Chiswick, A., & Simmonds, P. (1998). HIV encephalitis, proviral load and dementia in drug users and homosexuals with AIDS: Effect of neocortical involvement. *Brain, 121*(11), 2043–2052.

Bing, E. G., Burnam, M. A., Longshore, D., Fleishman, J. A., Sherbourne, C. D., London, A. S., et al. (2001). Psychiatric disorders and drug use among human immunodeficiency virus infected adults in the United States. *Arch Gen Psychiatry, 58,* 721–728.

Blume, J., Douglas, S. D., & Evans, D. L. (2011). Immune suppression and immune activation in depression. *Brain Behav Immun, 25*(2), 221–229.

Booth, R. E., Kwiatkowski, C. F., & Chitwood, D. D. (2000). Sex related HIV risk behaviors: Differential risks among injection drug smokers, crack mothers, and injection drug users who smoke crack. *Drug Alcohol Depend, 58,* 219–226.

Bredt, B. M., Higuera-Alhino, D., Shade, S. B., Hebert, S. J., McCune, J. M., & Abrams, D. I. (2002). Short-term effects of cannabinoids on immune phenotype and function in HIV-1-infected patients. *J Clin Pharmacol, 42*(Suppl. 11), 82S–89S.

Catania, J. A., Binson, D., Dolcini, M. M., Stall, R., Choi, K., Pollack, L. M., et al. (1995). Risk factors for HIV and other sexually transmitted diseases and prevention practices among U.S. heterosexual adults: Changes from 1990 to 1992. *Am J Public Health, 85,* 1492–1499.

Centers for Disease Control and Prevention (CDC). (2009). Guidelines for prevention and treatment of opportunistic infections in HIV infected adults and adolescents. *MMWR, 4*(58.RR), 84–85.

Centers for Disease Control and Prevention (CDC). (2012a). Estimated HIV Incidence in the United States, 2007–2010 (HIV Surveillance Supplemental Report). Retrieved October 20, 2010, from *www.cdc.gov/hiv/topics/surveillance/resources/reports/#supplemental.*

Centers for Disease Control and Prevention (CDC). (2012b). HIV infection and HIV-associated behaviors among injecting drug users—20 cities, United States, 2009. *MMWR, 61*(8), 133–138.

Centers for Disease Control and Prevention (CDC). (2012c). Recommendations for the identification of chronic hepatitis C virus infection among persons born during 1945–1965. *MMWR, 61*(4), 1–32.

Centers for Disease Control and Prevention (CDC). (2013). Statistics Center. HIV Surveillance Supplemental Report. Retreived September 5, 2012, from *www.cdc.gov/hiv/topics/surveillance/index.htm.*

Centers for Disease Control and Prevention (CDC). (2014). *U.S. public health service pre-exposure prophylaxis and prevention of HIV infection in United States, 2014; A clinical practice guideline.* Retrieved from *www.cdc.gov/hiv/guidelines/index.html.*

Chan, Y. F., Passetti, L. L., Garner, B. R., Lloyd, J. J., & Dennis, M. L. (2011). HIV risk behaviors: Risky sexual activities and needle use among adolescents in substance abuse treatment. *AIDS Behav, 15*(1), 114–124.

Chander, G., Lau, B., & Moore, R. D. (2006). Hazardous alcohol use: A risk factor for non-adherence and lack of suppression in HIV infection. *J Acquir Immune Defic Syndr, 43*(4), 411–417.

Chichinov, H., Wilson, K., & Enns, M. (1994). Prevalence of depression in the terminally ill: Effects of diagnostic criteria and symptom threshold judgments. *Am J Psychiatry, 151,* 1711–1713.

Colfax, G., Vittinghoff, E., Husnik, M. J., McKirnan, D., Buchbinder, S., Koblin, B., et al. (2004). Substance use and sexual risk: A participant- and episode-level analysis among a cohort of men who have sex with men. *Am J Epidemiol, 159,* 1002–1012.

Cook, R. T. (1998). Alcohol abuse, alcoholism, and damage to the immune system—a review. *Alcohol Clin Exp Res, 22,* 1927–1942.

Cooper, C. L., Giordano, C., Mackie, D., & Mills, E. J. (2010). Equitable access to HCV care in HIV–HCV co-infection can be achieved despite barriers to health care provision. *Ther Clin Risk Manag, 6,* 207–212.

Cruess, D. B., Evans, D. L., Repetto, M. J., Gettes, D., Douglas, S. D., & Petitto, J. M. (2003). Prevalence, diagnosis and pharmacologic treatment of mood disorders in HIV disease. *Biol Psychiatry, 54*, 307–316.

Danta, M., & Rodger, A. J. (2011). Transmission of HCV in HIV-positive populations. *Curr Opin HIV AIDS, 6*, 451–458.

Darrow, W. W., Biersteker, S., Geiss, T., Chevalier, K., Clark, J., Marrero, Y., et al. (2005). Risky sexual behaviors associated with recreational drug use among men who have sex with men in an international resort area: Challenges and opportunities. *J Urban Health, 82*, 601–609.

de Lédinghen, V., Barreiro, P., Foucher, J., Labarga, P., Castéra, L., Vispo, M. E., et al. (2008). Liver fibrosis on account of chronic hepatitis C is more severe in HIV-positive than HIV-negative patients despite antiretroviral therapy. *J Viral Hepat, 15*, 427–433.

DeRonchi, D., Faranca, I., Berardi, D., Scudellari, P., Borderi, M., Manfredi, R., et al. (2002). Risk factors for cognitive impairment in HIV-1 infected persons with different risk behaviors. *Arch Neurol, 59*(2), 812–818.

Des Jarlais, D. C., & Friedman, S. (1987). HIV infection among intravenous drug users: Epidemiology and risk reduction. *AIDS, 1*, 67–76.

Des Jarlais, D. C., Friedman, S. R., Choopanya, K., Varichseni, S., & Ward, T. (1992). International epidemiology of HIV and AIDS among injecting drug users. *AIDS, 6*, 1053–1068.

Des Jarlais, D. C., Wish, E., Friedman, S. R., Stoneburner, R., Yancovitz, S. R., Mildvan, D., et al. (1987). Intravenous drug use and the heterosexual transmission of the human immunodeficiency virus: Current trends in New York City. *NY State J Med, 3*, 283–286.

Donahue, R. M., & Vladhov, D. (1998). Opiates as potential cofactors in progression of HIV-1 infections to AIDS. *J Neuroimmunol, 15*(1–2),77–87.

Douaihy, A., Hilsabeck, R. C., Assam, P., Jain, A., & Daley, D. C. (2008). Neuropsychiatric aspects of coinfection with HIV and hepatitis C Virus. *AIDS Read, 18*, 425–432, 438–441.

Edlin, B. R., Irwin, K. L., Faruque, S., McCoy, C. B., Word, C., Serrano, Y., et al. (1994). Intersecting epidemics—crack cocaine use and HIV infection among inner city young adults: Multicenter crack cocaine and HIV infection study team. *N Engl J Med, 331*, 1422–1427.

Ellis, R. J., Childers, M. E., Cherner, M., Lazzaretto, D., Letendre, S., & Grant, I. (2003). Increased human immunodeficiency virus loads in active methamphetamine users are explained by reduced effectiveness of antiretroviral therapy. *J Infect Dis, 188*(12), 1820–1826.

Estrada, A. L. (2002). Epidemiology of HIV/AIDS, hepatitis B, hepatitis C, and tuberculosis among minority injection drug users. *Public Health Rep, 117*, S126–S134.

Evans, D. L., & Charney, D. S. (2003). Mood disorders and mental illness: A major public health problem. *Biol Psychiatry, 54*, 177–180.

Evans, D. L., Leserman, J., Perkins, D. O., Stern, R. A., Murphy, C., Tamul, K., et al. (1995). Stress-associated reductions of cytotoxic T-lymphocytes and natural killer cells in asymptomatic HIV infection. *Am J Psychiatry, 152*, 543–550.

Everall, I., Salaria, S., Roberts, E., Corbeil, J., Sasik, R., Fox, H., et al. (2005). Methamphetamine stimulates interferon inducible genes in HIV infected brain. *J Neuroimmunol, 170*(1–2), 158–171.

Feeney, E. R., & Chung, R. T. (2014) Antiviral treatment of hepatitis C. *BMJ, 349*, g3308.

Fisher, J. C., Bang, H., & Kapiga, S. H. (2007). The association between HIV infection and alcohol use: A systematic review and meta-analysis of African studies. *Sex Transm Dis, 34*(11), 856–863.

Folstein, M. F., Folstein, S. E., & McHugh, P. R. (1975). Mini-Mental State Exam: A practical method for grading the cognitive state of patients for the clinician. *J Psychiatr Res, 3*, 189–198.

Friedman, H., Newton, C., & Klein, T. W. (2003). Microbial infections, immuno-modulation, and drugs of abuse. *Clin Microbiol Rev, 16*, 209–219.

Furber, A. S., Maheswaran, R., Newell, J. N., & Carroll, C. (2007). Is smoking tobacco an independent risk factor for HIV infection and progression to AIDS?: A systemic review. *Sex Transm Infect, 83*, 41–46.

Galai, N., Safaeian, M., Vlahov, D., Bolotin, A., & Celentano, D. D. (2003). Longitudinal patterns of drug injection behavior in the ALIVE Study cohort, 1988–2000: Description and determinants. *Am J Epidemiol, 158*(7), 695–704.

Galvan, F. H., Burnam, M. A., & Bing, E. G. (2003). Co-occurring psychiatric symptoms and drug dependence or heavy drinking among HIV+ people. *J Psychoactive Drugs, 35*, 153–160.

Gekker, G., Hu, S., Sheng, W. S., Rock, R. B., Lokensgard, J. R., & Peterson, P. K. (2006). Cocaine-induced HIV-1 expression in microglia involves sigma-1 receptors and transforming growth factor-beta1. *Int J Immunopharmacol, 6*(6), 1029–1033.

Gekker, G., Lokensgard, J. R., & Peterson, P. K. (2001). Naltrexone potentiates anti-HIV-1 activity of antiretroviral drugs in CD4+ lymphocyte cultures. *Drug Alcohol Depend, 64*, 257–263.

Gerra, G., Zaimovic, A., Ferri, M., Zambelli, U., Timpano, M., Neri, E., et al. (2000). Long-lasting effects of (+/–)3,4-methylenedioxymethamphetamine (ecstasy) on serotonin system function in humans. *Biol Psychiatry, 47*(2), 127–136.

Giunta, B., Ehrhart, J., Townsend, K., Sun, N., Vendrame, M., Shytle, D., et al. (2004). Galantamine and nicotine have a synergistic effect on inhibition of microglial activation induced by HIV-1 gp120. *Brain Res Bull, 64*, 165–170.

Goforth, H. W., Lupash, D. P., Brown, M., Tan, J., & Fernandez, F. (2004). Role of alcohol and substances of abuse in the immunomodulation of human immunodeficiency virus disease: A review. *Addict Disord Ther Treat, 3*(4), 174–182.

Golub, E. T., Astemborski, J. A., Hoover, D. R., Anthony, J. C., Vlahov, D., & Strathdee, S. A. (2003). Psychological distress and progression to AIDS in a cohort of injection drug users. *J Acquir Immune Defic Syndr, 32*, 429–434.

Gomez-Flores, R., & Weber, R. J. (2000). Differential effects of buprenorphine and morphine on immune and neuroendocrine functions following acute administration in the rat mesencephalon periaqueductal gray. *Immunopharmacol, 48*, 145–156.

Gostin, L. O., Lazzarini, S., Jones, S., & Flaherty, K. (1997). Prevention of HIV/AIDS and other blood-borne diseases among injection drug users. *JAMA, 277*, 53–62.

Gouzoulis-Mayfrank, E., & Daumann, J. (2009). Neurotoxicity of drugs of abuse—the case of methylenedioxy amphetamines (MDMA, ecstasy), and amphetamines. *Dialogues Clin Neurosci, 11*(3), 305–317.

Govitrapong, P., Suttitum, T., Kotchabhakdi, N., & Uneklabh, T. (1998). Alterations of immune functions in heroin addicts and heroin withdrawal subjects. *J Pharmacol Exp Ther, 286*, 883–889.

Hayaki, J., Anderson, B., & Stein, M. (2006). Sexual risk behaviors among substance users: relationship to impulsivity. *Psychol Addict Behav, 20*(3), 328–332.

Health Insurance Portability Assurance Act. (2003). Office for Civil Rights. Retrieved October 12, 2012, from *www.hhs.gov/ocr/hipaa*.

Hebert, P., & Pruett, S. B. (2002). Ethanol suppresses polyinosinic: Polycytidylic acid-induced activation of natural killer cells primarily by acting on natural killer cells, not through effects on other cell types. *Alcohol, 28*, 75–81.

Hendershot, C. S., Stoner, S. A., Pantalone, D. W., & Simoni, J. M. (2009). Alcohol use and antiretroviral adherence: Review and meta-analysis. *J Acquir Immune Defic Syndr, 52*(2), 180–202.

Holmberg, S. D., Ly, K. N., & Xing, J. (2012). The increasing burden of mortality from viral hepatitis in the United States. *Ann Intern Med, 157*(2), 150.

Irwin, M., Caldwell, C., Smith, T. L., Brown, S., Schuckit, M. A., & Gillin, J. C. (1990). Major depressive disorder, alcoholism, and reduced natural killer cell cytotoxicity: Role of severity of depressive symptoms and alcohol consumption. *Arch Gen Psychiatry, 47*(8), 713–719.

Jenness, S. M., Neaigus, A., Hagan, H., Murrill, C. S., & Wendel, T. (2012). Heterosexual HIV and sexual partnerships between injection drug users and noninjection drug users. *AIDS Patient Care STDS, 24*(3), 175–181.

Kalokhe, A. S., Paranjape, A., Bell, C. E., Cardenas, G. A., Kuper, T., Metsch, L. R., et al. (2012). Intimate partner violence among HIV-infected crack cocaine users. *AIDS Patient Care STDS, 26*(4), 234–240.

Kennedy, C. A., Botwinick, G., Johnson, D., Ruranga, E., & Johnson, R. L. (2006, March). *PTSD and HIV: Is one a risk factor for the other?: A report on HIV positive adolescents and young adults.* Poster presented at the 64th annual meeting of the American Society for Psychosomatic Medicine Meeting, Denver, CO.

Kennedy, C. A., & Eckholdt, H. M. (1997). Diagnosis of AIDS in U.S. adolescents: 1983–1993. In L. Sherr (Ed.), *Adolescents and AIDS* (pp. 51–61). London: Harwood Academic.

Kennedy, C. A., & Hill, J. M. (1997, March). *Barriers to advance directives in hospitalized AIDS patients.* Paper presented at the annual meeting of the American Psychosomatic Association, Santa Fe, NM.

Kennedy, C. A., Holland, B., Sarwin, J. S., Mundy, D., & Jones, P. (2000). *Positive relationship with provider: An important factor in HAART Adherence.* Poster presented at the 13th annual conference on AIDS, Durban, South Africa.

Kennedy, C. A., Johnson, D., Botwinick, G., & Johnson, R. L. (2002, July). *High rates of depression, anxiety, past sexual and physical trauma prompt development of specialized mental health services for HIV+ adolescents and young adults.* Poster presented at the 14th international meeting on HIV/AIDS. Barcelona, Spain.

Kennedy, C. A., Skurnick, J. H., Foley, M., & Louria, D. (1995). Gender differences in HIV-related psychological distress in heterosexual couples. *AIDS Care, 7*, S33–S38.

Kennedy, C. A., Skurnick, J., Jaffee, M., Foley, M., & Louria, D. (1994, July). *Psychological distress is associated with lack of family support in female HIV+ heterosexual couples: A report from the HATS Study (W11.1).* Paper presented at AIDS Impact, Biopsychosocial Aspects of HIV Infection, Brighton, UK.

Kennedy, C. A., Skurnick, J. H., & Lintott, M. (1994, May). *Evaluation of factors related to retention of HIV positive patients in ambulatory psychiatric treatment.* Poster presented at the annual meeting of the American Psychiatric Association, Philadelphia, PA.

Kennedy, C. A., Skurnick, J., Wan, J. Y., Quattrone, G., Sheffet, A., Quinones, M., et al. (1993). Psychological distress, drug and alcohol use as correlates of condom use in HIV-serodiscordant heterosexual couples. *AIDS, 7*, 1493–1499.

Kjome, K. L., Lane, S. D., Schmitz, J. M., Green, C., Ma, L., Prasla, I., et al. (2010). Relationship between impulsivity and decision making in cocaine dependence (Research Support, NIH Extramural). *Psychiatry Res, 178*(2), 299–304.

Klitzman, R. L., Greenberg, J. D., Pollack, L. M., & Dolezal, C. (2002). MDMA ("ecstasy") use, and its association with high risk behaviors, mental health, and other factors among gay/bisexual men in New York City. (Comparative Study Research Support, U.S. Government, P.H.S.). *Drug Alcohol Depend, 66*(2), 115–125.

Knowlton, A. R., Hoover, D. R., Chung, S. E., Celentano, D. D., Vlahov, D., & Latkin, C. A. (2001). Access to medical care and service utilization among injection drug users with HIV/AIDS. *Drug Alcohol Depend, 64*, 55–62.

Korthuis, P. T., Fiellin, D. A., Fu, R., Lim, P. J., Altice, F. L., Sohler, N., et al. (2011). Improving adherence to HIV quality of care indicators in persons with opioid dependence: The role of buprenorphine. *J Acquir Immune Defic Syndr, 56*(Suppl. 1), S83–S90.

Koutsilieri, E., Scheller, C., Sopper, S., ter Meulen, V., & Riederer, P. (2002). The pathogenesis of HIV-induced dementia. *Mech Ageing Dev, 123*, 1047–1053.

Kraus, M. L., Alford, D. P., Kotz, M. M., Levounis, P., Mandell, T. W., Meyer, M., et al. (2011). Statement of the American Society of Addiction Medicine Consensus Panel on the use of buprenorphine in office-based treatment of opioid addiction. *J Addict Med, 5*, 254–263.

Kwiatkowski, C., Booth, R. E., & Lloyd, L. A.(2000) The effects of offering free treatment to street-recruited opioid injectors. *Addiction, 95,* 697–704

Ling, W., Compton, P., Rawson, R., & Wesson, D. (1996). Neuropsychiatry of alcohol and drug abuse. In B. Fogel, R. Schiffer, & S. Rao (Eds.), *Neuropsychiatry* (pp. 679–722). Baltimore, MD: Williams & Wilkins.

Lucas, G. M., Gebo, K. A., Chaisson, R. E., & Moore, R. D. (2002). Longitudinal assessment of the effects of drug and alcohol abuse on HIV-1 treatment outcomes in an urban clinic. *AIDS, 16,* 767–774.

Lurie, P., & Drucker, E. (1997). An opportunity lost: HIV infections associated with lack of a national needle-exchange programme in the USA. *Lancet, 349,* 604–608.

Massi, P., Vaccani, A., & Parolaro, D. (2006). Cannabinoids, immune system and cytokine network.*Curr Pharm Des, 12*(24), 3135–3146.

Matthews, G. V., Pham, S. T., Hellard, M., Grebely, J., Zhang, L., Oon, A., et al. (2011). Patterns and characteristics of hepatitis C transmission clusters among HIV-positive and HIV-negative individuals in the Australian trial in acute hepatitis C. *Clin Infect Dis, 52,* 803–811.

McArthur, J. C., Steiner, J., Sacktor, N., & Nath, A. (2010). Human immunodeficiency virus-associated neurocognitive disorders: Mind the gap. *Ann Neurol, 67,* 699–714.

McCarthy, L., Wetzela, M., Slikera, J. K., Eisenstein, T. K., & Rogers, T. J. (2001). Opioids, opioid receptors, and the immune response. *Drug Alcohol Depend, 62,* 111–123.

Meier, M. H., Caspi, A., Ambler, A., Harrington, H., Houts, R., Keefe, R. E., et al. (2012). Persistent cannabis users show neuropsychological decline from childhood to midlife. *Proc Nat Acad Sci USA, 109,* 2657–2664.

Metzger, D. S., Woody, G., McLellan, T., O'Brien, C. P., Druley, P., Navaline, H., et al. (1993). Human immunodeficiency virus seroconversion among intravenous drug users in- and out-of-treatment: An 18-month prospective follow-up. *J Acquir Immune Defic Syndr, 6,* 1049–1056.

Mofenson, L. M., & Flynn, P. M. (2000). *The challenge of adolescent HIV infection: From prevention to treatment.* Paper presented at the American Academy of Pediatrics Annual Meeting, Chicago, IL, Seminar S221.

Moore, R. D., Keruly, J. C., & Chaisson, R. E. (2004). Differences in HIV disease progression by injecting drug use in HIV-infected persons in care. *J Acquir Immune Defic Syndr, 35,* 46–51.

Nath, A., Hauser, K. F., Wojna, V., Booze, R. M., Maragos, W., Prendergast, M., et al. (2002). Molecular basis for interactions of HIV and drugs of abuse. *J Acquir Immune Defic Syndr, 31,* S62–S69.

National Institute of Allergy and Infectious Diseases (NIAID). (2012). HIV/AIDS. Retrieved May, 12, 2012, from *www.niaid.nih.gov/topics/HIV/AIDS.*

O'Leary, A., & Hatzenbuehler, M. (2009). Alcohol and AIDS. In P. Korsmeyer & H. R. Kranzler (Eds.), *Addictive behaviors* (3rd ed.). Detroit: Macmillian Reference.

Palepu, A., Tyndall, M., Yip, B., O'Shaughnessy, M. V., Hogg, R. S., & Montaner, J. S. (2003). Impaired virologic response to highly active antiretroviral therapy associated with ongoing injection drug use. *J Acquir Immnue Defic Syndr, 32,* 522–526.

Parsons, J. T., Grov, C., & Kelly, B. C. (2009). Club drug use and dependence among young adults recruited through time-space sampling (Research Support, NIH Extramural Research Support, Non-U.S. Government). *Public Health Rep, 124*(2), 246–254.

Pascal, C. B. (1987). Selected legal issues about AIDS for drug abuse treatment programs. *J Psychoactive Drugs, 19,* 1–12.

Persidsky, Y., Ho, W., Ramirez, S. H., Potula, R., Abood, M. E., Unterwald, E., et al. (2011). HIV-1.infection and alcohol abuse: Neurocognitive impairment, mechanisms of neurodegeneration and therapeutic interventions. *Brain Behav Immun, 25*(Suppl. 1), S61–S70.

Power, C., Selnes, O. A., Grim, J. A., & McArthur, J. C. (1995). HIV Dementia Scale: A rapid screening test. *J Acquir Immune Defic Syndr, 8*(3), 273–278.

Reger, M., Welsh, R., Razani, J., Martin, D. J., & Boone, K. B. (2002). A meta-analysis of the neuropsychological sequelae of HIV infection. *J Int Neuropsychol Soc, 8*, 410–424.

Reyes, M. G., Faraldi, F., Senseng, C. S., Flowers, C., & Fariello, R. (1991). Nigral degeneration in acquired immune deficiency syndrome (AIDS). *Acta Neuropathol, 82*, 39–44.

Rock, R. B., Gekker, G., Aravalli, R. N., Hu, S., Sheng, W. S., & Peterson, P. K. (2008). Potentiation of HIV-1 expression in microglial cells by nicotine: Involvement of transforming growth factor-beta 1. *J Neuroimmune Pharmacol, 3*(3), 143–149.

Roth, M. D., Tashkin, D. P., Choi, R., Jamieson, B. D., Zack, J. A., & Baldwin, G. C. (2002). Cocaine enhances human immunodeficiency virus replication in a model of severe combined immunodeficient mice implanted with human peripheral blood leukocytes. *J Infect Dis, 185*(5), 701–705.

Sacktor, N. C., Wong, M., Nakasujja, N., Skolasky, R. L., Selnes, O. A., Musisi, S., et al. (2005). The International HIV Dementia Scale: A new rapid screening test for HIV dementia. *AIDS, 19*(13), 1367–1374.

Sambamoorthi, U., Warner, L. A., Crystal, S., & Walkup, J. (2000). Drug abuse, methadone treatment and health services use among injection drug users with AIDS. *Drug Alcohol Depend, 60*, 77–89.

Schleifer, S. J., Keller, S., & Czaja, S. (2003, June). *Major depression, alcoholism and immunity in alcohol dependent persons.* Paper presented at the 10th annual meeting of the Psychoneuroimmunology Research Society, Amelia Island, FL.

Schleifer, S. J., Keller, S. E., Shiflett, S., Benton, T., & Eckholdt, H. (1999). Immune changes in alcohol-dependent patients without medical disorders. *Alcohol Clin Exp Res, 23*, 1199–1206.

Schmidt, A. J., Rockstroh, J. K., Vogel, M., An der Heiden, M., Balliot, A., Krznaric, I., et al. (2011). Trouble with bleeding: Risk factors for acute hepatitis C among HIV-positive gay men from Germany—a case–control study. *PLoS ONE, 6*, e17781.

Sidney, S., Beck, J. E., Tekawa, I. S., Quesenberry, C. P., & Friedman, G. D. (1997). Marijuana use and mortality. *Am J Public Health, 87*(4), 585–590.

Simioni, S., Cavassini, M., Annoni, J. M., Rimbault Abraham, A., Bourquin, I., Schiffer, V., et al. (2010). Cognitive dysfunction in HIV patients despite long-standing suppression of viremia. *AIDS, 24*(9), 1243–1250.

Singh, G. K., Kochaneck, K. D., & MacDorman, M. F. (1996). Advance report of final mortality statistics, 1994. *MVSR, 45*(3S), 1–13.

Skurnick, J. H., Abrams, J., Kennedy, C. A., Valentin, S., & Cordell, J. (1998). Maintenance of safesex behavior by HIV-serodiscordant heterosexual couples. *AIDS Educ Prev, 10*, 493–505.

Skurnick, J. H., Kennedy, C. A., Perez, G., Abrams, J., Vermund, S. H., Denny, T., et al. (1998). Behavioral and demographic risk factors for transmission of human immunodeficiency virus type 1 in heterosexual couples: Report from the heterosexual HIV transmission study. *Clin Infect Dis, 26*, 855–864.

Sopori, M. L., Kozak, W., Savage, S. M., Geng, Y., & Kluger, M. J. (1998). Nicotine-induced modulation of T cell function:. Implications for inflammation and infection. *Advances in Experimental Medical Biology, 437*, 279–289.

Spire, B., Lucas, G. M., & Carrieri, M. P. (2007). Adherence to HIV treatment among IDUs and the role of opioid substitution treatment (OST). *Int J Drug Policy, 18*(4), 262–270.

Szabo, G., & Zakhari, S. (2011). Mechanisms of alcohol-mediated hepatotoxicity in human-immunodeficiency-virus-infected patients. *World J Gastroenterol, 17*(20), 2500–2506.

Thompson, M. A., Aberg, J. A., Hoy, J. F., Telenti, A., Benson, C., Cahn, P., et al. (2012). Antiretroviral treatment of adult HIV infection: 2012 recommendations of the International Antiviral Society–USA panel. *JAMA, 308*(4), 387–402.

UNAIDS (Joint United Nations Programme on HIV/AIDS). (2014). *Gap report.* Geneva, Switzerland: Author.

U.S. Federal Drug Administration. (2012). News release: FDA approves first over-the-counter home-use rapid HIV test. Immediate release July 3, 2012.

U.S. General Accounting Office. (1993, March). *Report to the Chairman, Select Committee on Narcotics Abuse and Control, House of Representatives: Needle exchange, needle exchange programs research suggests promise as an AIDS prevention strategy.* Washington, DC: Author.

U.S. Government: Federal Funding Ban on Needle Exchange Programs. (2012). Retrieved from *www.whitehouse.gov/blog/2012/01/05/federal-funding-ban-needle-exchange-programs.*

Vance, D. E., Ross, L. A., & Downs, C. A. (2008). Self-reported cognitive ability and global cognitive performance in adults with HIV. *J Neurosci Nurs, 40*(1), 6–13.

Wang, X., Douglas, S. D., Peng, J. S., Metzger, D. S., O'Brien, C. P., Zhang, T., et al. (2006). Naltrexone inhibits alcohol-mediated enhancement of HIV infection of T lymphocytes. *J Leukoc Biol, 79*(6), 1162–1172.

Wang, X., & Ho, W. Z. (2011). Drugs of abuse and HIV infection/replication: Implications for mother–fetus transmission. *Life Sci, 88*(21–22), 972–979.

Watters, J. K., Estilo, M. J., Clark, G. L., & Lorvick, J. (1994). Syringe and needle exchange as HIV/AIDS prevention for injection drug users. *JAMA, 271,* 115–120.

Weber, R., Sabin, C. A., Friis-Moller, N., Reiss, P., El-Sadr, W. M., Kirk, O., et al. (2006). Liver-related deaths in persons infected with the human immunodeficiency virus: The D:A:D study. *Arch Intern Med, 166,* 1632–1641.

Wright, E. J., Nunn, M., Joseph, J., Robertson, K., Lal, L., & Brew, B. J. (2008). NeuroAIDS in the Asia Pacific Region. *J Neurovirol, 14*(6), 465–473.

Young, S. D., & Shoptaw, S. (2013). Stimulant use among African American and Latino MSM social networking users. *J Addict Dis, 32*(1), 39–45.

Yu, Q., Zhang, D., Walston, M., Zhang, J., Liu, Y., & Watson, R. R. (2002). Chronic methamphetamine exposure alters immune function in normal and retrovirus-infected mice. *Int J Immunopharmacol, 2*(7), 951–962.

Zhao, L., Li, F., Zhang, Y., Elbourkadi, N., Wang, Z., Yu, C., et al. (2010). Mechanisms and genes involved in enhancement of HIV infectivity by tobacco smoke. *Toxicol, 278*(2), 242–248.

CHAPTER 23

Women and Substance Abuse

DAWN E. SUGARMAN
CHRISTINA BREZING
SHELLY F. GREENFIELD

There is considerable evidence that substance use disorders (SUDs) have been a growing problem among girls and women in the United States (Grucza, Bucholz, Rice, & Bierut, 2008) and much of Europe (Allamani, 2008) over the past six decades. Converging data from numerous studies indicate that there are significant sex differences in the epidemiology, physiology, neurobiology, natural history, and treatment course of SUDs, and these differences have been the subject of several reviews (Greenfield & O'Leary, 2002), chapters (Greenfield, Back, Lawson, & Brady, 2010; Greenfield, Back, & Brady, 2011), and books (Brady, Back, & Greenfield, 2009). We focus in this chapter on women and SUDs, and highlight research from the last 10 years examining gender differences in the epidemiology, neurobiology, and substance-specific effects of alcohol and other drugs. We summarize studies on co-occurring medical and psychiatric disorders, as well as substance abuse treatment outcomes in women.

EPIDEMIOLOGY

Over the past two decades, several large-scale epidemiological studies have provided prevalence rates of substance use, such as the Epidemiologic Catchment Area Study (ECA), the National Comorbidity Survey (NCS), the National Survey on Drug Use and Health (NSDUH), and the National Epidemiologic Survey on Alcohol and Related Conditions (NESARC). In this chapter, we draw more heavily on data from the more recent studies (NSDUH and NESARC).

Telescoping

Recent research supports the notion that the gender gap in alcohol use and related disorders is narrowing. Although men consistently report more alcohol use and alcohol use disorders than women, research on birth cohort differences has found significant decreases in gender differences in heavy drinking, alcohol abuse, and alcohol dependence between older and younger birth cohorts (Keyes, Grant, & Hasin, 2008; Keyes, Li, & Hasin, 2011). In addition to this narrowing gender gap in the younger birth cohorts, the phenomenon in which women progress more rapidly from first use to the onset of dependence and first treatment compared to men has been labeled "telescoping" (Piazza, Vrbka, & Yeager, 1989; Randall et al., 1999). Evidence for the telescoping effect has been found with alcohol-, cannabis-, cocaine-, and opioid-dependent women (Ehlers et al., 2010; Haas & Peters, 2000; Hernandez-Avila, Rounsaville, & Kranzler, 2004). However, some studies that have examined this phenomenon have not found evidence to support the telescoping effect (Alvanzo et al., 2011; Keyes, Martins, Blanco, & Hasin, 2010). One reason may be that earlier studies were conducted on treatment samples, and these more recent studies surveyed the general population. There is some evidence that telescoping differs by age. Johnson, Richter, Kleber, McLellan, and Carise (2005) examined a large sample of substance users recruited from treatment programs and found evidence for telescoping in an older cohort of women (≥ 30 years) but not in a younger cohort (≤ 29 years).

Race and Ethnicity

The majority of research focused on gender and racial/ethnic differences in SUDs has focused on alcohol use. Overall, European American men and women are more likely to use alcohol, initiate alcohol use at an earlier age, and have higher prevalence of alcohol use disorder compared to African Americans or Hispanics (Alvanzo et al., 2011; Caetano, 2003; Hasin, Stinson, Ogburn, & Grant, 2007).

A large, multisite study of Hispanic Americans found that, consistent with other epidemiological studies, men reported more alcohol use (drinks per week) and binge drinking compared to women (Ramisetty-Mikler, Caetano, & Rodriguez, 2010). However, differences among Hispanic subgroups were noted for women, such that Puerto Rican females reported consuming more drinks per week and more binge drinking than women in other subgroups. Of note, in this study, among women of all Hispanic subgroups, number of drinks per week increased with level of acculturation, and binge-drinking rates were higher for women born in the United States compared to women born abroad. Although marijuana use in the general population has remained relatively stable over time, comparison of data from the 1992 National Longitudinal Alcohol Epidemiologic Survey (NLAES) and the 2001–2002 NESARC indicated increased rates of marijuana use among 18- to 29-year-old Hispanic and African American women (Compton, Grant, Colliver, Glantz, & Stinson, 2004).

Native Americans/Alaskan Natives have the highest rates of SUDs and alcohol-related mortality rates compared with all other ethnic groups in the United States (Compton, Thomas, Stinson, & Grant, 2007; Hasin et al., 2007). Overall, Native American/Alaskan Native women have lower rates of illicit drug use compared to men; however, one study found that in younger age groups, use of illicit drugs by women in some tribes was equivalent to rates in men (Young & Joe, 2009).

Asian Americans and Pacific Islanders (AAPI) have the lowest rates of substance use among ethnic groups in the United States (Compton et al., 2007; Hasin et al., 2007). In regard to gender differences, similar to the findings of Young and Joe (2009) data from the National Longitudinal Study of Adolescent Health indicated that in this young adult sample, there were very few gender differences in substance use (Hahm, Wong, Huang, Ozonoff, & Lee, 2008).

Special Populations

Pregnant Women

Although pregnant women report significantly less substance use than nonpregnant women, it is estimated that one in four women uses substances during pregnancy (Ebrahim & Gfroerer, 2003; Havens, Simmons, Shannon, & Hansen, 2009). Pregnant women who use illicit substances are less likely than non-substance-using pregnant women to receive prenatal care (El-Mohandes et al., 2003; Maupin et al., 2004). The most prevalent substances used by pregnant women who participated in the 2002 or 2003 NSDUH were cigarettes (19%), alcohol (10%), and marijuana (4%) (Havens et al., 2009). Similar to previous epidemiological studies, these data also indicated that white women were four times more likely to report substance use during pregnancy than nonwhite women. Moreover, current psychopathology, unemployment, and not being married were also associated with substance use during pregnancy for women in the NSDUH. With regard to use during pregnancy, substance use is reported as less prevalent during successive pregnancy trimesters (e.g., less prevalent in third trimester than in the first trimester) (Ebrahim & Gfroerer, 2003; Havens et al., 2009).

Sexual Minorities

Overall, the prevalence of substance use has been found to be higher in lesbians, gays, and bisexuals than in the general population (McKirnan & Peterson, 1989; Skinner & Otis, 1996). Sexual minority women may be especially vulnerable to the effects of alcohol. One study found that lesbian and bisexual women reported more alcohol-related problems than did heterosexual women; however, there were no differences between gay men and heterosexual men in the number of alcohol-related problems reported (Drabble, Midanik, & Trocki, 2005). Hahm and colleagues (2008) found a significantly higher rate of tobacco, binge drinking, marijuana, and other drug use among AAPI sexual minority women compared to heterosexual women. When compared to sexual minority men, women were also found to have a heightened risk of substance use (Hahm et al., 2008).

Older Adults

Rates of illicit substance use in older adults are higher than in previous generations (Grella & Lovinger, 2012). Older adults show similar gender differences for rates of binge drinking, with data from the NSDUH and NESARC studies indicating that men are more likely than women to report binge drinking (Blazer & Wu, 2009; Naimi et al., 2003). The NESARC study also found that among older females (> 50 years of age), African American women had a higher prevalence of binge drinking compared to European American women (Blazer & Wu, 2009). These data also indicated that binge drinking in older women was associated with nonmedical use of prescription drugs, whereas binge drinking in men was associated with illicit drug use.

NEUROBIOLOGY

Neuroactive Gonadal Steroid Hormones

Estrogen, progesterone, metabolites of progesterone, and dehydroepiandrosterone (DHEA) may all influence behavioral effects of drugs (Greenfield et al., 2010). The different phases of the menstrual cycle, when hormones such as estrogen and progesterone fluctuate, are thought to affect responses to substances. During the follicular phase, when estradiol is high and progesterone is low, women demonstrate a greater responsivity to stimulants (Sofuoglu, Dudish-Poulsen, Nelson, Pentel, & Hatsukami, 1999). It is unclear whether the elevated estradiol or low progesterone is responsible for this effect, but a different study showed that exogenous progesterone attenuates subjective response to smoking cocaine in women but not in men (Evans & Foltin, 2006). During the luteal phase, when progesterone levels are elevated, women report lower rates of feeling high compared to women in the follicular phase (low progesterone) and men (Sofuoglu et al., 1999). Studies of nicotine show greater saliency in the luteal phase (Perkins et al., 2000). Women tend to be less successful with smoking cessation during the late luteal phase, with greater craving and dysphoria than during the follicular phase (Carpenter, Upadhyaya, LaRowe, Saladin, & Brady, 2006) The effects of gonadal steroids on responses to other substances, such as alcohol, are less clear, and more research is needed (Holdstock & de Wit, 2000).

Sex Differences in Stress Reactivity and Relapse to Substance Abuse

Stress has been associated with increases in drug craving and contributes to relapse in substance abuse (Sinha, 2007). Gender differences in response to stress have been observed in both nonaddicted and substance-dependent samples (Fox et al., 2006; Kajantie & Phillips, 2006). Substance-dependent women have attenuated neuroendocrine stress response (decreased adrenocorticotropic hormone and cortisol) following exposure to stress and drug cues (Back et al., 2008). This dysregulation of the hypothalamic–pituitary–adrenocortical axis in women may play a role in the increased vulnerability to relapse in response to negative affect (Fox, Hong, Paliwal, Morgan, & Sinha, 2008).

Neuroimaging

Gender differences have been described in the roles of different brain regions, including the amygdala, striatum, prefrontal cortex and insula, in cravings, instrumental learning, habits, chronic cocaine abuse, stress, and reward tasks, which suggests that a gender-specific understanding of the neural mechanisms involved in drug craving and relapse is warranted in order to develop more effective behavioral and pharmacological treatments (Kilts, Gross, Ely, & Drexler, 2004; Li, Kosten, & Sinha, 2005; Munro et al., 2006). A recent functional magnetic resonance imaging (fMRI) study demonstrated that corticostriatal–limbic hyperactivity is linked to stress cues in cocaine-dependent women, which suggests that targeting stress reduction in the treatment of women with addiction should be taken into account (Potenza et al., 2012). A study using positron emission tomography (PET) imaging demonstrated greater reactivity to cocaine-cues in females as compared to males, without differences in subjective craving, suggesting that a mechanism not linked with craving could affect drug use. More deactivation of brain regions involved in cognitive inhibition (prefrontal, cingulate, inferior parietal cortices and thalamus) was found in women compared to men, suggesting an increase in vulnerability to relapse due to impairment in executive functioning (Volkow et al., 2011).

In addition to increased vulnerability to relapse, imaging has demonstrated that women are more susceptible to the negative physiological effects of chronic substance abuse. Women with alcohol dependence appear to develop brain atrophy, as measured by computed tomography, at an accelerated rate compared to men with alcohol dependence, suggesting a higher vulnerability to adverse consequences of alcoholism (Mann et al., 2005).

SPECIFIC SUBSTANCES

Alcohol

Epidemiological data indicate that the prevalence of alcohol use and related disorders is consistently higher in men (Hasin et al., 2007; Helzer, Burnam, & McEvoy, 1991). Recent data from the 2001–2002 NESARC study estimate the 12-month prevalence of alcohol use disorders at 12.4% for men and 4.9% for women, and the lifetime prevalence of alcohol use disorders at 42% for men and 19.5% for women (Hasin et al., 2007). Rates of binge drinking have also been shown to be more prevalent in men than in women (Naimi et al., 2003). Prior to 2004, the definition of "binge drinking" was often the same for men and women (consuming five or more drinks on one occasion); however, in order to control for physiological gender differences, the definition was revised to five or more drinks for men and four or more drinks for women on one occasion, and endorsed by the National Institute on Alcohol Abuse and Alcoholism (NIAAA, 2004; Chavez, Nelson, Naimi, & Brewer, 2011; Naimi et al., 2003). A recent examination revealed that this change in the definition of binge drinking has directly led to increased estimates in the prevalence rates of binge drinking in women (Chavez et al., 2011).

As discussed previously, there are gender differences in the course of alcohol use and related disorders (i.e., telescoping). In addition, there are also biological differences between men and women that make women more vulnerable to the effects of alcohol. Due to differences in body size, composition, and metabolism, women reach higher blood alcohol concentration (BAC) after consuming the same amount of alcohol as men (Mumenthaler, Taylor, O'Hara, & Yesavage, 1999). Women are also more likely to experience alcohol-related physical illness at lower levels of alcohol use compared to men (Nolen-Hoeksema, 2004). There are also gender differences in the types of alcohol-related problems that men and women report. Research suggests that alcoholic women develop cirrhosis faster than alcoholic men (Loft, Olesen, & Dossing, 1987), have accelerated brain atrophy (Mann et al., 2005), and earlier onset of cognitive deficits (Acker, 1986). Gender differences in psychosocial alcohol-related problems have also been noted. Women report more self-related problems (e.g., blacking out, passing out), whereas men report more antisocial behaviors (e.g., getting into fights, damaging property) (Sugarman, DeMartini, & Carey, 2009). These results were even stronger when researchers controlled for consumption and BAC, which suggests that when women drink equivalent amounts of alcohol as men, they are at heightened risk for alcohol-related personal harm (Sugarman et al., 2009). Men and women also report different reasons for using alcohol. Women more often report using alcohol to get away from problems and to deal with anger and frustration; men more often report using alcohol to get high, to fit in, to alleviate boredom, to sleep, and to moderate the effects of other drugs (Patrick et al., 2011).

The research results on treatment outcome for women with alcohol use disorders are mixed. There is some evidence that treatment outcome is better for women (Project MATCH Research Group, 1997; Timko, Moos, Finney, & Connell, 2002). However, other studies have found no difference between men and women in regard to treatment outcome (Diehl et al., 2007; Foster, Peters, & Marshall, 2000), or worse outcomes for women (Anton et al., 2006). It is important to note that the differences found in these studies may represent differing methods, outcome measures, and follow-up time period.

Nicotine

Worldwide, about 176 million women smoke tobacco daily; the majority of female smokers are in developed countries (Eriksen, Mackay, Schluger, Gomeshtapeh, & Drope, 2015). This has led to an increase in morbidity and mortality for women who may be at an increased risk for health problems compared to men. Women who smoke are twice as likely as men to have myocardial infarctions (Prescott, Hippe, Schnohr, Hein, & Vestbo, 1998), have faster lung deterioration, and are at increased risk for chronic obstructive pulmonary disease (Dransfield, Davis, Gerald, & Bailey, 2006) and lung cancer (Henschke, Yip, & Miettinen, 2006). Additionally, smoking-related deaths have increased in women and decreased in men (Centers for Disease Control and Prevention, 2002). Nicotine metabolism in women may provide a window into these gender differences. The genes for the cytochrome p450 enzymes responsible for metabolizing some of the chemicals in cigarette smoke are upregulated in females (Rahmanian, Diaz, & Wewers, 2011). This upregulation leads to increased metabolism of nicotine and increased toxic bioactive compounds, leading to adjusted dose consumption with increased exposure to toxins.

There are a number of barriers facing women when confronting tobacco cessation. The rate of decline of smoking in women is half that observed in men (25 vs. 50% rate reduction; Giovino, 2002). Several studies of self-quitters and treatment seekers demonstrate that women are less able to quit smoking than men, with or without treatment, nicotine replacement, or medication (Saladin et al., 2012). Women report shorter intervals between cigarettes and find it subjectively more difficult to quit smoking cigarettes than men (Lynch, Roth, & Carroll, 2002). Women appear to be more vulnerable than men to relapse to cigarette smoking with unaided cessation attempts (Perkins, 2001). This is thought to be due to differential sensitivity to nicotine, variation in responsiveness to social support, menstrual cycle effects, and gender-related differences in craving and reactivity to smoking cues (Saladin et al., 2012). Compared with men, women seem to be more influenced by nonpharmacological cues, such as the smell of the cigarette or people associated with smoking (Perkins et al., 2001), and less influenced by pharmacological factors, such as the dose of nicotine (Perkins et al., 2006; Perkins, Jacobs, Sanders, & Caggiula, 2002). Women's sensitivity to external cues associated with smoking leads to increased craving to smoke compared to men, suggesting that relapse prevention would be improved if treatments targeted reduction of cues associated with smoking by extinction training (Field & Duka, 2004). Relative to men, it has been shown that women have greater subjective craving for nicotine, stress, and arousal ratings in response to negative affect and stress (Saladin et al., 2012), suggesting that stress reduction may also aid in smoking cessation. Additionally, gonadal steroid hormones are thought to be associated with women's smoking cessation success or difficulty. Women who attempt to quit during the follicular phase are more likely to succeed than women who attempt to quit during the luteal phase (Newman & Mello, 2009; Perkins et al., 2000). Fears of weight gain also impede women's smoking cessation success. Women worry twice as much about weight gain caused by smoking cessation compared to men (Pirie, Murray, & Luepker, 1991) and relapse three times more often because of these concerns (Swan, Ward, Carmelli, & Jack, 1993).

There is inconclusive data regarding gender differences in the efficacy of nicotine replacement therapy (NRT); whereas some studies have found NRT equally effective in men and women (Munafo, Bradburn, Bowes, & David, 2004), others reveal that NRT is more effective in men than in women (Perkins & Scott, 2008). Non-nicotine medications such as bupropion and varenicline are equally effective in men and women, and bupropion is thought to have an added benefit in women of alleviating depression that contributes to its effectiveness in aiding smoking cessation (Gonzales et al., 2006; Scharf & Shiffman, 2004). Therapy and counseling, as adjunctive treatment to medication, may be more effective in women than in men (Cepeda-Benito, Reynoso, & Erath, 2004).

Cannabis

In 2010, marijuana was the illicit drug with the highest rate of past-year dependence or abuse, and the most common illicit drug of use among admissions to treatment in the United States (Substance Abuse and Mental Health Services Administration, 2011). Treatment was broadly defined as any location, including inpatient or outpatient treatment at a hospital or rehabilitation facility, mental health center, emergency department, doctor's office, prison or jail, or self-help groups. Marijuana use has been associated with several psychosocial problems, including low academic achievement, delinquency, legal problems, and unemployment (Sofuoglu, Sugarman, & Carroll, 2010). In addition, marijuana use is associated with dose-related impairments in verbal learning and memory, sustained attention, and executive functioning (Hart, van Gorp, Haney, Foltin, & Fischman, 2001; Heishman, Huestis, Henningfield, & Cone, 1990; McDonald, Schleifer, Richards, & de Wit, 2003; Solowij & Battisti, 2008).

Evidence indicates that women progress more rapidly from age of first use of marijuana to the development of cannabis dependence (Ehlers et al., 2010). Moreover, rates of marijuana use among 18- to 29-year-old African American and Hispanic women have increased over a 10 year period (Compton et al., 2004). Compared to nonusers, women who used marijuana were significantly more likely to have had vaginal intercourse and to have ever received treatment for a pelvic inflammatory disease (van Gelder, Reefhuis, Herron, Williams, & Roeleveld, 2011). Thus, compared with nonusers, female marijuana users seem to be engaging in higher rates of sexual behaviors that could put them at risk for sexually transmitted infections.

Stimulants

Women and female adolescents are equally, if not more, likely than their male counterparts to use and abuse methamphetamine and other stimulant drugs, and there is evidence that suggests females may be more vulnerable to the reinforcing effects of stimulants (Brady et al., 2009). Abstinent women report higher levels of craving following exposure to cocaine-related cues than men, which suggests that women may be more sensitive than men to addictive properties of cocaine (Gallop et al., 2007). Women are also three to four times more likely than men to become addicted within 24 months of first cocaine use (O'Brien & Anthony, 2005). Ovarian hormones, specifically estrogen and progesterone, are thought to play a role in mediating the initiation of drug use and reinforcing the effects of stimulants in females (Becker & Hu, 2008; Carroll, Lynch, Roth, Morgan, & Cosgrove, 2004; Sofuoglu, Mitchell, & Kosten, 2004). Estrogen is also thought to be neuroprotective, because women who abuse cocaine, crack cocaine, or methamphetamine have fewer perfusion abnormalities in the cortex and decreased neurotoxicity compared to men (Chang, Ernst, Strickland, & Mehringer, 1999; Dluzen & McDermott, 2002).

Few studies of treatment for methamphetamine addiction have focused on women or gender differences. One study offered methamphetamine-using women in prison standard outpatient treatment or a modified therapeutic community-based treatment prior to their release. There were modest gains in several outcomes (e.g., self-esteem, depression, among others) for both treatments, but the study treatment did not examine methamphetamine use following prison release (Rowan-Szal, Joe, Simpson, Greener, & Vance, 2009). While there are no approved pharmacological therapies, preclinical studies suggest that baclofen may help to decrease cocaine use among women (Campbell, Morgan, & Carroll, 2002; Hser, Evans, & Huang, 2005). In a few studies, bupropion for the treatment of methamphetamine use, and naltrexone for the treatment of cocaine use, have been shown to be more effective treatments in men than in women (Elkashef et al., 2008; Pettinati et al., 2008). Mirtazapine has been studied as a potential treatment of methamphetamine withdrawal because of its anxiolytic and sedative properties (Karila et al., 2010). A recent small randomized controlled trial of mirtazapine, in conjunction with substance use counseling, showed decreased methamphetamine use and associated decreases in risky sexual behaviors in methamphetamine-dependent sexually active men who have sex with men (Colfax et al., 2011). This study did not examine gender differences.

Opioids

Rates of heroin use are higher in men than in women (Back et al., 2011; Substance Abuse and Mental Health Services Administration, 2009). However, heroin dependence among women has been associated with higher rates of psychiatric problems and poorer physical health compared to men (Back et al., 2011; Grella & Lovinger, 2012; Shand, Degenhardt, Slade, & Nelson, 2011). Thus, although rates of heroin use are lower in women than in men, women present with more comorbidity and impairment. Conflicting evidence exists regarding gender differences in mortality rates associated with heroin use. Whereas one study found higher rates of mortality among male heroin users (Bauer et al., 2008), a longitudinal study that followed heroin-dependent patients 25 years postadmission to methadone maintenance treatment found no gender differences in mortality rates (Jimenez-Treviño et al., 2011). Jimenez-Treviño and colleagues also found that surviving women were more likely than men to be abstinent from heroin at the 25-year follow-up. With regard to treatment, one study found that women with heroin dependence are more likely than men to engage in methadone maintenance treatment (Coviello, Zanis, Wesnoski, Lynch, & Drapkin, 2011).

Prescription opioid misuse has increased dramatically in recent years (Back, Payne, Simpson, & Brady, 2010). In contrast to heroin use, women demonstrate equal or greater use of prescription opioids compared to men (Green, Serrano, Licari, Budman, & Butler, 2009). Findings from a large database study revealed that women more often reported past-30-day prescription opioid use, and the use of prescribed pain medication was the strongest factor for risk of abuse of prescription opioids (Green et al., 2009). Overall, studies that examine gender differences in prescription opioid use have found mixed results. Although some studies have shown that compared to men, women have greater nonmedical use of narcotic analgesics and are more likely to abuse prescription opioids, other studies have found either higher rates of nonmedical prescription opioid use in men or no gender difference in use patterns at all (for review, see Back et al., 2011). Similar to findings relative to heroin users, women who use prescription opioids report higher rates of psychological problems compared to men (Back et al., 2010).

CO-OCCURRENCE OF SUDs WITH HIV AND OTHER SEXUALLY TRANSMITTED INFECTIONS

It is well known that women with SUDs are susceptible to medical morbidity directly through toxic effects of the substances (carcinogenic effects, cytotoxic effects, etc.) and more indirectly by either contributing to transmission of infection or high-risk behavior. Women with SUDs are particularly vulnerable to sexually transmitted infections

(STIs) and blood-borne pathogens. Heterosexual contact is the primary transmission route of HIV in U.S. women of all ethnicities (Centers for Disease Control and Prevention, 2009). Heavy alcohol use and illicit drug use in women are markers for high-risk sexual behavior and have been shown to compromise use of preventive measures (e.g., use of condoms) and lead to an increase in heterosexual transmission of HIV and other STIs (El-Bassel, Witte, Wada, Gilbert, & Wallace, 2001; Samet et al., 2010; Weeks et al., 2010). Injection drug use and use of illegal drugs before or during sex are independent risk factors associated with viral hepatitis and syphilis infections in high-risk populations of women (Loza et al., 2010). Female injection drug users are even more susceptible given the dual risk of transmission via injection and sexual behavior. One study demonstrated that certain populations of vulnerable female injection drug users have developed a high-risk "altruistic" practice of sharing a syringe of blood drawn back immediately after initial heroin injection (flashblood), which contributes to the transmission of blood-borne infections (McCurdy, Ross, Williams, Kilonzo, & Leshabari, 2010). Women are more susceptible to transactional sex for substances, economic insecurity, and intimate partner violence. These factors may explain why some studies have shown that female injection drug users are at an elevated risk for HIV infection compared to men (Garfein, Vlahov, Galai, Doherty, & Nelson, 1996; Taran, Johnston, Pohorila, & Saliuk, 2011).

PSYCHIATRIC COMORBIDITY

Substance-abusing individuals show high rates of comorbid psychiatric disorders (Mann, Hintz, & Jung, 2004), and women evidence higher rates than men (Zilberman, Tavares, Blume, & el-Guebaly, 2003). Moreover, women are more likely than men to have multiple comorbid psychiatric diagnoses (Zilberman et al., 2003). This section covers the most common co-occurring disorders in women: mood and anxiety disorders, posttraumatic stress disorder, eating disorders, and borderline personality disorder.

Mood and Anxiety Disorders

As summarized by Zilberman and colleagues (2003), studies of treatment-seeking substance abusers indicate that women report higher rates of comorbid mood and anxiety disorders compared to men. Examination of the 2001–2002 NESARC data revealed that when gender differences occur, there are likely to be greater associations between SUDs and specific mood and anxiety disorders for women than for men (Conway, Compton, Stinson, & Grant, 2006). In particular, the high co-occurrence of depression and SUDs is well documented (Compton et al., 2007; Conway et al., 2006; Kessler et al., 1997). Women with SUDs are at twice the risk of having depression than men (Kessler et al., 1997). Depression has been linked to poor substance abuse treatment prognosis (Greenfield et al., 1998; Landheim, Bakken, & Vaglum, 2006). Substance-dependent women are also more likely than substance-dependent men to report suicide attempts (Zilberman et al., 2003). However, there is mixed evidence for gender differences in the effects of depression on substance use treatment outcomes. Some studies have found no gender differences in the effect of depression on treatment outcome (Greenfield et al., 1998; Kranzler, Del Boca, & Rounsaville, 1996). Another study found that women with co-occurring substance use and major depression had shorter periods of abstinence compared to women with only a substance use diagnosis, whereas dually diagnosed men had longer abstinence periods compared to men with only a substance use diagnosis (Westermeyer, Kopka, & Nugent, 1997). Thus, there is some evidence that depression may have greater significance in substance abuse treatment outcomes for women than for men. However, a few studies demonstrate that women with comorbid depression have better substance use treatment outcomes than men (Rounsaville, Dolinsky, Babor, & Meyer, 1987), and greater participation in treatment (Conner, Pinquart, & Duberstein, 2008).

A study of 100 substance-dependent individuals receiving inpatient treatment found that alcohol-dependent females had higher rates of all anxiety disorders and were three times more likely than men to be diagnosed with panic disorder (Brady, Grice, Dustan, & Randall, 1993). In this study, the authors also looked at course of the disorder and found that for women, onset of panic disorder preceded the SUD; whereas this was not the case for men (Brady et al., 1993). The finding of higher rates of anxiety disorders in females with SUDs has been replicated with larger samples as well (Grella, Karno, Warda, Niv, & Moore, 2009).

Posttraumatic Stress Disorder

The high comorbidity of posttraumatic stress disorder (PTSD) and substance use has been well established in the literature (Johnson, Cottler, O'Leary, & Abdallah, 2010; Zilberman et al., 2003). Individuals with comorbid PTSD and SUDs tend to have more severe psychiatric, medical, and psychosocial impairment as well (Peirce, Kindbom, Waesche, Yuscavage, & Brooner, 2008; Sonne, Back, Zuniga, Randall, & Brady, 2003). Research suggests that, compared to men, women more often develop PTSD after being exposed to trauma (Breslau, 2009; Kessler, Sonnega, Bromet, & Hughes, 1995), and women with PTSD are more likely to be drug dependent than women without PTSD (Kessler et al., 1995). Men and women differ in the type of trauma they experience. Women are more likely to report sexual assault, whereas men are more likely to report physical assault or combat-related trauma (Peirce et al., 2008; Sonne et al., 2003). Peirce and colleagues (2008) found that sexual assault trauma produced the highest rates of PTSD in a large sample of substance users. Women who have been exposed to trauma are also at a higher risk of developing an alcohol use disorder (Cottler, Compton, Mager, & Spitznagel, 1992). Sonne and colleagues (2003) investigated order of onset of PTSD and alcohol use disorders, and found that women were more likely than men to have a diagnosis of PTSD prior to developing alcohol dependence.

One treatment for comorbid substance abuse and PTSD in women is Seeking Safety (Hien et al., 2009; Najavits, 2002; Najavits, Weiss, Shaw, & Muenz, 1998), which is a cognitive-behavioral, integrated treatment for PTSD and SUDs. It has been shown to reduce substance use and PTSD symptoms in various populations of women (Hien, Cohen, Miele, Litt, & Capstick, 2004; Najavits, Gallop, & Weiss, 2006). Research comparing Seeking Safety to a women's health education control condition found that for more severe substance users, Seeking Safety was more effective than the control condition at reducing substance use (Hien et al., 2010).

Eating Disorders

Studies have shown that 30–50% of individuals with bulimia and 12–18% of individuals with anorexia had a concurrent diagnosis of an alcohol or drug use disorder (National Center on Addiction and Substance Abuse, 2003). Lifetime eating disorder behaviors co-occurred with SUDs in up to 40% of women (Holderness, Brooks-Gunn, & Warren, 1994). Additionally, a history of sexual or physical trauma is associated with greater rates of substance abuse among women with binge-eating disorder (Dohm et al., 2002).

Despite the significant rate of co-occurrence of eating disorders and SUDs in women, there are currently no integrated treatments. Additionally, a minority of publicly funded (Gordon et al., 2008) and privately funded (Killeen et al., 2011) addiction treatment programs screen for eating disorders. A randomized controlled trial of treatment-seeking woman with PTSD and SUDs found that the most common eating disorder behavior reported in this population was binge eating. In this group, women with binge-eating behaviors had worse substance abuse treatment outcomes than those without binge-eating behaviors (Cohen et al., 2010; Greenfield et al., 2011).

Borderline Personality Disorder

In clinical settings, 75% of patients with borderline personality disorder (BPD) are female (Gunderson, 2011; Lenzenweger, Lane, Loranger, & Kessler, 2007). BPD has a high rate of co-occurrence with SUDs, with some studies demonstrating that up to half or more patients with BPD have co-occurring alcohol or drug use disorders (Fenton et al., 2012; Zanarini et al., 1998). One study demonstrated that co-occurring BPD and drug use disorders significantly predicted prospective suicide attempts (Yen et al., 2003). It is thought that the high rate of co-occurring SUDs in BPD, compared with other personality disorders, may be related to poor impulse control in BPD (Walter et al., 2009). Individuals with BPD show higher responses to psychosocial stressors, specifically interpersonal stressors, compared to healthy individuals, and this may heighten vulnerability to new onset of, and relapse to an SUD (Walter et al., 2009).

BPD is a specific predictor of drug use disorder persistence over time (Fenton et al., 2012). A co-occurrence of SUD and BPD is associated with poor outcomes, resistance to treatment, and slowed time to remission of symptoms (Verheul, 2001; Zanarini et al., 2011). Remission of an SUD is sometimes followed by remission of BPD, and treatment of the SUD should be a priority in this patient population (Gunderson et al., 2003).

TREATMENT

Screening

Accurate identification, assessment, and diagnosis of SUDs are critical first steps to ensure successful treatment in both men and women. However, in light of data indicating an accelerated course of addiction in women compared with men, screening and early, prompt identification of SUDs may have additional importance in pre-venting adverse consequences of addiction in women. Also, because at least one-fourth of pregnant women use substances during pregnancy, and substance use dur-ing pregnancy can contribute to adverse pregnancy and neonatal outcomes, effective screening for SUDs in pregnant women or women who are planning pregnancies can be another important health intervention in this population. In conjunction with structured interviews, detailed history, physical examination, and biological mark-ers, standardized screening instruments are useful tools that enhance assessment and evaluation of severity. The CAGE (Cut down, Annoyed, Guilty, Eye-opener), the Alcohol Use Disorders Identification Test (AUDIT) and the Short Michigan Alcohol and Screening Test (S-MAST) can be used to assess for alcohol dependence in adults (Greenfield & Hennessy, 2008). The Michigan Alcohol Screening Test (MAST), Drug Abuse Screening Test (DAST) and Fagerstrom Test for Nicotine Dependence can be used to evaluate problem drinking, drug abuse and nicotine dependence, respectively, in adults and adolescents (Greenfield & Hennessy, 2008). The CRAFFT (Car, Relax, Alone, Forget, Friends, Trouble) consists of six questions designed to evaluate drug and alcohol abuse in an adolescent population. Additionally, there are two tests, the TWEAK (Tolerance, Worried, Eye-opener, Amnesia, Cut down) and the T-ACE (Tol-erance, Annoyed, Cut down, Eye-opener), designed to identify high-risk drinking in pregnant women. The TWEAK consists of five items and has been validated in both men and women. The T-ACE consists of four items and looks at quantities of alcohol that might be dangerous to the fetus (Greenfield & Hennessy, 2008).

Treatment Outcomes

Women with SUDs are less likely in the course of their lifetime than their male coun-terparts to enter treatment, but once in treatment, few or no gender differences in outcome exist (Greenfield, Brooks, et al., 2007). However, gender-specific predictors of outcome suggest that treatment approaches tailored to these characteristics matter. Some predictors of outcome that vary by gender include co-occurring psychiatric dis-orders, history of victimization, treatment retention and completion, and therapist–patient gender matching. Co-occurring psychiatric disorders and history of victim-ization have been shown to have a negative impact on substance abuse treatment response (Greenfield, Brooks, et al., 2007) and their greater prevalence in women compared with men may have greater salience for SUD treatment outcome. Some factors, including greater financial resources, fewer mental health problems, and less severe drug problems, are associated with more favorable treatment outcomes in both men and women (Green, Polen, Dickinson, Lynch, & Bennett, 2002; Greenfield, Brooks, et al., 2007). Better psychological functioning, higher levels of personal sta-bility and social support, lower levels of anger, treatment beliefs, and referral source are associated with retention in women-only samples (Greenfield, Brooks, et al., 2007; Kelly, Blacksin, & Mason, 2001; Loneck, Garrett, & Banks, 1997).

Men and women also differ in addiction treatment referral sources. Approxi-mately twice as many women are referred from community agencies (welfare, mental health, and other health care providers) as men (Schmidt & Weisner, 1995). Men are more likely than women to be referred through the criminal justice system; however, the number of female prisoners is growing, largely due to changes in sentencing for drug-related charges that have disproportionately affected women (Harrison & Beck, 2005). This suggests that the criminal justice system is increasingly more relevant to women with SUD.

Children can play a particularly important role in women's entrance to treatment. Most women who enter substance abuse treatment are mothers, and more than half of them have had contact with child welfare (Conners et al., 2004; Grella, Scott, Foss, Joshi, & Hser, 2003). One study of mothers on methadone maintenance found that women residing with their children were more likely to enter treatment than women not residing with their children (Lundgren, Schilling, Fitzgerald, Davis, & Amodeo, 2003), while other evidence suggests that residing with children can be an obstacle to entering treatment because the mothers fear losing custody (Haller, Miles, & Dawson, 2003). Once in treatment, women who are able to keep their children with them or retain custody are more likely to continue treatment (Chen et al., 2004).

In some studies, treatment effectiveness can be enhanced when treatment is directed toward a specific problem that is more common to substance abusing women or to a specific subgroup, such as older women (Greenfield, Brooks, et al., 2007). For example, adding a trauma-focused treatment component to women with PTSD and SUD led to PTSD symptom improvement. Sustained reductions in PTSD symptoms can be associated with subsequent substance use improvement (Greenfield et al., 2011).

Gender-Specific Treatment for Women with SUDs

Compared with mixed-gender treatment programs, gender-specific treatment programs for women address characteristics that are more prevalent in women, such as psychiatric comorbidity; history of trauma; differences in interaction styles; and other psychosocial issues that differentially affect women, such as parenting and child care, pregnancy, and the social stigma of substance use (for review, see Greenfield & Pirard, 2009). According to a meta-analysis by Orwin, Francisco, and Bernichon (2001), women's treatment programs are more likely to include services for women that enhance treatment outcomes, such as family planning, child care services, self-esteem and assertiveness training, and parent training. Such women-focused treatment is associated with greater satisfaction among women and provides a more comfortable treatment environment compared to mixed-gender treatment (Greenfield & Grella, 2009).

Single-gender group therapy for women has been shown to enhance comfort and promote communication, thereby enhancing treatment outcomes (Kauffman, Dore, & Nelson-Zlupko, 1995). One study indicated that women with low self-efficacy may have more enhanced treatment outcomes in a single-gender substance use treatment group than in mixed-gender group treatment (Cummings, Gallop, & Greenfield, 2010). Better retention rates, which have been associated with increased abstinence rates, have been found for women-only (WO) compared to mixed-gender (MG) programs (Claus et al., 2007; Grella, Joshi, & Hser, 2000; Grella, Polinsky, Hser, & Perry, 1999). Participation in WO treatment programs has also been associated with increased levels of continuity of care following discharge (Claus et al., 2007). The meta-analysis by Orwin and colleagues (2001) determined that, compared to MG treatment programs, WO treatment programs showed positive outcomes in six domains: alcohol use, drug use, psychiatric problems, attitudes and beliefs, psychological well-being, and criminal activity; however, five of the effect sizes for these outcomes were small (only psychiatric problems exceeded a small effect size), and the analysis was based on only four studies. Thus, these results should be interpreted with caution.

More recently, several quasi-experimental design studies have compared women in WO programs to those in MG programs (Claus et al., 2007; Hser, Evans, Huang, & Messina, 2011; Niv & Hser, 2007; Prendergast, Messina, Hall, & Warda, 2011). In general, these WO programs are not only all-female in patient and staff composition, but they also differ from MG programs in treatment philosophies and types of services provided (Prendergast et al., 2011). One study examined characteristics of women in WO programs compared to those in MG programs and found that the former had more severe alcohol, drug use, and psychiatric severity; were less educated and more likely to be white; were more likely to report physical abuse; and were engaged in more treatment services (Niv & Hser, 2007). In spite of higher scores on drug use and psychiatric severity, the results of this study also showed that women in WO programs had better drug use outcomes at 9-month follow-up and were less likely to report arrests (Niv & Hser, 2007). A recent study comparing 12 WO outpatient programs to eight MG outpatient programs found that women in the WO programs were less likely to report substance use and criminal activity at 12-month follow-up compared to women in the MG programs; however, women in the MG programs were more likely to be employed (Prendergast et al., 2011). Examination of long-term outcomes (8 years postadmission to treatment) for mothers in WO compared to those in MG treatment programs indicated that mothers in the MG programs showed increased rates of incarceration posttreatment, whereas mothers in the WO program had stable rates of incarceration (Hser et al., 2011). However, no other differences were found between the two types of programs in regard to long-term trajectories.

Few randomized controlled trials have compared WO and MG treatment. The majority of randomized controlled trials have focused on WO group therapies for SUDs and specific populations of women, such as pregnant women (Reynolds, Coombs, Lowe, Peterson, & Gayoso, 1995), women with comorbid PTSD (Hien et al., 2004), and women with comorbid borderline personality disorder (Linehan et al., 1999). One randomized controlled study examined women-specific group therapy for SUDs in a heterogeneous sample of women (Greenfield, Trucco, McHugh, Lincoln, & Gallop, 2007). This study compared the Women's Recovery Group (WRG) to mixed-gender Group Drug Counseling (GDC). The WRG is a manual-based, relapse prevention group therapy that uses a relapse prevention approach and has both women-focused content and an all-women group composition (Greenfield, in press). No differences were found between groups during the 12-week treatment phase of the study; however, at 6-months posttreatment, women in the WRG showed greater reductions in drug and alcohol use compared to women in the mixed-gender GDC group (Greenfield, Trucco, et al., 2007).

FUTURE DIRECTIONS

Although there have been several quasi-experimental studies of women-only treatment programs for SUDs, there have been relatively few randomized controlled trials of gender-specific treatments. Moreover, given the high rates of psychiatric comorbidity and SUDs in women, more research on combined treatments is necessary. Furthermore, it is also important to understand which subpopulations of women would benefit more from gender-specific treatment than standard treatment. Research on expanding treatment programs for women to community settings, primary care clinics, and urgent care centers is also a necessary next step. Additionally, there are limited studies on the neurobiological gender differences in substance abuse. Future efforts should focus on understanding gender differences in risk for developing SUDs, biomarkers for treatment response, and the neurobiological and molecular levels during intoxication, withdrawal, and craving across different substances in addition to potential psychopharmacological and psychotherapeutic targets.

ACKNOWLEDGMENTS

This work was supported in part by Grant No. K24 DA019855 (to Shelly F. Greenfield) from the National Institute on Drug Abuse and by the McLean Hospital Women's Mental Health Initiative. We wish to thank Sara Wigderson, BA, for her help with the preparation of this chapter.

REFERENCES

Acker, C. (1986). Neuropsychological deficits in alcoholics: The relative contributions of gender and drinking history. *Br J Addict, 81*(3), 395–403.

Allamani, A. (2008). Alcoholic beverages, gender and European cultures. *Subst Use Misuse, 43*(8–9), 1088–1097.

Alvanzo, A. A. H., Storr, C. L., La Flair, L., Green, K. M., Wagner, F. A., & Crum, R. M. (2011). Race/ethnicity and sex differences in progression from drinking initiation to the development of alcohol dependence. *Drug Alcohol Depend, 118*(2–3), 375–382.

Anton, R. F., O'Malley, S. S., Ciraulo, D. A., Cisler, R. A., Couper, D., Donovan, D. M., et al. (2006). Combined pharmacotherapies and behavioral interventions for alcohol dependence: The COMBINE Study. *JAMA, 295*, 2003–2017.

Back, S. E., Payne, R. L., Simpson, A. N., & Brady, K. T. (2010). Gender and prescription opioids: Findings from the National Survey on Drug Use and Health. *Addict Behav, 35*(11), 1001–1007.

Back, S. E., Payne, R. L., Wahlquist, A. H., Carter, R. E., Stroud, Z., Haynes, L., et al. (2011). Comparative profiles of men and women with opioid dependence: Results from a national multisite effectiveness trial. *Am J Drug Alcohol Abuse, 37*(5), 313–323.

Back, S. E., Waldrop, A. E., Saladin, M. E., Yeatts, S. D., Simpson, A., McRae, A. L., et al. (2008). Effects of gender and cigarette smoking on reactivity to psychological and pharmacological stress provocation. *Psychoneuroendocrinol, 33*(5), 560–568.

Bauer, S. M., Loipl, R., Jagsch, R., Gruber, D., Risser, D., Thau, K., et al. (2008). Mortality in opioid-maintained patients after release from an addiction clinic. *Eur Addict Res, 14*(2), 82–91.

Becker, J. B., & Hu, M. (2008). Sex differences in drug abuse. *Front Neuroendocrinol, 29*(1), 36–47.

Blazer, D. G., & Wu, L.-T. (2009). The epidemiology of at-risk and binge drinking among middle-aged and elderly community adults: National Survey on Drug Use and Health. *Am J Psychiatry, 166*(10), 1162–1169.

Brady, K. T., Back, S. E., & Greenfield, S. F. (2009). *Women and addiction: A comprehensive handbook.* New York: Guilford Press.

Brady, K. T., Grice, D. E., Dustan, L., & Randall, C. (1993). Gender differences in substance use disorders. *Am J Psychiatry, 150*(11), 1707–1711.

Breslau, N. (2009). The epidemiology of trauma, PTSD, and other posttrauma disorders. *Trauma Violence Abuse, 10*(3), 198–210.

Caetano, R. (2003). Alcohol-related health disparities and treatment related epidemiological findings among Whites, Blacks, and Hispanics in the United States. *Alcohol Clin Exp Res, 27*, 1337–1339.

Campbell, U. C., Morgan, A. D., & Carroll, M. E. (2002). Sex differences in the effects of baclofen on the acquisition of intravenous cocaine self-administration in rats. *Drug Alcohol Depend, 66*(1), 61–69.

Carpenter, M. J., Upadhyaya, H. P., LaRowe, S. D., Saladin, M. E., & Brady, K. T. (2006). Menstrual cycle phase effects on nicotine withdrawal and cigarette craving: A review. *Nicotine Tob Res, 8*(5), 627–638.

Carroll, M. E., Lynch, W. J., Roth, M. E., Morgan, A. D., & Cosgrove, K. P. (2004). Sex and estrogen influence drug abuse. *Trends Pharmacol Sci, 25*(5), 273–279.

Centers for Disease Control and Prevention. (2002). Annual smoking-attributable mortality, years of potential life lost, and economic costs—United States, 1995–1999. *MMWR, 51*(14), 300–303.

Centers for Disease Control and Prevention. (2009). Cases of HIV infection and AIDS in the United States and dependent areas by race/ethnicity, 2003–2007. *HIV AIDS Surveill Suppl Rep, 14*(2), 1–43.

Cepeda-Benito, A., Reynoso, J. T., & Erath, S. (2004). Meta-analysis of the efficacy of nicotine replacement therapy for smoking cessation: Differences between men and women. *J Consult Clin Psychol, 72*(4), 712–722.

Chang, L., Ernst, T., Strickland, T., & Mehringer, C. M. (1999). Gender effects on persistent cerebral metabolite changes in the frontal lobes of abstinent cocaine users. *Am J Psychiatry, 156*(5), 716–722.

Chavez, P. R., Nelson, D. E., Naimi, T. S., & Brewer, R. D. (2011). Impact of a new gender-specific definition for binge drinking on prevalence estimates for women. *Am J Prev Med, 40*(4), 468–471.

Chen, X., Burgdorf, K., Dowell, K., Roberts, T., Porowski, A., & Herrell, J. M. (2004). Factors associated with retention of drug abusing women in long-term residential treatment. *Eval Prog Plann, 27*(2), 205–212.

Claus, R. E., Orwin, R. G., Kissin, W., Krupski, A., Campbell, K., & Stark, K. (2007). Does gender-specific substance abuse treatment for women promote continuity of care? *J Subst Abuse Treat, 32*(1), 27–39.

Cohen, L. R., Greenfield, S. F., Gordon, S., Killeen, T., Jiang, H., Zhang, Y., et al. (2010). Survey of eating disorder symptoms among women in treatment for substance abuse. *Am J Addict, 19*(3), 245–251.

Colfax, G. N., Santos, G.-M., Das, M., Santos, D. M., Matheson, T., Gasper, J., et al. (2011). Mirtazapine to reduce methamphetamine use: A randomized controlled trial. *Arch Gen Psychiatry, 68*(11), 1168–1175.

Compton, W. M., Grant, B. F., Colliver, J. D., Glantz, M. D., & Stinson, F. S. (2004). Prevalence of marijuana use disorders in the United States: 1991–1992 and 2001–2002. *JAMA, 291*(17), 2114–2121.

Compton, W. M., Thomas, Y. F., Stinson, F. S., & Grant, B. F. (2007). Prevalence, correlates, disability, and comorbidity of DSM-IV drug abuse and dependence in the United States: Results from the National Epidemiologic Survey on Alcohol and Related Conditions. *Arch Gen Psychiatry, 64*(5), 566–576.

Conner, K. R., Pinquart, M., & Duberstein, P. R. (2008). Meta-analysis of depression and substance use and impairment among intravenous drug users (IDUs). *Addiction, 103*(4), 524–534.

Conners, N. A., Bradley, R. H., Mansell, L. W., Liu, J. Y., Roberts, T. J., Burgdorf, K., et al. (2004). Children of mothers with serious substance abuse problems: An accumulation of risks. *Am J Drug Alcohol Abuse, 30*(1), 85–100.

Conway, K. P., Compton, W., Stinson, F. S., & Grant, B. F. (2006). Lifetime comorbidity of DSM-IV mood and anxiety disorders and specific drug use disorders: Results from the National Epidemiologic Survey on Alcohol and Related Conditions. *J Clin Psychiatry, 67*(2), 247–257.

Cottler, L. B., Compton, W. M., Mager, D., & Spitznagel, E. L. (1992). Posttraumatic stress disorder among substance users from the general population. *Am J Psychiatry, 149*(5), 664–670.

Coviello, D. M., Zanis, D. A., Wesnoski, S. A., Lynch, K. G., & Drapkin, M. (2011). Characteristics and 9-month outcomes of discharged methadone maintenance clients. *J Subst Abuse Treat, 40*(2), 165–174.

Cummings, A. M., Gallop, R. J., & Greenfield, S. F. (2010). Self-efficacy and substance use outcomes for women in single gender versus mixed-gender group treatment. *J Groups Addict Recover, 5*(1), 4–16.

Diehl, A., Croissant, B., Batra, A., Mundle, G., Nakovics, H., & Mann, K. (2007). Alcoholism in women: Is it different in onset and outcome compared to men? *Eur Arch Psychiatry Clin Neurosci, 257*(6), 344–351.

Dluzen, D. E., & McDermott, J. L. (2002). Estrogen, anti-estrogen, and gender: Differences in methamphetamine neurotoxicity. In S. F. Ali (Ed.), *Cellular and molecular mechanisms of drugs of abuse: II. Cocaine, substituted amphetamines, GHB, and opiates* (pp. 136–156). New York: New York Academy of Sciences.

Dohm, F.-A., Striegel-Moore, R. H., Wilfley, D. E., Pike, K. M., Hook, J., & Fairburn, C. G. (2002). Self-harm and substance use in a community sample of black and white women with binge eating disorder or bulimia nervosa. *Int J Eat Disord, 32*(4), 389–400.

Drabble, L., Midanik, L. T., & Trocki, K. (2005). Reports of alcohol consumption and alcohol-related problems among homosexual, bisexual and heterosexual respondents: Results from the 2000 National Alcohol Survey. *J Stud Alcohol, 66*(1), 111–120.

Dransfield, M. T., Davis, J. J., Gerald, L. B., & Bailey, W. C. (2006). Racial and gender differences in susceptibility to tobacco smoke among patients with chronic obstructive pulmonary disease. *Respir Med, 100*(6), 1110–1116.

Ebrahim, S. H., & Gfroerer, J. (2003). Pregnancy-related substance use in the United States during 1996–1998. *Obstet Gynecol, 101*(2), 374–379.

Ehlers, C. L., Gizer, I. R., Vieten, C., Gilder, D. A., Stouffer, G. M., Lau, P., et al. (2010). Cannabis dependence in the San Francisco Family Study: Age of onset of use, DSM-IV symptoms, withdrawal, and heritability. *Addict Behav, 35*(2), 102–110.

El-Bassel, N., Witte, S. S., Wada, T., Gilbert, L., & Wallace, J. (2001). Correlates of partner violence among female street-based sex workers: Substance abuse, history of childhood abuse, and HIV risks. *AIDS Patient Care STDS, 15*(1), 41–51.

Elkashef, A. M., Rawson, R. A., Anderson, A. L., Li, S. H., Holmes, T., Smith, E. V., et al. (2008). Bupropion for the treatment of methamphetamine dependence. *Neuropsychopharmacol, 33*(5), 1162–1170.

El-Mohandes, A., Herman, A. A., Nabil El-Khorazaty, M., Katta, P. S., White, D., & Grylack, L. (2003). Prenatal care reduces the impact of illicit drug use on perinatal outcomes. *J Perinatol, 23*(5), 354–360.

Eriksen, M., Mackay, J., Schluger, N., Gomeshtapeh, F., & Drope, J. (2015). *The tobacco atlas* (5th ed.). Atlanta, GA: American Cancer Society.

Evans, S. M., & Foltin, R. W. (2006). Exogenous progesterone attenuates the subjective effects of smoked cocaine in women, but not in men. *Neuropsychopharmacol, 31*(3), 659–674.

Fenton, M. C., Keyes, K., Geier, T., Greenstein, E., Skodol, A., Krueger, B., et al. (2012). Psychiatric comorbidity and the persistence of drug use disorders in the United States. *Addiction, 107*(3), 599–609.

Field, M., & Duka, T. (2004). Cue reactivity in smokers: The effects of perceived cigarette availability and gender. *Pharmacol Biochem Behav, 78*(3), 647–652.

Foster, J. H., Peters, T. J., & Marshall, E. J. (2000). Quality of life measures and outcome in alcohol-dependent men and women. *Alcohol, 22*(1), 45–52.

Fox, H. C., Garcia, M., Jr., Kemp, K., Milivojevic, V., Kreek, M. J., & Sinha, R. (2006). Gender differences in cardiovascular and corticoadrenal response to stress and drug cues in cocaine dependent individuals. *Psychopharmacol, 185*(3), 348–357.

Fox, H. C., Hong, K. A., Paliwal, P., Morgan, P. T., & Sinha, R. (2008). Altered levels of sex and stress steroid hormones assessed daily over a 28-day cycle in early abstinent cocaine-dependent females. *Psychopharmacol, 195*(4), 527–536.

Gallop, R. J., Crits-Christoph, P., Ten Have, T. R., Barber, J. P., Frank, A., Griffin, M. L., et al. (2007). Differential transitions between cocaine use and abstinence for men and women. *J Consult Clin Psychol, 75*(1), 95–103.

Garfein, R. S., Vlahov, D., Galai, N., Doherty, M. C., & Nelson, K. E. (1996). Viral infections in short-term injection drug users: The prevalence of the hepatitis C, hepatitis B, human immunodeficiency, and human T-lymphotropic viruses. *Am J Public Health, 86*(5), 655–661.

Giovino, G. A. (2002). Epidemiology of tobacco use in the United States. *Oncogene, 21*(48), 7326–7340.

Gonzales, D., Rennard, S. I., Nides, M., Oncken, C., Azoulay, S., Billing, C. B., et al. (2006). Varenicline, an alpha$_4$beta$_2$ nicotinic acetylcholine receptor partial agonist, vs sustained-release bupropion and placebo for smoking cessation: A randomized controlled trial. *JAMA, 296*(1), 47–55.

Gordon, S. M., Johnson, J. A., Greenfield, S. F., Cohen, L., Killeen, T., & Roman, P. M. (2008). Assessment and treatment of co-occurring eating disorders in publicly funded addiction treatment programs. *Psychiatr Serv, 59*(9), 1056–1059.

Green, C. A., Polen, M. R., Dickinson, D. M., Lynch, F. L., & Bennett, M. D. (2002). Gender differences in predictors of initiation, retention, and completion in an HMO-based substance abuse treatment program. *J Subst Abuse Treat, 23*(4), 285–295.

Green, T. C., Serrano, J. M. G., Licari, A., Budman, S. H., & Butler, S. F. (2009). Women who abuse prescription opioids: Findings from the Addiction Severity Index–Multimedia Version® Connect prescription opioid database. *Drug Alcohol Depend, 103*(1–2), 65–73.

Greenfield, S. F. (in press). *Treating women with substance use disorders: The Women's Recovery Group*. New York: Guilford Press.

Greenfield, S. F., Back, S., & Brady, K. (2011). Women's issues. In P. Ruiz & E. Strain (Eds.), *Lowinson and Ruiz's substance abuse: A comprehensive textbook* (5th ed., pp. 847–870). Baltimore, MD: Lippincott, Williams & Wilkins.

Greenfield, S. F., Back, S. E., Lawson, K., & Brady, K. T. (2010). Substance abuse in women. *Psychiatr Clin N Am, 33*(2), 339–355.

Greenfield, S. F., Brooks, A. J., Gordon, S. M., Green, C. A., Kropp, F., McHugh, R. K., et al. (2007). Substance abuse treatment entry, retention, and outcome in women: A review of the literature. *Drug Alcohol Depend, 86*(1), 1–21.

Greenfield, S. F., & Grella, C. E. (2009). What is "women-focused" treatment for substance use disorders? *Psychiatr Serv, 60*(7), 880–882.

Greenfield, S. F., & Hennessy, G. (2008). Assessment of the patient. In M. Galanter & H. D. Kleber (Eds.), *The American Psychiatric Publishing textbook of substance abuse treatment* (4th ed., pp. 55–78). Arlington, VA: American Psychiatric Publishing.

Greenfield, S. F., & O'Leary, G. (2002). Sex differences in substance use disorders. In F. Lewis-Hall, T. S. Williams, J. A. Panetta, & J. M. Herrera (Eds.), *Psychiatric illness in women: Emerging treatments and research* (pp. 467–533). Arlington, VA: American Psychiatric Publishing.

Greenfield, S. F., & Pirard, S. (2009). Gender-specific treatment for women with substance use disorders. In K. T. Brady, S. E. Back, & S. F. Greenfield (Eds.), *Women and addiction: A comprehensive handbook*. New York: Guilford Press.

Greenfield, S. F., Rosa, C., Putnins, S. I., Green, C. A., Brooks, A. J., Calsyn, D. A., et al. (2011). Gender research in the National Institute on Drug Abuse National Treatment Clinical Trials Network: A summary of findings. *Am J Drug Alcohol Abuse, 37*(5), 301–312.

Greenfield, S. F., Trucco, E. M., McHugh, R. K., Lincoln, M., & Gallop, R. J. (2007). The women's recovery group study: A stage I trial of women-focused group therapy for substance use disorders versus mixed-gender group drug counseling. *Drug Alcohol Depend, 90*(1), 39–47.

Greenfield, S. F., Weiss, R. D., Muenz, L. R., Vagge, L. M., Kelly, J. F., Bello, L. R., et al. (1998). The effect of depression on return to drinking: A prospective study. *Arch Gen Psychiatry, 55*(3), 259–265.

Grella, C. E., Joshi, V., & Hser, Y.-I. (2000). Program variation in treatment outcomes among women in residential drug treatment. *Eval Rev, 24*(4), 364–383.

Grella, C. E., Karno, M. P., Warda, U. S., Niv, N., & Moore, A. A. (2009). Gender and comorbidity among individuals with opioid use disorders in the NESARC study. *Addict Behav, 34*(6–7), 498–504.

Grella, C. E., & Lovinger, K. (2012). Gender differences in physical and mental health outcomes among an aging cohort of individuals with a history of heroin dependence. *Addict Behav, 37*(3), 306–312.

Grella, C. E., Polinsky, M. L., Hser, Y. I., & Perry, S. M. (1999). Characteristics of women-only and mixed-gender drug abuse treatment programs. *J Subst Abuse Treat, 17*(1–2), 37–44.

Grella, C. E., Scott, C. K., Foss, M. A., Joshi, V., & Hser, Y.-I. (2003). Gender differences in drug treatment outcomes among participants in the Chicago Target Cities Study. *Eval Prog Plann, 26*(3), 297–310.

Grucza, R. A., Bucholz, K. K., Rice, J. P., & Bierut, L. J. (2008). Secular trends in the lifetime prevalence of alcohol dependence in the United States: A re-evaluation. *Alcohol Clin Exp Res, 32*(5), 763–770.

Gunderson, J. G. (2011). Borderline personality disorder. *N Engl J Med, 364*(21), 2037–2042.

Gunderson, J. G., Bender, D., Sanislow, C., Yen, S., Rettew, J. B., Dolan-Sewell, R., et al. (2003). Plausibility and possible determinants of sudden "remissions" in borderline patients. *Psychiatry, 66*(2), 111–119.

Haas, A. L., & Peters, R. H. (2000). Development of substance abuse problems among drug-involved offenders: Evidence for the telescoping effect. *J Subst Abuse, 12*(3), 241–253.

Hahm, H. C., Wong, F. Y., Huang, Z. J., Ozonoff, A., & Lee, J. (2008). Substance use among Asian Americans and Pacific Islanders sexual minority adolescents: Findings from the National Longitudinal Study of Adolescent Health. *J Adolesc Health, 42*(3), 275–283.

Haller, D. L., Miles, D. R., & Dawson, K. S. (2003). Factors influencing treatment enrollment by pregnant substance abusers. *Am J Drug Alcohol Abuse, 29*(1), 117–131.

Harrison, P. M., & Beck, A. J. (2005). *Prisoners in 2004* (Bureau of Justice Statistics Bulletin NCJ 210677). Washington, DC: U.S. Department of Justice, Office of Justice Programs.

Hart, C. L., van Gorp, W., Haney, M., Foltin, R. W., & Fischman, M. W. (2001). Effects of acute smoked marijuana on complex cognitive performance. *Neuropsychopharmacol, 25*(5), 757–765.

Hasin, D. S., Stinson, F. S., Ogburn, E., & Grant, B. F. (2007). Prevalence, correlates, disability, and comorbidity of DSM-IV alcohol abuse and dependence in the United States: Results from the National Epidemiologic Survey on Alcohol and Related Conditions. *Arch Gen Psychiatry, 64*(7), 830–842.

Havens, J. R., Simmons, L. A., Shannon, L. M., & Hansen, W. F. (2009). Factors associated with substance use during pregnancy: Results from a national sample. *Drug Alcohol Depend, 99*(1–3), 89–95.

Heishman, S. J., Huestis, M. A., Henningfield, J. E., & Cone, E. J. (1990). Acute and residual effects of marijuana: Profiles of plasma THC levels, physiological, subjective, and performance measures. *Pharmacol Biochem Behav, 37*(3), 561–565.

Helzer, J. E., Burnam, A., & McEvoy, L. T. (1991). Alcohol abuse and dependence. In L. N. Robins & D. A. Regier (Eds.), *Psychiatric disorders in America: The Epidemiological Catchment Area Study* (pp. 81–115). New York: Free Press.

Henschke, C. I., Yip, R., & Miettinen, O. S. (2006). Women's susceptibility to tobacco carcinogens and survival after diagnosis of lung cancer. *JAMA, 296*(2), 180–184.

Hernandez-Avila, C. A., Rounsaville, B. J., & Kranzler, H. R. (2004). Opioid-, cannabis- and alcohol-dependent women show more rapid progression to substance abuse treatment. *Drug Alcohol Depend, 74*(3), 265–272.

Hien, D. A., Cohen, L. R., Miele, G. M., Litt, L. C., & Capstick, C. (2004). Promising treatments for women with comorbid PTSD and substance use disorders. *Am J Psychiatry, 161*(8), 1426–1432.

Hien, D. A., Jiang, H., Campbell, A. N. C., Hu, M.-C., Miele, G. M., Cohen, L. R., et al. (2010). Do treatment improvements in PTSD severity affect substance use outcomes?: A secondary analysis from a randomized clinical trial in NIDA's Clinical Trials Network. *Am J Psychiatry, 167*(1), 95–101.

Hien, D. A., Wells, E. A., Jiang, H., Suarez-Morales, L., Campbell, A. N. C., Cohen, L. R., et al. (2009). Multisite randomized trial of behavioral interventions for women with co-occurring PTSD and substance use disorders. *J Consult Clin Psychol, 77*(4), 607–619.

Holderness, C. C., Brooks-Gunn, J., & Warren, M. P. (1994). Co-morbidity of eating disorders and substance abuse review of the literature. *Int J Eat Disord, 16*(1), 1–34.

Holdstock, L., & de Wit, H. (2000). Effects of ethanol at four phases of the menstrual cycle. *Psychopharmacol, 150*(4), 374–382.

Hser, Y.-I., Evans, E., & Huang, Y. C. (2005). Treatment outcomes among women and men methamphetamine abusers in California. *J Subst Abuse Treat, 28*(1), 77–85.

Hser, Y.-I., Evans, E., Huang, D., & Messina, N. (2011). Long-term outcomes among drug-dependent mothers treated in women-only versus mixed-gender programs. *J Subst Abuse Treat, 41*(2), 115–123.

Jimenez-Treviño, L., Saiz, P. A., García-Portilla, M. P., Díaz-Mesa, E. M., Sánchez-Lasheras, F., Burón, P., et al. (2011). A 25-year follow-up of patients admitted to methadone treatment for the first time: Mortality and gender differences. *Addict Behav, 36*(12), 1184–1190.

Johnson, P. B., Richter, L., Kleber, H. D., McLellan, A. T., & Carise, D. (2005). Telescoping of drinking-related behaviors: Gender, racial/ethnic, and age comparisons. *Subst Use Misuse, 40*(8), 1139–1151.

Johnson, S. D., Cottler, L. B., O'Leary, C. C., & Abdallah, A. B. (2010). The association of trauma and PTSD with the substance use profiles of alcohol- and cocaine-dependent out-of-treatment women. *Am J Addict, 19*(6), 490–495.

Kajantie, E., & Phillips, D. I. W. (2006). The effects of sex and hormonal status on the physiological response to acute psychosocial stress. *Psychoneuroendocrinol, 31*(2), 151–178.

Karila, L., Weinstein, A., Aubin, H. J., Benyamina, A., Reynaud, M., & Batki, S. L. (2010). Pharmacological approaches to methamphetamine dependence: A focused review. *Br J Clin Pharmacol, 69*(6), 578–592.

Kauffman, E., Dore, M. M., & Nelson-Zlupko, L. (1995). The role of women's therapy groups in the treatment of chemical dependence. *Am J Orthopsychiatry, 65*(3), 355–363.

Kelly, P. J., Blacksin, B., & Mason, E. (2001). Factors affecting substance abuse treatment completion for women. *Issues Ment Health Nurs, 22*(3), 287–304.

Kessler, R. C., Crum, R. M., Warner, L. A., Nelson, C. B., Schulenberg, J., & Anthony, J. C.

(1997). Lifetime co-occurence of DSM-III-R alcohol abuse and dependence with other psychiatric disorders in the National Comorbidity Study. *Arch Gen Psychiatry, 54,* 313–321.

Kessler, R. C., Sonnega, A., Bromet, E., & Hughes, M. (1995). Posttraumatic stress disorder in the National Comorbidity Survey. *Arch Gen Psychiatry, 52*(12), 1048–1060.

Keyes, K. M., Grant, B. F., & Hasin, D. S. (2008). Evidence for a closing gender gap in alcohol use, abuse, and dependence in the United States population. *Drug Alcohol Depend, 93*(1–2), 21–29.

Keyes, K. M., Li, G., & Hasin, D. S. (2011). Birth cohort effects and gender differences in alcohol epidemiology: A review and synthesis. *Alcohol Clin Exp Res, 35*(12), 2101–2112.

Keyes, K. M., Martins, S. S., Blanco, C., & Hasin, D. S. (2010). Telescoping and gender differences in alcohol dependence: New evidence from two national surveys. *Am J Psychiatry, 167*(8), 969–976.

Killeen, T. K., Greenfield, S. F., Bride, B. E., Cohen, L., Gordon, S. M., & Roman, P. M. (2011). Assessment and treatment of co-occurring eating disorders in privately funded addiction treatment programs. *Am J Addict, 20*(3), 205–211.

Kilts, C. D., Gross, R. E., Ely, T. D., & Drexler, K. P. G. (2004). The neural correlates of cue-induced craving in cocaine-dependent women. *Am J Psychiatry, 161*(2), 233–241.

Kranzler, H. R., Del Boca, F. K., & Rounsaville, B. J. (1996). Comorbid psychiatric diagnosis predicts three-year outcomes in alcoholics: A posttreatment natural history study. *J Stud Alcohol, 57*(6), 619–626.

Landheim, A. S., Bakken, K., & Vaglum, P. (2006). Impact of comorbid psychiatric disorders on the outcome of substance abusers: A six year prospective follow-up in two Norwegian counties. *BMC Psychiatry, 6,* 44.

Lenzenweger, M. F., Lane, M. C., Loranger, A. W., & Kessler, R. C. (2007). DSM-IV personality disorders in the National Comorbidity Survey Replication. *Biol Psychiatry, 62,* 553–564.

Li, C. S., Kosten, T. R., & Sinha, R. (2005). Sex differences in brain activation during stress imagery in abstinent cocaine users: A functional magnetic resonance imaging study. *Biol Psychiatry, 57*(5), 487–494.

Linehan, M. M., Schmidt, H., III, Dimeff, L. A., Craft, J. C., Kanter, J., & Comtois, K. A. (1999). Dialectical behavior therapy for patients with borderline personality disorder and drug-dependence. *Am J Addict, 8*(4), 279–292.

Loft, S., Olesen, K. L., & Dossing, M. (1987). Increased susceptibility to liver disease in relation to alcohol consumption in women. *Scand J Gastroenterol, 22*(10), 1251–1256.

Loneck, B., Garrett, J., & Banks, S. M. (1997). Engaging and retaining women in outpatient alcohol and other drug treatment: The effect of referral intensity. *Health Soc Work, 22*(1), 38–46.

Loza, O., Patterson, T. L., Rusch, M., Martinez, G. A., Lozada, R., Staines-Orozco, H., et al. (2010). Drug-related behaviors independently associated with syphilis infection among female sex workers in two Mexico–US border cities. *Addiction, 105*(8), 1448–1456.

Lundgren, L. M., Schilling, R. F., Fitzgerald, T., Davis, K., & Amodeo, M. (2003). Parental status of women injection drug users and entry to methadone maintenance. *Subst Use Misuse, 38*(8), 1109–1131.

Lynch, W. J., Roth, M. E., & Carroll, M. E. (2002). Biological basis of sex differences in drug abuse: Preclinical and clinical studies. *Psychopharmacol (Berl), 164*(2), 121–137.

Mann, K., Ackermann, K., Croissant, B., Mundle, G., Nakovics, H., & Diehl, A. (2005). Neuroimaging of gender differences in alcohol dependence: Are women more vulnerable? *Alcohol Clin Exp Res, 29*(5), 896–901.

Mann, K., Hintz, T., & Jung, M. (2004). Does psychiatric comorbidity in alcohol-dependent patients affect treatment outcome? *Eur Arch Psychiatry Clin Neurosci, 254*(3), 172–181.

Maupin, R., Jr., Lyman, R., Fatsis, J., Prystowiski, E., Nguyen, A., Wright, C., et al. (2004). Characteristics of women who deliver with no prenatal care. *J Matern Fetal Neonatal Med, 16*(1), 45–50.

McCurdy, S. A., Ross, M. W., Williams, M. L., Kilonzo, G. P., & Leshabari, M. T. (2010). Flash-blood: Blood sharing among female injecting drug users in Tanzania. *Addiction, 105*(6), 1062–1070.

McDonald, J., Schleifer, L., Richards, J. B., & de Wit, H. (2003). Effects of THC on behavioral measures of impulsivity in humans. *Neuropsychopharmacol, 28*(7), 1356–1365.

McKirnan, D. J., & Peterson, P. L. (1989). Alcohol and drug use among homosexual men and women: Epidemiology and population characteristics. *Addict Beh, 14*(5), 545–553.

Mumenthaler, M. S., Taylor, J. L., O'Hara, R., & Yesavage, J. A. (1999). Gender differences in moderate drinking effects. *Alcohol Health Res World, 23*, 55–64.

Munafo, M., Bradburn, M., Bowes, L., & David, S. (2004). Are there sex differences in transdermal nicotine replacement therapy patch efficacy?: A meta-analysis. *Nicotine Tob Res, 6*(5), 769–776.

Munro, C. A., McCaul, M. E., Wong, D. F., Oswald, L. M., Zhou, Y., Brasic, J., et al. (2006). Sex differences in striatal dopamine release in healthy adults. *Biol Psychiatry, 59*(10), 966–974.

Naimi, T. S., Brewer, R. D., Mokdad, A. L., Denny, C., Sefudla, M. K., & Marks, J. S. (2003). Binge drinking among US adults. *JAMA, 289*, 70–75.

Najavits, L. (2002). *Seeking Safety: A treatment manual for PTSD and substance abuse.* New York: Guilford Press.

Najavits, L. M., Gallop, R. J., & Weiss, R. D. (2006). Seeking Safety therapy for adolescent girls with PTSD and substance use disorder: A randomized controlled trial. *J Behav Health Serv Res, 33*(4), 453–463.

Najavits, L., Weiss, R., Shaw, S., & Muenz, L. (1998). "Seeking Safety": Outcome of a new cognitive-behavioral psychotherapy for women with posttraumatic stress disorder and substance dependence. *J Trauma Stress, 11*, 437–456.

National Center on Addiction and Substance Abuse. (2003). *Food for thought: Substance abuse and eating disorders.* New York: Columbia University.

National Institute of Alcohol Abuse and Alcoholism. (2004). NIAAA council approves definition of binge drinking. *NIAAA Newsletter, 3*, 3.

Newman, J. L., & Mello, N. K. (2009). Neuroactive gonadal steroid hormones and drug addiction in women. In K. T. Brady, S. E. Back, & S. F. Greenfield (Eds.), *Women and addiction: A comprehensive handbook* (pp. 35–64). New York: Guilford Press.

Niv, N., & Hser, Y.-I. (2007). Women-only and mixed-gender drug abuse treatment programs: Service needs, utilization and outcomes. *Drug Alcohol Depend, 87*(2–3), 194–201.

Nolen-Hoeksema, S. (2004). Gender differences in risk factors and consequences for alcohol use and problems. *Clin Psychol Rev, 24*(8), 981–1010.

O'Brien, M. S., & Anthony, J. C. (2005). Risk of becoming cocaine dependent: Epidemiological estimates for the United States, 2000–2001. *Neuropsychopharmacol, 30*(5), 1006–1018.

Orwin, R., Francisco, L., & Bernichon, T. (2001). *Effectiveness of women's substance abuse treatment programs: A meta-analysis.* Fairfax, VA: Center for Substance Abuse Treatment.

Patrick, M. E., Schulenberg, J. E., O'Malley, P. M., Maggs, J. L., Kloska, D. D., Johnston, L. D., et al. (2011). Age-related changes in reasons for using alcohol and marijuana from ages 18 to 30 in a national sample. *Psychol Addict Behav, 25*(2), 330–339.

Peirce, J. M., Kindbom, K. A., Waesche, M. C., Yuscavage, A. S. E., & Brooner, R. K. (2008). Posttraumatic stress disorder, gender, and problem profiles in substance dependent patients. *Subst Use Misuse, 43*(5), 596–611.

Perkins, K. A. (2001). Smoking cessation in women. Special considerations. *CNS Drugs, 15*(5), 391–411.

Perkins, K. A., Doyle, T., Ciccocioppo, M., Conklin, C., Sayette, M., & Caggiula, A. (2006). Sex differences in the influence of nicotine dose instructions on the reinforcing and self-reported rewarding effects of smoking. *Psychopharmacol (Berl), 184*(3–4), 600–607.

Perkins, K. A., Gerlach, D., Vender, J., Grobe, J., Meeker, J., & Hutchison, S. (2001). Sex differences in the subjective and reinforcing effects of visual and olfactory cigarette smoke stimuli. *Nicotine Tob Res, 3*(2), 141–150.

Perkins, K. A., Jacobs, L., Sanders, M., & Caggiula, A. R. (2002). Sex differences in the subjective and reinforcing effects of cigarette nicotine dose. *Psychopharmacol (Berl), 163*(2), 194–201.

Perkins, K. A., Levine, M., Marcus, M., Shiffman, S., D'Amico, D., Miller, A., et al. (2000). Tobacco withdrawal in women and menstrual cycle phase. *J Consult Clin Psychol, 68*(1), 176–180.

Perkins, K. A., & Scott, J. (2008). Sex differences in long-term smoking cessation rates due to nicotine patch. *Nicotine Tob Res, 10*(7), 1245–1250.

Pettinati, H. M., Kampman, K. M., Lynch, K. G., Suh, J. J., Dackis, C. A., Oslin, D. W., et al. (2008). Gender differences with high-dose naltrexone in patients with co-occurring cocaine and alcohol dependence. *J Subst Abuse Treat, 34*(4), 378–390.

Piazza, N. J., Vrbka, J. L., & Yeager, R. D. (1989). Telescoping of alcoholism in women alcoholics. *Int J Addict, 24*, 19–28.

Pirie, P. L., Murray, D. M., & Luepker, R. V. (1991). Gender differences in cigarette smoking and quitting in a cohort of young adults. *Am J Public Health, 81*(3), 324–327.

Potenza, M. N., Hong, K. I., Lacadie, C. M., Fulbright, R. K., Tuit, K. L., & Sinha, R. (2012). Neural correlates of stress-induced and cue-induced drug craving: Influences of sex and cocaine dependence. *Am J Psychiatry, 169*(4), 406–414.

Prendergast, M. L., Messina, N. P., Hall, E. A., & Warda, U. S. (2011). The relative effectiveness of women-only and mixed-gender treatment for substance-abusing women. *J Subst Abuse Treat, 40*(4), 336–348.

Prescott, E., Hippe, M., Schnohr, P., Hein, H. O., & Vestbo, J. (1998). Smoking and risk of myocardial infarction in women and men: Longitudinal population study. *BMJ, 316*(7137), 1043–1047.

Project MATCH Research Group. (1997). Matching alcohol treatments to client heterogeneity: Project MATCH posttreatment drinking outcomes. *J Studies Alcohol, 58*, 7–29.

Rahmanian, S. D., Diaz, P. T., & Wewers, M. E. (2011). Tobacco use and cessation among women: Research and treatment-related issues. *J Womens Health (Larchmt), 20*(3), 349–357.

Ramisetty-Mikler, S., Caetano, R., & Rodriguez, L. A. (2010). The Hispanic Americans Baseline Alcohol Survey (HABLAS): Alcohol consumption and sociodemographic predictors across Hispanic national groups. *J Subst Use, 15*(6), 402–416.

Randall, C. L., Roberts, J., DelBoca, F. K., Carroll, K. M., Connors, G. J., & Mattson, M. E. (1999). Telescoping of landmark events associated with drinking: A gender comparison. *J Stud Alcohol, 60*, 252–260.

Reynolds, K. D., Coombs, D. W., Lowe, J. B., Peterson, P. L., & Gayoso, E. (1995). Evaluation of a self-help program to reduce alcohol consumption among pregnant women. *Int J Addict, 30*(4), 427–443.

Rounsaville, B. J., Dolinsky, Z. S., Babor, T. F., & Meyer, R. E. (1987). Psychopathology as a predictor of treatment outcome in alcoholics. *Arch Gen Psychiatry, 44*, 505–513.

Rowan-Szal, G. A., Joe, G. W., Simpson, D. D., Greener, J. M., & Vance, J. (2009). During-treatment outcomes among female methamphetamine-using offenders in prison-based treatments. *J Offender Rehabil, 48*(5), 388–401.

Saladin, M. E., Gray, K. M., Carpenter, M. J., LaRowe, S. D., DeSantis, S. M., & Upadhyaya, H. P. (2012). Gender differences in craving and cue reactivity to smoking and negative affect/stress cues. *Am J Addict, 21*(3), 210–220.

Samet, J. H., Pace, C. A., Cheng, D. M., Coleman, S., Bridden, C., Pardesi, M., et al. (2010). Alcohol use and sex risk behaviors among HIV-infected female sex workers (FSWs) and HIV-infected male clients of FSWs in India. *AIDS Behav, 14*(Suppl. 1), S74–S83.

Scharf, D., & Shiffman, S. (2004). Are there gender differences in smoking cessation, with and without bupropion?: Pooled- and meta-analyses of clinical trials of Bupropion SR. *Addiction, 99*(11), 1462–1469.

Schmidt, L., & Weisner, C. (1995). The emergence of problem-drinking women as a special population in need of treatment. *Recent Dev Alcohol, 12*, 309–334.

Shand, F. L., Degenhardt, L., Slade, T., & Nelson, E. C. (2011). Sex differences amongst dependent heroin users: Histories, clinical characteristics and predictors of other substance dependence. *Addict Behav, 36*(1–2), 27–36.

Sinha, R. (2007). The role of stress in addiction relapse. *Curr Psychiatry Rep, 9*(5), 388–395.

Skinner, W. F., & Otis, M. D. (1996). Drug and alcohol use among lesbian and gay people in a southern U.S. sample: Epidemiological, comparative and methodological findings from the trilogy project. *J Homosexuality, 30*(3), 59–92.

Sofuoglu, M., Dudish-Poulsen, S., Nelson, D., Pentel, P. R., & Hatsukami, D. K. (1999). Sex and menstrual cycle differences in the subjective effects from smoked cocaine in humans. *Exp Clin Psychopharmacol, 7*, 274–283.

Sofuoglu, M., Mitchell, E., & Kosten, T. R. (2004). Effects of progesterone treatment on cocaine responses in male and female cocaine users. *Pharmacol Biochem Behav, 78*(4), 699–705.

Sofuoglu, M., Sugarman, D. E., & Carroll, K. M. (2010). Cognitive function as an emerging treatment target for marijuana addiction. *Exp Clin Psychopharmacol, 18*(2), 109–119.

Solowij, N., & Battisti, R. (2008). The chronic effects of cannabis on memory in humans: A review. *Curr Drug Abuse Rev, 1*, 81–98.

Sonne, S. C., Back, S. E., Zuniga, C. D., Randall, C. L., & Brady, K. T. (2003). Gender differences in individuals with comorbid alcohol dependence and post-traumatic stress disorder. *Am J Addict, 12*(5), 412–423.

Substance Abuse and Mental Health Services Administration. (2009). *The TEDS Report: Heroin and other opiate admissions to substance abuse treatment*. Rockville, MD: Office of Applied Studies.

Substance Abuse and Mental Health Services Administration. (2011). *Results from the 2010 National Survey on Drug Use and Health: Summary of national findings* (NSDUH Series H-41, HHS Publication No. SMA 11-4658). Rockville, MD: Author.

Sugarman, D. E., DeMartini, K. S., & Carey, K. B. (2009). Are women at greater risk?: An examination of alcohol-related consequences and gender. *Am J Addict, 18*(3), 194–197.

Swan, G. E., Ward, M. M., Carmelli, D., & Jack, L. M. (1993). Differential rates of relapse in subgroups of male and female smokers. *J Clin Epidemiol, 46*(9), 1041–1053.

Taran, Y. S., Johnston, L. G., Pohorila, N. B., & Saliuk, T. O. (2011). Correlates of HIV risk among injecting drug users in sixteen Ukrainian cities. *AIDS Behav, 15*(1), 65–74.

Timko, C., Moos, R. H., Finney, J. W., & Connell, E. G. (2002). Gender differences in help-utilization and the 8-year course of alcohol abuse. *Addiction, 97*(7), 877–889.

van Gelder, M. M., Reefhuis, J., Herron, A. M., Williams, M. L., & Roeleveld, N. (2011). Reproductive health characteristics of marijuana and cocaine users: Results from the 2002 National Survey of Family Growth. *Perspect Sex Reprod Health, 43*(3), 164–172.

Verheul, R. (2001). Co-morbidity of personality disorders in individuals with substance use disorders. *Eur Psychiatry, 16*(5), 274–282.

Volkow, N. D., Tomasi, D., Wang, G.-J., Fowler, J. S., Telang, F., Goldstein, R. Z., et al. (2011). Reduced metabolism in brain "control networks" following cocaine-cues exposure in female cocaine abusers. *PLoS ONE, 6*(2), e16573.

Walter, M., Gunderson, J. G., Zanarini, M. C., Sanislow, C. A., Grilo, C. M., McGlashan, T. H., et al. (2009). New onsets of substance use disorders in borderline personality disorder over 7 years of follow-ups: Findings from the Collaborative Longitudinal Personality Disorders Study. *Addiction, 104*(1), 97–103.

Weeks, M. R., Hilario, H., Li, J., Coman, E., Abbott, M., Sylla, L., et al. (2010). Multilevel social influences on female condom use and adoption among women in the urban United States. *AIDS Patient Care STDS, 24*(5), 297–309.

Westermeyer, J., Kopka, S., & Nugent, S. (1997). Course and severity of substance abuse among patients with comorbid major depression. *Am J Addict, 6*(4), 284–292.

Yen, S., Shea, M. T., Pagano, M., Sanislow, C. A., Grilo, C. M., McGlashan, T. H., et al. (2003). Axis I and Axis II disorders as predictors of prospective suicide attempts: Findings from the collaborative longitudinal personality disorders study. *J Abnorm Psychol, 112*(3), 375–381.

Young, R. S., & Joe, J. R. (2009). Some thoughts about the epidemiology of alcohol and drug use among American Indian/Alaska native populations. *J Ethn Subst Abuse, 8*(3), 223–241.

Zanarini, M. C., Frankenburg, F. R., Dubo, E. D., Sickel, A. E., Trikha, A., Levin, A., & Reynolds, V. (1998). Axis I comorbidity of borderline personality disorder. *Am J Psychiatry, 155*(12), 1733–1739.

Zanarini, M. C., Frankenburg, F. R., Weingeroff, J. L., Reich, D. B., Fitzmaurice, G. M., & Weiss, R. D. (2011). The course of substance use disorders in patients with borderline personality disorder and Axis II comparison subjects: A 10-year follow-up study. *Addiction, 106*(2), 342–348.

Zilberman, M. L., Tavares, H., Blume, S. B., & el-Guebaly, N. (2003). Substance use disorders: Sex differences and psychiatric comorbidities. *Can J Psychiatry, 48*(1), 5–13.

CHAPTER 24

Substance Use Disorders in Adolescence

YIFRAH KAMINER
OSCAR G. BUKSTEIN

Substance use by adolescents remains an important public health problem, because the early initiation of drug use is correlated with an increased risk of a range of problem behaviors, such as legal problems (e.g., selling drugs and violence-related charges); driving under the influence of a substance (Centers for Disease Control and Prevention [CDC], 2012); and physical, sexual, and emotional abuse. In addition, substance use problems in adolescence have been shown to increase the risk of later development of a substance use disorder (SUD; Briones, Wilcox, Mateus, & Boudjenah, 2006). Potential consequences of use include accidents; the possible progression of use into an SUD; and the persistence of the SUD into adulthood. Substance use is associated with the leading causes of adolescent morbidity and mortality in the United States, including motor vehicle accidents, suicidal behavior, violence, delinquency, drowning, and unprotected sexual behavior. Of those adolescents with SUDs, less than 10% receive treatment for the disorder (Dennis, Dawud-Noursi, & Muck, 2003). This treatment gap may be due to a variety of factors, including (but not limited to) poor health care coverage, low motivation of the youth or parents, a lack of specialized adolescent treatment programs, and inconsistent quality in adolescent treatment services. Our objective in this chapter is to review recent trends in adolescent substance use, nosology, etiology of substance use and its transition to adolescent SUD, psychiatric comorbidity, prevention, assessment, and treatment–aftercare continuum. As a point of clarification, the generic term "substance use" refers here to nonpathological use of any licit drug (tobacco, alcohol, and inhalants) or illicit drug (controlled substances, both those that are essentially legally proscribed for everyone and those that are available by prescription). We use the term "substance use disorder (SUD)" generically to indicate pathological use of any potential drug of abuse.

EPIDEMIOLOGY

Illicit Substance Use

A large number of youth use psychoactive substances. According to the 2011 Monitoring the Future (MTF) survey (Johnston, O'Malley, Bachman, & Schulenberg, 2011), the proportion of young people using any illicit drug has risen gradually over the past 4 years due largely to increased use of marijuana—the most widely used of all the illicit drugs. In 2011, 50% of high school seniors reported having tried an illicit drug at some time, 40% had used one or more drugs in the past 12 months, and 25% had used one or more drugs in the prior 30 days. The figures are lower for younger teens; among 10th graders, 38% reported having tried an illicit drug, 31% had used in the past 12 months, and 19% had used in the prior 30 days. Corresponding prevalences for eighth graders are 20, 15, and 8.5%, respectively. Marijuana accounts for most of high school use of illicit drugs. The annual prevalence rates for use of any illicit drug other than marijuana in the prior 12 months are 6, 11, and 18% in grades 8, 10, and 12; the corresponding lifetime prevalence rates are 10, 16, and 25%, respectively. Over-the counter (OTC) and prescription medication (ab)use are second in prevalence only to marijuana use among adolescents.

In terms of regular use, according to the 2011 National Survey on Drug Use and Health (Substance Abuse and Mental Health Services Administration [SAMHSA], 2012), 10.1% of youth ages 12–17 were current illicit drug users, with 7.9% current users of marijuana, 2.8% current nonmedical users of psychotherapeutic drugs, 0.9% current users of hallucinogens, 0.9% current users of inhalants, and 0.3% current users of cocaine. The rate of current illicit drug use was higher among males ages 12–17 than females ages 12–17 (10.8 vs. 9.3%).

Nationwide, 25.6% of students had been offered, sold, or given an illegal drug by someone on school property during the 12 months before the survey (CDC, 2012).

Alcohol

Across the United States, 70.8% of students had had at least one drink of alcohol on at least 1 day during their life (i.e., ever drank alcohol), and 21.9% of students had had five or more drinks of alcohol in a row (i.e., within a couple of hours) on at least 1 day during the 30 days before the survey (i.e., binge drinking) (SAMHSA, 2012). Among persons ages 12–20, past-month alcohol use rates in 2011 were 18.1% among blacks, 18.8% among Asians, 20.0% among Native Americans or Alaska Natives, 22.5% among Hispanics, 27.5% among those reporting two or more races, and 28.2% among whites (SAMHSA, 2012).

Tobacco

Over 10% of students had ever smoked at least one cigarette every day for 30 days (i.e., ever smoked cigarettes daily) (CDC, 2012). Nationwide, 6.4% of students had smoked cigarettes 20 or more days during the 30 days before the survey (i.e., current frequent cigarette use).

Diversion and Misuse

In a study of 1,086 public school students, opioid analgesics were the most widely prescribed and the most widely abused substances (Boyd, McCabe, & Teter, 2006). Stimulant and sedative or anxiety medications had the highest illicit–medical use ratios. Diversion of prescription medication was common; between 29 and 62% of 390 students with legal prescriptions had been approached to divert their medications within the previous year.

PREVALENCE

The prevalence of SUDs increases with age through young adulthood. National survey data indicate that very few youth met criteria for any past-year SUD prior to age 14 (less than 3%). In 2011, the rate of substance dependence or abuse among adults ages 18–25 (18.6%) was higher than that among youth ages 12–17 (6.9%) and among adults ages 26 or older (6.3%) (SAMHSA, 2012). Rates of substance dependence or abuse were associated with age. In 2011, the rate of substance dependence or abuse among adults ages 18–25 (18.6%) was higher than that among youth ages 12–17 (6.9%) and among adults age 26 or older (6.3%). In the National Comorbidity Survey Adolescent Supplement, SUDs were present in 11.4% of the sample, corresponding to 8.9% of adolescents with drug abuse/dependence and 6.4% with alcohol abuse/dependence (Merikangas et al., 2010). These disorders occurred more frequently in males, and a five- to 11-fold increase in prevalence was observed across increasing age groups. Fifty percent of those with SUDs reported onset by age 15 (Merikangas et al., 2010).

DIAGNOSTIC CRITERIA

The recently published DSM-5 criteria (American Psychiatric Association, 2013) eliminate the diagnosis of substance abuse and define a single SUD for various substance classes—using a set of 11 symptoms and requiring that two or more criteria be met before one receives an SUD diagnosis (with gradations of severity). DSM-5 criteria include some changes in definition of SUDs, including the use of a combined criterion set to diagnose a single entity—substance use disorder (Winters, Martin, & Chung, 2011). The criteria for DSM-IV abuse and dependence have overlapping conceptual content with those of DSM-5 and do not differ systematically in prevalence, sensitivity, specificity, severity, or age of onset (Martin, Chung, Kirisci, & Langenbucher, 2006). Factor and latent class analyses indicate a single dimension of substance problems (Martin et al., 2006).

The impact of the threshold of two out of 11 criteria for a SUD in youth requires further research. Because some of the proposed DSM-5 symptoms are mild, developmentally normative for teenagers, and/or easily misunderstood and overendorsed, those diagnosed may include many mild cases that do not fit the classic definition of a compulsive pattern of substance use. This may unnecessarily apply a stigmatized and loaded label to youth whose problem severity may be mild and whose substance use pattern may be more intermittent than regular, and more likely to remit (Winters et al., 2011).

ETIOLOGY, RISK, AND COURSE

Adolescence is a remarkably variable period of development. As with earlier developmental stages, changes emerge both within the individual and in the physical, relational, and social contexts within which the individual develops. The adolescent years are characterized by major role transitions in every domain of life, as well as continued physical and cognitive development (Brown et al., 2008). Normative changes center around taking increased responsibility for one's daily life, behavior, and future; moving toward less dependent and more mature relationships with members of the family of origin; exploring romantic and sexual relationships; and preparing for and initiating adult occupational roles, including pursuit of postsecondary education and/or employment. Preparation for adult relationships includes the development of romantic and sexual relationships for most and cohabitation, and/or childbearing for some. Preparation for occupational life includes completing (or leaving) high school, beginning formal paid work, and possibly initiating postsecondary training.

The popular conception of adolescent drama and angst can now be examined in light of broader understanding of cognitive and emotional development and the role of puberty in brain maturation. In many ways adolescence represents the interval between the beginning of sexual maturation and the attainment of adult roles and responsibilities in society. The transition from parental control to self-control is usually framed in social context. With adulthood, job, and marriage delayed, many young adolescents are faced with an enormous amount of freedom in which to navigate complex decision making. If the adolescent has preexisting deficits in executive functioning or an environment that predisposes him or her to early exposure, how he or she deals with substance use, sex, and other high-risk behaviors may be compromised. Because executive functions mediate the complex interplay between thinking, affect, and social judgment, it is not surprising that research has confirmed associations with alcohol and drug abuse. Poorly developed executive functions are prominent in adolescents who are, thereby, at high risk of developing alcohol/substance abuse problems, including those with conduct disorder.

Despite the seeming synchrony of the changes seen in adolescence, some of the brain changes precede pubertal increase in hormones and body changes, and others appear to be the consequence of pubertal processes (e.g., hormone effects feeding back on the brain); other brain maturation appears to be independent of pubertal processes. Adult functioning ultimately requires developing self-control of behavior and emotions, which center around the ability to inhibit or modify behaviors appropriately to avoid negative future consequences; to initiate, persist, and sequence steps toward goals; to navigate complex social situations despite strong affect; and to use skills in the self-regulation of affect and complex behavior to serve long-term goals. Many of these functions require brain maturation involving neurobehavioral systems in the prefrontal cortex (PFC), which unfortunately is among the last regions of the brain to achieve full functional maturation (Casey & Jones, 2010). In the meantime, the physical changes of puberty have occurred much earlier. Earlier timing of puberty results in several years with a sexually mature body and sexually activated brain circuits, but with relatively immature neurobehavioral systems necessary for self-control and affect regulation. The potential for a poor match between impulse and controls points to an increased risk for disorders of self-control and increases in risk taking, novelty/sensation seeking and, ultimately, difficulties navigating complex socioemotional situations.

That substance use is associated with adolescents is not surprising, because many adolescents associate substance use—particularly alcohol and tobacco—with adulthood. When the opportunity presents itself, depending on the individual teen's environment, the adolescent experiments and tries this adult behavior, but with a lesser ability to "handle it" or moderate the behavior relative to the circumstances. Unfortunately, the effects of substances have additional consequences relative to adolescents' decision making and other cognitive processes. Acute effects of alcohol, marijuana, and likely other drugs in interfering with cognitive function are well-known, hence the reason for "driving under the influence" (DUI) laws. Based on human and animal studies, adolescent alcohol use is also associated with damage to the brain and neurocognitive deficits, with implications for learning and other cognitive abilities that may continue to affect the individual into adulthood. For example, adolescents with an alcohol use disorder have deficits in memory retrieval and in visuospatial functioning (Spear, 2000). Research relating alcohol use to brain structure and functioning supports the conclusion that heavy alcohol use in adolescence can result in selective long-term cognitive impairments with a variety of cognitive abilities deteriorating for late adolescents and young adults who persist in heavy drinking (Hanson, Cummins, Tapert, & Brown, 2011). How extensive adolescent drinking must be and/or the effects of similar levels of other substance use before brain damage is significant and protracted, the extent of variation in vulnerability to alcohol-related brain damage, the rate and pattern of neurocognitive recovery, and the extent to which structural and functional changes are attributable solely to alcohol are not yet clear. Needless to say, alcohol and/or other drug use, particularly in the context of adolescence and adolescent development, is not good for optimal brain functioning.

While discontinuities in neurocognitive development may explain some of the risk for adolescent substance use and SUDs, the literature on the development of substance use and SUDs in adolescents has identified an assortment of individual, peer, family, and community risk factors (Kaminer & Bukstein, 2007; see Figure 24.1).

Within a developmental context, an individual adolescent's genetic predispositions toward affective, cognitive, and behavioral dysregulation are exacerbated by family and peer factors that increase the likelihood of substance use and even pathological use. Both temperament and social interactions (i.e., family, peer relations) play a critical role in adolescent SUD outcomes. First, experiences with substance use most often take place in a social context with the use of "gateway" substances such as alcohol and cigarettes, which are legal for adults and readily available to minors. Initial use may occur because of adolescent curiosity or simply the availability of a substance. Progressively fewer adolescents advance to later and more serious levels of substance use, but because high-risk youth are more likely to associated with deviant

---

Individual risk factors

- Early childhood characteristics
- Early conduct problems, aggression
- Poor academic performance/school failure
- Early onset of substance use
- Adolescent's attitudes and beliefs about substance use
- Risk-taking behaviors

Peer-related risk factors

- Peer substance use
- Peer attitudes about substance use
- Greater orientation (attachment) to peers
- Perception(s) of peer substance use/attitudes

Parent/family risk factors

- Parental substance use
- Parental beliefs/attitudes about substance use
- Parental tolerance of substance use/deviant behavior
- Lack of closeness/attachment with parents
- Lack of parental involvement in a youth's life
- Lack of appropriate supervision/discipline

FIGURE 24.1. Risk factors for adolescent SUDs.

peers and have less parental supervision, early exposure to substance use may be increased. Although drug consumption frequently follows a predictable sequence as per the "gateway hypothesis," the risk for and rate of progression to an SUD is the same whether consumption begins with a legal or illegal drug.

Early onset and a more rapid progression through the stages of substance use are among the risk factors for the development of SUDs. Initiation and early patterns of use are strongly influenced by social and familial environmental factors, while later levels of use are strongly influenced by genetic factors (Grant & Dawson, 1997). Finally, it is important to note that risks associated with use and abuse of different categories of drugs, alcohol, and tobacco share as much as 50–85% of their genetic variance; this indicates that common factors have largely been shown to account for the genetic risk for SUDs related to different categories of illicit drugs or that these factors largely underlie the genetic risk for most or all of the different SUDs (Kendler, Jacobson, & Prescott, 2003).

PSYCHIATRIC COMORBIDITY

In both community surveys of adolescents with SUD and samples of adolescents in addictions treatment, the majority have a co-occurring non-substance-related mental disorder (Hser, Grella, & Hubbard, 2001). More than half of adolescents treated for addictions who have a co-occurring mental illness have three or more co-occurring psychiatric disorders (Dennis et al., 2003). The most commonly comorbid psychiatric disorders among youth in addiction treatment include conduct problems, attention-deficit/hyperactivity disorder (ADHD), mood disorders (e.g., depression), and trauma-related symptoms (Grella, Hser, & Joshi, 2001). Comorbid psychopathology may precede, exacerbate, or follow the onset of heavy substance use. A review of adolescent community surveys indicated that childhood mental illness generally predicted earlier initiation of substance use and SUD onset, particularly in relation to conduct disorder (Armstrong & Costello, 2002). Co-occurring psychopathology also generally predicted a more persistent course of substance involvement over 1-year follow-up (Grella et al., 2001). Rather than type of diagnosis, the total number of psychiatric symptoms may predict relapse risk (McCarthy, Tomlinson, & Anderson, 2005). For a more detailed discussion of comorbidity, see Kaminer and Bukstein (2007).

SCREENING/ASSESSMENT

Given the multiple risk factors, frequent comorbidity, and multiple areas of possible dysfunction related to alcohol and other drug abuse, the comprehensive assessment of substance abuse and related problems in adolescents requires evaluation of many areas of functioning in the adolescent's life and possible psychopathology (Winters & Kaminer, 2008). Many screening and assessment instruments have followed a multilevel, multidomain model, wherein the optimal screening or assessment not only measures substance use variables but also identifies specific areas of dysfunction (Tarter, 1990). Each domain (see Figure 24.2) is then more thoroughly assessed by more detailed questions or use of standardized instrument(s) designed to assess that specific domain.

"Screening" refers to the initial, and usually brief, assessment of adolescents or other groups to identify the likely presence or absence of a given problem. Adolescents who screen positive for substance abuse or any other disorder should then be referred for or given a more detailed, comprehensive assessment. As demonstrated by the discussion on epidemiology and substance use patterns in adolescence (Sugarman, Brezing, & Greenfield, Chapter 23, this volume), one can expect a significant number of adolescents to report at least occasional use of substances; an overwhelming majority

- Substance use
- Psychiatric symptoms/disorders
- Family functioning
- School/vocational functioning
- School competency/peer relations
- Leisure/recreation
- Medical

FIGURE 24.2. Domain model of assessment.

will report some exposure to alcohol. Considering quantity and frequency information alone is also problematic. Use data will probably serve to identify a large population of adolescents for whom administering a more comprehensive evaluation would be impractical. In keeping with a useful definition of "substance abuse," screening should include inquiry about dysfunction and/or distress associated with levels of substance use. Most screens are based on a "use plus" concept. First, the adolescent has to have a pattern of use. One to two episodes of use of a specific substance would not meet this threshold standard. Once a threshold for frequency is met, a screen also includes a brief survey of direct consequences of use or salient drug use behaviors. The typical presentation of an adolescent with a potential SUD is one in which dysfunction is the initial concern. The teen is having difficulty with family relationshps, academic functioning, emotional problems, and antisocial or disruptive behavior. An optimal screen combines the elements of use and dysfunction in a brief series of questions. This is not the final word in determining the nature of the problem, but a method of decreasing the number of adolescents requiring a more detailed time- and cost-intensive comprehensive assessment.

With the exception of epidemiological studies or other research projects and primary care settings in which more universal screening is feasible, screening should target a population of adolescents at risk, that is, adolescents who, by virtue of their current behavior (e.g., disruptive behavior disorders, academic failure, and legal problems) and other characteristics (e.g., family history of addiction), have an elevated chance of having an SUD. The importance of being acquainted with such risk factors cannot be overemphasized. Screening often takes place in nonclinical settings (i.e., non-SUD or non-mental health settings), with the venue often determining who to screen and how screening is accomplished. While primary care physicians and other health care workers should briefly inquire about substance use and associated problems during routine visits, time constraints may limit both the extent of the inquiry and the reliability of the adolescent's response, especially when no other informant or additional information is available.

High-risk teens indirectly identify themselves through their high-risk behavior, such as possession of drug and alcohol, delinquency and other deviant social behavior, and school violations. Screening is then "for cause" and is based on adolescents' behavior rather than their universal status as students or teenagers.

The method of screening depends largely on the setting and the purpose for screening. In general clinical settings, the most common method is several questions in a clinical interview format. These questions should cover types of substances used, quantity and frequency, as well as a general screen for negative consequences of use. A list of major drug/alcohol categories is found in Figure 24.3. Similar to the more comprehensive assessment (discussed below), having sufficient clinical skills to screen during an oral interview appears reasonable, with the level of expertise commensurate with the setting. For example, school staff members may have less expertise than juvenile justice professionals and less than mental health and SUD treatment personnel. All, however, should have a minimal level of ability to deliver basic questions about substance use.

Primary medical care sites offer a practical setting for screening, as well as a model for screening in other settings, and lead to the development of a system consisting of

- Alcohol
    - Beer
    - Wine
    - Spirits
- Cannabis
    - Marijuana
    - Hashish
- Opiates/opioids
    - Heroin
    - Oral opiates
- Cocaine
    - Powder
    - Crack
- Hallucinogens
    - LSD
    - Psilocybin (mushroom)
    - PCP
    - Peyote/mescaline
- Sedatives/hypnotics
    - Benzodiazepines
    - GHB
    - Rohypnol
    - Barbiturates
- Stimulants
    - Amphetamines
    - Methamphetamine
    - Methylphenidate
- Steroids
- Inhalants
- Club drugs, miscellaneous
    - Ecstasy/MDMA
    - K2/Spice
    - *Salvia divinorum*
    - Bath salts

FIGURE 24.3. Major classes of drugs and alcohol.

screening, brief intervention, and referral to treatment (SBIRT) in non-drug/alcohol settings (e.g., emergency departments, primary care settings, health clinics; American Academy of Pediatrics, 2011). Over the past decade, adolescent models of SBIRT have been developed. One of principles underlying SBIRT is that screening may reveal varying levels of substance use involvement, ranging from abstinence to dependence. Although individuals who deal with adolescents should be particularly in tune with screening adolescents at high risk for the development of SUDs, providing universal screening and brief intervention within primary care settings is a promising strategy to reduce problems caused by substance abuse by identifying youth at an early stage of drug or alcohol involvement. Universal screening also helps to identify high-risk teens who require a referral to more intensive treatment.

The American Academy of Pediatrics (2011) recommends CRAFFT (Car, Relax, Alone, Forget, Friends, Trouble) for use with adolescents because of the tool's simplicity, practicality, and psychometrics. This six-item questionnaire quickly screens simultaneously for alcohol and other drug use disorders (Knight, Sherritt, & Shrier, 2002) CRAFFT is a mnemonic acronym in which each letter stands for a key word in the six screening questions (see Figure 24.4). The six-question CRAFFT screen is administered after a positive response to any of the opening questions regarding personal substance use (e.g., "Have you ever drunk alcohol?"; "Have you ever smoked marijuana?"; "Have you ever used a substance to get high?"). Each "yes" response on CRAFFT is 1 point. A score of 2 or greater is a positive screen and indicates that the adolescent is at high risk for having an alcohol- or drug-related disorder. The CRAFFT is reasonably sensitive, specific, and predictive, and the established validity is not significantly affected by age, gender, or race/ethnicity (Knight et al., 2002).

The comprehensive assessment of an adolescent with possible or likely SUD requires a broad view of the problems that predispose and maintain substance use

1. Have you ever ridden in a CAR driven by someone (including yourself) who was "high" or had been using alcohol or drugs?
2. Do you ever use alcohol or drugs to RELAX, feel better about yourself, or fit in?
3. Do you ever use alcohol or drugs while you are by yourself, or ALONE?
4. Do you ever FORGET things you did while using alcohol or drugs?
5. Do your FAMILY or FRIENDS ever tell you that you should cut down on your drinking or drug use?
6. Have you ever gotten into TROUBLE while you were using alcohol or drugs?

FIGURE 24.4. CRAFFT screen.

and also those that commonly coexist with SUDs. Symptoms, behaviors, social context, and functioning within multidomain contexts should all be examined. Although the emphasis is primarily on substance use behaviors, a comprehensive assessment of adolescents with SUDs will not be altogether different from assessments for depression, anxiety, or other behavioral or emotional problems.

When lifetime use of different substances has been determined, questions should become substance-specific. If use of a particular substance is endorsed, the clinician should proceed with a more detailed inquiry about the frequency, quantity, negative consequences, context, and control of use for each specific substance. Inquiry into control of use generally follows DSM-5 criteria for substance dependence. Despite the lower prevalence of physical sequelae of substance use and the rarity of overt physiological withdrawal symptoms, questions about these features are essential and, if answered in the affirmative, indicate a severe level of substance dependence for the adolescent.

Ideally, comprehensive assessment for SUDs, aside from an emphasis on the substance use domain, should not greatly differ from comprehensive assessments for other mental health problems in adolescents. The high prevalence of psychiatric comorbidity demands, at minimum, screening for depression, mania, psychosis, suicidal or homicidal ideation and/or behavior, aggressive behavior, anxiety disorders and posttraumatic stress disorder (PTSD), attention-deficit/hyperactivity disorder (ADHD), oppositional defiant disorder (ODD), conduct disorder (CD), and eating disorders. As previously discussed (Westermeyer, Chapter 2, this volume), these are psychiatric disorders or mental health problems that commonly co-occur in adolescents with substance use or SUDs. The remaining domains (family functioning, social/leisure activities, peer relationships, academic functioning, and medical problems) serve to provide a baseline for the level of overall functioning and help to determine whether substance use has been adversely affecting any specific domain(s).

The need for more thorough and complete assessment in the area of adolescent substance abuse in a variety of clinical and nonclinical settings has resulted in the creation of a wide range of instruments. The varied uses of such instruments include the diagnosis of substance abuse and dependence and other psychiatric disorders, rating the severity of substance use and related behaviors, and assessment of many of the specific domains related to adolescent substance use.

The value of instruments to the clinician is similar and includes the ability to obtain more consistent, reliable information; to obtain serial measures at regular intervals; and to define more homogenous patient populations to determine treatment needs. Instruments can assist in determining relevant outcome variables, adjunct clinical judgment, and potentially allow the user a less expensive and more efficient method of assessment.

Whether a researcher, a clinician, or both, administer the instrument, the attributes of a good instrument are the same. The instrument should be valid; that is, it should measure the concept it purports to measure. The instrument should be reliable (i.e., consistent in its results across time and across users). Finally, the instrument should also be practical; it should not demand too much time or effort.

There are two types of screening instruments: unidomain and multidomain. Unidomain instruments measure a specific area, most likely substance use and directly related behaviors. Multidomain instruments assess a wider range of variables, including behaviors, psychiatric symptoms, family and school functioning, and attitudes. Given the need for multidimensional or multidomain assessment of adolescent substance abuse, multidomain instruments are likely to be more useful to both clinicians and researchers. In addition to information about substance use, multidomain instruments assess other areas of adolescent functioning that may be affected by the adolescents' substance use.

Clinicians equate assessment with obtaining baseline information. They forget that assessment continues throughout treatment and beyond. Outcomes assessment usually consist of variables related to quantity and frequency of substance use, such as self-report of use and urine toxicology.

TREATMENT

Does Treatment Work?

Reviewers of the literature on adolescent treatment outcome have concluded that treatment is better than no treatment. In the year following treatment, on average, adolescents reported decreased heavy drinking, marijuana and other illicit drug use, and criminal involvement, as well as improved psychological adjustment and school performance. Although the majority of treated adolescents return to some substance use following treatment, treated adolescents generally show reductions in substance use and problems over both short and long-term follow-up (e.g., Williams & Chang, 2000). Considerable individual variability in the rate of return and extent of posttreatment substance use exists.

A number of variables predict outcome among adolescents attending SUD treatment (Williams & Chang, 2000). Pretreatment, during treatment, and posttreatment variables have been examined as predictors of clinical course. The most robust pretreatment characteristics predicting more persistent levels of substance involvement typically included the presence of co-occurring psychopathology (e.g., Grella et al., 2001). In-treatment factors associated with better outcomes included greater readiness to change, that is, higher motivation. In addition, longer duration of treatment (e.g., Hser et al., 2001) and family involvement in treatment predicted better outcomes. Posttreatment factors associated with better outcomes, including aftercare involvement (e.g., Winters et al., 2000), low levels of peer substance use (e.g., Winters et al., 2000), and continued commitment to abstain had a greater effect on outcome over 1-year follow-up than pre- and during treatment factors (Hsieh, Hoffman, & Hollister, 1998).

Improvements following treatment for SUDs extend beyond changes in substance use. Following treatment, teens with low substance involvement generally had better psychosocial functioning at young adult follow-up than did teens with moderate to high levels of posttreatment substance involvement (e.g., Brown et al., 2008). Worse outcomes among heavier users may reflect the impact of co-occurring psychopathology (e.g., conduct problems) on course. Changes in different domains of psychosocial functioning occurred at different rates: School functioning improved within the first year of follow-up, but improvements in family functioning generally emerged later (Chung, Maisto, & Cornelius, 2005). Thus, an adolescent-onset SUD, likely in combination with co-occurring psychopathology and other risk factors (e.g., negative environmental influences), appears to interfere with the achievement of some normative developmental tasks during adolescence despite post-SUD treatment success.

The most frequently reported alcohol or drug-related symptoms during 1-year follow-up included interpersonal problems due to use (e.g., parents' complaints about the teen's drinking) and symptoms related to impaired control over drinking behavior (Chung et al., 2005).

Unfortunately, only a small percentage of adolescents with SUDs actually receive treatment. In 2005, only 11.3% of youth ages 12–17 who needed SUD treatment received treatment at a specialty facility. For youth in publicly funded addictions treatment, most were referred by the criminal justice system, with smaller proportions referred by schools or family; rates of self-referral to treatment begin to increase only in young adulthood (Dennis et al., 2003).

Elements of Effective Treatment

Despite the identification of effective treatments for adolescents with SUDs, a substantial proportion of youth do not respond to these treatments. Currently, there are no empirical results to guide us in matching specific treatment modalities with specific types of adolescents. Nevertheless, the clinician deserves some guidance. Based on the combination of empirical research and current clinical consensus (American Academy of Child and Adolescent Psychiatry [AACAP], 2005), the clinician dealing with adolescents with SUDs should develop a treatment plan that uses modalities that target (1) motivation and engagement; (2) family involvement to improve supervision, monitoring, and communication between parents and adolescent; (3) improved problem solving, social skills, and relapse prevention; (4) comorbid psychiatric disorders through psychosocial and/or medication treatments; (5) social ecology in terms of increasing prosocial behaviors, peer relationships, and academic functioning,; and (6) adequate duration of treatment, including provision of follow-up care after acute treatment. Self-support groups can be encouraged as adjuncts to the previously mentioned modalities.

The primary goal of treatment of adolescents with SUDs for most professionals in the field is achieving and maintaining abstinence from substance use. While clinicians should explicitly endorse abstinence as the long-term goal of treatment, a realistic view recognizes both the chronicity of SUDs in many populations of youth and the developmental context of substance use and substance use–related problems in others. As noted by the majority of posttreatment adolescents who improve functioning and decrease their substance use without maintaining abstinence, harm reduction may be an interim, implicit goal of treatment. The concept of harm reduction proposes, as a goal, reduction in the use and adverse effects of substances, reduction in the severity and frequency of relapses, and improvement in one or more domains of the adolescent's functioning (e.g., academic performance or family functioning). While many adolescents initially may not be motivated to stop substance use or to be able accept the notion of lifelong abstinence, taking steps to reduce the consequences and severity of use may ultimately move the adolescent toward the goal of abstinence. Despite some implicit acceptance of harm reduction as an interim goal of treatment, "controlled use" of any nonprescribed substance of abuse should never be an explicit goal in the treatment of adolescents.

Control of substance use (i.e., abstinence or reduced use) should not be the only goal of treatment. A broad concept of rehabilitation involves targeting associated problems and domains of functioning for treatment. Integrated interventions that concurrently deal with coexisting psychiatric and behavioral problems, family functioning, peer and interpersonal relationships, and academic/vocational functioning should not only produce general improvement in psychosocial functioning but also be more likely to produce improved outcomes in the primary treatment goal of achieving and maintaining abstinence.

As many adolescents with SUDs have a multiplicity of psychosocial problems, many possible targets for many possible intervention exist. Triage decisions must be made about the importance of problems and sequence of interventions. Particularly in cases involving moderate to severe comorbid psychiatric disorders, clinicians can express confusion or disagreement about what problem to address first.

There are several problems with a sequential model. The first and perhaps most important is the effect that untreated or inadequately treated psychiatric problems have on SUD treatment success. Clinicians usually have a limited amount of time and resources to treat each adolescent. Some type of integrated or concurrent treatment seems to be the best goal for adolescents with comorbidity.

Psychosocial Interventions

Interventions Targeting Motivation

Recognition that adolescents rarely seek treatment on their own, show low motivation for treatment, and may see little problem with their use prompts clinicians to use interventions that increase motivation for treatment. Two such motivational interventions include motivational interviewing and contingency management, which are evidence-based interventions usually used as adjuncts to other treatment modalities in adolescent SUD treatment (AACAP, 2005).

Motivational interviewing (MI) is defined by its developers, Stephen Rollnick and William R. Miller (1995, p. 326) as "a directive, client-centered counseling style for eliciting behavior change by helping clients to explore and resolve ambivalence."

There are a number of variations, adaptations, and techniques used under the umbrella MI concept (e.g., motivational enhancement therapy [MET], a type of expanded version of MI). A meta-analytic review of MI interventions for substance use in adolescents (Jensen et al., 2011) found small but significant effect sizes at follow-up, suggesting that MI interventions for adolescent substance use retain their effectiveness over time. The review concluded that MI interventions are effective across a variety of substance use behaviors, varying session lengths, and different settings, and for interventions that used clinicians with different levels of education.

Contingency management (CM) interventions are based on evidence demonstrating that drug use and abuse are sensitive to systematically applied environmental consequences (i.e., reinforcement and punishment contingencies; Higgins, Silverman, & Heil, 2008). CM approaches have become one of the most thoroughly researched and effective behavioral procedures to increase drug abstinence and other treatment targets across SUDs in adults (Higgins et al., 2008). Increasingly CM procedures are being tested and integrated into adolescent SUD treatment (Stanger & Budney, 2010). CM procedures, coupled with certain psychosocial interventions such as cognitive-behavioral therapy (CBT), MET, and family therapy—including multisystemic family therapy—have been shown to increase retention in treatment and reduce drug use in adolescents and young adults with marijuana use disorders (Stanger & Budney, 2010).

CM involves the use of incentives (i.e., tangible positive reinforcers) to achieve and maintain abstinence or to increase behaviors (treatment compliance or attendance) that eventually facilitate abstinence. A program-based CM procedure may use a voucher system to increase motivation for abstinence. The targets usually are (1) urine and/or breath testing, (2) attendance at treatment sessions, and (3) the quality of participation in treatment sessions. Reinforcement of these targets involves monetary-based vouchers that are redeemable for goods and services deemed appropriate in achieving treatment goals of increasing prosocial, adaptive behaviors. These can include gift certificates or cards at department stores or other establishments, websites, restaurants, and movie theaters. This allows the adolescent to exercise some choice, further increasing reinforcement and potentially motivation. Selection of achievable targets (e.g., abstinence over a short period) is especially important earlier in treatment but becomes more difficult as the adolescent achieves his or her targets. The schedule of reinforcement is critical and involves minimizing the delay between achieving the target behavior and reinforcement, using more frequent reinforcement earlier in treatment (weekly or more often), and creative use of different schedules that are important for a successful CM program.

Skills-Based Interventions

CBT models adapted for adolescent with SUDs are well supported. CBT interventions seek to help adolescents replace their substance use with less risky behavior by recognizing antecedents of their use, avoiding those circumstances if possible, and coping more effectively with problems that lead to increased use (Waldron & Kaminer, 2004).

Researchers have developed several specific CBT adaptations for adolescents with SUDs that differ in the extent to which they emphasize changing behavior, modifying thoughts, and teaching new coping skills. Most models contain two key components: functional analysis and skills building. In a functional analysis, the therapist and adolescent(s) work collaboratively to identify the adolescent's specific thoughts, feelings, and circumstances before and after substance use. Such exercises help the adolescent to identify high-risk situations that lead to increased use, while gaining insight into why he or she uses substances in those situations. The therapist applies the information obtained through functional analysis to identify specific areas in which the adolescent would benefit from learning or practicing new skills. Skills in CBT commonly include questioning and testing the adolescent's assumptions about substance use, practicing assertiveness to resist peer pressure, building a social network that is supportive of recovery, increasing pleasant activities, problem solving during high-risk situations, and gradually trying out new ways of behaving and reacting. CBT is often combined with other interventions, such as MI or family therapy. Both individual and group models of CBT have been tested in well-controlled clinical trials. Several studies have also examined CBT in combination with MI adaptations and functional family therapy. Waldron and Turner (2008), in a recent meta-analysis of evidence-based psychosocial treatments for adolescents with SUDs, classified group CBT as a well-established intervention and noted that individual CBT (which has been studied less extensively than group-based CBT) appears promising. In another review of the quality of evidence in support of outpatient interventions for adolescents with SUDs, CBT was the outpatient intervention supported by the highest proportion of methodologically stronger studies (Becker & Curry, 2008).

Family Interventions

Several family therapy approaches have a significant evidence base (Williams & Chang, 2000). Family interventions for substance abuse treatment have common goals: providing psychoeducation about SUDs, which decreases familial resistance to treatment and increases motivation and engagement; assisting parents and family members to initiate and maintain efforts to get the adolescent into appropriate treatment and achieve abstinence; helping parents and family members to establish or reestablish structure with consistent limit -setting and careful monitoring of the adolescent's activities and behavior; improving communication among family members; and getting other family members into treatment and/or support programs. Family therapeutic approaches are also generally covered by Kaufman (Chapter 29, this volume).

Among the forms of family therapy with support based on controlled studies are functional family therapy (FFT), brief strategic family therapy (BSFT), multisystemic therapy (MST), and multidimensional family therapy (MDFT) (Waldron & Turner, 2008). Based on the quality of the studies and replications in the field, two family-based approaches, MDFT and FFT, are well established for adolescent SUD treatment (Waldron & Turner, 2008). Other family models, including MST, BSFT, and brief family therapy (BFT), are probably efficacious, pending replications by independent research teams. Despite the collective evidence, however, no clear pattern emerged for the superiority of one treatment model over another.

Peer-Oriented Interventions

While many of the evidenced-based interventions described earlier can be delivered in a group format, several less evidenced-based practices deserve mention. Twelve-step approaches have often been used as a basis for treatment. Attendance at Alcoholics Anonymous (AA) and Narcotics Anonymous (NA) groups is an adjunct to professional treatment of SUDs and should be encouraged. Twelve-step approaches, using AA and NA as a basis for treatment, are perhaps the most common approaches for treatment and treatment programs in the United States. Attendance in aftercare treatment or self-support groups (e.g., AA or NA) is related to positive outcomes in several studies of adolescent SUD treatment (Williams & Chang, 2000). Twelve-step programs can be defined as having adolescents work on specific steps toward recovery, attendance at self-support groups (AA or NA), and obtaining the assistance of a sponsor, another person in recovery from substance use problems. Although 12-step programs may be effective for many adolescents, they have not been subject to controlled clinical trials. Alternative peer group programs and "Sober" high schools are 12-step-based programs using the peer support model.

Because posttreatment relapse rates at 3 to 6 months amount to 60% (Kaminer & Godley, 2010), continuity of care is imperative. Randomized clinical trials (RCTs) indicate that active aftercare (continued care) interventions showed efficacy in slowing the expected relapse (Kaminer & Godley, 2010).

Psychopharmacological Interventions

Although a number of family-based, behavioral, and cognitive-behavioral interventions have been shown to have efficacy in the treatment of adolescent SUDs, there is a paucity of controlled treatment outcome research evaluating the effectiveness of pharmacotherapies in the combined or integrated treatment of psychiatric comorbidity and SUDs (Kaminer & Bukstein, 2007). The limited pharmacotherapy research using well-controlled studies is confined to two areas: (1) targeting comorbid psychopathology such as mood disorders (including major depressive disorder [MDD] and bipolar disorder), and ADHD; and (2) substitution therapy with buprenorphine.

Mood Disorders

For adolescents, there are only four well-controlled trials of agents for mood disorders coexisting with SUDs. One small study ($n = 22$) supported the safety and efficacy (measured by fewer positive drug screens but not self-report of drug use) of lithium carbonate for bipolar disorder in adolescents with concurrent SUD (Geller et al., 1998). There are three trials using fluoxetine for MDD and SUDs. Two show no difference between placebo and fluoxetine for either depression or SUDs measures, whereas one reported fewer depressive symptoms with fluoxetine but no difference in substance use.

In two placebo-controlled studies of fluoxetine in adolescents with MDD and alcohol use disorders and SUDs, respectively (Cornelius, Maisto, & Martin, 2004; Findling et al., 2009), no differences were noted between the fluoxetine and placebo groups either on depression or drug use outcomes. In the third study (Riggs, Mikulich-Gilbertson, & Davies, 2007) of adolescents with either a current MDD or a depressive disorder and a comorbid SUD randomized to receive either fluoxetine or placebo in a single site, 8-week double-blind, placebo-controlled study, both patients who received fluoxetine or placebo had a reduction in depressive symptoms. However, there was no significant difference in mean change in depressive symptoms in subjects treated with fluoxetine and those who received placebo, and no significant difference in rates of positive urine drug toxicology results between treatment groups at any postrandomization visit. The results of these studies suggest that comorbid depression and SUDs in adolescents may remit without antidepressant pharmacotherapy or abstinence in the context of individual outpatient CBT for SUDs (but not precluding the use of CBT for depression). However, if depression does not remit, their drug use may not decrease even if they continue with substance treatment. Thus, in dually diagnosed adolescents, if depression does not appear to be improving early in the course of substance treatment (e.g., within the first several weeks of treatment) it appears to be safe, efficacious, and reasonable to initiate a selective serotonin reuptake inhibitor (SSRI, fluoxetine) with careful monitoring, even if the adolescent is not yet abstinent, because ongoing depression may prevent further improvements in substance use.

Attention-Deficit/Hyperactivity Disorder

For ADHD, there are three controlled trials, including two by Riggs and colleagues (Szobot & Bukstein, 2008; Riggs, Hall, & Mikulich-Gilbertson, 2004; Riggs, Winhusen, & Davies, 2011). Riggs et al. (2004) evaluated the safety and efficacy of pemoline (a Schedule IV psychostimulant) for ADHD in 69 out-of-treatment adolescents with active SUDs. Results showed that pemoline had a good safety profile and a comparable effect size to that reported for ADHD in adolescents without an SUD despite nonabstinence in most study adolescents. However, in the absence of specific behavioral treatment for SUD, pharmacotherapy for ADHD had no impact on drug use, which did not significantly decrease in either treatment group. Another study followed 16 male adolescents (mean age 17.5 years) with ADHD for 6 weeks using a crossover design in which half of the sample received active medication for 3 weeks, while the other half received placebo. After 3 weeks, the groups were switched. The main outcome measures for ADHD were parent report of ADHD symptoms and the Clinician Global Impression of Severity (CGI-S). The main outcome measure for substance use was the number of days of drug or alcohol use in the past week. Results showed a greater improvement in ADHD symptoms (ADHD outcome) and in CGI-S scores with active medication compared to placebo. There was no between-group difference in substance use change. In a double-blind, placebo-controlled study of osmotic-release oral system (OROS) methylphenidate (MPH) in 18-year-old adolescents with ADHD and a nonopiate SUD, Riggs and colleagues (2011) administered

CBT treatment for SUD to all subjects. Results showed that both groups improved on ADHD and SUD measures, although there were no differences between groups in adolescent report of ADHD symptoms or substance use (number of days used in past month). However, the OROS MPH group had lower ADHD scores than the placebo group on parent report. There were few significant adverse events. In a randomized, double-blind trial of atomoxetine and placebo treatment in 70 adolescents with ADHD and SUD, with both groups receiving MI/CBT for SUD, Thurstone, Riggs, Salomonsen-Sautel, and Mikulich-Gilbertson (2010) reported no difference between the atomoxetine + MI/CBT and placebo + MI/CBT groups in ADHD or SUD variables.

Overall, these results suggest that pharmacological treatment in comorbid adolescents (e.g., with SUDs and MDD or ADHD) may result in improvements in the psychiatric target but have little, if any, effect on the substance use, especially without concurrent and specific therapy for the SUD. However, there appears to be little medical risk or increase in adverse effects of treatment, and no evidence of abuse or diversion.

Opiate Dependence

Buprenorphine is a partial agonist. It is difficult to overdose on buprenorphine, and its combination with naloxone (opiate antagonist) makes it difficult to abuse intravenously. Naloxone is not absorbed orally; hence, it is not active if the combination is taken sublingually (e.g., buprenorphine is taken sublingually). In case someone tries to inject the medication, naloxone blocks the opiate receptors; hence, no euphoric effects of buprenorphine are experienced. In a recent double-blind, double-dummy trial of buprenorphine versus clonidine detoxification in a 28-day outpatient clinic with 36 adolescents with opiate dependence, buprenorphine had almost double the retention and half the number of positive urine tests for opiates compared to clonidine (Marsch, Bickel, & Badger, 2005). In another study of buprenorphine, opioid-dependent adolescents in the 12-week buprenorphine–naloxone group were prescribed up to 24 mg per day for 9 weeks, then tapered until Week 12; patients in the detox group were prescribed up to 14 mg per day, then tapered until day 14 (Woody et al., 2008). All were offered weekly individual and group counseling. Continuing treatment with buprenorphine–naloxone improved outcome compared with short-term detoxification.

In an 8-week, double-blind, randomized, placebo-controlled trial, 116 cannabis-dependent adolescents ages 15–21 received N-acetylcysteine (NAC) or placebo twice daily, each added to a CM intervention and brief weekly cessation counseling (Gray et al., 2012). Adolescents receiving NAC had more than twice the odds, when compared with placebo participants, of having negative urine tests during treatment.

Integrated Interventions

In both community surveys of adolescents with SUDs and samples of adolescents in addictions treatment, the majority have a co-occurring non-substance-related mental disorder (Hser et al., 2001). More than half of those adolescents in addictions treatment who have a co-occurring mental illness have three or more co-occurring psychiatric disorders (Dennis et al. 2003).

In order to develop a more integrated conceptual framework for intervention with comorbid disorders to aid in understanding co-occurring conditions and the level of coordination needed between service systems that address them, the basis of treatment should be the severity of impairments rather than diagnosis. The model recommends moving toward integration as the severity of the co-occurring disorder increases, and it delineates a continuum of care based on provider behavior that spans minimal coordination consultation, collaboration, and integration. A survey of evidence-based practices reveals a paucity of interventions developed to treat mental health and SUDs concurrently in adolescents. The existing integrated practices consist of two general approaches. The first is treatment planning and care coordination, which helps create a system of care in which individual services are provided, usually separately, to best meet the needs of each adolescent and his or her family. The second approach includes evidenced-based interventions that concurrently address both psychiatric and SUDs.

Recently, several attempts at developing integrated treatments for adolescents with SUDs and depression, PTSD, bipolar disorder, and suicidal behavior have provided models for both investigators and clinicians (Goldston et al., 2009). Generally, these involved extending an existing evidenced-based treatment for one aspect of the comorbidity to another. For example, CBT for depression was expanded to include modules on substance use, or family therapy for SUDs was extended to include other deviant behaviors. Of course, existing evidenced-based treatments, such as family therapy that targets monitoring and supervision or CBT that targets problem solving, already target general factors that increase risk for multiple problems.

Critical elements of integrated treatment appear to be attention to motivation, family involvement, and the development of cognitive-behavioral skills. Recent emerging research and experience suggest that pharmacotherapy can be used safely and effectively in adolescents with SUDs, although not all studies have been consistently positive. However, pharmacotherapy has its limits, and all adolescents will need treatment targeting their substance use and related behaviors.

CONCLUSION

Our understanding of the development, assessment, and treatment of adolescents with SUDs continues to advance progressively. A number of evidence-based interventions reflecting several types of treatment modalities are available to the clinician. In order to best treat adolescents, clinicians should be familiar with factors affecting the risk and maintenance of SUDs, screening and assessment, and specific modalities. Evidence-based practices for SUDs include specific family therapies, CBT, and MI/MET. Of particular importance is the presence of comorbidity with other psychiatric disorders as the rule rather than the exception in adolescents with SUDs. Ideally, comorbid psychiatric disorders should be treated concurrently with SUDs. Aftercare and involvement in prosocial activities with nondeviant peers are critical following an acute treatment episode.

REFERENCES

American Academy of Child and Adolescent Psychiatry (AACAP). (2005). Practice parameters for the assessment and treatment of children and adolescents with substance use disorders. *J Am Acad Child Adolesc Psychiatry, 44*, 609–621.

American Academy of Pediatrics. (2011). Substance use screening, brief intervention, and referral to treatement for pediatricians. *Am Acad Pediatr, 128*(5), 1330–1340.

American Psychiatric Association. (2013). *Diagnostic and statistical manual of mental disorders* (5th ed.). Arlington, VA: Author.

Armstrong, T. D., & Costello, E. J. (2002). Community studies of adolescent substance use, abuse, or dependence and psychiatric comorbidity. *J Consult Clin Psychol, 70*(6), 1224–1239.

Becker, S. J., & Curry, J. F. (2008). Outpatient interventions for adolescent substance abuse: A quality of evidence review. *J Consult Clin Psychol, 76(4)*, 531–544.

Boyd, C. J., McCabe, S. E., & Teter, C. J. (2006). Medical and nonmedical use of prescription pain medication by youth in a Detroit area public school district. *Drug Alcohol Depend, 81*, 37–45.

Briones, D. F., Wilcox, J. A., Mateus, B., & Boudjenah, D. (2006). Risk factors and prevention in adolescent substance abuse: A biopsychosocial approach. *Adolesc Med Clin, 17*(2), 335–352.

Brown, S. A., McGue, M., Maggs, J., Schulenberg, J., Hingson, R., Swartzwelder, S., et al. (2008). A developmental perspective on alcohol and youths 16 to 20 years of age. *Pediatrics, 121*, 290–310.

Casey, B. J., & Jones, R. M. (2010), Neurobiology of adolescent brain and behavior: Implications for substance use disorders. *J Am Acad Child Adolesc Psychiatry, 49*(12), 1189–1201.

Centers for Disease Control and Prevention. (2012). Retrieved from *www.cdc.gov/publications*.

Chung, T., Maisto, S. A., & Cornelius, J. R. (2005). Joint trajectory analysis of treated adolescents' alcohol use and symptoms over 1 year. *Addict Behav, 30*(9), 1690–1701.

Cornelius, J. R., Maisto, S. A., & Martin, C. S. (2004). Major depression associated with earlier alcohol relapse in treated teens with AUD. *Addict Behav, 29*, 1035–1038.

Dennis, M. L., Dawud-Noursi, S., & Muck, R. D. (2003). The need for developing and evaluating adolescent treatment models. In S. J. Stevens & A. R. Morral (Eds.), *Adolescent substance abuse treatment in the United States: Exemplary models from a National Evaluation Study* (pp. 3–34). Binghamton, NY: Haworth Press.

Findling, R. L., Pagano, M. E., McNamara, N. K., Stansbrey, R. J., Faber, J. E., Lingler, J., et al. (2009). The short-term safety and efficacy of fluoxetine in depressed adolescents with alcohol and cannabis use disorders: A pilot randomized placebo-controlled trial. *Child Adolesc Psychiatry Ment Health, 3*, 11.

Geller, B., Cooper, T., Sun, K., Zimerman, B., Frazier, J., Williams, M., & Heath, J. (1998). Double-blind and placebo-controlled study of lithium for adolescent bipolar disorders with secondary substance dependency. *J Am Acad Child Adolesc Psychiatry, 37*(2),171–178.

Goldston, D. B., Esposito-Smythers, C., Curry, J., Wells, K, Spirito, A., & Kaminer, Y. (2009, October). *Psychosocial treatment of suicidal adolescents with substance use*. Paper presented at the meeting of the American Academy of Child and Adolescent Psychiatry (AACAP), Honolulu, HI.

Grant, B., & Dawson, D. (1997). Age at onset of alcohol use and its associated DSM-IV alcohol abuse and dependence: Results from the National Longitudinal Alcohol Epidemiologic Survey. *J Subst Abuse Treat, 9*, 103–110.

Gray, K. M., Carpenter, M. J., Baker, N. L., DeSantis, S. M., Kryway, E., Hartwell, K. J., et al. (2012). A double-blind randomized controlled trial of N-acetylcysteine in cannabis-dependent adolescents. *Am J Psychiatry, 169*(8), 805–812.

Grella, C., Hser, Y. I., & Joshi, V. (2001). Drug treatment outcomes for adolescents with comorbid mental and substance use disorders. *J Nerv Ment Dis, 189*, 384–392.

Hanson, K. L., Cummins, K., Tapert, S. F., & Brown, S. A. (2011). Changes in neuropsychological functioning over 10 years following adolescent substance abuse treatment. *Psychol Addict Behav, 25*(1), 127–142.

Higgins, S. T., Silverman, K., & Heil, S. H. (2008). *Contingency management in substance abuse treatment.* New York: Guilford Press.

Hser, Y. I., Grella, C. E., & Hubbard, R. L. (2001). An evaluation of drug treatments for adolescents in four U.S. cities. *Arch Gen Psychiatry, 58*(7), 689–695.

Hsieh, S., Hoffman, N. G., & Hollister, C. D. (1998). The relationship between pre-, during-, and post-treatment factors and adolescent substance abuse behaviors. *Addict Behav, 23*, 477–488.

Jensen, C. D., Cushing, C. C., Aylward, B. S., Craig, J. T., Sorell, D. M., & Steele, R. G. (2011). Effectiveness of motivational interviewing interventions for adolescent substance use behavior change: A meta-analytic review. *J Consult Clin Psychol, 79*(4), 433–440.

Johnston, L. D., O'Malley, P. M., Bachman, J. G., & Schulenberg, J. E. (2011, December 14). *University of Michigan News Service* (National press release). Retrieved from *www.monitoringthefuture.org/pressreleases/11drugpr_complete.pdf.*

Kaminer, Y., & Bukstein, O. G. (Eds.). (2007). *Adolescent substance abuse: Psychiatric comorbidity and high risk behaviors.* New York: Routledge.

Kaminer, Y., & Godley, M. (2010). From assessment reactivity to aftercare for adolescent substance abuse: Are we there yet? *Child Adolesc Psychiatr Clin N Am, 19*, 577–590.

Kendler, K. S., Jacobson, K. C., & Prescott, C. A. (2003). Specificity of genetic and environmental risk factors for use and abuse/dependence of cannabis, cocaine, hallucinogens, sedatives stimulants, and opiates in male twins. *Am J Psychiatry, 160*, 687–695.

Knight, J. R., Sherritt, L., & Shrier, L. A. (2002). Validity of the CRAFFT substance abuse screening test among adolescent clinic patients. *Arch Pediatr Adolesc Med, 156*, 607–614.

Marsch, L. A., Bickel, W. K., & Badger, G. J. (2005). Comparison of pharmacological treatments for opioid-dependent adolescents: A randomized controlled trial. *Arch Gen Psychiatry, 62*, 1157–1164.

Martin, C. S., Chung, T., Kirisci, L., & Langenbucher, J. W. (2006). Item response theory analysis of diagnostic criteria for alcohol and cannabis use disorders in adolescents: Implications for DSM-V. *J Abnorm Psychol, 115*(4), 807–814.

McCarthy, D. M., Tomlinson, K. L., & Anderson, K. G. (2005). Relapse in alcohol- and drug-disordered adolescents with comorbid psychopathology: Changes in psychiatric symptoms. *Psychol Addict Behav, 19*, 28–34.

Merikangas, K. R., He, J. P., Burstein, M., Swanson, S. A., Avenevoli, S., Cui, L., et al. (2010). Lifetime prevalence of mental disorders in U.S. adolescents: Results from the National Comorbidity Survey Replication—Adolescent Supplement (NCS-A). *J Am Acad Child Adolesc Psychiatry, 49*(10), 980–989.

Riggs, P. D., Hall, S. K., & Mikulich-Gilbertson, S. K. (2004). A randomized controlled trial of pemoline for attention-deficit/hyperactivity disorder in substance-abusing adolescents. *J Am Acad Child Adolesc Psychiatry, 43*, 420–429.

Riggs, P. D., Mikulich-Gilbertson, S. K., & Davies, R. D. (2007). A randomized controlled trial of fluoxetine and cognitive behavioral therapy in adolescents with major depression, behavior problems, and substance use disorders. *Arch Pediatr Adolesc Med, 161*, 1026–1034.

Riggs, P., Winhusen, T., & Davies, R. D. (2011). Randomized controlled trial of osmotic-release methylphenidate with cognitive-behavioral therapy in adolescents with attention-deficit/hyperactivity disorder and substance use disorders. *J Am Acad Child Adolesc Psychiatry, 50*(9), 903–914.

Rollnick, S., & Miller, W. R. (1995). What is motivational interviewing? *Behav Cogn Psychother, 23*(4), 325–334.

Spear, L. P. (2000). The adolescent brain and age-related behavioral manifestations. *Neurosci Biobehav Rev, 24*, 417–463.

Stanger, C., & Budney, A. J. (2010). Contingency management approaches for adolescent substance use disorders. *Child Adolesc Psychiatr Clin N Am, 19*(3), 547–562.

Substance Abuse and Mental Health Service Administration. (2012). *Results from the 2011 National Survey on Drug Use and Health.* Rockville, MD: Author.

Szobot, C. M., & Bukstein, O. G. (2008). Attention deficit hyperactivity disorder and substance use disorders. *Child Adolesc Psychiatr Clin N Am, 17*(2), 309–323.

Tarter, R. (1990). Evaluation and treatment of adolescent substance abuse: A decision tree method. *Am J Drug Alcohol Abuse, 16*, 1–46.

Thurstone, C., Riggs, P. D., Salomonsen-Sautel, S., & Mikulich-Gilbertson, S. K. (2010). Randomized, controlled trial of atomoxetine for attention-deficit/hyperactivity disorder in adolescents with substance use disorder. *J Am Acad Child Adolesc Psychiatry, 49*(6), 573–582.

Waldron, H. B., & Kaminer, Y. (2004). On the learning curve: The emerging evidence supporting cognitive-behavioral therapies for adolescent substance abuse. *Addiction, 99*(2), 93–105.

Waldron, H. B., & Turner, C. W. (2008). Evidence-based psychosocial treatments for adolescent substance abuse. *J Clin Child Adolesc Psychology, 37*(1), 238–261.

Williams, R. J., & Chang, S. Y. (2000). A comprehensive and comparative review of adolescent substance abuse treatment outcome. *Clin Psychol Sci Pract, 7*(2), 138–166.

Winters, K. C., & Kaminer, Y. (2008). Screening and assessing adolescent substance use disorders in clinical populations. *J Am Acad Child Adolesc Psychiatry, 47*(7), 740–744.

Winters, K. C., Martin, C. S., & Chung, T. (2011). Substance use disorders in DSM-V when applied to adolescents. *Addiction, 106*(5), 882–884.

Woody, G. E., Poole, S. A., Subramaniam, G., Dugosh, K., Bogenschutz, M., Abbott, P., et al. (2008). Extended vs. short-term buprenorphine–naloxone for treatment of opioid-addicted youth: A randomized trial. *JAMA, 330*(17), 2003–2011.

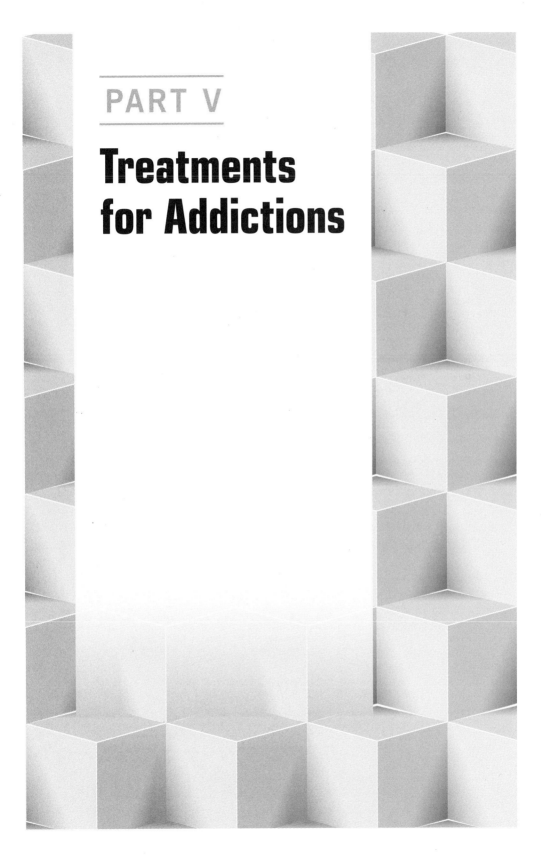

PART V

Treatments for Addictions

CHAPTER 25

Matching and Differential Therapies
Providing Substance Abusers with Appropriate Treatment

KATHLEEN M. CARROLL
BRIAN D. KILUK

Broadly defined, matching individuals to treatment means providing the individual with the treatment approach that is likely to maximize outcome. As seen in the earlier chapters in this volume, the past 20 years have been marked by both tremendous progress and increasing methodological rigor in substance abuse research, and therefore the development of a much wider range of empirically supported pharmacotherapies and behavioral therapies. Availability of a broader range of therapies has likewise heightened interest in differential treatment research, whether it be matching individuals to specific treatment approaches, matching patients to different levels of services, or identifying predictors of response to specific therapies (Insel, 2012).

To date however, empirical evidence supporting specific, a priori matching strategies has been modest at best (Magura et al., 2003; McKay, Cacciola, McLellan, Alterman, & Wirtz, 1997; McLellan & McKay, 1998; Project MATCH Research Group, 1993, 1997; UKATT Research Team, 2008), in part due to the complexity of treatment decisions for many patients, who typically present for treatment with a complex array of substance use, psychiatric, legal, medical, and social problems, as well as limits of the service delivery system in accommodating the needs of diverse patients (Gastfriend, Lu, & Sharon, 2000; McLellan, 2006). There is a bit more consistency in the literature, however, regarding prognostic variables that have emerged across patient populations. Briefly, greater severity of substance dependence, presence and severity of comorbid psychiatric problems, lower levels of social support, and unemployment have consistently related to outcome (reviewed in McLellan & McKay, 1998). Larger scale studies have also demonstrated with some consistency that addressing comorbid issues and problems in treatment is generally associated with improved outcome (McLellan, Arndt, Metzger, Woody, & O'Brien, 1993; McLellan, Grissom, Zanis, & Randall, 1997).

Thus, for our purposes in this chapter, rather than "matching" per se, we instead focus on strategies tailoring treatments to meet the needs of the individual. In general, appropriate treatment tailoring implies adequate provision of an effective, empirically supported therapy with adjunct therapies that are appropriate to the specific co-occurring problems as dictated by careful, thorough assessment of the patient functioning and status across a range of domains. Thus, this review summarizes empirically supported therapies across the most common substance use disorders (SUDs), with special emphasis on how pharmacological and behavioral therapies can be combined to enhance outcome. When available, data regarding the types of individuals who may respond particularly well or poorly to specific approaches are reviewed.

First, however, it is important to understand the respective roles of pharmacotherapy and behavioral approaches in terms of how these may be tailored, or combined, to meet the needs of specific individuals.

PHARMACOTHERAPY IN THE TREATMENT OF SUDs

The target symptoms addressed and roles typically played by pharmacotherapy differ from those of behavioral treatments in their course of action, time to effect, target symptoms, and durability of benefits (Elkin, Pilkonis, Docherty, & Sotsky, 1988). In general, pharmacotherapies have a much more narrow application than do most behavioral treatments for SUDs; that is, most of the behavioral therapies described below are applicable across a range of treatment settings (e.g., inpatient, outpatient, residential), modalities (e.g., group, individual, family), and a wide variety of populations, and are therefore readily tailored to the needs and preferences of specific individuals. For example, disease model, behavioral, or motivational approaches have been used, with relatively minor modifications, regardless of whether the patient is an opiate, alcohol, cocaine, or marijuana user. On the other hand, most available pharmacotherapies tend to be applicable only to a single class of substance use and exert their effects over a narrow band of symptoms. For example, methadone produces cross-tolerance for opioids but has little effect on concurrent cocaine abuse; disulfiram produces nausea after alcohol ingestion but not after ingestion of other illicit substances. A notable exception is naltrexone, which is used to treat both opioid and, more recently, alcohol dependence (Bouza, Angeles, Munoz, & Amate, 2004; Johansson, Berglund, & Lindgren, 2006; Oslin et al., 2008).

Common roles and indications for pharmacotherapy in the treatment of substance dependence disorders include the following (Carroll, 2001; Rounsaville & Carroll, 1997).

Detoxification

For those classes of substances that produce substantial physical withdrawal syndromes (e.g., alcohol, opioids, sedatives/hypnotics), medications are often needed to reduce or control the often-dangerous symptoms associated with withdrawal. Benzo-diazepines are often used to manage symptoms of alcohol withdrawal. Agents such as methadone, clonidine, naltrexone, and buprenorphine are typically used for the management of opioid withdrawal. Typically, the role of behavioral treatments during detoxification is typically extremely limited due to the level of discomfort, agitation, and confusion the patient may experience. However, recent studies have suggested the effectiveness of behavioral strategies in increasing retention and abstinence in the course of longer-term outpatient detoxification protocols (Bickel, Amass, Higgins, Badger, & Esch, 1997; Tuten, Defulio, Jones, & Stitzer, 2012).

Stabilization and Maintenance

A widely used example of the use of a medication for long-term stabilization of drug users is methadone maintenance for opioid dependence, a treatment strategy that involves the daily administration of a long-acting opioid (methadone) as a substitute for the illicit use of short-acting opioids (typically heroin). Methadone maintenance permits the patient to function normally, without experiencing withdrawal symptoms, craving, or side effects. The large body of research on methadone maintenance confirms its importance in fostering treatment retention, providing the opportunity to evaluate and treat other problems and disorders that often coexist with opioid dependence (e.g., medical, legal, and occupational problems), reducing the risk of HIV infection and other complications by reducing intravenous drug use, and providing a level of stabilization that permits the inception of psychotherapy and other aspects of treatment (Ball & Ross, 1991; Lowinson, Marion, Joseph, & Dole, 1992; Sees et al., 2000).

However, methadone maintenance in and of itself is rarely sufficient treatment for most chronic heroin-addicted individuals. Multiple studies indicate that addition of empirically supported therapies can broaden and strengthen the effectiveness of maintenance therapies (McLellan et al., 1993; Woody et al., 1983). As described at greater length in the later sections on behavioral therapies, specific behavioral therapies can be used to tailor treatment for specific individuals with specific co-occurring problems. For example, contingency management has been shown in multiple studies to be effective in reducing concurrent cocaine dependence among methadone-maintained cocaine users, a group with particularly poor outcomes (Peirce et al., 2006; Silverman, Higgins, et al., 1996). Behavioral therapies can also target other problems among agonist-maintained populations, such as Silverman's model of work-based therapy, in which individuals are provided access to paid work that is contingent on regular submission of cocaine-free urine specimens (Silverman, 1999; Silverman et al., 2002).

Antagonist and Other Behaviorally Oriented Pharmacotherapies

A more recent pharmacological strategy is the use of antagonist treatment, that is, the use of medications that block the effects of specific drugs. An example of this approach is naltrexone, an effective, long-acting opioid antagonist. Naltrexone is nonaddicting, does not have the reinforcing properties of opioids, has few side effects and, most important, effectively blocks the effects of opioids. Therefore, naltrexone treatment represents a potent behavioral strategy: As opioid ingestion will not be reinforced while the patient is taking naltrexone, unreinforced opioid use allows extinction of relationships between conditioned drug cues and drug use. For example, a naltrexone-maintained patient, anticipating that opioid use will not result in desired drug effects, may be more likely to learn to live in a world full of drug cues and high-risk situations without resorting to drug use.

On the other hand, the efficacy of naltrexone treatment, particularly for the treatment of opioid dependence, has been undercut by problems of adherence since its inception (Anton, Hogan, Jalali, Riordan, & Kleber, 1981; Grabowski et al., 1979; Rounsaville, 1995). Thus, for many years, clinical use of naltrexone was limited to groups such as professionals (e.g., medical care providers) who agreed to supervised naltrexone treatment as a condition of their continued licensure or employment (Rounsaville, 1995). Longer acting depot formulations of naltrexone have addressed this issue to a large extent; however, attrition still remains a problem (Kranzler, Wesson, & Billot, 2004; Krupitsky & Blokhina, 2010). Again, behavioral therapies such as contingency management (Carroll et al., 2001) and family therapy (Fals-Stewart & O'Farrell, 2003) may have utility in facilitating adherence and outcome with naltrexone treatment, as well as other medication approaches in which efficacy is limited by problems in compliance (Carroll & Rounsaville, 2007a).

Treatment of Coexisting Disorders

Another important role of pharmacotherapy in addictive disorders is as treatment for coexisting psychiatric syndromes that may precede or play a role in the maintenance or complications of drug dependence. The frequent co-occurrence of psychiatric disorders, particularly affective and anxiety disorders, with SUDs is well documented in a variety of populations and settings (Kessler et al., 1997; Regier et al., 1990). Given that psychiatric disorders often precede development of SUDs, several researchers have hypothesized that individuals with primary psychiatric disorders may be attempting to self-medicate their psychiatric symptoms with drugs and alcohol. Thus, effective pharmacological treatment of the underlying psychiatric disorder may improve not only the psychiatric disorder but also the perceived need for and therefore the use of illicit drugs. Overall, however, studies evaluating the effect of antidepressant treatment on comorbid depressive disorders and SUDs have shown very modest effects on levels of substance use (reviewed in Nunes & Levin, 2004).

Fostering Compliance with Pharmacotherapy

The difficulties of fostering adequate levels of treatment compliance with substance users is well known (Skolnick & Volkow, 2012), so much so that substance users are typically excluded from clinical trials of treatments for other disorders. Thus, when pharmacotherapies are used in the treatment of substance use, it is not surprising to see high rates of noncompliance. A major role that behavioral treatments play when pharmacotherapies are used in the treatment of substance use is in fostering compliance, because most strategies to improve compliance are inherently psychosocial.

These include, for example, regular monitoring of medication compliance through pill counts and medication serum levels; encouragement of patient self-monitoring of compliance (e.g., through medication logs or diaries); clear communication between patient and staff about the study medication, its expected effects, side effects and benefits; repeatedly stressing the importance of adherence; contracting with the patients for adherence; directly reinforcing adherence through incentives or rewards; providing telephone or written reminders about appointments or taking medication; preparing and educating patients about the disorder and its treatment; and frequent contact and the provision of extensive support and encouragement to the patient and his or her family (Haynes, McDonald, & Garg, 2002; Haynes, McDonald, Garg, & Montague, 2000; Weiss, 2004).

BEHAVIORAL TREATMENTS FOR SUDs

We present in the following sections a brief overview of the major categories of behavioral therapies that are typically considered to be evidence based (Carroll & Onken, 2005; DeRubeis & Crits-Christoph, 1998; Dutra et al., 2008; National Institute on Drug Abuse, 2007; Roth & Fonagy, 2005). These focus on categories that have been found to be effective in multiple randomized clinical trials and on the major types of SUDs (alcohol, opioid, cocaine, and marijuana dependence). Many of these were described in more detail in earlier chapters in this volume; they are discussed here primarily in terms of their focus (e.g., earlier vs. later phases of treatment) and how they can be tailored to improve outcomes in specific individuals.

Motivational Interviewing and Brief Approaches

Motivational and brief approaches tend to be those best suited for the initial phases of treatment and those with lower levels of problem substance use (e.g., nondependent users in ambulatory settings). As such, they are an excellent "first-line" approach in a number of settings, so that more intensive resources can be reserved for individuals who do not respond to brief motivational interventions (Carroll & Rounsaville, 2007b). They are often delivered in settings in which problems related to SUDs are addressed but the individual is not necessarily seeking treatment for a substance use problem. These include screening and brief intervention approaches in emergency and primary care departments (Babor et al., 2007; D'Onofrio et al., 2008; Saitz et al., 2007).

Motivational approaches are brief treatments that are designed to produce rapid, internally motivated change in addictive behavior and other problem behaviors. Motivational interviewing (MI), developed by William Miller and his colleagues, best represents these types of treatment approaches. Grounded in principles of motivational psychology and client-centered counseling, MI (Miller & Rollnick, 1991, 2002) arose out of several recent theoretical and empirical advances (Miller, 2000). First, several studies of problem drinking indicated that very brief interventions (e.g., one or two sessions in duration) were associated with reductions in drinking that were as robust and enduring as those associated with much more intensive treatments

(Bien, Miller, & Tonigan, 1993). These studies highlighted that change in addictive behavior can happen with relatively little treatment. Second, research on how people change problem behaviors led to greater interest in natural recovery and the transtheoretical model (Prochaska, DiClemente, & Norcross, 1992), also called the stages of change model, in which individuals who are attempting to change problem behaviors move through a reliable sequence of stages, from precontemplation (associated with individuals who are not considering changing their behavior) to contemplation (recognition of the need to change and consideration of the costs and feasibility of behavior change) to determination (making the decision to take action and change) to action and maintenance. Motivation for change was seen as a critical variable for understanding how people move from one stage to another (DiClemente, Bellino, & Neavins, 1999). Likewise, the model emphasized the need for developing interventions matched to different stages of change. MI was seen as very well suited for the early stages (DiClemente & Velasquez, 2002). Third, research on substance users indicated that patient drinking outcomes were associated with therapist style, with high levels of therapist confrontation associated with poorer outcomes, and high levels of empathy associated with better outcomes (Miller, Benefield, & Tonigan, 1993). Empathic listening became a central feature in the development of MI. MI typically occurs over the course of one to four sessions, with earlier work focusing on building the patient's motivation for change and subsequent work strengthening the patient's commitment to change. The core of each of these phases is the therapist's consistent use of MI techniques, summarized by the acronym OARS (Open-ended questions, Affirming, Reflecting, and Summarizing; Miller & Rollnick, 2002).

MI has a high level of empirical support across a wide range of SUDs, with particularly strong support among alcohol-abusing and -dependent populations (Miller & Wilbourne, 2002; Swanson, Pantalon, & Cohen, 1999; Wilk, Jensen, & Havighurst, 1997) and good support for adolescent substance users and smokers (Heckman, Egleston, & Hofmann, 2010; Jensen et al., 2011). Although some studies have suggested the effectiveness of brief motivational approaches for enhancing engagement and outcome among users of illicit drugs, there have been several negative studies in this area, suggesting more mixed support for MI as a sole treatment for more severely dependent drug-using populations (Budney, Roffman, Stephens, & Walker, 2007; Burke, Arkowitz, & Menchola, 2003; Dunn, Deroo, & Rivara, 2001; Miller, Yahne, & Tonigan, 2003; Rubak, Sandbaek, Lauritzen, & Christensen, 2005). Some meta-analyses also suggest larger effect sizes among members of ethnic/minority groups (Hettema, Steele, & Miller, 2005). Thus, for patients seeking treatment for marijuana, cocaine, or alcohol dependence, MI is typically used in the early phases of treatment or combined with another behavioral (often cognitive-behavioral therapy [CBT]) or pharmacological approach for more severely dependent populations.

Cognitive-Behavioral and Skills Training Therapies

As a next line of treatment for those who do not respond to brief motivational approaches, a reasonable next step would be those approaches that seek to improve skills and control over use. These approaches may also be useful after more intensive approaches (e.g., inpatient programs, detoxification) to prevent relapse.

Cognitive-behavioral approaches have also been demonstrated to be compatible with pharmacotherapies and are often combined with medication-assisted therapies such as methadone or naltrexone maintenance.

Cognitive-behavioral approaches are grounded in social learning theories and principles of operant conditioning. The defining features of these approaches are (1) an emphasis on functional analysis of drug use (i.e., understanding drug use within the context of its antecedents and consequences) and (2) skills training, through which the individual learns to recognize the situations or states in which he or she is most vulnerable to drug use, avoid those high-risk situations whenever possible, and use a range of behavioral and cognitive strategies to cope effectively with those situations if they cannot be avoided. Meta-analyses and extensive reviews of the literature have established that cognitive-behavioral approaches have strong empirical support for use in treatment of alcohol use disorders and several non-substance-related psychiatric disorders, and that these approaches have been demonstrated to be effective in drug-using populations as well (Tolin, 2010). Several research groups have demonstrated the efficacy of CBT in the treatment of cocaine-dependent outpatients, particularly depressed and more severely dependent cocaine users, and have shown that CBT is compatible and possibly has additive effects when combined with pharmacotherapies such as disulfiram.

Furthermore, CBT is characterized by an emphasis on the development of skills that not only can be used initially to foster abstinence but can also be applied to a range of co-occurring problems. This feature may be a factor in emerging evidence for the long-term durability of the effects of CBT. Several studies have demonstrated that CBT's effects are durable and that continuing improvement may occur even after the end of treatment. These findings are consistent with evidence that CBT may have enduring effects for other disorders, such as panic disorder and depression (Hollon, 2003; Tolin, 2010). Delayed emergence of the effects of CBT was highlighted in two studies that directly compared group CBT and contingency management among cocaine-dependent patients in a methadone maintenance program. Although end-of-treatment outcomes favored contingency management over CBT, 1-year follow-up indicated significant continuing improvement for patients assigned to CBT, in contrast to weakening effects for contingency management, which resulted in comparable, or slightly better, outcomes for CBT at the end of follow-up (Epstein, Hawkins, Covi, Umbricht, & Preston, 2003; Rawson et al., 2006). Data suggest that acquisition of specific coping skills conveyed through a computerized CBT program mediated continued improvements in outcome through a 6-month follow-up in a mixed group of substance users (Kiluk, Nich, Babuscio, & Carroll, 2010). Another multisite study involving 450 marijuana-dependent individuals demonstrated that a nine-session individual approach that integrated CBT and MI was more effective than a two-session MI approach, which in turn was more effective than a delayed-treatment control condition (MTP Research Group, 2004).

Despite the emerging empirical support for use of CBT in drug-dependent populations, additional research is needed to address its limitations. There are few data on specific patient predictors of outcome for CBT, although completion of homework assignments is emerging as a marker of better long-term response (Addis & Jacobson, 2000; Bryant, Simons, & Thase, 1999; Burns & Spangler, 2000; Carroll, Nich, &

Ball, 2005; Gonzalez, Schmitz, & DeLaume, 2006; Kazantzis, Deane, & Ronan, 2000). In addition, there are several reports of poorer response to CBT among substance users with higher levels of difficulty in cognitive functioning (Aharonovich et al., 2006; Aharonovich, Nunes, & Hasin, 2003). Thus, when the individual has problems in maintaining attention, and following and remembering explanations and tasks, adaptations of CBT may be needed (repetition, simplification on concepts). CBT is also a comparatively complex approach, and training clinicians to implement this approach effectively can be challenging (Sholomskas et al., 2005). Strategies for addressing these issues include greater emphasis on understanding CBT's mechanisms of action, so that ineffective components can be removed, and treatment delivery can be simplified, shortened, and perhaps even accomplished by computer or other automated means.

Contingency Management Therapies

As a next-level approach for individuals who have more severe substance use or social problems, contingency management, in which patients receive incentives or rewards for meeting specific behavioral goals (e.g., verified abstinence), has particularly strong, consistent, and robust empirical support across a range of types of drug use. Contingency management approaches are based on principles of behavioral pharmacology and operant conditioning, in which behavior that is followed by positive consequences is more likely to be repeated. For example, allowing a patient the privilege of taking home methadone doses, contingent on the patient's providing drug-free urine specimens, is associated with significant reductions in illicit drug use, and this strategy can be used address a number of other problems, such as benzodiazepine use, that are common in methadone maintenance programs. This body of work also supports the view that positive incentives (e.g., rewards for desired behaviors) are more effective in producing improved substance use outcomes and in retaining patients in treatment than negative consequences (e.g., methadone dose reductions, restriction of clinic privileges, or termination of treatment). Despite consistent findings on the efficacy of contingent take-home privileges in methadone maintenance programs, contingency management procedures proved difficult to implement outside of methadone programs until the early 1990s, when Budney, Higgins, and their colleagues demonstrated the efficacy of vouchers redeemable for goods and services, contingent on the patient's providing cocaine-free urine specimens, in reducing targeted drug use and enhancing retention in treatment (Higgins, Budney, Bickel, & Hughes, 1993; Higgins et al., 1991; Higgins & Silverman, 1999).

Voucher-based incentives have been shown to be effective in improving retention and abstinence in outpatient opioid detoxification (Chutuape, Silverman, & Stitzer, 1999), in reducing illicit substance use among opioid addicts in a methadone maintenance program (Stitzer, Iguchi, Kidorf, & Bigelow, 1993), in reducing the frequency of marijuana use (Budney, Higgins, Radonovich, & Novy, 2000), and in improving medication compliance among opioid-dependent individuals treated with naltrexone maintenance (Carroll et al., 2001). Iguchi and colleagues (1996) expanded voucher-based contingency management to outcomes other than drug-negative urine specimens, demonstrating that reinforcement of tasks outlined in an individualized, verifiable treatment plan was associated with greater reductions in illicit drug use than reinforcement of drug-free urine specimens. Voucher-based contingency management has also been shown to reduce cocaine and opioid use in the context of methadone maintenance, thus extending the availability of contingency management procedures to methadone programs in which the ability to offer take-home privileges is restricted. Silverman and colleagues (1998; Silverman, Higgins, et al., 1996) demonstrated the efficacy of a therapeutic workplace for pregnant and postpartum drug-abusing women in a methadone maintenance program. Access to the therapeutic workplace, which provided job training and a salary, was linked to abstinence and was contingent on the participants' producing drug-free urine specimens (Silverman, Chutuape, Bigelow, & Stitzer, 1996; Silverman, Svikis, Robles, Stitzer, & Bigelow, 2001; Silverman et al., 2002).

Despite these findings, questions have arisen regarding the applicability and sustainability of contingency management in clinical practice, especially in community-based treatment programs in which the cost of the vouchers and the need for frequent urine monitoring can be prohibitive. These issues have been addressed in part by the work of Petry et al., who developed a lower-cost contingency management procedure in which vouchers are not given but participants receive the opportunity to draw prizes of varying value, contingent on verifiable target behaviors such as provision of drug-free urine specimens (Petry, 2000; Petry, Alessi, Marx, Austin, & Tardif, 2005; Petry et al., 2004). This approach has been effective in reducing drug use among both methadone maintenance patients and cocaine-dependent outpatients (Petry, Kolodner, et al., 2006; Petry, Peirce, et al., 2006).

Although the consistent findings of effectiveness in contingency management interventions are compelling, some limitations have been noted. First, the effects tend to weaken after the contingencies are terminated. This problem might be addressed by evaluating combinations of contingency management with approaches that have more enduring effects, for example, by transferring rewards from monetary reinforcers to behaviors that, in and of themselves, are reinforcing, or by exploring novel discontinuation strategies, such as lengthening periods between reinforcement or offering more intermittent reinforcements. Also, because a substantial proportion of substance users do not respond to contingency management, there is a need to understand and address individual differences in response to these approaches. In general, contingency management appears to be effective for individuals with a wide range of demographic characteristics (race, education, employment status); for more severely dependent individuals, higher levels of rewards may be necessary to achieve good outcomes (Barry, Sullivan, & Petry, 2009; Rash, Alessi, & Petry, 2008a, 2008b).

Couple and Family Treatments

A final class of empirically validated therapies that can be applied in a large range of settings includes couple and family treatments, described in more detail by Kaufman (Chapter 29, this volume). The defining feature of family and couple treatments is that they treat drug-using individuals in the context of family and social systems in which substance use may develop or be maintained. The engagement of the individual's social networks in treatment can be a powerful predictor of change; thus, the inclusion of family members in treatment may be helpful in reducing attrition (particularly among adolescents) and addressing multiple problem areas. Meta-analyses have strongly supported the efficacy of these approaches for both adult and adolescent substance users (Baldwin, Christian, Berkeljon, & Shadish, 2012; Stanton & Shadish, 1997). It is important to note that family-based approaches are quite diverse, and it is unlikely that all are equally effective. Moreover, many family-based approaches combine a variety of techniques, including family and individual therapies, skills training, and communication training.

Behavioral couple therapy and behavioral family counseling combine abstinence contracts and behavioral principles to reinforce abstinence from drugs; these approaches require the participation of a non-substance-abusing spouse or cohabitating partner (O'Farrell & Fals-Stewart, 2006). Several family therapies have been demonstrated to be effective among drug-using adolescents. Azrin's family behavior therapy, which combines behavioral contracting with contingency management, was found to be more effective than supportive counseling in a series of comparisons involving adolescents with SUDs, with and without conduct disorder (Azrin et al., 1996). Multisystemic therapy, a manual-based approach that addresses multiple determinants of drug use and antisocial behavior and is intended to promote fuller family involvement by engaging family members as collaborators in treatment, emphasizes the strengths of youth and their families, and addresses a broad and comprehensive array of barriers to attaining treatment goals (Henggeler et al., 2008; Henggeler, Melton, Brondino, Scherer, & Hanley, 1997; Henggeler, Pickrel, Brondino, & Crouch, 1996). Henggeler and colleagues have demonstrated the efficacy and durability of multisystemic therapy in retaining patients and broadly improving outcomes among substance-using juvenile offenders, compared with similar juvenile offenders who received the usual community treatment services. Brief strategic family therapy has also received a substantial level of empirical support. In contrast to the other family therapies for adolescents reviewed here, brief strategic family therapy is somewhat less intensive, as it targets fewer systems and can be delivered through once-weekly office visits. Brief strategic family therapy has been associated with improved retention, as well as significant reductions in the frequency of externalizing behaviors (e.g., aggression, delinquency) (Robbins et al., 2011; Santisteban et al., 2003; Szapocznik & Williams, 2000). Multidimensional family therapy (MFT) is a multicomponent, staged family therapy that incorporates both individual and family formats, and targets the substance-using youth, the family members, and their interactions. Liddle and colleagues (2001) demonstrated that MFT is more effective than group therapy or multifamily education among substance-using adolescents referred to treatment by the criminal justice system or by schools.

CONCLUSIONS

Recent years have been marked by enormous progress in the identification of a wide range of empirically validated pharmacological and behavioral therapies for SUDs. Important new treatment options, such as naltrexone and acamprosate for alcohol use disorders, and buprenorphine for opioid dependence, were unavailable 25 years ago, as were behavioral therapies including contingency management, behavioral marital counseling, MI, and CBT, all of which have demonstrated efficacy across a range of SUDs and populations. Equally promising are results demonstrating that combining pharmacotherapies with behavioral therapies can extend, strengthen, and make treatment effects more durable. Increasing attention to adaptive therapies (Murphy, Collins, & Rush, 2007), as well as the promise of developing treatment-matching algorithms based on markers such as genetic or cognitive characteristics (Kranzler & McKay, 2012; Ray & Hutchison, 2007) may result in more effective, personalized treatments (McMahon & Insel, 2012). Nevertheless, the recent progress in the identification of efficacious therapies has not been matched by identification of moderating variables or consistent patient predictors of response to specific treatment approaches that can guide researchers' and clinicians' efforts to match individuals to optimal treatment strategies. Identification of moderators of response to efficacious therapies, as well as identification of the specific mechanisms by which those treatments achieve their effects, should be a primary focus among clinical researchers in the years that lie ahead.

ACKNOWLEDGMENTS

Support was provided by National Institute on Drug Abuse Grant No. P50-DA09241.

REFERENCES

Addis, M. E., & Jacobson, N. S. (2000). A closer look at the treatment rationale and homework compliance in cognitive-behavioral therapy for depression. *Cogn Ther Res, 24*, 313–326.

Aharonovich, E., Hasin, D. S., Brooks, A. C., Liu, X., Bisaga, A., & Nunes, E. V. (2006). Cognitive deficits predict low treatment retention in cocaine dependent patients. *Drug Alcohol Depend, 81*(3), 313–322.

Aharonovich, E., Nunes, E. V., & Hasin, D. (2003). Cognitive impairment, retention and abstinence among cocaine abusers in cognitive-behavioral treatment. *Drug Alcohol Depend, 71*, 207–211.

Anton, R. F., Hogan, I., Jalali, B., Riordan, C. E., & Kleber, H. D. (1981). Multiple family therapy and naltrexone in the treatment of opioid dependence. *Drug Alcohol Depend, 8*, 157–168.

Azrin, N. H., Acierno, R., Kogan, E. S., Donohue, B., Besalel, V. A., & McMahon, P. T. (1996). Follow-up results of supportive versus behavioral therapy for illicit drug use. *Behav Res Ther, 34*, 41–46.

Babor, T. F., McKee, B. G., Kassenbaum, P. A., Grimaldi, P. L., Ahmed, K., & Bray, J. (2007). Screening, Brief Intervention, and Referral to Treatment (SBIRT): Toward a public health approach to the management of substance abuse. *Subst Abuse, 28*, 7–30.

Baldwin, S. A., Christian, S., Berkeljon, A., & Shadish, W. R. (2012). The effects of family therapies for adolescent delinquency and substance abuse: A meta-analysis. *J Marital Fam Ther, 38*(1), 281–304.

Ball, J. C., & Ross, A. (1991). *The effectiveness of methadone maintenance treatment*. New York: Springer-Verlag.

Barry, D., Sullivan, B., & Petry, N. M. (2009). Comparable efficacy of contingency management for cocaine dependence among African American, Hispanic, and White methadone maintenance clients. *Psychol Addict Behav, 23*(1), 168–174.

Bickel, W. K., Amass, L., Higgins, S. T., Badger, G. J., & Esch, R. A. (1997). Effects of adding behavioral treatment to opioid detoxification with buprenorphine. *J Consult Clin Psychol,* *65,* 803–810.

Bien, T. H., Miller, W. R., & Tonigan, J. S. (1993). Brief interventions for alcohol problems: A review. *Addiction, 88,* 315–335.

Bouza, C., Angeles, M., Munoz, A., & Amate, J. M. (2004). Efficacy and safety of naltrexone and acamprosate in the treatment of alcohol dependence: A systematic review. *Addiction, 99*(7), 811–828.

Bryant, M. J., Simons, A. D., & Thase, M. E. (1999). Therapist skill and patient variables in homework compliance: Controlling an uncontrolled variable in cognitive therapy outcome research. *Cogn Ther Res, 23,* 381–399.

Budney, A. J., Higgins, S. T., Radonovich, K. J., & Novy, P. L. (2000). Adding voucher-based incentives to coping skills and motivational enhancement improves outcomes during treatment for marijuana dependence. *J Consult Clin Psychol, 68,* 1051–1061.

Budney, A. J., Roffman, R., Stephens, R. S., & Walker, D. (2007). Marijuana dependence and its treatment. *Addict Sci Clin Pract, 4*(1), 4–16.

Burke, B. L., Arkowitz, H., & Menchola, M. (2003). The efficacy of motivational interviewing: A meta-analysis of controlled clinical trials. *J Consult Clin Psychol, 71*(5), 843–861.

Burns, D. D., & Spangler, D. L. (2000). Does psychotherapy homework lead to improvements in depression in cognitive-behavioral therapy or does improvement lead to increased homework compliance? *J Consult Clin Psychol, 68,* 46–56.

Carroll, K. M. (2001). Combined treatments for substance dependence. In M. T. Sammons & N. B. Schmidt (Eds.), *Combined treatments for mental disorders: Pharmacological and psychotherapeutic strategies for intervention* (pp. 215–238). Washington, DC: American Psychiatric Association Press.

Carroll, K. M., Ball, S. A., Nich, C., O'Connor, P. G., Eagan, D., Frankforter, T. L., et al. (2001). Targeting behavioral therapies to enhance naltrexone treatment of opioid dependence: Efficacy of contingency management and significant other involvement. *Arch Gen Psychiatry, 58,* 755–761.

Carroll, K. M., Nich, C., & Ball, S. A. (2005). Practice makes progress?: Homework assignments and outcome in treatment of cocaine dependence. *J Consult Clin Psychol, 73*(4), 749–755.

Carroll, K. M., & Onken, L. S. (2005). Behavioral therapies for drug abuse. *Am J Psychiatry, 162,* 1452–1460.

Carroll, K. M., & Rounsaville, B. J. (2007a). A perfect platform: Combining contingency management with medications for drug abuse. *Am J Drug Alcohol Abuse, 33*(3), 343–365.

Carroll, K. M., & Rounsaville, B. J. (2007b). A vision of the next generation of behavioral therapies research in the addictions. *Addiction, 102*(6), 850–862; discussion 863–859.

Chutuape, M. A., Silverman, K., & Stitzer, M. (1999). Contingent reinforcement sustains postdetoxification abstinence from multiple drugs: A preliminary study with methadone patients. *Drug Alcohol Depend, 54*(1), 69–81.

DeRubeis, R. J., & Crits-Christoph, P. (1998). Empirically supported individual and group psychological treatments for adult mental disorders. *J Consult Clin Psychol, 66,* 37–52.

DiClemente, C. C., Bellino, L. E., & Neavins, T. M. (1999). Motivation for change and alcoholism treatment. *Alcohol Health Res World, 23,* 86–92.

DiClemente, C. C., & Velasquez, M. M. (2002). Motivational interviewing and the stages of change. In W. R. Miller & S. Rollnick (Eds.), *Motivational interviewing: Preparing people for change* (2nd ed., pp. 201–216). New York: Guilford Press.

D'Onofrio, G., Pantalon, M. V., Degutis, L. C., Fiellin, D. A., Busch, S. H., Chawarski, M. C., et al. (2008). Brief intervention for hazardous and harmful drinkers in the emergency department. *Ann Emerg Med, 51*(6), 742–750.

Dunn, C., Deroo, L., & Rivara, F. P. (2001). The use of brief interventions adapted from motivational interviewing across behavioral domains: A systematic review. *Addiction, 96*(12), 1725–1742.

Dutra, L., Stathopoulou, G., Basden, S. L., Leyro, T. M., Powers, M. B., & Otto, M. W. (2008). A meta-analytic review of psychosocial interventions for substance use disorders. *Am J Psychiatry, 165*(2), 179–187.

Elkin, I., Pilkonis, P. A., Docherty, J. P., & Sotsky, S. M. (1988). Conceptual and methodologic issues in comparative studies of psychotherapy and pharmacotherapy: I. Active ingredients and mechanisms of change. *Am J Psychiatry, 145*, 909–917.

Epstein, D. E., Hawkins, W. E., Covi, L., Umbricht, A., & Preston, K. L. (2003). Cognitive behavioral therapy plus contingency management for cocaine use: Findings during treatment and across 12-month follow-up. *Psychol Addict Behav, 17*, 73–82.

Fals-Stewart, W., & O'Farrell, T. J. (2003). Behavioral family counseling and naltrexone for male opioid-dependent patients. *J Consult Clin Psychol, 71*, 432–442.

Gastfriend, D. R., Lu, S. H., & Sharon, E. (2000). Placement matching: Challenges and technical progress. *Subst Use Misuse, 35*, 2191–2213.

Gonzalez, V. M., Schmitz, J. M., & DeLaume, K. A. (2006). The role of homework in cognitive behavioral therapy for cocaine dependence. *J Consult Clin Psychol, 74*, 633–637.

Grabowski, J., O'Brien, C. P., Greenstein, R. A., Long, M., Steinberg-Donato, S., & Ternes, J. (1979). Effects of contingent payments on compliance with a naltrexone regimen. *Am J Drug Alcohol Abuse, 6*, 355–365.

Haynes, R. B., McDonald, H. P., & Garg, A. X. (2002). Helping patients follow prescribed treatment: Clinical applications. *JAMA, 288*(22), 2880–2883.

Haynes, R. B., McDonald, H. P., Garg, A. X., & Montague, P. (2000). Interventions for helping patients to follow prescriptions for medications. *Cochrane Database Syst Rev, 2*, CD000011.

Heckman, C. J., Egleston, B. L., & Hofmann, M. T. (2010). Efficacy of motivational interviewing for smoking cessation: A systematic review and meta-analysis. *Tob Control, 19*(5), 410–416.

Henggeler, S. W., Chapman, J. E., Rowland, M. D., Halliday-Boykins, C. A., Randall, J., Shackelford, J., et al. (2008). Statewide adoption and initial implementation of contingency management for substance-abusing adolescents. *J Consult Clin Psychol, 76*(4), 556–567.

Henggeler, S. W., Melton, G. B., Brondino, M. J., Scherer, D. G., & Hanley, J. H. (1997). Multisystemic therapy with violent and chronic juvenile offenders and their families: The role of treatment fidelity. *J Consult Clin Psychol, 65*, 821–833.

Henggeler, S. W., Pickrel, S. G., Brondino, M. J., & Crouch, J. L. (1996). Eliminating (almost) treatment dropout of substance abusing or dependent delinquents through home-based multisystemic therapy. *Am J Psychiatry, 153*(3), 427–428.

Hettema, J., Steele, J., & Miller, W. R. (2005). Motivational interviewing. *Annu Rev Clin Psychol, 1*, 91–111.

Higgins, S. T., Budney, A. J., Bickel, W. K., & Hughes, J. R. (1993). Achieving cocaine abstinence with a behavioral approach. *Am J Psychiatry, 150*, 763–769.

Higgins, S. T., Delany, D. D., Budney, A. J., Bickel, W. K., Hughes, J. R., Foerg, F., et al. (1991). A behavioral approach to achieving initial cocaine abstinence. *Am J Psychiatry, 148*, 1218–1224.

Higgins, S. T., & Silverman, K. (1999). *motivating behavior change among illicit-drug abusers.* Washington, DC: American Psychological Association.

Hollon, S. D. (2003). Does cognitive therapy have an enduring effect? *Cogn Ther Res, 27*, 71–75.

Iguchi, M. Y., Lamb, R. J., Belding, M. A., Platt, J. J., Husband, S. D., & Morral, A. R. (1996). Contingent reinforcement of group participation versus abstinence in a methadone maintenance program. *Exp Clin Psychopharmacol, 4*, 1–7.

Insel, T. R. (2012). Next-generation treatments for mental disorders. *Sci Transl Med, 4*(155), 155ps119.

Jensen, C. D., Cushing, C. C., Aylward, B. S., Craig, J. T., Sorell, D. M., & Steele, R. G. (2011). Effectiveness of motivational interviewing interventions for adolescent substance use behavior change: A meta-analytic review. *J Consult Clin Psychol, 79*(4), 433–440.

Johansson, B. A., Berglund, M., & Lindgren, A. (2006). Efficacy of maintenance treatment with naltrexone for opioid dependence: A meta-analytical review. *Addiction, 101*(4), 491–503.

Kazantzis, N., Deane, F. P., & Ronan, K. R. (2000). Homework assignments in cognitive and behavioral therapy: A meta-analysis. *Clin Psychol Sci Pract, 7*, 189–202.

Kessler, R. C., Crum, R. M., Warner, L. A., Nelson, C. B., Schulenberg, J., & Anthony, J. C. (1997). Lifetime co-occurence of DSM-III-R alcohol abuse and dependence with other psychiatric disorders in the National Comorbidity Study. *Arch Gen Psychiatry, 54*, 313–321.

Kiluk, B. D., Nich, C., Babuscio, T., & Carroll, K. M. (2010). Quality versus quantity: Acquisition of coping skills following computerized cognitive-behavioral therapy for substance use disorders. *Addiction, 105*(12), 2120–2127.

Kranzler, H. R., & McKay, J. R. (2012). Personalized treatment of alcohol dependence. *Curr Psychiatry Rep, 14*(5), 486–493.

Kranzler, H. R., Wesson, D. R., & Billot, L. (2004). Naltrexone depot for treatment of alcohol dependence: A multicenter, randomized, placebo-controlled clinical trial. *Alcohol Clin Exp Res, 28*(7), 1051–1059.

Krupitsky, E. M., & Blokhina, E. A. (2010). Long-acting depot formulations of naltrexone for heroin dependence: A review. *Curr Opin Psychiatry, 23*(3), 210–214.

Liddle, H. A., Dakof, G. A., Parker, K., Diamond, G. S., Barrett, K., & Tejeda, M. (2001). Multidimensional family therapy for adolescent drug abuse: Results of a randomized clinical trial. *Am J Drug Alcohol Abuse, 27*(4), 651–688.

Lowinson, J. H., Marion, I. J., Joseph, H., & Dole, V. P. (1992). Methadone maintenance. In J. H. Lowinson, P. Ruiz, & R. B. Millman (Eds.), *Substance abuse: A comprehensive textbook* (2nd ed., pp. 550–561). Baltimore, MD: Williams & Wilkins.

Magura, S., Staines, G., Kosanke, N., Rosenblum, A., Foote, J., DeLuca, A., et al. (2003). Predictive validity of the ASAM Patient Placement Criteria for naturalistically matched vs. mismatched alcoholism patients. *Am J Addict, 12*, 386–397.

McKay, J. R., Cacciola, J. S., McLellan, A. T., Alterman, A. I., & Wirtz, P. W. (1997). An initial evaluaiton of the psychosocial dimensions of the American Society of Addiction Medicine criteria for inpatient versus outpatient substance abuse rehabilitation. *J Consult Clin Psychol, 58*, 239–252.

McLellan, A. T. (2006). What we need is a system: Creating a responsive and effective substance abuse treatment system. In W. R. Miller & K. M. Carroll (Eds.), *Rethinking substance abuse: What the science shows and what we should do about it* (pp. 275–292). New York: Guilford Press.

McLellan, A. T., Arndt, I. O., Metzger, D., Woody, G. E., & O'Brien, C. P. (1993). The effects of psychosocial services in substance abuse treatment. *JAMA, 269*, 1953–1959.

McLellan, A. T., Grissom, G. R., Zanis, D., & Randall, M. (1997). Problem-service "matching" in addiction treatment: A prospective study in four programs. *Arch Gen Psychiatry, 54*, 730–735.

McLellan, A. T., & McKay, J. R. (1998). The treatment of addiction: What can research offer practice? In S. Lamb, M. R. Greenlick, & D. McCarty (Eds.), *Bridging the gap between practice and research: Forging partnerships with community based drug and alcohol treatment* (pp. 147–185). Washington, DC: National Academy Press.

McMahon, F. J., & Insel, T. R. (2012). Pharmacogenomics and personalized medicine in neuropsychiatry. *Neuron, 74*(5), 773?776.

Miller, W. R. (2000). Rediscovering fire: Small interventions, large effects. *Psychol Addict Behav, 14*, 6–18.

Miller, W. R., Benefield, R. G., & Tonigan, J. S. (1993). Enhancing motivation for change in problem drinking: A controlled comparison of two therapist styles. *J Consult Clin Psychol, 61*, 455–461.

Miller, W. R., & Rollnick, S. (1991). *Motivational interviewing: Preparing people to change addictive behavior.* New York: Guilford Press.

Miller, W. R., & Rollnick, S. (2002). *Motivational interviewing: Preparing people for change* (2nd ed). New York: Guilford Press.

Miller, W. R., & Wilbourne, P. L. (2002). Mesa Grande: A methodological analysis of clinical trials of treatments for alcohol use disorders. *Addiction, 97,* 265–277.

Miller, W. R., Yahne, C. E., & Tonigan, J. S. (2003). Motivational interviewing in drug abuse services: A randomized trial. *J Consult Clin Psychol, 71*(4), 754–763.

MTP Research Group. (2004). Brief treatments for cannabis dependence: Findings from a randomized multisite trial. *J Consult Clin Psychol, 72,* 455–466.

Murphy, S. A., Collins, L. M., & Rush, A. J. (2007). Customizing treatment to the patient: Adaptive treatment strategies. *Drug Alcohol Depend, 88*(Suppl. 2), S1–S3.

National Institute on Drug Abuse. (2007). *Principles of drug addiction treatment: A research based guide.* Bethesda, MD: Author.

Nunes, E. V., & Levin, F. R. (2004). Treatment of depression in patients with alcohol or other drug dependence: A meta-analysis. *JAMA, 291*(15), 1887–1896.

O'Farrell, T. J., & Fals-Stewart, W. (2006). *Behavioral couples therapy for alcoholism and drug abuse.* New York: Guilford Press.

Oslin, D. W., Lynch, K. G., Pettinati, H. M., Kampman, K. M., Gariti, P., Gelfand, L., et al. (2008). A placebo controlled randomized clinical trial of naltrexone in the context of different levels of psychosocial intervention. *Alcohol Clin Exp Res, 32*(7), 1299–1308.

Peirce, J. M., Petry, N. M., Stitzer, M. L., Blaine, J. D., Kellog, S., Satterfield, F., et al. (2006). Effects of lower-cost incentives on stimulant abstinence in methadone maintenance treatment: A National Drug Abuse Treatment Clinical Trials Network study. *Arch Gen Psychiatry, 63,* 201–208.

Petry, N. M. (2000). A comprehensive guide to the application of contingency management procedures in clinical settings. *Drug Alcohol Depend, 58,* 9–25.

Petry, N. M., Alessi, S. M., Marx, J., Austin, M., & Tardif, M. (2005). Vouchers versus prizes: Contingency management treatment of substance abusers in community settings. *J Consult Clin Psychol, 73*(6), 1005–1014.

Petry, N. M., Kolodner, K. B., Li, R., Peirce, J. M., Roll, J. M., Stitzer, M. L., et al. (2006). Prize-based contingency management does not increase gambling. *Drug Alcohol Depend, 83*(3), 269–273.

Petry, N. M., Peirce, J. M., Stitzer, M. L., Blaine, J. D., Roll, J. M., Cohen, A., et al. (2006). Effect of prize-based incentives on outcomes in stimulant abusers in outpatient psychosocial treatment programs: A national drug abuse Clinical Trials Network study. *Archives of General Psychiatry, 62,* 1148–1156.

Petry, N. M., Tedford, J., Austin, M., Nich, C., Carroll, K. M., & Rounsaville, B. J. (2004). Prize reinforcement contingency management for treating cocaine users: How low can we go, and with whom? *Addiction, 99,* 349–360.

Prochaska, J. O., DiClemente, C. C., & Norcross, J. C. (1992). In search of how people change: Applications to addictive behaviors. *Am Psychol, 47,* 1102–1114.

Project MATCH Research Group. (1993). Project MATCH: Rationale and methods for a multisite clinical trial matching alcoholism patients to treatment. *Alcohol Clin Exp Res, 17,* 1130–1145.

Project MATCH Research Group. (1997). Matching alcohol treatments to client heterogeneity: Project MATCH posttreatment drinking outcomes. *J Stud Alcohol, 58,* 7–29.

Rash, C. J., Alessi, S. M., & Petry, N. M. (2008a). Cocaine abusers with and without alcohol dependence respond equally well to contingency management treatments. *Exp Clin Psychopharmacol, 16*(4), 275–281.

Rash, C. J., Alessi, S. M., & Petry, N. M. (2008b). Contingency management is efficacious for cocaine abusers with prior treatment attempts. *Exp Clin Psychopharmacol, 16*(6), 547–554.

Rawson, R. A., McCann, M. J., Flammino, F., Shoptaw, S., Miotto, K., Reiber, C., et al. (2006). A comparison of contingency management and cognitive-behavioral approaches for stimulant-dependent individuals. *Addiction, 101,* 267–274.

Ray, L. A., & Hutchison, K. E. (2007). Effects of naltrexone on alcohol sensitivity and genetic moderators of medication response: A double-blind placebo-controlled study. *Arch Gen Psychiatry, 64*(9), 1069–1077.

Regier, D. A., Farmer, M. E., Rae, D. S., Locke, B. Z., Keith, S. J., Judd, L. L., et al. (1990). Comorbidity of mental disorders with alcohol and other drug abuse: Results from the Epidemiologic Catchment Area (ECA) study. *JAMA, 264,* 2511–2518.

Robbins, M. S., Feaster, D. J., Horigian, V. E., Rohrbaugh, M., Shoham, V., Bachrach, K., et al. (2011). Brief strategic family therapy versus treatment as usual: Results of a multisite randomized trial for substance using adolescents. *J Consult Clin Psychol, 79*(6), 713–727.

Roth, A., & Fonagy, P. (2005). *What works for whom?: A critical review of the psychotherapy literature* (2nd ed.). New York: Guilford Press.

Rounsaville, B. J. (1995). Can psychotherapy rescue naltrexone treatment of opioid addiction? In L. S. Onken & J. D. Blaine (Eds.), *Potentiating the efficacy of medications: Integrating psychosocial therapies with pharmacotherapies in the treatment of drug dependence* (pp. 37–52). Rockville, MD: National Institute on Drug Abuse.

Rounsaville, B. J., & Carroll, K. M. (1997). Individual psychotherapy for drug abusers. In J. H. Lowinsohn, P. Ruiz, & R. B. Miller (Eds.), *Comprehensive textbook of substance abuse* (3rd ed., pp. 430–439). New York: Williams & Wilkins.

Rubak, S., Sandbaek, A., Lauritzen, T., & Christensen, B. (2005). Motivational interviewing: A systematic review and meta-analysis. *Br J Gen Pract, 55*(513), 305–312.

Saitz, R., Palfai, T. P., Freedner, N., Winter, M. R., MacDonald, A., Lu, J., et al. (2007). Screening and brief intervention online for college students: The iHealth study. *Alcohol Alcohol, 42,* 28–36.

Santisteban, D. A., Coatsworth, J. D., Perez-Vidal, A., Kurtines, W. M., Schwartz, S. J., LaPerriere, A., et al. (2003). Efficacy of brief strategic family therapy in modifying Hispanic adolescent behavior problems and substance use. *J Fam Psychol, 17*(1), 121–133.

Sees, K. L., Delucchi, K. L., Masson, C., Rosen, A., Clark, H. W., Robillard, H., et al. (2000). Methadone maintenance vs 180-day psychosocially enriched detoxification for treatment of opioid dependence: A randomized controlled trial. *JAMA, 283*(10), 1303–1310.

Sholomskas, D. E., Syracuse-Siewert, G., Rounsaville, B. J., Ball, S. A., Nuro, K. F., & Carroll, K. M. (2005). We don't train in vain: A dissemination trial of three strategies of training clinicians in cognitive-behavioral therapy. *J Consult Clin Psychol, 73*(1), 106–115.

Silverman, K. (1999). Voucher-based reinforcement of cocaine abstinence in treatment-resistant methadone patients: Effects of reinforcer magnitude. *Psychopharmacol (Berl), 146*(2), 128–138.

Silverman, K., Chutuape, M. A., Bigelow, G. E., & Stitzer, M. L. (1996). Voucher-based reinforcement of attendance by unemployed methadone patients in a job skills training program. *Drug Alcohol Depend, 41*(3), 197–207.

Silverman, K., Higgins, S. T., Brooner, R. K., Montoya, I. D., Cone, E. J., Schuster, C. R., et al. (1996). Sustained cocaine abstinence in methadone maintenance patients through voucher-based reinforcement therapy. *Arch Gen Psychiatry, 53,* 409–415.

Silverman, K., Svikis, D., Robles, E., Stitzer, M. L., & Bigelow, G. E. (2001). A reinforcement-based therapeutic workplace for the treatment of drug abuse: Six-month abstinence outcomes. *Exp Clin Psychopharmacol, 9*(1), 14–23.

Silverman, K., Svikis, D. S., Wong, C. J., Hampton, J., Stitzer, M. L., & Bigelow, G. E. (2002). A reinforcement-based therapeutic workplace for the treatment of drug abuse: Three year abstinence outcomes. *Exp Clin Psychopharmacol, 10,* 228–240.

Silverman, K., Wong, C. J., Umbricht-Schneiter, A., Montoya, I. D., Schuster, C. R., & Preston, K. L. (1998). Broad beneficial effects of cocaine abstinence reinforcement among methadone patients. *J Consult Clin Psychol, 66,* 811–824.

Skolnick, P., & Volkow, N. D. (2012). Addiction therapeutics: Obstacles and opportunities. *Biol Psychiatry, 72,* 890–891.

Stanton, M. D., & Shadish, W. R. (1997). Outcome, attrition, and family-couples treatment for drug abuse: A meta-analysis and review of the controlled, comparative studies. *Psychol Bull, 122*(2), 170–191.

Stitzer, M. L., Iguchi, M. Y., Kidorf, M., & Bigelow, G. E. (1993). Contingency management in methadone treatment: The case for positive incentives. In L. S. Onken, J. D. Blaine, & J. J. Boren (Eds.), *Behavioral treatments for drug abuse and dependence* (pp. 19–36). Rockville, MD: National Institute on Drug Abuse.

Swanson, A. J., Pantalon, M. V., & Cohen, K. R. (1999). Motivational interviewing and treatment adherence among psychiatric and dually diagnosed patients. *J Nerv Ment Dis, 187,* 630–635.

Szapocznik, J., & Williams, R. A. (2000). Brief strategic family therapy: Twenty-five years of interplay among theory, research and practice in adolescent behavior problems and drug abuse. *Clin Child Fam Psychol Rev, 3*(2), 117–134.

Tolin, D. F. (2010). Is cognitive-behavioral therapy more effective than other therapies?: A meta-analytic review. *Clin Psychol Rev, 30*(6), 710–720.

Tuten, M., Defulio, A., Jones, H. E., & Stitzer, M. (2012). Abstinence-contingent recovery housing and reinforcement-based treatment following opioid detoxification. *Addiction, 107*(5), 973–982.

UKATT Research Team. (2008). UK Alcohol Treatment Trial: Client-treatment matching effects. *Addiction, 103*(2), 228–238.

Weiss, R. D. (2004). Adherence to pharmacotherapy in patients with alcohol and opioid dependence. *Addiction, 99*(11), 1382–1392.

Wilk, A. I., Jensen, N. M., & Havighurst, T. C. (1997). Meta-analysis of randomized controlled trials addressing brief interventions in heavy alcohol drinkers. *J Gen Intern Med, 12,* 274–283.

Woody, G. E., Luborsky, L., McLellan, A. T., O'Brien, C. P., Beck, A. T., Blaine, J. D., et al. (1983). Psychotherapy for opiate addicts: Does it help? *Arch Gen Psychiatry, 40,* 639–645.

CHAPTER 26

Individual Psychodynamic Psychotherapy

LANCE M. DODES
EDWARD J. KHANTZIAN

Individual psychotherapy is widely used in treatment of addicted individuals, though it is perhaps still less common than group modalities in inpatient and clinic programs. While many addicted patients benefit from a combination of individual and group treatments (Khantzian, 1986), a significant number can be treated successfully *only* with individual psychotherapy, This chapter rearticulates and extends ideas that we and others have developed, based on our understanding and treatment experience with addicted individuals over many years (Khantzian, Dodes, & Brehm, 2003; Dodes, 1984, 1988, 1990, 1996, 2002, 2003, 2009, 2011; Dodes & Khantzian, 1991; Flores, 2003; Kaufman, 1994; Khantzian, 1980, 1986, 1995, 1999a, 1999b, 2001, 2003, 2012; Walant, 1995; Weegmann & Khantzian, 2011).

The rationale for individual psychotherapy with addicts arises from an understanding that with the exception of simple states of physical addiction, addictive behaviors are powerfully rooted in psychological factors that lead them both to arise and to return. The fact that nondrug addictions (compulsive gambling, Internet use, etc.) regularly substitute for drug addictions, and vice versa, and that other compulsive behaviors, such as housecleaning, may also substitute for addictions of all sorts, is evidence that addictions, as one of us (L. M. D.) has proposed, are a subset of psychologically based compulsions generally.

Contemporary psychodynamic formulations have stressed the role of conflict, the object meaning of alcohol or drugs, deficits and dysfunctions in ego functioning, narcissistic deficits, and the function of addictive behavior to reverse overwhelming feelings of helplessness. These factors contribute to self-regulation disturbances involving affects, self-esteem maintenance, and the capacity for self-care and self–other relations. These psychological factors contribute significantly to addictions and are targeted in psychotherapy (Khantzian, 1986, 1995, 1999a, 2001; Dodes, 2002,

2011). Patients come to psychotherapy via referral from other professionals, as well as self-referral (perhaps especially with patients who are more psychologically oriented). Others start individual psychotherapy after first attempting treatment through self-help groups or a more educationally based treatment program, such as that offered in many inpatient settings and outpatient clinics. Regardless of how they come to therapy, once having begun to explore their emotional issues, patients begin to understand the way their substance abuse arises from key aspects of their emotional lives. This understanding addresses not only the reasons for their continued problems even when drug-free but also, by placing the substance problem in the context of their emotional lives, it provides a strong internal basis for avoiding relapse.

Some patients seek individual psychotherapy following repeated treatment failure in less introspective settings. Typically, these patients have repeatedly relapsed despite clear and conscious motivation to abstain, because they are unaware of the internal emotional factors that led them to resume substance use. Failing to recognize these factors contributes to patients' attributing their behavior to lack of willpower, adding to their self-devaluation. Learning about themselves in individual psychotherapy thereby contributes not only to a more stable drug-free state and to overall general improvement in emotional function but also to less shame about their addiction.

Many addicted individuals also successfully pursue individual psychotherapy in conjunction with other treatment (e.g., professionally led group therapy or a self-help group). In such cases, the individual work aims for the usual goals of insight and emotional growth, while the other modalities focus on supporting the patient's drug-free state.

The experience of many psychotherapists, including ourselves, has conclusively shown that psychodynamic psychotherapy is effective with substance use disorders (SUDs). Shedler (2010) has reviewed the efficacy of psychodynamic psychotherapy as an effective model for understanding and treating a wide range of psychiatric disorders, and a number of empirical studies substantiate the value of the psychodynamic paradigm with addicted individuals. Woody et al. (1983) noted that in seven studies with methadone-treated patients, in which patients were randomly assigned to psychotherapy or a different treatment (most often drug counseling), five of the studies showed better outcome in the psychotherapy group. Woody's own group also found that patients who received psychotherapy and drug counseling had better results than did patients who received drug counseling alone, when measured in terms of number of areas of improvement, less use of illicit opiates, and lower doses of methadone required. This group (Woody, McLellan, Luborsky, & O'Brien, 1986) also found that the patients with the most disturbed global psychiatric ratings benefited particularly from psychotherapy, as compared with drug counseling. A number of investigators have documented a high correlation between psychiatric disorders, especially depression, and addiction (Rounsaville, Weissman, Kleber, & Wilber, 1982; Khantzian & Treece, 1985; Carroll & Rounsaville, 1992; Halikas, Crosby, Pearson, Nugent, & Carlson, 1994; Kessler et al., 1997; Kleinman, Miller, & Millman, 1990; Penick et al., 1994; Regier et al., 1990; Rounsaville et al., 1991; Wilens, Biederman, Spencer, & Frances, 1994; Schuckit & Hesselbrock, 1994; Schuckit, Irwin, & Brown, 1990).

Brown (1985) found that 45% of a group of abstinent alcoholics in Alcoholics Anonymous (AA) sought psychotherapy, and more than 90% of them found it helpful.

Rounsaville, Gawin, and Kleber (1985) also reported positive results in a preliminary treatment of outpatient cocaine abusers with a modified interpersonal psychotherapy, along with medication trials. Woody et al. (1986) reported that when psychotherapists were integrated in the treatment team, the stress of the entire staff was reduced as a result of successful management of the most psychiatrically troubled patients. More recently, Woody, McLellan, Luborsky, and O'Brien (1995) validated the benefit of psychotherapy in community programs. In contrast, Carroll et al. (1994), as well as Kang et al. (1991), reported less benefit from psychotherapy in ambulatory cocaine abusers. In the latter studies, the authors underscored the importance of the severity of illness, stages of recovery, and level of care. When psychotherapy was added to paraprofessional drug counseling in an inpatient setting (Rogalski, 1984), patients improved in compliance with treatment as measured in decreased number of discharges against medical advice, disciplinary discharges, or unauthorized absences.

In addition to these studies that statistically examined effects of psychotherapy, a significant psychodynamic literature has reported on the treatability of addicted patients with psychodynamic or psychoanalytically oriented psychotherapy (Brown, 1985; Dodes, 1984, 1988, 1990, 1996, 2002, 2003, 2011; Johnson, 1992; Kaufman, 1994; Khantzian, 1986, 1999a, 1997, 2001, 2012; Krystal, 1982; Krystal & Raskin, 1970; Flores, 2003; Silber, 1974; Treece & Khantzian, 1986; Wurmser, 1974; Woody, Luborsky, McLellan, & O'Brien, 1989; Walant, 1995; Weegmann & Khantzian, 2011). The experience of treating addicted individuals in psychodynamic therapy has also provided our best information about the psychology of addiction, which in turn serves as the theoretical basis for technical approaches to therapy with these patients. Indications for psychodynamic psychotherapy depend on both the patient's capacity to benefit and his or her motivation. People with addictions who are able to achieve and maintain sobriety with substance abuse counseling and/or self-help groups, and are inattentive to their emotional lives (or who defensively avoid knowing about it), are less likely to seek psychotherapy. Patients who have at least some capacity to be moderately introspective and develop a therapeutic alliance, and who are aware of emotional suffering, are candidates for psychotherapy as much as are nonaddicted patients with similar characteristics. These patients use psychotherapy to help them to achieve and maintain abstinence and improve their overall emotional health as they achieve abstinence.

PSYCHODYNAMIC BASIS FOR PSYCHOTHERAPY OF ADDICTED PATIENTS

There have been a number of major contributions to understanding the psychology of addiction over the past 40 years (Khantzian et al., 2005). One of the earliest of these formulations described substance use as an effort to manage intolerable or overwhelming affect. The idea that certain substances are preferentially chosen on the basis of their specific ability to address (ameliorate, express) certain affective states is termed the "self-medication hypothesis" (Khantzian, 1985a, 1997). A number of authors have described connections between certain affects and the use of particular drugs, for example, use of narcotics to manage rage or loneliness, and use of cocaine and other stimulants to manage depression and emptiness or to provide a sense of grandeur (Khantzian, 1985a; Wurmser, 1974; Milkman & Frosch, 1973). Earlier, Krystal and Raskin (1970) spoke of a "defective stimulus barrier" in addicts that causes them to be susceptible to flooding with intolerable affective states that are traumatic. They described a normal process of affective development in which affects are differentiated, desomatized, and verbalized, and they pointed to defects in this development in some addicted individuals. In these cases, such defects can lead to an inability to use affects as signals—a critical capacity for managing affects.

Others have noted the quality of addicts' relatedness to their drugs as being akin to human object relationships. A substance may become a substitute for a longed-for or needed figure—one that has omnipotent properties or is completely controllable and available (Krystal & Raskin, 1970; Wieder & Kaplan, 1969; Wurmser, 1974).

Other investigators have focused on narcissistic pathology in addicted individuals. Wurmser (1974) described a "narcissistic crisis" in which collapse of a grandiose self or of an idealized object provides the impetus for substance use in an effort to resolve feelings of narcissistic shame and rage. Kohut (1971) referred to the narcissistic function of drugs in addiction as a replacement for defective psychological structure, particularly that arising from an inadequate idealized self-object.

From another perspective, Khantzian (1978, 1995, 1999a) and Khantzian and Mack (1983) described defective self-care functions in addicts—the group of ego functions involved with anticipation of danger, appropriate modulated response to protect oneself, and sufficient positive self-esteem to care about oneself. Such defective self-care functions may be a factor in substance abusers who place themselves and their health in danger, beyond the risks of their addiction itself. In turn, this problem may have originated in patients' early experiences of overprotective or inadequate attention to their safety by parents, resulting in failure to internalize robust self-care functions.

Some investigators have focused on a subpopulation of addicts who also suffer with "alexithymia" (an inability to name or describe emotions in words; Krystal, 1982). Krystal felt that substance use in this group of patients could be seen as a search for an external agent to soothe them, in response to their lack of ability to soothe themselves. McDougall (1984) similarly described patients whose use of words and ideas is without affective meaning, and who use substances to disperse emotional arousal, avoiding affective flooding. Although the final appearance of this affective intolerance has the quality of an incapacity or deficit, its underlying basis is understood by McDougall to be a defensive avoidance of intolerable feelings.

Khantzian (1999b) wrote about the preverbal origins of distress found in some substance abusers. Very early experience that remains out of conscious awareness may create a nameless pain that recurs in response to a current stimulus, leading to an addictive relapse. He offered an example in which a patient's early experience of abandonment, which became clear in the course of a psychodynamic group therapy, instead of being managed through substance abuse, could be interpreted, understood, and borne. Walant (1995) similarly stressed infantile origins of problems with interpersonal contact and interdependence that could predispose an individual to an addictive adaptation. Flores (2003) has likewise described addictions as an attachment disorder for some patients.

Dodes (1990, 1996, 2002, 2011) has suggested that many of these observations may be understood to be instances of a more general formulation of addiction as a compulsive behavior in which addictive acts serve to reverse states of overwhelming helplessness. In this view, the key moment in addiction occurs well before ingesting a drug or placing a bet. It is when a person decides to perform an addictive act—a moment that can occur hours to days before the event. At this moment, people with addictions are making a decision that they believe will make them feel better and, most importantly, a decision over which they have complete control. These decisions are emotionally compelled, because they reverse a sense of overwhelming helplessness. For any single individual, the factors that make a situation overwhelming are unique and determined by that person's individual psychology. This fact is a major reason that treatment of people with addictions must not be of the "one-size-fits-all" variety. Knowing the individual nature of the emotional factors precipitating experiences of overwhelming helplessness—hence, the addictive urges—is essential to treating both the addiction and the patient in general, because whatever psychological vulnerabilities produce the overwhelming helplessness that precipitates addictive acts are also those close to the heart of a patient's greatest emotional difficulty.

When people feel overwhelmingly helpless, it is a narcissistic injury. Serious challenges to narcissism always produce an enraged response—an essentially normal survival mechanism. Dodes notes that this narcissistic rage is precisely what arises when the urge to perform an addictive act occurs (Dodes 1990, 1996, 2002, 2011), and that the central presence of this rage in addiction helps to explain the distinctive quality of addictive acts: their intense, driven, apparently irrational nature that seems to override a person's ordinary concerns for his or her own welfare or that of others.

A final element of this formulation offers an explanation of the particular forms taken by addiction. In addiction, the reassertion of power against helplessness and the narcissistic rage that drives it are not expressed in a direct, appropriate action. They are expressed in *displacement*. The substitute or displaced action is what we call the addiction. For instance, Dodes (1996) described a man who had an alcoholic binge after he was unable to fire his son from his company, despite the fact the son had embezzled a large amount of money. This man believed it was morally wrong to fire his son, even though he felt a strong impetus to do so and, as a consequence, he rendered himself helpless. This was intolerable, but since he could not allow himself to act directly (fire his son), he displaced his need to be empowered to his drinking, which therefore acquired a compulsive character. His addictive behavior, then, reflected a psychological compromise: He had to do something but forbade himself from acting directly. He compromised (unconsciously) by acting, but in a substitute (displaced) way—drinking compulsively.

The fact that addictions are inherently psychological compromises is important, because it makes the psychology of addictions identical to the psychology of other compulsive behaviors, which are also displaced enactments of forbidden behaviors. The critical implication of this finding is that addictions should be seen as being treatable in traditional psychodynamic psychotherapy as much as are compulsions, which have traditionally been understood to be amenable to a psychodynamic or psychoanalytic approach (Dodes, 1996, 2003). Director (2005) has drawn on Dodes's emphasis on states of helplessness in maintaining addictive behavior. She describes a patient for whom the feelings of helplessness and rage are converted into defensive attitudes of omnipotence and invincibility.

TECHNICAL ASPECTS OF PSYCHOTHERAPY WITH ADDICTS

There are a number of special considerations in the psychodynamic psychotherapy of addicted individuals (Dodes & Khantzian, 1991). Based on the formulations discussed previously, it is clear that various meanings and roles of drugs (or nondrug addictive behaviors) need to be considered in understanding patients with addictions. From a practical standpoint, however, when addicts are still abusing substances at the time they are first seen, it is necessary to assess the immediate threat to their emotional and physical health, their relationships, and their overall capacity to function. Especially when this threat is severe, it is necessary to address the question of abstinence from substance use when beginning treatment.

The first step here is diagnosing addiction and informing the patient of the diagnosis, since he or she may fail to perceive the extent of the problem or may present with overt denial or minimization. The manner in which this is accomplished is an important beginning in the establishment of a positive therapeutic relationship, a basic element for all subsequent phases of treatment. In this respect, given the common feelings of shame, confusion, and being overwhelmed, especially when first encountered, one of us (E. J. K.) recently detailed essential elements of psychotherapeutic work with addicted patients, such as kindness, empathy, patience, support, and instruction, which ensure the development of a positive therapeutic relationship (Khantzian, 2012).

To make the diagnosis and clearly have a basis for showing it to the patient, it is necessary to take a detailed history of the problems that have been caused by the patient's use of drugs. It is useful to inquire systematically about trouble in the areas of work, medical health, relationships with friends, relationships with family (adults and children), legal problems, and intrapsychic problems (depression, shame, anxiety). It may be helpful to ask what the patient is like when he or she drinks or uses another drug and the details of what happens at these times, as well as the effects the patient seeks from substance use. This involves exploring both the "positive" and negative effects he or she experiences from the use of drugs. In the first instance, it is often reassuring and alliance building to ask, "What does the drug do for you?" Inquiring in this way makes the patient more apt to feel understood and not judged. Both the patient and therapist are provided an opportunity to appreciate how drugs became important. On the maladaptive side, does he or she become more belligerent, moody, withdrawn, or sad? Might the patient have had more or better relationships with friends if he or she had never had a drug? Patients sometimes deny trouble in their marriages, but when the matter is explored in detail, they acknowledge that their spouses would prefer that they drink, smoke, or take pills less often or have asked them on more than one occasion to stop. Upon reflection, they may recognize that their use of drugs has silently become a source of chronic tension in their relationships. Once the patient clarifies or even lists the areas of difficulties that are due to his or her addictive behavior, it is often possible to acknowledge the global impact of this on his or her life.

Focusing on the diagnosis is more than a merely cognitive process. The realization that he or she is out of control in this area of life is a significant psychological step in itself. Mack (1981) felt that an alcoholic's recognition of failure to be in control of his or her drinking is a first step in the assumption of responsibility. Brown (1985), in her work with alcoholic patients, stressed loss of control as a core issue and focus of psychotherapy. This acknowledgment is a blow to the narcissistic potency of the patient; as such, it may be useful to investigate it, because it has a bearing on the patient's important feelings and issues concerning powerlessness and mastery (Dodes, 1988).

Through all this early diagnostic and at times even confrontational work, as in therapy in general, the therapist's attitude must be exploratory without being judgmental. The patient's denial or minimization is often closely connected with his or her shame, and it is good to keep in mind that throughout this initial evaluation, the patient is simultaneously evaluating the therapist, especially the therapist's attitude toward the patient, and his or her addictive problem. The patient is faced with his or her own projections onto the therapist, and it is important that a therapist not accede to the role of a harsh or punitive conscience that might be invisibly attributed to the therapist.

Common countertransference difficulties with substance abusers revolve around frustration, anger and guilt, because patients' failures to abstain challenge the therapeutic potency of the treatment professional. These countertransference feelings may result in a therapist's withdrawal, inappropriately critical attitudes, or overinvolvement (when therapists defensively act to reverse their desire to withdraw).

The severe nature of the risks facing addicts makes work with them both challenging and rewarding. It is important for therapists to be able to view both the overt behavior and the inner psychopathology of their addicted patients with the same combination of objectivity and compassion that is brought to any patient.

However, developing a therapeutic alliance early in therapy may be difficult because of patients' ambivalence about abstention from substance use. It may be ineffective and even counterproductive for a therapist to be seen as requiring (vs. suggesting) complete abstinence. The psychological issues in abstention are in fact complex (Dodes, 1984; Khantzian, 1980). Patients' achievement of abstinence hinges on both the place of substance use in their psychological equilibrium and the alliance with, and transference to, the therapist. Many patients quickly achieve abstinence upon beginning psychotherapy, in spite of the evident importance to them of their substances. Others may continue to use drugs but not in a way that is malignantly out of control or that creates an emergency. In a number of these cases, we have helped patients establish abstinence over time, psychotherapeutically. When a therapist focuses on the patient's failure to perceive the danger to him- or herself that is contained in continued abuse, the therapist's caring concern may be internalized by the patient, providing a nucleus for the internalization of a healthy "self-care" function (Dodes, 1984). However, patients' ability to perceive their therapists in a benign way that may be internalized depends on absence or resolution of negative transference feelings at the beginning of treatment.

For some patients, early achievement of abstinence is possible because of a genuine therapeutic alliance with a therapist. In other cases, abstinence may be achieved early in treatment because of unconscious wishes to merge with, or be held by, a therapist who is idealized, or because of a compliant identification with the aggressor (Dodes, 1984). When patients do not initially abstain, subsequent confrontation may produce abstention, because patients perceive this confrontation as a longed-for message of caring that was absent or insufficient in their childhoods. (Khantzian and Mack [1983] described this kind of parental insufficiency in their discussion of the origin of self-care deficits.) From a practical standpoint, the clinical choices involved must depend on the immediate risks to the patient. If patients use substances only intermittently and are able to participate genuinely in the process of psychotherapy, we have found that the psychotherapy can continue. Indeed, psychotherapy provides an opportunity to explore the issues causing continued substance use, including the underlying issues that led to addiction in the first place, problems with self-care, and the transference implications of a failure to abstain. However, when drinking becomes continually destructive, patients are generally unable to participate in the process, and require early confrontation around the need to be hospitalized or in rare cases even to interrupt therapy. Over the course of an ongoing psychotherapy, the capacity for abstinence may vary, depending in part on shifts in the therapeutic relationship (Dodes, 1984).

We have described an approach that follows from a close understanding of the individual patient. Some authors writing about alcoholism, however, have recommended a kind of preordained staging of therapy (Prochaska & DiClemente, 1985). Based on a cognitive-behavioral paradigm, these authors introduced a "stages of change" model in which patients are encouraged to shift from "a precontemplative" stage (denial) to a "contemplative" (acknowledgement) stage, to initiate a process of engaging in treatment and preventing relapse. Not inconsistent with a psychodynamic approach, the first phase is directed toward helping patients develop an identity as an alcoholic (Brown, 1985), with a focus on drinking, on ways to stay sober, and on mourning the losses incurred as a result of drinking (Bean-Bayog, 1985). Kaufman (1994) similarly stressed the importance of abstinence, stabilization, and relapse prevention by addressing issues of intimacy and autonomy. In our experience, however, it is generally unnecessary and potentially counterproductive to attempt to direct the therapeutic process according to a preconceived agenda. As is the case with any patient, imposing one's own focus risks interfering with learning patients' deeper, more personal issues, which can be seen when patients are allowed to speak freely and move naturally from thought to thought. In our opinion, although some people with addictions (like some patients in general) require a more supportive rather than an exploratory approach, this decision should be based on an individual assessment of the patient's psychology rather than a generalization about steps suitable for all substance abusers.

The idea of imposing structure in psychotherapy with addicts arose in part from concerns about the ability of such patients to tolerate the process of psychotherapy.

At the heart of this thought is the worry that exploring the important issues in their lives will lead addicts to resume their substance abuse. Actually, the reverse is often the case—patients who do not deal with the emotional problems that trouble them are at greater risk of continued substance use or relapse.

Nonetheless, there may be difficulties with pursuing psychotherapy. At times, therapists fail to attend appropriately to the life-threatening nature of continued substance abuse (Bean-Bayog, 1985) or fail to make the diagnosis (Brown, 1985), overlooking the ongoing deterioration of their patients' lives. Some patients may try to use psychotherapy to deny the importance of addressing their addictive behavior. However, these concerns largely hinge on failures by the therapist and may be avoided (Dodes, 1988, 1991). For instance, attention must be paid initially to the question of abstinence (whether or not it can be achieved). If a patient misuses treatment to rationalize continued substance use, an appropriately responsive therapist would recognize this misuse and bring it into the treatment process for therapist and patient to identify and think through together. People with addictions have a wide variety of characterological structures, strengths, and weaknesses, and in general are as capable of dealing with the issues and strong transference feelings that may arise in psychotherapy as patients with other presenting problems. Part of the advantage of psychotherapy with addicts is that it offers an ongoing opportunity for patients to take firmer control over their addiction, based on understanding and tolerating the feelings and issues that contribute to it. A therapist's continual attentiveness to improving understanding of the patient's drug use protects against the problem of distracting a patient from his or her addiction.

Of course, any therapist can be fooled—patients who deny, minimize, or distort the facts about their substance use may render its diagnosis and treatment impossible for any therapist. This is a limitation to every treatment, including psychotherapy.

For some patients it is particularly important to attend to the object-substitute meanings of substances. In others, narcissistic vulnerabilities are of paramount importance, for instance, the collapse of idealized objects, as described by Wurmser (1974), or the role of particular affective states in precipitating substance use, mentioned by a number of authors. With some patients, self-care deficits, as described by Khantzian and Mack (1983), are of great significance. Tthe active nature of addictive behavior in seizing control against an intolerable feeling of helplessness, as described by Dodes (1990), is usually an important focus. With patients whose affect management and self-care are seriously impaired (Khantzian, 1986, 1995), it is necessary for the therapist to be especially active. Excessive passivity with such patients can be dangerous. It is necessary in these cases to draw the patients' attention empathically to ways in which they render themselves vulnerable as a result of their self-care deficits, and to underscore how these self-care deficits render them susceptible to addictive behavior and all the associated risks. Khantzian (2012) emphatically suggests that the therapist should be ready to use the alarm patients evoke in them (by dangerous behaviors) to help such patients appreciate how their emotions are absent or inoperative in guiding their behaviors. Likewise with these patients, it is necessary to explore the details of current life situations to help them recognize their feelings and use them as "guides to appropriate reactions and self-protective behavior rather than signals for impulsive action" (Khantzian, 1986, p. 217). Patients with a serious lack of self-care capacity may require that a therapist serve as a "primary care" physician—especially at the start of treatment, when the therapist must often play multiple roles to ensure that patients receive appropriate care from a number of sources (Khantzian, 1985b, 1988). This task may include decisions about (and active involvement in arranging) hospitalization and detoxification, professionally led group treatments, pharmacological treatment, and other supportive measures. Such an active approach, although possibly lifesaving, may interfere with the later development of a traditional psychotherapeutic relationship because of the transference and countertransference issues it induces, particularly with regard to the patient's realistic gratitude. If this gratitude becomes a prominent interfering factor (e.g., a patient might never feel justified about any negative reactions to the therapist), referral to another therapist for continued psychotherapy may be required (Khantzian, 1985b).

Just as with the initial attention to abstinence, therapy must focus on relapses when they occur. Relapses (or patients' awareness that they feel a greater urge to repeat their addictive behaviors) provide an opportunity to learn about the factors leading to these behaviors. Frequently patients are unaware of these factors. Their lack of awareness contributes to their feelings of frustration and helplessness, and leaves them unprepared for further relapses. A careful, even microscopic, investigation of the feelings, relationships, and events that preceded a relapse is often revealing. As we described earlier, knowledge of the precipitating emotional factors to a relapse contributes to understanding both the addiction and the patient's psychology in general, since they center on areas felt to be intolerable by the patient.

Patients commonly bring up their increased thinking about drugs when there is an impending relapse, but at other times, the therapist may infer an increased risk based on what he or she knows of the patient's history and emotional life. Conveying this perception to patients is one way to help them learn to attend to their affects, thoughts, and behaviors, and utilize them as signals. Often, abstinent addicts have dreams about drugs that indicate something current in their lives is reviving the association with substance use, warning of the risk of relapse.

A concern sometimes expressed about treating addicts in psychotherapy is that they may be too cognitively impaired as a result of drug abuse ("wet brain") until there has been a lengthy period of abstinence. Certainly, some patients exhibit impaired memory and capacity for skilled cognitive functions immediately after stopping drug use. However, in our experience, this limitation is frequently mild or not significant for all but the most severely affected addicts (e.g., alcoholics with hepatic failure and elevated blood ammonia levels). Indeed, it is regularly observed in inpatient treatment centers that patients can do significant work to understand themselves and the dynamic issues in their families, as well as return to complex tasks within a week or so following detoxification. It is therefore rarely necessary to wait an extended time to begin psychotherapy because of organic brain factors. Patients who are truly impaired because their drug use is so continuous that they are always either high/drunk or withdrawing should not be in psychotherapy to begin with, since they require hospitalization to break this pattern before they will be able to attend to the work of the treatment.

PSYCHOTHERAPY AND SELF-HELP GROUPS

Patients in a combined treatment of psychotherapy and a 12-step group engage differently with each element. They often split their transference projections, expectations, and attachments (Dodes, 1988). Attachment to AA may provide needed internalization of self-care and self-valuing, with AA serving as a valuing, idealized object (or transitional object). Here, important elements of a narcissistic (idealizing and mirroring) transference are assigned to AA. The degree to which the transference is split in this way varies in different patients. It is critical for therapists to be aware of this split, because a patient's sobriety may hinge on an idealization of AA or its "Higher Power" concept, and this sobriety may be lost if the idealization is prematurely challenged (Dodes, 1988). Consequently, therapists may first have to help patients to increase their tolerance of affects and "await internalization of sufficient narcissistic potency" (Dodes, 1988, p. 289) before too closely examining the emotional functions assigned by patients to AA or Narcotics Anonymous (NA).

In our opinion, the need for a nondynamic, supportive approach through AA may lessen eventually either as a consequence of a patient's growth, including internalization of a sense of adequate narcissistic strength, or as a consequence of greater insight into the psychology of his or her addictive behavior. However, this does not always occur, leading to the need to attend AA meetings indefinitely (Dodes, 1984). Sometimes, patients remain involved in AA because of social and interpersonal factors, or because of their interest in helping others, even though they may not require AA for sobriety. Rosen (1981) noted the striking fact that AA, unlike psychodynamic psychotherapy, provides no mechanism for termination. He saw a critical aspect of the role of psychotherapy as helping to work out separation and termination from AA. Such termination, we have found, is best initiated by patients rather than therapists, and is important only when allegiance to AA ideas is interfering with self-awareness or AA precepts are actively causing harm (e.g., producing shame because patients' are told they must view themselves as back to zero [in days of sobriety] if they have a slip).

While there is a risk of disrupting the idealizing transference to AA (and consequently losing the sobriety that is dependent on this transference), a careful therapist will avoid this pitfall. Overall, the combination of psychodynamic psychotherapy and AA or NA is useful for many patients who are already engaged with a 12-step group (Dodes, 1988; Khantzian, 1985b, 1988). However, it should be kept in mind that AA has an overall 5-10% success rate, so referring patients to 12-step treatments when they are not already usefully engaged with them will not be helpful 90% of the time (Dodes & Dodes, 2014). Consequently, patients who are referred but do not like or do well in 12-step programs should be reassured that this is not their fault, and they should not be encouraged to "work the program harder." If additional support beyond psychotherapy is felt to benecessary, many non-12-step programs are available.

The disease concept is closely linked with self-help groups and has traditionally been difficult to reconcile with psychoanalytically oriented psychotherapy. Mack (1981) noted that this concept led to "oversimplified physiological models and a territorial smugness . . . which . . . precludes a sophisticated psychodynamic understanding of the problems of the individual alcoholic" (p. 129). The term "disease" itself has not been well or clearly defined (Shaffer, 1985). However, some patients (and treaters) are deeply attached to the "disease" idea regardless of its lack of scientific meaning. This is another area therapists may need to approach carefully. If it is necessary for treatment of a particular patient, the disease concept can be integrated with a psychodynamic approach (Dodes, 1988). A "disease" (e.g., of alcoholism) could be defined to a patient as having two parts: the patient's history of alcoholism, and the patient's being at permanent risk of repeating this behavior in the future. This definition does not impede psychological exploration of the meanings of the patient's drinking. The concept of permanent risk that is so central to the disease idea is troublesome for dynamic exploration only if it has the quality of something that is inexplicable in dynamic terms. Indeed, a central problem with the disease idea is precisely that it encourages a "black box" mentality, implying that beyond the word "disease" there is nothing to understand. However, the existence of a permanent risk to return to addictive behavior is actually the same as the regressive potential in any patient. Addicts, like all other individuals, never totally eliminate the potential of regression (resuming old pathological defenses and behaviors). Acknowledging their risk of resuming substance abuse is therefore just an example of this general rule and is not antithetical to psychological understanding.

CONCLUSION

In this chapter, we have described individual psychodynamic psychotherapy with addicted individuals, based on a contemporary psychological understanding of their vulnerabilities and disturbances. We have emphasized the defensive function, narcissistic vulnerabilities, and possible self-regulatory problems that contribute to addictive behavior. A major psychotherapeutic task for addicted patients is to bring into their awareness their emotional difficulties and the way their problems predispose them to relapse into substance abuse. We have reviewed implications for technique with regard to characteristic central issues for patients with addictions and the need in certain cases for active intervention. We have explored issues in establishing abstinence. Finally, we have emphasized a flexible approach with regard to the timing, sequencing, and integration of psychotherapy in relation to other interventions and needs based on patient characteristics and clinical considerations.

REFERENCES

Bean-Bayog, M. (1985). Alcoholism treatment as an alternative to psychiatric hospitalization. *Psychiatr Clin North Am, 8*, 501–512.

Brown, S. (1985). *Treating the alcoholic: A developmental model of recovery.* New York: Wiley.

Carroll, K. M., & Rounsaville, B. J. (1992). Contrast of treatment seeking and untreated cocaine abusers. *Arch Gen Psychiatry, 49*, 464–471.

Carroll, K. M., Rounsaville, B. J., Gordon, L. T., Nich, C., Jatlow, P., Bisighini, R. M., et al. (1994). Psychotherapy and pharmacotherapy for ambulatory cocaine abusers. *Arch Gen Psychiatry, 51*, 177–187.

Director, L. (2005). Encounters with omnipotence in the psychoanalysis of substance users. *Psychoanal Dialogues, 15*, 567–586.

Dodes, L. M. (1984). Abstinence from alcohol in long-term individual psychotherapy with alcoholics. *Am J Psychother, 38,* 248–256.

Dodes, L. M. (1988). The psychology of combining dynamic psychotherapy and Alcoholics Anonymous. *Bull Menninger Clin, 52,* 283–293.

Dodes, L. M. (1990). Addiction, helplessness, and narcissistic rage. *Psychoanal Q, 59,* 398–419.

Dodes, L. M. (1991). Psychotherapy is useful, often essential, for alcoholics. *Psychodynamic Lett, 1*(2), 4–7.

Dodes, L. M. (1996) Compulsion and addiction. *J Am Psychoanal Assoc, 44,* 815–835.

Dodes, L. M. (2002). *The heart of addiction.* New York: HarperCollins.

Dodes, L. M. (2003). Addiction and psychoanalysis. *Can Journal Psychoanal,* 11, 123–134.

Dodes, L. M. (2009). Addiction as a psychological symptom. *Psychodynamic Pract, 15,* 381–393.

Dodes, L. M. (2011). *Breaking addiction: A 7-step handbook for ending any addiction.* New York: HarperCollins.

Dodes, L., & Dodes, Z. (2014). *The sober truth: Debunking the bad science behind 12-step treatment and the rehab industry.* Boston: Beacon Press.

Dodes, L. M., & Khantzian, E. J. (1991). Psychotherapy and chemical dependence. In D. Ciraulo & R. Shader (Eds.), *Clinical manual of chemical dependence* (pp. 345–358). Washington, DC: American Psychiatric Press.

Flores, P. (2003). *Addiction as an attachment disorder.* Northvale, NJ: Jason Aronson.

Halikas, J. A., Crosby, R. D., Pearson, V. L., Nugent, S. M., & Carlson, G. A. (1994). Psychiatric comorbidity in treatment seeking cocaine abusers. *Am J Addict, 3,* 25–35.

Johnson, B. (1992) The psychoanalysis of a man with active alcoholism. *J Subst Abuse Treat, 9,* 111–123.

Kang, S. Y., Kleinman, P. H., Woody, G. E., Millman, R. B., Todd, T. C., Kemp, J., et al. (1991). Outcome for cocaine abusers after once-a-week psychosocial therapy. *Am J Psychiatry, 148,* 630–635.

Kaufman, E. (1994). *Psychotherapy of addicted persons.* New York: Guilford Press.

Kessler, R. C., Crum, R. M., Warner, L. A., Nelson, C. B., Schulenberg, J., & Anthony, J. C. (1997). Lifetime co-occurrence of DSM-III-R alcohol abuse and dependence with other psychiatric disorders in the National Comorbidity Survey. *Arch Gen Psychiatry, 54,* 313–321.

Khantzian, E. J. (1978). The ego, the self and opiate addiction: Theoretical and treatment considerations. *Int Rev Psychoanal, 5,* 189–198.

Khantzian, E. J. (1980). The alcoholic patient: An overview and perspective. *Am J Psychother, 34,* 4–19.

Khantzian, E. J. (1985a). The self-medication hypothesis of addictive disorders: Focus on heroin and cocaine dependence. *Am J Psychiatry, 142,* 1259–1264.

Khantzian, E. J. (1985b). Psychotherapeutic interventions with substance abusers: The clinical context. *J Subst Abuse Treat, 2,* 83–88.

Khantzian, E. J. (1986). A contemporary psychodynamic approach to drug abuse treatment. *Am J Drug Alcohol Abuse, 12,* 213–222.

Khantzian, E. J. (1988). The primary care therapist and patient needs in substance abuse treatment. *Am J Drug Alcohol Abuse, 14*(2), 159–167.

Khantzian, E. J. (1995). Self-regulation vulnerabilities in substance abusers: Treatment implications. In S. Dowling (Ed.), *The psychology and treatment of addictive behavior* (pp. 17–41). New York: International Universities Press.

Khantzian, E. J. (1997). The self-medication hypothesis of substance use disorders: A reconsideration and recent applications. *Harv Rev Psychiatry, 4,* 231–244.

Khantzian, E. J. (1999a). *Treating addictions as a human process.* Northvale, NJ: Jason Aronson.

Khantzian, E. J. (1999b). Preverbal origins of distress: Substance use disorders and psychotherapy In E. J. Khantzian (Ed.), *Treating addictions as a human process* (pp. 629–637). Northvale, NJ: Jason Aronson.

Khantzian, E. J. (2001). Reflections on group treatment as corrective experiences for addictive vulnerability. *Int J Group Psychother, 51*, 11 –20.

Khantzian, E. J. (2003). Understanding addictive vulnerability: An evolving psychodynamic perspective. *Neuropsychoanal, 5*, 5 –21.

Khantzian, E. J. (2012). Reflections on treating addictive disorders—a psychodynamic perspective. *Am J Addict, 21*(3), 274–279.

Khantzian, E. J., Dodes, L. M., & Brehm, N. M. (2005). Determinants and perpetuators of substance abuse: Psychodynamics. In J. H. Lowinson, P. Ruiz, R. B. Millman, & J. G. Langrod (Eds.), *Substance abuse: A comprehensive textbook* (4th ed., pp. 97–107). Baltimore, MD: Lippincott/Williams & Wilkins.

Khantzian, E. J., & Mack, J. (1983). Self-preservation and the care of the self. *Psychoanal Study Child, 38*, 209–232.

Khantzian, E. J., & Treece, C. (1985). DSM-III psychiatric diagnosis of narcotic addicts. *Arch Gen Psychiatry, 42*, 1067–1071.

Kleinman, P. K., Miller, A. B., & Millman, R. B. (1990). Psychopathology among cocaine abusers entering treatment. *J Nerv Ment Dis, 178*, 442–447.

Kohut, H. (1971). *The analysis of the self.* Madison, CT: International Universities Press.

Krystal, H. (1982). Alexithymia and the effectiveness of psychoanalytic treatment. *Int J Psychoanal Psychother, 9*, 353–378.

Krystal, H., & Raskin, H. (1970). *Drug dependence: Aspects of ego function.* Detroit, MI: Wayne State University Press.

Mack, J. (1981). Alcoholism, A.A., and the governance of the self. In M. H. Bean & N. E. Zinberg (Eds.), *Dynamic approaches to the understanding and treatment of alcoholism* (pp. 128–162). New York: Free Press.

McDougall, J. (1984). The "disaffected" patient: Reflections on affect pathology. *Psychoanal Q, 53*, 386–409.

Milkman, H., & Frosch, W. A. (1973). On the preferential abuse of heroin and amphetamines. *J Nerv Ment Dis, 156*, 242–248.

Penick, E. C., Powell, B. J., Nickel, E. J., Bingham, S. F., Rieseenmy, K. R., Read, M. R., et al. (1994). Co-morbidity of lifetime psychiatric disorder among male alcoholic patients. *Alcohol Clin Exp Res, 18*, 1289–1293.

Prochaska, J. O., DiClemente, C. C. (1985). Common processes of change in smoking, weight control, and psychological distress. In S. Shiffman & T. A. Willis (Eds.), *Coping and substance abuse* (pp. 345–363). New York: Academic Press.

Regier, D. A., Farmer, M. E., Rae, D. S., Locke, B. Z., Keith, S. J., Judd, L. L., et al. (1990). Comorbidity of mental disorders with alcohol and other drug abuse: Results from the Epidemiologic Catchment Area (ECA) study. *JAMA, 264*, 2511–2518.

Rogalski, C. J. (1984). Professional psychotherapy and its relationship to compliance in treatment. *Int J Addict, 19*, 521–539.

Rosen, A. (1981). Psychotherapy and Alcoholics Anonymous: Can they be coordinated? *Bull Menninger Clin, 45*, 229–246.

Rounsaville, B. J., Anton, S. F., Carroll, K., Budde, D., Prusoff, B., & Gawin, F. (1991). Psychiatric diagnosis of treatment-seeking cocaine-abusers. *Arch Gen Psychiatry, 48*, 43–51.

Rounsaville, B. J., Gawin, F., & Kleber, H. (1985). Interpersonal psychotherapy adapted for ambulatory cocaine abusers. *Am J Drug Alcohol Abuse, 11*(3–4), 171–191.

Rounsaville, B. J., Weissman, M., Kleber, H., & Wilber, C. (1982). Heterogeneity of psychiatric diagnosis in treated opiate addicts. *Arch Gen Psychiatry, 39*, 161–166.

Schuckit, M. A., & Hesselbrock, V. (1994). Alcohol dependence and anxiety disorders: What is the relationship? *Am J Psychiatry, 151*, 1723–1734.

Schuckit, M. A., Irwin, M., & Brown, S. A. (1990). The history of anxiety symptoms among 171 primary alcoholics. *J Stud Alcohol, 51*, 34–41.

Shaffer, H. J. (1985). The disease controversy: Of metaphors, maps and menus. *J Psychoactive Drugs, 17,* 65–76.

Shedler, J. (2010) The efficacy of psychodynamic psychotherapy. *Am Psychologist, 65*(2), 98–109.

Silber, A. (1974). Rationale for the technique of psychotherapy with alcoholics. *Int J Psychoanal Psychother, 3,* 28–47.

Treece, C., & Khantzian, E. J. (1986). Psychodynamic factors in the development of drug dependence. *Psychiatr Clin North Am, 9,* 399–412.

Walant, K. B. (1995). *Creating the capacity for attachment: Treating addictions and the alienated self.* Northvale, NJ: Jason Aronson.

Weegman, M., & Khantzian, E. J. (2011). Envelopments: Immersion in and emergence from drug misuse. *Am J Psychother, 65,* 163–177.

Wieder, H., & Kaplan, E. (1969). Drug use in adolescents. *Psychoanal Study Child, 24,* 399–431.

Wilens, T. E., Biederman, J., Spencer, T. J., & Frances, R. J. (1994). Comorbidity of attention deficit hyperactivity and psychoactive substance use disorders. *Hosp Community Psychiatry, 45,* 421–435.

Woody, G. E., Luborsky, L., McLellan, A. T., & O'Brien, C. P. (1989). Individual psychotherapy for substance abuse. In T. B. Karasu (Ed.), *Treatment of psychiatric disorders: A task force report of the American Psychiatric Association* (pp. 1417–1430). Washington, DC: American Psychiatric Press.

Woody, G. E., Luborsky, L., McLellan, A. T., O'Brien, C. P., Beck, A. T., Blaine, J., et al. (1983). Psychotherapy for opiate addicts: Does it help? *Arch Gen Psychiatry, 40,* 639–645.

Woody, G. E., McLellan, A. T., Luborsky, L., & O'Brien, C. P. (1986). Psychotherapy for substance abuse. *Psychiatr Clin North Am, 9,* 547–562.

Woody, G. E., McLellan, A. T., Luborsky, L., & O'Brien, C. P. (1995). Psychotherapy in community methadone programs. *Am J Psychiatry, 152,* 1302–1308.

Wurmser, L. (1974). Psychoanalytic considerations of the etiology of compulsive drug use. *J Am Psychoanal Assoc, 22,* 820–843.

CHAPTER 27

Cognitive Therapy

JUDITH S. BECK
BRUCE S. LIESE
LISA M. NAJAVITS

Kim is a 32-year-old woman with a complex history of substance abuse that began when she was 13 years old. At various times, Kim has experimented with many illicit substances (including marijuana, heroin, lysergic acid diethylamide [LSD], Ecstasy, and cocaine), and she has been dependent on nicotine, alcohol, amphetamines, and barbiturates. She also suffers from chronic depression. She has been treated intermittently for depression since age 15 and has cycled in and out of substance treatment programs since age 19. Kim has never been married. She works as a night janitor at a fast-food restaurant.

Currently, Kim smokes marijuana several times daily. She says, "I smoke so much, I don't even get high anymore." She smokes to try to feel "normal" and to deal with feelings of depression, emptiness, and loneliness. She views herself as hopeless but says she has no plans to kill herself, because she is afraid of dying. She has gained over 50 pounds in the last few years and she says she wants to "do nothing but sit around the house all day."

Kim meets criteria for avoidant personality disorder with dependent and borderline features. She describes constant boredom and isolation. Nonetheless, she refuses to take social or occupational risks, saying, "If I put myself out there, I'll only get burned." She has a history of numerous failed relationships and jobs.

Eventually Kim joins a self-help group for women with depression, where she admits to daily marijuana use. Another group member, Jenna, explains that she, too, was a heavy marijuana smoker at one time. Jenna warns Kim that she will only feel better when she quits smoking marijuana. After listening, Kim feels motivated to stop but finds it impossible to quit. After only a few days of abstinence, she feels more depressed and anxious, and she resumes smoking pot.

For more than 20 years, cognitive-behavioral therapy (CBT) has been adapted and refined to help people like Kim, who are addicted to a variety of substances, including alcohol, cocaine, opioids, marijuana, prescription medications, nicotine, and other psychoactive substances (A. T. Beck, Wright, Newman, & Liese, 1993; Carroll, 1998, 1999; Liese & Beck, 1997; Liese & Franz, 1996; Najavits, Liese, & Harned, 2004; Newman & Ratto, 1999). CBT has also been adapted for compulsive gambling, shopping, and sexual behaviors. Applications of CBT to substance-abusing adolescents (Fromme & Brown, 2000; Waldron, Slesnick, Brody, Turner, & Peterson, 2001), dual diagnosis patients (e.g., Barrowclough et al., 2001; Najavits, 2002a; Weiss, Najavits, & Greenfield, 1999), older patients (Schonfeld et al., 2000), and other important subgroups are additional recent developments. Patients like Kim have taught us a great deal about the development, maintenance, and treatment of addictive behavior (Liese & Franz, 1996). Currently, CBT approaches to substance abuse are considered among the most empirically-studied, well-defined, and widely used treatment modalities (Carroll, 1999; Thase, 1997).

There are many CBT approaches for substance abuse (Utley & Najavits et al., 2015), and a variety of major empirical studies have been published in the past several years (e.g., Crits-Christoph et al., 1999; Maude-Griffin et al., 1998; Project MATCH Research Group, 1997; Rawson et al., 2002; Waldron et al., 2001). In this chapter, we focus primarily on the cognitive therapy (CT) model defined by Aaron T. Beck and colleagues, which is often incorporated into other cognitive-behavioral therapies

CT for substance abuse shares similarities to CT for other psychiatric disorders and psychological problems, including depression (A. T. Beck, Rush, Shaw, & Emery, 1979), anxiety (A. T. Beck & Emery, with Greenberg, 1985), and personality disorders (A. T. Beck, Freeman, & Associates, 1990; J. S. Beck, 2005; Young, 1999). Each places emphasis on the *therapeutic alliance, collaboration, case conceptualization, structure, patient education,* and the application of standard *cognitive-behavioral techniques.* In addition, when working with patients with substance use disorders (SUDs), cognitive therapists focus on the cognitive and behavioral sequences leading to substance use, management of cravings, avoidance of high-risk situations, case management, mood regulation (i.e., coping), and lifestyle change. CT for substance abuse is an integrative, collaborative endeavor. Patients are encouraged to seek adjunctive services (e.g., 12-step and other programs) to reinforce their progress.

In CT for substance abuse, thoughts are viewed as playing a major role in addictive behavior (e.g., substance use), negative emotions (e.g., anxiety and depression), and physiological responses (including some withdrawal symptoms). Although strategies and interventions vary based on the individual and the particular substance, the basic conceptualization of the patient in cognitive terms remains constant (A. T. Beck et al., 1993; Wenzel, Liese, Beck, & Friedman-Wheeler, 2012; see Figure 27.1 for the basic cognitive model of substance abuse).

Cognitive therapists assess the development of their patients' beliefs about themselves, their early life experiences, their exposure to substances, the development of substance-related beliefs, and their eventual reliance on substances (Liese & Franz, 1996; see Figure 27.2). An important assumption is that substance abuse is in large part learned and can be modified by changing cognitive-behavioral processes.

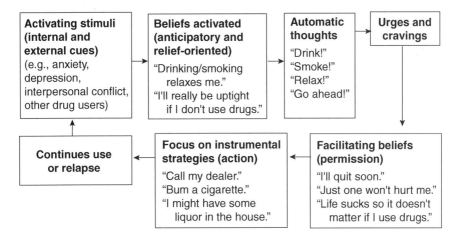

FIGURE 27.1. The cognitive model of substance abuse. Adapted with permission from A. T. Beck et al. (1993, p. 47).

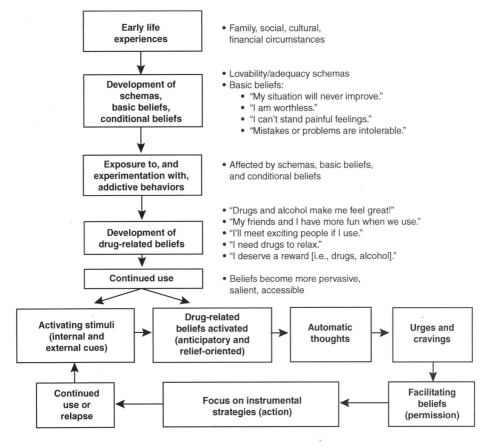

FIGURE 27.2. The cognitive developmental model of substance abuse. Adapted with permission from Liese and Franz (1996, p. 482).

Our model for CT of substance abuse has been substantially influenced by other cognitive behaviorists. For example, Marlatt and colleagues (Marlatt & Gordon, 1985; Dimeff & Marlatt, 1998) presented a profoundly important model of relapse prevention that has contributed greatly to our own work. Identifying high-risk situations, understanding the decision chain leading to substance use, modification of substance users' dysfunctional lifestyles, and learning from lapses to prevent full-fledged relapses are all integral to the relapse prevention model and the cognitive models of addiction.

In this chapter, we address four key topics: cognitive case conceptualization; principles of treatment; treatment planning (including specific cognitive and behavioral interventions); and comparison to other major psychosocial treatments for substance abuse. Our patient, Kim, is used as an example throughout.

THE COGNITIVE CONCEPTUALIZATION DIAGRAM

CT begins with a formulation of the case, using a standardized form for structuring the case conceptualization (J. S. Beck, 2011). An example using Kim's current difficulties is provided in Figure 27.3. She holds fundamental beliefs that she is helpless and incompetent, bad, unlovable, and vulnerable. These beliefs originated in childhood and became stronger and stronger as time went on. The next to last of eight children in a poor family, Kim was emotionally neglected by a depressed, alcoholic mother. Her father was cold, distant, and uninterested in Kim. He abandoned the family when Kim was 7 and never made contact them again. Kim had few friends, felt rejected by her family, did poorly in school, and dropped out when she was halfway through 11th grade.

Kim's core beliefs of helplessness, badness, and vulnerability have caused her great pain, and over the years she has developed rules (i.e., conditional assumptions) for survival. One such conditional assumption is, "If I avoid challenges, I won't have to face failure." Thus, Kim uses a typical coping strategy: She avoids applying for any but the most menial jobs. She then quits these jobs when small problems arise, believing she is helpless to solve problems. Likewise, she tries only halfheartedly in substance abuse treatment programs and drops out prematurely, believing she cannot abstain from using substances. She also avoids conflicts with others, believing that she does not deserve getting what she wants.

Kim's core beliefs of badness and unlovability permeate virtually all of her relationships. In addition to her conditional belief, "If I try to get what I want from a relationship, I'll fail" (which stems from a core belief of helplessness), she also believes, "If I assert myself or let others get too close, they'll reject me because nobody could possibly love me." Therefore, she uses coping strategies such as isolating herself, avoiding assertiveness and intimacy, and, perhaps most obvious, taking substances. Most of her social contacts are with other substance abusers who tend to manipulate and take advantage of her.

Kim also has a core belief that she is vulnerable, especially to negative emotion. Her conditional assumption is, "If I start to feel bad, my emotions will get out of control and overwhelm me." She avoids even mildly challenging situations in which she

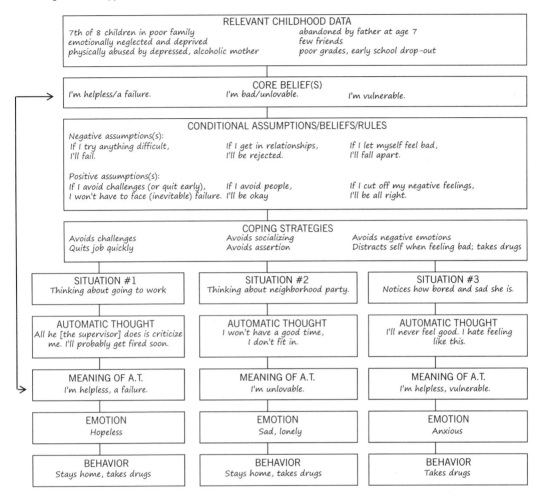

FIGURE 27.3. Cognitive conceptualization diagram. Adapted with permission from J. S. Beck (2011, p. 200).

predicts she will feel sad, rejected, or helpless. Avoidance itself, however, often leads to boredom and frustration, which increases her sense of failure and helplessness.

Kim discovered at an early age that she could feel better by drinking alcohol and taking substances. As a result, she failed to develop healthier coping strategies (e.g., learning to tolerate bad moods, solving problems, asserting herself, or looking at situations more realistically). For much of her life, she has tried to cope with a combination of avoidance and substance use.

The cognitive conceptualization diagram in Figure 27.3 demonstrates how Kim's thinking in specific situations leads to substance use. In situation #1, for example, Kim thinks about going to work. She has a mental image of her supervisor looking at her "with a mean face," and she thinks, "All he ever does is criticize me. I'll probably get fired soon." This is an *automatic thought,* because it seems to pop into Kim's mind spontaneously. Prior to receiving therapy, Kim had little awareness of her automatic thoughts; she was much more aware of her subsequent negative emotions. As a result, she felt helpless and her behavioral response was to stay home and take substances.

Why does Kim consistently have these thoughts of failure and helplessness? Kim's negative core beliefs about herself influence her perception of her experiences. She *assumes* she will fail, never thinking to question such beliefs about herself. Given this tendency, it is no surprise that Kim avoids challenges. She thinks it is just a matter of time until her failure becomes apparent.

In situation #2 (see Figure 27.3), Kim considers whether to attend a party given by neighbors. Because of her core belief that she is unlovable, she automatically thinks, "I won't have a good time. I don't fit in." Accepting these thoughts as true, she feels sad and chooses to stay home and get high. Whereas many automatic thoughts have some validity, they are usually distorted in some way. Had Kim evaluated her thoughts critically, she might have concluded that she could not predict the future with certainty, that several neighbors had seemed pleasant in the past, and that the reason for the neighbors' party was to get to know others better. Kim's core belief of unlovability once again leads her to accept negative thoughts as true and to use her dysfunctional strategies of avoidance and substance use.

In situation #3 (Figure 27.3), Kim becomes aware of how bored and sad she feels. She thinks, "I'll never feel good. I *hate* feeling like this." Her negative prediction and intolerance of dysphoria are again linked to her core beliefs of helplessness and vulnerability. Again, she copes with her anxiety by turning to substances.

The cognitive conceptualization diagram (Figure 27.3) can serve as a valuable aid to identify quickly the most central beliefs and dysfunctional strategies of substance abusers, to recognize how their beliefs influence their perceptions of current situations, and to explain why they respond emotionally and behaviorally in such ineffective ways. An important part of the cognitive approach is to help patients begin to question the validity of their perceptions and the accuracy of automatic thoughts that lead to substance abuse.

One important initial step in therapy is to help patients recognize that many of their negative automatic thoughts are not completely valid. When they test their thinking and modify it to resemble reality more closely, they generally feel better. A later step is to help them use the same kind of evaluative process with their core beliefs, to guide them in understanding that such beliefs are ideas, not necessarily truths. Once they see themselves in a more realistic light, they begin to perceive situations differently, feel better emotionally, and use more functional behavioral strategies learned in treatment. When this occurs, they become less likely to "need" substances for mood regulation, because they have developed internal strategies for coping.

CT for substance abuse therefore aims to modify thoughts associated with substance use (both surface-level "automatic thoughts" and deeper-level "core beliefs"). The goal is to develop new behaviors to take the place of dysfunctional ones. An additional focus, described later in this chapter, is practical problem solving and modifying the patient's lifestyle to decrease the likelihood of relapse. The modification of patients' long-term negative beliefs about the self is crucial to their ability to see alternative explanations for distressing events, to use more functional coping strategies learned in therapy, and to create better lives.

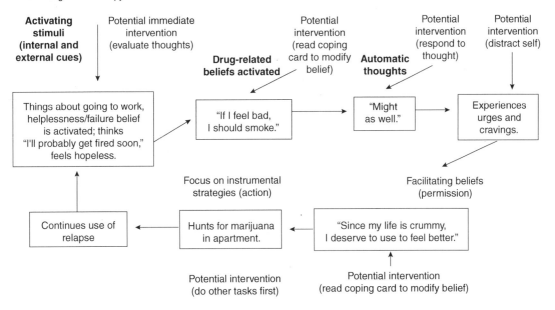

FIGURE 27.4. Cognitive model of substance abuse applied to case example.

At some point, cognitive therapists may explore childhood issues that relate to patients' core beliefs and addictive behavior. Such exploration helps both clinicians and patients understand how patients developed and maintained such rigid, global, and inaccurate negative ideas about themselves (J. S. Beck, 2005).

Figure 27.4 reflects the basic cognitive model of substance abuse as applied to Kim's substance abuse behavior. It illustrates the cyclical nature of substance abuse. Kim, like most substance abusers, believes that taking substances is an automatic process, beyond her control. This diagram helps her identify the sequence of events leading to an incident of substance use and identifies potential points of intervention in the future. In this example, Kim feels hopeless, because she predicts she will lose her job. As she searches for a way to cope with her dysphoria, a basic substance-related belief emerges ("If I feel bad, I should smoke") and she thinks, "I might as well use." She then experiences cravings and gives herself permission to use ("My life is crummy. I deserve to feel better"); she hunts for her marijuana and smokes a joint. This typical sequence of events takes place in seconds, and Kim initially believes it is automatic. By breaking it down into a series of steps, Kim can learn a variety of ways to intervene at each stage along the way.

PRINCIPLES OF TREATMENT

A cognitive therapist may use hundreds of interventions with any given patient at any given time. In this section, we discuss CT principles that apply to all patients, using substance abuse examples.

1. CT is based on a unique cognitive conceptualization of each patient.
2. A strong therapeutic alliance is essential.
3. CT is goal-oriented.
4. The initial focus of therapy is on the present.
5. CT is time sensitive.
6. Therapy sessions are structured, with active participation by both patient and therapist.
7. Patients are taught to identify and respond to dysfunctional thoughts and beliefs.
8. CT emphasizes psychoeducation and relapse prevention.

Principle 1: CT Is Based on a Unique Cognitive Conceptualization of Each Patient

Conceptualization of the case includes analysis of the current problematic situations of substance abusers and their associated thoughts and reactions (emotional, behavioral, and physiological). Therapists and patients look for meanings expressed in patients' automatic thoughts to identify their most basic dysfunctional core beliefs about themselves, their world, and other people (e.g., "I am weak," "The world is a hostile place").

They also identify patterns of behavior that patients develop to cope with these negative ideas. Such patterns might include taking substances, preying on people, and distancing themselves from others. The connection between their core beliefs and coping strategies becomes clearer when therapists and patients identify the conditional assumptions that drive patients' behavior (e.g., "If I try to do anything difficult, I'll probably fail because I'm so weak").

Cognitive therapists and patients consider patients' developmental histories to understand how they came to hold such strong, rigid, negative core beliefs. They also explore how these beliefs might not be true today and, in some cases, were not completely true even in childhood. They look at patients' enduring patterns of interpretation that have caused them to process information so negatively.

Therapists also draw diagrams of scenarios in which patients take substances (Figure 27.4) to illustrate the cyclical process of substance use and the many opportunities to intervene and avert a relapse.

Principle 2: A Strong Therapeutic Alliance Is Essential

Successful treatment relies on a caring, collaborative, respectful therapeutic relationship. Effective therapists explain their therapeutic approach, encourage patients to express skepticism, help them test the validity of their doubts, provide explanations for their interventions, share their cognitive formulation to make sure they have an accurate understanding of the patient, and consistently ask for feedback.

Therapists who are very collaborative typically find that they can establish sound therapeutic relationships with most patients with substance abuse. However, even the most skilled therapists, who embody the essential characteristics of warmth, empathy, caring, and genuine regard, find it challenging to develop good relationships with occasional patients who are suspicious, manipulative, or avoidant. Therapists are encouraged to examine relationship problems with the same careful cognitive exploration of session-related behavior they use for all other behaviors. See Figure 27.5, for example, for a cognitive conceptualization diagram of missed sessions and dropout.

An effective cognitive therapist seeks to avoid activating patients' core beliefs through his or her own behavior in therapy and helps patients test the validity of their ideas about the therapist. For example, Kim's therapist asked for evidence when Kim said she believed the therapist was judging her as "bad" for having a substance abuse problem. Of course, effective therapists need to examine their own thoughts, feelings, and behaviors periodically to ensure that they are *not* viewing their patients in a negative light. When therapists maintain truly nonjudgmental attitudes, they can

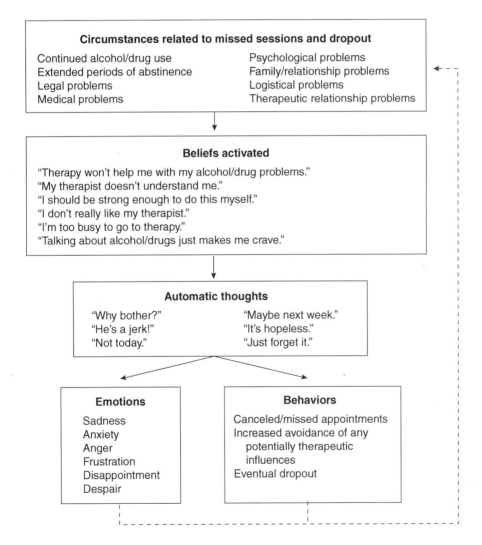

FIGURE 27.5. Cognitive conceptualization of missed sessions and dropout. From Liese and Beck (1997, p. 212).

sincerely tell patients that they are *not* negatively evaluating them. They can further explain that they view patients as using substances to try to cope with the difficulties inherent in their lives.

At times a persistent problem in the therapeutic relationship arises from a clash of patient and therapist beliefs. Therapists are advised to do conceptualization diagrams of patients and of themselves to identify dysfunctional ideas they may have about interacting with difficult people.

For example, one patient with substance abuse held the core belief, "If I show any weakness, others will hurt me," and a related assumption, "If I listen to my therapist, he'll see me as weak." As a result, the patient was very controlling in session, kept criticizing the therapist, and would not do any self-help assignments suggested by the therapist. The problem persisted, at least in part, because the *therapist* also had a broad assumption, "If people don't listen to me, it means they don't value me, and therefore don't deserve my best effort." The therapist became irritated with the patient, expressing dissatisfaction through body language and tone of voice. The patient, already hypervigilant for possible harm from others, perceived the therapist's negative attitude and dropped out of therapy prematurely.

Liese and Franz (1996) have identified common dysfunctional beliefs of therapists that interfere with delivering therapy to patients with substance abuse. Although many patients minimize their substance use, confronting them in a harsh manner is likely to result in diminished therapeutic efficacy and dropping out. When patients report no substance use during the previous week, it is often useful to inquire about times when they felt cravings. By doing so, therapists can obtain relevant cognitive material to help patients continue effective responses in the coming week.

Because patients with substance problems have high dropout rates (Simpson, Joe, Rowan Szal, & Greener, 1997), it is essential to build a strong therapeutic relationship. Liese and Beck (1997) describe how CT skills can maximize retention in treatment. Figure 27.5 presents their model for missed sessions and dropout.

Therapists strengthen the alliance by emphasizing that they and the patient are on the same team, working toward the patient's long-term goals. The patient can learn that therapy is not an adversarial relationship. The therapist and patient collaboratively make most of the decisions about therapy. However, therapists should know that a common coping strategy of patients with substance abuse is avoidance (e.g., minimizing difficulties in abstaining from substances). It is important, therefore, to help patients examine (in a nonconfrontational manner) the advantages and disadvantages of avoidance.

Principle 3: CT Is Goal Oriented

At the first session and periodically thereafter, therapists ask patients to set goals. They identify objectives in specific behavioral terms by asking, "How would you like to be different by the end of therapy?" It is important to give patients feedback about their goals, because they sometimes harbor unrealistic expectations. Therapists also help to identify short-term goals and propose ways the patient can meet those goals.

For example, Kim's therapist helped her specify her goal of "being happy" in behavioral terms: getting a job she enjoyed, entering into a romantic relationship, getting along with her family, and staying abstinent. He helped her set smaller goals along the way. A first step in getting a new job was to improve her attendance at her current job so she could get a good letter of reference.

Therapists also question patients about the degree to which they *really* want to meet their goals. A helpful technique is the advantage–disadvantage analysis (Figure 27.6), adapted from Marlatt and Gordon (1985). In this exercise, the therapist explores the benefits of achieving a goal while also reframing the disadvantages.

For some patients, a goal of harm reduction is more acceptable and achievable than complete abstinence (Fletcher, 2001; Marlatt, Tucker, Donovan, & Vuchinich, 1997). While abstinence is generally the safest goal, a decrease in substance use is more desirable than early dropout from treatment, which can occur if the therapist tries too early or too strongly to impose a total ban on all substances.

Principle 4: The Initial Focus of Therapy Is on the Present

Therapists initially emphasize current and specific problems that are distressing to the patient. When the patient has a comorbid diagnosis, it is important to address problems related to both. For example, Kim needed help in interacting with a critical supervisor at work and in learning alternate coping strategies (instead of using substances) when she was distressed about a work problem. She and her therapist discussed how to respond to the hurt she felt when the supervisor rebuked her for lateness, how to decrease her anger by rehearsing a coping statement addressing her

Advantages of Abstinence	Advantages of Taking Drugs (with reframe)
1. Feel better about myself. 2. Feel more in control. 3. Get to work on time. 4. More likely to keep my job. 5. Save money. 6. Better for my health. 7. Not get so criticized by my sister. 8. Not hang around other "druggies" so much. 9. Spend my time better.	1. Escape from feeling bad (**BUT** it's only a temporary escape and I don't really solve my problems). 2. Have people to hang out with (**BUT** they're druggies and I don't really like them). 3. It's hard work to quit (**BUT** I'll do it step-by-step with my therapist).
Disadvantages of Abstinence (with reframe)	**Disadvantages of Taking Drugs**
1. I may feel bored and anxious (**BUT** it's only temporary and it's good to learn to stand bad feelings). 2. I don't know what to do with my time (**BUT** I can learn in therapy how to spend time better). 3. I won't be able to hang out with my "friends" (**BUT** I do want to meet new "nondruggie" friends).	1. Seems to make me depressed. 2. Costs money. 3. Bad for my health. 4. Makes me feel like I'm not in control of my life. 5. Makes me feel unmotivated. 6. Hard to solve my real problems. 7. May make me lose my job. 8. Makes relationship with my sister worse. 9. Stops me from going out and making new friends. 10. Makes me feel like I'm wasting time. 11. Makes me feel stuck, like I'm not getting anywhere.

FIGURE 27.6. Advantages/disadvantages analysis.

activated core belief, how to use anger management techniques such as controlled breathing and time out, and how to talk to the supervisor in a reasonable manner.

The therapist also helped Kim respond to automatic thoughts. Through a combination of guided discovery and modeling, Kim learned to change the thought, "I should tell my supervisor off" with "He's just trying to do his job; I want to keep this job; I can just say 'OK' for now and stay calm." Toward the middle of therapy, the therapist and Kim began discussing her past as well—to see how she developed her ideas about relationships and how they related to her current difficulties.

Principle 5: CT Is Time Sensitive

The course of therapy for patients with substance abuse varies, depending on the severity of the substance use. Weekly or even twice-weekly sessions are recommended until symptoms are significantly reduced. With effective treatment, patients stabilize their moods, learn more tools, and gain confidence in using alternate coping strategies. At this point therapist and patient may experiment with decreasing the frequency of sessions. In a major study of CT for cocaine dependence (Crits-Christoph et al., 1997), the frequency of sessions went from once a week to once every 2 weeks, then to once every 3 or 4 weeks. After termination, an "open door" approach is helpful, in which patients are invited to return to therapy if they use (or are tempted to use) substances again.

Principle 6: Therapy Sessions Are Structured, with Active Participation by Both Patient and Therapist

Typically, cognitive therapists use a structured format, unless it interferes with the therapeutic alliance. They usually first check their patients' mood and recent amount and type of substance use (including, if possible, objective assessments), and frequency and intensity of cravings. They explore patients' progress or lack thereof, and elicit patients' feelings about coming to therapy that day. Next they set an agenda and decide with the patient which problems to focus on in the session. Standard items include the successes and difficulties the patient experienced during the past week and upcoming situations that could lead to substance use or dropout.

The therapist then makes a bridge from the previous session, asking the patient to recall the important things they discussed. If the patient has difficulty remembering the content, they problem-solve to help the patient make better use of future sessions. Encouraging patients to review notes (taken by therapist or patient) helps them integrate the lessons of therapy throughout the week. Also, during this part of the session, the therapist reviews the therapy homework completed during the week. If therapists suspect that patients have reacted badly to their previous meeting, they may ask for feedback about that session.

Next, they address specific topics of most concern to the patient. As they discuss a problem, they collect information about it and conceptualize how it arose. They may evaluate thoughts about the problem, modify relevant beliefs, and/or engage in problem solving. In the context of discussing a problem, the therapist may teach the patient skills in various domains: interpersonal (e.g., assertiveness), mood management (e.g., relaxation, anger management), behavioral (e.g., alternate behaviors when cravings start), and cognitive (e.g., worksheets evaluating dysfunctional cognitions).

Homework is customized to the patient. Typically, it includes monitoring substance use and mood, responding to automatic thoughts and beliefs, practicing new skills, and implementing solutions to problems discussed in session.

Throughout the session, the therapist summarizes the material the patient has presented, and after they have finished discussing a problem, asks the patient what he or she thinks will be important to remember during the week. The therapist ensures that these "main messages" (responses to dysfunctional cognitions, potential solutions to problems, new behavioral skills, etc.) are written down. At the end of the session, they summarize what occurred, checking to see that the patient understands and is highly likely to do the homework. Finally, the therapist asks for feedback. Skillful questioning to elicit the patient's honest reactions and nondefensive problem solving by the therapist promote progress and decrease the likelihood of dropout.

Adhering to this structure has many benefits: The most important issues are discussed, there is continuity between sessions, substance use is monitored, and problems are directly addressed. In addition, patients learn new skills and are more likely to use these in the coming week. The structure also ensures that patient and therapist understand the lessons of the session and that the patient is given the opportunity to provide feedback so treatment can be modified if needed.

Principle 7: Patients Are Taught to Identify and Respond to Dysfunctional Thoughts

The therapist emphasizes the cognitive model at each session—that the patients' thoughts influence how they react emotionally, physiologically, and behaviorally, and that by correcting their dysfunctional thinking, they can feel and behave better. The therapist does not assume that automatic thoughts are distorted; instead, therapist and patient investigate to what degree a given thought is valid. When thoughts *are* accurate (e.g., "I want a fix"), they either problem-solve (discuss ways to respond to the thought) or explore the validity of the conclusion the patient has drawn (e.g., "If I have an urge, there is nothing I can do but give in to it"). When evaluating thoughts, the therapist primarily uses questioning (and refrains from trying to persuade the patient), and may employ standard tools such as the Thought Record or Testing Your Thoughts worksheet (J. S. Beck, 2006).

Principle 8: CT Emphasizes Psychoeducation and Relapse Prevention

From the first session, the goal is to maximize patients' learning. The therapist encourages patients to write down important points during the session or does the writing for them, if they so desire. When patients have limited reading skills, the therapist uses ingenuity to create a system for helping patients remember (e.g., audiotaping the session, a brief summary of the session, or brainstorming about whom the patient might ask to read therapy notes).

The therapist teaches patients how to best use the new strategies. The goal is to make the patient his or her own "cognitive therapist." For example, the therapist teaches Kim how to identify her negative thoughts when she feels upset, respond to these thoughts, examine her behaviors, use coping strategies when she has cravings, solve problems, communicate effectively, avoid high-risk situations, and use many more cognitive, behavioral, mood-stabilizing, and general life skills.

Prior to termination, relapse prevention is emphasized. The therapist and patient review skills, predict difficulties, note early warning signs of relapse, and discuss how to prevent a lapse from becoming a relapse. They agree on when the patient needs to return to therapy, that is, if a lapse is imminent (instead of after it occurs). Finally, they develop a plan for patients to continue to work on their goals, preferably with the support of friends and family.

TREATMENT PLANNING

The first step in treatment planning is completing a thorough diagnostic assessment based on the criteria of the *Diagnostic and Statistical Manual of Mental Disorders* (American Psychiatric Association, 2013). It is essential to evaluate comorbid disorders, as well as medical complications.

According to research (e.g., Kessler et al., 1996), many patients with an SUD have a co-occurring psychiatric disorder. Treatment plans should address both. For example, Kim's therapist conceptualized that she was medicating her depression with marijuana. In addition to treating her substance use, the therapist focused on the depression itself, using standard CT strategies to reduce her depressive symptoms: activity scheduling, responding to negative cognitions (e.g., "I can't do anything right"), and problem solving (e.g., about work problems and loneliness), among others (see A. T. Beck et al., 1979; J. S. Beck, 2011). She was also referred to a psychiatrist for a medication consult.

Kim also had avoidant personality disorder with dependent and borderline features. One important implication of any personality disorder is the strong likelihood that associated dysfunctional beliefs (e.g., "I am helpless; I am bad") might become activated in the therapy session itself. Her therapist planned treatment to avoid intense activation of these very painful, rigid, overgeneralized dysfunctional ideas early in therapy that could have led to premature dropout. Adding elements from CT for personality disorders may be helpful for some issues (J. S. Beck, 2005; Beck, Freeman, & Associates, 1990; Young, 1999)

A second key step in treatment planning is identifying the patient's motivation for change. Prochaska, DiClemente, and Norcross (1992) described five stages of change: the *precontemplation* stage (in which they are only minimally, if at all, distressed about their problems and have little motivation to change), the *contemplation* stage (in which they have sufficient motivation to consider their problems and think about change, although not necessarily enough to take action), the *preparation* stage (in which they want help to make changes but may not feel they know what to do), the *action* stage (in which they start to change their behavior), or the *maintenance* stage (in which they are motivated to continue to change).

Kim, for example, was at the contemplation stage when she entered therapy. Her therapist helped her identify the problems associated with her substance use, some of which she had avoided focusing on before therapy. Her therapist also helped her do an advantage–disadvantage analysis of marijuana use (Figure 27.6). Her therapist helped her "reframe" or find a functional response to her dysfunctional ideas of not changing. These techniques helped move Kim from the contemplation to the preparation stage. Had her therapist started with a treatment plan that emphasized immediate change of substance use behaviors, it is likely that Kim would have resisted, tried only halfheartedly, or dropped out of therapy altogether.

Part of every treatment plan involves socializing patients to the cognitive model, so that they begin to view their reactions as stemming from their (often distorted) perceptions of situations. Once her therapist taught her to ask herself what was going through her mind just before she reached for a joint, Kim could understand how her automatic thoughts influenced her emotional and behavioral reactions. Later her therapist taught her how to identify the more complex sequence (Figure 27.5) leading to substance use and helped her identify how she could intervene at each stage.

An essential element in treatment planning is evaluating the strength of the therapeutic alliance. Substance abuse patients often enter treatment with dysfunctional beliefs about therapy, such as the following:

"My therapist may try to force me to do things I don't like."
"This therapy may do more harm than good."
"He probably thinks he knows everything."
"She'll think I'm a failure if I use again."
"I'm better off without therapy."

The treatment plan should include the identification and testing of these dysfunctional beliefs. Otherwise, patients may drop out prematurely. A good treatment plan also specifies patients' problems (or, positively framed, their goals) and the concrete steps needed to ameliorate them. Kim and her therapist discussed her work problems. They combined problem solving and correcting distortions related to aspects of the problem, such as getting to work on time, feeling bored, fearing criticism, and relating to coworkers. Eventually Kim sought a new job, when it became clear that the disadvantages of the job (low pay and lack of stimulation) still outweighed the advantages. Her therapist encouraged and aided her in the job search.

Difficulty at work was one of the first problems they tackled, because Kim was motivated to address it, it was closely connected to her marijuana use, and it seemed that they might make improvements on it in a short period. Later in therapy they addressed situations that were more difficult: getting along with her family, meeting new friends, and developing broader interests.

Her therapist continuously assessed Kim's readiness to change her substance abuse by measuring the strength of her beliefs. At the beginning of therapy, Kim believed that her marijuana use might contribute to her work problems, her social isolation, and her lack of motivation. However, she also believed that nothing, including therapy, could help. After several weeks, she began to see things differently, especially when she recognized that some initial behavioral activation and responding to automatic thoughts improved her mood. Now she was ready to explore how she came to use marijuana, to start monitoring her substance use, to learn strategies to manage cravings, to avoid high-risk situations, to respond to substance-related beliefs, to join a self-help group, and to make some lifestyle changes. These strategies are described next.

Teaching Patients to Observe Substance Use Sequences

Kim's therapist used a blank version of Figure 27.5, and together they filled in the boxes about a recent episode of marijuana use. For the first time, it became clear to Kim that her behavior was at least somewhat voluntary. Previously, she had believed that her use was completely outside her control.

The therapist reviewed how a typical activating stimulus gave rise to negative thoughts, which led to feelings of hopelessness. They discussed how Kim could learn to intervene. First, she could respond to her negative thoughts to reduce her dysphoria. If that did not work well enough, she could still respond to her substance-related beliefs. Kim agreed, for example, to read a coping card they developed in session. Such a card might list activities of "what to do if I want to smoke." These coping cards are not affirmations but jointly composed statements that the patient endorses in session. They might include the following:

1. Go for a walk.
2. Call (a specific friend, sponsor, or family member).
3. Go out for coffee.
4. Watch a compelling movie.
5. Read a chapter from a relevant self-help book.
6. Write e-mails.
7. Surf the Web.
8. Play a video game.

If Kim's automatic thoughts about substance use continued, she would have still more opportunities to respond. Upon experiencing cravings, she could tell herself to ignore these sensations and read a coping card that said:

If I feel cravings, *they are just cravings*. I don't have to pay attention to them. They'll go away. I can stand them. I've stood cravings in the past. I'll be *very* glad in a few minutes that I ignored them. When I ignore them, I get stronger!"

If she recognized her permission-giving beliefs, she could read another coping card that she and her therapist composed in session: "Don't reach for a joint. Set a timer and wait 5 minutes. You are strong enough to wait. In the meantime, do what's on my 'to do' list."

If she found herself focusing on strategies to get substances, she could try another waiting period or do other tasks outlined in therapy. A careful analysis of the substance-taking sequence, along with potential interventions, gave Kim hope that she could conquer this problem.

Kim and her therapist developed the coping cards over several sessions. First they discussed what Kim wished she could tell herself at each stage. Before writing the cards, the therapist asked Kim how much she believed each statement. When the strength of her belief was less than 90–100%, they reworded the statement or discussed it further to increase its validity. They observed that if Kim did not believe an idea strongly in the session, it was unlikely to work in "real life"; therefore, they needed more compelling statements.

Monitoring Progress

Progress is monitored in several ways. Most obvious is the patient's report of substance use, obtained at each session. Urine and Breathalyzer tests can motivate a decrease in use and an increase in the validity of self-reports. When patients do use, they are encouraged to see it not as an indication of failure, but rather as an opportunity to learn from the experience and to make future abstinence more likely. A variety of self-report instruments exist for substance abuse, such as the Timeline Followback (Sobell & Sobell, 1993). For substance abuse instruments that can be downloaded directly from the Web, see Table 27.1. Reports from others, such as family members or probation officers, may also be particularly important for patients with low motivation or a history of lying about their use.

When a patient has a comorbid depression or a personality disorder, progress is also measured by instruments such as the Beck Depression Inventory (A. T. Beck & Steer, 1993b), the Beck Anxiety Inventory (A. T. Beck & Steer, 1993a), the Brief Symptom Inventory (Derogatis, 1992), and other instruments relevant to particular

TABLE 27.1. Substance Abuse Assessment Resources

Resource	Website	Phone
National Institute on Alcohol Abuse and Alcoholism	*www.niaaa.nih.gov/publications*	—
Substance Abuse and Mental Health Services Administration	*www.store.samhsa.gov*	877-726-4727
National Institute on Drug Abuse	*www.drugabuse.gov* (Click "publications")	—
Free screening online for alcoholism	*www.alcoholscreening.org*	—
University of New Mexico Center on Alcoholism, Substance Abuse, and Addictions	*http://casaa.unm.edu*	
To locate substance abuse home test kits	*www.thomasnet.com* (Enter "alcohol drug test" for list of companies that provide home test kits for substance abuse)	—

Note. Adapted with permission from Najavits (2004).

symptoms. Improvements in scores provide an opportunity to reinforce positive changes patients have made in their thinking and behavior in the past week. Worsening scores raise a red flag, and careful questioning about recent events and perceptions often reveals agenda items to prevent the resumption of substance use in the coming week.

It is also important to monitor how patients spend their time. Kim, for example, made some changes early in therapy: less time watching television alone and fewer visits to substance-using friends. Had her therapist not been vigilant about checking weekly on these improvements, he might have missed significant backsliding many weeks later, which could have led to a relapse.

Another aspect of monitoring is assessment of old, dysfunctional beliefs versus newer, more functional ideas. At each session, the therapist assessed how much Kim believed substance-related ideas, such as "I can't stand to feel bored" and "Smoking marijuana is the only way to feel better," and how much she believed the new ideas they had developed, such as "My life will improve if I don't use" and "I can feel better by answering my negative thoughts and completing my 'to do' list." This monitoring helped the therapist intervene early when Kim's dysfunctional beliefs occasionally resurfaced strongly.

Dealing with High-Risk Situations

Marlatt and Gordon (1985) observed that exposure to activating stimuli, or triggers, makes substance use more likely. In high-risk situations, activating stimuli trigger substance-related beliefs, leading to cravings. These stimuli are idiosyncratic; what triggers one patient may not trigger another.

Triggers can be internal or external. Internal cues include negative mood states, such as depression, anxiety, loneliness, and boredom, or physical factors, such as pain, hunger, or fatigue. Although many patients use substances to regulate negative moods, many also use substances when they already feel good to "celebrate" or keep the good mood going.

External cues occur outside the individual: people, places, or things related to substance use, such as relationship conflicts or seeing substance paraphernalia. In one study, Cummings, Gordon, and Marlatt (1980) found that 35% of relapses were precipitated by negative emotional states, 20% by social pressure, and 16% by interpersonal conflict.

Therapists help patients identify the high-risk situations in which their substance-related beliefs and cravings occur. They are encouraged to avoid these situations and are taught relationship skills to handle conflict and pressure. For example, they might role-play how Kim could respond when a friend offers her a drink.

Dealing with Cravings and Urges

In CT, patients learn cognitive techniques to handle cravings. The therapist can help patients identify beliefs that encourage the use of substances to deal with cravings, for example, "I can't stand cravings"; "If I have cravings, I have to give in." Socratic questioning that examines past experiences of resisting craving, reflecting on the relative difficulty versus impossibility of tolerating cravings, and other cognitive techniques can modify these dysfunctional ideas.

Othere diverse methods can also be helpful for cravings, which are used in some cognitive and/or behavioral therapies. Distraction is often helpful, and patients are encouraged to devise a list of things they can easily do (e.g., exercise, read, and talk on the telephone). Snapping a rubber band and yelling "Stop!" while envisioning a stop sign helped Kim manage her craving. Grounding is another strategy that aids distraction from cravings and intense negative emotions; one can teach mental, physical, and soothing grounding methods (see Najavits, 2002a, for a description).

Case Management and Lifestyle Change

Helping patients solve their real-life problems is an essential part of CT. Patients who abuse substances often have complex medical, legal, employment, housing, and/ or family difficulties. Therapists should refer patients for assistance when needed. Therefore, they need to be aware of community resources and social services. Sometimes they can help patients identify specific people in their social network who might assist in working through such practical problems.

In some cases, however, it is necessary to help patients directly in session to take steps to improve their lives. Examining employment ads, for example, or completing forms (e.g., for public housing) with the patient may be an important part of treatment. For examples of case management for substance abuse, including dual diagnosis, see Drake and Noordsy (1994), Najavits (2002b), and Ridgely and Willenbring (1992).

Some lifestyle change is usually necessary to help patients eliminate substance use and maintain progress. Often the therapist needs to help the patient repair important relationships and to develop new relationships with people who do not use. Many substance abusers are deficient in relationship skills and need to learn these through discussion and role plays. Patients often have dysfunctional beliefs about relationships, and modification of these beliefs is a necessary step in learning to relate well to others. In addition, they may need help figuring out how they can build a new network of nonusing friends. The therapist can discuss contact with nonusers in the patient's environment, as well as encourage activities to help the patient meet new people.

Self-help groups can be a valuable adjunct to therapy—for meeting new abstinent individuals, reinforcing functional beliefs, and building a healthier lifestyle. Therapists should be aware of self-help groups in their area and encourage patients to attend. Alcoholics Anonymous, Narcotics Anonymous, SMART Recovery, and Moderation Management are a few examples of groups that can be of significant benefit to patients. See Table 27.2 for websites and phone numbers. Therapists can help patients who are reluctant to attend self-help groups by eliciting their automatic thoughts and aiding them in responding to these thoughts. Problem solving may be needed to help the patient choose groups or activities, find transportation, and manage anxiety about new experiences.

TABLE 27.2. Substance Abuse Recovery Resources

Resource	Website	Phone/e-mail
Substance Abuse and Mental Health Services Administration	*www.samhsa.gov*	877-726-4727
Alcoholics Anonymous	*www.alcoholics-anonymous.org*	212-870-3400
Cocaine Anonymous	*www.ca.org*	Varies by state and region—see website
Narcotics Anonymous	*www.na.org*	818-773-9999, Ext. 771
Marijuana Anonymous	*www.marijuana-anonymous.org*	800-766-6779
Nicotine Anonymous	*www.nicotine-anonymous.org*	877-879-6422
Smart Recovery	*www.smartrecovery.org*	866-951-5357
Secular Organization for Sobriety/ Save Our Selves	*www.secularsobriety.org*	323-666-4295
Harm Reduction Coalition	*www.harmreduction.org*	East coast: 212-213-6376 West coast: 510-444-6969
Moderation Management Network	*www.moderation.org*	*mm@moderation.org*
Women for Sobriety	*www.womenforsobriety.org*	215-536-8026

Note. Based on Najavits (2002b).

Reducing Dropout

Studies have shown that approximately 30 to 60% of substance abuse patients drop out of therapy (Wierzbicki & Pekarik, 1993). Many factors account for this high rate, including continued substance use; legal, medical, relationship, or psychological problems; practical problems (e.g., transportation, finances); dissatisfaction with therapy; and problems with the therapeutic alliance (Liese & Beck, 1997). Early in treatment, therapist and patient should predict potential difficulties that might interfere with regular attendance in therapy and either problem-solve in advance or collaboratively develop a plan for contact (usually by phone) if the patient misses a session.

Kim's therapist, for example, helped her with difficulties such as a changing her work schedule and transportation, which otherwise would have impeded her attendance. Both straightforward problem solving and responding to negative thinking ("I'll be too tired to come after work"; "It's not worth taking two buses") were necessary to avert missed sessions.

To maximize regular attendance, the therapist needs to monitor the strength of the therapeutic relationship at each session. Negative changes in patients' body language, voice, and degree of openness usually signal that dysfunctional beliefs (about themselves, the therapist, or therapy) have been activated. A list of 50 common beliefs leading to missed sessions and dropout (Liese & Beck, 1997) is a valuable guide for therapists.

Testing negative thoughts immediately can prevent a negative reaction that otherwise might result in missing the next session. Kim had many such cognitions, especially early in treatment: "I'm not smart enough for this therapy"; "I can't do this." A therapist who still suspects a patient may miss the next session may be able to turn the tide by phoning the patient the day before the session and demonstrating care and concern.

Formulating an accurate cognitive conceptualization of the patient from the start enables the therapist to plan interventions to avoid inadvertent activation of dysfunctional beliefs in and between sessions. Kim's therapist, for example, recognized how overwhelmed Kim became when faced with even minor challenges. The therapist therefore took care to explain concepts simply, to limit the amount of material each session, to check her understanding frequently, and to suggest homework that she could do. Thus, the therapist avoided undue activation of Kim's beliefs in her own inadequacy and helped to maintain her regular attendance in therapy.

COMPARISON WITH OTHER MODELS

It may be helpful to compare CT for substance abuse with two other widely-known approaches, specifically, motivational enhancement therapy (MET) and dialectical behavior therapy (DBT).

MET, originated by Miller, Zweben, DiClemente, and Rychtarik (1995) derives from several different theories, including client-centered, cognitive-behavioral, systems, and the social psychology of persuasion. The treatment is guided by five principles: The therapist should express empathy, develop discrepancy between the patient's goals and current problem behavior, avoid argumentation, roll with resistance rather than opposing it directly, and support self-efficacy by emphasizing personal responsibility and the hope of change. Specific strategies include reflective listening, affirmation, open-ended questions, summarizing, and eliciting self-motivational statements (e.g., asking evocative questions, inquiring about pros and cons of behavior, and exploring goals). The therapist also addresses ambivalence that may interfere with motivation and uses assessment instruments that are presented to the patient to increase motivation for change (e.g., alcohol/drug use, functional analysis of behavior, readiness to change, life problems, and biomedical impact).

MET differs from CT for substance abuse in several ways. First, MET is primarily designed as a process-oriented method to increase motivation. It was not designed to teach specific new skills or coping strategies (e.g., CT skills of identifying dysfunctional cognitions, rehearsal of new responses to cognitions, identification of alternative coping strategies, mood monitoring, social skills training, and lifestyle changes). Second, and likely because of the latter difference in goals, MET is typically much shorter. For example, in Project MATCH, MET was four sessions. Indeed, MET is primarily thought of as a precursor to other therapies for substance abuse, including CT (e.g., Barrowclough et al., 2001).

DBT, originated by Linehan, is a CBT designed for borderline personality disorder (BPD). It comprises twice-weekly group sessions and weekly individual sessions, and as-needed phone coaching. DBT teaches a variety of skills, in part inspired by

Eastern philosophy, including mindfulness, distress tolerance, emotion regulation, interpersonal effectiveness, and self-management (Linehan, 1993).

After positive outcomes in patients with BPD, DBT was adapted for substance abuse patients with BPD in the late 1990s (Dimeff, Rizvi, Brown, & Linehan, 2000; Linehan et al., 1999, 2002). The adaptation for substance abuse includes several new skills, including alternative rebellion, adaptive denial, burning bridges to drug use, and building a life worth living.

DBT differs from CT in several ways. First, CT for substance abuse was designed for a very broad spectrum of patients who abuse substances, whereas DBT focuses on patients with the dual diagnosis of BPD and substance abuse. Thus, some precepts that may be especially helpful for BPD may not apply to the typical substance abuse patient without BPD. For example, under the "four-session rule" in DBT, if a client misses four or more sessions, he or she loses access to the therapy. Also, a patient in DBT must agree to a lengthy course of treatment (e.g., two full rounds of the DBT skills modules, and a dose of three sessions per week). In CT, such imperatives are not required.

Second, and likely again due to the nature of BPD, DBT therapists use a team or community-of-therapists approach, and therapists are asked to be available after hours for phone coaching of clients. CT follows more traditional therapist roles. Finally, whereas both DBT and CT focus on teaching new coping skills, the skills themselves differ to some degree. For example, CT focuses much more formally on changing cognitions through the use of structured tools for cognitive change such as the Thought Record.

CONCLUSION

CT can be an effective treatment for patients with SUDs. It requires accurate conceptualization of the patient, a sound treatment plan based on this case formulation, a strong therapeutic relationship, and specialized interventions. Structuring the therapy session, problem solving of current difficulties, education about the sequence of substance use, planning for high-risk situations, monitoring of substance use, lifestyle change, and intensive case management are important facets of treatment.

Kim could easily have become an unemployed "revolving door" user and a burden to family, friends, and society. CT helped her to engage in therapy, work through dysfunctional beliefs about herself and the therapist, develop functional goals, learn new skills to solve problems, tolerate negative emotion, persist when she felt hopeless, engage in alternative behaviors when she craved substances, and develop a healthier lifestyle. Hard work by therapist and patient is likely to result in satisfying outcomes.

REFERENCES

American Psychiatric Association. (2013). *Diagnostic and statistical manual of mental disorders* (5th ed.). Arlington, VA: Author.
Barrowclough, C., Haddock, G., Tarrier, N., Lewis, S. W., Moring, J., O'Brien, R., et al. (2001).

Randomized controlled trial of motivational interviewing, cognitive behavior therapy, and family intervention for patients with comorbid schizophrenia and substance use disorders. *Am J Psychiatry, 158,* 1706–1713.

Beck, A. T., & Emery, G., with Greenberg, R. L. (1985). *Anxiety disorders and phobias: A cognitive perspective.* New York: Basic Books.

Beck, A. T., Freeman, A., & Associates. (1990). *Cognitive therapy of personality disorders.* New York: Guilford Press.

Beck, A. T., Rush, A. J., Shaw, B. F., & Emery, G. (1979). *Cognitive therapy of depression.* New York: Guilford Press.

Beck, A. T., & Steer, R. A. (1993a). *Beck Anxiety Inventory manual.* San Antonio, TX: Psychological Corporation.

Beck, A. T., & Steer, R. A. (1993b). *Beck Depression Inventory manual.* San Antonio, TX: Psychological Corporation.

Beck, A. T., Wright, F. D., Newman, C. F., & Liese, B. S. (1993). *Cognitive therapy of substance abuse.* New York: Guilford Press.

Beck, J. S. (2005). *Cognitive therapy for challenging problems: What to do when the basics don't work.* New York: Guilford Press.

Beck, J. S. (2006). *Cognitive therapy worksheet packet.* Bala Cynwyd, PA: Beck Institute for Cognitive Behavior Therapy.

Beck, J. S. (2011). *Cognitive behavior therapy: Basics and beyond* (2nd ed.). New York: Guilford Press.

Carroll, K. (1998). *A cognitive-behavioral approach: Treating cocaine addiction* (NIH Publication 98-4308). Rockville, MD: National Institute on Drug Abuse.

Carroll, K. M. (1999). Behavioral and cognitive behavioral treatments. In B. S. McCrady & E. E. Epstein (Eds.), *Addictions: A comprehensive guidebook* (pp. 250–267). New York: Oxford University Press.

Crits-Christoph, P., Siqueland, L., Blaine, J., Frank, A., Luborsky, L., Onken, L. S., et al. (1997). The NIDA Cocaine Collaborative Treatment Study: Rationale and methods. *Arch Gen Psychiatry, 54,* 721–726.

Crits-Christoph, P., Siqueland, L., Blaine, J., Frank, A., Luborsky, L., Onken, L. S., et al. (1999). Psychosocial treatment for cocaine dependence: The National Institute on Drug Abuse Collaborative Cocaine Treatment Study. *Arch Gen Psychol, 56,* 493–502.

Cummings, C., Gordon, J. R., & Marlatt, G. A. (1980). Relapse: Prevention and prediction. In W. R. Miller (Ed.), *The addictive behaviors: Treatment of alcoholism, substance abuse, smoking and obesity* (pp. 291–321). Oxford, UK: Pergamon Press.

Derogatis, L. R. (1992). *Brief Symptom Inventory.* Clinical Psychometric Research, Inc.

Dimeff, L. A., & Marlatt, G. A. (1998). Preventing relapse and maintaining change in addictive behaviors. *Clin Psychol Sci Pract, 5,* 513–525.

Dimeff, L., Rizvi, S. L., Brown, M., & Linehan, M. M. (2000). Dialectical behavior therapy for substance abuse: A pilot application to methamphetamine-dependent women with borderline personality disorder. *Cog Behav Pract, 7,* 457–468.

Drake, R. E., & Noordsy, D. L. (1994). Case management for people with coexisting severe mental disorder and substance use disorder. *Psychiatr Ann, 24,* 427–431.

Fletcher, A. (2001). *Sober for good: New solutions for drinking problems—advice from those who have succeeded.* Boston: Houghton Mifflin.

Fromme, K., & Brown, S. A. (2000). Empirically based prevention and treatment approaches for adolescent and young adult substance use. *Cogn Behav Pract, 7,* 61–64.

Kessler, R. C., Nelson, C. B., McGonagle, K. A., Edlund, M. J., Frank, R. G., & Leaf, P. J. (1996). The epidemiology of co-occurring addictive and mental disorders: Implications for prevention and service utilization. *Am J Orthopsychiatry, 66*(1), 17–31.

Liese, B. S., & Beck, A. T. (1997). Back to basics: Fundamental cognitive therapy skills for keeping substance-dependent individuals in treatment. In L. S. Onken, J. D. Blaine, & J. J. Boren

(Eds.), *Beyond the therapeutic alliance: Keeping substance-dependent individuals in treatment* (NIDA Research Monograph No. 165, DHHS Publication No. 97-4142, pp. 207–230). Washington, DC: U.S. Government Printing Office.

Liese, B. S., & Franz, R. A. (1996). Treating substance use disorders with cognitive therapy: Lessons learned and implications for the future. In P. Salkovskis (Ed.), *Frontiers of cognitive therapy* (pp. 470–508). New York: Guilford Press.

Linehan, M. M. (1993). *Skills training for treating borderline personality disorder.* New York: Guilford Press.

Linehan, M. M., Dimeff, L. A., Reynolds, S. K., Comtois, K. A., Welch, S. S., Heagerty, P., et al. (2002). Dialectal behavior therapy versus comprehensive validation therapy plus 12-step for the treatment of opioid dependent women meeting criteria for borderline personality disorder. *Drug Alcohol Depend, 67,* 13–26.

Linehan, M. M., Schmidt, H., Dimeff, L. A., Craft, J. C., Kanter, J., & Comtois, K. A. (1999). Dialectical behavior therapy for patients with borderline personality disorder and drug-dependence. *Am J Addict, 8,* 279–292.

Marlatt, G. A., & Gordon, J. R. (Eds.). (1985). *Relapse prevention: Maintenance strategies in the treatment of addictive behavior.* New York: Guilford Press.

Marlatt, G. A., Tucker, J., Donovan, D., & Vuchinich, R. (1997). Help-seeking by substance abusers: The role of harm reduction and behavioral–economic approaches to facilitate treatment entry and retention. In L. Onken, J. Blaine, & J. Boren (Eds.), *Beyond the therapeutic alliance: Keeping the drug-dependent individual in treatment* (pp. 44–84). Rockville, MD: U.S. Department of Health and Human Services.

Maude-Griffin, P. M., Hohenstein, J. M., Humfleet, G. L., Reilly, P. M., Tusel, D. J., & Hall, S. M. (1998). Superior efficacy of cognitive-behavioral therapy for urban crack cocaine abusers: Main and matching effects. *J Consult Clin Psychol, 66,* 832–837.

Miller, W. R., Zweben, A., DiClemente, C. C., & Rychtarik, R. G. (Eds.). (1995). *Motivational enhancement therapy manual* (Vol. 2). Rockville, MD: U.S. Department of Health and Human Services.

Najavits, L. M. (2002a). *Seeking Safety: A treatment manual for PTSD and substance abuse.* New York: Guilford Press.

Najavits, L. M. (2002b). *A woman's addiction workbook.* Oakland, CA: New Harbinger.

Najavits, L. M. (2004). Assessment of trauma, PTSD, and substance use disorder: A practical guide. In J. P. Wilson & T. M. Keane (Eds.), *Assessment of psychological trauma and PTSD.* New York: Guilford Press.

Najavits, L. M., Liese, B. S., & Harned, M. (2004). Cognitive-behavioral therapy. In J. H. Lowinson, P. Ruiz, R. B. Millman, & J. G. Langrod (Eds.), *Substance abuse: A comprehensive textbook* (4th ed.). Baltimore, MD: Williams & Wilkins.

Newman, C. F., & Ratto, C. L. (1999). Cognitive therapy of substance abuse. In E. T. Dowd & L. Rugle (Eds.), *Comparative treatments of substance abuse* (Vol. 1, pp. 96–126). New York: Springer.

Prochaska, J. O., DiClemente, C. C., & Norcross, J. C. (1992). In search of how people change: Applications to addictive behaviors. *Am Psychol, 47,* 1102–1114.

Project MATCH Research Group. (1997). Matching alcoholism treatments to client heterogeneity: Project MATCH posttreatment drinking outcomes. *J Stud Alcohol, 58,* 7–29.

Rawson, R. A., Huber, A., McCann, M., Shoptaw, S., Farabee, D., Reiber, C., et al. (2002). A comparison of contingency management and cognitive-behavioral approaches during methadone maintenance treatment for cocaine dependence. *Arch Gen Psychiatry, 59,* 817–824.

Ridgely, M. S., & Willenbring, M. L. (1992). Application of case management to drug abuse treatment: Overview of models and research issues. In R. S. Ashery (Ed.), *NIDA Research Monograph* (Vol. 127, pp. 12–33). Rockville, MD: U.S. Department of Health and Human Services.

Schonfeld, L., Dupree, L. W., Dickson-Fuhrmann, E., Royer, C. M., McDermott, C. H., Rosansky,

J. S., et al. (2000). Cognitive-behavioral treatment of older veterans with substance abuse problems. *J Geriatr Psychiatry Neurol, 13*, 124–129.

Simpson, D. D., Joe, G. W., Rowan Szal, G. A., & Greener, J. M. (1997). Drug abuse treatment process components that improve retention. *J Subst Abuse Treat, 14*(6), 565–572.

Sobell, M. B., & Sobell, L. C. (1993). *Problem drinkers: Guided self-change treatment.* New York: Guilford Press.

Thase, M. E. (1997). Cognitive-behavioral therapy for substance abuse disorders. In L. J. Dickstein, M. B. Riba, & J. M. Oldham (Eds.), *American Psychiatric Press review of psychiatry* (Vol. 16, pp. 145–171). Washington, DC: American Psychiatric Press.

Utley, J., & Najavits, L. M. (2015). Addiction treatments. In R. Cautin & S. Lilienfeld (Eds.), *The encyclopedia of clinical psychology* (pp. 1–10). New York: Wiley-Blackwell.

Waldron, H. B., Slesnick, N., Brody, J. L., Turner, C. W., & Peterson, T. R. (2001). Treatment outcomes for adolescent substance abuse at 4- and 7-month assessments. *J Consult Clin Psychol, 69*, 802–813.

Weiss, R. D., Najavits, L. M., & Greenfield, S. F. (1999). A relapse prevention group for patients with bipolar and substance use disorders. *J Subst Abuse Treat, 16*(1), 47–54.

Wenzel, A., Liese, B. S., Beck, A. T., & Friedman-Wheeler, D. G. (2012). *Group cognitive therapy for addictions.* New York: Guilford Press.

Wierzbicki, M., & Pekarik, G. (1993). A meta-analysis of psychotherapy dropout. *Prof Psychol Res Pract, 24*, 190–195.

Young, J. E. (1999). *Cognitive therapy for personality disorders: A schema-focused approach* (3rd ed.). Sarasota, FL: Professional Resource Press.

CHAPTER 28

Group Therapy, Self-Help Groups, and Network Therapy

MARC GALANTER

Treatment modalities that employ social networks, such as group therapy, self-help programs, and adaptations of individual office-based psychotherapy (e.g., network therapy, described below), are of particular importance in treating alcoholism and drug abuse. Family therapy is described elsewhere in this volume (Kaufman, Chapter 29). One reason is that the addictions are characterized by massive denial of illness, and rehabilitation must begin with a frank acknowledgment of the nature of the patient's addictive process. The consensual validation and influence necessary to achieve such pronounced attitude change are most effectively gained through group influence. Indeed, for this purpose, a fellow addict carries the greatest amount of credibility. Another reason for employing social networks is that they provide an avenue for maintaining ties to the patient beyond the traditional therapeutic relationship. Furthermore, therapists are not in the position to confront, cajole, support, and express feeling in a manner that can influence the abuser to return to abstinence; a group of fellow addicts or members of the patient's family can do so quite directly.

This chapter explores the impact of group treatment in a number of disparate settings. I examine therapy groups directed specifically at the treatment of addiction, at 12-step programs such as Alcoholics Anonymous (AA) and Narcotics Anonymous (NA), and at institution-based self-help for substance abusers. The role of the clinician varies considerably in relation to each of these modalities; in each case, the mental health professional is provided with an unusual opportunity to step out of the traditional role of the psychodynamic therapist or the psychopharmacologist and examine the ways in which social influence is wrought through the group setting.

GROUP THERAPY FOR ALCOHOLISM AND DRUG ABUSE

How to Refer a Patient to Group Therapy

It is important to match the treatment needs of an addicted individual adequately with the most appropriate group therapy format. Psychotherapeutic groups for alcoholics, for example, generally fare better when all members are alcoholics and the focus of the group is on the characteristic behaviors and consequences of this problem. Usually, each group includes from five to 12 members who meet from one to three times a week. Criteria for exclusion include severe sociopathy or lack of motivation for treatment, acute or poorly controlled psychotic disorders, and the presence of transient or permanent severe cognitive deficits. Those patients who, because of their dual problems—addiction and mental illness—cannot be integrated into single-problem group formats must be treated within specialized dual-diagnosis groups and treatment settings (Galanter, Casteñeda, & Ferman, 1988; Minkoff & Drake, 1991). Vannicelli (1982) observed that often patients are eventually excluded from the addiction group if they are unable to commit themselves to working toward abstinence. Polyaddicted individuals frequently are better integrated within multifocused groups. While dependent and nonsociopathic individuals are more easily engaged in interactional group models, individuals with sociopathic and other character problems are better retained in coping-skills groups (Cooney, Kadden, Litt, & Getter, 1991; Poldrugo & Forti, 1988).

Group Treatment Modalities

Group treatment for alcoholism and other addictions developed out of general disappointment with the results of individual therapy (Cooper, 1987). Table 28.1 presents brief descriptions of different group modalities for treatment of addicted individuals.

Leadership Style and Group Aims

The optimum style for a leader conducting a group for substance abusers appears to be one in which the focus is group- rather than leader-determined, in which the leader not only is knowledgeable about substance abuse but also acts as a facilitator of interpersonal process, and in which the group members seek to understand each other from their own perspective.

Groups differ in their aims and the styles of their leaders. Some groups allow for discussion of issues other than addiction in the hope that group members will identify the association between the addictive behavior and all other problems. Other groups focus primarily on relapse prevention through the identification and discussion of all problems, even if unrelated to the addictive behavior. Groups also vary according to the degree of support offered to members—from confrontational groups that give support only when a patient espouses the views of the group leader, to supportive groups that accept and explore individual attitudes and beliefs.

Despite the obvious importance of group style and the need for clearly described group techniques, little has been written that provides group leaders with specific group strategies (Vannicelli, Canning, & Griefen, 1984). The question of the group's

TABLE 28.1. Different Group Modalities for Treatment of Alcoholics

Category	Technique	Goals	Curative factors
Interactional	Interpretation of interactional process; promotion of self-disclosure and emotion expression	Promotion of understanding and resolution of interpersonal problems	Increased awareness of own relatedness
Modified interactional	Processing of interactional problems, but strong emphasis on ancillary supports for abstinence, such as AA and Antabuse	Promotion of abstinence and improvement of interpersonal difficulties	Incorporation of specific resources to support abstinence and improve interpersonal relatedness
Behavioral	Reinforcement of abstinence-promoting behaviors; punishment of undesirable behaviors	Specific behavior modification	Prevention of specific responses
Insight-oriented psychotherapy	Exploration and interpretation of group and individual processes	Promotion of ability to tolerate distressing feelings without resorting to alcohol	Increased insight and improved ability to tolerate stress
Supportive	Specific support offered to individuals, to enable them to draw on their own resources	Promotion of adaptation to alcohol-free living	Improved self-confidence and incorporation of specific recommendations

"style" (defined as the way in which the group's goals and processes are linked) is not merely one of academic importance. For example, Harticollis (1980) found that psychoanalytical groups are widely regarded as inadequate and are not recommended for active substance abusers because of the counterproductive degree of anxiety they generate. An early study by Ends and Page (1957) demonstrated that the style of a group of alcoholics predicted treatment outcome. In this study, alcoholics were assigned to one of several groups with different designs. Group styles varied from one group, described as relatively unfocused and "client-centered," whose leader avoided a dominant role and instead promoted interpersonal processes among the group members, to another group based on learning theory, whose leader assumed a dominant role, offered only conditional support, and focused strongly on punishment and reward. At follow-up, those alcoholics treated in the client-centered group fared far better than those in the confrontational group.

Descriptions of Some Representative Group Models

Exploratory and Supportive Groups

An interesting model, the modified dynamic group psychotherapy, developed by Khantzian, allows for the identification of individuals' vulnerabilities and problems within a context of "safety." Abstinence is strongly endorsed, and the group, which requires an active style of leadership, promotes mutual support and outreach, and constantly strives to identify and manage contingencies for relapse. According to Cooper (1987), psychotherapeutic groups based on exploration and interpretation aim at forging members' increased ability to tolerate higher levels of distressing feelings without resorting to mood-altering substances. In contrast, purely supportive treatment groups' aim is to help addicted group members tolerate abstinence and assist them in remaining chemical-free, without necessarily understanding the determinants of their addiction.

The Interactional Group Model

Yalom (1985) described an important group style in which therapy is conducted in weekly 90-minute meetings of eight to 10 members who, under the leadership of two trained group therapists, are encouraged to explore their interpersonal relationships with the group leaders and the other members. An effort is made to create an environment of safety, cohesion, and trust, in which members engage in in-depth self-disclosure and affective expression. The goal of the group is not abstinence but the understanding and working through of interpersonal conflicts. (However, "improvement" without abstinence is often illusory.) In fact, groups of alcoholics are oriented away from an explicit discussion of drinking. The leaders emphasize that they do not see the group as the main instrument for achieving abstinence, and patients are encouraged to attend AA or to seek other forms of treatment for this purpose. Within this format, a group member can be described as "improved" along a series of 19 possible areas of growth, irrespective of the severity of his or her drinking.

This interactional model was further developed by Vannicelli (1982; Vannicelli et al., 1984), who, unlike Yalom (1985), recommends that the group leaders strongly support abstinence as essential to the patient's eventual emotional stability. The group leaders firmly endorse simultaneous use of other supports, such as AA and Antabuse (disulfiram) therapy. In contrast to working with neurotics, whose anxieties provide motivation and direction for treatment, the leaders of such a group of alcoholics are forced to intervene to provide limits and focus without generation of more anxiety than necessary. The group therapists resist members' inquiries into the leaders' drinking habits by instead exploring patients' underlying concerns about whether they will be helped and understood. Patients who miss early group sessions are actively sought out and brought back into the group. Confrontation (particularly of actively drinking members) is used sparingly and only with the aim of providing better understanding of the behavior, thus promoting growth and the necessary goal of activity changes.

Interpersonal Problem-Solving Skills Group

According to Jehoda (1958), interpersonal problem-solving skills groups are based on the premise that the capacity to solve problems in life determines quality of mental health. Several empirical studies lend some support to this assumption, suggesting that there is a relation between cognitive interpersonal problem-solving skills and psychological adjustment. These groups have been implemented for alcoholics (Intagliata, 1978) and heroin addicts (Platt, Scura, & Hannon, 1973) with some degree of success. Usually problem-solving skill groups are run for a limited number of sessions (frequently 10) and are organized to teach a several-step approach to interpersonal problem solving. Most often, such steps include the following: (1) recognize that a problem exists, (2) define the problem, (3) generate several possible solutions, and (4) select the best alternative after determining the likely consequences of each of the available possible solutions to the problem. Follow-up studies determined that groups with this format were effective in generating specific skills such as anticipating and planning ahead for problems, even following discharge from the treatment programs. The value of problem-solving skills groups with respect to other primary modalities of addiction treatment, however, remains to be determined. It is unclear, for instance, whether these groups contribute to the overall rates of abstinence achieved in inpatient and outpatient treatment programs.

Educational Groups

Educational groups represent important ancillary treatment modalities in substance abuse treatment, not only for addicts but for their relatives and other social contacts. The obvious purpose of these groups is to provide information on issues relevant to specific addictions, such as the natural course and medical consequences of alcoholism, the implications of intravenous addiction for sexual contacts and the family, the availability of community resources, and so forth. Often, educational groups provide opportunities for cognitive reframing and behavioral changes along specific guidelines. These groups are often welcomed by some treatment-resistant addicts and alcoholics who cannot cooperate with other forms of therapy. More often than not, educational groups offer structured, group-specific, didactic material delivered by different means, including videotapes, audiocassettes, or lectures; these presentations are followed by discussions led by an experienced and knowledgeable leader.

Activity Groups

Like educational groups, activity groups constitute another important ancillary modality in the treatment of alcoholics and other addicts. Unlike educational groups, however, patient participation is the main goal of activity groups, which can evolve around a variety of occupational and recreational avenues. In a safe and sober context, the addict can expedite socialization, recreation, and self- and group expression. Activity groups are often the source of valuable insight into patients' deficits and assets, both of which may go undetected by treatment staff members concerned with more narrowly focused treatment interventions, such as psychotherapists and nurses. When appropriately designed, activity groups may constitute invaluable sources of self-discovery, self-esteem, and newly acquired skills that facilitate sober social interactions.

Other groups also promote the acquisition of specific skills, such as those devoted to reviewing relapse prevention techniques and those aimed at building social skills. These groups are particularly helpful in the early stages of the rehabilitation process of the alcoholic patient.

Groups with Methadone-Maintenance Patients

Groups with methadone-maintenance patients experience problems that relate more to the structure of the therapy than to the group content. Encouragement is always needed for patients to participate in these groups. Often, groups for these patients are an efficient way of coping with problems under professional guidance and peers' support (Ben-Yehuda, 1980). These groups generally go through several stages: the development of esprit de corps, the division of labor, the establishment of group cohesion, and the development of outside-the-group relations.

Relationship of Group Therapy to Individual Treatment

It is not a surprise that group therapists maintain that group treatment is the treatment of choice for alcoholics and other addicts (Matano & Yalom, 1991). In support of this, group therapists such as Kanas (1982) invoke not only the difficulty that these patients have in developing an "analyzable transference neurosis" in individual therapy but also their tendency to act out impulsively—characteristics that are better addressed in the anxiety-diffusing context of a group setting. Alcoholics, for example, are often seen as being orally fixated with resulting "narcissistic, passive–dependent, and depressive personality traits" (Feibel, 1960). Platt et al. (1973) and Feibel (1960) pointed out that individual insight-oriented psychotherapy is often said to be contraindicated in addicts, because the following problems often present in these patients: intolerance of anxiety, episodes of rage and self-destructive behavior as a result of frustrated infantile needs, poor impulse control, and (probably most importantly) the tendency to develop a primitive transference toward the therapist.

Pfeffer, Friedland, and Wortis (1949) describe an undeniable advantage of group therapy over individual treatment—namely, the easily generated peer pressure, which can often promote behavioral changes and a reduction of denial of addiction and interpersonal difficulties. In addition, peer-generated support often satisfies narcissistic and dependency needs. Primitive, intense transferences are often avoided in the group setting because of diffusion among the other members of the group. The tendency to leave treatment prematurely in individual therapy is often countered by the group's ability to promote a reduction of anxiety and to generate a therapeutic alliance with not only the leader but also the other group members. As stated previously, it is important when deciding between group and individual therapy to assess both the patient's ability to tolerate and benefit from social interactions and his or her level of cognitive and psychological functioning. Patients with moderate cognitive deficits, or paranoid or other psychotic disorders are likely to become isolated or hostile and to leave the group setting prematurely.

What follows is a clinical example of the success of group therapy in a case in which individual therapy had no impact.

> At the time of referral, "A" was a 45-year-old white male, employed as an administrator. He was married and had children. His chief complaints were frequent mood changes of many years' duration and unprovoked bouts of anger often directed at his wife, children, and coworkers. Although he had no history of psychiatric or medical

problems, he reluctantly acknowledged that his wife thought he drank too much and that his boss had strongly demanded that he do something about his angry outbursts and poor job attendance. The patient was referred for individual therapy, but initial attempts at establishing a therapeutic relationship failed. He displayed markedly narcissistic personality traits, which resulted in an often disruptive relationship with the therapist, and he had difficulty in recognizing any interpersonal and mood problems associated with his alcohol consumption. The patient, however, acknowledged drinking more and more often than what was "healthy" for him. His motivation for treatment derived from his determination to maintain his current employment and his interest in learning how to avoid depressive thinking.

Both the patient and the therapist felt that no progress was being made in individual therapy, and the therapist then referred the patient to alcoholism group treatment. In the group, the patient was exposed to other group members' descriptions of their problems with mood and social relations. On two occasions during the beginning phases of his involvement with the group, he came to the group while intoxicated. The threat of expulsion from the group in the face of these intoxications brought into focus the similar situation he faced at work, where his drinking was also jeopardizing his ability to remain employed. Confronted by group members and therapists alike, he eventually identified a relationship between his drinking and his angry outbursts at home and at work. From the outset, his drinking was interpreted by other group members as a reflection of his alcoholism rather than the expression of psychological conflicts. After a few months in treatment, this patient finally felt that he indeed was an alcoholic. The absence of drinking was associated with a total remission of depressive moods. He eventually made a commitment to abstinence, and he has remained in group treatment for several years.

Management of Group Members Who Do Not Remain Abstinent

Drinking by some group members is to be expected in alcoholic groups. Full-blown slips or covert drinking by any group member interrupts the group process, elicits drinking-related thoughts and behaviors in other members, and requires specific and prompt intervention by the group leader. Often, however, a well-managed drinking episode represents an invaluable learning opportunity for all group members. A slip is not in itself cause for dismissal from the group. A resumption of drinking illustrates to all members the importance of prompt identification and interruption of denial and the need to constantly ensure the effectiveness of selected measures for maintaining abstinence. Responsibility for the slip should be defined to the group as resting entirely on the patient who is drinking and not on any past event or interaction between other group members.

Drinking can assume different forms, depending on whether it is acknowledged or denied by the person and whether, despite the drinking, the group member professes adherence to the group norms regarding abstinence and self-disclosure. Those patients who keep drinking and express no intention to stop should be asked to leave the group. Dismissal from the group is best explained to the patient and to the other group members as justified by the person's present drinking behavior. Readmission into the group once the patient is willing to accept the group norms, including a commitment to achieving abstinence, should always be offered to a patient who is leaving the group. A different approach should be adopted with patients who express a desire to end the relapse and agree to participate in a discussion within the group of their active drinking. Initially, any information from any source (within or outside the group) that a group member is drinking should be immediately shared with all members. If the patient is intoxicated, he or she needs to be asked to leave the group and to return sober to the following session. The next meeting should serve as an occasion to explore feelings about drinking behavior and denial. At this point, the group norms are reiterated; if necessary, specific contingency contracts with the drinking member are drawn up.

Another presentation of the problem is the patient who drinks yet refuses to acknowledge it. It should be part of the group contract that any important information concerning drinking behavior by a group member should be shared with the group. In the face of contrasting versions of a patient's behavior, clarification should be sought from the patient in a way that facilitates "voluntary" disclosure. Eventually, it may be necessary to confront the patient directly; if denial persists, the patient should leave the group.

Other Group Treatment Considerations

Group psychotherapy based on interpersonal and interpretive approaches rests in part on the self-medication hypothesis, which contends that substance abuse should be understood as the outcome of efforts at self-medication of distressing symptoms (Cooper, 1987; Khantzian, 1989). Recent challenges to this theory, however, suggest that drug abuse (particularly abuse of cocaine) may not necessarily be related to attempts at self-medication (Castañeda, Galanter, & Franco, 1989). Accordingly, it is advisable that group leaders be knowledgeable about addiction and able to anticipate that addicted group members may display drug-seeking behaviors that can best be regarded as conditioned responses (triggered by specific internal or environmental cues, such as the sight of a bottle or feelings of euphoria and celebration) rather than attempts on the part of the addict at dealing with emotional conflict (Galanter & Castañeda, 1985).

SELF-HELP, 12-STEP GROUPS, AND 12-STEP FACILITATION

Role of Self-Helps Groups in Addiction Treatment

Self-help groups represent a widely available resource for the treatment of alcoholism, as well as other forms of chemical dependency. AA and other 12-step organizations such as NA and Cocaine Anonymous (CA) have not only provided a large population of addicts with support and guidance but also have contributed conceptually to the field of understanding and treating substance abuse. However, important questions for the clinician and the researcher need to be answered before the proper role of 12-step programs in the treatment of addicts can be established. In what ways are such self-help programs compatible with professional care? In what ways do these groups achieve their effects? For which patients are they most useful? Familiarity with self-help groups is essential both for the clinician providing care for substance abusers and the researcher attempting to understand psychosocial factors involved in the outcome of addictions.

History of Self-Help Programs

Self-help groups can be understood as a grassroots response to a perceived need for services and support (Levy, 1976; Tracy & Gussow, 1976). In this sense, AA is the prototypical organization; it provided a model for the other successful groups, such as NA and CA, as well as its more closely related offspring such as Al-Anon, Alateen, and Children of Alcoholics. Levy (1976) proposed a rough division of self-help groups in two types of organizations: type I groups, which are truly mutual help organizations and include all 12-step programs, and type II groups, which more frequently operate as foundations and place more emphasis on promoting biomedical research, fundraising, public education, and legislative and lobbying activities. Type I and type II groups are by no means totally exclusive, as type I associations promote public education, and type II groups sometimes provide direct services.

The development of AA has exerted a major influence on the self-help movement in general. The next section is concerned only with the development of AA and related 12-step programs for addictions, which are clearly defined as type I associations.

Origins and Growth of Alcoholics Anonymous

AA's principal founder, "Bill W.," in accordance with the AA tradition of anonymity, was himself an alcoholic. Bill was spiritually influenced by a drinking friend, Edwin Thatcher, who belonged to the Oxford Group, an evangelical religious sect (Kurtz, 1982). Thatcher, usually referred to as Ebby, attributed his abstinence to his involvement with the Oxford Group, which displayed many of the characteristics later adopted by AA, such as open confessions and guidance from members of the group. Bill W. continued to drink despite his encounter with Ebby in 1934, but he felt that there was a kinship of common suffering among alcoholics. During his final hospital detoxification, he experienced an altered state of consciousness characterized by a strong feeling of proximity with God, which gave him a sense of mission to help other alcoholics achieve sobriety.

Bill's initial efforts to influence other alcoholics were unsuccessful until May 1935, when he met another member of the Oxford Group, "Dr. Bob," who a month later achieved sobriety and became the cofounder of AA. The number of alcoholics who experienced spiritual recovery and achieved sobriety in AA progressively increased; in 1939, when group membership reached 100, they published *Alcoholics Anonymous*, the book that became the bible for the movement (Galanter, 1989). AA institutionalized practices such as a 90-day induction period, sponsorship relationships, the "12 Steps," and recruitment for the fellowship. The expansion and stability of the organization resulted from its "12 Traditions," which avoid concentration of power within the organization, prevent involvement of AA with other causes, maintain the anonymity of its membership, and preserve the neutrality of the association in relation to controversial issues. Its membership continued to grow; AA is now a global organization, reported to have more than 75,000 informal groups in the United States and 114 other countries, with a membership estimated at 1.5 million. The birth and development of NA illustrate how AA provided a model to other self-help programs for addictions.

History and Approach of Narcotics Anonymous

Although the NA program was first applied to drug addiction at the U.S. Public Health Service Hospital at Lexington, Kentucky, in 1947, an NA group, independent of any institution and formed by AA members who were addicts in Sun Valley, California in 1953, expanded and gave NA its current form (Peyrot, 1985). The Sun Valley NA group did not identify itself with a program organized in New York City in 1948 by Dan Carlson, an addict formerly exposed to the Lexington program, because the Sun Valley founders felt that NA should strictly adhere to AA's 12 steps and 12 traditions by not identifying itself with any specific agency and by not accepting government funds.

There are a few differences between AA and NA. NA members usually use illegal drugs, in contrast to most AA members who, until recently, could be described as traditional alcoholics. Also, instead of using the term "alcoholism," NA refers to its problem as "addiction" and addresses the entire range of abusable psychoactive substances. There is, however, a clear overlap of approach and membership between the organizations, despite their complete independence of each other. Following in the footsteps of AA, NA has experienced fast-paced growth. It became an international organization, present in at least 36 countries, with a probable membership of 250,000. According to the NA World Service Office, which publishes NA literature and centralizes information within NA, the growth rate of the organization's membership has been 30–40% a year (Wells, 1987). The growth of NA and other 12-step programs demonstrates the organizational strength and appeal of the AA model.

How 12-Step Programs Work

Participation in a 12-step program can start at the moment the addict meets a member of an organization, reads its literature, or simply attends meetings (e.g., an open meeting or an institutional meeting run by AA or NA speakers; Galanter, 1989). A desire to stop drinking and/or abusing other drugs is the only requirement for membership. Total abstinence becomes a goal from the outset of the participation in the fellowship. Initial participation turns into an induction period, which, in the case of AA, for instance, lasts 90 days and encourages daily attendance at meetings. The member is exposed to the 12-step approach to recovery; the First Step consists of admitting powerlessness over the addiction, and consequently breaking with denial. Seeking sponsorship from another member who has been sober for months (preferably more than a year) is also encouraged. Sponsors are usually of the same sex if the group is large enough, so that emotional entanglements can be avoided to keep from distracting the members from the purpose of attaining and maintaining sobriety. Open meetings usually consist of talks by a leader and two or three speakers, who share their experiences of how the 12-step program related to their recovery.

The 12-step program is an attempt to effect changes in addicts' lives that go beyond just stopping the use of substances—changes in personal values and interpersonal behavior, as well as continued participation in the fellowship. The 12 steps are studied and followed with the guidance of a sponsor and participation in meetings focused on each step. Each step involves changes in behavior and attitudes that may profoundly affect the addict's life. To achieve the Ninth Step, for instance, the addict makes amends to people formerly harmed by his or her behavior. These amends may result in changes in the way in which the person relates to others and interprets the problems that have affected past and present relationships. For instance, an alcoholic man may "talk" to the deceased father he or she formerly hated and attempt a "conciliation" with the image of his or her dead father. The Twelfth Step encourages propagation of the group's philosophy and consequently fosters the individual's recovery by providing opportunities to others to recover and expand the fellowship.

Traditionally, 12-step meetings are open to all members, but they may be directed to special interest groups (e.g., gays, women, minority groups, and physicians). Meetings can be of different types, such as discussions, study of the 12 steps, and testimonials; some are open to nonmembers, and others are for members only. If the recovery progresses, the member learns strategies to avoid relapse (e.g., "One day at a time"), obtains help from other members, and eventually helps fellow addicts in their recovery. By helping other addicts and by sponsoring newcomers to the program, the individual is helping him- or herself by becoming more involved with the recovery process and the organization's philosophy.

Why 12-Step Programs Work

It is still unclear why 12-step programs can help people exposed to them. From an existential perspective, AA, for instance, encourages acceptance of one's finitude and essential limitation by conveying the idea of powerlessness over alcohol. On the other hand, one can go beyond this limitation by relating to others and sharing some of the painful aspects of human existence. Kurtz (1982) emphasized that consistency in thought and action is crucial to maintaining a conscious effort to be honest with oneself and others. This effort produces an increased awareness of one's own needs for growth. AA stresses the need for consistency in thought and action in all stages of its recovery program.

From a learning theory perspective, the group selectively reinforces social and cognitive behaviors that usually are incompatible with the addictive behavior. Attendance at meetings is basically incompatible with using the same time to drink or abuse other drugs. Achievements resulting from sobriety are generously praised, and strategies of self-monitoring and self-control are constantly reinforced through constant interactions with others attempting to remain sober. Self-monitoring of emotions and behaviors is enhanced by helping the addict to detect reactions to certain internal and external stimuli (craving, distress with interpersonal problems, denial in the presence of depressive feelings, unrealistic goals when under pressure, etc.). In addition to self-monitoring, self-control is enhanced by learning a new repertoire of cognitive and social behaviors, such as attending more meetings when craving increases, using the 12 steps to cope with stressful life events, and obtaining group support to face painful feelings about oneself and others. Other theoretical perspectives used to understand 12-step programs include operant and social learning views; however, because experimentation with the processes involved in participation in 12-step programs is an almost impossible proposition, the use of learning models remains largely descriptive and speculative.

OUTCOME STUDIES

Group Treatment Outcomes

The immense popularity of group treatment and self-help for alcoholics and other substance abusers preceded the availability of significant numbers of controlled outcome studies (Bowers & al-Rheda, 1990; Cooney et al., 1991; Kang, Kleinman, & Woody, 1991; Poldrugo & Forti, 1988; Yalom, 1985). Yalom (1985) reported significant improvement at 8-month and 1-year follow-ups of both alcoholics and neurotics treated in weekly interactional group therapy. Improvement was measured along specific variables, however, and not according to the quality of abstinence eventually attained by the group members. In an early report, Ends and Page (1957) compared the outcome effects on alcoholics of several group therapy designs, including groups based on learning theory, client-centered (supportive) groups, psychoanalytical groups, and nonpsychotherapy discussion groups. They found that both client-centered and psychoanalytical groups yielded better outcomes than did discussion groups and groups based on learning theory, as measured by improvement in self-concept at a 1-year follow-up. Client-centered groups also were associated with lower rates of readmission than all other groups in this and a subsequent study. Mindlin and Belden (1965) studied the attitudes of hospitalized alcoholics before and after participation in group psychotherapy, occupational groups, or no-group treatment and found that group psychotherapy significantly improved motivation for treatment and attitude toward alcoholism.

The 1998 report by the Institute of Medicine, "Bridging the Gap between Research and Practice," has spurred on the development and evaluation of evidence-based therapies (Marinelli-Casey, Domier, & Rawson, 2002). The past 10 years have seen a large increase in the number and quality of clinical trials (e.g., Magura et al., 2003; Meyers, Miller, Smith, & Tonigan, 2002; Petry, Martin, & Finocche, 2001; Marques & Formigoni, 2001; Ouimett et al., 2001; Charney, Paraherakis, & Gill, 2001). Many of these studies examine heretofore understudied populations, such as those with co-occurring substance dependence and other major mental illness, serious medical conditions, and or polysubstance dependence. Studies have been designed to test the effectiveness of a variety of group treatment approaches. The feasibility of both their transfer from research to clinical settings, and from individual to group formats, has been investigated (Petry & Simcic, 2002; Carroll et al., 2002; Hanson, Leshner, & Tai, 2002; Carise, Cornely, & Gurel, 2002; Van Horn & Bux, 2001; Foote et al., 1999). While some of the more ambitious protocols, such as those developed via the Clinical Trials Network (CTN), are still undergoing various phases of implementation, there is widespread optimism that group therapy will soon be established on a much firmer empirical foundation than was true in the past.

Some of the approaches that have been receiving significant attention in terms of adaptation to group format, standardization, and dissemination include motivational enhancement therapy (MET; see Miller, Zweben, DiClemente, & Rychtarik, 1994), cognitive-behavioral coping skills therapy (CBST; often referred to as "relapse prevention"; see Kadden et al., 1995; for an update, see Longabaugh & Morgenstern, 1999), and 12-step facilitation (TSF, discussed below).

Self-Help and Treatment Outcome

AA Outcome

AA has received more attention from investigators studying outcome variables than other 12-step programs. Consequently, most of our knowledge about the impact of 12-step programs on the lives of addicts is limited to the effects of AA on some samples of alcoholics. The structure of 12-step organizations and their emphasis on anonymity make scientific research on these groups a very difficult task (Glaser & Osborne, 1982). Investigators have studied outcome variables related to participation in AA, such as severity of drinking, personality traits, attendance at meetings, total abstinence versus controlled drinking as a therapeutic goal, and concomitance of AA attendance with professional care (Elal-Lawrence, Slade, & Dewey, 1987; Seixas, Washburn, & Eisen, 1988; Thurstin, Alfano, & Nerviano, 1987; Thurstin, Alfano, & Sherer, 1986).

The first variable to deserve attention is that those alcoholics who join AA are not representative of the total population of alcoholics receiving treatment (Emrick, 1987). AA members tend to be, as common sense would indicate, more sociable and affiliative. Studies also suggest that AA members have more severe problems resulting from their drinking and experience more guilt regarding their behavior. Attendance at meetings has been associated in some studies (Emrick, 1987) with better outcome, although the nature of this association remains unclear. Thurstin et al. (1986) found no clear personality traits that might seem to be associated with AA membership, but they reported that success among members appears to be related to less depression, less anxiety, and better sociability. AA seems not to benefit those who can become nonproblem users and may actually be detrimental to patients who can learn to control their drinking (Emrick, 1987). AA members who receive other forms of treatment concomitantly with their participation in AA meetings probably do better.

As noted earlier, several problems make it difficult to study outcome factors related to participation in 12-step programs. One is the changing composition of AA membership: more women, younger people, and multiply addicted alcoholics that have been joining the organization. The heterogeneity of addictive disorders, the anonymity of membership, the impossibility of experimentation with components of the programs, the self-selection factor in affiliation, and the lack of appropriate group controls all impose serious methodological difficulties in evaluating outcome variables. For clinical purposes, the benefit of membership in self-help groups has to be empirically evaluated for each individual patient.

12-Step Facilitation

TSF is a manualized individual counseling method that was developed for use in Project MATCH (Anonymous, 1997), a large multicenter study of the effect of customizing alcoholism treatment to individual needs. It describes a type of therapy in which the goal is to engender patients' active participation in AA. It regards such active involvement as the main treatment element promoting sobriety. The study found it to be effective, and equal to other treatments employed, namely, MET and CBST (Nowinski, Baker, & Carroll, 1995).

Institutional Self-Help Treatment Groups

Most ambulatory programs for substance abuse treatment are modeled after ones used in general psychiatric clinics. They rely primarily on professionally conducted individual and small-group therapy. Whether there are more cost-effective options or more potent ones has yet to be fully explored. One alternative approach to conventional institutional treatment is based on psychological influence in a self-help group context and is designed to allow for decreased staffing. Such an approach to group treatment is designed to draw on the principles of zealous group psychology observed in freestanding self-help approaches to addictive illness, such as those of AA and the drug-free therapeutic communities, but at the same time serves as the primary group-based modality employed in an institutional treatment setting. In other words, it can be employed in institutional settings such as hospitals and clinics and still capture the psychological effect of freestanding self-help groups.

In a study of this treatment model (Galanter, 1982, 1983), primary therapists were social workers and paraprofessionals experienced in alcoholism treatment, supervised by attending psychiatrists. There was one social worker and one paraprofessional treating patients in the experimental self-help treatment program, and two members of each of the latter disciplines treating the controls; the self-help program therefore operated at half the usual staffing level. The program included an alcohol clinic attached to an inpatient detoxification unit.

The control and the experimental self-help programs illustrate the contrast between institution-based self-help groups and conventional care. In the study (Galanter, 1982, 1983), the programs operated simultaneously and independently in the outpatient department. Therapists in each program were encouraged to perfect their respective clinical approaches, and each group of therapists received clinical supervision appropriate to its own needs and experience. Differences between the two programs are outlined here to illustrate the operation of institutionally grounded self-help group care.

ORIENTATION PROGRAM

In the control (traditional) group setting, two primary therapists served as co-leaders of a group for their own patients, and attendance in each session ranged between eight and 15 participants. In the self-help program, the same format was used, but groups were led by patients of the primary therapists who had established sobriety and had demonstrated a measure of social stability over several months. These "senior patients" monitored the progress of patients in the orientation group and were supervised by the primary therapists, who attended the orientation for part of each session, participating in a limited fashion only. A patient in crisis might be invited to return to the orientation group if this invitation was seen as helpful.

GROUP THERAPY

Weekly group meetings were oriented toward practical life issues among controls, but insight was encouraged; progress toward abstinence was a major theme. The two primary therapists served as facilitators for the group, using their own empathic manner to encourage mutual acceptance and support. When confrontation was necessary, the therapists undertook it in a forthright but supportive manner. In the self-help program, groups met with the same frequency, but senior patients assumed the leadership role. Primary therapists attended part of each session and participated intermittently; they served, however, primarily in a coordinating capacity for these groups and supervised the senior patients. Patients were encouraged to deal with unusual problems by recourse to their peers in the program, either in their therapy group or through senior patients.

PEER THERAPY

Self-help program patients were made aware that the primary source of support in the clinic was the peer group. New patients were encouraged to seek out peers and senior patients who would be available to assist them throughout the program. Senior patients were supervised in assisting with crises when this assistance was judged clinically appropriate by the primary therapists. The senior patient program was operated in the self-help modality. Potential senior patients were screened for sobriety and social stability, and assisted in patient management of the program for a time-limited period. Those who served as group leaders met weekly as a group with the primary therapists, focusing on their therapeutic functions in the unit. Under supervision of the therapists, they directed orientation, therapy, and activity groups. Their interventions in more difficult patients' problems were reviewed with the primary therapists, and they referred self-help patients to their respective primary therapists for more troublesome problems. Other senior patients had administrative functions in the program.

Meetings of the full patient complement also took place in the self-help program. A monthly evening meeting, open to all patients, served as a focus for group spirit and as a context for organizing recreational activities. The meetings were run collaboratively by staff and senior patients, with programwide activities and patients' progress as the focus. Socialization at the time of these meetings focused on the status of patients' recovery.

OUTCOME AND COMMENTS

Two outcome studies (Galanter, 1982, 1983) of this project found that the experimental program, with half the staffing of the traditional modality, was quite viable in a municipal hospital alcoholism treatment program. Furthermore, retention of inpatients upon transfer to the alcohol clinic was 38% greater than in the control (non-self-help) program; rates of abstinence in outpatients were no less, and social adjustment over the course of a 12-month follow-up was enhanced. Therefore, the self-help format appears to offer a format for institutional treatment that is less expensive and potentially more effective.

This case example that follows illustrates the ethos of the self-help program.

A 36-year-old outpatient came to the clinic intoxicated, without a scheduled visit, and asked to speak with a senior patient he knew well. He had been in outpatient treatment for 8 months and had been abstinent for the last 4 months. Five days earlier, he had begun drinking subsequent to a crisis in his family and had missed his group meeting. He gave a history of falling down a staircase earlier in the day, bruising his head. The senior patient he had asked to see and another were present, and they encouraged him to seek a medical evaluation. The case was then reviewed with the primary therapist, who saw him briefly, wrote a referral for medical assessment, and returned him to the two senior patients' care. After an hour, the senior patients prevailed on him to go with one of them to the emergency service. The other took him on the following afternoon to a meeting of an AA group he had previously attended. The patient was able to maintain abstinence until his next weekly group therapy meeting, at which time a group member offered to get together with him during the ensuing week to provide him with some encouragement.

Given a need for increased substance abuse treatment services, it is important to note that counseling staff members (social workers and counselors) comprise 66% of the personnel in all federally assisted alcoholism treatment facilities, which constitute the bulk of publicly supported programs (Vischi, Jones, Shank, & Lima, 1980). The question then arises as to whether these counseling staffers are used in the most cost-effective way. One problematic aspect of this issue is illustrated by Paredes and Gregory's (1979) finding that in alcoholism treatment programs, the economic resources invested in alcoholism treatment are not positively correlated with outcome. They concluded that the type and quantity of therapeutic resources invested are related to the characteristics of the agencies themselves rather than to a treatment strategy conceived for optimal cost-effectiveness.

Two issues common to most small-group therapies for substance abuse in the clinic setting are relevant here. In the first place, whether behavioral, insight-oriented, or directive, they all focus on the concerns of a relatively small number of patients involved in the therapy group (typically six to 10), to the exclusion of other program participants. Second, it is generally agreed that such small-group therapy for alcoholics offers a better outcome when conducted in the context of a multimodal program. Such a program may integrate treatment components to implement a carefully structured plan, as described by Hunt and Azrin (1973).

These two aspects of small-group therapy may be considered in relation to a self-help–oriented treatment program such as the one described previously. With regard to group size, such a program introduces the option of the patients' strong identification with and sense of cohesion in a treatment network of many more than six to 10 patients. In fact, it encourages affiliative feelings among the full complement of self-help patients, providing an experience of a large, zealous group (Galanter, 1989). This cohesion is promoted by therapeutic contact with a number of senior patients who are involved in the therapy groups; by programwide patient-run activities, such as the orientation groups open to patients in crisis; and in monthly large-group meetings, also open to all patients. This broader identification forms the bulwark of a self-help orientation.

Self-Help Groups and the Clinician

The relationship between professional treatment and membership in a 12-step group has been less than systematically addressed. Clark (1987) proposed guidelines to orient the clinician. Clearly, acquaintance with 12-step programs is essential for the clinician to orient patients regarding their needs and response to possible conflicts between the nature and goals of professional care, and the demands of participation in self-help organizations. Clinicians treating addicts can learn about 12-step programs by attending local meetings, by becoming familiar with fellowship literature, and by exploring patients' experiences in the context of their membership in these organizations.

One point deserving emphasis is that physicians should be aware of the danger of prescribing habit-forming substances to addicts because of not only the inherent dangers involved in the use of these substances, but also the goals of programs that demand complete avoidance of chemical solutions for life's problems (Zweben, 1987). When psychotropic medication is strongly recommended, the benefits and risks involved in their use should be carefully discussed with the patient in the context of the 12-step program goals. An occasional sponsor may be opposed to any medication, even when a patient clearly needs pharmacological treatment to alleviate disabling behavioral or physical conditions. In this situation, the clinician has to address the nature of the conflict involved in the treatment by making the needed medical treatment compatible with the program philosophy. This desirable goal can only be achieved when the clinician is well informed about the nature of 12-step programs and can help the patient to integrate the rationale for medical treatment with the general goals of his or her membership in the self-help program. Avoidance of prescribing drugs with habit-forming potential, willingness to educate patients about the nature of their problems, and a positive attitude toward 12-step organizations make it easier for clinicians to integrate their interventions with the orientation of the fellowship. Candidates for controlled drinking should not be encouraged to participate in abstinence-oriented programs, because the incompatibility of the goals of professional treatment with a 12-step orientation may prove to be very detrimental to therapy (Emrick, 1987).

Clinicians should, in general, encourage their patients' exposure to 12-step programs, but they should remember that a large number of addicts who never participate in these organizations can make good use of professional treatment and successfully recover. Because the composition of the membership of self-help groups continually changes, it is possible for patients treated with psychotropic medication, including methadone, to benefit from participation in these groups (Obuchowsky & Zweben, 1987).

THE NETWORK THERAPY TECHNIQUE

Overview

This approach can be useful in addressing a broad range of addicted patients characterized by the following clinical hallmarks of addictive illness. When they initiate consumption of their addictive agent, be it alcohol, cocaine, opiates, or depressant drugs, they frequently cannot limit that consumption to a reasonable and predictable level; this phenomenon has been termed "loss of control" by clinicians who treat alcohol- or drug-dependent persons (Jellinek, 1963). Second, they consistently demonstrate relapse to the agent of abuse, that is, they attempted to stop using the drug for varying periods of time but returned to it, despite a specific intent to avoid it.

This treatment approach is not necessary for those abusers who can, in fact, learn to set limits on their use of alcohol or drugs; their abuse may be treated as a behavioral symptom in a more traditional psychotherapeutic fashion. Nor is it directed at those patients for whom the addictive pattern is most unmanageable (e.g., addicted people with unusual destabilizing circumstances such as homelessness, severe character pathology, or psychosis). These patients may need special supportive care (e.g., inpatient detoxification or long-term residential treatment).

Key Elements of Network Therapy

Three elements are essential to the network therapy technique. The first is a cognitive-behavioral approach to relapse prevention, independently reported to be valuable in addiction treatment (Marlatt & Gordon, 1985). Emphasis in this approach is placed on triggers to relapse and behavioral techniques for avoiding them rather than on exploring underlying psychodynamic issues.

Second, support of the patient's natural social network is engaged in treatment. Peer support in AA has long been shown to be an effective vehicle for promoting abstinence, and the idea of the therapist's intervention with family and friends at the start of treatment was employed in one of the early ambulatory techniques specific to addiction (Johnson, 1986). The involvement of spouses (McCrady, Stout, Noel, Abrams, & Fisher-Nelson, 1991) has since been shown to be effective in enhancing the outcome of professional therapy.

Third, the orchestration of resources to provide community reinforcement suggests a more robust treatment intervention by providing support for drug-free rehabilitation (Azrin, Sisson, & Meyers, 1982). In this relation, Khantzian (1988) points to the "primary care therapist" as one who functions in direct coordinating and monitoring roles in order to combine psychotherapeutic and self-help elements. It is this overall management role over circumstances outside, as well as inside, the office session that is presented to trainees to maximize the effectiveness of the intervention.

Starting a Network

Patients should be asked to bring their spouse or a close friend to the first session. Alcoholic patients often dislike certain things they hear when they first come for treatment and may deny or rationalize even if they voluntarily sought help. Because of their denial, a significant other is essential to both history taking and implementing a viable treatment plan. A close relative or spouse can often cut through the denial in a way that an unfamiliar therapist cannot and may therefore be invaluable in setting a standard of realism in dealing with the addiction.

Once the patient comes for an appointment, establishing a network is a task undertaken with active collaboration of patient and therapist. The two, aided by those parties who join the network initially, must search for the right balance of members. The therapist must carefully promote the choice of appropriate network members, however, just as the platoon leader selects those who will go into combat.

Defining the Network's Task

As conceived here, the therapist's relationship to the network is like that of a task-oriented team leader rather than that of a family therapist oriented toward insight. The network is established to implement a straightforward task: aiding the therapist in sustaining the patient's abstinence. It must be directed with the same clarity of purpose that a task force is directed in any effective organization. Competing and alternative goals must be suppressed or at least prevented from interfering with the primary task.

Unlike family members involved in traditional family therapy, network members are not led to expect symptom relief for themselves or self-realization. This lack of expectation prevents the development of competing goals for the network's meetings. It also provides the members protection from having their own motives scrutinized and thereby supports their continuing involvement without the threat of an assault on their psychological defenses.

Adapting Individual Therapy to the Network Treatment

Of primary importance is the need to address exposure to substances of abuse or to cues that might precipitate alcohol or drug use (Galanter, 1993). Both patient and therapist should be sensitive to this matter and explore these situations as they arise. Second, a stable social context in an appropriate social environment—one that is conducive to abstinence with minimal disruption of life circumstances—should be supported. Considerations of minor disruptions in place of residence, friends, or job need not be a primary issue for the patient with a character disorder or neurosis, but they cannot go untended here. For a considerable period, the substance abuser is highly vulnerable to exacerbations of the addictive illness and, in some respects, must be viewed with the considerable caution with which one treats the recently compensated psychotic.

Study on Training Naïve Therapists

A course of training for psychiatric residents who are naive to addiction and ambulatory treatments was undertaken over a period of 2 academic years. Before beginning treatment, the residents were given a structured treatment manual for network therapy and participated in a 13-session seminar on application of the network therapy technique. Cocaine-abusing patients were eligible for treatment in this study if they could come for evaluation with a friend or family member who could participate in their treatment. In all, 22 patients were enrolled. The treating psychiatric residents were able to establish requisite networks for 20 of these patients (i.e., a network with at least one member). The networks had an average of 2.3 members, and the most typical configuration included family members and friends. Supervisors' evaluation of videotapes of the network sessions employing standardized instruments indicated good adherence to the manualized treatment, with effective use of network therapy techniques. The outcome of treatment (Galanter, Keller, & Dermatis, 1997; Galanter, Dermatis, Keller, & Trujillo, 2002; Keller, Galanter, & Weinberg, 1997) reflected retention and abstinence rates as good as, or better than, comparable ambulatory care carried out by therapists experienced in addiction treatment. The study demonstrated the feasibility of teaching the network technique to therapists naive to addiction treatment.

Research on the Network Approach

Copello et al. (2002) combined elements of network therapy with social aspects of the community reinforcement approach and relapse prevention, referred to as social behavior and network therapy (SBNT), in the treatment of persons with alcohol drinking problems. A number of social skills training strategies are incorporated into the treatment, especially those involving social competence in relation to the development of positive social support for change in alcohol use. Every individual involved in treatment is considered a client in his or her own right, and the person with alcohol problems is referred to as the focal client. The core element of the approach is mobilizing the support of the network, even though this may involve network sessions that are conducted in the absence of the focal client.

This approach was extended to a large sample of alcoholics in the U.K. Alcohol Treatment Trial (UKATT) project. The UKATT team evaluated the cost-effectiveness of network therapy (NT) relative to MET. SBNT resulted in a fivefold cost savings in health, social, and criminal justice service expenditures and was similar to cost-effectiveness estimates obtained for MET. The UKATT Research Team (2008) tested a priori hypotheses concerning client–treatment matching effects similar to those tested in Project MATCH. The findings were consistent with Project MATCH in that no hypothesized matching effects were significant. Orford et al. (2009) interviewed a subset of clients ($n = 397$) who participated in this trial to assess their views concerning whether any positive changes in drinking behavior had occurred and to what they attributed those changes. Three months after randomization to treatment, NT clients made more social attributions (e.g., involvement of others in supporting behavior change), and MET clients made more motivational attributions (e.g., awareness of the consequences of drinking).

Galanter et al. (2004) evaluated the impact of NT relative to a control condition (medical management, MM) among 66 patients inducted into buprenorphine treatment for 16 weeks, then tapered to zero dose. NT resulted in a greater percentage of opioid-free urines than did MM (65 vs. 45%). By the end of treatment, NT patients were more likely to experience a positive outcome relative to secondary heroin use (50 vs. 23%). The use of NT in office practice may enhance the effectiveness of eliminating secondary heroin use during buprenorphine maintenance.

REFERENCES

Anonymous. (1997). Matching alcoholism treatments to client heterogeneity: Project MATCH posttreatment drinking outcomes. *J Stud Alcohol, 58,* 7–29.

Azrin, N. H., Sisson, R. W., & Meyers, R. (1982). Alcoholism treatment by disulfiram and community reinforcement therapy. *J Behav Ther Exp Psychiatry, 13,* 105–112.

Ben-Yehuda, N. (1980). Group therapy with methadone-maintained patients: Structural problems and solutions. *Int J Group Psychother, 30,* 331–345.

Bowers, T. G., & al-Rheda, M. R. (1990). A comparison of outcome with group/marital and standard/individual therapies with alcoholics. *J Stud Alcohol, 51,* 301–309.

Carise, D., Cornely, W., & Gurel, O. (2002) A successful researcher–practitioner collaboration in substance abuse treatment. *J Subst Abuse Treat, 23,* 157–162.

Carroll, K. M., Nich, C., Sifry, R. L., Nuro, K. F., Frankforter, T. L., Ball, S. A., et al. (2002). A general system for evaluating therapist adherence and competence in psychotherapy research in the addictions. *Drug Alcohol Depend, 57,* 225–238.

Castañeda, R., Galanter, M., & Franco, H. (1989). Self-medication among addicts with primary psychiatric disorders. *Compr Psychiatry, 30,* 80–83.

Charney, D. A., Paraherakis, A. M., & Gill, K. J. (2001). Integrated treatment of comorbid depression and substance use disorders. *J Clin Psychiatry, 62,* 672–677.

Clark, H. W. (1987). On professional therapists and Alcoholics Anonymous. *J Psychoactive Drugs, 19,* 233–242.

Cooney, N. L., Kadden, R. M., Litt, M. D., & Getter, H. (1991). Matching alcoholics to coping skills or interactional therapies: Two-year follow-up results. *J Consult Clin Psychol, 59,* 598–601.

Cooper, D. E. (1987). The role of group psychotherapy in the treatment of substance abusers. *Am J Psychother, 41,* 55–67.

Copello, A., Orford, J., Hodgson, R., Tober, G., Barrett, C., & UKATT Research Team Alcohol Treatment Trial. (2002). Social behavior and network therapy: Basic principles and early experiences. *Addict Behav, 27,* 345–366.

Elal-Lawrence, G., Slade, P. D., & Dewey, M. E. (1987). Treatment and follow-up variables discriminating abstainers, controlled drinkers and relapsers. *J Stud Alcohol, 48,* 39–46.

Emrick, C. D. (1987). Alcoholics Anonymous: Affiliation processes and effectiveness as treatment. *Alcohol Clin Exp Res, 11,* 416–442.

Ends, E. J., & Page, C. W. (1957). A study of three types of group psychotherapy with hospitalized male inebriates. *Q J Stud Alcohol, 18,* 263–277.

Feibel, C. (1960). The archaic personality structure of alcoholics and its indications for therapy. *Int J Group Psychother, 10,* 39–45.

Foote, J., DeLuca, A., Magura, S., Warner, A., Grand, A., Rosenblum, A., et al. (1999). A group motivational treatment for chemical dependency. *J Subst Abuse Treat, 17,* 181–192.

Galanter, M. (1982). Overview: Charismatic religious sects and psychiatry. *Am J Psychiatry, 139,* 1539–1548.

Galanter, M. (1983). Engaged members of the Unification Church: The impact of a charismatic group on adaptation and behavior. *Arch Gen Psychiatry, 40,* 1197–1202.

Galanter, M. (1989). *Cults: Faith, healing and coercion.* New York: Oxford University Press.

Galanter, M. (1993). Network therapy for addiction: A model for office practice. *Am J Psychiatry, 150,* 28–36.

Galanter, M., & Castañeda, R. (1985). Self-destructive behavior in the substance abuser. *Psychiatr Clin North Am, 8,* 251–261.

Galanter, M., Castañeda, R., & Ferman, J. (1988). Substance abuse among general psychiatric patients: Place of presentation, diagnosis and treatment. *Am J Drug Alcohol Abuse, 14,* 211–235.

Galanter, M., Dermatis, H., Glickman, L., Maslanksy R., Sellers, M. B., Neumann, E., et al. (2004). Network therapy: decreased secondary opioid use during buprenorphine maintenance. *J Subst Abuse Treat, 26,* 313–318.

Galanter, M., Dermatis, H., Keller, D., & Trujillo, M. (2002). Network therapy for cocaine abuse: Use of family and peer supports. *Am J Addict, 11,* 161–166.

Galanter, M., Keller, D., & Dermatis, H. (1997). Network therapy for addiction: Assessment of the clinical outcome of training. *Am J Drug Alcohol Abuse, 23,* 355–367.

Glaser, F. B., & Osborne, A. (1982). Does AA really work? *Br J Addict, 77,* 123–129.

Hanson, G. R., Leshner, A. I., & Tai, B. (2002). Putting drug abuse research to use in real-life settings. *J Subst Abuse Treat, 23,* 69–70.

Harticollis, P. (1980). Alcoholism, borderline and narcissistic disorders: A psychoanalytic overview. In W. Fann (Ed.), *Phenomenology and treatment of alcoholism* (pp. 93–110). New York: Spectrum.

Hunt, G. M., & Azrin, N. H. (1973). A community-reinforcement approach to alcoholism. *Behav Res Ther, 11,* 91–104.

Intagliata, J. C. (1978). Increasing the interpersonal problem-solving skills of an alcoholic population. *J Consult Clin Psychol, 46,* 489–498.

Jehoda, M. (1958). *Current concepts in positive mental health.* New York: Basic Books.

Jellinek, E. M. (1963). *The disease concept of alcoholism.* New Haven, CT: Hillhouse.

Johnson, V. E. (1986). *Intervention: How to help someone who doesn't want help.* Minneapolis, MN: Johnson Institute.

Kadden, R., Carroll, K. M., Donovan, D., Cooney, N., Monti, P., Abrams, D., et al. (1995). *Cognitive-behavioral coping skills therapy manual: A clinical research guide for therapists treating individuals with alcohol abuse and dependence.* Rockville, MD: National Institute on Alcohol Abuse and Alcoholism.

Kanas, N. (1982). Alcoholism and group psychotherapy. In E. Kauffman & M. Pattison (Eds.), *Comprehensive textbook of alcoholism* (pp. 1011–1021). New York: Gardner Press.

Kang, S. Y., Kleinman, P. H., & Woody, G. E. (1991). Outcomes for cocaine abusers after once-a-week psychosocial therapy. *Am J Psychiatry, 131,* 160–164.

Keller, D. S., Galanter, M., & Weinberg, S. (1997). Validation of a scale for network therapy: A technique for systematic use of peer and family support in addition treatment. *Am J Drug Alcohol Abuse, 23,* 115–127.

Khantzian, E. J. (1988). The primary care therapist and patient needs in substance abuse treatment. *Am J Drug Alcohol Abuse, 14*(2), 159–167.

Khantzian, E. J. (1989). The self-medication hypothesis for substance abusers. *Am J Psychiatry, 30,* 81–83.

Kurtz, E. (1982). Why AA works. *J Stud Alcohol, 43,* 38–80.

Levy, L. H. (1976). Self-help health groups: Types and psychological processes. *J Appl Behav Sci, 12,* 310–322.

Longabaugh, R., & Morgenstern, J. (1999). Cognitive-behavioral coping-skills therapy for alcohol dependence. Current status and future directions. *Alcohol Res Health, 23,* 78–85.

Magura, S., Laudet, A. B., Mahmood, D., Rosenblum, A., Vogel, H. S., & Knight, E. L. (2003). Role of self-help processes in achieving abstinence among dually diagnosed persons. *Addict Behav, 28,* 399–413.

Marinelli-Casey, P., Domier, C. P., & Rawson, R. A. (2002). The gap between research and practice in substance abuse treatment. *Psychiatr Serv, 53,* 984–987.

Marlatt, G. A., & Gordon, J. R. (Eds.). (1985). *Relapse prevention: Maintenance strategies in the treatment of addictive behaviors.* New York: Guilford Press.

Marques, A. C., & Formigoni, M. L. (2001). Comparison of individual and group cognitive-behavioral therapy for alcohol and/or drug-dependent patients. *Addiction, 96,* 835–846.

Matano, R. N., & Yalom, I. D. (1991). Approaches to chemical dependency: Chemical dependency and interactive group therapy—a synthesis. *Int J Group Psychother, 41,* 269–293.

McCrady, B. S., Stout, R., Noel, N., Abrams, D., & Fisher-Nelson, H. (1991). Effectiveness of three types of spouse-involved behavioral alcoholism treatment. *Br J Addict, 86,* 1415–1424.

Meyers, R. J., Miller, W. R., Smith, J. E., & Tonigan, J. S. (2002). A randomized trial of two methods for engaging treatment-refusing drug users through concerned significant others. *J Consult Clin Psychol, 70,*1182–1185.

Miller, W. R., Zweben, A., DiClemente, C. C., & Rychtarik, R. G. (1994). *Motivational enhancement therapy manual: A clinical research guide for therapists treating individuals with alcohol abuse and dependence.* Rockville MD: National Institute on Alcohol Abuse and Alcoholism.

Mindlin, D. F., & Belden, E. (1965). Attitude changes with alcoholics in group therapy. *CA Ment Health Rev Digest, 3,* 102–103.

Minkoff, K., & Drake, R. E. (Eds.). (1991). *Dual diagnosis of major mental illness and substance abuse disorder.* San Francisco: Jossey-Bass.

Nowinski, J., Baker, S., & Carroll, K. M. (1995). *Twelve step facilitation therapy manual: A clinical research guide for therapists treating individuals with alcohol abuse and dependence.* Rockville, MD: National Institute on Alcohol Abuse and Alcoholism.

Obuchowsky, M. A., & Zweben, J. E. (1987). Bridging the gap: The methadone client in 12-step programs. *J Psychoactive Drugs, 19,* 301–302.

Orford, J., Hodgson, R., Copello, A., Wilton, S., Slegg, G., & UKATT Research Team. (2009). To what factors do clients attribute change?: Content analysis of follow-up interviews with clients of the UK treatment trial. *J Subst Abuse Treat, 36,* 49–58.

Ouimette, P., Humphreys, K., Moos, R. H., Finney, J. W., Cronkite, R., & Federman. B. (2001). Self-help group participation among substance use disorder patients with posttraumatic stress disorder. *J Subst Abuse Treat, 20,* 25–32.

Paredes, A., & Gregory, D. (1979). Therapeutic impact and fiscal investment in alcoholism services. In M. Galanter (Ed.), *Currents in alcoholism* (Vol. 4, pp. 441–456). New York: Grune & Stratton.

Petry, N. M., Martin, B., & Finocche, C. (2001). Contingency management in group treatment: A demonstration project in an HIV drop-in center. *J Subst Abuse Treat, 21,* 89–96.

Petry, N. M., & Simcic, F., Jr. (2002). Recent advances in the dissemination of contingency management techniques: Clinical and research perspectives. *J Subst Abuse Treat, 23,* 81–86.

Peyrot, M. (1985). Narcotics Anonymous: Its history, structure, and approach. *Int J Addict, 20,* 1509–1522.

Pfeffer, A. Z., Friedland, P., & Wortis, S. B. (1949). Group psychotherapy with alcoholics. *Q J Stud Alcohol, 10,* 198–216.

Platt, J. J., Scura, W., & Hannon, J. R. (1973). Problem-solving thinking of youthful incarcerated heroin addicts. *J Community Psychol, 1,* 278–281.

Poldrugo, F., & Forti, B. (1988). Personality disorders and alcoholism treatment outcome. *Drug Alcohol Depend, 21,* 171–176.

Seixas, F., Washburn, S., & Eisen, S. V. (1988). Alcoholism, Alcoholics Anonymous attendance, and outcome in a prison system. *Am J Drug Alcohol Abuse, 14,* 515–524.

Thurstin, A. H., Alfano, A. M., & Nerviano, V. J. (1987). The efficacy of AA attendance for aftercare of inpatient alcoholics: Some follow-up data. *Int J Addict, 22,* 1083–1090.

Thurstin, A. H., Alfano, A. M., & Sherer, M. (1986). Pretreatment MMPI profiles of AA members and non-members. *J Stud Alcohol, 47,* 468–471.

Tracy, G. S., & Gussow, Z. (1976). Self-help health groups: A grass roots response to a need for services. *J Appl Behav Sci, 12,* 381–396.

UKATT Research Team. (2008). UK Alcohol Treatment Trial: Client treatment matching effects. *Addiction, 103,* 223–238.

Van Horn, D. H., & Bux, D. A. (2001). A pilot test of motivational interviewing groups for dually diagnosed inpatients. *J Subst Abuse Treat, 20,* 191–195.

Vannicelli, M. (1982). Group psychotherapy with alcoholics: Special techniques. *J Stud Alcohol, 43,* 17–37.

Vannicelli, M., Canning, D., & Griefen, M. (1984). Group therapy with alcoholics: A group case study. *Int J Group Psychother, 34,* 127–147.

Vischi, T. R., Jones, K. R., Shank, E. L., & Lima, L. H. (1980). *The alcohol, drug abuse and mental health national data book* (DHHS Publication No. 80-983). Washington, DC: U.S. Government Printing Office.

Wells, B. (1987). Narcotics Anonymous (NA): The phenomenal growth of an important resource [Editorial]. *Br J Addict, 82,* 581–582.

Yalom, I. D. (1985). *The theory and practice of group psychotherapy* (3rd ed.). New York: Basic Books.

Zweben, J. E. (1987). Can the patient on medication be sent to 12-step programs? *J Psychoactive Drugs, 19,* 299–300.

CHAPTER 29

Family Therapy Approaches

EDWARD KAUFMAN

Drug abuse has a profound effect on the family, and the family is a critical factor in the treatment of drug abuse.

This chapter presents definitions of typologies of families, as well as an integrative approach to the multiple forms of family treatment and outcome studies of these different types of treatment as currently practiced. Families may be traditional, extended, or elected. Family systems and dynamics are greatly influenced by many factors, including age, gender, ethnicity, culture, social class, and choice of substances of abuse. Family therapy may include the substance abuser and his or her partner, the entire family or part of it, or groups of families, or it may be family-focused with any individual in the family. Types of family therapy described include structural–strategic, cognitive-behavioral, multidimensional, and my structural–psychodynamic system.

Dealing with the family also represents involvement with the patient's ecosystem, which may include the treatment team, 12-step groups, sponsors, peers, employers, employee assistance program (EAP) counselors, managed care workers, parole officers, and other members of the legal system. Upon entering treatment, the family is generally the most critical part of this ecosystem. In family therapy, I have defined three basic phases of the family's involvement in treatment: (1) developing a system for establishing and maintaining a drug-free state, (2) establishing a workable method of family therapy, and (3) dealing with the family's readjustment after the cessation of drug abuse. I discuss these three phases, with an emphasis on variations in treatment techniques to meet the needs of different types of drug-abusing individuals.

EFFICACY OF FAMILY THERAPY IN DRUG ABUSE TREATMENT

Family therapy outcome studies, including my own, began in the 1970s with little sophistication, but they indicate that even multiple-family therapies may reduce recidivism by 50% (Kaufman, 1985).

Stanton and Todd (1982) provided the field with an early controlled study of family therapy for drug abuse. They emphasized concrete behavioral changes, including a focus on family rules about drug-related behavior and the use of weekly urine tests to give tangible indications of progress. They focused on interrupting and altering the repetitive family interactional patterns that maintain drug taking. In their family therapy groups, Stanton and Todd found at 1-year follow-up that days free of methadone, illegal opioids, and marijuana all shifted favorably, compared with non-family-therapy groups. McCrady et al. (1986) compared the effect of family therapy on drinking behavior and life satisfaction in three treatment groups: (1) minimal spouse involvement, with interventions directed toward the drinker, although the spouse was present; (2) alcohol-focused spouse involvement emphasizing coping skills for alcohol-related situations; and (3) alcohol-focused behavioral marital therapy addressing the need to modify the marital relationship. Results showed better compliance, a faster decrease in drinking, greater likelihood of staying in treatment, and more marital satisfaction posttreatment in the subjects receiving alcohol-focused behavioral marital therapy.

Cognitive-behavioral skills training has continued to be successful, as evaluated in several studies of family treatment of drug abuse (Maisto, McKay, & O'Farrell, 1995; Monti et al., 1990; Nakamura & Takano, 1991). Inclusion of the family, particularly in the treatment of drug abuse in adolescents, has been associated consistently with greater improvement relative to drug abuse and family function (Alexander & Gwyther, 1995; Enders & Mercier, 1993) that is sustained and enhanced 2 years after completion of treatment.

Positive family function predicts success in drug abuse treatment, particularly to the extent to which family members are encouraged to be assertive and self-sufficient (Friedman, Utada, & Morrissey, 1987). Home-based multisystemic therapy with drug-abusing delinquents greatly enhanced completion of a full course of therapy (98%) compared to treatment through usual community services, in which completion was minimal (Henggeler, Pickrel, Brondino, & Crouch, 1996).

In the first decade of the 21st century, family-based treatment became the most thoroughly studied behavioral treatment modality for substance abuse, particularly with adolescents. Many randomized, well-controlled, long-term studies utilizing standardized manuals have been reported from that period and are summarized by Hogue and Liddle (2009).

Significant effects have been found for multidimensional, cognitive-behavioral, and functional family therapy, while brief strategic, behavioral, and multisystemic therapies were all classified as "probably efficacious." Notably, important influences on success were ethnicity-based treatment, therapeutic alliance, treatment fidelity (to model), and targeting problematic parent–adolescent interactions (e.g., actively blocking, diverting, or working through negative emotions; amplifying feelings of

sadness, regret, and loss; and prompting parent–adolescent conversation on important topics were associated with successful resolution of family impasses observed in
treatment sessions; Hogue & Liddle, 2009).

DEVELOPING A SYSTEM FOR ACHIEVING
AND MAINTAINING ABSTINENCE

The family treatment of drug abuse begins with development of a system to achieve
and maintain abstinence. This system, together with specific family therapeutic techniques and knowledge of patterns commonly seen in families with a drug-abusing
member (also known as the identified patient, or IP), provides a workable therapeutic
approach to drug abuse.

Family treatment of drug abuse must begin with an assessment of the extent of
drug dependence and the difficulties it presents for the individual and the family. The
quantification of the individual's drug abuse history can take place with the entire
family present; the IP often will be honest in this setting, and "confession" is a helpful way to begin communication. Moreover, other family members often provide
more accurate information that the IP. However, some IPs give an accurate history
only when interviewed alone. In taking a drug abuse history, the clinician should
determine the IP's current and past use of every type of abusable drug, including
alcohol. Other past or present drug-abusing family members may be identified, and
their drug use and its consequences should be quantified without putting the family
on the defensive. It is also essential to document the family's patterns of reactivity,
codependency, and enabling of drug use and abuse. The specific method necessary to
achieve abstinence can be decided on only after the extent and nature of drug abuse
are quantified.

Establishing a System for Achieving Abstinence

It is critical to establish a system for enabling the IP to become a drug free, so that
effective family therapy can take place. The specific methods used to achieve abstinence vary according to the extent of use, abuse, and dependence. Mild to moderate
abuse in adolescents can often be controlled if both parents agree on clear limits and
expectations, and on how to enforce them. Older abusing individuals may sometimes
stop if they are made aware of the medical or psychological consequences to themselves or the effects on their families.

If drug abuse is moderately severe or intermittent and without physical dependence, such as intermittent use of hallucinogens or weekend cocaine abuse, then the
family can be offered a variety of measures, such as regular attendance at Narcotics
Anonymous (NA) or Cocaine Anonymous (CA) for the IP, and Al-Anon, Co-Anon,
or Nar-Anon for family members.

If the abuse pattern is severe, then hospitalization or, as established more recently,
community–residential high-intensity treatment programs should be set as a requirement very early in therapy.

Establishing a System for Maintaining Abstinence

The family is urged to adopt some system that will enable the IP to continue to stay drug free. The system is part of the therapeutic contract made early in treatment. A lifetime commitment to abstinence is not required. Rather, the "one day at a time" approach of AA is recommended. The patient is asked to establish a system for abstinence, which is renewed daily using the basic principles of NA and CA. When the patient has a history of drug dependence, therapy is most successful when total abstinence is advocated.

Many individuals initially have to shop around for 12-step groups in which they personally feel comfortable. Every recovering patient is strongly encouraged to attend small study groups that work on the 12 Steps, and larger meetings that often feature inspirational speakers and are open to anyone, including family members. Abstinence can also be achieved in heroin-addicted individuals by drug-aided measures such as methadone maintenance, Suboxone, Vivitrol, or naltrexone blockade. These medications work quite well in conjunction with family therapy, because work with the family enhances compliance, and the blocking effects on the primary drug of abuse help to calm the family system so that family and individual therapy can take place. Institutionalization also calms an overreactive family system. Another advantage of this modality is that it provides an intensive 24-hour per day orientation to treatment.

Individuals who have been dependent on illicit drugs for more than a few years generally do not do well in short-term programs, although these programs may buy time so that effective individual and family therapy can occur. For drug-dependent patients who fail in outpatient and short-term hospital programs, insistence on long-term residential treatment is the only workable alternative. Most families, however, will not accept this approach until other methods have failed. To accomplish this end, a therapist must be willing to maintain long-term ties with the family, even through multiple treatment failures. However, it may be more helpful to terminate treatment if the patient continues to abuse drugs, because continued family treatment implies that change is occurring when it is not. Families that believe therapy is being terminated in their best interest often return a few months or years later, ready and willing to commit to abstinence from drugs of abuse (Kaufman, 1985).

WORKING WITH FAMILIES IN WHICH DRUG ABUSE CONTINUES

The family therapist is in a unique position in regard to continued drug abuse and other manifestations of the IP's resistance to treatment, including total nonparticipation. The family therapist still has a workable and highly motivated patient: the family. A technique that can be used with an absent or highly resistant patient is the *intervention* (Johnson, 1980), which was developed for use with alcoholic patients but can be adapted readily for drug-abusing patients, particularly those who are middle class, employed, involved with their nuclear families, and not acutely paranoid.

FAMILY DIAGNOSIS

Accurate diagnosis is as important a cornerstone in family therapy as it is in individual therapy. In family diagnosis, we examine familial interactional and communication patterns and relationships. In assessing a family, we examine the family rules, boundaries, and adaptability. We look for coalitions (particularly transgenerational ones), shifting alliances, splits, cutoffs, and triangulation. We observe communication patterns, confirmation and disconfirmation, unclear messages, and conflict resolution. We note the family's stage in the family life cycle. We note *mind reading* (i.e., predicting reactions and reacting to them before they happen, or knowing what someone thinks or wants), double binds, and fighting styles. It is often helpful to obtain an abbreviated three-generation genogram that focuses on the IP, his or her parents and progeny, and the IP's spouse's parents.

OVERVIEW OF FAMILY THERAPY TECHNIQUES

Structural–Strategic Family Therapy

In structural–strategic family therapy, the structural and strategic types of family therapy are combined, because they were developed by many of the same practitioners, and these therapists, depending on the family's needs, frequently shift between the two therapy types. The thrust of structural family therapy is to restructure the system by creating interactional change within the session. The therapist actively becomes a part of the family yet retains sufficient autonomy to restructure the family (Stanton, 1981).

According to strategic therapists, symptoms are maladaptive attempts to deal with difficulties that develop a homeostatic life of their own and continue to regulate family transactions. The strategic therapist works to substitute new behavior patterns for the destructive repetitive cycles. The therapist is responsible for planning a strategy to solve the family's problems. Techniques used by strategic therapists include the following (Stanton, 1981):

- Putting the problem in solvable form.
- Placing considerable emphasis on change outside the sessions.
- Learning to take the path of least resistance, so that the family's existing behaviors are used positively.
- Using the paradox (described later in this chapter), including restraining change and exaggerating family roles.
- Allowing the change to occur in stages. The therapist may create a new problem, so that solving it leads to solving the original problem. The family hierarchy may be shifted to a different, abnormal one before reorganizes into a new functional hierarchy.
- Using metaphorical directives in which the family members do not know they have received a directive.

Stanton and Todd (1982) successfully used an integrated structural–strategic approach with heroin-addicted patients who were receiving methadone maintenance.

Case Example: Joining and Establishing Boundaries

THE FAMILY

The client, a 22-year-old white female who abused prescribed medication and had problems with depression and a thought disorder, is the younger of two children whose parents divorced when the client was age 3. She stayed with her mother, while her brother (age 7 at the time) went with their father. Both parents remarried within a few years. Initially, the families lived near each other; both parents were actively involved with both children, despite ill feelings between the parents. When the client was 7, her stepfather was transferred to a location 4 hours away, and the client's interactions with her father and stepmother were curtailed. Animosity between the parents escalated. When the client was 8, she chose to live with her father, brother, and stepmother, and the mother agreed. The arrangement almost completely severed ties between the parents. When the client entered a psychiatric unit for detoxification, the parents had no communication at all. The initial family contact was with the father and stepmother. As the story unfolded, it became clear that the client had constructed different stories for the two family subsystems of parents. She has artfully played one against the other. This was possible because the birth parents did not communicate.

TREATMENT

The first task was to persuade the father to contact the mother and request that she attend a family meeting. He, along with the stepmother, agreed, though it took great courage to make the request, because the father believed his daughter's negative stories about her relationship with the mother. In the next session, the older brother (the intermediary for the past 4 years) and his wife also attended. Because the relationship between the counselor and the paternal subsystem had already been established, it was critical also to join with the maternal subsystem before attempting any family system work. The counselor knew that nothing could be accomplished until the mother and stepfather felt they had equal parental status in the group. This goal was reached, granting the mother free rein to tell the story as she saw it and express her beliefs about what was happening. A second task was to establish appropriate boundaries in the family system. Specifically, the counselor sought to join the separate parental subsystems into a single subsystem of adult parents and to remove the client's brother and sister-in-law as part of that subsystem. The exclusion was accomplished by leaving them and the client out of the first part of the meeting. This procedural action realigned the family boundaries, placing the client and her brother in a subsystem different from that of the parents. This activity proved to be positive and productive. By the end of the first hour of a 3-hour session, the parents were comparing information, noting incorrect assumptions about each other's beliefs and behaviors, and forming a healthy, reliable, and cooperative support system that would work for the good of their daughter. This outcome would have been impossible without taking the time to join with the mother and father in a way that allowed them to feel equal as parents. Removing the brother from the parental subsystem required the client to deal directly with the parents, who had committed themselves to communicating with each other and to speaking to their daughter in a single voice (Center for Substance Abuse Treatment, 2004).

Cognitive-Behavioral Family Therapy

McCrady et al. (1986) developed seven steps in the therapy of couples with alcoholism that can be applied to married, drug-abusing adults and their families:

1. Functional analysis. Families are taught to understand the interactions that maintain drug abuse.
2. Stimulus control. Drug use is viewed as a habit triggered by certain antecedents and maintained by certain consequences. The family is taught to avoid or change these triggers.
3. Rearranging contingencies. The family is taught techniques to provide reinforcement for efforts at achieving a drug-free state by frequent review of positive and negative consequences of drug use by self-contracting for goals and specific rewards for achieving these goals. Covert reinforcement is accomplished by rehearsing fantasy a scene in which the IP resists a strong urge to use drugs.
4. Cognitive restructuring. IPs are taught to question their self-derogatory, retaliatory, or guilt-related thoughts and replace them with more rational ideation.
5. Planning alternatives to drug use. IPs are taught techniques for refusing drugs through role playing and covert reinforcement.
6. Problem solving and assertion. IPs and their families are helped to decide whether a situation calls for an assertive response, then, through role-playing, develop effective assertive techniques.
7. Maintenance planning. The entire course of therapy is reviewed, and the new armamentarium of skills is emphasized. IPs are encouraged to practice these skills regularly and to reread handout materials that explain and reinforce these skills.

Families can also be taught through behavioral techniques to become aware of their nonverbal communication, to make the nonverbal message concordant with the verbal, and to learn to express interpersonal warmth nonverbally and verbally (Stuart, 1971).

Case Example

THE FAMILY

Peter, a 17-year-old white male, was referred for substance abuse treatment. He acknowledged that he drank and smoked marijuana but minimized his substance use. Peter's parents reported that he had come home 1 week earlier with a strong smell of alcohol on his breath. The following morning, when the parents confronted Peter about drinking and drug use, he denied using marijuana steadily, declaring, "It's not a big deal. I just tried marijuana once."

Despite Peter's denial, his parents found three marijuana cigarettes in his bedroom. For at least a year, they had suspected that Peter abused drugs. Their concern was based on Peter's falling grades, his appearance (from meticulous grooming to poor hygiene), and his unprecedented borrowing without repaying.

Peter, his older sister Nancy, age 18, and their parents attended the first two family sessions. During the sessions, Peter revealed that he resented his father's favoritism toward Nancy, an honor student and popular athlete in her school, and the related conflict between the parents about the unequal treatment of Peter and Nancy. The father was often sarcastic and hostile toward Peter, disparaging about his attitude and problems. Peter viewed himself as a failure and experienced depression, frustration, anger, and low self-esteem. Furthermore, Peter wanted to retaliate against his father by causing problems in the family. His substance abuse and falling grades had created a hostile environment at home.

TREATMENT

The counselor used cognitive-behavioral therapy to focus on Peter's irrational thoughts (e.g., viewing himself as a total failure) and to teach Peter and other family members communication and problem-solving skills. The counselor also used behavioral family therapy to strengthen the marital relationship between Peter's parents and to resolve conflicts between family members. Positive treatment outcomes included an improved relationship between Peter and his father, improved academic performance, and cessation of drug use (Center for Substance Abuse Treatment, 2004).

Multidimensional Family Therapy

Liddle and Hogue (2001) developed multidimensional family therapy. Their view of substance abuse is that it is a multidetermined and multidimensional disorder. They use an integrative developmental, environmental, and contextual framework to conceptualize the beginning, progression, and cessation of drug use and abuse. They use knowledge about risk and protective factors to arrive at a case conceptualization that includes and integrates individual, familial, and environmental factors. Both normative (failure to meet developmental challenges and transitions) and non-normative (abuse, trauma, mental health, and substance abuse in the family) crises are instrumental in starting and maintaining adolescent drug problems.

The goals of multidimensional family therapy are

- To facilitate restoring or creating a process of adaptation to the youth's and family's developmentally appropriate functioning.
- To enhance and bolster psychosocial functioning in several realms, including individual developmental adaptation, coping skills relative to drug and problem-solving situations, peer relations, and family relationships.
- To improve adolescent functioning in several realms, including individual developmental adaptation, coping skills relative to drug and problem-solving situations, peer relations, and family relationships.

- To improve parents' functioning in several realms, including their own personal functioning (e.g., substance abuse or mental health issues) and parenting practices.
- To improve family functioning, as evidenced by changes in day-to-day family environment and family transactional patterns.
- To improve adolescent and parent functioning with key extrafamilial systems (e.g., school and juvenile justice systems).

Strategies and Techniques

- The overall therapeutic strategy calls for multilevel, multidomain, multicomponent interventions.
- Treatment is flexible; multidimensional family therapy (MDFT) is a therapy system rather than a one-size-fits-all model. As such, therapy length, number, and frequency of the sessions is determined by the treatment setting, provider, and family.
- Treatment format includes individual and family sessions, and sessions with various and extrafamilial sessions.
- Treatment begins with an in-depth, multisystem assessment that uses a developmental/ecological and risk and protective factor framework.
- Case conceptualization individualizes the treatment system and pinpoints areas of strengths and deficits.

Psychodynamic Family Therapy

A psychodynamic family therapy approach has rarely been applied to IPs, because such patients usually require a more active, limit-setting emphasis on the here and now than is usually associated with psychodynamic techniques. However, if certain basic limitations are kept in mind, psychodynamic principles can be extremely helpful in the family therapy of drug abuse.

The implementation of psychodynamic techniques has three cornerstones: the therapist's self-knowledge, developing an awareness of the therapeutic alliance, and a detailed family history. Family members internalize a therapist's good qualities, such as warmth, trust, trustworthiness, assertion, empathy, and understanding. Likewise, they may incorporate less desirable qualities, such as aggression, despair, and emotional distancing. It is essential that a therapist thoroughly understand his or her own emotional reactions and those of the family.

The following are important elements of psychodynamic family therapy.

Countertransference

A fundamental difference in work with families is that the therapist may have a countertransference problem toward the entire family. We may particularly rally to the defense of our IPs against "oppressive" family members; this can set up power struggles between the therapist and the family.

Judicious expression of countertransference feelings may be helpful in breaking fixed family patterns. For example, sharing anger at a controlling patient may give the family members enough support to express their anger at that patient in a manner that finally has an effect.

Family therapists view their emotional reactions to families in a systems framework and in a countertransference context. Thus, they must be aware of how families replay their problems in therapy by attempting to detour or triangulate their problems onto the therapist. The therapist must be particularly sensitive about becoming an enabler who, like the family, protects or rejects the IP.

The Therapist's Role in Interpretation

Interpretations can be extremely helpful if they are made in a complimentary way, without blaming, inducing guilt, or dwelling on the hopelessness of long-standing, fixed patterns. The therapist can point out to each family member repetitive patterns and their maladaptive aspects, and give tasks to these individuals to help them change these patterns. Some families need interpretations before they can fulfill tasks. An emphasis on mutual responsibility when making any interpretation is an example of a beneficial fusion of structural and psychodynamic therapy (Kaufman, 1985).

Other valuable psychodynamic techniques include awareness and utilization of resistance countertransference and the importance of thoroughly working through conflicts as opposed to the transient, exciting change in high-impact, short-term family therapy so often practiced in residential and hospital 30-day programs.

Case Example of My Integrated System as Used in Multifamily Therapy

A family seen only in multifamily therapy (MFT) included the IP, a 34-year-old Irish male, and a younger sister and brother. The mother had been quite active in MFT but did not attend this session because the family had moved further away. The father had never been present but was frequently discussed because of his pattern of severe withdrawal. The father had not left his bedroom in 3 years and never came out when his son visited. In this session, the son realized how much he had identified with his father's emotional isolation, even to the point of duplicating his posture. He was helped to recognize and experience this rigid control system. His anger toward his father would be a subject for future group work. He also realized how he had attempted to be a "father" to his younger siblings to the point of neglecting his own needs. The sister reached out to him and partially broke though his isolation with her poignant plea for adult intimacy. At this point, another resident began to sob and talk about not being closer to his own sister. He was asked to talk to the first resident's sister as if she were his own. In doing so, he reached a deep level of yearning and anguish. His mother reached out to him and began to rock him. To diminish the infantilization, the therapist asked the mother to not rock him. Freed from his mother, he was able to sob heavily about missing his sister and his guilt in pushing her away. We then returned to the Irish family but were still unable to break though the IP's emotional isolation. It was pointed out that it was difficult for him to express feelings because of his identification with his father and his need to stay in the role of the big brother who had no weaknesses.

Unfortunately, this man repeated his family role in the Therapeutic Community and became a leader before he had worked through his own problems. Several months later he used drugs again and had to begin the program over from the beginning so thathe could recognize and meet his own needs rather than assuming a caretaking "parental sibling" role. This time he more slowly emerged as a leader in the program, but with greater self-knowledge (Kaufman & Kaufmann, 1977).

Case Example of Integrative Individual and Psychodynamic Family Therapy, as Told by the Patient

"We began with private sessions every week and family sessions (my parents and me) once every few weeks. I didn't emote very much in the private sessions, but I would leave feeling a little better than when I came in. In the family sessions, though, I would begin to cry within the first few minutes. I was filled with a pain I had never felt before—not the empty pain I felt while bottoming out on drugs; no, this pain was full and round and great inside of me. I felt worthless; I thought they felt I was worthless. Worthlessness and feeling judged led to anger, but I didn't know how to express anger, particularly with my parents, and so I turned it back on myself. I would judge myself and believe everything they said; I left these sessions feeling terrible, as if my self-esteem had been smashed. I felt lonely, worthless, afraid, hurt.

"I decided I could not participate in family therapy any more. I went to my private session that week and told Ed I couldn't handle another session with my parents; it was undermining my sobriety.

"Ed's reply was the single, most important event in my first year of therapy. He told me I had the mistaken idea that family therapy was a tool only to bring families together. He said my family was dysfunctional and that I needed to break away from them. I was amazed and relieved. I knew intellectually that my parents had problems relating to me, but in my heart I thought the problem was me. If only I could change, the problem would be solved; yet every time I tried to do what they wanted, I invariably felt hurt or angry.

"When Ed planted the 'breaking away' message, I knew he wasn't lying. He validated my feelings and, because of that validation, I not only felt better but I also drew closer to him. I trusted him a little bit more than I had before.

"His validation gave me a new freedom: I could allow myself to feel real anger toward my parents.

"The rest of the first year, I stayed angry with my parents. I took baby steps in not seeking their approval, support, and love, and I started to accept that they were going to continue to hurt me every so often. This education took the form of not calling them all the time. They live 50 miles away, but I would turn to them for what I thought was approval or love. Every week Ed would ask if I had called them, and I would invariably answer, 'Yes'; then he would ask me to recount these conversations. After some time, I realized that my parents always hurt my feelings in these discussions.

"Communicating openly not only helped me to relieve whatever feeling I was experiencing at the time but it also forced me to be myself. I stopped acting out my mother's form of expression of feelings, namely, anger at my father, and began to learn what was appropriate for me.

"My last lesson involves issues I learned about in family therapy. I call these the present issue, the expectation issue, and the showing love issue. The first, the present issue, is my personal favorite. This one depicts my sick family at its best. As an adult, almost all the gifts I have received from my parents have been cultured pearls, even though I *hate* cultured pearls. In fact, I told them this in family therapy.

"However, 3 years after family therapy, my parents returned from a trip to Thailand and Singapore. Thailand is the ruby capital of the world. Before they left for this trip, I said often, 'A ruby ring or little bracelet would really be nice, hint, hint. After all, you'll be back just in time for my birthday.' Well, my parents came back from Thailand and Singapore and what did they get me? A cultured pearl pendant!

"I first learned about false expectations in the family therapy sessions. I learned that sometimes my expectations of my parents are unrealistic and vice versa, but I have had to work diligently at keeping that knowledge alive. Often I have seen myself fall into the expectation trap not only with my parents but also with men in relationships, girlfriends, bosses, and all sort of people with whom I come in contact. My expectations of people can become either unrealistically high or unrealistically low because, I believe, I learned this behavior from my parents. Their expectations of me are either too high or too low.

"My parents expected me to get straight A's all through school and couldn't accept that possibly I was a B student in math. I can remember being tutored by my algebra teacher every day at lunch in the eighth grade because I had a B in his class. If I didn't improve my grade, I couldn't take a dance class I wanted desperately to take. All through high school and college, grades were almost more important to me than the classes. Driven by my parents to excel, I went to one of the finest universities in the country. Even though I was a practicing drug addict there, I still achieved over a B average. The expression of love issue was the easiest problem to resolve. Basically, my father had a great deal of trouble showing love or affections. Ed brought this out openly in family therapy, and I simply asked for more attention. My father immediately took to expressing love and now hugs and kisses me when he sees me; occasionally, he will even hold my hand if we are walking together. This has helped our relationship immensely and he has, to some extent, helped me to express my feelings.

"I believe that I too had trouble expressing love, particularly to my female friends. I was not conscious of it before, but I think my father's attempts at correcting something he felt uncomfortable about helped me to do the same. I can now say, 'I love you,' to my friends, something I always shuddered at before.

"On a deeper level, I think my going through therapy has enabled my father to express his feelings more openly in a number of ways. During my first and second years of therapy, I was asked to speak at several different types of AA and CA meetings and panels. On one of these occasions, I thought it would be nice to invite my parents, Ed, and my sponsor and her husband to hear me speak. I consider it an honor to be asked to tell my story, and I wanted to share this occasion with some of the people I felt close to. I had no idea the experience would be so enlightening.

"On the day I was supposed to speak, my mother got sick with a cold, and my father drove from Los Angeles to Orange County (50 miles in rush hour traffic) without her. At the meeting my father sat near Ed and my sponsor and her husband. My mother called me to tell me how proud she was of herself because she had been sick and had stayed home; I wanted to scream at her over the phone. When I went to see Ed, he began the session by reinforcing my good feelings about speaking. He told me I was great. Then he asked what my parents had said. I told him I thought my father was proud of me and I told him what my mother had said. He commented that it sounded right to him and I asked him why. That was the day I remember learning exactly what a dysfunctional family is all about.

"My mother vies with my sister and me for my father's attention. She cannot handle his giving us more attention than her, so she got sick in order to turn the family attention back to herself. That day I not only learned that my father was capable of feeling pride for his children but that for some reason, either while growing up or throughout my parents' marriage, my mother felt so ignored that she needed to have the family's attention on her constantly. I had to make two decisions: The first was to let my parents know I would no longer accept any kind of money from them; the second was not to sleep in their house.

"After the trip to New York with my parents, I had decided not to accept any more money from them even in the form of paying for air-fare or hotel bills at family weddings. However, I had never actually told them I would no longer accept their money. I let them know this before our trip to Chicago for a cousin's wedding. I don't think I ever enjoyed myself more at a family function than at that wedding, and I am sure it was because I felt no guilt and no pressure about money or doing what everyone else wanted me to do because "they" were paying the bill.

"The second decision—not to sleep at my parent's house—has been difficult. The reason why I cannot stay in their home, really, it's them. They are very critical and negative, and they know no boundaries. In addition, my mother constantly picks on my father. He shuts off his feelings and it all slides off his back. Frustrated, my mother starts to pick on me. Because I experience my feelings today, I become irritated. A friend of mine who came over for dinner one night said afterward that I had learned to build a strong ego because my mother was always attacking me. What he didn't know was how very weak my ego really is.

"In the last year of therapy I came to accept myself—my good traits and my bad traits. I no longer feel at odds with myself because at times I can be very aggressive, loud, and self-obsessed. I know that I am a good person with a lot to give but, like anyone, sometimes my less attractive traits get in the way of that. Today, I am comfortable with who I am.

"It didn't happen in one room, for 1 hour of the week. It was a process of living life as a trial ground for a new person. It was really a process for which AA has coined the perfect phrase: uncover, discover and discard. In therapy I did one more thing: build. Not only did I rid myself of the unnecessary baggage I was carrying around, but I added a wealth of knowledge and happiness to my life" (Kaufman & Kaufmann, 1992).

VARIATIONS IN FAMILY TREATMENT FOR DIFFERENT TYPES OF DRUG-ABUSING PATIENTS

In this section, the modification of treatment typologies necessary for optimal results with abusers of various types of drugs and their families is considered. In family treatment we must consider the needs of at least one other individual and in most cases many others, as we adapt our treatment techniques to each individual family. It is not the drug of abuse per se that demands modification in techniques but rather other variables such as extent and severity of drug abuse, psychopathology, ethnicity, family reactivity, stage of disease, gender, and life cycle (Kaufman, 1985).

Drug Type

Most of the modifications in family treatment that are based on drug type occur in the first phase of treatment, when a system is developed for establishing and maintaining a drug-free state. The more extensive the medical, social and legal history of the consequences of drug and alcohol abuse, the more intensive the system required for abstinence.

Family Reactivity

Drug-abusing families have been categorized according to four types: functional, enmeshed, disintegrated, and absent, each with different needs for family therapy (Kaufman & Pattison, 1981).

Functional Families

Functional families have minimal overt conflict and a limited capacity for insight as they protect their working homeostasis. Thus, the therapist should not be too ambitious about cracking the defensive structure of the family, which is likely to be resistant. The initial use of family education is often well received.

Enmeshed Families

The therapeutic approach used with enmeshed families is much more difficult and prolonged than that used with functional families. Educational and behavioral methods may provide some initial relief but are not likely to have much effect on enmeshed neurotic relationships. Often these families are resistant to ending drug abuse, and the therapist is faced with working with the family while drug abuse continues. The more hostile the enmeshed family interactions, the poorer the prognosis.

Although initial hospitalization or detoxification may achieve temporary abstinence, the IP is highly vulnerable to relapse. Therefore, long-term family therapy with substantial restructuring is required to develop an affiliated family system free of drug abuse. An integrated synthesis of several schools of family therapy techniques may be required.

Because of the enmeshment and explosiveness of these families, the therapist usually must reinforce boundaries, define personal roles, and diminish reactivity. The therapist must be active and directive to keep the emotional tensions within workable limits. Getting family members involved with external support groups can assist disengagement.

Disintegrated Families

Disintegrated families have a history of reasonable vocational function and family life but a progressive deterioration of family function and, finally, separation from the family. The use of family intervention might seem irrelevant in such a case; however, many of these marriages and families have fallen apart only after severe drug-related behavior. Furthermore, there is often only pseudo-individuation (i.e., false individuation by rebellion, which keeps children close to their family of origin through failure) of the patient from marital, family, and kinship ties.

These families cannot and will not reconstitute during the early phases of rehabilitation. When abstinence and personal stability have been achieved over several months, the therapist can work with the family to reestablish family ties, but reconstitution of the family unit is often not a necessary goal.

Absent Families

In absent families systems, there is a total loss of the family of origin and a lack of other permanent relationships. Nevertheless, two types of social network interventions are possible. The first is the elaboration of still-existing friend and relative contacts. Often these social relationships can be revitalized and provide meaningful social support. Second, younger patients have a positive response to peer-group approaches, such as long-term therapeutic communities, NA, church fellowships, and recreational and avocational clubs that draw them into social relationships and vocational rehabilitation.

Gender

Drug abuse treatment in the United States has traditionally been male oriented. In countering this one-sided approach, family therapists must be aware that the families of chemically dependent women demonstrate much greater disturbance than those of male patients seeking treatment. These disturbances include great incidence of chemical dependency of other family members, mental illness, suicide, violence, and physical and sexual abuse. Family-related issues also bring far more women than men into treatment: Potential loss of custody of minor children heads the list (Sutker, 1981).

Because of the difference between the families of drug-abusing men and those of women, family intervention strategies with women must differ from those for men. Family therapy may be more essential for drug-abusing women because of symbolic or often actual losses of spouse and children. The therapist should not impose a stereotyped view of femininity on female patients; this could intensify the conflicts that may have precipitated the drug use (Sandmaier, 1980). The therapist should be sensitive to the specific problems of women and drug-abusing women in our society and should address these issues in treatment.

Drug-abusing women have special concerns about caring for their children. Family therapy may help them see how the parenting role fits into their lives and how to establish parenting skills, perhaps for the first time. Many women have been victimized, including through incest, battering, and rape. Catharsis and understanding these feelings may be essential before a woman can build new relationships or improve her current ties (Kaufman, 1985). Several studies have demonstrated that drug abuse treatment programs that address women's needs and accommodate children have better program retention and treatment outcomes.

For male patients, special issues such as pride and acceptance of their own dependency strivings often need to be addressed (Metsch et al., 1995).

Ethnicity

Ethnicity exerts a powerful effect on family function, styles, roles, and communication patterns, which supersede the differential effects of various drugs. The effects of ethnicity depend on how many generations of the family have lived in the United States and the homogeneity of the neighborhood in which they live. The reader is referred to McGoldrick, Giordano, and Garcia-Preto (2005) for a detailed and comprehensive review of the effects of ethnicity on family systems and family therapy.

Life-Cycle Phase of the Family

Often therapists must deal with several phases of the family cycle simultaneously because of the high frequency of substance abuse in many generations of the same family. The therapy of 15-year-olds will be quite similar regardless of the substance being abused. The treatment of a 45-year-old alcoholic corporate executive may be quite different from that of a 45-year-old heroin-addicted individual because their individual styles and family systems have evolved so differently over a long period of time.

Family therapy with an adolescent IP differs from that with an adult in the following ways: less chronicity and severity, peer group involvement that is not susceptible to parental influence, less criminal activity, and fewer involvements in extrafamilial systems. Families with an adolescent IP invariably experience difficulties in setting appropriate limits on adolescent individuation. The major therapeutic thrust in these families is to help the parents remain unified when setting limits, while permitting flexibility in their negotiating these limits (Fishman, Stanton, & Rossman, 1982).

For a drug-abusing young adult offspring, separation from the family is often a more desirable goal. To achieve this, the therapist must create intensity, escalate stress, and use other strategic unbalancing techniques. In dealing with older adults, the structural–dynamic techniques I described at the beginning of this chapter are more often indicated.

The family therapy of substance-abusing grandparents has barely been addressed. Here it may be critical to involve their children and grandchildren to facilitate the IP's entry into treatment. Once a substance-free state is achieved, the IP grandparent can work toward achieving or reestablishing an executive or consultant position in the hierarchy (Kaufman & Kaufmann, 1992).

REFERENCES

Alexander, D., & Gwyther, R. (1995). Alcoholism in adolescents and their families. *Pediatr Clin North Am, 42*, 217–234.

Center for Substance Abuse Treatment. (2004). Substance abuse treatment and family therapy (DHHS Tip #39). Rockville, MD: Substance Abuse and Mental Health Administration.

Enders, L., & Mercier, J. (1993). Treating chemical dependence: The need for including the family. *Int J Addict, 28*, 507–519.

Fishman, H. C., Stanton, M. D., & Rossman, B. L. (1982). Treating families of adolescent drug abusers. In M. D. Stanton & T. C. Todd (Eds.), *The family therapy of drug abuse and addiction.* New York, Guilford Press.

Friedman, A. S., Utada, A., & Morrissey, M. R. (1987). Families of adolescent drug abusers are "rigid": Are these families either "disengaged" or "enmeshed" or both? *Fam Process, 26,* 131–148.

Henggeler, S., Pickrel, S., Brondino, M., & Crouch, J. L. (1996). Eliminating (almost) treatment dropout of substance abusing or dependent delinquents through home-based multisystemic therapy. *Am J Psychiatry, 153,* 427–428.

Hogue, A., & Liddle, H. A. (2009). Family based treatment for adolescent substance abuse: Controlled trials and new horizons in services research. *J Fam Ther, 31*(2), 126–154.

Johnson, V. A. (1980). *I'll quit tomorrow.* San Francisco: Harper & Row.

Kaufman, E. (1985). *Substance abuse and family therapy.* New York: Grune & Stratton.

Kaufman, E., & Kaufmann, P. (1977). Multiple family therapy: A new direction in the treatment of drug abusers. *Am J Drug Alcohol Abuse, 4,* 467–468.

Kaufman, E., & Kaufmann, P. (1992). *Family therapy of drug and alcohol abuse* (2nd ed.). Boston: Allyn & Bacon.

Kaufman, E., & Pattison, E. M. (1981). Different methods of family therapy in the treatment of alcoholism. *J Stud Alcohol, 42,* 951–971.

Liddle, H. A., & Hogue, A. T. (2001). Multidimensional family therapy: Pursuing empirical support through planful treatment development. In E. Wagner & H. Waldron (Eds.), *Adolescent substance abuse* (pp. 227–259). New York: Elsevier.

Maisto, S., McKay, J., & O'Farrell, T. (1995). Relapse precipitants and behavioral marital therapy. *Addict Behav, 20,* 383–393.

McCrady, B., Noel, N. E., Abrams, D. B., et al. (1986). Comparative effectiveness of three types of spousal involvement in outpatient behavioral alcoholism treatment. *J Stud Alcohol, 47*(6), 459–467.

McGoldrick, M., Giordano, J., & Garcia-Preto, N. (2005). *Ethnicity and family therapy.* New York: Guilford Press.

Metsch, L., Rivers, J., Miller, M., et al. (1995). Implementation of a family centered treatment program for substance abusing women and their children. *J Psychoactive Drugs, 27,* 73–83.

Monti, P., Abrams, D., Binkoff, J., et al. (1990). Communication skills training with family and cognitive behavioral mood management training for alcoholics. *J Stud Alcohol, 51,* 263–270.

Nakamura, K., & Takano, T. (1991). Family involvement for improving the abstinence rate in the rehabilitation process of female alcoholics. *Int J Addict, 26,* 1055–1064.

Sandmaier, M. (1980). *The invisible alcoholics: Women and alcohol abuse in America.* New York: McGraw-Hill.

Stanton, M. D. (1981). An integrated structural/strategic approach to family therapy. *J Marital Family Ther, 7,* 427–439.

Stanton, M. D., & Todd, T. C. (1982). *Family therapy of drug abuse and addiction.* New York: Guilford Press.

Stuart, R. B. (1971). Behavioral contracting within the families of delinquents. *J Behav Ther Exp Psy, 2,* 1–11.

Sutker, P. B. (1981). *Drug dependent women: An overview of the literature* (DHHS Publication No. 81-1177). Washington, DC: National Institute on Drug Abuse.

CHAPTER 30

Motivational Interviewing

JENNIFER L. SMITH
KENNETH M. CARPENTER
R. MORGAN WAIN
EDWARD V. NUNES

This chapter provides a brief overview of the counseling style known as motivational interviewing (MI). MI is an essential skill for clinicians, as it provides a way of working with clients who are ambivalent about changing their behavior, seeking help, or following treatment recommendations—a typical scenario with substance-abusing clients. As clinicians, and particularly as physicians, we are trained to take a history, make a diagnostic assessment, formulate a treatment plan, and prescribe it to the client (e.g., "I recommend that you stop drinking and attend AA meetings"). Unfortunately, if this client is struggling with drinking (wanting to stop on the one hand, but wanting a drink on the other), which is often the case with substance dependent clients, this approach is not likely to engender change. The clinician–client interaction becomes a standoff, or, worse, confrontational ("Come back when you are ready to do something about your problem"). It is frustrating for both parties—the client who does not feel understood, and the clinician who does not know what else to do. MI provides a way of talking with clients that is more collaborative (as opposed to prescriptive or authoritative), more conducive to building a treatment alliance, and ultimately a more supportive context for change.

MI is a complex skill that cannot be fully conveyed by an overview. Ongoing study, training (e.g., participation in workshops), and, ideally, continued supervision and feedback are needed to develop this skill (de Roten, Zimmermann, Ortega, & Despland, 2013; Martino, Canning-Ball, Carroll, & Rounsaville, 2011; Miller & Rose, 2009; Miller, Sorensen, Selzer, & Brigham, 2006; Miller, Yahne, Moyers, Martinez, & Pirritano, 2004; Schoener, Madeja, Henderson, Ondersma, & Janisse, 2006; Smith et al., 2012). A chapter like this one provides an introduction and encourages the reader to pursue further training. Readers are encouraged to study the work of Miller and Rollnick (1991, 2002, 2013), which presents more in-depth discussions of how MI was developed, its implementation, and how it can be utilized in different clinical contexts. Detailed descriptions and guidelines for implementing, mentoring, and supervising MI in clinical settings are provided in the manual, *Motivational Interviewing Assessment: Supervisory Tools for Enhancing Proficiency* (MIA:STEP; Martino et al., 2006). Internet-based resources can be accessed on, for example, the websites of two organizations, each promoting the development and dissemination of MI-related materials: the Motivational Interviewers Network of Trainers (MINT; *motivationalinterviewing.org*) and the Center on Alcoholism, Substance Abuse, and Addictions at the University of New Mexico (CASAA; *http://casaa.unm.edu*).

MI was originally developed to treat nicotine and other substance dependencies. However, it is equally applicable to supporting other psychiatric or medical treatments and other health behaviors related to clients' struggles with changing their behavior (e.g., diet, exercise, medication adherence, or treatment plan adherence more generally) (Hettema, Steele, & Miller, 2005).

A significant challenge in the substance abuse treatment field is creating a context for promoting and maintaining clients' committed action toward change. All too often, clients and professionals embrace the hopefulness associated with the initiation of a treatment episode only to experience the disappointment and frustration of clients' broken resolutions and the resurgence of troubling behaviors. The change process is often characterized by peaks and valleys and by periods of motivation for change interspersed with periods of reverting to old behaviors. However, the familiarity of this changing landscape offers little to the clinician in terms of how to effectively guide individuals attempting to make a behavior change. A conceptual framework that elucidates the factors that influence the change process, and highlights how they are manifested during clinical interactions, can provide an important clinical lens for the health care professional. Furthermore, the utility of such a conceptual framework is best demonstrated by how well it can effectively guide clinician behavior to influence the outcomes of clinical interactions.

MI, which has been an evolving practice over the past three decades, offers such a conceptual framework for understanding the process of change and recognizing indicators of a client's movement toward or away from change during clinical encounters. MI also identifies specific skills a clinician may utilize to facilitate a client's movement toward change when ambivalence about behavior change is a central issue. Together, the conceptual framework of behavior change and the specific MI skills can provide clinicians an effective mechanism for guiding clients during their pursuit of important lifestyle changes.

In this chapter we provide an overview of the MI counseling style. This discussion will highlight the factors that influenced its development, as well as the specific elements that define the behavior of a clinician during an MI guided clinical interaction. To place MI in the broader context of psychological theories of motivation, we touch on some of the processes that may account for the effectiveness of MI. Furthermore, we outline some of the important parameters for successfully learning and becoming proficient in the MI counseling style.

MI BORN OF UTILITY RATHER THAN THEORY

Traditional conceptualizations of motivation and treatment failure have utilized theories that emphasize the importance of a client's dispositional characteristics (Miller, 1985). This class of theories attributes poor motivation to defense mechanisms, such as denial, that prevent an individual from seeing that he or she has a substance use problem or needs to change. Intervention strategies from this perspective view motivation for change as arising from events that override or undermine the substance user's elaborate defense system. "Hitting bottom," or experiencing a significant number of negative substance-related events, is seen as a process and as a place from which a substance abuser's defense systems can be broken down, and in which he or she may recognize and accept that there is a problem. In the field of addiction counseling, confrontational techniques have been utilized to accelerate the dismantling of elaborate defense mechanisms. This approach, although promoting change for some individuals, has not garnered empirical support over time (Miller, 1985; White & Miller, 2007). In contrast, the MI counseling style was initially formalized by examining and drawing from the characteristics and styles of counseling that promote better treatment outcomes. MI differs from traditional confrontational treatment approaches and offers guidelines for interacting with individuals in a manner that helps to promote treatment engagement and resolve ambivalence about change.

DEFINING MI

MI is an empirically supported counseling style that has been employed as a standalone brief behavioral intervention, as part of structured interactions that focus on the provision of medical and behavioral feedback, and as a precursor to longer term treatment programs (e.g., Brown & Miller, 1993; Burke, Dunn, Atkins, & Phelps, 2004; Lundahl, Kunz, Brownell, Tollefson, & Burke, 2010; Miller & Rollnick, 2002, 2009, 2013; Rubak, Sandbaek, Lauritzen, & Christensen, 2005; Vasilaki, Hosier, & Cox, 2006; Wain et al., 2011). It has demonstrated efficacy across a range of health related issues and behaviors, such as managing hypertension, diabetes, and reducing illicit drug use (Burke, Arkowitz, & Menchola, 2003; Hettema et al., 2005; Rubak et al., 2005).

MI has been described as a "collaborative conversational style for strengthening a person's own motivation and commitment to change" (Miller & Rollnick, 2013, p. 12). More technically, "MI is a collaborative, goal-oriented style of communication with particular attention to the language of change. It is designed to strengthen personal motivation for and commitment to a specific goal by eliciting and exploring the person's own reasons for change within an atmosphere of acceptance and compassion" (p. 29). While MI adopts a person-centered therapeutic stance, the goal-oriented framework and the special emphasis on change talk differentiate MI from more traditional person-centered counseling approaches.

Miller and Rollnick (2013) have identified four processes underlying discussions about change: engaging, focusing, evoking, and planning. "Engaging" highlights the process of developing a helping relationship. "Focusing" is the process by which a clear direction of change is developed or clarified. Engaging and focusing occur in many clinical consultations and therapeutic styles, and are not unique to an MI approach. "Evoking" is a means of educing change talk, recognizing it when it occurs during an interaction, and skillfully responding to it when it is present. Evoking is central to the MI approach. "Planning" is what happens when a discussion about change transitions from evoking an individual's motivation for making change to developing a specific change plan that can be carried out. The MI counseling style and skills outlined in this chapter can be employed throughout all four processes of a clinical discussion (i.e., engaging, focusing, evoking, and planning). The directional components of MI are more evident during the evoking process.

Prochaska and DiClemente's (1983) transtheoretical model (TTM) of change, while not directly related to MI (Miller & Rollnick, 2009), provides a useful heuristic for conceptualizing the normative process of change. It describes the process individuals go through while considering change, independent of the type of problem. Decisions about change can be as simple as "Do I want to go back to school?" or as complex as "Can I give up heroin use?" For the purposes of MI, it is helpful to keep in mind where the client is in terms of stages of change. This frame of reference can help to sensitize the clinician to the particular process that may be most applicable (e.g., engaging vs. focusing or evoking). For example, a client in the precontemplation stage is not yet considering change. During the process of engagement, a clinician employing an MI style may begin to build a treatment alliance and guide the conversation toward a focusing process that explores the client's reasons for attending the consultation. A person in the contemplation stage may already be experiencing a lot of ambivalence, which may be moved in the direction of change by the clinician during the evoking process. An MI style may be employed to explore what has worked in the past, to evoke change talk, and to support self-efficacy. MI is intended to help guide clients toward making a commitment to important and personally valued lifestyle changes. If individuals have already committed to change or have already started to make that change, MI skills may be useful for developing a change plan and outlining the steps needed to meet the goals of the individual. However, it should be kept in mind that commitment to change is a dynamic phenomenon and a solidly committed client today may not necessarily feel the same tomorrow. Thus, the clinician may need to revisit the processes of focusing or evoking to meet the client where he or she is at during any given moment and help guide the session back to a path of meaningful change. While the goals of the interaction may vary depending on the client's stage of change, the MI counseling style is applicable throughout all four processes.

THE SPIRIT AND PRINCIPLES OF MI

The spirit of MI is fundamental and defines the overarching context in which a clinician practices MI techniques. The spirit in which MI is implemented is what defines the MI approach and differentiates it from being merely a collection of techniques. The spirit of MI also dictates that the clinician ultimately lets the client set the goals and that MI is not used in an attempt to manipulate the client into doing what the clinician thinks is best. MI spirit consists of four interrelated elements: partnership, acceptance, compassion, and evocation.

Partnership

An MI counseling style is based on a collaborative partnership between the clinician and client. From this perspective, clinician and client are viewed as each possessing valuable expertise. It is through a collaborative process and partnership with the clinician that clients can explore their reasons for change and utilize their expertise to activate their own motivation for change. The clinician does not adopt an expert stance or communicate that he or she has the right or best answer. Instead the clinician provides an atmosphere that is conducive to change rather than coercive. The collaborative stance of an MI clinician is best exemplified in the use of open questions and strong listening skills to help him or her understand the world from the client's perspective.

Acceptance

Acceptance stems from the humanistic, person-centered nature of the MI counseling style that is significantly influenced by the work of Carl Rogers (Miller & Rollnick, 2013). This element of MI spirit refers to the clinician's openness to what the client brings to the interaction. Acceptance consists of four elements that are realized in the clinician's view of others and in his or her counseling behaviors. First, from an accepting stance, the clinician views clients as being fundamentally trustworthy and having worth (i.e., absolute worth). Clinicians do not counsel from a place of judgment or conditional acceptance. It is from a place of genuine acceptance that MI fosters a context for change. Second, the expression of accurate empathy is essential for developing good rapport with a client. To be empathic is to have an appreciation of another's perspective; it does not mean the clinician necessarily agrees with the client's perspective, nor does it mean the clinician feels one way or the other about the person's situation (i.e., it is not sympathy). It refers to an objective appreciation of the person's perspective. It takes a very nonjudgmental stance to be truly empathic. In MI, being empathic is not enough; it is the expression of empathy that makes the clinical interaction so moving. When the clinician can accurately summarize the client's meaning from verbal and nonverbal communication, the client is more likely to feel understood and, in turn, develop self-understanding. Third, acceptance involves respecting and supporting a client's autonomy. Ultimately, it is the client who decides to change, and an MI counseling style supports the individual's freedom to choose. The MI counseling style does not coerce, control, or force change on an individual. It is through the process of explicitly acknowledging an individual's freedom to choose a direction that MI reduces defensiveness and opens up the possibility of change. Finally, MI explicitly acknowledges a client's strengths, efforts, and successes. Affirming an individual's strengths and efforts distances an MI counseling style from counseling strategies more closely aligned with deficit models. From the deficit perspective, clinical interactions focus on delineating shortcomings and failures, then attempting to develop a plan to fix these problems. The aim of MI is to mobilize the strength and wisdom assumed to reside within the individual.

Compassion

The clinician utilizing the compassion component of MI spirit acknowledges that the process of counseling is ultimately for the client's benefit, not the clinician's. The clinician explicitly embraces the commitment to pursue what is in the best interests of the client and gives priority to the client's needs. Thus, MI is not implemented as a counseling strategy to influence an individual's behavior in order to meet the goals or desires of others.

Evocation

MI embraces the idea that the individual often has the motivation and resources to change under the right circumstances (e.g., the resolution of ambivalence). Thus, the individual is not deficient and does not need fixing. Instead, MI operates from a strengths-focused perspective; the resources and motivation for change are considered to reside within the client, and the clinician's role is to evoke the client's wisdom and motivation during clinical interactions. Discussions about change that draw on the client's own perceptions, goals, and values are seen as being central to enhancing intrinsic motivation to change. Individuals know what they are willing to do and what they are not willing to do, what they have tried, and what has not worked in the past. Thus, while the clinician evokes the client's perspective, the client does most of the talking and builds his or her own case for making behavior change.

MI TECHNIQUE: DEFINING THE MICROSKILLS

MI spirit defines the therapeutic stance, overarching context, or mindset of the clinician adopting this counseling style. The technical implementation of MI is characterized by the strategic use of several communication skills: open-ended questions, affirmations, reflective listening, and summary statements (OARS; Table 30.1). These core communication skills are initially employed during the processes of engaging and focusing. Once the client has identified a target behavior (the outcome of the focusing process), the OARS skills are utilized to educe a client's motivation and commitment to change (evoking process) and to develop a change strategy (planning process).

Open-Ended Questions

Open-ended questions have a large variety of potential responses, as opposed to closed-ended questions that have a very limited number of answers (e.g., yes or no; number of hours sleeping; number of days using). Closed-ended questions yield

TABLE 30.1. Microskills of Motivational Interviewing

Microskill	Definition
Open-ended questions	Questions with an unlimited set of possible responses
Affirmations	Clinician statements pointing out positive behavior or trait of client
Reflections	Clinician statements that echo client statements and may add meaning to client statements
Summaries	Clinician statements that tie together important points or themes shared by client

limited information and run the risk setting a more passive role for the client during a clinical discussion. Open-ended questions are useful in an MI counseling style because they garner more information and are more likely to invite the client to be an active collaborator during a clinical discussion. The strategic use of open-ended questions can help guide a discussion toward what is particularly important about making a change or help to clarify the client's life goals or values (e.g., "What are the most important reasons why you want to stop using?" or "How is your drug use a problem for you?"). Discussing the discrepancy between where clients are in their lives, and where they would like to be, can help build intrinsic motivation for change and may help to guide individuals toward resolving their ambivalence about making a commitment to change.

Affirmations

Clinicians adopting an MI counseling style strive to support and encourage individuals throughout the process of change. "Affirmations" are statements that accentuate the positive, help build self-efficacy, and acknowledge the worth of an individual. Affirmations may involve pointing out something positive an individual does, even if it is as simple as coming to the appointment, and may offer hope and support to clients considering behavior change. Clinicians need to be sincere; an affirmation is not a patronizing falsehood. A good affirmation reflects something the clinician has observed or heard, supports the client's autonomy, and is not a value judgment. For example, "I'm proud of you for getting a clean urine" is not an affirmation but an expression of the clinician's judgment and it exemplifies the differential between clinician and client. An example of an MI-consistent affirmation might be "You've really worked hard to comply with parole so that you can see your children again." It is easy to neglect the use of affirmations if the clinician tends to think in terms of problems and solutions; however, affirmations can help clients see their own potential for change. For example, an individual has left an abusive relationship but may ask, "How did I get myself into this?" The clinician can choose to affirm the change: "You got yourself out of a very difficult situation." It is important for individuals to hear and take away a positive message, so that they continue to strive for positive change. It should be noted that affirmations are not used to bypass difficult situations; if a client is grappling with a difficulty, it should be not overlooked in the clinician's effort to find something to affirm. It is up to the clinician to find a therapeutic balance between being present with the client and affirming strengths and capacities the client may have difficulty recognizing in him- or herself.

Reflective Listening

Listening skills are fundamental to the practice of MI. A counselor utilizes reflective listening to develop a deeper understanding of a client's perspective, to help clarify the meaning of what a client has said, and to guide the discussion strategically toward the resolution of ambivalence. There are two levels of reflective listening statements: simple and complex. A simple reflection can be either a straight repeat or a paraphrase of what the client has said. Simple reflections do not significantly alter the meaning of what was said. Why make simple reflections? Simple reflections demonstrate to the client that the clinician is listening and offer the client an opportunity to correct the clinician, if the clinician misunderstood. A client is more likely to share information if he or she feels heard. Simple reflections can also serve to set the pace of the session; simple reflections help to slow the client down, which can be useful when working with manic or anxious individuals. Clinicians can use simple reflections throughout the conversation to make certain that they are "on the same page" as the client.

Complex reflections are higher-level reflective statements that add to or change the meaning of what the client has said in a significant way. There are several different types of complex reflection (Table 30.2). Complex reflections express empathy; they convey to the client that the clinician understands at perhaps a deeper level than what was communicated by the words the client used.

Summary Statements

Summarizing allows the clinician to bring together what the client has said over the course of a discussion in a meaningful, effective narrative. A summary statement is a particular type of reflection that encompasses more of what the client has said than just what was in the immediately preceding statement. Summaries serve to juxtapose several ideas expressed by the individual. As with reflections, summaries are useful for keeping the clinician and client on the same page. Furthermore, they may frame things in a way that can extend the client's understanding of the situation. For example, a summary juxtaposing some of what the client has said regarding substance use, along with some difficulties the client is currently experiencing, may help the client to see a relationship between those two things. When creating a summary statement, it is not necessary to list every bit of information discussed over a period of time. Bill Miller describes the summary as a bouquet that the clinician presents to the client, and the flowers in the bouquet are bits of information the individual has shared throughout the session. An example of a summary might be "You are concerned about your increased alcohol use in recent weeks, and also about the fights you have been having with your wife and about your boss confronting you over days missed at work."

TABLE 30.2. Complex Reflection Examples

Complex reflection	Example
Continuing the paragraph	The clinician states the next thought or idea that the client has not yet said. For example, if the client has finished talking about a troubling interaction with a significant other, the clinician could *continue the paragraph* and say, "That conversation really upset you and almost served as a trigger for relapse, which was scary for you." This is done to lead the client to see connections between emotions and behaviors.
Metaphor and simile	The clinician might say, "It seemed as though the rug was pulled out from under you." Metaphors may convey to the client that the clinician has heard beyond the client's words, to the client's meaning.
Double-sided reflection	A double-sided reflection is a type of complex reflection that contains two ways of thinking or feeling in one statement: "On the one hand, the alcohol helps you to sleep, and on the other hand, you wake up groggy and confused every day." This is done to reduce ambivalence. Or "On the one hand, you feel you're a good son, and on the other, you've taken your parent's meds." This is done to highlight the discrepancy between values and behaviors.
Reflection of feeling	This involves describing emotions and other feelings that that client has not yet stated directly. Many clients do not readily identify their feelings, perhaps because they are reluctant to admit their emotions or because they are unaware of their emotions. For example, the client may describe a number of barriers he or she experienced in getting to the clinic that day, and the counselor might reflect: "It was a frustrating morning." When the clinician labels the client's emotions, those emotions may no longer feel so overwhelming. It can also be an expression of empathy for a clinician to reflect an emotion about which the client has not yet spoken.
Amplified reflection	This occurs when the clinician alters a client's statement so that the client hears an exaggerated reflection: For example, the clinician might respond to the client's statement that his drinking is under control by reflecting "Your alcohol use isn't a problem for you at all." This is done to prompt the client to argue the opposite. It is important that the clinician not deliver the amplified reflection with any trace of sarcasm or disbelief.

THE EVOKING PROCESS: STRENGTHENING CHANGE TALK

How clients talk about their behavior and their commitment to making change is an important indicator for assessing the level of ambivalence and motivation in a given moment. From an MI perspective, client speech offers the clinician real-time feedback about the motivation-enhancing or motivation-depleting effects of the clinician's style and responses. Client talk also helps guide the clinician's responses throughout the course of a clinical discussion.

From the perspective of MI, it is assumed that individuals may be ambivalent about change. This ambivalence can be expressed as either sustain talk or change talk. Sustain talk, the non-change side of ambivalence, presents arguments against change (i.e., pro-status quo), may highlight the pros of engaging in a problem behavior and the cons of change, may defend the client's actions, and may signal a commitment for maintaining current behavioral patterns. Decreasing the frequency of sustain talk is a goal of the evoking process. However, an increase in sustain talk may signal to the clinician that the current approach is not working and he or she should try something else. Change talk is an argument in favor of change; it highlights the pros of alternative actions and the cons of inaction, and signals a commitment to change. Increasing the frequency and strength of change talk is a central goal of the evoking process, and an increase in change talk offers the clinician important feedback on the effectiveness of the interaction. Identifying, evoking, and selectively responding to change talk (using the OARS skills) is central to the goal-oriented aspect of an MI approach.

Several coding schemes have been developed to categorize client language during MI interventions (CLEAR; Glynn & Moyers, 2012; The Motivational Interviewing Skill Code [MISC]; Miller, Moyers, Ernst, & Amrhein, 2008). Amrhein, Miller, Yahne, Palmer, and Fulcher (2003) outlined a psycholinguistic framework that categorizes the type and quantifies the strength of different categories of change and sustain talk. Client change talk can be conceptualized as preparatory change talk or mobilizing change talk (Miller & Rollnick, 2013). Preparatory change talk consists of statements expressing Desire, Ability, Reasons, and Need to change. Mobilizing change talk consists of statements of Commitment, Activation, and Taking steps to change (the acronym for both is DARN-CAT). It is important to note that preparatory language (DARN) and mobilizing language (CAT) may be associated with both change and sustain talk. For example, individuals may express strong reasons for continuing their substance use ("Smoking really helps me cope with the stress of my day": sustain talk), as well as reasons for altering their behavior ("I want to stop smoking so I can live longer and see my kids grow up": change talk). The goal of the evoking process is to implement the OARS skills to increase the frequency and strength of change talk and guide the discussion toward the planning process.

Identifying preparatory talk as it occurs during a discussion about change is an important skill. Preparatory change talk signals an increased likelihood that mobilizing change talk will occur. Mobilizing change talk predicts positive treatment outcome (Amerhein et al., 2003; Table 30.3). Thus, clinicians should strive to strengthen preparatory and mobilizing change talk during a clinical interaction. A clinician who can effectively discriminate between change talk and sustain talk is in the position to selectively reinforce change talk when it occurs. If client change talk is not responded to or is directly challenged, the client may shift toward sustain talk. For example, operating from a deficit model may bias the clinician to evoke sustain talk by probing what is not going well or focusing on the reasons for current behavior problems. It is the skillful discrimination between change talk and sustain talk, and the differential response to change talk within the spirit of MI, that defines a proficient MI style throughout the evoking process.

Preparatory Change Talk (DARN)

Desire statements indicate something the client wants, wishes for, or is willing to do. Usually they express a general level of desire rather than contain specific reasons. "I really want to lose weight (e.g., "I want . . . ," "I wish . . . ," "I would like to . . ."). A useful tool to generate desire talk in a session is the "Desire Ruler." The clinician asks the client, "On a scale of 1 to 10, with 10 being the highest, how much do you

TABLE 30.3. Change Talk

Element	Definition
Preparatory change talk	
Desire	Client desire related to target behavior (*Note.* This could be the desire to stop or the desire to continue target behavior)
Ability	Client sense of ability to change target behavior
Reasons	Client reasons related to target behavior (to continue or to stop)
Need	Client-identified needs related to target behavior
Mobilizing change talk	
Commitment to change	Client statements describing expected future behavior
Action	Client statements indicating a shift toward action but not a commitment to do it
Taking steps	Client statements indicating that the client has already started to move in the direction of change

want to make this change?" When the client responds with a number, the clinician explores that further. If the client responds with, for example, a 5, the clinician asks, "Why are you at a 5 instead of a 3?" This gets the client thinking about why the change is important, and about why his or her desire is as high as it is. Then the clinician asks, "What would it take to get you from a 5 to, say, an 8 or a 9?" The client may then respond by talking about what it would take to increase the importance of the change. Note that these questions are worded carefully so as *not* to evoke sustain talk; a question such as "Why are you only at a 5 and not an 8?" would focus the client on deficits or problems, and this type of question is ill-advised. The clinician elicits specific information from the client to help build a case for change.

Ability statements indicate perceptions of capability or possibility of change. Usually they do not contain specifics; rather, they express a general level of ability or inability. For example, "I know I can do this. I will start exercising again." Strategic open-ended questions from the clinician can elicit statements of optimism from clients (e.g., "What have you done in the past that led to sobriety?"; "What other challenges in your life were you able to overcome?"; "What do you think would work for you if you decided to change?"). The clinician then listens to the client's response and finds key elements to reflect or affirm. Another way to elicit statements of ability from the client would be to use the "Confidence Ruler." In the course of the MI session, the clinician guides the client to identify a SMART goal (Small, Measurable, Achievable, Relevant, and Timed). Once the SMART goal has been identified, the clinician asks, "On a scale of 1 to 10, with 10 being the highest, how confident are you in being able to make this change?" The strategic open-ended follow-up question ("Why are you at a 5 and not a 3?") elicits statements of ability from the client. The client responds with all the strengths and resources he or she has within him- or herself. The clinician can then ask, "What would it take to get that 5 up to an 8?" This prompts the client to think about what is needed for an increase in confidence to occur.

Reasons are a particular rationale, justification, or motive for making the behavior change (e.g., "It's important for me to lose weight for my health"). Reasons are elicited throughout the therapeutic interview by getting the cons of the target behavior (e.g., possibility of arrest, cost), the pros of change (e.g., ability to save money, improved health), problem recognition through open-ended questions (e.g., "Why is your wife worried about you?" or "In what ways has your drug use been a problem for you?"), the client's intentions regarding the target behavior (e.g., "What are you thinking about your drug use at this point?"), and exploring the client's goals and values (e.g., "What matters to you? How do you see yourself? What do you hope for?").

Need statements indicate necessity, urgency, or requirement for change. They do not usually contain specific reasons but instead express a general level of need (e.g., "I really need to lose weight" or "I must stop eating this way or I'm going to give myself another heart attack"). The clinician can elicit statements of need by exploring problem recognition (e.g., "What makes you think you need to make this change?").

Mobilizing Change Talk (CAT)

Commitment statements imply agreement, intention, or obligation regarding future target behavior change, and client commitment language has been correlated with positive clinical outcomes. Commitment statements vary in strength and direction. For example, "I am stopping my use" is a very strong statement of positive change; "I will try to stop using" is a weaker statement of positive change. When eliciting statements of change from a client, the clinician should strive for the strongest level of commitment. Questions that ask for small and clear commitments often can evoke commitment statements (e.g., "What will you do this week?").

Activation statements indicate movement toward change but do not necessarily reflect a solid commitment to make change. A client may state a willingness or readiness to change ("I'm ready to stop drinking") but may not express a commitment (e.g., "I will not drink this week"). The clinician may reflect the client's readiness ("You have decided to stop") or probe how the client may accomplish this ("You have made up your mind. What do you have to do to make this happen?"), which may help guide the client from activation to commitment.

Statements about taking steps highlight behaviors in which the client engages that are in the direction of change, although a commitment to change has not yet occurred. For example, looking at Alcoholics Anonymous (AA) meeting locations is a step toward a change in drinking behavior, even though it does not include a commitment to stop drinking. From an MI perspective, taking steps signals the process of resolving ambivalence in the direction of change, and the clinician may want to further reflect, probe, or affirm this activity.

Evidence suggests that the relative distribution of change talk and sustain talk during a conversation about change has prognostic significance. A discussion that includes more client sustain talk or equitable levels of sustain and change talk is predictive of poor outcome. In contrast, discussions that include a greater proportion of client change talk predict future behavior change (Moyers, Martin, Houck,

Christopher, & Tonigan, 2009). Thus, the strategic use of MI skills to increase change talk during a clinical discussion has direct relevance to the overall efficacy of an MI counseling session.

The process of evoking change talk involves the strategic use of the MI microskills (OARS). One of the simplest ways to elicit change talk is to use open-ended questions to explore a client's perceptions or concerns. It is assumed that a certain amount of ambivalence is associated with change, and open-ended questions can set the occasion for probing this assumption. It is important to note the need for elaboration. Indeed, once a reason for change has been elicited, it is often the clinician's tendency to move on and find other reasons for change. It can be quite useful to ask the client to elaborate further on a topic before moving on. The clinician can also reflect the client's stated reasons, which may also elicit elaboration and further change talk, making the possibility of change more realistic for the client.

Several other strategies can be used to generate change talk. Clinicians can employ a decisional balance exercise during which clients discuss the positive, as well as the negative, aspects of a target behavior. In this exercise, the client lists the positives of the behavior (e.g., benefits of drug use) first, followed by the downsides (e.g., negative consequences of drug use). Note that ending the exercise on the negatives of the problematic behavior is advised as it will prompt the client to remember that portion of the exercise more strongly. In contrast, ending with a discussion of the positives of the problem behavior is not recommended as it increases the probability that the client will focus on that portion of the exercise and engage in sustain talk. It can also be useful for clients to discuss the positives and negatives of both staying the same and making the behavior change; this may help prepare the client for the struggles that giving up a certain behavior may entail. In such a discussion, the clinician would want to start by exploring the positives of staying the same, and end with exploring the negatives of staying the same. This type of decisional balance should always end with the side of the argument that the clinician most wants the client to adopt. Exploring goals and values with the person can be another useful strategy. Inviting the client to discuss what is important in life and to envision how to achieve those things can help increase change talk and motivation. Reflective listening can be very helpful for highlighting a client's change talk.

UNPACKING RESISTANCE: SUSTAIN TALK AND DISCORD

Early formulations of MI conceptualized client resistance as a function of the clinical interaction (Miller & Rollnick, 1991, 2002). This framework differed from more traditional theoretical perspectives that viewed resistance as a characteristic of the client or of the clinical condition (e.g., denial in substance dependence). However, a more recent formulation of MI (Miller & Rollnick, 2013) has moved to deconstruct the concept of resistance further. From this perspective, resistance comprises two distinct processes: sustain talk and discord. It is important to note that counseling style influences both processes. Thus, the clinician's stance and communication skills are important parameters in understanding and influencing what has traditionally been labeled as "resistance."

As previously noted, sustain talk represents one side of ambivalence. From an MI perspective, ambivalence is a natural part of the change process and is to be expected to occur as clients contemplate change. It is not pathological. However, sustain talk is predictive of poor outcome, and the more individuals engage in sustain talk, the greater the chance that they will talk themselves out of change. Thus, recognizing sustain talk and responding to it effectively has important treatment implications. Reflective listening, reinforcing autonomy, and reframing can help minimize the chances of a confrontational interaction, guide the discussion fruitfully toward reduced sustain talk, and begin to evoke change talk.

Discord signals the disruption of a collaborative relationship (low MI spirit). The presence of discord may provide feedback to the clinician that his or her therapeutic stance or style has shifted away from an MI-adherent position. Discord can arise at any stage during the processes of engaging, focusing, evoking, and planning. The client may feel coerced into change; the client may disagree with the clinician about the target for change; the clinician may directly challenge sustain talk; or the clinician may be overly instructive about what the client needs to do. These are but a few examples of occurrences that can disrupt the collaborative nature of the interaction and promote an increase in client defensiveness, disengagement, and verbal jousting (interrupting, arguing). Significantly, an increase in discord may be accompanied by a decrease in motivation. A clinician can effectively respond to discord and shift the session back to a more collaborative process. The use of reflective listening, affirming, reinforcing client autonomy, shifting the focus of the conversation, and reframing can be utilized to rebuild a more effective working alliance. While there is no single correct response to discord or sustain talk, the overarching goal of the clinician is to establish a collaborative working relationship that reinforces the client's autonomy in the change process, makes clear the nonjudgmental stance of the clinician, and reduces the client's defense of the status quo.

Formulation of a Theory

MI has been developed and refined over the past three decades. A significant amount of writing has been devoted to outlining the therapeutic stance and the MI microskills (Miller & Rollnick, 1991, 2002, 2013), testing MI's efficacy in numerous randomized clinical trials (e.g., Brown & Miller, 1993: Burke et al., 2004; Hettema et al., 2005; Lundahl et al., 2010; Miller & Rollnick, 2002, 2009, 2013; Rubak et al., 2005; Vasilaki et al., 2006: Wain et al., 2011), and highlighting the predictors of change during MI sessions (Amrhein et al., 2003). The increasing body of evidence that supports MI as an effective counseling style has also prompted formal discussions about the theoretical underpinnings of the strategy and the mechanisms by which MI may guide behavior (Miller & Rose, 2009).

MI explicitly acknowledges three fundamentally important parameters of discussions about change: the clinician's interpersonal stance, the clinician's verbal behavior, and the client's verbal behavior. All three parameters are proposed to be important mechanisms or signals by which clinicians can influence conversations about change that in turn help to resolve ambivalence and promote lifestyle changes (Miller & Rose, 2009).

The spirit of MI has been hypothesized to play a central role in the efficacy of MI (Rollnick & Miller, 1995; Miller & Rose, 2009). Evidence supports a positive link between therapist empathy and treatment outcome (Miller, Taylor, & West, 1980), as well as a link between clinician interpersonal skills and client engagement during MI sessions (Moyers, Miller, & Hendrickson, 2005). Furthermore, clinician behavior that is consistent with MI is more likely to engender change talk, while a counseling style that is inconsistent with MI (e.g., directing, confronting) is associated with sustain talk (Moyers & Martin, 2006). Other studies have examined the relative importance of clinicians' microskills versus the more global elements of MI (empathy and spirit). These findings suggest that the global elements of MI may be more powerful than the specific skills in engendering client engagement and treatment alliance (Moyers et al., 2005; Boardman, Catley, Grobe, Little, & Ahluwalia, 2006). Thus, the general pattern of findings to date supports the contention that therapist style is an active ingredient in the overall efficacy of this counseling approach.

Psycholinguistic studies of client speech during MI-guided discussions about change demonstrate that the way individuals talk about their behavior during an MI session (i.e., commitment language or change talk) predicts treatment outcome (Amrhein et al., 2003; Moyers et al., 2007). Furthermore, the relationship between change talk and drug treatment outcome has been demonstrated in counseling styles other than MI (cognitive-behavioral therapy [CBT]; Aharonovich, Amrhein, Bisaga, Nunes, & Hasin, 2008) and for other behavioral problems (Gaume, Gmel, & Daeppen, 2008; Hodgins, Ching, & McEwen, 2009; Strang & McCambridge, 2004). Overall, the increasing evidence has supported an important link between client talk and future behavior change.

The significant relationships between (1) counseling style and client change talk and (2) client change talk and treatment outcome suggest an important mediating role of change talk. That is, the clinician's counseling style influences treatment, because it increases change talk. However an important, although unanswered, question remains. How does increasing change talk help resolve ambivalence and promote changes in behavior? Several psychological theories have been utilized to understand how the process of MI engenders change. Bem's (1972) self-perception theory hypothesizes that the beliefs one develops about oneself result from observing oneself: "As I hear myself talk, I learn what I believe." In MI, the client's verbal commitment to change serves as a precursor to change. Thus, when a clinician evokes change talk, which is understood to be an important and facilitative part of the change process, he or she may enhance the client's motivation to change. Festinger's cognitive dissonance theory (1957) states that when a person is enticed to speak in a new way, some discomfort is experienced due to the discrepancy between the newly voiced beliefs and long-held thought and behavior patterns. An individual's beliefs and values tend to shift in the same direction as the spoken words to help reduce this "dissonance." Accordingly, in the process of focusing and evoking, clients may offer statements about what is important to them and how their current behavior interferes with a lifestyle that is consistent with their values and goals. Engaging in this process may motivate individuals to reduce this discrepancy. Also apparent in MI is decisional conflict theory from Janis and Mann (1977), in which "ambivalence" is defined as a cognitive conflict. Clients struggling with addiction are almost always struggling with ambivalence about change. In order to address and resolve the ambivalence, clinicians engage clients in a rational decision-making process rather than avoid, or attempt to avoid, the ambivalence.

In summary, increasing empirical evidence has highlighted the mechanistic links between a clinician's style and skills and in-session client speech. In turn, in-session client speech has predicted treatment outcome. These investigations have provided the empirical scaffolding upon which a deeper understanding of the relationship between change talk and behavior change can be investigated. This knowledge has the potential to yield a comprehensive understanding of how MI influences the process of change.

A NOTE ON LEARNING MI

MI has been described as a "simple but not easy" counseling style to learn (Miller & Rollnick, 2009). It is a complex combination of therapeutic stance and behavioral practice, for which it is difficult to develop sustained competence (Forsberg, Berman, Kallmen, Hermansson, & Helgason, 2008; Hettema et al., 2005; Smith et al., 2012). Training formats can vary from brief educational lectures that provide an overview of the counseling style to more in-depth training workshops that are followed by a supervised practice schedule. Interactive training workshops remain the primary context for learning MI. However, an increasing body of evidence suggests that while training workshops (approximately 16 hours of training) can facilitate the acquisition of an MI counseling style, they do not promote long-term proficiency (Miller & Mount, 2001; Walters, Matson, Baer, & Ziedonis, 2005). Evidence generally supports combining training workshops with postworkshop supervision that includes opportunities to practice MI with the provision of objective feedback and coaching (Miller et al., 2004; Smith et al., 2012). Thus, it is recommended that in the process of learning MI, clinicians both receive didactic instruction and participate in supervised practice that includes constructive feedback on their clinical interaction. The resources presented at the beginning of this chapter provide important didactic and supervisory resources that can facilitate the development of a proficient MI counseling style.

CLINICAL CORNER: THE "MI SANDWICH"

Medical clinicians may find it challenging to implement MI due to the factual data collection that is necessary for clinical practice and record keeping. Medical personnel also frequently feel pressed for time and find it difficult to add "one more thing" to an already pressured schedule. However, there are times when a doctor may wish to incorporate an MI counseling style. This style may be particularly useful if there is a history of substance abuse or other behavior patterns that are negatively impacting an individual's health and ability to comply with health care recommendations. In these circumstances, the physician may choose to use the "MI sandwich," which refers to opening and closing a clinical encounter with MI and gathering the more factual data in the middle. In a collaborative atmosphere, one that supports a stance consistent with the spirit of MI, the physician can begin a discussion by asking the client open-ended questions, respecting the client's perspective, and offering reflections. The middle of the session does not need to be a true MI session; this is when the physician may ask a lot of closed-ended questions for differential diagnostic purposes, discuss prescriptions, and collect other factual data. Then, the physician resumes the MI stance for the closing minutes of the session. During the opening and the closing of the medical appointment, the physician assumes the role of MI therapist to build rapport, to engage the client, and to increase the client's motivation for making change. The client should feel empowered by the experience and may be more willing to consider making the identified behavior change. The client needs to know that, whether he or she succeeds or fails at making the change, the physician will remain receptive and supportive.

ACKNOWLEDGMENTS

This work was supported in part by the National Institute on Drug Abuse Grant Nos. R01 DA016950 (to Edward V. Nunes), K24 DA022412 (to Edward V. Nunes), and K23 DA021850 (to Kenneth M. Carpenter).

REFERENCES

Aharonovich, E., Amrhein, P. C., Bisaga, A., Nunes, E. V., & Hasin, D. S. (2008). Cognition, commitment language, and behavioral change among cocaine-dependent patients. *Psychol Addict Behav, 22,* 557–562.

Amrhein, P. C., Miller, W. R., Yahne, C. E., Palmer, M., & Fulcher, I. (2003). Client commitment language during motivational interviewing predicts drug use outcomes. *J Consult Clin Psychol, 71*(5), 862–878.

Bem, D. J. (1972). Self-perception theory. In L. Berkowitz (Ed.), *Advances in experimental social psychology* (Vol. 6, pp. 1–62). New York: Academic Press

Boardman, T., Catley, D., Grobe, J., Little, T., & Ahluwalia, J. (2006). Using motivational interviewing with smokers: Do therapist behaviors relate to engagement and therapeutic alliance? *J Subst Abuse Treat, 31,* 329–339.

Brown, J. M., & Miller, W. R. (1993). Impact of motivational interviewing on participation and outcome in residential alcoholism treatment. *Psychology of Addictive Behaviors, 7*(4), 211–218.

Burke, B. L., Arkowitz, H., & Menchola, M. (2003). The efficacy of motivational interviewing: A meta-analysis of controlled clinical trials. *J Consult Clin Psychol, 71*(5), 843–861.

Burke, B. L., Dunn, C. W., Atkins, D. C., & Phelps, J. S. (2004). The emerging evidence base for motivational interviewing: A meta-analytic and qualitative inquiry. *J Cogn Psychother, 18*(4), 309–322.

de Roten, Y., Zimmermann, G., Ortega, D., & Despland, J.-N. (2013). Meta-analysis of the effects of MI training on clinicians' behavior. *J Subst Abuse Treat, 45*(2), 155–162.

Festinger, L. (1957). *A theory of cognitive dissonance.* Evanston, IL: Row, Peterson.

Forsberg, L., Berman, A. H., Kallmen, H., Hermansson, U., & Helgason, A. R. (2008). A test of the validity of the Motivational Interviewing Treatment Integrity Code. *Cogn Behav Ther, 37*(3), 183–191.

Gaume, J., Gmel, G., & Daeppen, J. B. (2008). Brief alcohol interventions: Do counsellors' and patients' communication characteristics predict change? *Alcohol Alcohol, 43,* 62–69.

Glynn, L. H., & Moyers, T. B. (2012). Manual for client language Easy rating (CLEAR) Coding System: Formerly "Motivational Interviewing Skill Code (MISC) 1.1." Retrieved from *http://casaa.unm.edu/download/CLEAR.pdf*.

Hettema, J., Steele, J., & Miller, W. R. (2005). Motivational interviewing. *Annu Rev Clin Psychol, 1*(1), 91–111.

Hodgins, D. C., Ching, L. E., & McEwen, J. (2009). Strength of commitment language in motivational interviewing and gambling outcomes. *Psychol Addict Behav, 23*, 122–130.

Janis, I. L., & Mann, L. (1977). *Decision making: A psychological analysis of conflict, choice, and commitment.* New York: Free Press.

Lundahl, B. W., Kunz, C., Brownell, C., Tollefson, D., & Burke, B. L. (2010). A meta-analysis of motivational interviewing: Twenty-five years of empirical studies. *Res Social Work Prac, 20*(2), 137–160.

Martino, S., Ball, S. A., Gallon, S. L., Hall, D., Garcia, M., Ceperich, S., et al. (2006). *Motivational Interviewing Assessment: Supervisory tools for enhancing proficiency.* Salem, OR.

Martino, S., Canning-Ball, M., Carroll, K. M., & Rounsaville, B. J. (2011). A criterion-based stepwise approach for training counselors in motivational interviewing. *J Subst Abuse Treat, 40*(4), 357–365.

Miller, W. R. (1985). Motivation for treatment: A review with with special emphasis on alcoholism. *Psychol Bull, 98*, 84–107.

Miller, W. R., & Mount, K. A. (2001). A small study of training in motivational interviewing: Does one workshop change clinician and client behavior? *Behav Cogn Psychother, 29*, 457–471.

Miller, W. R., Moyers, T. B., Ernst, D. B., & Amrhein, P. C. (2008). *Manual for the Motivational Interviewing Skill Code (MISC) Version 2.1.* New Mexico: Center on Alcoholism, Substance Abuse, and Addictions, The University of New Mexico.

Miller, W. R., & Rollnick, S. (1991). *Motivational interviewing: Preparing people to change addictive behavior.* New York: Guilford Press.

Miller, W. R., & Rollnick, S. (2002). *Motivational interviewing: Preparing people for change* (2nd ed.). New York: Guilford Press.

Miller, W. R., & Rollnick, S. (2009). Ten things that motivational interviewing is not. *Behav Cogn Psychother, 37*(2), 129–140.

Miller, W. R., & Rollnick, S. (2013). *Motivational interviewing: Helping people change* (3rd ed.). New York: Guilford Press.

Miller, W. R., & Rose, G. S. (2009). Towards a theory of motivational interviewing. *Am Psychol, 64*, 527–537.

Miller, W. R., Sorensen, J. L., Selzer, J. A., & Brigham, G. S. (2006). Disseminating evidence-based practices in substance abuse treatment: A review with suggestions. *J Subst Abuse Treat, 31*(1), 25–39.

Miller, W. R., Taylor, C. A., & West, J. C. (1980). Focused versus broad spectrum behavior therapy for problem drinkers. *J Consult Clin Psychol, 48*, 590–601.

Miller, W. R., Yahne, C. E., Moyers, T. B., Martinez, J., & Pirritano, M. (2004). A randomized trial of methods to help clinicians learn motivational interviewing. *J Consult Clin Psychol, 72*(6), 1050–1062.

Moyers, T. B., & Martin, T. (2006). Therapist influence on client language during motivational interviewing sessions. *J Subst Abuse Treat, 30*, 245–251.

Moyers, T. B., Martin, T., Christopher P. J., Houck, J. M., Tonigan, J. S., & Amrhein, P. C. (2007). Client language as a mediator of motivational interviewing efficacy: Where is the evidence? *Alcohol Clin Exp Res, 10*(Suppl.), 40s–47s.

Moyers, T. B., Martin, T., Houck, J. M., Christopher, P. J., & Tonigan, J. S. (2009). From in-session behaviors to drinking outcomes: A causal chain for motivational interviewing. *J Consult Clin Psychol, 77*, 1113–1124.

Moyers, T. B., Miller, W. R., & Hendrickson, S. M. L. (2005). How does motivational interviewing work?: Therapist interpersonal skill predicts client involvement with motivational interviewing sessions. *J Consult Clin Psychol, 73,* 590–598.

Prochaska, J. O., & DiClemente, C. C. (1983). Stages and processes of self-change of smoking: Toward an integrative model of change. *J Consult Clin Psychol, 51,* 390–395.

Rollnick, S. & Miller, W. R. (1995). What is motivational interviewing? *Behav Cogn Psychother, 23,* 325–334.

Rubak, S., Sandbaek, A., Lauritzen, T., & Christensen, B. (2005). Motivational interviewing: A systematic review and meta-analysis. *Br J Gen Pract, 55,* 305–312.

Schoener, E. P., Madeja, C. L., Henderson, M. J., Ondersma, S. J., & Janisse, J. J. (2006). Effects of motivational interviewing training on mental health therapist behavior. *Drug Alcohol Depend, 82*(3), 269–275.

Smith, J. S., Carpenter, K. M., Amrhein, P, Brooks, A, Levin, D., Schreiber E. A., et al. (2012). Training subsatnce abuse clinicians in motivational interviewing using live supervision via tele-conferencing technology. *J Consult Clin Psychol, 80,* 450–464.

Strang, J., & McCambridge, J. (2004). Can the practitioner correctly predict outcome in motivational interviewing? *J Subst Abuse Treat, 27,* 83–88.

Vasilaki, E. I., Hosier, S. G., & Cox, W. M. (2006). The efficacy of motivational interviewing as a brief intervention for excessive drinking: A meta-analytic review. *Alcohol Alcoholism, 41*(3), 328–335.

Wain, R. M., Wilbourne, P. L., Harris, K. W., Pierson, H., Teleki, J., Burling, T. A., et al. (2011). Motivational interview improves treatment entry in homeless veterans. *Drug Alcohol Depen, 115*(1–2), 113–119.

Walters, S. T., Matson, S. A., Baer, J. S., & Ziedonis, D. M. (2005). Effectiveness of workshop training for psychosocial addiction treatments: A systematic review. *J Subst Abuse Treat, 29,* 283–293.

White, W. L., & Miller, W. R. (2007). The use of confrontation in addiction treatment: History, science, and time for a change. *The Counselor, 8,* 12–30.

CHAPTER 31

Dialectical Behavior Therapy for Individuals with Borderline Personality Disorder and Substance Use Disorders

DORIAN HUNTER
M. ZACHARY ROSENTHAL
THOMAS R. LYNCH
MARSHA M. LINEHAN

Dialectical behavior therapy for substance use disorders (DBT-SUD) is a comprehensive psychosocial intervention for substance users with borderline personality disorder (BPD) (Linehan, 2014a, 2014b). DBT-SUD is an extension of standard dialectical behavior therapy (DBT; Linehan, 1993a, 1993b), a treatment for BPD that has been investigated to the extent that the treatment can be considered "well-established" according to criteria outlined by Chambless and Hollon (1998). It is the subject of several well-controlled randomized clinical trials (RCTs) for the treatment of BPD, and efficacy has been demonstrated across independent research teams (Koons et al., 2001; Linehan, Armstrong, Suarez, Allmon, & Heard, 1991; Linehan et al., 1999, 2002, 2006; Verheul et al., 2003). Across studies, the evidence suggests that standard DBT is an efficacious treatment for reducing a variety of problems associated with BPD, including self-injurious behavior, suicide attempts, suicidal ideation, hopelessness, depression, and bulimia.

This chapter provides an overview of the modifications of standard dialectical behavior therapy that comprise DBT-SUD. We outline the philosophy and theory behind DBT-SUD, the biosocial model of BPD, as well as the treatment modes and functions, skills modules, and treatment strategies in DBT-SUD. We conclude with a description of treatment outcome studies supporting DBT-SUD and future applications of the treatment. For a comprehensive description of this treatment approach, interested readers are referred to the DBT treatment manual and group skills training manual (Linehan, 1993a, 1993b) and the DBT-SUD treatment manual (Linehan, Dimeff, & Sayrs, 2004).

WHY IS A TREATMENT FOR SUBSTANCE USERS WITH BPD NEEDED?

Separately, substance use disorders (SUDs) and BPD are serious public health problems associated with significant psychosocial impairment. However, they frequently co-occur (Trull, Sher, Minks-Brown, Durbin, & Burr, 2000). Estimates of prevalence of current SUDs among patients being treated for BPD range from 21 to 67% (Becker, Grilo, Anez, Paris, & McGlashan, 2005; Darke, Williamson, Ross, Teesson, & Lynskey, 2004; Dulit, Fyer, Haas, Sullivan, & Frances, 1990; Miller, Belkin, & Gibbons, 1994; Skinstad & Swain, 2001; Swadi & Bobier, 2003; Zanarini, Frankenburg, Hennen, Reich, & Silk, 2004), and it has been estimated that between 5 and 32% of individuals with SUDs meet criteria for BPD (Brooner, King, Kidorf, Schmidt, & Bigelow, 1997; Weiss, Mirin, Griffin, Gunderson, & Hufford, 1993). The two disorders share core features (e.g., impulsivity; Trull et al., 2000); however, overlap in criteria does not appear to account for the high correlation between the disorders, because dropping substance use as a criterion for BPD has not been shown to lead to a significant reduction in diagnosis of BPD (Dulit et al., 1990).

The combination of BPD and SUDs results in complex and difficult-to-treat behavioral problems, and is associated with greater problems than substance abuse alone (Links, Heslegrave, Mitton, van Reekum, & Patrick, 1995), including significantly more behavioral, legal, psychological, and medical problems (Cacciola, Alterman, McKay, & Rutherford, 2001; Cacciola, Alterman, Rutherford, & Snider, 1995; Leshner & Koob, 1999; McKay, Alterman, Cacciola, Mulvaney, & O'Brien, 2000; Nace, Davis, & Gaspari, 1991; Rutherford, Cacciola, & Alterman, 1994), and poorer treatment prognosis (Moos, Moos, & Finney, 2001). The presence of BPD specifically may lead to a number of impediments in standard substance abuse treatments. A diagnosis of BPD among opiate addicts treated with methadone was found to predict greater psychiatric impairment and alcoholism following treatment (Kosten, Kosten, & Rounsaville, 1989). BPD remission is negatively predicted by co-occurring SUDs (Zanarini et al., 2004). The extension of DBT from clients with BPD to those with BPD and SUD can be attributed in part to the high severity and comorbidity of the two separate presentations, along with the evidence that standard DBT is efficacious for individuals with BPD.

TARGET POPULATION FOR DBT-SUD

DBT-SUD was originally developed and tested with female clients meeting full DSM-IV diagnostic criteria for BPD and polysubstance abuse or SUD for opiates, cocaine, amphetamines, sedatives/hypnotics, hallucinogens, or anxiolytics. In our most recent clinical trial, DBT was found to perform equally well with both male and female opiate-dependent clients. Individuals with mental retardation, schizophrenia, schizoaffective disorder, bipolar affective disorder, and psychotic disorder not otherwise specified (NOS) also have been excluded from studies evaluating the efficacy of DBT-SUD. As a result, DBT-SUD has been tested in a relatively specific population. Although it may be impossible to limit the use of DBT-SUD to such a specific population in clinical practice, it is recommended that DBT-SUD be used with clients similar to the population from DBT-SUD clinical trials, until future outcome studies support the efficacy of DBT-SUD in different populations.

EMPIRICAL SUPPORT

Three randomized trials examining DBT-SUD were conducted. Linehan et al. (1999) compared DBT-SUD to treatment as usual (TAU) in the community in a sample of 28 women diagnosed with BPD and either SUD or polysubstance use disorder. Participants received 1 year of treatment, and were assessed 4, 8, 12, and 16 months after treatment. Participants were matched at pretreatment on age, severity of drug dependence, readiness to change, and global adjustment. Those in the DBT-SUD condition attended significantly more individual psychotherapy sessions during treatment, dropped out of treatment less, and, importantly, evidenced significantly less drug use as indicated by urine analyses. At 16-month follow-up, individuals in the DBT-SUD condition had higher scores on measures of global and social adjustment compared to those in the TAU condition.

In a second study, 23 participants with BPD and heroin dependence were randomly assigned to receive 1 year of DBT-SUD or comprehensive validation therapy, a treatment consisting of therapist validation coupled with 12 step (Linehan et al., 2002). Participants also concurrently received ORLAAM (an opiate replacement medication). Participants were matched at pretreatment on age, cocaine dependence, antisocial personality disorder, and global functioning. Although participants in both conditions had a small proportion of positive urinary analyses at follow-up, in the last 4 months of treatment, participants in the DBT-SUD condition maintained treatment gains, whereas those in the comprehensive validation condition had a significant increase in opiate use during this period. In addition, participants in both conditions reported greater social adjustment and general adjustment following treatment. Taken together, these studies suggest that DBT-SUD is an efficacious treatment for substance users with BPD.

In a third study that selected highly suicidal and self-injurious participants meeting criteria for BPD, patients in DBT with substance dependence disorders (SDD) had a SDD remission rate of 78% in the one-year treatment and were were more likely to achieve full remission, spend more time in partial remission, spend less time meeting full criteria, and report more drug and alcohol abstinent days than subjects in the community therapy-by-experts control condition. These findings suggest that improvements in co-occurring SDD among suicidal BPD patients are specific to DBT and cannot be attributed to general factors associated with nonbehavioral expert psychotherapy. Further, group differences in SDD remission were not explained by either psychotropic medication usage or changes in BPD criterion behaviors (Harned et al., 2009).

PHILOSOPHY AND THEORY

Philosophers such as Hegel and Kant discussed dialectics as a means of understanding or synthesizing apparent contradictions. Dialectics includes both a worldview and a process of change in DBT-SUD. From a dialectical worldview, behavior is conceptualized as interrelated, contextually determined, and systemic. The dialectical process of change is guided by the fundamental notions that (1) for every point an opposite position can be held, and (2) natural tensions can be resolved and adaptive change can occur when workable syntheses emerge from the consideration of contradicting polarities or opposing ideas. For example, a client might insist that substance use helps him or her feel less bored, whereas the therapist might insist that substance use is the problem. Using a dialectical perspective, therapist and client could jointly create a synthesis by discussing how substance use is understandable as a means of reducing boredom *and* simultaneously a cause of much long-term suffering. Working together, therapist and client would look for ways to relieve boredom and feel better without creating long-term suffering.

There are many dialectical tensions in DBT-SUD. However, the central dialectic is that of *acceptance and change*. For the therapist, this entails balancing acceptance of clients as they are in the present moment with an explicit long-term goal of meaningful change. For a client, changing one's own behaviors must be balanced by accepting unpleasant thoughts, emotions, or the reality that unpleasant events have occurred. As an example, in DBT-SUD, clients are encouraged to accept the reality that painful emotions will occur, while concurrently working to prevent unnecessary emotional suffering caused by dysfunctional behavior. A compromise between acceptance and change is not necessarily the goal. Instead, a synthesis of polarities may be more acceptance-based in one moment and more change-focused in another depending on the context and what is likely to be effective. This is similar to how a golfer might hit the ball toward one side of the fairway or the other, depending on the direction and strength of the wind in the present moment, the shape of the fairway, and the obstacles that lie to the side. The target is to hit the ball as close to the putting green or cup as possible without having the ball going out of play, not to hit the ball down the exact middle of the fairway.

BIOSOCIAL MODEL

Linehan (1993a, 1993b) suggests that BPD is fundamentally a disorder of the emotion regulation system, and results from a reciprocal transaction between an emotional vulnerability, an invalidating environment, and emotional dysregulation (see Figure 31.1). Emotional vulnerability is considered to be the key diathesis, environmental invalidation is the primary socially mediated process, and emotional dysregulation is the multidimensional construct thought to underlie BPD criterion behaviors.

Emotional Vulnerability

According to Linehan (1993a), BPD is characterized by emotional vulnerability, a biologically mediated predisposition for affective instability involving genetic, intrauterine, and temperamental factors that is defined by heightened emotional sensitivity, heightened emotional reactivity, and a slow return to baseline level of emotional arousal. That is, individuals with BPD respond quickly to stimuli, respond with a

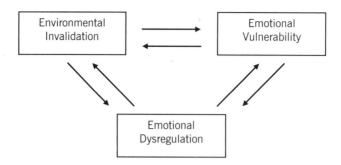

FIGURE 31.1. Components of the biosocial theory of BPD.

high magnitude of arousal, and take a long time before arousal decreases to baseline. Similar to the intense physical pain felt when someone with a serious lower back injury tries to walk, emotionally vulnerable individuals feel acute emotional pain in response to what appear to others to be ordinary events.

The Invalidating Environment

Broadly put, the invalidating environment is described by Linehan (1993a) as being characterized by pervasive criticizing, minimizing, trivializing, punishing, or erratically reinforcing communication of internal experiences (e.g., thoughts and emotions), and oversimplifying the ease of problem solving. For example, a parent may pervasively communicate, "You're not hurt, you just think you are" or "This is easy; just deal with it!" In addition, verbal communication is indiscriminately rejected and the individual is chronically pathologized as having undesirable personality traits (e.g., too sensitive, paranoid, lazy, or unmotivated). Because appropriate emotional expression is chronically punished and extreme emotional displays are intermittently reinforced, escalation of emotional expressions (e.g., suicidal behavior) may occur. In addition to emotional invalidation, prototypical examples of invalidation are childhood sexual or physical abuse (Wagner & Linehan, 1997).

Emotional Dysregulation

In the context of environmental invalidation and emotional vulnerability, the biosocial model suggests that emotional dysregulation occurs, leading to problems with behavioral–motoric, physiological, and cognitive–experiential emotional systems. Such problems with emotion are hypothesized by Linehan (1993a) to underlie BPD criterion behaviors, and, as shown in Table 31.1, can be organized across domains of functioning (emotional, behavioral, cognitive, and interpersonal). Linehan suggests that emotional dysregulation in BPD is characterized by problems with up- and down-regulation of physiological arousal, inhibition of mood-dependent behavior, excessive reliance on avoidant coping strategies, attentional control, processing emotional information, self-soothing, and self-validation. For example, an inability to

TABLE 31.1. Summary of DSM-5 Criteria for BPD

Emotion dysregulation
    Affective instability
    Problems with anger

Behavioral dysregulation
    Impulsive behavior
    Self-injurious behavior

Cognitive dysregulation
    Dissociation
    Paranoia

Interpersonal dysregulation
    Chaotic relationships
    Fears of abandonment

Self-dysregulation
    Identity disturbances
    Chronic feelings of emptiness

decrease intense physiological arousal may precede the behavioral dyscontrol that is a hallmark of BPD, such as self-injury or impulsive substance use. Although substance use may occur in response to dysregulated emotional systems, in DBT-SUD, substance use also can be conceptualized as a means of emotion regulation. That is, substance use can function as an attempt to regulate emotions or as the outcome of emotional dysregulation.

TREATMENT

DBT-SUD is a principle-driven, flexible, and comprehensive treatment. As a behavioral therapy, it is change-focused. As an acceptance-based therapy, DBT-SUD incorporates strategies for when changing behavior may not be possible or effective. Treatment begins by orienting clients to the therapeutic assumptions, agreements, levels and modes of treatment, and includes obtaining a commitment to treatment.

Assumptions and Agreements

In DBT-SUD, assumptions and agreements are openly delineated with clients in the first few "pre-treatment" sessions (see Tables 31.2 and 31.3). During these sessions, the therapist discusses the requirement that clients commit to treatment. Although standard DBT often uses a variety of commitment strategies during pretreatment sessions, in DBT-SUD, clients must, at a minimum, agree to work toward abstinence from all illicit drugs. Because commitment to treatment often ebbs and flows, it is necessary to monitor ongoing changes in committed behavior throughout treatment.

TABLE 31.2. Patient and Therapist Assumptions in DBT

Patient
1. Patients are doing the best they can.
2. Patients want to improve.
3. Patients need to do better, try harder, and be more motivated to change.
4. Patients must solve their current problems, regardless of who caused these problems.
5. Patients are living lives that are unbearable as they are currently being lived.
6. Patients must learn new behaviors in all relevant contexts.

Therapist
1. Patients cannot fail in DBT, but the therapy or therapist can fail the patient.
2. Helping patients work toward their ultimate goals in life is the most caring thing a therapist can do.
3. DBT therapists need support.
4. The therapeutic relationship is a relationship of two equals.
5. Principles of behavior are universal, affecting both patients and therapists alike.

TABLE 31.3. Patient and Therapist Agreements in DBT

Patient agreements
1. Stay in therapy for a specified period of time, usually 1 year.
2. Attend all therapy sessions.
3. Therapy will be discontinued if four consecutive sessions are missed.
4. Work toward terminating self-injurious behavior and other therapeutic targets.
5. Participate in skills training.
6. Abide by relevant research conditions of therapy.
7. Pay agreed upon fees for service.

Therapist agreements
1. Maintain competence and effort.
2. Provide ethical and professional treatment.
3. Be available for weekly sessions and phone consultation.
4. Treat patients humanely, with respect and integrity.
5. Maintain confidentiality.
6. Seek appropriate consultation.

Treatment Targets

Clients with BPD often present for treatment with severe behavioral dyscontrol (e.g., self-injurious behavior), treatment-interfering behaviors (e.g., not showing up for treatment), and problems affecting physical (e.g., sleep problems), emotional (e.g., excessive emotionality), and cognitive (e.g., hopelessness) functioning. To treat this range of therapeutic targets consistently, a hierarchy of problem behaviors is used in DBT-SUD: (1) Reduce acute life-threatening and self-injurious behaviors; (2) reduce treatment-interfering behaviors; and (3) reduce quality-of-life interfering behaviors, such as drug use, eating disorders, anxiety, depression, and physical health problems.

In the earliest iterations of DBT-SUD, complete and total cessation of all problematic drug use was the primary treatment target. However, we have found this to be problematic in working with substance abusers, who frequently have other primary goals that are personally more important to them. While suicide, self-harm, and therapy-interfering behaviors remain prioritized over clients' individual goals, owing to the fact that it is critical for clients to be alive and in therapy to work on such goals, substance abuse is still targeted within quality-of-life interfering behavior, but is not necessarily prioritized over other behaviors. It is targeted when it is interfering with the client's own goals, as it often does.

Within the larger treatment hierarchy, DBT-SUD outlines the "path to clear mind" in order to provide specific treatment targets addressing substance use. In accomplishing this, the next target in the path to clear mind is to maintain an adequate dose of drug replacement medications, when relevant, and more generally to decrease the physical discomfort associated with abstinence. Physical pain and psychological distress are targeted for change when possible. However, acceptance skills are used to tolerate pain that cannot be reduced directly.

Clients also learn how to monitor cravings, evaluate the intensity of cravings, identify when cravings are particularly likely to increase drug use, reduce cravings, and avoid using drugs once cravings occur. On the one hand, clients learn that cravings should be expected to occur; on the other hand, they learn how to actively problem-solve ways to cope with cravings without using. Unlike standard DBT, in which clients are frequently encouraged to turn their attention toward the experience of aversive emotions, DBT-SUD clients are encouraged to use skills to turn their attention *away from* cravings and urges to use. As coping skills are acquired and generalized, DBT-SUD emphasizes community reinforcement of "non-addict wisemind" behaviors. That is, clients increase activities associated with a decreased likelihood for drug use, such as AA/NA meetings, gaining steady and legitimate employment, and socializing whenever possible with nonaddicts in mainstream settings.

Next, "apparently unimportant behaviors" are targeted. Patterned after Marlatt's work on apparently irrelevant decisions (Marlatt & Gordon, 1985), in DBT-SUD behaviors (both observable events and privately experienced events, such as thoughts) that are links on the chain towards drug use are targeted. Examples range from obvious (e.g., selling drugs) to less obvious (e.g., going into an environment with many cues associated with drug use). Finally, on the path to clear mind, DBT-SUD targets closing options to use drugs, for example, by ending contacts and throwing away contact information with those who sell and use drugs, getting rid of all drug paraphernalia, and not lying about drug use.

Dialectical Abstinence

The goal of DBT-SUD is to stop using drugs, with the ideal outcome of treatment being complete and indefinite abstinence. However, the cold reality suggested by clinical observation and supported by treatment outcome studies is that even in the best treatments for substance use, abstinence may not last indefinitely. Harm reduction approaches take into account the likelihood of lapse following treatment (e.g., Marlatt & Gordon, 1985), with the aim of reducing the impact of substance use rather than focusing exclusively on abstinence. In DBT-SUD, abstinence is the goal, not harm reduction. However, the synthesis between complete abstinence and a harm reduction approach is struck. The resulting perspective, "dialectical abstinence," refers to the position of targeting complete abstinence on the one hand, while being prepared for and responding effectively to drug lapse on the other. That is, dialectical abstinence is achieved through the therapist targeting 100% abstinence with the client, while also planning for the possibility of relapse by developing a relapse management plan.

Attachment Strategies

Although similar to clients with BPD without substance use problems, those presenting with co-occurring BPD and SUD appear to have important differences. Linehan (1993a) characterizes individuals with BPD either as "attached" or as "butterflies." Whereas attached clients with BPD communicate often with therapists, rarely miss appointments, and appear closely affiliated to their therapists, butterfly clients do the opposite. Substance-abusing clients with BPD are often butterflies, possibly because their drug use has become more reinforcing than social interactions, and this clinical observation has led to the addition of a set of attachment strategies in DBT-SUD. For example, to develop rapport, the first several sessions include a large amount of therapist validation, with less emphasis on immediate change and/or interpersonal aversive contingencies than in standard DBT. In addition, because these clients tend to come into and out of therapy, therapists may become easily demoralized. Thus, a strong emphasis is made on remoralizing and motivating therapists during consultation team meetings. Other attachment strategies include orienting the client to this problem, increasing contact with clients toward the beginning of treatment, frequent contacts with clients via voice mail, *in vivo* therapy sessions, decreasing or increasing session length as needed, family and friends network meetings, calling clients when they are avoiding treatment, and finding clients when they repeatedly do not show up or respond to telephone calls.

Modes and Functions of Treatment

DBT-SUD includes methods for learning adaptive coping skills, generalizing such skills into all relevant contexts, enhancing commitment to treatment, and preventing demoralization of both the therapist and client. There are four standard modes of treatment: group skills training, individual therapy, phone consultation, and consultation team. Because of the need for replacement medication, and the frequent comorbidity of other psychological disorders, DBT-SUD also can incorporate a pharmacotherapy mode. Next, the function, process, and structure of treatment modes are briefly reviewed.

Skills Training

Weekly 2.5-hour skills training classes occur in a group format. The primary function of skills training classes is the acquisition of new behavioral and cognitive skills.

Skills training classes are co-led by two skills trainers, and include both homework review of previously learned skills and didactic presentation of new skills from the skills training manual (Linehan, 1993b). Specifically, there are separate skill modules for mindfulness, distress tolerance, emotion regulation, and interpersonal effectiveness.

MINDFULNESS

Derived from Eastern meditative and Western contemplative prayer traditions, "mindfulness" is the practice of paying attention in a particular way: on purpose, in the present moment, and without judgment. In this module, clients learn that their behavior is a function of current emotions (emotion mind) or logical analysis (reasonable mind). "Wise mind" knowing and behavior is emphasized as a synthesis of emotion and reasonable minds, such that decisions and actions are both effective and remain within personal values. In teaching wise mind, clients also are taught to learn how to identify the distinction between "addict mind" and "nonaddict mind," or the difference between making decisions as an addict or as a nonaddict.

Mindfulness skills specifically include the ability to observe, describe, and participate fully in one's actions and experiences, in a nonjudgmental, one-mindful, and effective manner. "Observing" refers to noticing experiences without becoming attached, allowing thoughts or other internal experiences to flow freely with full awareness. "Describing" follows observing and involves labeling or putting words on experiences. "Participating" is somewhat different and involves entering fully into the present moment, without observing and describing internal experiences (e.g., an athlete at peak performance). Being nonjudgmental, including being aware of judgments and letting go of their literal truth, is a central skill repeatedly practiced by DBT clients and therapists. Being one-mindful entails a sharpening of attentional focus on one thing or activity at a time. This skill involves staying in the present moment and not becoming distracted by thoughts about the past or future. Finally, the focus on effectiveness is a key aspect of mindfulness. "Effectiveness" refers to behaving in a way that is consistent with one's values and long-term goals. The emphasis on effectiveness as a DBT skill illustrates how mindfulness is a behavioral, psychological, and spiritual practice, extending beyond formal meditation practice.

Additional mindfulness skills specific to DBT-SUD include "urge surfing" and "alternate rebellion." Urge surfing stems from Marlatt's treatment for alcohol abuse (Marlatt & Gordon, 1985) and involves awareness of urges to use, coupled with the use of imagery of a wave as the urge is "surfed." As is always the case with waves, urges eventually cease. For many, use of this skill helps considerably in preventing substance use following cravings to use. "Alternate rebellion" refers to identifying ways to rebel against society in a skillful way that does not involve drug use. This skill is relevant for those drug users whose identity as an addict functions as a way to be different or unique. As a mindfulness skill, alternate rebellion is linked to being effective and value-driven, and might include dyeing one's hair, getting a tattoo, or wearing unusual clothes.

DISTRESS TOLERANCE

The distress tolerance module is designed to teach clients how to tolerate aversive emotional experiences without behaving maladaptively (or ineffectively). A list of crisis management skills is taught, including strategies for effective temporary distraction, such as activities, eliciting opposite emotions, and squeezing ice or a rubber ball. Self-soothing skills are introduced, whereby clients learn to soothe themselves intentionally during periods of crisis with calming visual stimuli, sounds, smells, tastes, and objects to touch. In addition, other skills, such as imaginal and relaxation exercises, are taught to improve the current moment in order to avert crises. Other distress tolerance skills include awareness, breathing, and half-smile exercises, as well as radical acceptance of reality as it is in the present moment. Overall, distress tolerance skills are intended to interrupt and change habitual, problematic, and often context-insensitive responses to emotional distress, allowing the opportunity for new responses to aversive stimulation and the emergence of a broader repertoire of skillful responses.

There are two new skills added to the distress tolerance module: "adaptive denial" and "burning your bridges." When a strong urge occurs, clients can use the adaptive denial skill to convince themselves adamantly that they actually do not want to engage in the addictive behavior, or that the addictive behavior is not a possibility. Adaptive denial may include deliberately replacing thoughts of strong urges for one behavior with strong urges for another. As an example, a client with an intense urge to use heroin might say, "I just have to have an ice-cream cone, right now; I must" and focus on obtaining ice cream rather than heroin. This behavior functions to divert attention away from thinking about heroin. Because such attempts to control thinking can, at times, have paradoxical effects, leading to an increase in unwanted thoughts (e.g., Abramowtiz, Tolin, & Street, 2001; Purdon, 1999), adaptive denial is a skill that can only be used by individuals for whom it is effective, and it should be used only in the midst of an actual crisis (e.g., when a person cannot tolerate sitting with the urge). In mentally denying access to certain thoughts, substance use may, in some contexts, be averted. In other contexts, adaptive denial would not be effective; instead, the client might focus attention on unpleasant thoughts. The point is that, depending on the context, it may or may not be effective to attempt to deny entry into awareness of thoughts that may lead to drug use. Thus, awareness of the context and an ability not to avoid thoughts chronically is the key to this skill.

"Burning your bridges" is a skill that is derived from the notion of radical acceptance. In order to help tolerate distress associated with no longer using drugs, "burning your bridges" includes behaviors that function to cut off all previous links to drug use and the identity of being a drug user. This skill is compatible with the target on the path to clear mind described as eliminating options to use drugs (e.g., telling the truth).

EMOTION REGULATION

The emotion regulation skills module is designed to help clients better understand their emotions, reduce emotional vulnerability, and decrease emotional suffering.

Specific skills taught include an increased awareness of emotions, identifying and challenging distorted ways of thinking about emotions, learning how emotions are related to problem behaviors, accurately labeling emotions, understanding the functions of emotions, reducing emotional vulnerability, increasing pleasant emotions, and *acting opposite* to behavioral urges associated with emotions. Although all of these skills are useful, the opposite action skill is particularly helpful, because it can be applied in many contexts to change a variety of problem behaviors.

The opposite action skill uses an algorithm for knowing when to change emotion. This includes first determining whether the emotion is justified based on the facts of the situation. Next, it is important to know the action urge of the emotion being experienced. Each emotion has its own urging component (e.g., anger—attack, fear—run, sadness—withdraw, guilt—repair, shame—hide). When the client is experiencing an unjustified emotion that he or she wishes to change, the skill is to go opposite to the action urge of the emotion. For example, if a client is feeling guilty for disagreeing with a friend, the opposite action skill would be to teach the client first to ask him- or herself whether the behavior was egregious according to his or her own value system. If the disagreement was done in a manner inconsistent with the client's values (e.g., disrespectfully and judgmentally disagreeing), then a repair (e.g., apology) would be suggested as a way to lower justified guilt. However, if the disagreement did not violate the client's values and guilt was unjustified (i.e., respectfully and nonjudgmentally disagreeing), then the client would be instructed not to repair but to repeat the behavior (i.e., effective opinion giving) multiple times. As the client learns that giving opinions does not always result in negative outcomes, over time the unjustified guilt response to disagreeing effectively would extinguish. Similarly, for individuals who have unjustified fear, opposite action for fear is to engage in the feared behavior, or approach the feared stimulus, over and over again.

INTERPERSONAL EFFECTIVENESS

Because chaotic interpersonal relationships are a key characteristic of BPD, the development of interpersonal skills is crucial. This skills module teaches clients how to identify factors interfering with interpersonal effectiveness, challenge common cognitive distortions associated with interpersonal situations, and determine the appropriate level of intensity for making requests or saying no a given situation. Specific guidelines for being taken seriously, attending to relationships, and preserving self-respect are taught, and clients are instructed to practice developing new interpersonal skills based on these guidelines in a wide variety of situations, including frequent rehearsal and role playing during group and individual sessions. When teaching interpersonal effectiveness in DBT-SUD, specific skills are taught that are designed to avoid drug-using contexts (e.g., drug refusal interpersonal skills) and to respond effectively when such contexts can not be avoided (e.g., craving tolerance skills).

Individual Therapy

Individual therapy sessions with a DBT-SUD therapist are typically for 50–60 minutes once per week. The individual therapist provides psychoeducational information to the client early in treatment, including handouts that describe the pros and cons of participating in DBT-SUD compared to other treatments, and facts about drug addiction. However, a primary function of individual therapy is to develop and maintain client motivation to overcome obstacles to change. A validating environment is created, whereby clients are treated with compassion and acceptance in the context of targeting behavioral change. Factors interfering with progress in treatment are discussed, preventing problems that might interfere with the development of new skills, and helping clients remain in treatment despite urges to drop out. Episodes of emotional dysregulation from the previous week are discussed in light of skills that could have been used. In addition, skills are practiced during session and are woven into plans in anticipation of upcoming events.

DIARY CARDS

In order to monitor a variety of targets, a daily diary card is used. For example, clients rate their mood and monitor the frequency of self-injurious urges and behavior, drug use urges and behavior, HIV risk behaviors, and other relevant and personalized emotion and behavior targets. The diary card is reviewed at the beginning of each session, and the therapy session is organized around targets evident on the diary card. Given the plethora of treatment targets and the possibility that clients will not remember salient events over the week, the diary card is instrumental in directing therapy sessions toward highly relevant targets.

BEHAVIORAL ANALYSIS

To change dysfunctional behaviors, DBT-SUD uses a number of problem-solving strategies. Behavioral analysis is frequently used to identify problem behaviors and understand the relevant context in which these behaviors occur. Behavioral analysis involves an active, directive effort by the therapist to identify specific antecedents and consequences associated with the problem behavior. A thorough elaboration of events before, during, and after problem behaviors facilitates the selection of appropriate treatment interventions. Based on a functional-analytic approach to behavioral assessment, the goal of behavioral analysis is prediction and control of functional classes of problem behavior rather than traditional diagnostic assessment of disease entities (Hayes & Follette, 1992; Kanfer & Saslow, 1969). In other words, in DBT-SUD, borderline symptoms are conceptualized as problem *behaviors*. These may be external, publicly observable behaviors, such as self-mutilation or impulsive aggression, or internal, publicly unobservable experiences, such as self-judgmental thoughts or urges to use substances.

Because behavioral analysis in DBT-SUD involves explicating the links in a chain of events, it is often referred to as a "chain analysis," during which the topography, intensity, duration, and frequency of the target problem is discussed. As links in the chain are explored, the therapist considers the role of classical and instrumental conditioning. Classically conditioned (respondent) behaviors are under the control of an antecedent stimulus, and instrumentally conditioned (operant) behaviors are under the control of consequent events. For example, strong urges to use substances may be classically conditioned to occur after interpersonal conflicts. On the other hand, substance use may be instrumentally conditioned by the consequences that follow, such as less hostility or increased attention from others. Knowing the controlling variables (i.e., antecedent or consequent) of a problem behavior informs the choice of interventions. Strategies for changing antecedents include behavioral exposure (e.g., to rehearse saying no to a drug dealer) or stimulus control (e.g., to avoid drug dealers). In addition, other behavioral principles used during chain analyses are positive and negative reinforcement, punishment, extinction, and shaping.

Dysfunctional links uncovered in a chain analysis are examined and replaced with more adaptive responses during a *solution analysis*. Typically, this is guided by three questions:

1. Can the client change the circumstance (e.g., flush the drugs down the toilet, quit the job)?
2. Can the client change an emotional reaction (e.g., go opposite to the emotion action urge)?
3. Can the client better tolerate the pain associated with the problem (e.g., radically accept the problem)?

Together, client and therapist collaboratively develop strategies to replace problematic links, then commit to using new solutions the next time the problem behavior emerges.

SKILLS ENHANCEMENT

A primary goal of individual therapy is to enhance skills learned during group. One way to do this is to ask clients to rehearse behavior in session. Behavioral rehearsal may occur in the form of covert rehearsing of challenges to distorted cognitions or by role playing of interpersonal scenarios. Therapists provide reinforcement and coaching during rehearsals and role plays, with an emphasis on skills use. Whenever skillful behavior occurs in session, the therapist reinforces such behavior. Ineffective behavior during session, on the other hand, is often ignored or punished. In addition, positive regard is applied contingently. For example, when the client is behaving inappropriately (e.g., threatening self-injury), the therapist remains cool and matter-of-fact, while skillful behavior (e.g., commitment not to self-injure and to using skills) is greeted with therapist warmth. In this way, the therapist is actively involved in contingency management.

Another method of facilitating skills use is to use behavioral exposure and response prevention in session. Clients often become angry, ashamed, or fearful in session, and a range of behaviors may be evoked in response to these emotions. Clients with BPD who feel angry may lash out, while those who feel ashamed may look down or dissociate, and clients feeling fearful may suddenly leave a session. Behavioral exposure and response prevention applied to these emotions in session target paying attention to these emotions nonjudgmentally, observing urges to behave ineffectively, and blocking these urges by helping clients not to lash out, to keep eye contact, or to remain in the therapy room.

VALIDATION

Verification of what the client does effectively and disconfirmation of what is ineffective is a commonality across many psychotherapies. Although validation of clients may be defined in various ways, in DBT-SUD, validation is a core strategy that is operationalized on several levels (see Table 31.4). Validation may be explicitly verbal or it may occur more implicitly and functionally, such as when the therapist offers a tissue when an emotionally inhibited client appears on the verge of tears. Validation may be used as pure acceptance, with no directed effort toward change. However, therapist validation of client behaviors is contingent on the legitimacy, effectiveness, or validity of these behaviors. DBT-SUD therapists attempt to validate what is valid, and, at times, to invalidate what is invalid. This requires the DBT therapist to discern carefully what is valid, and to apply validation contingently and in accordance with the conceptualization of each client's problem behaviors. In DBT-SUD, validation is essential, because clients often come and go from treatment and may not be as attached to therapists as standard DBT clients with BPD and no substance use problems. Consequently, aversive interpersonal contingencies are held to a minimum, unless, of course, such contingencies assist in reducing problem behaviors.

DIALECTICAL STRATEGIES

In DBT, dialectical strategies are fundamentally based around acceptance (e.g., validation) and change (e.g., problem solving). When dialectical reasoning is pursued, the therapist helps the client move from a polarized position of "either–or" to a dialectical synthesis of "both–and." There are a number of specific dialectical strategies used with clients (see Table 31.5). Importantly, in order to be effective, these strategies must be used in a manner that is genuine, and not as simple techniques. In addition, from a dialectical perspective, the therapist must be willing to let go of the truth or rightness of any dialectical strategy, instead continually searching for ways to help clients change problem behaviors.

TABLE 31.4. Levels of Validation in DBT

1. Listening and observing

2. Accurate reflection of patient experiences

3. Helping patients articulate unverbalized emotions, thoughts, and patterns of behavior

4. Communicating an understanding of behavior as valid given past learning history or biological vulnerability

5. Communicating an understanding of behavior as valid given a current context or what is deemed normative

6. Therapist provides radical genuineness, treating the individual as an equal and not as a sick and fragile patient

Note. Adapted with permission from Linehan (1993a).

Telephone Consultation

To enhance generalization of skills, clients may contact their individual therapists for telephone consultation between sessions. Because these individuals may experience unrelenting crises, it is crucial that therapists observe personal limits associated with telephone consultation. Telephone calls are intended to be brief and usually last approximately 5–10 minutes. Clients are oriented during pretreatment to the purpose of skills calls and are told to call when they are nable to implement skills in necessary situations, but before crises occur. In order to reduce inadvertent reinforcement of self-injurious behavior using warmth and validation over the telephone, a 24-hour rule is applied. This rule states that clients will not receive skills help from their individual therapists until 24 hours after any self-injurious behavior, or have contact that is not already scheduled. Instead, early in treatment, a contingency plan is created for occasions when clients self-injure, and therapists may refer clients to this plan in the event that they call after self-injuring. In all consultation calls, therapists assess for immediate danger and provide appropriate assistance if a client is deemed to be in imminent danger of harming him- or herself or others.

Consultation Team

As mentioned earlier, a consultation team is a necessary mode of treatment. Team members commit to weekly meetings and agree to a team structure and process (see Table 31.6). In important ways, team members treat each other by providing validation, support, and motivation. This support is invaluable and can help DBT-SUD therapists with a more balanced approach toward their clients. The consultation team also provides opportunities for fresh perspectives and new solutions, helping

TABLE 31.5. Dialectical Strategies Used in DBT

1. Acceptance and change-focused interventions.
2. Nurture the patient and demand that patients help themselves.
3. Being stable and persistent as well as flexible.
4. Highlight patient's strengths and deficits.
5. Structure session with an agenda, and respond to in-session patient behaviors as they occur.
6. Highlight both ends of continua, and make synthesizing statements.
7. Point out paradoxes when present (e.g., patient's behavior, therapeutic process).
8. Use metaphors.
9. Play devil's advocate.
10. Extend the seriousness or implications of the patient's communication.
11. Help the patient activate "wise mind."
12. Help make lemonade out of lemons.
13. Allow natural changes in therapy.

Note. Adapted with permission from Linehan (1993a, p. 206).

therapists get unstuck and remain hopeful. It is not uncommon for DBT-SUD therapists to periodically become rigid in their thinking and behavior with a client. The consultation team offers problem solving and validation for the therapist, and team members actively use a dialectical process to help find effective syntheses between polarized positions. For example, the team can help remind the therapist to continue managing contingencies in session appropriately (e.g., not being warm in response to client hostility). If possible, it is extremely helpful to videotape therapy sessions and watch important segments of the therapy session during the consultation team meeting, as this engenders a full appreciation for the difficulty a therapist may be having and allows the team to ensure that all members are indeed adhering to the treatment.

Pharmacotherapy

There are five principles that organize the management of psychotropic medications in DBT-SUD. First, and most important, safe and nonlethal medications must be prescribed and used in a safe manner. This principle is considered in light of each individual. For those with a history of medication abuse, the DBT-SUD pharmacotherapist observes the medication being ingested and provides the client with a small supply of take-home medications. Second, simple medication regimens are used in order to mitigate problems with side effects and drug interactions, both of which can interfere with treatment. Third, specific symptoms are targeted first, rather than general problems, such as affective instability. Fourth, choice of medications is guided by controlled efficacy studies. Finally, speed of clinical improvement is imperative, with, for example, opiate replacement rapidly induced to the desirable therapeutic maintenance dose.

DBT-SUD Case Management

Because substance users with BPD often encounter problems obtaining and maintaining adequate food, housing, and employment, case management can be added

TABLE 31.6. Consultation Team Agreements in DBT

1. Meet weekly for 1–2 hours.
2. Discuss cases according to the treatment hierarchy (i.e., self-injurious/life-threatening behavior, treatment-interfering behavior, and quality-of-life interfering behavior).
3. Accept a dialectical philosophy.
4. Consult with the patient on how to interact with other therapists and do not tell other therapists how to interact with the patient.
5. Consistency of therapists with one another (even across the same patient) is not expected.
6. All therapists observe their own limits without fear of judgmental reactions from other consultation group members.
7. Search for nonpejorative empathic interpretation of patient's behavior.
8. All therapists are fallible.

to DBT-SUD. Unlike standard case management approaches that intervene directly in the environment (e.g., making a phone call on behalf of a client), however, DBT-SUD case management emphasizes actively coaching the client to intervene on his or her own behalf. The DBT-SUD case manager does not manage the client's resources; instead, clients manage their resources with skills coaching from the case manager or individual therapist. The case manager is utilized by the individual therapist on an ad hoc basis in one of the following ways: (1) as a resource to the therapist for referrals or advice, (2) to provide information or referrals directly to the client, or (3) to provide *in vivo* skills coaching in the client's natural environment.

FUTURE DIRECTIONS

To date, the efficacy of DBT-SUD has been demonstrated in two small clinical trials, and a Stage II efficacy trial. These studies suggest that DBT-SUD is a promising manual-based treatment for substance users with BPD. There are two major future directions for DBT-SUD.

The corresponding pharmacotherapy protocol for opiate dependence should be modified. The clinical trial utilized Suboxone, which we would be wary of using again for several reasons. First, Suboxone is administered sublingually (it is placed under the patient's tongue to dissolve), and is only bioavailable using this route of administration. As such, it is relatively easy to pretend to take it. Second, it is very valuable on the street, greatly increasing the probability of diversion. Third, it does not have many of the physiological benefits of methadone and is more beneficial for less severely dependent users.

We are currently adapting DBT-SUD for use with individuals with alcohol use disorders (AUDs). The major differences between DBT-SUD and DBT-AUD include the development of moderation materials, modification of the motivational elements of DBT, and an alcohol-specific pharmacotherapy protocol.

SUMMARY

DBT-SUD is a comprehensive psychosocial treatment designed to treat substance users with BPD. The philosophy, theory, structure, skills modules, treatment modes and functions, and treatment strategies are equivalent to those of standard DBT. However, notable additions to DBT-SUD include (1) treatment targets that aim to reduce drug-related behaviors, (2) new coping skills for managing drug cravings and withdrawal, (3) new wise mind skills, (4) attachment strategies, (5) increased use of validation and less aversive interpersonal contingencies, (6) increased use of case management to assist in housing and other crises via direct environmental intervention, and (7) a pharmacotherapy mode. Overall, DBT-SUD is a promising new treatment that is grounded in philosophy and theory, supported by preliminary empirical findings and, importantly, offering hope for substance users with BPD.

REFERENCES

Abramowitz, J. S., Tolin, D. F., & Street, G. P. (2001). Paradoxical effects of thought suppression: A meta-analysis of controlled studies. *Clin Psychol Rev, 21,* 683–703.

Becker, D. F., Grilo, C. M., Anez, L. M., Paris, M., & McGlashan, T. H. (2005). Discriminant efficiency of antisocial and borderline personality disorder criteria in Hispanic men with substance use disorders. *Compr Psychiatry, 46,* 140–146.

Brooner, R. K., King, V. L., Kidorf, M., Schmidt, C. W., & Bigelow, G. E. (1997). Psychiatric and substance use comorbidity among treatment-seeking opioid abusers. *Arch Gen Psychiatry, 54,* 71–80.

Cacciola, J. S., Alterman, A. I., McKay, J. R., & Rutherford, M. J. (2001). Psychiatric comorbidity in patients with substance use disorders: Do not forget Axis II disorders. *Psychiatr Ann, 31,* 321–331.

Cacciola, J. S., Alterman, A. I., Rutherford, M. J., & Snider, E. C. (1995). Treatment response of antisocial substance abusers. *J Nerv Ment Dis, 183*(3), 166–171.

Chambless, D. L., & Hollon, S. D. (1998). Defining empirically supported therapies. *J Consult Clin Psychol, 66,* 7–18.

Darke, S., Williamson, A., Ross, J., Teesson, M., & Lynskey, M. (2004). Borderline personality disorder, antisocial personality disorder, and risk-taking among heroin users: Findings from the Australian Treatment Outcome Study (ATOS). *Drug Alcohol Depend, 74,* 77–83.

Dulit, R. A., Fyer, M. R., Haas, G. L., Sullivan, T., & Frances, A. J. (1990). Substance use in borderline personality disorder. *Am J Psychiatry, 147,* 1002–1007.

Harned, M. S, Chapman, A., Mazza, E. T., Murray, A., Comtois, K. A. & Linehan, M. M. (2009). Treating co-occurring Axis I disorders in recurrently suicidal women with borderline personality disorder: A two-year randomized trial of dialectical behavior therapy vs. community treatment by experts. Retrieved from *www.psycontent.com/index/P77V88284K231376.pdf.*

Hayes, S. C., & Follette, W. C. (1992). Can functional analysis provide a substitute for syndromal classification? *Behav Assess, 14,* 345–365.

Kanfer, F. H., & Saslow, G. (1969). Behavioral diagnosis. In C. M. Franks (Ed.), *Behaviortherapy: Appraisal and status.* New York: McGraw-Hill.

Koons, C. R., Robins, C. J., Tweed, J. L., Lynch, T. R., Gonzalez, A. M., Morse, J. Q., et al. (2001). Efficacy of dialectical behavior therapy in women veterans with borderline personality disorder. *Behav Ther, 32,* 371–390.

Kosten, R. A., Kosten, T. R., & Rousaville, B. J. (1989). Personality disorders in opiate addicts show prognostic specificity. *J Subst Abuse Treat, 6,* 163–168.

Leshner, A. I., & Koob, G. F. (1999). Drugs of abuse and the brain. *Proc Assoc Am Physicians, 111,* 99–108.

Linehan, M. M. (1993a). *Cognitive-behavioral treatment of borderline personality disorder.* New York: Guilford Press.

Linehan, M. M. (1993b) *Skills training manual for treating borderline personality disorder.* New York: Guilford Press.

Linehan, M. M. (2014a). *DBT skills training manual* (2nd ed.). New York: Guilford Press.

Linehan, M. M. (2014b). *DBT skills training handouts and worksheets* (2nd ed.). New York: Guilford Press.

Linehan, M. M., Armstrong, H. E., Suarez, A., Allmon, D., & Heard, H. L. (1991). Cognitive-behavioral treatment of chronically parasuicidal borderline patients. *Arch Gen Psychiatry, 48,* 1060–1064.

Linehan, M. M., Comtois, K. A., Murray, A. M., Brown, M. Z., Gallop, H. L., Heard, H. L., et al. (2006). Two-year randomized controlled trial and follow-up of dialectical behavior therapy vs. therapy by experts for suicidal behaviors and borderline personality disorder. *Arch Gen Psychiatry, 63,* 757–766.

Linehan, M. M., Dimeff, L. A., Reynolds, S. K., Comtois, K. A., Welch, S. S., Heagerty, P., et al. (2002). Dialectical behavior therapy versus comprehensive validation therapy plus 12-step for the treatment of opioid dependent women meeting criteria for borderline personality disorder. *Drug Alchohol Depend, 67,* 13–26.

Linehan, M. M., Dimeff, L. A., & Sayrs, J. H. R. (2004). *Dialectical behavior therapy for substance abusers with borderline personality disorder: An extension of standard DBT.* Unpublished manuscript.

Linehan, M. M., Schmidt, H., III, Dimeff, L. A., Craft, J. C., Kanter, J., & Comtois, K. A. (1999). Dialectical behavior therapy for patients with borderline personality disorder and drug-dependence. *Am J Addict, 8,* 279–292.

Links, P. S., Heslegrave, R. J., Mitton, J. E., van Reekum, R., & Patrick, J. (1995). Borderline personality disorder and substance use: Consequences of comorbidity. *Can J Psychiatry, 40,* 9–14.

Marlatt, G. A., & Gordon, J. R. (1985). *Relapse prevention: Maintenance strategies in the treatment of addictive behaviors.* New York: Guilford Press.

McKay, J. R., Alterman, A. I., Cacciola, J. S., Mulvaney, F. D., & O'Brien, C. P. (2000). Prognostic significance of antisocial personality disorders in cocaine-dependent patients entering continuing care. *J Nerv Ment Dis, 188*(5), 287–296.

Miller, N. S., Belkin, B. M., & Gibbons, R. (1994). Clinical diagnosis of substance use disorders in private psychiatric populations. *J Subst Abuse Treat, 11,* 387–392.

Moos, R. H., Moos, B. S., & Finney, J. W. (2001). Predictors of deterioration among patients with substance-use disorders. *J Clin Psychol, 57,* 1403–1419.

Nace, E. P., Davis, C. W., & Gaspari, J. P. (1991). Axis II comorbidity in substance abusers. *Am J Psychiatry, 148,* 118–120.

Purdon, C. (1999). Thought suppression and psychopathology. *Behav Res Ther, 37,* 1029–1054.

Rutherford, M. J., Cacciola, J. S., & Alterman, A. I. (1994). Relationships of personality disorders with problem severity in methadone patients. *Drug Alcohol Depend, 35,* 69–76.

Skinstad, A., & Swain, A. (2001). Comorbidity in a clinical sample of substance abusers. *Am J Drug Alcohol Abuse, 27,* 45–64.

Swadi, H., & Bobier, C. (2003). Substance use disorder comorbidity among inpatient youths with psychiatric disorder. *Austr N Z J Psychiatry, 37,* 294–298.

Trull, T. J., Sher, K. J., Minks-Brown, C., Durbin, J., & Burr, R. (2000). Borderline personality disorder and substance use disorders: A review and integration. *Clin Psychol Rev, 20,* 235–253.

Verheul, R., van den Bosch, L. M. C., Koeter, M. W. J., de Ridder, M. A. J., Stijnen, T., & van den Brink, W. (2003). Dialectical behaviour therapy for women with borderline personality disorder: 12-month, randomised clinical trial in The Netherlands. *Br J Psychiatry, 182,* 135–140.

Wagner, A. W., & Linehan, M. M. (1997). Biosocial perspective on the relationship of childhood sexual abuse, suicidal behavior, and borderline personality disorder. In M. C. Zanarini (Ed.), *Role of sexual abuse in the etiology of borderline personality disorder* (pp. 203–224). Washington, DC: American Psychiatric Press.

Weiss, R. D., Mirin, S. M., Griffin, M. L., Gunderson, J. G., & Hufford, C. (1993). Personality disorders in cocaine dependence. *Compr Psychiatry, 34,* 145–149.

Zanarini, M. C., Frankenburg, F. R., Hennen, J., Reich, D. B., & Silk, K. R. (2004). Axis I comorbidity in patients with borderline personality disorder: 6-year follow-up and prediction of time to remission. *Am J Psychiatry, 161,* 2108–2114.

CHAPTER 32

Psychopharmacological Treatments

LARISSA J. MOONEY
ELINORE F. McCANCE-KATZ

This chapter reviews pharmacological treatment options for substance use disorders (SUDs), including nicotine, alcohol, sedatives/hypnotics, opioids, methamphetamine, and cocaine. Pharmacotherapies for SUDs have been developed to address two broad treatment categories: (1) acute withdrawal and the initial attainment of abstinence and (2) chronic maintenance and the prevention of relapse. There are medications approved by the U.S. Food and Drug Administration (FDA) for the treatment of nicotine, opioid, and alcohol use disorders. Despite clinical trials demonstrating the benefit of some medications in ameliorating cravings and preventing relapse, no medication has been proven effective as a pharmacotherapy for stimulant or cannabis use disorders.

Medications for acute withdrawal are particularly relevant to dependence on opioids, alcohol, and benzodiazepines, all of which produce physical dependence. Maintenance pharmacotherapies may be broadly classified as either blocking or substitution agents. For example, the competitive opioid antagonist naltrexone blocks the effects of heroin, including the subjective euphoria and the production of physiological dependence from repeated heroin use. In contrast, substitution agents help to prevent illicit drug use by reducing drug craving and withdrawal symptoms, as well as by producing, to some degree, cross-tolerance to another drug from the same pharmacological class (e.g., methadone and heroin, which are both opioids). Examples of substitution agents that produce cross-tolerance to heroin and have been shown to be effective in reducing illicit opioid use are methadone, levo-alpha-acetylmethadol (LAAM), and buprenorphine. Blocking and substitution are not necessarily incompatible, and partial agonists provide a pharmacological tool to combine both approaches in treating drug dependence. At low doses, partial agonists such as buprenorphine and varenicline suppress withdrawal symptoms in dependent patients and produce some subjective reinforcing properties, whereas at higher dosages these same medications block the reinforcement from full agonists.

The following sections review a variety of standard treatments for SUDs, as well as several new agents. The goal is to provide an overview of current pharmacological treatments for nicotine, alcohol, sedatives/hypnotics (e.g., benzodiazepines), opioid, and cocaine use disorders. Ideally, these pharmacotherapies should be administered in the context of psychosocial interventions to encourage adherence to medications and to facilitate the rehabilitation that is a necessary component of any successful treatment.

PHARMACOTHERAPIES FOR TOBACCO USE DISORDER

A variety of pharmacotherapies are FDA-approved for the treatment of tobacco use disorder, including nicotine replacement therapy, the antidepressant bupropion, and varenicline, a nicotine receptor partial agonist. These medications have demonstrated efficacy in clinical trials in diminishing nicotine withdrawal symptoms and at least doubling the odds of quitting smoking relative to placebo in general populations. Second-line agents for smoking cessation include clonidine (Covey & Glassman, 1991) and nortriptyline (Hall et al., 1998), and are not FDA-approved for this indication. Overall, 6- and 12-month quit rates observed in clinical trials remain low, with less than 25% abstinence observed in individuals receiving approved pharmacotherapies and 10% for placebo (McNeil, Piccenna, & Ioannides-Demos, 2010).

Nicotine Replacement Therapy

Five nicotine replacement therapy (NRT) products have been approved by the FDA for smoking cessation treatment: transdermal patch, gum, lozenge, nasal spray, and vapor inhaler. The use of NRT has been shown in clinical trials to improve quit rates relative to placebo (17 vs. 10%, respectively; Stead, Perera, Bullen, Mant, & Lancaster, 2008) and to increase the odds of quitting smoking by 1.77 (95% confidence interval [CI] 1.66–1.88; Silagy, Lancaster, Stead, Mant, & Fowler, 2004). NRT works by partially replacing the nicotine obtained from tobacco, in turn ameliorating cravings and withdrawal symptoms upon cessation of smoking. According to the 2008 U.S. Clinical Practice Guideline Update, the use of most NRT products should be limited to 12 weeks or less (Fiore et al., 2008). Side effects common to all NRT formulations include nausea, dizziness, and headache. Current guidelines recommend starting NRT on the target quit date (Raupach & van Schayck, 2011), although recent research suggests that starting NRT earlier than the quit date may be associated with improved abstinence rates (Rose, Herskovic, Behm, & Westman, 2009).

Transdermal nicotine patches are available without a prescription and are the most commonly used NRT formulation. Several marketed patch formulations are available in a range of doses that deliver nicotine through the skin at a relatively stable rate over a 16- or 24-hour period (Henningfield, Fant, Ruchhalter, & Stitzer, 2005). It is recommended that individuals who smoke more than 10 cigarettes daily use the highest dose nicotine patch (21 mg), while those who smoke fewer than 10 cigarettes per day may use the lower dose patches. The recommended duration of patch use is generally 10 weeks, beginning with 6 weeks at the highest dose, followed by 2 weeks each at the lower doses prior to discontinuation. A meta-analysis reported that continuation of the nicotine patch beyond 8 weeks is not associated with improvement in smoking cessation, and tapering of the dose may not improve outcomes relative to abrupt cessation of the patch (Stead et al., 2008). In contrast, a clinical trial reported improved nicotine abstinence rates in individuals randomized to receive transdermal nicotine for 6 months relative to those who received the patch for only 8 weeks (Schnoll et al., 2010), suggesting that prolonged treatment may confer additional benefit. Transdermal nicotine patches are generally well tolerated, with minor side effects including local irritation at the application site, mild gastric disturbances, and sleep disturbances, which may be reduced by alternating patch sites and using the shorter, 16-hour formulation (McNeil et al., 2010).

Nicotine polacrilex (nicotine gum) is also available over the counter in two doses: 2 or 4 mg; about 50% of the dose (1 and 2 mg of nicotine, respectively) is absorbed through the buccal mucosa, with peak nicotine concentrations reached in 15–30 minutes. Recommended dosing is one piece every 1–2 hours for the first 6 weeks, followed by a taper in dosing frequency every 3 weeks thereafter. The 4-mg dose is superior to the 2-mg one in more highly dependent smokers (over 25 cigarettes per day), and extra pieces may be taken between doses as needed to target acute cravings. Buccal absorption of nicotine is decreased in an acidic environment, and patients should be instructed not to consume acidic beverages such as coffee, juices, and soda immediately before, during, or after use of the gum. In addition, the "park and chew" method is recommended to reduce jaw soreness, whereby users rest the gum between the cheek and gum for about a minute after first chewing to release the nicotine (Henningfield et al., 2005).

The nicotine lozenge is also available without a prescription in 2 and 4 mg doses, chosen according to how soon the first cigarette of the day is smoked upon awakening. When using the lozenge, nicotine is absorbed slowly through the buccal mucosa at levels somewhat higher than those delivered by the gum (Henningfield et al., 2005).

Other nicotine delivery systems used less frequently in clinical practice include a nasal spray and an inhaler, which are both available only by prescription. The nasal spray permits more rapid delivery of nicotine than other NRTs, and the inhaler delivers nicotine via a mouthpiece and plastic cartridge, which releases a vapor in the mouth when "puffed." Use of the inhaler mimics the familiar hand-to-mouth ritual of smoking cigarettes that some users miss when they quit (Henningfield et al., 2005).

Bupropion

The observed relationship between tobacco use and mood disorders led to research examining the potential for antidepressant medications as effective pharmacotherapies for cigarette smoking cessation (Glassman, 1997). Sustained-release (SR) bupropion, an antidepressant with dopaminergic and noradrenergic properties, has demonstrated anti-smoking properties in multiple randomized clinical trials (RCTs; Hurt et al., 1997; Hughes, Stead, & Lancaster, 2007). The effectiveness of bupropion treatment is at least equivalent to NRT, with an approximate doubling of quit rates relative to placebo. A recent meta-analysis of 36 RCTs reported 1.7 times greater odds of abstinence following at least 6 months of treatment with bupropion than placebo (95% CI 1.53–1.85; Hughes et al., 2007). The mechanism of action of bupropion in smoking cessation is not fully understood, but it may be related to amelioration of nicotine withdrawal symptoms, including dysphoria (Henningfield et al., 2005), and inhibition of brain nicotinic receptor activity that may interfere with reinforcing effects of nicotine (Slemmer, Martin & Damaj, 2000). The dose of bupropion SR used for smoking cessation is the same as that for depression (150 mg twice a day), and it is recommended to begin medication 7-14 days prior to the target quit date. The duration of treatment is typically up to 12 weeks but may be extended. The most common side effects of bupropion include headache, insomnia, and dry mouth. Bupropion also lowers the seizure threshold and should not be used in individuals with a prior history of seizures, anorexia or bulimia nervosa, or other medical conditions that increase seizure risk. Like other antidepressants, warnings have been added about potential increased risk of suicidal thoughts and behaviors (McNeil et al., 2010).

Varenicline

Varenicline is a partial agonist at the $alpha_4beta_2$ nicotinic acetylcholine receptor approved by the FDA for smoking cessation in 2006. As a partial agonist, varenicline alleviates nicotine craving and withdrawal symptoms while simultaneously inhibiting nicotine binding and diminishing the rewarding effects of smoking (McNeil et al., 2010). In prior clinical trials, varenicline has demonstrated greater efficacy in reducing cigarette smoking than both bupropion and NRT. A recent meta-analysis reported a 2.3 times greater likelihood of abstinence from smoking at 6 months or longer with varenicline than with placebo (95% CI 2.02–2.55), and a 1.5 times greater likelihood of quitting at 1 year with varenicline compared to bupropion (95% CI 1.22–1.88). Analysis of two open-label trials also suggested more improved nicotine abstinence rates at 6 months with varenicline than with NRT (Cahill, Stead, & Lancaster, 2012).

Though the standard duration of varenicline therapy is 12 weeks, improved outcomes have been observed in clinical investigations of extended therapy, with approximately two times greater smoking cessation rates after 24 weeks of treatment compared to 6 weeks (Lee, Jones, Bybee, & O'Keefe, 2008). Recommended dosing of varenicline is 0.5 mg daily titrated gradually to 1 mg twice a day over 8 days, starting 7 days prior to the target quit date. The most common side effects include nausea, dizziness, and headache, which may be minimized by gradual dose titration (McNeil et al., 2010). Serious adverse reactions, including cardiovascular events and neuropsychiatric symptoms, have been reported to the FDA, prompting a safety warning issued in 2008 to report increased risk of suicidal ideation and behaviors, agitation, and behavioral changes associated with varenicline use. However, subsequent literature on the causality of varenicline with serious cardiovascular events and neuropsychiatric symptoms has been inconclusive (Hays, Croghan, Baker, Cappelleri, & Bushmakin, 2012).

Combination Therapy

Medications for smoking cessation may be combined to improve treatment outcomes in some individuals. The nicotine patch, for example, may be combined with acute dosing products (e.g., gum or lozenge) to provide increased nicotine levels and the ability to relieve cravings or breakthrough withdrawal symptoms. Results from clinical trials suggest improvement in smoking abstinence and quit rates when the patch is combined with other NRT products compared to the use of either therapy alone (e.g., Fagerstrom, Schneider, & Lunell, 1993; Kornitzer, Boutsen, Dramaix, Thisjs, & Gustavsson, 1995; Piper et al., 2009). In addition, prior literature supports the combination of bupropion with different forms of NRT to improve smoking cessation success, at least in the short-term (e.g., Jorenby et al., 1999; Shah, Wilken, Winkler, & Lin, 2003). Though an open-label, one-arm Phase II study has supported the safety and potential efficacy of combining varenicline with bupropion for smoking cessation (Ebbert et al., 2009), dual administration of other anti-smoking medications with varenicline is not currently recommended and may increase the risk of side effects, including nausea (McNeil et al., 2010).

Anti-Nicotine Vaccines

There are several nicotine vaccines under investigation for smoking cessation, including Nicotine-Qb (NicQb), TA-NIC, and NicVax. The goal of vaccine therapy is to stimulate production of antibodies that bind nicotine in the plasma and limit its entry into the central nervous system (CNS). Though preliminary results have been encouraging, development has been limited by variable antibody production and abstinence rates (Henningfield et al., 2005; McNeil et al., 2010).

PHARMACOTHERAPIES FOR ALCOHOL USE DISORDER

Medications for Acute Withdrawal

Acute withdrawal from alcohol is characterized by hyperactivity of the autonomic nervous system related to compensatory changes in brain receptors and neurotransmitter systems, including gamma-aminobutyric acid (GABA) and glutamate, after long-term use. Common symptoms of alcohol withdrawal include autonomic hyperactivity (e.g., tachycardia or diaphoresis), tremulousness, anxiety, and insomnia; more serious complications include seizures or delirium tremens, a condition with up to 15% mortality when left untreated (Kosten & O'Connor, 2003). Alcohol withdrawal may require pharmacological treatment depending on the severity of symptoms. The current standard approach to treating alcohol withdrawal involves administration of tapering dosages of benzodiazepines, such as chlordiazepoxide or lorazepam, which are effective in relieving autonomic hyperactivity and reducing risk of seizures and delirium. Benzodiazepines are initially made available on an as-needed basis, with parameters for dosing based on appearance and severity of withdrawal symptoms, including diaphoresis, tremor, hypertension, and tachycardia.

Withdrawal symptoms can be assessed over the course of the detoxification using the Clinical Institute Withdrawal Assessment of Alcohol Scale, revised (CIWA-Ar) (Sullivan, Sykora, Schneiderman, Naranjo, & Sellers, 1989). This extensively studied scale has been shown to have good reliability, reproducibility, and validity. The scale measures 10 symptoms associated with withdrawal, each of which can be scored in increasing severity on a scale of 0–7 (with the exception of orientation and clouding of sensorium which is scored on a scale of 0–4). Summed scores above 10 indicate a need for medication to treat withdrawal symptoms. Furthermore, the CIWA-Ar predicts that those with a score greater than 15 are at increased risk for severe alcohol withdrawal, with higher scores conveying higher risk. Although detoxification schedules must be individualized, a benzodiazepine taper can usually be accomplished in 3–4 days. Patients with hepatic disease should be detoxified with lorazepam or oxazepam, shorter-acting drugs that, unlike the other benzodiazepines, have no metabolites requiring hepatic clearance.

Anticonvulsants have also been studied in the treatment of alcohol withdrawal (Malcolm, Myrick, Brady, & Ballenger, 2001; Eyer et al., 2011) and may be considered safe alternatives to benzodiazepines in mild to moderate withdrawal states given their limited ability for abuse or potentiation of sedating and cognitive effects of alcohol (Ait-Doud, Malcolm, & Johnson, 2006). Prior research supports the efficacy of sodium valproate (e.g., Hillbom et al., 1989; Roy-Byrne, Ward, & Donnelly, 1989) to ameliorate alcohol withdrawal symptoms and reduce the need for benzodiazepines in detoxification protocols (Reoux, Saxon, Malte, Baer, & Sloan, 2001). Carbamazepine has also been widely used to treat alcohol withdrawal and has demonstrated superiority to placebo in rapid relief of symptoms, including tremor, sweating, palpitations, sleep disturbances, depression, anxiety, and anorexia (Björkqvist, Isohanni, Mäkelä, & Malinen, 1976). When compared to a benzodiazepine in the treatment of alcohol withdrawal, carbamazepine was at least as effective as oxazepam in reducing withdrawal symptoms over a 7-day period (Stuppaeck et al., 1992). In an outpatient randomized clinical trial comparing a 5-day fixed-dose taper of carbamazepine starting at 600–800 mg versus lorazepam 6–8 mg on day 1, both drugs effectively suppressed withdrawal symptoms. Less posttreatment drinking was observed in the carbamazepine group, especially among individuals with multiple prior withdrawal treatment episodes (Malcolm et al., 2002). Carbamazepine has common side effects of dizziness, nausea and vomiting. It may induce the metabolism of drugs that are substrates of hepatic cytochrome P450-3A4 and should not be used in patients with severe hepatic or hematological conditions.

The combination of anticonvulsants with moderate doses of benzodiazepines can facilitate successful alcohol detoxification in patients with a history of previous alcohol withdrawal seizures or head trauma (Kasser, Geller, Howell, & Wartenberg, 1997). In these cases, the anticonvulsant should be administered concomitantly with benzodiazepines in dosages that will provide therapeutic anticonvulsant blood levels. The anticonvulsant should be tapered within a week of completion of the benzodiazepine-assisted detoxification, as there is no indication for continuation of anticonvulsant therapy in individuals who have experienced generalized, nonfocal seizures secondary to alcohol withdrawal. Despite an emerging body of literature investigating the role of anticonvulsants in alcohol withdrawal treatment, a recent meta-analysis suggests that evidence is insufficient to support the routine use of anticonvulsant monotherapy to prevent seizures during alcohol detoxification, suggesting the need for further comparative research (Amato, Minozzi, & Davoli, 2011).

Other anticonvulsants, including vigabatrin and gabapentin, have been examined as adjunctive therapies for the treatment of alcohol withdrawal (Malcolm et al., 2001). Open-label studies have provided preliminary support for the use of levetiracetam in relieving alcohol withdrawal symptoms (Müller et al., 2010). Gabapentin has been shown to ameliorate alcohol withdrawal symptoms but may not be indicated in cases of severe withdrawal (Bonnet et al., 2010). In a study comparing two doses of gabapentin with lorazepam in the treatment of alcohol withdrawal, symptoms were reduced in all three groups but were most effectively treated with the highest dose of gabapentin (1,200 mg); furthermore, individuals who received gabapentin were less likely to drink alcohol in the week following treatment than those who received lorazepam (Myrick et al., 2009). Recent evidence also supports the use of gabapentin in combination with naltrexone, an opioid antagonist, to ameliorate symptoms of early abstinence and improve drinking outcomes in alcohol-dependent individuals (Anton et al., 2011). Gabapentin in doses up to 1800 mg per day was associated with improved abstinence rates and reduced symptoms of insomnia, cravings, and dysphoria in alcohol dependent individuals relative to placebo (Mason et al., 2014).

Medications for Alcohol Use Disorder

Four medications have been approved by the FDA for the treatment of alcohol use disorder: disulfiram, oral naltrexone, extended-release intramuscular naltrexone (XR-NTX), and acamprosate. Various other agents have demonstrated at least preliminary efficacy in reducing relapse to alcohol use, including topiramate, ondansetron, and quetiapine. Selective serotonin reuptake inhibitors (SSRIs) have also been studied, and effects on drinking outcomes have been mixed depending on the target population.

Disulfiram is a relatively nonspecific irreversible inhibitor of sulfhydryl-containing enzymes (Wright & Moore, 1990). The pharmacological effect of disulfiram in the treatment of alcohol use disorder is due to inhibition of aldehyde dehydrogenase, an enzyme that converts acetaldehyde to acetate in the alcohol metabolism pathway. Alcohol consumption in the presence of disulfiram leads to an aversive physical reaction secondary to accumulation of acetaldehyde. Typical alcohol–disulfiram reactions last about an hour and include the following symptoms: flushing, headache, nausea or vomiting, palpitations, and sweating (Wright & Moore, 1990). A more severe reaction may include respiratory depression, hypotension, and cardiovascular collapse. Treatment of the disulfiram reaction is primarily supportive and includes hydration and oxygen (Elenbaas, 1977).

In prior research trials, disulfiram has been shown to have limited effectiveness in facilitating abstinence or preventing relapse due to problems with medication compliance (Fuller & Gordis, 2004). However, in motivated patients and with monitoring of ingestion, disulfiram may be beneficial in reducing alcohol consumption. Some patients use disulfiram on an as-needed basis in high-risk situations (Garbutt, West,

Carey, Lohr, & Crews, 1999; Allen & Litten, 1992). Disulfiram must not be initiated until alcohol is completely eliminated (usually within 24 hours after the last drink). Standard dosing is 250 mg orally daily, with a maximum of 500 mg per day. The time to onset of aldehyde dehydrogenase inhibition sufficient to result in an alcohol reaction is 12 hours, and aldehyde dehydrogenase recovery is complete within 1–2 weeks of the last disulfiram dose (Helander & Carlsson, 1990). Patients taking disulfiram must be warned to avoid alcohol-containing foods and products, such as hand sanitizer. Disulfiram is associated with a variety of potential side effects, such as metallic aftertaste, hepatotoxicity, and peripheral and optic neuropathies. It is not recommended in individuals with severe cardiovascular or pulmonary disease, psychosis, renal failure, or diabetes, and it is contraindicated after recent alcohol ingestion or use of metronidazole (Williams, 2005).

Naltrexone, a mu-opioid receptor antagonist approved for the treatment of alcohol use disorder, is available in daily oral and monthly extended-release injectable formulations. By blocking opioid receptors, naltrexone is postulated to diminish the pleasurable and reinforcing effects of alcohol. In clinical trials, naltrexone has been shown to reduce alcohol consumption, alcohol craving, and relapse to heavy drinking, defined as at least four drinks per day for women and at least five for men (Bouza, Angeles, Munoz, & Amate, 2004; Srisurapanont & Jarusuraisin, 2005). Side effects of naltrexone are typically mild and transient, and include nausea, vomiting, dizziness, fatigue, and headache. (Srisurapont & Jarusuraisin, 2005). Naltrexone is also associated with dose-related hepatotoxicity and carries a black box warning for this effect. Though hepatotoxicity is not typically seen at recommended doses, naltrexone should be avoided in individuals with severe liver disease (Williams, 2005).

Volpicelli, Alterman, Hayashida, and O'Brien (1992) conducted a double-blind, controlled study in which 70 male veterans were randomized to naltrexone tablets (50 mg daily) or placebo. Compared to placebo, naltrexone significantly reduced alcohol craving, days of drinking per week, and the rate of relapse among those who drank. A 6-month follow-up study reported on the persistence of naltrexone and psychotherapy effects following discontinuation after 12 weeks of treatment for alcohol use disorder (O'Malley et al., 1996). Subjects who received naltrexone were less likely than those who received placebo to drink heavily or to meet criteria for alcohol use disorders, but only through the first month of follow-up, suggesting that some patients may benefit from a period of naltrexone treatment exceeding 12 weeks. Multiple other studies have also demonstrated a modest but consistent effect of naltrexone treatment in combination with psychosocial support on short-term drinking outcomes (e.g., Anton et al., 1999, 2006; Volpicelli et al., 1997; O'Malley et al., 1992); findings related to longer-term treatment outcomes with naltrexone have been mixed (Krystal et al., 2001; West et al., 1999). A meta-analysis by Srisurapanont and Jarusuraisin (2005) reported a 36% reduction in risk of relapse to alcohol in the first 12 weeks for individuals taking naltrexone compared to placebo (28 vs. 43% relapse rate, respectively), and 36% ($n = 302/841$) of individuals in this analysis discontinued naltrexone treatment before 12 weeks.

Response to naltrexone is variable, and improved treatment outcomes have been demonstrated in subgroups of individuals, including those with a family history of alcoholism and with higher levels of alcohol craving (Monterosso et al., 2001), and in individuals with an earlier age of onset of alcohol use (Rubio et al., 2005). Heterogeneity of response to naltrexone is likely related in part to genetic factors that affect response of the endogenous opioid system to alcohol (O'Brien, 2005). Genetic polymorphisms related to differential treatment response are being actively studied; the Asp40 allele of the mu-opioid receptor gene (*OPRM1*), for example, has been associated with improved response to naltrexone relative to placebo (Oslin et al., 2003). The 118G single-nucleotide polymorphism is associated with tighter binding of beta-endorphin, and carriers of this polymorphism have been shown to exhibit improved response to naltrexone compared to carriers of the AA allele in some studies (Kim et al., 2003; Anton et al., 2008) but not all (Gelernter et al., 2007). Findings from a meta-analysis support the moderating role of the A118G polymorphism in the effect of naltrexone in alcohol use disorder treatment and an increased response to naltrexone in carriers of the G allele (Chamorro et al., 2012).

The clinical utility of oral naltrexone has been limited by problems with adherence. To address this problem, an extended-release injectable formulation of naltrexone (XR-NTX) was developed and approved in 2006 by the FDA for the treatment of alcohol dependence. XR-NTX is administered as a once-monthly 380 mg injection in the gluteal muscle. XR-NTX maintains steady state blood levels of naltrexone for approximately 28 days (Dunbar et al., 2006). Potential side effects are similar to those for oral naltrexone but also include injection site reactions, which may involve pain, erythema, bruising, induration, or, rarely, tissue necrosis requiring surgical intervention. Site reactions are more likely when XR-NTX is inadvertently injected subcutaneously or into fatty tissue (Center for Substance Abuse Treatment, 2009). In a Phase III trial, XR-NTX administered over 24 weeks in combination with psychosocial support was more effective than placebo in reducing heavy drinking, and treatment effects were greatest in individuals who had maintained at least 7 days of abstinence prior to initiation of medication (Garbutt et al., 2005). A subsequent post hoc analysis revealed that improved drinking outcomes associated with XR-NTX, including time to first drink, number of drinking days per month, and rate of continuous abstinence, also extend to the subgroup of participants who had maintained at least 4 days of abstinence (O'Malley, Garbutt, Gastfriend, Dong, & Kranzler, 2007).

Acamprosate is a synthetic analogue of homocysteic acid with a chemical structure similar to GABA and, as such, has been reported to stimulate inhibitory GABA transmission and inhibit glutamate neurotransmitter systems (Williams, 2005). As a result of these properties, acamprosate may act by reducing symptoms of protracted abstinence, including restlessness, anxiety, and insomnia, which may predispose alcoholics to relapse (Littleton, 1995). Standard dosing of acamprosate is 666 mg three times a day. Acamprosate has no abuse potential and is excreted unchanged by the kidneys, which means it is safe to use in persons with liver impairment. Side effects are typically mild and transient, and include gastrointestinal symptoms, especially diarrhea (Wilde & Wagstaff, 1997).

Multiple clinical trials in Europe have demonstrated efficacy of acamprosate in reducing relapse and prolonging abstinence in recently abstinent alcohol-dependent individuals; this finding was confirmed in a meta-analysis of 17 studies that reported significantly improved continuous abstinence rates at 6 months in individuals treated with acamprosate compared to those treated with placebo (26 vs. 23%, respectively;

Mann, Lehert, & Morgan, 2004). Two large U.S. studies, however, have failed to demonstrate benefits of acamprosate in improving drinking outcomes (Anton et al., 2006; Mason, Goodman, Chabac, & Lehert, 2006), although a greater percentage of abstinent days was observed in a post hoc analysis of the subgroup reporting a desire for abstinence at baseline (Mason et al., 2006). Purported explanations for discrepant findings between U.S. and European acamprosate studies include longer periods of lead-in abstinence and greater severity of alcohol use disorder among subjects enrolled in the European trials (National Institute of Alcohol Abuse and Alcoholism [NIAAA], 2008).

Several studies have compared naltrexone and acamprosate treatment for alcohol use disorder. In a 1-year follow-up study, no differences were observed in time to first drink, but time to first relapse was shorter in acamprosate-treated patients, while those treated with naltrexone were found to have a greater cumulative number of days of abstinence, to consume fewer drinks at one time, and to have less craving for alcohol (Rubio et al., 2001). In a study comparing naltrexone, acamprosate, the combination of naltrexone and acamprosate, and placebo, both active drugs and the combination were associated with significantly longer time to first drink and relapse to alcohol use relative to placebo. Additionally, there was a trend for more positive outcomes in the naltrexone-treated group relative to the acamprosate-treated group. The combination was more effective than placebo or acamprosate, but not naltrexone (Kiefer et al., 2003). The nine-arm Combined Pharmacotherapies and Behavioral Interventions for Alcohol Dependence (COMBINE) study examined naltrexone and acamprosate alone and in combinations with cognitive-behavioral treatment in alcoholics recently abstinent from alcohol and found that acamprosate was not effective alone or in combination with naltrexone; naltrexone, while effective at early stages of follow-up, did not work better when combined with acamprosate (Anton et al., 2006).

Although not FDA-approved for the treatment of alcohol dependence, topiramate has been shown to be effective in reducing relapse to alcohol, diminishing alcohol craving, and improving abstinence rates among alcoholics in two RCTs (B. A. Johnson et al., 2003, 2007). Topiramate is believed to reduce the reinforcing effects of alcohol by diminishing glutamatergic activity and facilitating GABA function, resulting in inhibition of mesocorticolimbic dopamine release (B. A. Johnson et al., 2003). The dose of topiramate is titrated slowly to minimize side effects, which may include dizziness, confusion, fatigue, paresthesias, and ataxia (Williams, 2005).

Serotonergic dysfunction has been implicated in the pathogenesis of alcohol use disorder. Serotonergic agents including buspirone, a serotonin receptor (5HT-1_A) agonist indicated for the treatment of anxiety (Kranzler et al., 1994), ondansetron, an antinausea medication that antagonizes 5-HT3 receptors (Sellers et al., 1994; B. A. Johnson et al., 2000), and SSRI antidepressants (Kranzler et al., 1995; Cornelius et al., 1997; Pettinati et al., 2000) have been studied as treatment agents for alcohol dependence, but results have been mixed. Ondansetron has been shown to reduce self-reported drinking and improve abstinence in people with early-onset alcoholism; differential outcomes between early- and late-onset alcoholism may be related to prevalence rates of a 5-HT gene polymorphism (B. A. Johnson et al., 2000). The SSRI fluoxetine demonstrated no effect on drinking outcomes in a prior study

(Kranzler et al., 1995), and in a subgroup of alcoholics with more severe dependence (i.e., Type B alcoholics) was associated with worse outcomes relative to placebo (Kranzler, Burleson, Brown, & Babor, 1996). The study by Pettinati and colleagues (2000) confirmed findings that differential treatment response to SSRIs may be associated with alcoholic subtypes; in this study, however, treatment with sertraline was associated with reduced drinking and a greater likelihood of continuous abstinence among less severely dependent (i.e., Type A) alcoholics, whereas a significant effect on outcomes was not demonstrated among Type B alcoholics. Interest in improving medication efficacy by identifying preferential response among alcoholic subtypes has been extended to research involving alternate medication classes. In a pilot study of quetiapine as a treatment for alcohol use disorder, reduced drinking and alcohol craving were observed in Type B alcoholics who received quetiapine but not in Type A alcoholics (Kampman et al., 2007).

PHARMACOTHERAPIES FOR SEDATIVE, HYPNOTIC, OR ANXIOLYTIC USE DISORDERS

Medications for Overdose

Benzodiazepines have sedative/hypnotic (sleep-inducing), anxiolytic, anticonvulsant, and muscle relaxant properties and are some of the most frequently prescribed medications in the United States for the treatment of anxiety and insomnia. Benzodiazepines bind to a subunit of the GABA-A receptor and enhance the effects of the neurotransmitter GABA. They have a rapid onset of action and relatively low risk of toxicity relative to other medications used for such indications. In cases of benzodiazepine overdose leading to respiratory depression and coma, flumazenil may be administered in 0.1–0.3 mg boluses. Flumazenil is a competitive antagonist at the benzodiazepine receptor and causes reversal of benzodiazepine effects. Precipitation of benzodiazepine withdrawal symptoms, including seizures may occur after flumazenil administration (Veriaiah, Dyas, Cooper, Routledge, & Thompson, 2012); thus, use with caution and slow dose titration is advised (Weinbroum, Flaishon, Sorkine, Szold, & Rudick, 1997).

Medications for Acute Withdrawal

Benzodiazepines may be used in the treatment of some anxiety disorders (e.g., panic disorder, generalized anxiety disorder), insomnia (short-term; i.e., for 4 weeks or less), or for other indications, and many benefit from treatment with this class of medication. However, benzodiazepines have abuse and dependence liability in a subset of individuals. Tolerance and physiological dependence may occur with longer term use (greater than 30 days), leading to escalating dosages. Symptoms of benzodiazepine withdrawal are similar to those of alcohol and other sedatives/hypnotics and include autonomic hyperactivity, anxiety, insomnia, tremor, and, in severe cases, seizures or delirium tremens. Interestingly, severity of the withdrawal syndrome does not always correlate significantly with the ability to taper off benzodiazepines successfully; personality traits and psychopathology appear to contribute to taper outcomes (Rickels et al. 1999).

The process of medical withdrawal from benzodiazepines may be challenging, particularly in those who have escalated their doses. Furthermore, as with alcohol withdrawal, complications that occur may be life-threatening, such as seizures, should taper occur too rapidly. The issue of outpatient benzodiazepine taper has been reviewed (Denis, Fatseas, Lavie, & Auriacombe, 2006), and multiple studies have reported on different approaches. Briefly, all individuals were receiving a stable dose of benzodiazepine from which taper was undertaken. Reports of taper using both long-acting (e.g., diazepam) and various short-acting benzodiazepines (e.g., lorazepam) showed no superiority of one medication over another. Tapers of 20–50% every 1–2 weeks over durations of 4–12 weeks were reported. Adjunctive medications were generally shown not to be effective, or studies that used such ancillary medications were poorly controlled. Medications included hydroxyzine, progesterone, propanolol, buspirone, and a tricyclic antidepressant, dothiepin. Carbamazepine has been shown to have some promise in treatment of benzodiazepine withdrawal.

When tapering low therapeutic doses of benzodiazepines in an outpatient setting, the taper may be conducted slowly to minimize withdrawal symptoms. Tapers are generally completed within 4–12 weeks and typically should not last more than 6 months. As one example, to taper higher dosages in an outpatient setting, short-acting benzodiazepines may be converted to longer acting forms (e.g., diazepam), and the dosage may be reduced by 10–25% every week (Cloos, 2010). Patients with significant underlying anxiety or depression should be treated with antidepressants or other medications as necessary in order to stabilize their psychiatric condition both during the taper and posttaper (Rickels, DeMartinis, Rynn, & Mandos, 1999). Adjuvant medications that have demonstrated benefit in improving taper outcomes after long-term benzodiazepine therapy in outpatient settings, but not in diminishing withdrawal severity, include trazodone, valproic acid (Rickels, Schweizer, et al., 1999), and carbamazepine (Schweizer, Rickels, Case, & Greenblatt, 1991). Emerging evidence also supports newer anticonvulsants, such as pregabalin (Rubio et al., 2011), gabapentin (Himmerich, Nickel, Dalal, & Müller, 2007), and oxcarbazapine (Croissant, Grosshans, Diehl, & Mann, 2008) in the treatment of benzodiazepine withdrawal.

PHARMACOTHERAPIES FOR OPIOID USE DISORDER

Medications for Overdose

Opioid agonist activity at the mu-opioid receptor causes multiple effects, including analgesia, sedation, euphoria, nausea, miosis, and decreased bowel motility. Opioid overdose is a medical emergency that can be life-threatening due to potential complications of respiratory depression and loss of consciousness. Naloxone is an injectable opioid antagonist that rapidly reverses effects of opioid overdose by displacing opioids from mu receptors in the brain. Naloxone may be administered intravenously or, in patients without venous access, by subcutaneous or intramuscular injection.

A dosage of 0.4–0.8 mg should reverse most opioid overdoses. In opioid-dependent patients, lower doses (0.1–0.2 mg) may be sufficient to minimize precipitated withdrawal and may be increased as clinically indicated. Once the symptoms of overdose have abated, it is important to continue to monitor level of consciousness and respiratory status, because long-acting opioids may require prolonged naloxone treatment that can be administered by intravenous infusion. Patients with opioid overdose should react within minutes to naloxone treatment. Failure to do so should call into question the working diagnosis and prompt additional evaluation.

Medications for Acute Withdrawal

Opioid withdrawal, while not life-threatening, causes significant discomfort and increased risk of relapse. Opioid withdrawal symptoms include muscle aches, lacrimation, abdominal pain, nausea, vomiting, diarrhea, anxiety, yawning, and autonomic hyperactivity (i.e., hypertension, tachycardia). Symptoms typically start between 6 and 49 hours after last use of opioids, depending on the half-life of the opioid; drugs with longer half-lives have a longer time to onset of withdrawal and slower symptom resolution (Beswick et al., 2003). Withdrawal from opioids or "detoxification" may be accomplished using long-acting opioids, including methadone or buprenorphine, or nonopioid medications, such as clonidine or lofexidine. The goal of detoxification is to alleviate withdrawal symptoms and facilitate the transition to abstinence-based treatment. Relapse rates after detoxification are high, and treatment should be supplemented with psychosocial therapy that targets relapse prevention or rehabilitation (Lobmaier, Gossop, Waal, & Bramness, 2010). Those with chronic, relapsing opioid use disorder should be considered for initiation of naltrexone treatment following medical withdrawal. Naltrexone will block reinforcing effects of opioids and can be helpful in maintaining sobriety following cessation of opioid abuse.

Methadone, a full mu agonist with a half-life of approximately 24 hours, has been traditionally used for ambulatory opioid detoxification, but stringent federal regulations, including the requirement that ambulatory use of the drug for this indication only occur in licensed narcotic treatment programs, and the potential for rebound withdrawal, tolerance, or dependence limit its use (Kreek, 2000). Methadone can be administered in starting doses of 10- to 30-mg daily, with the goal of blocking withdrawal symptoms, which can be accomplished with doses of methadone in the 40-mg daily range and gradually tapering the dose over 10–28 days (Gossop, Griffiths, Bradley, & Strang, 1989; Lobmaier et al., 2010; van den Brink, Goppel, & van Ree, 2003).

Clonidine, an alpha$_2$-adrenergic agonist, reduces the severity of acute withdrawal symptoms related to sympathetic nervous system stimulation, including hypertension, tachycardia, restlessness, nausea, diarrhea, and sweating. It does not reduce other symptoms, including muscle aches, insomnia, or cravings. The potential for sedation or postural hypotension, particularly at higher doses, may be a limitation to the use of clonidine (Lobmaier et al., 2010). To treat opioid withdrawal, clonidine is usually started at a dose of 0.1 mg three times a day; for patients in inpatient settings, the dose may be adjusted upward as necessary for symptom relief and tapered over 5–7 days. Additional supportive medications may be given to target ongoing or breakthrough withdrawal symptoms, such as nonsteroidal anti-inflammatory drugs (NSAIDs) for muscle aches, antinausea agents, antidiarrheals, and non-benzodiazepine sleep medications. Like clonidine, lofexidine is an alpha$_2$-adrenergic agonist that has been used primarily in the United Kingdom to treat opioid withdrawal but has not yet been approved for use in the United States (Yu et al., 2008; Strang, Bearn, & Gossop, 1999).

"Ultrarapid" detoxification is a technique involving withdrawal of opioids while maintaining individuals under heavy sedation or general anesthesia to ease symptoms precipitated by opioid antagonists. Using this procedure, individuals may become opioid-free within a few hours to days due to the masking of withdrawal symptoms. Ultrarapid detoxification has been associated with serious and potentially life-threatening adverse events, including complications of anesthesia, severe withdrawal symptoms lasting for several days following the procedure, and, rarely, death (e.g., Rabinowitz, Cohen, & Atias, 2002; Badenoch, 2002; O'Connor & Kosten, 1998). Furthermore, this procedure has not been associated with better long-term treatment outcomes including opioid relapse, calling into question the expense and risk of the procedure relative to other strategies for opioid withdrawal (Collins, Kleber, Whittington, & Heitler, 2005; Lawental, 2000; Rabinowitz et al., 2002).

Withdrawal from opioids can also be undertaken with buprenorphine, a partial agonist at the mu opioid receptor (Lobmaier et al., 2010). Prior studies have demonstrated superiority of buprenorphine to clonidine in reducing opioid withdrawal symptoms (Fingerhood, Thompson, & Jasinski, 2001; Oreskovich et al., 2005). Findings were confirmed in a recent meta-analysis that reported greater efficacy of buprenorphine than clonidine or lofexidine in managing opioid withdrawal symptoms and improving retention in treatment. Furthermore, compared to methadone, buprenorphine treatment may be associated with a shorter duration of opioid withdrawal and a greater likelihood of completing detoxification (Gowing, Ali, & White, 2009). Success rates for detoxification treatments have generally assessed only short-term outcomes, either becoming opioid-free or becoming opioid-free with concomitant naltrexone treatment, the latter of which has not been widely adopted. Ling and colleagues (2009) showed low rates of opioid abstinence following completion of either a 7- or a 28-day buprenorphine–naloxone taper in opioid-dependent individuals. Such results are common with other methods of opioid withdrawal as well when ongoing pharmacotherapy is not utilized. Consideration should be given to maintaining recently detoxified patients on an opioid antagonist medication such as naltrexone, because relapse rates of illicit opioid use following medical withdrawal are very high ($\geq 90\%$) over a 6- to 12-month period without sustained outpatient treatment (Kleber, 1981; Kosten & Kleber, 1984). Methods for transferring those who are medically withdrawn from opioids using buprenorphine to naltrexone have been reviewed (Sigmon et al., 2012). In a study of methadone maintenance versus a 180-day methadone detoxification program with enhanced psychosocial treatment services, methadone maintenance therapy resulted in greater treatment retention and lower heroin use than did the enhanced detoxification treatment (Sees et al., 2000). Similarly, Kakko, Svanborg, Kreek, and Heilig (2003) compared buprenorphine maintenance to buprenorphine medical withdrawal, with both groups having access to enhanced psychosocial services. The entire sample of those randomized to buprenorphine medical withdrawal had dropped out of the study by 60 days and four individuals in this sample died, although the cause of death was not described. These observations underscore the difficulty of successfully undertaking opiate detoxification in opioid-addicted patients. Moreover, such observations speak to the need to increase the availability of opiate therapy programs that can provide long-term opioid pharmacotherapy to this population.

Maintenance Medications

There have been four medications approved for the maintenance treatment of opioid dependence: naltrexone, methadone, and levomethadyl acetate (LAAM), and buprenorphine. LAAM is no longer produced in the United States due to concerns about prolongation of the cardiac QT interval. These medication treatments are summarized below.

Naltrexone, an opioid antagonist that is administered orally and can be used in patients who do not want to be maintained on opioid agonist medication, should not be initiated until the patient is completely opioid-free to avoid precipitating withdrawal. An abstinence period of 7–10 days from short-acting opioids (e.g., heroin) and 10 days from long-acting opioids (e.g., methadone) is usually required. If doubt exists as to the opioid history, a "naloxone challenge" may be given—lack of withdrawal symptoms indicates the absence of current physiological opioid dependence and naltrexone can then be safely administered. To perform a naloxone challenge, 2-ml naloxone (0.4 mg/ml) solution is prepared, and an initial dose of approximately 0.5 ml of this solution (0.2 mg of naloxone) is administered intravenously. Symptoms of opioid withdrawal (mydriasis, dysphoria, diaphoresis, and gastrointestinal discomfort) appearing in approximately 30 seconds indicate that the patient remains dependent. If no withdrawal is observed, the remaining naloxone solution is administered and observation continued. If intravenous access is not available, naloxone may be administered subcutaneously with an observation period of 45 minutes (Galloway & Hayner, 1993).

For maintenance therapy with an opioid antagonist, naltrexone in either daily oral form or monthly XR-NTX intramuscular injection may be used. The standard dosing of oral naltrexone is 50 mg daily, although this medication can also be administered less frequently at larger doses (100 mg every other day, or 150 mg every third day). Naltrexone will block opioid agonist effects and thereby inhibit relapse. Naltrexone should be administered for at least 6 months and discontinuation should be carefully planned. Naltrexone side effects are few, but hepatotoxicity has been reported at higher doses, and hepatic function should be monitored before and during treatment. The greatest problem with naltrexone has been a lack of patient and clinician acceptance of the treatment and poor adherence rates (e.g., Kosten & Kleber, 1984; Azatian, Papiasvilli, & Joseph, 1994). Patients should be warned that the use of naltrexone eliminates any prior tolerance they may have had to opioids, and use of large doses of opioids that they may have tolerated when physically dependent on opioids in the past now would place them at risk for opioid toxicity, including overdose, were they to ingest significant amount of opioids following naltrexone treatment.

XR-NTX was approved by the FDA in 2010 to prevent relapse in opioid-dependent individuals after complete withdrawal from opioids. XR-NTX is administered as a monthly gluteal injection of 380 mg and maintains steady therapeutic levels of naltrexone for approximately 28 days. Treatment is associated with side effects including nausea, injection site reactions, and potential hepatotoxicity, as described earlier. Prior studies have demonstrated safety and efficacy of XR-NTX treatment for opioid dependence (Comer et al., 2002, 2006). In a large, multicenter trial in Russia, opioid-dependent participants were randomized to receive XR-NTX or placebo for 6 months. Significantly greater opioid abstinence rates were observed in the XR-NTX group than in the placebo group, and XR-NTX was generally well-tolerated (Krupitsky et al., 2011).

For patients who chronically relapse to opioid use, the treatment of choice is maintenance with a long-acting opioid agonist. The goal of treatment with any long-acting opioid is to achieve a stable dose that reduces or, ideally, eliminates illicit opioid craving and use, and that facilitates the engagement of the patient in a comprehensive program that promotes rehabilitation and recovery. Because treatment with long-acting opioids results in physical dependence, it is important to restrict such treatment to patients who have a history of prolonged addiction (greater than 1 year) and demonstrate physiological dependence (a positive urine toxicology screen for opioids and evidence of opiate withdrawal prior to initiation of treatment).

Methadone is the most widely used of these long-acting opioids. It is effective in decreasing psychosocial consequences and medical morbidity associated with opioid use disorder. Long-acting opioid therapies such as methadone are also important tools in decreasing the spread of human immunodeficiency virus (HIV) infection in and by injection drug users. Methadone is given once daily and can accumulate with rapid dose increases. Therefore, the starting dose of methadone in opioid-tolerant patients is 20–30 mg and the dose on the first day cannot exceed 40 mg. Methadone dose should not be rapidly escalated; dose increases should be approximately every 5 days as clinically indicated. The efficacy of methadone spans a wide range of doses, and each patient's dose must be individually titrated. Methadone 40–60 mg daily will block opioid withdrawal symptoms, but doses of 70–80 mg daily are more often needed to curb craving. Generally, doses of at least 60–100 mg daily are associated with better retention in treatment and less illicit opioid use (Ball & Ross, 1991; Bao et al., 2009; Faggiano, Vigna-Taglianti, Versino, & Lemma, 2003).

LAAM, a methadone congener that was thought to have potential advantages over methadone primarily in terms of duration of effects, has been associated with cardiac electrophysiological complications in some patients. LAAM labeling received a "black box" warning recommending that a cardiogram be performed prior to treatment, 12–14 days after initiation of LAAM, then periodically thereafter to rule out any alterations in the QT interval (Orlaam Package Insert, 2001). LAAM was removed as a first-line treatment for opioid dependence based on the finding that LAAM and its metabolites, norLAAM and dinorLAAM exert negative chronotropic effects and negative ionotropic responses in cardiac tissue, compounded by the association of LAAM with several lethal cardiac arrhythmias, including torsade de pointes (Deamer, Wilson, Clark, & Prichard, 2001). LAAM was removed from the market in the European Union in 2001, followed by a decision by the manufacturer to stop making the drug for the U.S. market in 2003.

The Drug Addiction Treatment Act of 2000 significantly expanded treatment options for opioid use disorder by permitting waivered physicians to prescribe buprenorphine in office-based settings. Buprenorphine, a mu-opioid receptor partial agonist, was approved for use as a treatment for opioid dependence in October 2002. Buprenorphine, formulated as a sublingual tablet, is available as a monoproduct or as a combination tablet or film containing buprenorphine and naloxone in a ratio of 4:1. The latter combination product was designed to prevent the drug from being diverted to injection drug use. Whereas naloxone is not absorbed sublingually, the injection of buprenorphine/naloxone in those physically dependent on full mu-opioid receptor agonists and who have recently ingested such drugs (e.g., heroin, methadone, oxycodone) will produce opioid withdrawal symptoms due to the antagonist activity of naloxone.

Buprenorphine has been shown to be a safer drug than methadone, in that a plateau has been observed for dose effects in terms of subjective responses and respiratory depression (Walsh, Preston, Stitzer, Cone, & Bigelow, 1994). Several clinical trials have been reported in which buprenorphine showed comparable efficacy to other opioid therapies. R. E. Johnson and colleagues (2000) reported that in a 17-week randomized study, compared to low-dose methadone maintenance (20 mg daily), high-dose methadone maintenance (60–100 mg daily), LAAM (75–100 mg daily), and buprenorphine (16–32 mg daily) substantially reduced the use of illicit opioids. Although the FDA-approved maximum daily dose of buprenorphine is 24 mg, many patients can be effectively maintained on lower dosages.

Induction with buprenorphine is a straightforward clinical procedure in which the patient is instructed to abstain from short-acting opioid use for at least 12 hours (for long-acting opioids such as methadone, required abstinence is 36–72 hours), then initiate treatment once mild to moderate withdrawal symptoms have emerged. An initial dose of buprenorphine–naloxone 4/1 mg is administered sublingually, and the dose may be titrated by 2–4 mg approximately every 2 hours as needed for ongoing withdrawal symptoms with a dose of up to 8/2 mg on the first day (McNicholas, 2004). Typically, on the second day, administration of a dose of 12–16 mg is based on patient report of the course of response to buprenorphine and degree of opiate withdrawal experienced on Day 1 following dosing. Dose adjustments up or down should be based on clinical examination with the goal of suppressing withdrawal symptoms and reducing opioid craving. Buprenorphine should be administered once per day, and because of its high affinithy for and slow dissociation from opioid receptors, doses may be taken as infrequently as three times per week to maintain effectiveness (Schottenfeld et al. 2000). A study of outcomes after 1 year of buprenorphine treatment (16 mg daily) or placebo given with psychosocial interventions showed a highly significant positive treatment effect of buprenorphine both in terms of retention in treatment and reduction in the use of illicit drugs (opiates, stimulants, cannabinoids, and benzodiazepines; Kakko et al. 2003). Findings from multiple clinical trials have confirmed the effectiveness of buprenorphine as a pharmacotherapy for opioid use disorder (e.g., Ling et al., 1998; Ling & Wesson, 2003; Mattick, Kimber, Breen, & Davoli, 2008).

Drug–Drug Interactions

Individuals with SUDs are frequently diagnosed with comorbid medical or mental disorders that require pharmacotherapy. The prescribing of multiple medications to the same patient can result in adverse interactions between medications, leading to adverse events and, in many cases, nonadherence to medication regimens, increased use of illicit drugs, drug toxicities, and lack of therapeutic benefit of treatment regimens. These interactions can be especially difficult in the opioid-dependent patient who is maintained on an opiate therapy. These patients are at risk for opiate withdrawal syndromes when prescribed medications that induce the metabolism of opioids (e.g., inducers of cytochrome P450-3A4) and for opiate toxicity should a coadministered medication inhibit opioid metabolism. Similarly, if an opioid delays absorption of a medication or inhibits the metabolism of the drug, toxicity from that drug may occur. Table 32.1, which summarizes currently known drug interactions of clinical significance that have been described in methadone- or buprenorphine-maintained individuals treated with medications for comorbid medical or psychiatric disorders, is by no means exhaustive, and the effect of drugs on metabolic pathways may need to be determined before multiple medications are prescribed.

PHARMACOTHERAPIES FOR STIMULANT USE DISORDERS

Medications for Acute Intoxication and Withdrawal

Stimulant drugs such as cocaine, methamphetamine, and other amphetamine-type stimulants increase levels of brain catecholamines, including dopamine and norepinephrine. Acute intoxication may cause anxiety, insomnia, agitation, or psychosis in some individuals. Increased noradrenergic tone may also result in sympathetic nervous system activation (i.e., tachycardia, hypertension). Anxiolytics and sleep medications may be used on a short-term basis to target anxiety and insomnia, respectively. In addition, benzodiazepines and/or antipsychotics may be used to reduce symptoms of heightened agitation or psychosis (e.g., Shoptaw, Kao, & Ling, 2009; Leelahanaj, Kongsakon, & Netrakom, 2005).

Anxiety, depression, insomnia, and fatigue are characteristic symptoms of acute withdrawal from stimulants, and such symptoms typically resolve without medication-assisted therapy (Newton, Kalechstein, Duran, Vansluis, & Ling, 2004). However, antidepressants or other anxiolytics may be used to treat persistent depression or anxiety, and sleep medications may be prescribed for insomnia. Behavioral therapy and possibly pharmacotherapy may be useful to address long-lasting cravings or to reduce relapse risk. No medications have yet been approved by the FDA for the treatment of cocaine or methamphetamine use disorder, although evidence from research studies suggests that some drugs may be useful, as described below, based on the rationale of amending neurotransmitter deficits caused by stimulant use and target symptoms associated with withdrawal, with the goal of initiating abstinence or reducing relapse (Kampman, 2008).

TABLE 32.1. Drug Interactions between Methadone or Buprenorphine and Medications Used to Treat Other Common Medical Conditions in Opioid-Dependent Patients

	Methadone	Buprenorphine
HIV medications		
Zidovudine (AZT)	Increase in AZT concentrations; possible AZT toxicity	No clinically significant interaction
Lamivudine	No clinically significant interaction	No clinically significant interaction
Tenofovir	No clinically significant interaction	No clinically significant interaction
Didanosine	Tablet: Significant decrease in didanosine concentrations; enteric coated: no interaction	No clinically significant interaction
Stavudine	Significant decrease in stavudine concentrations	Not studied in human pharmacokinetics studies
Delavirdine	Increased methadone (and LAAM) concentrations; no cognitive impairment	Increased buprenorphine concentrations; no cognitive impairment
Nevirapine	Opiate withdrawal may occur	No clinically significant interaction
Efavirenz	Opiate withdrawal may occur	No clinically significant interaction
Atazanavir	Not associated with increased levels of methadone	Significant increases in buprenorphine and clinical report of cognitive dysfunction
Darunavir	Opiate withdrawal may occur	No clinically significant interaction (Gruber et al., 2012)
Fosamprenavir	Data suggest that the pharmacokinetic (PK) interaction is not clinically relevant; however, patients should be monitored for opiate withdrawal symptoms	No clinically significant interaction (McCance-Katz et al., 2012)
Ritonavir (at boosting doses given with protease inhibitors; 100–200 mg/day)	No clinically significant interaction	No clinically significant interaction
Nelfinavir	Methadone levels are decreased; opiate withdrawal may occur	No clinically significant interaction
Lopinavir/ritonavir	Opiate withdrawal may occur	No clinically significant interaction
Tipranavir	Decrease in methadone concentrations; dose increase may be needed	No clinically significant interaction
Tuberculosis medications		
Rifampin	Opiate withdrawal may occur	Opiate withdrawal may occur (McCance-Katz et al. 2011)
Rifabutin	No clinically significant interaction	No clinically significant interaction (McCance-Katz et al., 2011)

(continued)

TABLE 32.1. *(continued)*

	Methadone	Buprenorphine
Hepatitis C medications		
Interferon	No clinically significant interaction	Not examined in human PK studies
Ribavirin	Not examined in human PK studies	Not examined in human PK studies
Medications for other infections		
Fluconazole	Increased methadone plasma concentrations	Not examined in human PK studies
Voriconazole	Increased methadone plasma concentrations	Not examined in human PK studies
Ciprofloxacin	Increased methadone plasma concentrations	Not examined in human PK studies
Clarithromycin	Increased methadone plasma concentrations	Not examined in human PK studies
Antidepressants		
Fluoxetine	Reported association with increased levels of methadone	Not examined in human PK studies
Fluvoxamine	May cause increased methadone plasma levels; discontinuation has been associated with onset of opioid withdrawal	Not examined in human PK studies
Paroxetine	Shown to increase methadone levels	Not examined in human PK studies
Sertraline	No reported adverse drug interaction	No clinically significant interaction
Citalopram/ escitalopram	No reported significant interaction; but citalopram is associated with prolongation of QT interval, so co-administration could lengthen QT interval	No reported clinically significant interaction; but citalopram is associated with prolongation of QT interval, so co-administration could lengthen QT interval
Mirtazapine	Not examined in human PK studies	Not examined in human PK studies
Duloxetine	May potentially lead to increased duloxetine exposure, but not studied in humans	Not examined in human PK studies
Amitriptyline	Could be associated with increases in plasma methadone concentrations	Not examined in human PK studies
St. John's wort	Increased metabolism and elimination of methadone	Increased metabolism and elimination of buprenorphine
Desipramine	Associated with increased desipramine levels	Not examined in human PK studies
Dextromethorphan	Associated with delirium	Not examined in human PK studies
Antipsychotics		
Quetiapine	Increased plasma methadone concentrations	Not examined in human PK studies
Risperidone	Not examined in human PK studies	Not examined in human PK studies
Clozapine	Not examined in human PK studies	Not examined in human PK studies

(continued)

TABLE 32.1. *(continued)*

	Methadone	Buprenorphine
Antipsychotics *(continued)*		
Aripiprazole	Not examined in human PK studies	Not examined in human PK studies
Olanzapine	Not examined in human PK studies	Not examined in human PK studies
Ziprasidone	Not examined in human PK studies	Not examined in human PK studies
Anxiolytics		
Diazepam	Associated with increased sedation and impaired performance on psychological tests	Associated with increased sedation and impaired performance on psychological tests
Alprazolam	Fatalities have been associated with combined use	Fatalities have been associated with combined use
Anticonvulsants		
Carbamazepine	Associated with opiate withdrawal	No clinically significant interaction reported
Phenytoin	Associated with opiate withdrawal	Not examined in human PK studies
Phenobarbital	Associated with opiate withdrawal	Not examined in human PK studies
Oxcarbazepine	No clinically significant interaction reported	No clinically significant interaction reported
Lamotrigine	No clinically significant interaction reported	No clinically significant interaction reported
Topiramate	No clinically significant interaction reported	No clinically significant interaction reported
Psychostimulants		
Methylphenidate	Not examined in human PK studies	Not examined in human PK studies
Pemoline	Not examined in human PK studies	Not examined in human PK studies
Modafinil	Not examined in human PK studies	Not examined in human PK studies
Antihistamines		
Promethazine	May have a synergistic depressant effect	Not examined in human PK studies
Diphenhydramine	May have synergistic depressant effect	Not examined in human PK studies
Cardiac and pulmonary disease medications		
Digoxin	Not examined in human PK studies	Not examined in human PK studies
Quinidine	Not examined in human PK studies	Not examined in human PK studies
Verapamil	Not examined in human PK studies	Not examined in human PK studies

(continued)

TABLE 32.1. *(continued)*

	Methadone	Buprenorphine
Cardiac and pulmonary disease medications *(continued)*		
Heparin	Not examined in human PK studies	Not examined in human PK studies
Theophylline	Not examined in human PK studies	Not examined in human PK studies
Aspirin	No clinically significant interaction reported	Not examined in human PK studies
Illicit stimulants		
Cocaine	Decrease in trough methadone concentrations	Increased metabolism and diminished plasma concentrations
Methamphetamine	Not examined in human PK studies	Not examined in human PK studies
Alcohol	Pharmacodynamic interaction with adverse events possible	Pharmacodynamic interaction with adverse events possible

Note. Based on McCance-Katz, Sullivan, and Nallani (2010).

Medications for Cocaine Use Disorder

Cocaine is a stimulant that blocks reuptake and enhances release of catecholamines, including dopamine, norepinephrine, and serotonin (Dackis, 2004). Multiple medications, including antidepressants, anticonvulsants, and dopaminergic agents, have been studied as potential treatments for cocaine use disorder. No medication has been consistently effective in improving treatment outcomes for cocaine dependence in RCTs, and no medication has been approved by the FDA for this indication (e.g., Boyarsky & McCance-Katz, 2000; de Lima et al., 2002; Jin & McCance-Katz, 2003).

The neurobiology of the reinforcing effects produced by cocaine and other stimulants involves central mesolimbic and mesocortical dopamine (DA) functioning (Jentsch & Taylor, 1999). Initial efforts to develop a medication for cocaine dependence focused on counteracting effects on DA functioning (de Lima et al., 2002), including agents that enhance or block dopaminergic activity. Although trials of DA agonists have not shown efficacy (Amato, Minozzi, Pani, et al., 2011), research has examined additional strategies to alter the reinforcing effects produced by cocaine, including the use of GABA system modulators (Dewey et al., 1998; Cousins, Roberts, & de Wit, 2002). Activation of GABA-ergic neurons inhibits activation of the dopaminergic reward system. In prior studies, the GABA-B agonist baclofen treatment attenuated cocaine-induced DA release in the nucleus accumbens (Fadda, Scherma, Fresu, Collu, & Fratta, 2003) and attenuated conditioned locomotion to cues associated with cocaine (Hotsenpiller & Wolf, 2003). One double-blind, placebo-controlled study revealed that baclofen-treated patients exhibited statistically significant reductions in cocaine use compared to those who received placebo (Shoptaw et al., 2003). A more recent investigation of baclofen in severely dependent cocaine users, however, did not demonstrate a significant difference in cocaine use in baclofen- compared to placebo-treated individuals (Kahn et al., 2009).

Other GABA-ergic medications that have been studied for the treatment of cocaine use disorder include the anticonvulsants topiramate, gabapentin, tiagabine, and gamma-vinyl GABA. Topiramate has demonstrated preliminary efficacy in a 13-week RCT in which individuals in the the topiramate group were more likely to be abstinent from cocaine than those in the placebo group after full dose titration at Week 8 (Kampman et al., 2004), and findings were extended in a recent RCT in which topiramate was associated with a greater weekly proportion of cocaine non-use days than placebo (B. A. Johnson et al., 2013). Gamma-vinyl GABA (GVG), a GABA transaminase inhibitor, is not approved for use in the United States due to an associated risk of visual field deficits. GVG has shown promise in preclinical trials, including the ability to inhibit cocaine self-administration in rodents (Kushner, Dewey, & Kornetsky, 1999). It has also demonstrated positive effects on cocaine use in preliminary, open-label trials in stimulant users (Brodie, Figueroa, & Dewey, 2003; Brodie Figueroa, Laska, & Dewey, 2005), and findings were replicated in a subsequent 9-week RCT in which end-of trial abstinence was significantly greater in GVG-treated subjects compared to subjects receiving placebo (Brodie et al., 2009). Tiagabine, a GABA reuptake inhibitor, has been associated with decreased cocaine use relative to placebo (Gonzalez et al., 2003) and to both gabapentin and placebo (Gonzalez et al., 2007) in RCTs in methadone-maintained individuals.

Evidence from prior literature suggests that disulfiram, a medication approved for the treatment of alcohol dependence, may have efficacy in reducing cocaine use. Disulfiram inhibits DA beta-hydroxylase, causing increased DA levels and possibly enhancing the aversive effects of cocaine (Dackis, 2004). In a randomized, clinical investigation of disulfiram 250 mg daily, administered in combination with psychotherapy in cocaine-dependent, alcohol-using individuals, disulfiram was associated with significantly reduced cocaine and alcohol use relative to placebo, and few adverse events were observed (Carroll, Nich, Ball, McCance, & Rounsaville, 1998); a 1-year follow-up evaluation with 96 participants demonstrated that effects on cocaine and alcohol were sustained (Carroll et al., 2000). The benefits of disulfiram in reducing cocaine use have been found to be independent of its effects on alcohol use (Carroll et al., 2004). Petrakis et al. (2000) reported that disulfiram treatment decreased cocaine and alcohol use in methadone-maintained patients who were also cocaine-dependent. Similar findings were observed in a study of buprenorphine-maintained opioid-addicted patients who were also cocaine-dependent (George et al., 2000). One study comparing three doses of disulfiram (62.5, 125, or 250 mg/day) with placebo in cocaine-dependent methadone-maintained patients, showed increased cocaine use over time in individuals who received doses less than 250 mg, and decreased cocaine use was observed in the 250 mg and placebo groups (Oliveto et al., 2011). Results of a meta-analysis indicate a trend for improved outcomes with disulfiram treatment over placebo or naltrexone in cocaine-dependent individuals, but additional clinical trials were recommended to investigate fully its possible effectiveness (Pani et al., 2010). Human laboratory studies have shown a statistically significant decrease in cocaine-associated "high" and "rush" in those receiving chronic disulfiram treatment, either 62.5 mg/day or 250 mg/day in combination with intravenous doses of cocaine. Additionally, disulfiram treatment is associated with decreased cocaine clearance and increased plasma levels of cocaine (Baker, Jatlow, & McCance-Katz, 2007). Though no adverse events occurred in this study, reduced cocaine metabolism in the presence of disulfiram treatment could potentially result in cocaine accumulation and related medical effects. The opioid antagonist naltrexone has also has been examined as a treatment for cocaine use disorder. Although results of earlier studies in individuals with comorbid cocaine and alcohol use disorder were not encouraging, Oslin et al. (1999) reported that doses of naltrexone 150 mg daily in individuals who were dependent on cocaine and alcohol were associated with decreased cocaine and alcohol use. Naltrexone 50 mg daily was also associated with significantly less cocaine use when administered in combination with relapse prevention therapy (Schmitz, Stotts, Rhoades, & Grabowski, 2001). Results from these studies suggest that the effectiveness of naltrexone may depend on multiple factors, including other substance comorbidity, dose of naltrexone, length of treatment, and type of psychotherapeutic intervention. Naltrexone will need to be examined in larger, controlled, clinical trials to determine its efficacy as a cocaine pharmacotherapy.

Cocaine-dependent individuals exhibit reduced dopaminergic function, which may increase dysphoria and relapse risk (Little et al., 2009). Elevated activity of endogenous kappa opioid receptor agonist systems after chronic drug use may contribute to this process (Spanagel, Herz, & Shippenberg, 1992) and promote stress-induced relapse (Beardsley, Pollard, Howard, & Carroll, 2010). As such, kappa-antagonists are under development as potential pharmacotherapies for cocaine use disorder. Recent evidence suggests that oral naltrexone in combination with buprenorphine largely blocks the mu effects of buprenorphine, creating a functional kappa-antagonist that may have efficacy in reducing cocaine use (Rothman et al., 2000; Gerra, Fantoma, & Zaimovic, 2006).

Also of interest is modafinil, a non-amphetamine-type stimulant with wakefulness-promoting properties that is approved for the control of daytime sleepiness in patients with narcolepsy, obstructive sleep apnea, and shift work sleep disorder. Though its exact mechanism of action is unknown, modafinil enhances glutamatergic activity and may ameliorate cocaine withdrawal symptoms due to its stimulating effects (Dackis, Kampman, Lynch, Pettinati, & O'Brien, 2005). Findings from RCTs of modafinil have yielded mixed results. A preliminary investigation of 400 mg/day modafinil versus placebo suggested benefit in reducing cocaine use and prolonging abstinence (Dackis et al., 2005), but findings were not replicated in a larger study comparing doses of 200 mg, 400 mg, and placebo (Dackis et al., 2012). Anderson et al. (2009) reported no difference in the primary outcome of change in weekly cocaine use over time between individuals receiving modafinil 200 mg, modafinil 400 mg, and placebo, but the 200-mg group demonstrated reduced cravings and maximum number of consecutive cocaine-free days relative to the other two groups. Additionally, significant treatment effects of modafinil were demonstrated in a post hoc analysis of individuals without comorbid alcohol dependence (Anderson et al., 2009).

A cocaine vaccine is also under investigation in clinical trials. Anti-cocaine antibodies have been developed that limit cocaine entry into the brain and have been shown in animal studies to inhibit self-administration. The presence of antibody has also been shown to reduce brain cocaine levels following intravenous or intranasal cocaine administration (Fox et al., 1996). The vaccine is structurally similar to cocaine but is coupled to a carrier protein that prevents rapid metabolism, thus making it possible to mount an immune response to cocaine (Fox, 1997). The results of clinical trials for efficacy in humans have demonstrated excellent safety and few side effects. The levels of antibody response to the vaccine have been variable, but individuals who develop sufficient antibodies have demonstrated significant reductions in cocaine use in some studies (Kosten et al., 2002; Shen, Orson, & Kosten, 2011), while in another study only 38% made antibody at protective levels, and these antibodies provided only 2 months of adequate cocaine blockade indicating the need for further refinement of the vaccine to maximize effectiveness (Martell et al., 2009).

Medications for Methamphetamine Use Disorder

Methamphetamine (MA) is a synthetic stimulant that increases intrasynaptic levels of dopamine and norepinephrine, primarily by facilitating the release of newly formed intravesicular catecholamines and blocking their reuptake. Medications that have been studied for the treatment of MA use disorder include antidepressants, dopaminergic agents, naltrexone, and stimulants, but researchers have yet to establish robust evidence for the efficacy of any medication, whether for initiating abstinence or preventing relapse to drug use. Studies of compounds such as selegilene, sertraline, gabapentin, risperidol, ondansetron, and rivastigmine, for example, have failed to demonstrate efficacy as potential treatments for MA use disorder (Ling, Rawson, & Shoptaw, 2006). Similar to cocaine, other medications that have been tested in pilot studies for the treatment of MA use disorder include baclofen and GVG, an epilepsy medication. Baclofen demonstrated potential benefit in reducing MA use relative to placebo in a post hoc analysis in subjects who reported taking a higher percentage of study medication (Heizerling et al., 2006). GVG was associated with reduced stimulant use in two open-label trials (Brodie et al., 2003, 2005). In a recent RCT, the antidepressant mirtazapine also demonstrated more efficacy than placebo in reducing MA use (Colfax et al., 2011).

Recent studies have indicated some promise for bupropion, an antidepressant with noradrenergic and dopaminergic effects, as a treatment for MA use disorder. A Phase I study demonstrated efficacy of bupropion in reducing subjective effects of MA and cue-induced craving (Newton et al., 2006). In a subsequent RCT of 72 adults with MA use disorder, bupropion treatment in combination with cognitive-behavioral group therapy was associated with reduced MA use at the trend level ($p = .09$) and was associated with significant reductions in MA use relative to placebo ($p = .03$) in individuals reporting fewer than 18 days of MA use in the past month (Elkashef et al., 2008). Similar findings were reported in another clinical trial in which post-hoc analysis found that subjects with less severe MA use at baseline had a greater response to bupropion than placebo (Shoptaw et al., 2008). Reanalysis of data from a multisite trial demonstrated a stronger signal for the efficacy of bupropion in achieving abstinence from MA (McCann & Li, 2012).

Another approach under investigation is stimulant replacement therapy (Grabowski, Shearer, Merrill, & Negus, 2004) akin to methadone or buprenorphine "substitution" for opioid use disorder. Methylphenidate, a stimulant approved for the treatment of attention-deficit/hyperactivity disorder that acts primarily as a DA reuptake inhibitor (e.g., Sandoval, Riddle, Hanson, & Fleckenstein, 2002; Volkow et al., 2002), has shown preliminary efficacy in reducing relapse in newly abstinent MA users (Tiihonen et al., 2007). A recent clinical trial demonstrated reductions in self-reported MA use associated with methylphenidate relative to placebo, particularly in individuals who reported heavier MA use at baseline (Ling et al., 2014). However, in a recent randomized, placebo-controlled trial of dextroamphetamine 60 mg/day, no difference was observed in MA-negative urines between the two groups. Given that diminished craving and withdrawal symptoms were observed in the dextroamphetamine group relative to placebo, the authors suggest that higher doses of medication might be more effective (Galloway et al., 2011).

Similar to the rationale behind its investigation as a potential treatment for cocaine use disorder, modafinil has stimulant properties that may counter dysphoria and fatigue produced by MA withdrawal, and may thereby be potentially useful in curtailing the reinforcing effects of MA when relapse occurs (Shearer et al., 2009). Modafinil improves cognitive performance in both healthy volunteers and clinical populations (Turner, Clark, Dowson, Robbins, & Sahakian, 2004; Turner, Clark, Pomarol-Clotet, et al., 2004) and improves impulse control (Turner, Clark, Dowson, et al., 2004), properties that may benefit MA-dependent patients striving to cease MA use. Recent research, however, demonstrated no benefit of modafinil 400 mg daily compared to placebo in reducing stimulant use in a sample of MA users, although there was a trend toward reduction of use in the group of modafinil-treated participants who reported a higher frequency MA use at baseline (Heinzerling et al., 2010). Another study comparing 200 mg modafinil, 400 mg modafinil or placebo for the treatment of MA use disorder failed to demonstrate significant differences in MA use between groups, though inadequate medication adherence could have contributed to these findings (Anderson et al., 2012).

There has been recent interest in the use of naltrexone as a treatment for MA use disorder. As an opioid receptor antagonist, naltrexone may function to modulate the dopaminergic neural systems involved in craving and drug-seeking behavior that may increase vulnerability to relapse. Naltrexone tolerability and adherence were established in an open-label trial in which reduced amphetamine use was observed (Jayaram-Lindström, Wennberg, Beck, & Franck, 2005). In a subsequent study led by Jayaram-Lindström et al. (2007), naltrexone reduced subjective effects of amphetamine and blocked cravings. Findings were replicated in a placebo-controlled trial of oral naltrexone, in which reductions in MA use and cravings were observed (Jayaram-Lindström, Hammarberg, Beck, & Franck, 2008).

SUMMARY

Substantial progress has been made in the development of pharmacotherapies for the treatment of SUDs. FDA-approved medications are now available for the treatment of nicotine, alcohol, and opioid use disorders. These treatments, utilized in conjunction with a program addressing the psychosocial needs of the patient, represent the most effective regimens available to treat addictive disorders. Ongoing research continues to broaden the number of pharmacotherapies available for these disorders.

The search continues for effective medication treatments for other SUDs, such as stimulant use disorders, including consideration of combination pharmacotherapies as potential treatments.

ACKNOWLEDGMENTS

This work was supported by National Institute on Drug Abuse Grant No. K24 DA 023359 (toElinore F. McCance-Katz).

REFERENCES

Ait-Doud, N., Malcolm, R. J., & Johnson, B. A. (2006). An overview of medications for the treatment of alcohol withdrawal and alcohol dependence with an emphasis on the use of older and newer anticonvulsants. *Addict Behav, 31*(9), 1628–1649.

Allen, J. P., & Litten, R. Z. (1992). Techniques to enhance compliance with disulfiram. *Alcohol Clin Exp Res, 16*(6), 1035–1041.

Amato, L., Minozzi, S., & Davoli, M. (2011). Efficacy and safety of pharmacological interventions for the treatment of Alcohol Withdrawal Syndrome. *Cochrane Database of Systematic Reviews, June 15*(6), CD008537.

Amato, L., Minozzi, S., Pani, P. P., et al. (2011). Dopamine agonists for the treatment of cocaine dependence. *Cochrane Database Syst Rev, 7*(12), CD003352.

Anderson, A. L., Li, S. H., Biswas, K., et al. (2012). Modafinil for the treatment of methamphetamine dependence. *Drug Alcohol Depend, 120*(1–3), 135–141.

Anderson, A. L., Reid, M. S., Li, S. H., et al. (2009). Modafinil for the treatment of cocaine dependence. *Drug Alcohol Depend, 104*(1–2), 133–139.

Anton, R. F., Moak, D. H., Waid, L. R., et al. (1999). Naltrexone and cognitive behavioral therapy for the treatment of outpatient alcoholics: Results of a placebo-controlled trial. *Am J Psychiatry, 156*(11), 1758–1764.

Anton, R. F., Myrick, H., Wright, T. M., et al. (2011). Gabapentin combined with naltrexone for the treatment of alcohol dependence. *Am J Psychiatry, 168*(7), 709–717.

Anton, R. F., O'Malley, S. S., Ciraulo, D. A., et al. (2006). Combined pharmacotherapies and behavioral interventions for alcohol dependence: The COMBINE study: A randomized controlled trial. *JAMA, 295*(17), 2003–2017.

Anton, R. F., Oroszi, G., O'Malley, S., et al. (2008). An evaluation of mu-opioid receptor (OPRM1) as a predictor of naltrexone response in the treatment of alcohol dependence: Results from the Combined Pharmacotherapies and Behavioral Interventions for Alcohol Dependence (COMBINE) study. *Arch Gen Psychiatry, 65*(2), 135–144.

Azatian, A., Papiasvilli, A., & Joseph, H. (1994). A study of the use of clonidine and naltrexone in the treatment of opioid addiction in the former USSR. *J Addict Dis, 13*(1), 35–52.

Badenoch, J. (2002). A death following ultra-rapid opiate detoxification: The General Medical Council adjudicates on a commercialized detoxification. *Addiction, 97*(5), 475–477.

Baker, J. R., Jatlow, P., & McCance-Katz, E. F. (2007). Disulfiram effects on responses to cocaine administration. *Drug Alcohol Depend, 87*(2–3), 202–209.

Ball, J., & Ross, A. (Eds.). (1991). *The effectiveness of methadone maintenance treatment.* New York: Springer-Verlag.

Bao, Y. P., Liu, Z. M., Epstein, D. H., Du, C., Shi, J., & Lu, L. (2009). A meta-analysis of retention in methadone maintenance by dose and dosing strategy. *Am J Drug Alcohol Abuse, 35*(1), 28–33.

Beardsley, P. M., Pollard, G. T., Howard, J. L., & Carroll, F. I. (2010). Effectiveness of analogs of the kappa opioid receptor antagonist (3R)-7-hydroxy-N-((1S)-1-{[(3R,4R)-4-(3-hydroxyphenyl)-3,4-dimethyl-1-piperidinyl]methyl}-2-methylpropyl)-1,2,3,4-tetrahydro-3-isoquinolinecarboxamide (JDTic) to reduce U50,488-induced diuresis and stress-induced cocaine reinstatement in rats. *Psychopharmacol (Berl), 210*(2), 189–198.

Beswick, T., Best, D., Bearn, J., Gossop, M., Rees, S., & Strang, J. (2003). The effectiveness of combined naloxone/lofexidine in opiate detoxification: Results from a double-blind randomized and placebo-controlled trial. *Am J Addict, 12*(4), 295–305.

Björkqvist, S. E., Isohanni, M., Mäkelä, R., & Malinen, L. (1976). Ambulant treatment of alcohol withdrawal symptoms with carbamazepine: A formal multicentre, double-blind comparison with placebo. *Acta Psychiatr Scand, 53*(5), 333–342.

Bonnet, U., Hamzavi-Abedi, R., Specka, M., Wiltfang, J., Lieb, B., & Scherbaum, N. (2010). An open trial of gabapentin in acute alcohol withdrawal using an oral loading protocol. *Alcohol Alcohol, 45*(2), 143–145.

Bouza, C., Angeles, M., Munoz, A., & Amate, J. M. (2004). Efficacy and safety of naltrexone and acamprosate in the treatment of alcohol dependence: A systematic review. *Addiction, 99*(7), 811–828.

Boyarsky, B. K., & McCance-Katz, E. F. (2000). Improving the quality of substance abuse dependency treatment with pharmacotherapy. *Subst Use Misuse, 35*(12–14), 2095–2125.

Brodie, J. D., Case, B. G., Figueroa, E., et al. (2009). Randomized, double-blind, placebo-controlled trial of vigabatrin for the treatment of cocaine dependence in Mexican parolees. *Am J Psychiatry, 166*(11), 1269–1277.

Brodie, J. D., Figueroa, E., & Dewey, S. L. (2003). Treating cocaine addiction: From preclinical to clinical trial experience with gamma-vinyl GABA. *Synapse, 50*, 261–265.

Brodie, J. D., Figueroa, E., Laska, E. M., & Dewey, S. L. (2005). Safety and efficacy of {gamma}-vinyl GABA (GVG) for the treatment of methamphetamine and/or cocaine addiction. *Synapse, 55*(2), 122–125.

Cahill, K., Stead, L. F., & Lancaster, T. (2012). Nicotine receptor partial agonists for smoking cessation. *Cochrane Database Syst Rev, 18*(4), CD006103.

Carroll, K. M., Fenton, L. R., Ball, S. A., et al. (2004). Efficacy of disulfiram and cognitive behavior therapy in cocaine-dependent outpatients: A randomized placebo-controlled trial. *Arch Gen Psychiatry, 61*(3), 264–272.

Carroll, K. M., Nich, C., Ball, S. A., McCance, E., Frankforter, T. L., & Rounsaville, B. J. (2000). One-year follow-up of disulfiram and psychotherapy for cocaine-alcohol users: Sustained effects of treatment. *Addiction, 95*(9), 1335–1349.

Carroll, K. M., Nich, C., Ball, S. A., McCance, E., & Rounsaville, B. J. (1998). Treatment of cocaine and alcohol dependence with psychotherapy and disulfiram. *Addiction, 93*(5), 713–727.

Center for Substance Abuse Treatment. (2009). *Incorporating alcohol pharmacotherapies into medical practice* (Treatment Improvement Protocol [TIP] Series 49; DHHS Publication No. [SMA] 00-4380). Rockville, MD: Substance Abuse and Mental Health Services Administration.

Chamorro, A. J., Marcos, M., Mirón-Canelo, J. A., Pastor, I., González-Sarmiento, R., & Laso, F. J. (2012). Association of μ-opioid receptor (OPRM1) gene polymorphism with response to naltrexone in alcohol dependence: A systematic review and meta-analysis. *Addict Biol, 17*(3), 505–512.

Cloos, J. M. (2010, August). Benzodiazepines and addiction: Long-term use and withdrawal (Part 2). *Psychiatric Times*, pp. 34–36.

Colfax, G. N., Santos, G. M., Das, M., et al. (2011). Mirtazapine to reduce methamphetamine use: A randomized controlled trial. *Arch Gen Psychiatry, 68*(11), 1168–1175.

Collins, E. D., Kleber, H. D., Whittington, R. A., & Heitler, N. E. (2005). Anesthesia-assisted vs. buprenorphine-or clonidine-assisted heroin detoxification and naltrexone induction: A randomized trial. *JAMA, 294*(8), 903–913.

Comer, S. D., Collins, E. D., Kleber, H. D., Nuwayser, E. S., Kerrigan, J. H., & Fischman, M.

W. (2002). Depot naltrexone: Long-lasting antagonism of the effects of heroin in humans. *Psychopharmacol (Berl), 189*(1), 37–46.

Comer, S. D., Sullivan, M. A., Yu, E., et al. (2006). Injectable, sustained-release naltrexone for the treatment of opioid dependence: A randomized, placebo-controlled trial. *Arch Gen Psychiatry, 63*(2), 210–218.

Cornelius, J. R., Salloum, I. M., Ehler, J. G., et al. (1997). Fluoxetine in depressed alcoholics: A double-blind, placebo-controlled trial. *Arch Gen Psychiatry, 54*(8), 700–705.

Cousins, M. S., Roberts, D. C., & de Wit, H. (2002). GABA(B) receptor agonists for the treatment of drug addiction: A review of recent findings. *Drug Alcohol Depend, 65*(3), 209–220.

Covey, L. S., & Glassman, A. H. (1991). A meta-analysis of double-blind placebo-controlled trials of clonidine for smoking cessation. *Br J Addict, 86*(8), 991–998.

Croissant, B., Grosshans, M., Diehl, A., & Mann, K. (2008). Oxcarbazepine in rapid benzodiazepine detoxification. *Am J Drug Alcohol Abuse, 34*(5), 534–540.

Dackis, C. A. (2004). Recent advances in the pharmacotherapy of cocaine dependence. *Curr Psychiatry Rep, 6*(5), 323–331.

Dackis, C. A., Kampman, K. M., Lynch, K. G., et al. (2012). A double-blind, placebo-controlled trial of modafinil for cocaine dependence. *J Subst Abuse Treat, 43*(3), 303–312.

Dackis, C. A., Kampman, K. M., Lynch, K. G., Pettinati, H. M., & O'Brien, C. P. (2005). A double-blind, placebo-controlled trial of modafinil for cocaine dependence. *Neuropsychopharmacol, 30*(1), 205–211.

Deamer R. L., Wilson, D. R., Clark, D. S., & Prichard, J. G. (2001). Torsades de pointes associated with high dose levomethadyl acetate (ORLAAM). *J Addict Dis, 20*(4), 7–14.

de Lima, M. S., de Olivereiro Soares, B. G., Reisser, A. A., & Farrell, M. (2002). Pharmacological treatment of cocaine dependence: A systematic review. *Addiction, 97*(8), 931–949.

Denis, C., Fatseas, M., Lavie, E., & Auriacombe, M. (2006). Pharmacological interventions for benzodiazepine mono-dependence management in outpatient settings. *Cochrane Database Syst Rev, 3*, CD005194.

Dewey, S. L., Morgan, A. E., Ashby, C. R., Jr., et al. (1998). A novel strategy for the treatment of cocaine addiction. *Synapse, 30*(2), 119–129.

Dunbar, J. D., Turncliff, R. Z., Dong, Q., Silverman, B. L., Ehrich, E. W., & Lasseter, K. C. (2006). Single- and multiple-dose pharmacokinetics of long-acting naltrexone. *Alcohol Clin Exp Res, 30*(3), 480–490.

Ebbert, J. O., Croghan, I. T., Sood, A., Schroeder, D. R., Hays, J. T., & Hurt, R. D. (2009). Varenicline and bupropion sustained-release combination therapy for smoking cessation. *Nicotine Tob Res, 11*(3), 234–239.

Elenbaas, R. M. (1977). Drug therapy reviews: Management of the disulfiram–alcohol reaction. *Am J Hosp Pharm, 34*(8), 827–831.

Elkashef, A., Rawson, R., Anderson, A., et al. (2008). Bupropion for the treatment of methamphetamine dependence. *Neuropsychopharmacol, 33*(5), 1162–1170.

Eyer, F., Schreckenberg, M., Hecht, D., et al. (2011). Carbamazepine and valproate as adjuncts in the treatment of alcohol withdrawal syndrome: A retrospective cohort study. *Alcohol Alcohol, 46*(2), 177–184.

Fadda, P., Scherma, M., Fresu, A., Collu, M., & Fratta, W. (2003). Baclofen antagonizes nicotine-, cocaine-, and morphine-induced dopamine release in the nucleus accumbens of rats. *Synapse, 50*(1), 1–6.

Fagerstrom, K. O., Schneider, N. G., & Lunell, E. (1993). Effectiveness of nicotine patch and nicotine gum as individual versus combined treatments for tobacco withdrawal symptoms. *Psychopharmacol, 111*, 271–277.

Faggiano, F., Vigna-Taglianti, F., Versino, E., & Lemma, P. (2003). Methadone maintenance at different dosages for opioid dependence. *Cochrane Database Syst Rev, 3*, CD002208.

Fingerhood, M. I., Thompson, M. R., & Jasinski, D. R. (2001). A comparison of clonidine and buprenrophine in the outpatient treatment of opiate withdrawal. *Subst Abuse, 22*(3), 193–199.

Fiore, M. C., Jaen, C. R., Baker, T. B., et al. (2008, May). *Clinical practice guidelines: Treating tobacco use and dependence: 2008 update.* Rockville, MD: U.S. Department of Health and Human Services, Public Health Service.

Fox, B. S. (1997). Development of a therapeutic vaccine for the treatment of cocaine addiction. *Drug Alcohol Depend, 48*(3), 153–158.

Fox, B. S., Kantak, K. M., Edwards, M. A., et al. (1996). Efficacy of a therapeutic cocaine vaccine in rodent models. *Nat Med, 2*(10), 1129–1132.

Fuller, R. K., & Gordis, E. (2004). Does disulfiram have a role in alcoholism treatment today? *Addiction, 99*(1), 21–24.

Galloway, G., Buscemi, R., Coule, J., et al. (2011). A randomized, placebo-controlled trial of sustained-release dextroamphetamine for treatment of methamphetmine addiction. *Clin Pharmacol Ther, 89*(2), 276–282.

Galloway, G., & Hayner, G. (1993). Haight-Ashbury Free Clinics' drug detoxification protocols: Part 2. Opioid blockade. *J Psychoactive Drugs, 25*(3), 251–252.

Garbutt, J. C., Kranzler, H. R., O'Malley, S. S., et al. (2005). Efficacy and tolerability of long-acting injectable naltrexone for alcohol dependence: A randomized controlled trial. *JAMA, 293*(13), 1617–1625.

Garbutt, J. C., West, S. L., Carey, T. S., Lohr, K. N., & Crews, F. T. (1999). Pharmacological treatment of alcohol dependence: A review of the evidence. *JAMA, 281*(14), 1318–1325.

Gelernter, J., Gueorguieva, R., Kranzler, H. R., et al. (2007). Opioid receptor gene (OPRM1, OPRK1, and OPRD1) variants and response to naltrexone treatment for alcohol dependence: Results from the VA Cooperative Study. *Alcohol Clin Exp Res, 31*(4), 555–563.

George, T. P., Chawarski, M. C., Pakes, J., Carroll, K. M., Kosten, T. R., & Schottenfeld, R. S. (2000). Disulfiram versus placebo for cocaine dependence in buprenorphine-maintained subjects: A preliminary trial. *Biol Psychiatry, 47*(12), 1080–1086.

Gerra, G., Fantoma, A., & Zaimovic, A. (2006). Naltrexone and buprenorphine combination in the treatment of opioid dependence. *J Psychopharmacol, 20*(6), 806–814.

Glassman, A. H. (1997). *Cigarette smoking and its comorbidity* (NIDA Research Monograph No. 172). Washington, DC: U.S. Government Printing Office.

González, G., Desai, R., Sofuoglu, M., et al. (2007). Clinical efficacy of gabapentin versus tiagabine for reducing cocaine use among cocaine dependent methadone-treated patients. *Drug Alcohol Depend, 87*(1), 1–9.

González, G., Sevarino, K., Sofuoglu, M., et al. (2003). Tiagabine increases cocaine-free urines in cocaine-dependent methadone-treated patients: Results of a randomized pilot study. *Addiction, 98*(11), 1625–1632.

Gossop, M., Griffiths, P., Bradley, B., & Strang, J. (1989). Opiate withdrawal symptoms in response to 10-day and 21-day methadone withdrawal programmes. *Br J Psychiatry, 154*, 360–363.

Gowing, L., Ali, R., & White, J. M. (2009). Buprenorphine for the management of opioid withdrawal. *Cochrane Database Syst Rev, 8*(3), CD002025.

Grabowski, J., Shearer, J., Merrill, J., & Negus, S. (2004). Agonist-like, replacement pharmacotherapy for stimulant abuse and dependence. *Addict Behav, 29*(7), 1439–1464.

Hall, S. M., Reus, V. I., Munoz, R. F., et al. (1998). Nortriptyline and cognitive-behavioral therapy in the treatment of cigarette smoking. *Arch Gen Psychiatry, 55*, 683–690.

Hays, J. T., Croghan, I. T., Baker, C. L., Cappelleri, J. C., & Bushmakin, A. G. (2012). Changes in health-related quality of life with smoking cessation treatment. *Eur J Pub Health, 22*(2), 224–229.

Heinzerling, K., Shoptaw, S., Peck, J., et al. (2006). Randomized, placebo-controlled trial of baclofen and gabapentin for the treatment of methamphetamine dependence. *Drug Alcohol Depend, 85*(3), 177–184.

Heinzerling, K., Swanson, A. N., Kim, S., et al. (2010). Randomized, double-blind, placebo-controlled trial of modafinil for the treatment of methamphetamine dependence. *Drug Alcohol Depend, 109*(1–3), 20–29.

Helander, A., & Carlsson, S. (1990). Use of leukocyte aldehyde dehydrogenase activity to monitor inhibitory effect of disulfiram treatment. *Alcohol Clin Exp Res, 14*(1), 48–52.

Henningfield, J. E., Fant, R. V., Ruchhalter, A. G., & Stitzer, M. L. (2005). Pharmacotherapy for nicotine dependence. *CA Cancer J Clin, 55*(5), 281–299.

Hillbom, M., Tokola, R., Kuusela, V., et al. (1989). Prevention of alcohol withdrawal seizures with carbamazepine and valproic acid. *Alcohol, 6*(3), 223–226.

Himmerich, H., Nickel, T., Dalal, M. A., & Müller, M. B. (2007). Gabapentin treatment in a female patient with panic disorder and adverse effects under carbamazepine during benzodiazepine withdrawal [German]. *Psychiatrische Praxis, 34*(2), 93–94.

Hotsenpiller, G., & Wolf, M. E. (2003). Baclofen attenuates conditioned locomotion to cues associated with cocaine administration and stabilizes extracellular glutamate levels in rat nucleus accumbens. *Neuroscience, 118*(1), 123–134.

Hughes, J. R., Stead, L. F., & Lancaster, T. (2007). Antidepressants for smoking cessation. *Cochrane Database Syst Rev, 1,* CD000031.

Hurt, R. D., Sachs, D. P., Glover, E. D., et al. (1997). A comparison of sustained-release bupropion and placebo for smoking cessation. *N Engl J Med, 337,* 1195–1202.

Jayaram-Lindström, N., Hammarberg, A., Beck, O., & Franck, J. (2008). Naltrexone for the treatment of amphetamine dependence: A randomized, placebo-controlled trial. *Am J Psychiatry, 165*(11), 1442–1448.

Jayaram-Lindström, N., Konstenius, M., Eksborg, S., Beck, O., Hammarberg, A., & Franck, J. (2007). Naltrexone attenuates the subjective effects of amphetamine in patients with amphetamine dependence. *Neuropsychopharmacol, 33*(8), 1856–1863.

Jayaram-Lindström, N., Wennberg, P., Beck, O., & Franck, J. (2005). An open clinical trial of naltrexone for amphetamine dependence: Compliance and tolerability. *Nord J Psychiatry, 59*(3), 167–171.

Jentsch, J. D., & Taylor, J. R. (1999). Impulsivity resulting from frontostriatal dysfunction in drug abuse: Implications for the control of behavior by reward-related stimuli. *Psychopharmacol (Berl), 146*(4), 373–390.

Jin, C., & McCance-Katz, E. F. (2003). Cocaine use disorders. In A. Tasman, J. Kay, & J. A. Lieberman (Eds.), *Psychiatry* (2nd ed.). Philadelphia: Saunders.

Johnson, B. A., Ait-Daud, N., Bowden, C., et al. (2003). Oral topiramate for treatment of alcohol dependence: A randomized controlled trial. *Lancet, 361*(9370), 1677–1685.

Johnson, B. A., Ait-Daud, N., Wang, X. Q., et al. (2013). Topiramate for the treatment of cocaine addiction: A randomized controlled clinical trial. *JAMA Psychiatry, 70*(12), 1338–1346.

Johnson, B. A., Roache, J. D., Javors, M. A., DiClemente, C. C., Cloninger, C. R., Prihoda, T. J., et al. (2000). Ondansetron for reduction of drinking among biologically predisposed alcoholic patients: A randomized controlled trial. *JAMA, 284*(8), 963–971.

Johnson, B. A., Rosenthal, N., Capece, J. A., et al. (2007). Topiramate for treating alcohol dependence: A randomized controlled trial. *JAMA, 298*(14), 1641–1651.

Johnson, R. E., Chutaupe, M. A., Strain, E. C., Walsh, S. L., Stitzer, M. L., & Bigelow, G. E. (2000). A comparision of levomethadyl acetate, buprenorphine, and methadone for opioid dependence. *N Engl J Med, 343*(18), 1290–1297.

Jorenby, D. E., Leischow, S. J., Nides, M. A., et al. (1999). A controlled trial of sustained-release bupropion, a nicotine patch, or both for smoking cessation. *N Engl J Med, 340,* 685–691.

Kahn, R., Biswas, K., Childress, A. R., et al. (2009). Multi-center trial of baclofen for abstinence initiation in severe cocaine-dependent individuals. *Drug Alcohol Depend, 103*(1–2), 59–64.

Kakko, J., Svanborg, K. D., Kreek, M. J., & Heilig, M. (2003). 1-year retention and social function after buprenorphine-assisted relapse prevention treatment for heroin dependence in Sweden: A randomized, placebo-controlled trial. *Lancet, 361*(9358), 662–668.

Kampman, K. M. (2008). The search for medications to treat stimulant dependence. *Addict Sci Clin Pract, 4*(2), 28–35.

Kampman, K. M., Pettinati, H., Lynch, K. G., et al. (2004). A pilot trial of topiramate for the treatment of cocaine dependence. *Drug Alcohol Depend, 75*(3), 233–240.

Kampman, K. M., Pettinati, H. M., Lynch, K. G., et al. (2007). A double-blind, placebo-controlled pilot trial of quetiapine for the treatment of Type A and Type B alcoholism. *J Clin Psychopharmacol, 27*(4), 344–351.

Kasser, C., Geller, A., Howell, E., & Wartenberg, A. (1997). *Detoxification: Principles and protocols: Topics in addiction medicine.* Chevy Chase, MD: American Society of Addiction Medicine.

Kiefer, F., Jahn, H., Tarnaske, T., et al. (2003). Comparing and combining naltrexone and acamprosate in relapse prevention of alcoholism: A double-blind, placebo-controlled study. *Arch Gen Psychiatry, 60*(1), 92–99.

Kim, D. J., Kim, W., Yoon, S. J., et al. (2003). Effects of alcohol hangover on cytokine production in healthy subjects. *Alcohol, 31*(3), 167–170.

Kleber, H. D. (1981). Detoxification from narcotics. In J. H. Lowinson & P. Ruiz (Eds.), *Substance abuse: Clinical problems and perspectives* (pp. 317–338). Baltimore, MD: William & Wilkins.

Kornitzer, M., Boutsen, M., Dramaix, M., Thisjs, J., & Gustavsson, G. (1995). Combined use of nicotine patch and gum in smoking cessation: A placebo-controlled trial. *Prev Med, 24*(1), 41–47.

Kosten, T. R., & Kleber, H. D. (1984). Strategies to improve compliance with narcotic antagonists. *Am J Drug Alcohol Abuse, 10*(2), 249–266.

Kosten, T. R., & O'Connor, P. G. (2003). Management of drug and alcohol withdrawal. *N Engl J Med, 348*(18), 1786–1795.

Kosten, T. R., Rosen, M., Bond, J., et al. (2002). Human therapeutic cocaine vaccine: Safety and immunogenicity. *Vaccine, 20*(7–8), 1196–1204.

Kranzler, H. R., Burleson, J. A., Brown, J., & Babor, T. F. (1996). Fluoxetine treatment seems to reduce the beneficial effects of cognitive-behavioral therapy in Type B alcoholics. *Alcohol Clin Exp Res, 20*(9), 1534–1541.

Kranzler, H. R., Burleson, J. A., Del Boca, F. K., et al. (1994). Buspirone treatment of anxious alcoholics: A placebo-controlled trial. *Arch Gen Psychiatry, 51*(9), 720–731.

Kranzler, H. R., Burleson, J. A., Korner, P., et al. (1995). Placebo-controlled trial of fluoxetine as an adjunct to relapse prevention in alcoholics. *Am J Psychiatry, 152*(3), 391–397.

Kreek, M. J. (2000). Methadone-related opioid agonist pharmacotherapy for heroin addiction. History, recent molecular and neurochemical ressearch and future in mainstream medicine. *Ann NY Acad Sci, 909,* 186–216.

Krupitsky, E., Nunes, E. V., Ling, W., Illeperuma, A., Gastfriend, D. R., & Silverman, B. L. (2011). Injectable extended-release naltrexone for opioid dependence: A double-blind, placebo-controlled, multicentre randomised trial. *Lancet, 377*(9776), 1506–1513.

Krystal, J. H., Cramer, J. A., Krol, W. F., et al. (2001). Naltrexone in the treatment of alcohol dependence. *N Engl J Med, 345*(24), 1734–1739.

Kushner, S. A., Dewey, S. L., & Kornetsky, C. (1999). The irreversible gamma-aminobutyric acid (GABA) transaminase inhibitor gamma-vinyl-GABA blocks cocaine self-administration in rats. *J Pharmacol Exp Ther, 290*(2), 797–802.

Lawental, E. (2000). Ultra rapid opiate detoxification as compared to 30-day inpatient detoxification program—a retrospective follow-up study. *J Subst Abuse, 11*(2), 173–181.

Lee, J. H., Jones, P. G., Bybee, K, & O'Keefe, J. H. (2008). A longer course of varenicline therapy improves smoking cessation rates. *Prev Cardiol, 11*(4), 210–214.

Leelahanaj, T., Kongsakon, R., & Netrakom, P. (2005). A 4-week, double-blind comparison of olanzapine with haloperidol in the treatment of amphetamine psychosis. *J Med Assoc Thai, 88*(Suppl. 3), S43–S52.

Ling, W., Chang, L., Hillhouse, M., et al. (2014). Sustained-release methylphenidate in a randomized trial of treatment of methamphetamine use disorder. *Addiction, 109*(9), 1489–1500.

Ling, W., Charuvastra, C., Collins, J. F., et al. (1998). Buprenorphine maintenance treatment of opiate dependence: A multicenter, randomized clinical trial. *Addiction, 93*(4), 475–486.

Ling, W., Hillhouse, M., Domier, C., et al. (2009). Buprenorphine tapering schedule and illicit opioid use. *Addiction, 104*(2), 256–265.

Ling, W., Rawson, R., & Shoptaw, S. (2006). Management of methamphetamine abuse and dependence. *Curr Psychiatry Rep, 8*(5), 345–354.

Ling, W., & Wesson, D. R. (2003). Clinical efficacy of buprenorphine: Comparisons to methadone and placebo. *Drug Alcohol Depend, 70*(Suppl. 2), S49–S57.

Little, K. Y., Ramssen, E., Welchko, R., Volberg, V., Roland, C. J., & Cassin, B. (2009). Decreased brain dopamine cell numbers in human cocaine users. *Psychiatry Res, 168*(3), 173–180.

Littleton, J. (1995). Acamprosate in alcohol dependence: How does it work? *Addiction, 90*(9), 1179–1188.

Lobmaier, P., Gossop, M., Waal, H., & Bramness, J. (2010). The pharmacological treatment of opioid addiction—a clinical perspective. *Eur J Clin Pharmacol, 66*(6), 537–545.

Malcolm, R., Myrick, H., Brady, K. T., & Ballenger, J. C. (2001). Update on anticonvulsants for the treatment of alcohol withdrawal. *Am J Addict, 10*(Suppl.), 16–23.

Malcolm, R., Myrick, H., Roberts, J., Wang, W., Anton, R. F., & Ballenger, J. C. (2002). The effects of carbamazepine and lorazepam on single versus multiple previous alcohol withdrawals in an outpatient randomized trial. *J Gen Intern Med, 17*(5), 349–355.

Mann, K., Lehert, P., & Morgan, M. Y. (2004). The efficacy of acamprosate in the maintenance of abstinence in alcohol-dependent individuals: Results of a meta-analysis. *Alcohol Clin Exp Res, 28*(1), 51–63.

Martell, B. A., Orson, F. M., Poling, J., et al. (2009). Cocaine vaccine for the treatment of cocaine dependence in methadone-maintained patients: A randomized, double-blind, placebo-controlled efficacy trial. *Arch Gen Psychiatry, 66*(10), 1116–1123.

Mason, B. J., Goodman, A. M., Chabac, S., & Lehert, P. (2006). Effect of oral acamprosate on abstinence in patients with alcohol dependence in a double-blind, placebo-controlled trial: The role of patient motivation. *J Psychiatr Res, 40*(5), 383–393.

Mason, B. J., Quello, S., Goodell, V., Shadan, F., Kyle, M., & Begovic, A. (2014). Gabapentin treatment for alcohol dependence: A randomized clinical trial. *JAMA Int Med, 174*(1), 70–77.

Mattick, R. P., Kimber, J., Breen, C., & Davoli, M. (2008). Buprenorphine maintenance versus placebo or methadone maintenance for opioid dependence. *Cochrane Database Syst Rev, 16*(2), CD002207.

Maxwell, J., & McCance-Katz, E. F. (2010). Indicators of methadone and buprenorphine use and abuse: What do we know? *Am J Addict, 19*, 73–88.

McCance-Katz, E. F. (2012). *Drug–drug interactions in opioid therapy: A focus on buprenorphine and methadone* (7th ed.). London: PCM Healthcare.

McCance-Katz, E. F., Moody, D. E., Prathikanti, S., Friedland, G. H., & Rainey, P. M. (2011). Rifampin, but not rifabutin may produce opiate withdrawal in buprenorphine-maintained patients. *Drug Alcohol Depend, 118*(2–3), 326–334.

McCance-Katz, E. F., Sullivan, L. S., & Nallani, S. (2010). Drug interactions of clinical importance between the opioids, methadone and buprenorphine, and frequently prescribed medications: A review. *Am J Addict, 19*, 4–16.

McCann, D. J., & Li, S. H. (2012). A novel, nonbinary evaluation of success and failure reveals bupropion efficacy versus methamphetamine dependence: Reanalysis of a multisite trial. *CNS Neurosci Ther, 18*(5), 414–418.

McNeil, J. J., Piccenna, L., & Ioannides-Demos, L. L. (2010). Smoking cessation—recent advances. *Cardiovasc Drug Ther, 24*(4), 359–367.

McNicholas, L. (2004). *Clinical guidelines for the use of buprenorphine in the treatment of opioid addiction: A treatment improvement protocol* (TIP 40). Rockville, MD: US Department of Health and Human Services, Substance Abuse and Mental Health Services Administration, Center for Substance Abuse Treatment.

Monterosso, J. R., Flannery, B. A., Pettinati, H. M., et al. (2001). Predicting treatment response to naltrexone: The influence of craving and family history. *Am J Addict, 10*(3), 258–268.

Müller, C. A., Schäfer, M., Schneider, S., et al. (2010). Efficacy and safety of levetiracetam for outpatient alcohol detoxification. *Pharmacopsychiatry, 43*(5), 184–189.

Myrick, H., Malcolm, R., Randall, P. K., et al. (2009). A double-blind trial of gabapentin versus lorazepam in the treatment of alcohol withdrawal. *Alcohol Clin Exp Res, 33*(9), 1582–1588.

National Institute of Alcohol Abuse and Alcoholism (NIAAA). (2008). Helping patients who drink too much: A clinician's guide (October 2008 Update: *Prescribing medications for alcohol dependence [NIH Publication 07-3769]). Retrieved from www.niaaa.nih.gov/guide.*

Newton, T. F., Kalechstein, A. D., Duran, S., Vansluis, N., & Ling, W. (2004). Methamphetamine abstinence syndrome: Preliminary findings. *Am J Addict, 13*(3), 248–255.

Newton, T. F., Roache, J. D., De La Garza, R., II, et al. (2006). Bupropion reduces methamphetamine-induced subjective effects and cue-induced craving. *Neuropsychopharmacol, 31*(7), 1537–1544.

O'Brien, C. P. (2005). Anticraving medications for relapse prevention: A possible new class of psychoactive medications. *Am J Psychiatry, 162*(8), 1423–1431.

O'Connor, P. G., & Kosten, T. R. (1998). Rapid and ultrarapid opioid detoxification techniques. *JAMA, 279*(3), 229–234.

Oliveto, A., Poling, J., Mancino, M. J., et al. (2011). Randomized, double blind, placebo-controlled trial of disulfiram for the treatment of cocaine dependence in methadone-stabilized patients. *Drug Alcohol Depend, 113*(2–3), 184–191.

O'Malley, S. S., Garbutt, J. C., Gastfriend, D. R., Dong, Q., & Kranzler, H. R. (2007). Efficacy of extended-release naltrexone in alcohol-dependent patients who are abstinent before treatment. *J Clin Psychopharmacol, 27*(5), 507–512.

O'Malley, S. S., Jaffe, A. J., Chang, G., Schottenfeld, R. S., Meyer, R. E., & Rounsaville, B. J. (1992). Naltrexone and coping skills therapy for alcohol dependence: A controlled study. *Arch Gen Psychiatry, 49*(11), 881–887.

O'Malley, S. S., Jaffe, A. J., Chang, G., et al. (1996). Six-month follow-up of naltrexone and psychotherapy for alcohol dependence. *Arch Gen Psychiatry, 53*(3), 217–224.

Oreskovich, M. R., Saxon, A. J., Ellis, M. L., Malte, C. A., Reoux, J. P., & Knox, P. C. (2005). A double-blind, double-dummy, randomized, prospective pilot study of the partial mu opiate agonist, buprenorphine, for acute detoxification from heroin. *Drug Alcohol Depend, 77*(1), 77–79.

Orlaam Package Insert. (2001, May, revised). Columbus, OH: Roxane Laboratories.

Oslin, D. W., Berrettini, W., Kranzler, H., et al. (2003). A functional polymorphism of the mu-opioid receptor gene is associated with naltrexone response in alcohol dependent patients. *Neuropsychopharmacol, 28*(8), 1546–1552.

Oslin, D. W., Pettinati, H. M., Volpicelli, J. R., Wolf, A. L., Kampman, K. M., & O'Brien, C. P. (1999). The effects of naltrexone on alcohol and cocaine use in dually addicted patients. *J Subst Abuse Treat, 16*(2), 163–167.

Pani, P. P., Trogu, E., Vacca, R., Amato, L., Vecchi, S., & Davoli, M. (2010). Disulfiram for the treatment of cocaine dependence. *Cochrane Database Syst Rev, 20*(1), CD007024.

Petrakis, I. L., Carroll, K. M., Nich, C., et al. (2000). Disulfiram treatment for cocaine dependence in methadone-maintained opioid addicts. *Addiction, 95*(2), 219–228.

Pettinati, H. M., Volpicelli, J. R., Kranzler, H. R., Luck, G., Rukstalis, M. R., & Cnaan, A. (2000). Sertraline treatment for alcohol dependence: Interactive effects of medication and alcoholic subtype. *Alcohol Clin Exp Res, 24*(7), 1041–1049.

Piper, M. E., Smith, S. S., Schalm, T. R., et al. (2009). A randomized placebo-controlled clinical trial of 5 smoking cessation pharmacotherapies. *Arch Gen Psychiatry, 66*, 1253–1262.

Rabinowitz, J., Cohen, H., & Atias, S. (2002). Outcomes of naltrexone maintenance following ultra rapid opiate detoxification versus intensive inpatient detoxification. *Am J Addict, 11*(1), 52–56.

Raupach, T., & van Schayck, C. P. (2011). Pharmacotherapy for smoking cessation: Current advances and research topics. *CNS Drugs, 25*(5), 371–382.

Reoux, J. P., Saxon, A. J., Malte, C. A., Baer, J. S., & Sloan, K. L. (2001). Divalproex sodium in alcohol withdrawal: A randomized double-blind placebo-controlled clinical trial. *Alcohol Clin Exp Res, 25*(9), 1324–1329.

Rickels, K., DeMartinis, N., Rynn, M., & Mandos, L. (1999). Pharmacologic strategies for discontinuing benzodiazepine treatment. *J Clin Psychopharmacol, 19*(6, Suppl. 2), 12S–16S.

Rickels, K., Schweizer, R., Garcia España, F., Case, G., DeMartinis, N., & Greenblatt, D. (1999). Trazodone and valproate in patients discontinuing long-term benzodiazepine therapy: Effects on withdrawal symptoms and taper outcomes. *Psychopharmacol (Berl), 141*(1), 1–5.

Rose, J. E., Herskovic, J. E., Behm, F. M., & Westman, E. C. (2009). Precessation treatment with nicotine patch significantly increases abstinence rates relative to conventional treatment. *Nicotine Tob Res, 11*(9), 1067–1075.

Rothman, R. B., Gorelick, D. A., Heishman, S. J., et al. (2000). An open-label study of a functional opioid kappa antagonist in the treatment of opioid dependence. *J Subst Abuse Treat, 18*(3), 277–281.

Roy-Byrne, P. P., Ward, N. G., & Donnelly, P. J. (1989). Valproate in anxiety and withdrawal syndromes. *J Clin Psychiatry, 50*(Suppl.), 44–48.

Rubio, G., Bobes, J., Cervera, G., et al. (2011). Effects of pregabalin on subjective sleep disturbance symptoms during withdrawal from long-term benzodiazepine use. *Eur Addict Res, 17*(5), 262–270.

Rubio, G., Jiménez-Arriero, M. A., Ponce, G., & Palomo, T. (2001). Naltrexone versus acamprosate: One year follow-up of alcohol dependence treatment. *Alcohol Alcohol, 36*(5), 419–425.

Rubio, G., Ponce, G., Rodriguez-Jiménez, R., Jiménez-Arriero, M. A., Hoenicka, J., & Palomo, T. (2005). Clinical predictors of response to naltrexone in alcoholic patients: Who benefits most from treatment with naltrexone? *Alcohol Alcohol, 40*(3), 227–233.

Sandoval, V., Riddle, E., Hanson, G., & Fleckenstein, A. (2002). Methylphenidate redistributes vesicular monoamine transporter-2: Role of dopamine receptors. *J Neurosci, 22*(19), 8705–8710.

Schmitz, J. M., Stotts, A. L., Rhoades, H. M., & Grabowski, J. (2001). Naltrexone and relapse prevention treatment for cocaine-dependent patients. *Addict Behav, 26*(2), 167–180.

Schnoll, R. A., Patterson, F., Wileyto, E. P., et al. (2010). Effectiveness of extended-duration transdermal nicotine therapy: A randomized trial. *Ann Intern Med, 152*(3), 144–151.

Schottenfeld, R. S., Pakes, J., O'Connor, P., Chawarski, M., Oliveto, A., & Kosten, T. R. (2000). Thrice-weekly versus daily buprenorphine maintenance. *Biol Psychiatry, 47*(12), 1072–1079.

Schweizer, E., Rickels, K., Case, W. G., & Greenblatt, D. J. (1991). Carbamazepine treatment in patients discontinuing long-term benzodiazepine therapy: Effects on withdrawal severity and outcome. *Arch Gen Psychiatry,48*(5), 448–452.

Sees, K. L., Delucci, K. L., Masson, C., et al. (2000). Methadone maintenance vs. 180-day psychosocially enriched detoxification for treatment of opioid dependence: A randomized controlled trial. *JAMA, 283*(10), 1303–1310.

Sellers, E. M., Toneatto, T., Romach, M. K., Somer, G. R., Sobell, L. C., & Sobell, M. B. (1994). Clinical efficacy of the 5HT-3 antagonist ondansetron in alcohol abuse and dependence. *Alcohol Clin Exp Res, 18*(4), 879–885.

Shah, S. D., Wilken, L. A., Winkler, S. R., & Lin, S. J. (2003). Systematic review and meta-analysis of combination therapy for smoking cessation. *J Am Pharm Assoc, 48*(5), 659–665.

Shearer, J., Darke, S., Rodgers, C., et al. (2009). A double-blind, placebo-controlled trial of modafinil (200 mg/day) for methamphetamine dependence. *Addiction, 104*(2), 224–233.

Shen, X. Y., Orson, F. M., & Kosten, T. R. (2011). Vaccines against drug abuse. *Clin Pharmacol Therapeut, 91*(1), 60–70.

Shoptaw, S., Heinzerling, K. G., Rotheram-Fuller, E., et al. (2008). Randomized, placebo-controlled trial of bupropion for the treatment of methamphetamine dependence. *Drug Alcohol Depend, 96*(3), 222–232.

Shoptaw, S., Kao, U., & Ling, W. (2009). Treatment for amphetamine psychosis. *Cochrane Database Syst Rev, 21*(1), CD003026.

Shoptaw, S., Yang, X., Rotheram-Fuller, E. J., et al. (2003). Randomized placebo-controlled trial of baclofen for cocaine dependence: Preliminary effects for individuals with chronic patterns of cocaine use. *J Clin Psychiatry, 64*(12), 1440–1448.

Sigmon, S. C., Bisaga, A., Nunes, E. V., O'Connor, P. G., Kosten, T., & Woody, G. (2012). Opioid detoxification and naltrexone induction strategies: Recommendations for clinical practice. *Am J Drug Alcohol Abuse, 38*(3), 187–199.

Silagy, C., Lancaster, T., Stead, L., Mant, D., & Fowler, G. (2004). Nicotine replacement therapy for smoking cessation. *Cochrane Database Syst Rev, 3*, CD000146.

Slemmer, J. E., Martin, B. R., & Damaj, M. I. (2000). Bupropion is a nicotinic antagonist. *J Pharmacol Exp Therapeut, 295*(1), 321–327.

Spanagel, R., Herz, A., & Shippenberg, T. S. (1992). Opposing tonically active endogenous opioid systems modulate the mesolimbic dopaminergic pathway. *Proc Natl Acad Sci USA, 89*(6), 2046–2050.

Srisurapanont, M., & Jarusuraisin, N. (2005). Naltrexone for the treatment of alcoholism: A meta-analysis of randomized controlled trials. *Int J Neuropsychopharmacol, 8*(2), 267–280.

Stead, L. F., Perera, R., Bullen, C., Mant, D., & Lancaster, T. (2008). Nicotine replacement therapy for smoking cessation. *Cochrane Database Syst Rev, 23*(1), CD000146.

Strang, J., Bearn, J., & Gossop, M. (1999). Lofexidine for opiate detoxification: Review of recent randomised and open controlled trials. *Am J Addict, 8*(4), 337–348.

Stuppaeck, C. H., Pycha, R., Miller, C., Whitworth, A. B., Oberbauer, H., & Fleischhacker, W. W. (1992). Carbamazepine versus oxazepam in the treatment of alcohol withdrawal: A double-blind study. *Alcohol Alcohol, 27*(2), 153–158.

Sullivan, J. T., Sykora, K., Schneiderman, J., Naranjo, C. A., & Sellers, E. M. (1989). Assessment of alcohol withdrawal: The revised Clinical Institute Withdrawal Instrument for Alcohol Scale (CIWA-Ar). *Br J Addict, 84*(11), 1353–1357.

Tiihonen, J., Kuoppasalmi, K., Föhr, J., et al. (2007). A comparison of aripiprazole, methylphenidate, and placebo for amphetamine dependence. *Am J Psychiatry, 164*(1), 160–162.

Turner, D. C., Clark, L., Dowson, J., Robbins, T. W., & Sahakian, B. J. (2004). Modafinil improves cognition and response inhibition in adult attention-deficit/hyperactivity disorder. *Biol Psychiatry, 55*(10), 1031–1040.

Turner, D. C., Clark, L., Pomarol-Clotet, E., McKenna, P., Robbins, T. W., & Sahakian, B. J. (2004). Modafinil improves cognition and attentional set shifting in patients with chronic schizophrenia. *Neuropsychopharmacol, 29*(7), 1363–1373.

van den Brink, W., Goppel, M., & van Ree, J. M. (2003). Management of opioid dependence. *Curr Opin Psychiatry, 16*, 297–304.

Veriaiaih, A., Dyas, J., Cooper, G., Routeledge, P. A., & Thompson, J. P. (2012). Flumazenil use in benzodiazepine overdose in the UK: A retrospective survey of NPIS data. *Emerg Med J, 29*(7), 565–569.

Volkow, N. D., Wang, G. J., Fowler, J. S., et al. (2002). Brain DA D2 receptors predict reinforcing effects of stimulants in humans: Replication study. *Synapse, 46*(2), 79–82.

Volpicelli, J., Alterman, A. I., Hayashida, M., & O'Brien, C. P. (1992). Naltrexone in the treatment of alcohol dependence. *Arch Gen Psychiatry, 49*(11), 867–880.

Volpicelli, J., Rhines, K., Rhines, J., Volpicelli, L. A., Alterman, A. I., & O'Brien, C. P. (1997). Naltrexone and alcohol dependence: Role of subject compliance. *Arch Gen Psychiatry, 54*(8), 737–742.

Walsh, S. L., Preston, K. L., Stitzer, M. L., Cone, E. J., & Bigelow, G. E. (1994). Clinical pharmacology of buprenorphine: Ceiling effects at high doses. *Clin Pharmacol Therapeut, 55*(5), 569–580.

Weinbroum, A. A., Flaishon, R., Sorkine, P., Szold, O., & Rudick, V. (1997). A risk-benefit assessment of flumazenil in the management of benzodiazepine overdose. *Drug Safety, 17*(3), 181–196.

West, S. L., Garbutt, J. C., Carey, T. S., et al. (1999). *Pharmacotherapy for alcohol dependence* (Evidence Report No. 3, AHCPR Publication No. 99-E004). Rockville, MD: U.S. Department of Health and Human Services, Public Health Service, Agency for Health Care Policy and Research.

Wilde, M. I., & Wagstaff, A. J. (1997). Acamprosate: A review of its pharmacology and clinical potential in the management of alcohol dependence after detoxification. *Drugs, 53*(6), 1038–1053.

Williams, S. H. (2005). Medications for treating alcohol dependence. *Am Fam Physician, 72*(9), 1775–1780.

Wright, C., & Moore, R. D. (1990). Disulfiram treatment of alcoholism. *Am J Med, 88*(6), 647–655.

Yu, E., Miotto, K., Akerele, E., et al. (2008). A phase 3 placebo-controlled, double-blind, multisite trial of the alpha-2-adrenergic agonist, lofexidine, for opioid withdrawal. *Drug Alcohol Depend, 97*(1–2), 158–168.

Index